ORAL *and* MAXILLOFACIAL INFECTIONS

ORAL *and* MAXILLOFACIAL INFECTIONS

4th edition

Richard G. Topazian, DDS

Professor
Department of Oral and Maxillofacial Surgery
School of Dental Medicine
Professor of Surgery
School of Medicine
Formerly Chairman
Department of Oral and Maxillofacial Surgery
University of Connecticut Health Center
Farmington, Connecticut

Morton H. Goldberg, DMD, MD

Clinical Professor of Oral and Maxillofacial Surgery
School of Dental Medicine
University of Connecticut
Farmington, Connecticut;
Formerly Director, Department of Dentistry
Hartford Hospital
Hartford, Connecticut

James R. Hupp, DMD, MD, JD, MBA, FACS, FACD

Professor and Chair
Department of Oral-Maxillofacial Surgery
University of Maryland Dental School
Chair, Department of Dental and Maxillofacial Surgery
University of Maryland Medical Center
Baltimore, Maryland

W.B. SAUNDERS COMPANY
An Imprint of Elsevier Science
Philadelphia   London   New York   St. Louis   Syndey   Toronto

W.B. SAUNDERS COMPANY
An Imprint of Elsevier Science
The Curtis Center
Independence Square West
Philadelphia, Pennsylvania 19106-3399

NOTICE

Pharmacology is an ever-changing field. Standard safety precautions must be followed, but as new research and clinical experience broaden our knowledge, changes in treatment and drug therapy may become necessary or appropriate. Readers are advised to check the most current product information provided by the manufacturer of each drug to be administered to verify the recommended dose, the method and duration of administration, and contraindications. It is the responsibility of the treating physician, relying on experience and knowledge of the patient, to determine dosages and the best treatment for each individual patient. Neither the publisher nor the editor assumes any liability for any injury and/or damage to persons or property arising from this publication.

Library of Congress Cataloging in Publication Data

Oral and maxillofacial infections / [edited by] Richard G. Topazian, Morton H. Goldberg, James R. Hupp.—4th ed.
    p. ; cm.
    Includes bibliographical references and index.
    ISBN 0-7216-9271-0
    1. Mouth—Infections. 2. Jaws—Infections. I. Topazian, Richard G. II. Goldberg, Morton H., 1933-III. Hupp, James R.
    [DNLM: 1. Infection. 2. Jaw Diseases. 3. Mouth Diseases. WU 140 0625 2002]
RK325 .073 2002
617.5'22—dc21

                                              2001055136

Publishing Director: Linda Duncan

Senior Acquisitions Editor: Penny Rudolph

Developmental Editor: Jaime Pendill

Editorial Assistant: Courtney Sprehe

Project Manager: Linda McKinley

Production Editor: Judy Ahlers

Designer: Julia Dummitt

Cover Design: Julia Dummitt

ORAL AND MAXILLOFACIAL INFECTIONS, 4TH EDITION   ISBN: 0-7216-9271 0

Printed in the United States of America

02 03 04 05 06 TG/MV 9 8 7 6 5 4 3 2 1

CONTRIBUTORS

Leon A. Assael, DMD
Professor and Dean
Department of Oral Health Science
University of Kentucky College of Dentistry
Lexington, Kentucky

Ali Behnia, DMD, MS
Assistant Professor
Director of Predoctoral Endodontics
Department of Endodontics
Baltimore College of Dental Surgery
University of Maryland Dental School
Baltimore, Maryland

Jeffrey D. Bennett, DMD
Associate Professor
Department of Oral and Maxillofacial Surgery
School of Dental Medicine
University of Connecticut Health Center
Farmington, Connecticut

Stewart A. Bergman, DDS, MS
Professor
Department of Oral and Maxillofacial Surgery
Baltimore College of Dental Surgery
University of Maryland Dental School
Baltimore, Maryland

Remy H. Blanchaert, Jr., MD, DDS
Assistant Professor
Department of Oral and Maxillofacial Surgery
Baltimore College of Dental Surgery
University of Maryland Dental School
Assistant Professor
Marlene & Stuart Greenebaum Cancer Center
Attending Surgeon
University of Maryland Medical Center and RA Cowley
    Shock Trauma Center
Baltimore, Maryland

George R. Deeb, DDS, MD
Chief Resident
Department of Oral and Maxillofacial Surgery
Oregon Health Sciences University
Portland, Oregon

Angelo M. DelBalso, MD, DDS, FACD
Professor and Chairman
Department of Radiology
State University of New York at Buffalo School of
    Medicine and Biomedical Sciences
Director of Radiology
Department of Diagnostic Radiology
Veteran's Administration Hospital Western New York
Buffalo, New York

Eric J. Dierks, MD, DMD, FACS
Clinical Professor
Department of Oral and Maxillofacial Surgery
Oregon Health Sciences University
Director of Fellowship in Head and Neck Surgery
Legacy Emanuel Hospital
Portland, Oregon

Thomas R. Flynn, DMD
Assistant Professor
Director of Predoctoral Oral and Maxillofacial Surgery
    Education
Department of Oral and Maxillofacial Surgery
Harvard School of Dental Medicine
Associate Visiting Surgeon
Department of Oral and Maxillofacial Surgery
Massachusetts General Hospital
Boston, Massachusetts

Morton H. Goldberg, DMD, MD
Clinical Professor of Oral and Maxillofacial Surgery
School of Dental Medicine
University of Connecticut
Farmington, Connecticut;
Formerly Director, Department of Dentistry
Hartford Hospital
Hartford, Connecticut

Richard E. Hall, DDS, MD, PhD, FACS
Professor and Chairman
Department of Oral and Maxillofacial Surgery
Professor, Department of Oral Biology
State University of New York at Buffalo School of
    Dental Medicine
Clinical Director
Department of Oral and Maxillofacial Surgery
Kalieda Health System
Buffalo, New York

Richard H. Haug, DDS
Professor and Director
Oral and Maxillofacial Surgery
Head
Department of Hospital Dentistry
Assistant Dean for Hospital Affairs
University of Kentucky College of Dentistry
Lexington, Kentucky

Marc J. Hirschbein, MD
Attending Oculoplastic Surgeon
Department of Ophthalmology
Sinai Hospital of Baltimore
Instructor
Department of Ophthalmology
Wilmer Eye Institute–Johns Hopkins University
Baltimore, Maryland

James R. Hupp, DMD, MD, JD, MBA, FACS, FACD
Professor and Chair
Department of Oral-Maxillofacial Surgery
University of Maryland Dental School
Chair, Department of Dental and Maxillofacial Surgery
University of Maryland Medical Center
Baltimore, Maryland

Julie M. Jameson, PhD
Research Associate
Department of Immunology
The Scripps Research Institute
La Jolla, California

James W. Karesh, MA, MS, MD, FACS
Associate Professor
The Johns Hopkins Medical Institutions
The Wilmer Eye Institute
Associate Clinical Professor
Department of Oral-Maxillofacial Surgery
University of Maryland Dental School
Zanyl and Isabelle Krieger Chairman
The Krieger Eye Institute
The Sinai Hospital of Baltimore
Baltimore, Maryland

Jeffrey Kingsbury, DDS, MD
Assistant Professor
Department of Oral and Maxillofacial Surgery
School of Dental Medicine
University of Connecticut Health Center
Farmington, Connecticut

Stuart E. Lieblich, DMD
Associate Clinical Professor
Department of Oral and Maxillofacial Surgery
School of Dental Medicine
University of Connecticut Health Center
Farmington, Connecticut;
Private Practice
Avon, Connecticut

Eufronio G. Maderazo, MD
Private Practice
Norwich, Connecticut

Yvette S. McCarter, PhD, DABMM
Clinical Associate Professor
Department of Pathology
University of Florida College of Medicine
Director
Clinical Microbiology Laboratory
University of Florida Health Science Center/Jacksonville
Jacksonville, Florida

Samuel J. McKenna, DDS, MD
Associate Professor
Department of Oral and Maxillofacial Surgery
Vanderbilt University
Chief
Department of Oral and Maxillofacial Surgery
Nashville VA Medical Center
Nashville, Tennessee

Michael Miloro, DMD, MD
Associate Professor
Director
Oral and Maxillofacial Surgery
University of Nebraska Medical Center
Omaha, Nebraska

Larry J. Peterson, DDS, MS
Professor
Department of Oral and Maxillofacial Surgery
The Ohio State University College of Dentistry
Private Practice
Columbus, Ohio

Joseph F. Piecuch, DMD, MD
Clinical Professor
Department of Oral and Maxillofacial Surgery
School of Dental Medicine
University of Connecticut Health Center
Farmington, Connecticut;
Director
Department of Oral and Maxillofacial Surgery Service
Hartford Hospital
Hartford, Connecticut

George S. Schuster, DMD, MS, PhD
Ione and Arthur Merritt Professor and Chairman
Department of Oral Biology and Maxillofacial Pathology
Medical College of Georgia School of Dentistry
Augusta, Georgia

David M. Shafer, DMD
Associate Professor, Head, and Residency Program
    Director
Department of Oral and Maxillofacial Surgery
School of Dental Medicine
University of Connecticut Health Center
Assistant Professor
Department of Surgery
School of Medicine
University of Connecticut Health Center
Farmington, Connecticut

Richard H. Simon, MD
Professor
Department of Surgery
Division of Neurosurgery
School of Medicine
University of Connecticut Health Center
Farmington, Connecticut

Richard G. Topazian, DDS
Professor and Formerly Chairman
Department of Oral and Maxillofacial Surgery
School of Dental Medicine
Professor of Surgery
School of Medicine
University of Connecticut Health Center
Farmington, Connecticut

Clarence L. Trummel, DDS, PhD
Professor and Head
Department of Periodontology
School of Dental Medicine
University of Connecticut Health Center
Farmington, Connecticut

John R. Werther, DMD, MD, FACS
Private Practice
Staff Surgeon
Department of Oral and Maxillofacial Surgery
Nashville Veterans Affairs Hospital
Nashville, Tennessee

Brett A. Weyman, DDS, MD
Resident, Oral Maxillofacial Surgery
School of Dental Medicine
University of Connecticut Health Center
Farmington, Connecticut

Iftach Yassur, MD
Attending Surgeon
Ophthalmic Plastic and Reconstructive Service
Department of Ophthalmology
Rabin Medical Center
Tel Aviv University School of Medicine
Petach Tikva, Israel

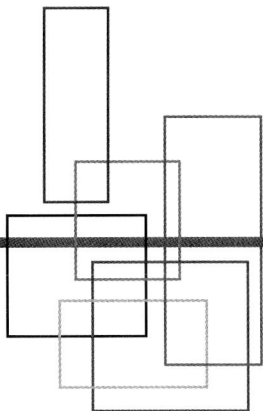

PREFACE TO THE FOURTH EDITION

Two decades after the first edition of this book and nearly a decade since the last edition, infections of the oral and maxillofacial region remain more challenging than ever. The object of the first edition in 1981 was to provide a one-volume reference source of contemporary information on all aspects of infections of the jaws and face. In subsequent editions, many changes were necessary to reflect the evolving flora of orofacial infections, the newest drugs for therapy, and the application of the advancing technology of soft and hard tissue imaging.

Today, infections continue to evolve while therapy, rather than being simplified, has become increasingly complex. The glory that is modern surgery and all of its subspecialties rests on the historical triumph over pain, bleeding, and infection. Although anesthesia and hemostasis continue to progress as success stories, infection remains today as the common threat to all surgery and the bane of all surgeons. Although our knowledge of microbiology and the spread of infection has grown, increased virulence and antibiotic resistance remain as constant liabilities to surgical success and create unacceptable levels of morbidity and mortality 60 years after the introduction of antibiotic therapy.

The following major questions loom over both patients and professionals for the foreseeable future: are we approaching the end of the antibiotic era, and are all diseases, in one sense, infections? Although the answer to both questions is probably a qualified "no," it is obvious that both questions relate to the realities of contemporary clinical microbiology. The overuse, abuse, and misuse of antibiotics has led to the emergence of resistant strains of streptococci, *Bacteroides, Escherichia coli,* staphylococci, and enterococci, and even the best pharmacological defenses have been breached as vancomycin-resistant organisms are threatening a return to the surgical sepsis of the preantibiotic era.

The realization that microorganisms are either causal agents or responsible for immune reactions that trigger illness is leading to a revolutionary change in concepts of human disease. Peptic ulcer disease, gastritis, Crohn's disease, juvenile diabetes, Burkitt's lymphoma, nasopharyngeal carcinoma, some leukemias, and some Bell's palsies now are recognized in association with transmissible agents, bacterial or viral. The possible relationship of periodontal pathogens in coronary artery disease has recently launched a major renewal in interest and research in oral microbiology. Cardiac valve infection, after decades of prophylaxis, remains a threat to life. This year, a friend of one of the authors died of prosthetic valve endocarditis from an oral organism that does not respond to the recommended dose of pretreatment amoxicillin.

This fourth edition addresses these issues and new antibiotics, therapy schedules, drug-drug interactions, and costs to both inpatients and outpatients. Although principles and therapeutic philosophy remain basically unaltered, the application, the nuts and bolts of therapy, are less constant. All chapters have been updated, including much new illustrative material, while maintaining essential data from previous editions.

Surgical anatomy has been clarified, laboratory diagnosis made practical, implant (xenographic) osteomyelitis described, and the differential diagnosis of salivary gland infections elucidated. New authors have contributed to this text and new chapters have been added, including pediatric infections and the infection risk of facial esthetic surgery. This text covers the full spectrum from localized dentoalveolar infection, to osteomyelitis, to death from sepsis of dental origin. To aid the practitioner, as much essential data as possible have been included for all mild to major infections.

Because the information database has grown and continues to change so rapidly, contradicting or even conflicting data and opinions inevitably occur, especially in a multiauthored text. The absence of unanimity and the variances in the authors' experience are not inconsistent with contemporary or competent practice but rather reflect the limitations of knowledge in a changing environment. We feel confident that this book will ultimately serve the needs of the many patients who are the beneficiaries of these efforts.

The senior editors welcome the addition of a third editor, James R. Hupp, former resident, former faculty associate, and current and much valued colleague.

As a special feature for readers of this book, an e-mail address is available to pose questions or provide comments to Dr. James Hupp. He will reply directly to your query or comment, or solicit others with the needed expertise to provide feedback to you. Any suggestions for improvement or notification of any errors in the book's content are welcome. Please note the speed of response cannot be guaranteed; if an emergency clinical situation exists, please try others means of gaining needed information.

The following e-mail address should be used to contact Dr. Hupp: jrhupp@mosby.com.

Richard G. Topazian
Morton H. Goldberg
James R. Hupp
Farmington, Connecticut, and
Baltimore, Maryland

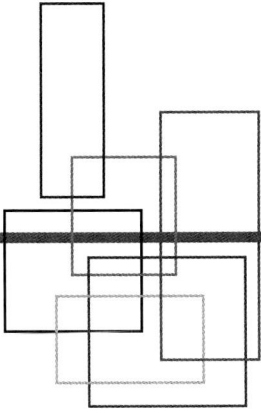

PREFACE TO THE FIRST EDITION

"To study the phenomena of disease without books is to sail an uncharted sea, while to study books without patients is not to go to sea at all."

SIR WILLIAM OSLER (1849-1919)

Nowhere in modern medicine or surgery has there been a more rapidly changing field of knowledge than in the diagnosis and treatment of clinical infections. Since the advent of antibiotics a little more than thirty-five years ago, there has been an almost exponential growth in the numbers of pathogenic species invading the human host and in the types of drugs and techniques available for defense against these pathogens.

Prior to the 1940's, infections of the head and neck were commonplace and often lethal. Ludwig's angina was a potential threat to every dental patient, and whole wards of large municipal hospitals were reserved for the care of osteomyelitis of the jaws. Erysipelas carried a 60 percent mortality, and bone grafting to the jaws frequently failed because of sepsis.

Today, deep fascial space infections, while still drained surgically by time-tested techniques, often require the most advanced laboratory diagnostic testing and intense antibiotic therapy administered by a variety of routes. Osteomyelitis remains a chronic debilitating disease, which is the bane of the oral and maxillofacial surgeon, despite new techniques for its management. Erysipelas, because it is so uncommon today, causes diagnostic confusion for many practitioners. In this modern era of grafting and implantation, infection remains the greatest cause of failure.

The constantly evolving flora of human infection, the advent of the opportunistic and nosocomial infections, the plethora of currently available antibiotics, and newer surgical techniques demand the doctor-in-training, the clinical practitioner, and the academician keep abreast of contemporary advances in this field. The need to understand the anatomic and microbiologic factors unique to the region adds to the complexity of dealing with oral and maxillofacial infections.

The clinician will find many sources of information to increase his knowledge of management of infections, but much of it is fragmentary. It is the purpose of this book to collect and collate information on many contemporary aspects of infections in order to aid the clinician in dealing more effectively with infections of the oral and maxillofacial regions.

RICHARD G. TOPAZIAN
MORTON H. GOLDBERG
Farmington, Connecticut
1981

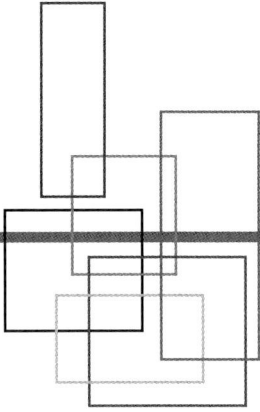

ACKNOWLEDGMENTS

The editors wish to express their appreciation to the many colleagues who contributed ideas, photographs and clinical case reports to this book, as well as to those who critiqued past editions and others who have made constructive suggestions over the years.

We acknowledge, with gratitude, the expert assistance, patience, and support of the staff of our publisher, the W.B. Saunders Company: Penny Rudolph, Senior Acquisitions Editor, Judy Ahlers, Project Manager, Jamie Pendill, Developmental Editor, Courtney Sprehe, Editorial Assistant, and Julia Dummitt, Senior Designer.

Richard G. Topazian
Morton H. Goldberg
James R. Hupp

CONTENTS

CHAPTER 1
Infections and the Host 1
Eufronio G. Maderazo
Julie M. Jameson

CHAPTER 2
Microbiology of the Orofacial Region 30
George S. Schuster

CHAPTER 3
Laboratory Microbiological Diagnostic
Techniques 43
Yvette S. McCarter

CHAPTER 4
Diagnostic Imaging of Maxillofacial and Fascial
Space Infections 62
Angelo M. DelBalso
Richard E. Hall

CHAPTER 5
Principles of Surgical and Antimicrobial
Infection Management 99
Larry J. Peterson

CHAPTER 6
Antimicrobial Pharmacology for Maxillofacial
Infections 112
James R. Hupp

CHAPTER 7
Periodontal and Pulpal Infections 126
Clarence L. Trummel
Ali Behnia

CHAPTER 8
Odontogenic Infections and Deep Fascial Space
Infections of Dental Origin 158
Morton H. Goldberg
Richard G. Topazian

CHAPTER 9
Anatomy of Oral and Maxillofacial
Infections 188
Thomas R. Flynn

CHAPTER 10
Osteomyelitis of the Jaws 214
Richard G. Topazian

CHAPTER 11
Fungal, Viral, and Protozoal Infections of the
Maxillofacial Region 243
Stewart A. Bergman

CHAPTER 12
Salivary Gland Infections 279
Michael Miloro
Morton H. Goldberg

CHAPTER 13
Infections of Soft Tissues of the Maxillofacial
and Neck Regions 294
James R. Hupp

CHAPTER 14
Ear, Nose, and Throat Infections 313
Eric J. Dierks
George R. Deeb

CHAPTER 15
Ophthalmic Considerations in Oral and
Maxillofacial Infections 328
Iftach Yassur
Marc J. Hirschbein
James W. Karesh

CHAPTER 16
Neurological Considerations in Oral and
Maxillofacial Infections 347
Richard H. Simon

CHAPTER 17
Infection in the Maxillofacial Trauma Patient 359
Richard H. Haug
Leon A. Assael

CHAPTER 18
Microbiological Considerations with Dental Implants 381
Stuart E. Lieblich
Joseph F. Piecuch

CHAPTER 19
Esthetic Facial Surgery and Infections 392
John R. Werther

CHAPTER 20
Identification, Management, and Prevention of Infections after Head and Neck Surgery 399
Remy H. Blanchaert, Jr.

CHAPTER 21
Pediatric Maxillofacial Infections 410
Jeffrey Kingsbury
David M. Shafer
Brett A. Weyman

CHAPTER 22
Uncommon Inflammatory Conditions and Infections of the Orofacial Region 423
Richard G. Topazian

CHAPTER 23
Anesthetic Considerations in Orofacial Infections 439
Jeffrey D. Bennett
Thomas R. Flynn

CHAPTER 24
Immunocompromised Host and Infection 456
Samuel J. McKenna

CHAPTER 25
Control and Prevention of Infection in the Surgical Patient 468
Morton H. Goldberg

CHAPTER 26
Medicolegal Aspects of Infection 484
James R. Hupp
Morton H. Goldberg

ORAL *and* MAXILLOFACIAL INFECTIONS

Infections and the Host

Eufronio G. Maderazo
Julie M. Jameson

Humans are subject to various infections; some are mild, others severe. Although infections often are self-limiting, many require the attention of the clinician, who first must make a diagnosis and then prescribe treatment. In establishing the presence of an infection, interaction occurs among three factors: the host, the environment, and the organism. In a state of homeostasis, a balance exists among these three. Disease occurs when an imbalance exists. For example, in a patient who has been burned, the host defenses are altered, allowing organisms that previously were kept in check to become pathogens, thus causing an infection. Similarly, in the patient with damaged muscle from a crush injury, the environment is altered, tetanus spores germinate in the anaerobic environment, and disease results. The clinician always must be aware of the role of these three factors to properly assess their importance in a particular patient. This chapter discusses the first of these factors, the host.

Host defense mechanisms are the major factor in determining the outcome of an infection; the environment and the microbe play important but usually secondary roles. The adversarial relationship between infectious microorganisms and the host is expressed best by imagining a balance on which the pathogenic attributes of the microbes are weighed against the protective mechanisms of the host (Figure 1-1). The pathogenic potential of microbes is favored by two major attributes: virulence and quantity. *Virulence* refers to all the qualities of the microbe that are harmful to the host, including invasiveness and a multitude of toxins, enzymes, and other harmful products. The *quantity* of microbes refers to the number of organisms that initially infect the host; in addition, an increase in quantity raises the concentration of the virulence factors. Under normal conditions, host factors predominate. The more host factors predominate, the greater is the host reserve. If microbial factors increase or protective host factors decrease (or as occurs more frequently, a com-

bination of both), the pathogenic potential increases. As this imbalance occurs, host reserve diminishes until microbial factors predominate and clinical infection supervenes. These relationships are not static; each day, microbes with various harmful qualities may invade the host or the host may acquire breaks in defenses. The scale therefore swings, continuously changing the amount of host reserve. In oral and facial surgery the surgeon first may attempt to reduce the quantity of the local microorganisms by disinfection of the oral cavity. This action decreases the pathogenic potential in anticipation of an extensive break in the local defenses when the surgeon cuts through the oral mucosa into the deeper tissues. During the operative procedure, microorganisms find themselves in inadequately protected tissues because of the break in

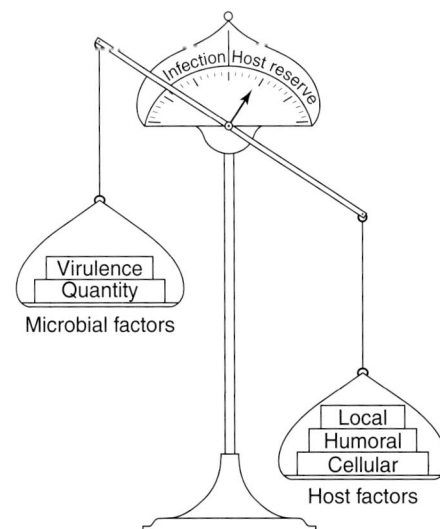

Figure 1-1 Host versus microbe relationship and its effects on host reserve and susceptibility to infection.

the local barrier. At this time the microbes have the advantage. As tissues are injured and microbes increase, a variety of signals in the host mobilize humoral and cellular factors. The mobilization and local accumulation of these protective factors generally are sufficient to contain the pathogens, prevent their dissemination, and allow prompt healing. Sometimes infection can develop and persist because of continued microbial dominance and subtle problems of the host. In many instances the latter is caused by a breakdown in local defenses produced by the presence of foreign bodies, failure to provide for adequate drainage, or elimination of indigenous microbial flora, followed by colonization by resistant microorganisms resulting from the inappropriate use of broad-spectrum antibiotics.

MAJOR ARMS OF THE HOST DEFENSE SYSTEM

The host defense system is composed of a multitude of smaller subsystems and factors that relate and interact to provide a coherent singular purpose: protection of the host. No subsystem or factor is a truly independent entity.

The rapid advances in molecular biological techniques have resulted in a virtual explosion of knowledge on this subject. A detailed review of the various components of the host defense system is beyond the scope of this chapter, but it does provide knowledge of the subject. Another result of this swift pace of research in host defenses is the rapid outdating of some generally accepted views. To minimize this problem, this chapter emphasizes general concepts and directs readers to recent reviews[14,15,36,37,46] of standards being questioned.

Division of the host defense system into three major components facilitates a general overview of its function. The major components are local, humoral, and cellular; in actuality, no boundaries exist, and overlaps and interrelating links exist to provide a unified protective mechanism for the host (Figure 1-2).

LOCAL DEFENSES

The epithelial lining, local epithelial antibiotic peptides, the secretion and drainage system, the microbial flora (interference), and local humoral and cellular defenses (mucosal immune system) compose local defenses.

Epithelial Lining   Lining epithelial cells physically hinder the penetration of surface bacteria into deeper tissues. This function is best illustrated by the loss of skin in patients who have been burned. Such patients constantly are at risk of serious systemic infections by bacteria that easily migrate through the burn area into the unprotected deeper tissues. The usual treatment approach in these patients is to replace the lost skin cover with sterile dressings, skin grafts, or skin substitutes. The mechanical function of the epithelial barrier is enhanced by the keratin of the skin and secretory and drainage capabilities (ciliary action, peristaltic motion, and flushing and emptying actions) of the mucous membrane and the organs lined by it. The keratin layer allows the skin to become relatively dry without injury to the deeper epithelial layers. Dryness limits the growth of certain organisms and limits bacterial population on the skin surface. Adherence of bacteria to epithelial cells by way of specific re-

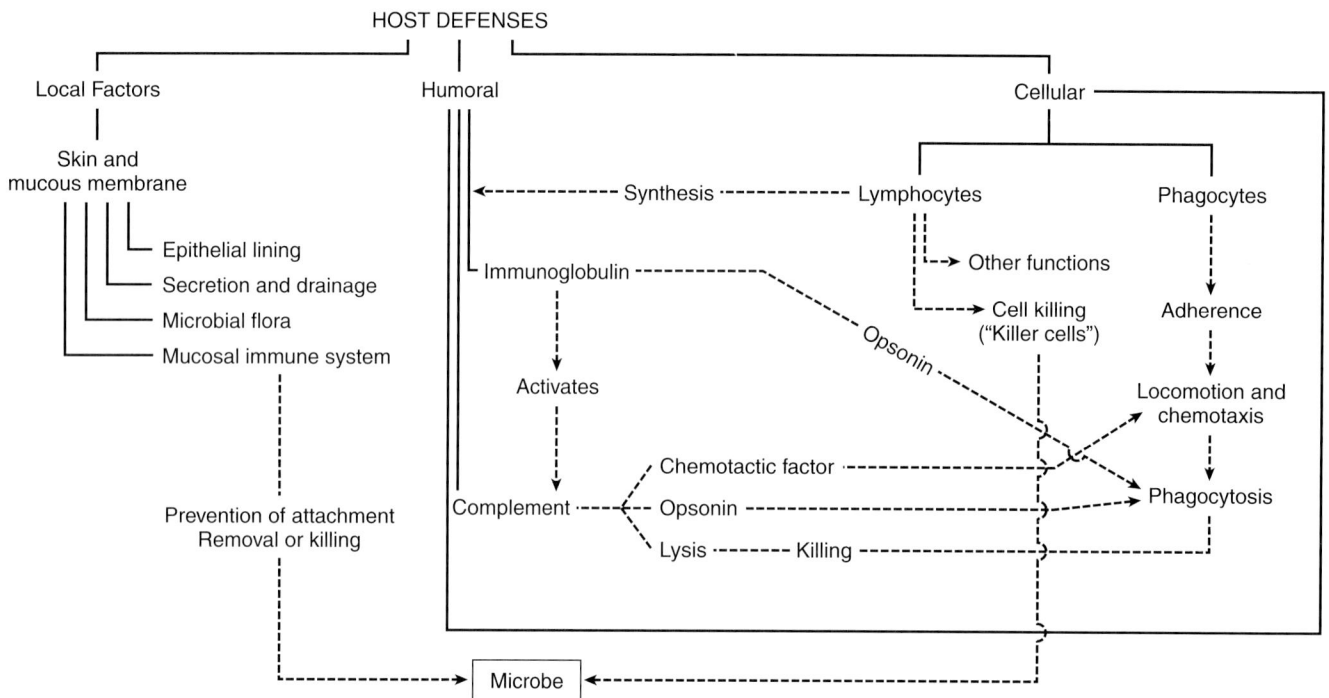

Figure 1-2 The interrelationships among the three major components of host defenses. *Solid lines,* subcomponents; *broken lines,* function.

ceptors is important in the potential pathogenicity of microorganisms.

Epidermal cells, primarily keratinocytes and to a lesser extent melanocytes and Langerhans cells, release a variety of regulatory proteins (cytokines), which may assist local defenses by recruitment and enhancement of phagocytic functions and promotion of wound healing.[30] Regulatory proteins produced by epidermal cells include colony-stimulating factors (CSFs) such as granulocyte CSF (G-CSF), granulocyte-macrophage CSF (GM-CSF), macrophage CSF, and interleukin (IL)-3; other growth factors such as transforming growth factor (TGF)-α, TGF-β, tumor necrosis factor (TNF)-α, basic fibroblast growth factor, and platelet-derived growth factors; and activating factors such as IL-1α, IL-lβ, IL-6, and IL-8. Epithelial cells also produce locally protective antimicrobial peptides.

Antimicrobial Peptides Numerous antimicrobial peptides have been described.[18] These peptides are synthesized either nonribosomally (most clinically useful antibiotics being derivatives of these) or ribosomally. Most living organisms with ribosomes can produce antimicrobial peptides, now considered an important part of the innate host defense system. These peptides are heterogeneous and show little sequence homology, suggesting that they separately evolved primarily to optimize local effects against locally harmful agents. Most antimicrobial peptides are synthesized by epithelial cells, but other sentries of the host defense system such as mobile phagocytes, platelets, and endothelial cells produce and use antimicrobial peptides as part of their complex arsenal. Some antimicrobial peptides are degradation products of proteins. For example, lactoferrin, which is primarily an iron-binding protein, has an antimicrobial peptide moiety that can be released by gastric pepsin digestion. The lactoferrin-derived antimicrobial peptides may then act in the distal bowel.

Although antimicrobial peptides have little sequence homology, a few chemical structural themes recur. These patterns include amphipathic hairpinlike β-structures with disulfide bridges and α-helices. Antimicrobial peptides generally are cationic with excess positively charged amino acids (arginine and lysine) and are hydrophobic. Both cationic and hydrophobic properties promote microbial membrane interaction, resulting in disruption of the phospholipid bilayer and pore formation and membrane depolarization and collapse of the energy gradient across the cell membrane. Both processes lead to increased membrane permeability, leakage of intracellular contents (in some instances, further uptake of antimicrobial peptides into the microbe and exertion of other antimicrobial peptides effects inside the microbe), and microbial death. Other antimicrobial peptides do not permeate membranes and are assumed to kill microbes by other means such as interference with microbial biosynthetic pathways and disruption of energy metabolism. In addition to their antibacterial, antifungal, and antiviral effects, antimicrobial peptides also have antitoxic (e.g., antiendotoxin), antitumor, antibiotic-enhancing, and regulatory effects on the

adaptive immune system. An example of the interaction between the innate and the adaptive immune systems is the cooperative relationship between antimicrobial peptides and IL-8. IL-8 produced by the epithelial cells in response to infection attracts neutrophils to the site. The arriving neutrophils then unload their α-defensins, which in turn attack the infectious agents, recruit T cells, and cause more IL-8 to be produced.

An increasing number of these peptides have been characterized. The three best studied groups are the defensins, histatins, and bacteriocins. Human defensins are composed of six α- (classic) and two β-defensins. The most studied are the α-defensins. In addition to their antimicrobial effects, other roles of defensins have been described such as chemotactic, mitogenic and apoptotic stimulation, and induction of histamine release. Of the α-defensins, human neutrophil peptides 1 to 4 are produced by neutrophils and stored in cytoplasmic granules, whereas human defensins 5 and 6 are produced by epithelial cells of the female genital tract and Paneth's cells of the small intestines. β-Defensins are produced in various epithelial cells, including the gingival epithelia, and are found in saliva. Both α- and β-defensins are salt sensitive; one proposed reason for frequent airway infections in cystic fibrosis is inhibition of defensin activity in lung fluid with high salinity.[54]

Histatins are a group of small, cationic histidine-rich peptides first described in human saliva.[53] At least 16 histatins have been reported; a few are degradation products of other histatins. Histatin-5, one of the major salivary histatins, assumes a random coiled structure in aqueous solution but adopts an α-helical conformation in nonaqueous conditions, such as when bound to bacterial membrane. Among the many functions ascribed to histatins are (1) high affinity to hydroxyapatite and dental enamel surfaces and inhibitory activity on hydroxyapatite crystal growth in supersaturated calcium phosphate solutions, suggesting importance in formation of acquired enamel pellicle and maintenance of tooth integrity; (2) antibacterial effects (bacterial inhibitory, bactericidal, and antiendotoxin effects); and (3) antifungal effects. The mechanism of antimicrobial effects of histatins is not well understood. The α-helical structure is not sufficiently amphipathic for pore formation or disruption of membrane. However, histatins are sufficiently cationic that they could competitively displace the major cations in fungal membranes to cause membrane permeability by their bulky structures or electrostatic mechanisms. Histatins are effective even against bacteria protected by oral biofilm, such as dental plaque bacteria.[19] Antifungal activity had been described as "azolelike," but histatins are fungicidal even against azole-resistant fungi. Histatins are being studied for possible clinical use as antifungal agents.

Another group of important antimicrobial peptides are those derived from bacteria that inhabit human epithelial surfaces. The best studied peptides are the bacteriocins, which are derived from lactic acid bacteria.[31] Bacteriocins, like other antimicrobial peptides, differ from most classic antibiotics by their protein nature and their narrow range of antibacterial activity; thus although the bacteriocinogenic strain may not be affected by the bacteriocin it produces, the bacteriocin may kill a narrow range of bacterial strains similar to the producer strain. This specificity is related to the presence of highly selective membrane receptors on susceptible bacteria. Because organisms that make up human mucocutaneous flora can synthesize bacteriocins, their importance as regulators of growth of potentially more pathogenic strains can be appreciated. As expected, categorization of substances with similar activity into one classification is difficult; bacteriocins are widely heterogeneous in not only their chemical structure but also their mode of action. Most bacteriocins are active against gram-positive bacteria because these organisms possess abundant membrane anionic lipids. Two classes of bacteriocins exist. Class I bacteriocins contain the uncommon peptide, lanthionine, and are referred to as *lantibiotics,* form intramolecular thioether rings, possess a broader spectrum of activity, and form unstable pores according to a wedgelike model.[18] Nisin, a 34-residue bacteriocin that has received considerable attention in applied research for fermented food preservation, belongs in this group. Class II bacteriocins are numerous, small, usually narrow-spectrum peptides, many with excellent activity against *Listeria* spp., and form pores of the "barrel stave" or "carpet" models.[18]

Secretion and Drainage System   The secretion and drainage system assists host defenses by physical and chemical action. The mucociliary activity, peristaltic motion, and flushing action all result in drainage and mechanical removal of bacteria. Obstruction or impairment of drainage almost always results in infections. For example, in the immotile-cilia syndrome, mucociliary clearance is impaired, resulting in chronic sinus and pulmonary infections.[13,50] The importance of ureteral dyskinesia in the causation and aggravation of urinary tract infections is well accepted. The lack of flushing action in the neurogenic bladder produces a situation that resembles an obstructive phenomenon, again predisposing to urinary tract infections. In addition to its flushing action, emptying of the urinary bladder increases microplicae formation of the bladder luminal cells. This action increases entrapment and uptake of bacteria by these cells and enhances the intrinsic antibacterial function of the urinary bladder.[32]

The effects of impaired drainage in the oral region are evident in patients who are unable to swallow or expectorate oral secretions; they have a higher frequency of bacterial parotitis and pneumonia. Movements of the lips, cheeks, and tongue may aid further in removal of bacteria. The chemical properties of secretions and other products of mucocutaneous surfaces also are important. Growth medium pH is important for the growth of certain bacteria; consequently, the maintenance of pH in certain bodily secretions may be important for the control of the bacterial population. The pH changes in vaginal and cervical secretions during pregnancy and menstruation

may be partly responsible for the higher frequency of dissemination of gonococcal infections during these periods. The nature and function of many of the chemical constituents of epithelium and secretions other than antimicrobial peptides are less well understood. For example, certain acetone-extractable lipids from skin selectively inhibit the growth of staphylococci, micrococci, and *Candida* organisms but not streptococci, *Pseudomonas,* and diphtheroid organisms. In addition to antimicrobial peptides, most secretions, including sweat, airway secretions, and saliva, contain lysozyme, lactoferrin, and other substances that are microbicidal; thus lysozyme can lyse bacteria by splitting sugars from the peptidoglycan polymers of the bacterial cell wall, and lactoferrin deprives bacteria of one of their vital enzyme cofactors (iron), in addition to its antimicrobial peptide moiety. A peroxidase-mediated antimicrobial system has been described in saliva and uterine fluid.[25] In this system, the H_2O_2 produced by bacteria such as *Streptococcus viridans* inhibits or kills other potentially pathogenic bacteria in the presence of peroxidase and thiocyanate or iodide ions.

Microbial Interference   *Microbial interference* refers to the inhibitory effect exerted by one microorganism on the growth and proliferation of another. As early as 1909, the observation was made that patients with staphylococcal infections of the pharynx who were mistakenly placed in diphtheria wards did not become colonized or infected with *Corynebacterium diphtheriae.* This finding led to experiments designed to determine whether staphylococci sprayed into the pharynxes of diphtheria carriers would have an inhibitory effect on the diphtheria organism. Good results were claimed. The protective influence on the host exerted by the normal mucocutaneous microflora in preventing colonization by potential pathogens now is generally accepted. This protective influence is demonstrated clinically when antibiotics are given, causing suppression of susceptible bacteria and subsequent proliferation of resistant ones. Thus administration of cephalosporins, for instance, eliminates oral gram-positive bacteria and allows emergence of resistant gram-negative aerobes and *Candida* organisms. If oropharyngeal or pulmonary infection occurs in these patients, a resistant gram-negative organism or *Candida* is usually the causative agent.

Although normal microflora produce bacteriocins and other antimicrobial peptides, other mechanisms involved in microbial interference still are not fully defined, but they may include (1) interference of microbial binding to epithelial cells, (2) competition for nutrients, and (3) release of by-products in addition to antimicrobial peptides that are toxic to other microbes. Lipoteichoic acid is responsible for the adherence of group A streptococci to oral epithelial cells. For most microorganisms, attachment is mediated by binding of mannose-containing ligands to mannose receptors on the epithelial cell surface. Therefore one possible mechanism for bacterial interference is competition for these binding sites. For example, less pathogenic normal oral bacteria could interfere with binding to these receptors and exclude pathogenic bacteria from attachment and colonization. Another mechanism for interference of one microorganism by another is competition for nutrients. Finally, ample evidence indicates that a major function of secretory immunoglobulins A (IgA) and E (IgE) is inhibition of the attachment of bacteria and parasites, respectively, to epithelial cells.

Mucosal Immune System   Large numbers of immunocompetent mononuclear cells are found beneath the basement membrane of epithelium, particularly that of the skin, gastrointestinal tract, and respiratory tract. The B lymphocytes and plasma cells, with the help of certain T lymphocytes, locally synthesize IgA, some IgE, and small amounts of IgG and IgM. In addition, the secretory (transport) piece is synthesized locally. This transport piece becomes covalently linked to IgA, and the complex appears in the secretory fluid on the mucosal surfaces as secretory IgA. (See later discussion of immunoglobulins.) The immunoglobulins in secretions, together with other local protective factors, compose an immensely important component of the first-line defenses (Table 1-1). Immunoglobulins may function by neutralization of toxins and viruses and by preventing the attachment of bacteria (IgA) or parasites (IgE) to mucosal epithelium.

In an assay of gingival fluid and serum, IgG concentration in gingival fluid was 85% of serum concentration and IgA and IgM were 72% and 75% of serum concentration, respectively.[44] Although gingival fluid levels are 15% to 30% lower than serum levels, these concentrations are sufficient to mount an immune response. In the normal mucosa, IgA-producing lymphoid cells predominate, and IgA is the major immunoglobulin in secretions. This predominance of IgA occurs only in the normal mucous membrane because the relative concentrations of secretory immunoglobulins can change during inflammation; thus IgG may increase dramatically during infections. Because of the large surface area of the mucous membrane, the mucosal immune system (in particular, the IgA system) is extensive and of great significance for the defense of the host. Although parenteral immunization (as with poliovirus) produces am increase in the serum antibody level and protects against the systemic manifestations of an infection, it does not stimulate mucosal immunity and the mucosa may still be susceptible to colonization and the host becomes a carrier of the organism. Mucosal immunity and improved protection can be produced by local administration of the vaccine to enhance specific secretory immunoglobulin production. Such a practice has been used widely for immunization against the poliovirus and typhoid fever.

In addition to IgA, IgE is present in relatively high concentration in secretions compared with the amount found in serum. This predominance of IgE in mucous membranes and the selective distribution of mast cells in the respiratory and gastrointestinal tracts partly explain the frequency of immediate hypersensitivity reactions manifested in these locations.

TABLE 1-1

Content of Immunoglobulins in External Fluids and Numbers of Lymphoid Plasma Cells in the Corresponding Mucous Membrane

Organ of Secretion	CONCENTRATION OF IMMUNOGLOBULINS (mg/100 mL)		CONCENTRATION RATIO		Cell Count
	IgG	IgA	IgM	IgG/IgA	IgG/IgA
Serum	1000	160	100	6	—
Colostrum	10	1234	61	0.008	—
Breast milk*	30	600	50	0.05	—
Parotid	0.03	10	0.04	0.003	1:50
Whole saliva	7	37	0.8	0.2	—
Nasal†	10	20	0-Trace	0.5	1:6
Lacrimal (tears)	0-Trace	20	—	<0.1	1:12
Bronchial†	20	28	—	0.7	1:5
Gastric	—	—	—	—	1:16
Duodenum	10	31	21	0.3	—
Jejunum	34	28	—	1.2	1:22
Ileum	30	35	—	0.9	—
Colon	86	83	—	1	1:23
Rectum	—	—	—	—	1:16
Appendix	—	—	—	—	1:1
Gallbladder (bile)	143	160	—	0.9	—

From Tomasi TB Jr: *The immune system of secretions,* Englewood Cliffs, NJ, 1976, Prentice-Hall.
*Average value in first 3 days. Concentration of all immunoglobulins decreases as lactation proceeds.
†Fluids obtained by irrigation of nasal mucosa and tracheobronchial tree.

TABLE 1-2

Properties of Different Human Immunoglobulin Classes

	IgG	IgA	IgM	IgD	IgE
Mean serum concentration (mg/100 mL)	1,000	160	100	3	0.03
Heavy chain designation	γ	α	μ	δ	ϵ
Sedimentation coefficient	7S	7S(10,13,15,18)	19S	7S	8S
Molecular weight	152,000	160,000	950,000	180,000	200,000
Carbohydrate (approximate %)	2.5	7.5	10	10	10
Sensitivity to sulfhydryl reagents	0	±	+	0	±
$t_{1/2}$ (days)	22*	6	5	2.8	2.3
Synthetic rate (g/70 kg/day)	2.3	2.7	0.4	0.03	0.0014
% intravascular	40	40	75	75	50
Placental transfer	+†	0	0	0	0
Association with secretory component	0	+	±	0	0
Complement fixation‡	+	0	+	0	0
Reagin activity	0	0	0	0	+
Passive cutaneous anaphylaxis	+	0	0	0	0
Blocking activity	+	0§	0	0	0
Relative hemagglutinating efficiency (per μg N)	1	2-10	10-25	—	—
Relative hemolytic efficiency (per μg N)	1	0	5-10	0	0
Reaction with rheumatoid factor‖	+	0	0	0	0
Reaches adult levels	1-3 yr	4-14 yr	6-12 mo	—	—

From Tomasi TB Jr: *The immune system of secretions,* Englewood Cliffs, NJ, 1976, Prentice-Hall.
$t_{1/2}$, Half-life.
*$t_{1/2}$ for IgG1, IgG2, and IgG4 subclasses. IgG3 has mean $t_{1/2}$ of 9 days.
†IgG2 subclass is poorly transported.
‡Refers to complement fixation by the classic pathway. IgA and IgE may fix complement by the alternative or C3 shunt pathway.
§IgA may have blocking activity in external secretions.
‖Refers only to classic rheumatoid factor. The sera of patients who have received multiple transfusions, are IgA deficient, or have allergies may have antigammaglobulin antibodies directed toward other classes.

HUMORAL DEFENSES

Immunoglobulins The host synthesizes specific protein molecules with antibody activities in response to antigenic stimulation. These proteins, or immunoglobulins, share many similar structural, biological, and antigenic properties, but their significant molecular differences permit highly specific antibody function. Immunoglobulins are derived from sensitized B lymphocytes or plasma cells.

In humans, five classes of immunoglobulins are known; each has distinct chemical and biological characteristics (Table 1-2). Although chemically different, the molecular structures of all immunoglobulin classes have certain similarities; for example, each molecule has two light chains, which are designated kappa (κ) and lambda (λ), and two heavy chains, which are different for each class of immunoglobulin. The heavy chains are identified by the Greek letter equivalent of their class name (γ for IgG, α for IgA, μ for IgM, δ for IgD, and ϵ for IgE). Each light chain occurs in association with a heavy chain. With 2 types of light chains and 5 known types of heavy chains, 10 possible combinations of light and heavy chains exist, and all combinations occur naturally in all individuals.

For IgG, the amino group (NH_2) terminal is the antigen-binding or the antibody-active portion, whereas the carboxyl group (COOH) terminal contains the binding portion to cell receptors and the complement-fixing active portion of the molecule. With the application of various proteolytic enzymes, IgG molecules can be broken into several well-defined fragments. For example, papain splits the heavy chains at the hinge region (Figure 1-3) into two Fab fragments, both of which retain their antibody-binding activity, and one Fc fragment, which also retains its complement-fixing and cell-binding activities. Pepsin digests the Fc portion but spares the interchain disulfide bands that link the heavy chains near the hinge region to produce a single F(ab)$_2$ fragment containing two antigen-combining sites. Finally, various products can be obtained with trypsin depending on the length of treatment. On short treatment, it acts like papain, producing two Fab fragments and one Fc fragment. On prolonged treatment, areas of the chain next to every arginine and lysine amino acid are split to produce small peptides. In addition to these fragments, the immunoglobulin molecule is divided into the variable and constant domains depending on the variability or constancy of its amino acid sequence. Each heavy chain has one variable domain closest to the amino terminal and three (or four for the μ chain) constant domains; the light chain has one variable and one constant domain. The variable domains for the heavy and light chains are in close apposition in the intact four-chain molecule. These domains have important molecular, genetic, and evolutionary implications.[38] IgG, IgD, and IgE usually

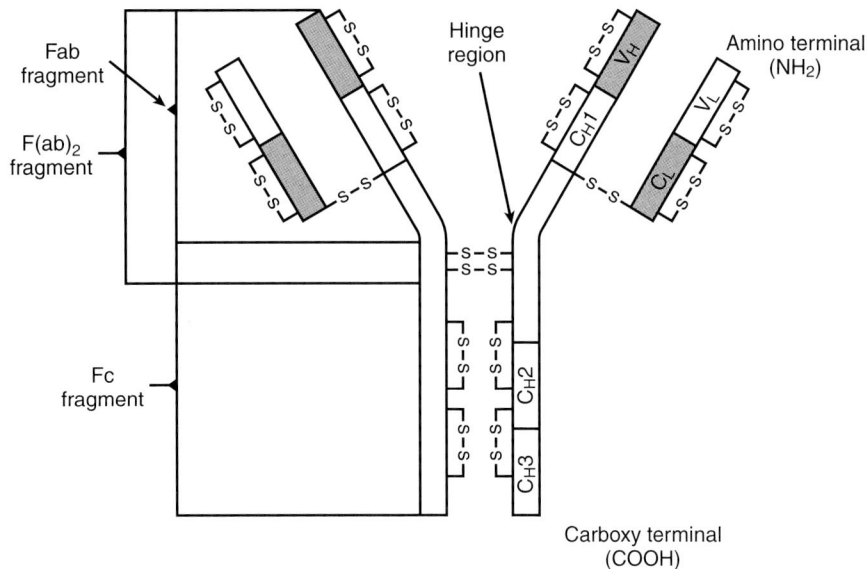

Figure 1-3 IgG molecule showing the relative positions of the light and heavy chains, the intrachain and interchain disulfide bonds *(-s-s-)*, the variable *(H)* and constant *(C)* domains, and the degradation fragments that result from enzyme treatment (see text). C_H1, C_H2, C_H3, heavy-chain constant domains; V_H, heavy-chain variable region; C_L, light-chain constant domain; V_L, light-chain variable region.

exist as monomers (i.e., single four-chain structural units containing two light and two heavy chains). IgA, IgM, and occasionally IgG occur as polymers of the basic four-chain unit. In serum, polymers of IgA and IgM occur with the participation of the J chain, which is a small nonimmunoglobulin molecule with high sulfhydryl content, whereas in secretory fluids, IgA polymers are formed with the participation of the J chain and the secretory component. Secretory component is a low molecular weight polypeptide chain. Unlike the light and heavy chains of the immunoglobulin molecule, it contains no methionine but contains high amounts of glycine, is not produced by lymphoid cells but rather by epithelial cells, and is present in secretions of newborns and individuals with agammaglobulinemia.

Of the five classes of immunoglobulins, IgG is the most abundant and is present in significant concentrations in intravascular and extravascular fluids. The four subclasses of IgG are IgGl, IgG2, IgG3, and IgG4. All have long half-lives (22 days for IgGl, IgG2, and IgG4 and 9 days for IgG3), fix complement by the classic pathway except IgGl, and cross the placental barrier except IgG2, which crosses poorly. The relative concentrations of the various IgG subclasses are IgGl, 70%; IgG2, 20%; IgG3, 7%; and IgG4, 3%. The IgG subtypes function as protective antibodies against most bacteria and neutralize antibodies against viruses and bacterial toxins. The secondary or late response to antigen stimulation is produced mainly by IgG. Major IgG synthesis occurs in plasma cells in lymph nodes and the spleen. Isolated absence or marked deficiency of IgGl, IgG2, or IgG3 has been reported in apparently healthy individuals with no symptoms, suggesting that other immunoglobulins can completely or partially compensate for one IgG

subclass deficiency.[20] Similar to the other IgG subtypes, isolated deficiency of IgG4 is compatible with health. Its complete absence, however, almost always is associated with increased susceptibility to infectious diseases, usually severe, recurrent, or chronic sinopulmonary infections.

IgA is the second most abundant serum immunoglobulin and, as mentioned previously, is the normally predominant immunoglobulin in secretions. The majority of immunoglobulin-producing cells in the lamina propria of the gastrointestinal, genitourinary, and respiratory tracts synthesize IgA. Some IgA produced in these areas may reach the systemic circulation and contribute to IgA concentration in serum. Two subclasses of IgA are known: IgAl and IgA2. IgAl predominates in serum, whereas IgA2 is the dominant IgA subclass present in secretions. IgA is synthesized as the monomeric form by plasma cells in the subepithelial zones that also produce the J protein. The J protein binds two or more monomeric IgA molecules to form polymeric IgA. During its passage through the epithelium on its way to secretions, the polymeric IgA acquires the secretory component, which is produced by the epithelial cells. Although the importance of the J protein is not clear, the secretory component conveys to the molecule the ability to resist digestion by proteolytic enzymes that may be present in secretions. IgA does not fix complement through the classic pathway, but aggregates of IgA may do so through the alternative pathway. IgA is the chief immunoglobulin involved in mucosal immunity by binding to microorganisms, thereby interfering with their ability to bind to mucosal cell receptors.[60] IgA also may limit the absorption or immune response to food allergens because patients with IgA deficiency have high levels of antibodies against food antigens.

IgM is the third most abundant immunoglobulin in serum and the largest of the immunoglobulin molecules. The molecular size is the result of the binding of five four-chain basic units into a pentamer with the participation of the J protein. After primary antigenic stimulation, synthesis of IgM and IgG commences simultaneously, but IgM production peaks within a few days and declines as the level of IgG increases. If IgG production is curtailed, the synthesis of IgM can proceed for a longer period, suggesting the possible regulatory function of IgG on IgM production. Because of its large size, IgM occurs mostly in the intravascular compartment and is not transferred by the placenta. Mole for mole, IgM fixes complement more efficiently than IgG. Antibodies against gram-negative bacteria, cold agglutinins, heterophile antibodies, hemolysins, rheumatoid factors, and isohemagglutinins are mostly, if not all, IgM.

The fourth class of immunoglobulin is IgD. Specific biological activity of IgD is not defined. However, naive B cells express both IgM and IgD heavy chains and cell surface specificity to IgD molecules is identical to IgM molecules, but IgD expression is switched off during primary immune response to antigen. Constitutively elevated levels of serum IgD occur in the hyperimmunoglobulinemia D and periodic fever syndrome, an autosomal recessive disease resulting from a missense mutation of the mevalonate kinase gene in the long arm of chromosome 12.[22] The disease is characterized by recurrent attacks of fever, abdominal pain, lymphadenopathy, and skin rash and arthralgias and is associated with mevalonic aciduria. Studies of patients with this disease eventually may allow understanding of the role of IgD in host defense.

The last class of immunoglobulins and the least abundant of all in serum is IgE. IgE includes the reaginic antibodies able to bind to skin, mast cells, basophils, and other cells; it is involved in the development of immediate hypersensitivity reactions. Akin to IgA, IgE is a secretory immunoglobulin, synthesized by lymphoid cells in the subepithelial regions of the skin and the respiratory, genitourinary, and gastrointestinal tracts.

Immunoglobulins are important components of host defenses against infectious agents. Secretory IgA and IgE antibodies directly prevent the attachment of pathogenic bacteria and parasites, respectively, to epithelial cell receptors. This activity appears crucial in preventing colonization and subsequent infection. Also by direct action, serum antibodies can neutralize viruses (antiviral activity) and microbial toxins (antitoxic activity). Other than these examples, however, antibody by itself is not protective or bactericidal. Rather, it relies on the complement system and phagocytes to destroy pathogenic microbes. Antibody and complement act as opsonins, coating the microbe and promoting phagocytosis by neutrophils or macrophages.

Complement System   The complement system consists of a group of serum proteins that, by a series of reactions, produce and release by-products initiating inflammatory reactions, regulating and enhancing phagocytic functions, and attacking bacterial cell membrane. All actions result in the destruction of the potentially pathogenic microbial invader. The complement system is activated by one of three pathways: (1) the classic pathway, (2) the alternative pathway, and (3) the mannose-binding lectin pathway (Figure 1-4). The classic pathway is initiated by IgG (IgG3, IgG1, and IgG2) and IgM immune complexes, by plasmin, or a variety of harmful microbes or agents that can convert C1 into its active form, C1 esterase ($\overline{C1}$). C1 esterase in turn reacts with C4 and with C2 to form C3 convertase (C4b2a), an enzyme that cleaves C3 into its active fragments, C3a (with anaphylatoxic activity) and C3b (opsonin). C3b at-

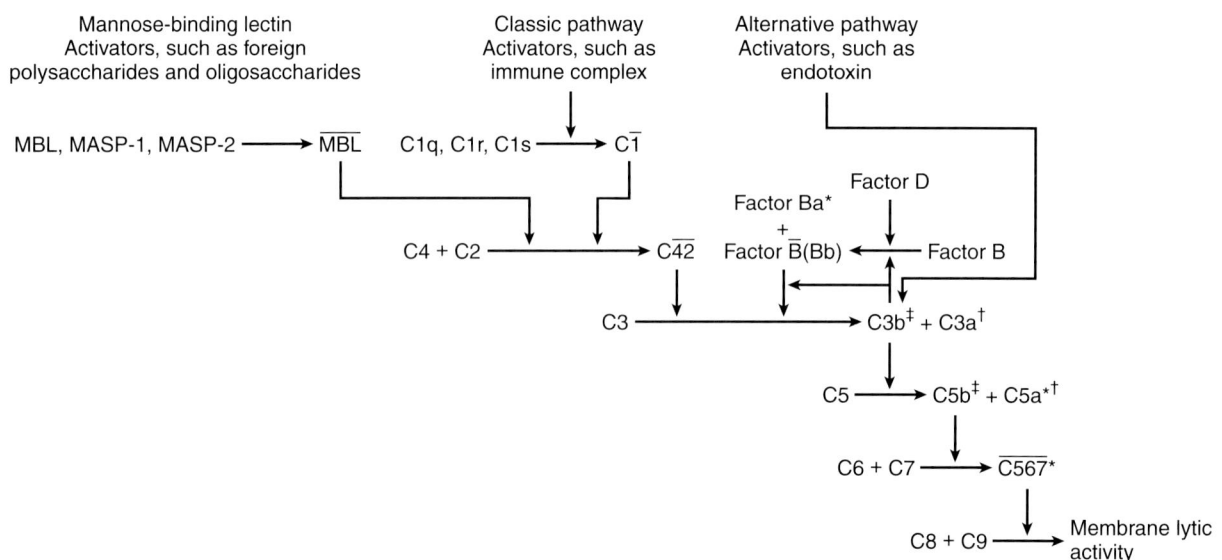

Figure 1-4 Complement system activation through the classic and alternative pathways. *MBL*, Mannose-binding lectin; *MASP-1*, MBL-associated serine protease-1; *MASP-2*, MBL-associated serine protease 2; $\overline{MBL}$, activated mannose-binding lectin. *, Chemotactic; †, anaphylatoxic; ‡, phagocytosis-enhancing.

taches to C4b2a complex to form the C5 binding and cleaving enzyme, C4b2a3b. This cleaves C5 to form C5a anaphylatoxin (which is highly chemotactic) and C5b, a phagocytosis-enhancing fragment. From this point, the sequence proceeds to activate the C6 to C9 components to generate C5b-9, the membrane attack complex.

The alternative pathway consists of several proteins: C3; factors B, D, H, and I, and properdin. This pathway bypasses the C142 steps and splits C3 directly by way of two enzymes: the priming C3 convertase (C3,Bb) and the amplifying C3 convertase (C3b,Bb). C3,Bb is formed through cleavage by factor D of a portion of factor B bound to a reconfigured C3 molecule. Structural reconfiguration of C3 occurs as a result of hydrolysis of the internal thioester bond that holds the hydrophobic portion of the structure into a strained bend. C3,Bb splits more C3 to C3a and C3b. The C3b then binds factor B in the presence of Mg^{++} to form C3b,B. Factor D cleaves the bound factor B portion to form C3b,Bb, the amplifying C3 convertase. Properdin stabilizes the C3 convertase. C3b is regulated by factor H, which binds to C3b and allows its inactivation by factor I. C3 bound to certain cell surfaces may interfere with this regulatory mechanism. For example, attachment of C3b to zymosan decreases affinity to factor H, increases affinity to factor B, and activates the alternative pathway, whereas its attachment to surfaces rich in sialic acid does the reverse. Because most host cells contain sialic acid, which most bacteria lack, this phenomenon may be an important triggering mechanism for the cytolytic defense system while keeping the host cells relatively immune from attack. Beyond C3, the alternative pathway is identical to that of the classic pathway with the formation of the C5b-9 membrane attack complex.

The mannose-binding lectin pathway consists of mannose-binding lectin (a C-type lectin or collectin), mannose-binding lectin–associated serine protease-1 and -2, which are distinct but partially homologous to C1q, C1r, and C1s, respectively. Mannose-binding lectin is the recognition unit that binds to foreign polysaccharides and oligosaccharides. Activated mannose-binding lectin complex, as with aC1, in turn reacts with C4 and C2 to form C3 convertase (C4b2a), and then cascades further as with the classic pathway.

Aside from factors H and I, membrane proteins regulate complement activation on cell surfaces. Similar to the potential protective effect of sialic acid on mammalian cell surfaces, these membrane proteins also may protect host cells from damage by complement. These proteins include the C3 and C5 receptors, decay-accelerating factor and membrane cofactor protein, S-protein, and the factor C8-binding protein (also known as the *homologous restriction factor* because it recognizes C8 and C9 of homologous species but not C8 and C9 of other species). Decay-accelerating factor and membrane cofactor protein prevent membrane activation of both complement pathways by reacting with C4b and C3b, thereby preventing C3 convertase formation, whereas S-protein and C8-binding protein prevent formation of C5b-9, the membrane attack complex.

Complement activation by any pathway results in (1) generation of membrane lytic (bacteriolytic) activity that is important in the killing of certain microbes, such as gram-negative bacteria (particularly *Neisseria*); (2) production of chemotactic factors that locally mobilize leukocytes; (3) formation of factors that control or enhance phagocytic function; and (4) production of peptides that mediate other components of the inflammatory process. In addition to assisting phagocyte function indirectly by the fixation of complement, antibody also may directly enhance phagocytosis by its opsonic activity. (Readers interested in greater detail are referred to reviews.[33,56])

CELLULAR COMPONENTS

If the invading microbe escapes the first-line defenses afforded by the local and humoral factors, containment becomes the responsibility of the phagocytic cells and lymphocytes. Activation of phagocytes and lymphocytes requires binding of the signal or ligand to a cell surface receptor. Formation of the signal-receptor complex then is followed by a cascade of reactions that eventually result in translation of signal to cell function.

Cell Surface Receptors Phagocytes and lymphocytes possess cell surface receptors that are anchored to the cell surface on one end and bound to its ligand on the other end. When the cell surface receptors form complexes with their specific ligands, a series of processes follows that signals initiation of cell function, regardless of purpose: cell protection, recognition, proliferation, cytotoxicity, or other regulatory functions. Cell surface receptors may be classified into (1) those that identify and bind microbial ligands and identify modified proteins and other chemically altered host substances (e.g., apoptotic cells) targeted for elimination and (2) those that bind host ligands to their two ends to initiate host cell-cell interaction and communication. The former recognize mainly pathogen-associated molecular patterns and are referred to as *pattern recognition receptors*. In humans, pattern recognition receptors appear to follow a hierarchy from the most primitive, simple, and less specific (e.g., scavenger receptors) to the more advanced, complex, and highly specific systems (e.g., complement and immunoglobulin receptors).

Although mannose, complement, and immunoglobulin receptors bind foreign ligands, they also are configured to bind to host cells to initiate cell-cell interactions. For example, cell-associated mannose receptors (found on macrophages, dendritic cells, and some endothelial cells) consist of five distinct domains, two of which (a cysteine-rich *N*-terminus and a fibronectin type II–like domain) do not bind carbohydrates but rather bind to ligands on surfaces of subsets of macrophages and B lymphocytes, in keeping with the known macrophage cell-cell interactive function for antigen processing and presentation to specifically reactive lymphocytes. Complement receptors are found mainly on polymorphonuclear neutrophils (PMNs) and monocytes and subserve certain cell functions (e.g.,

C3a subserves secretion; C5a subserves chemotaxis and secretion); CR1 and CR3 (C3b/C4b and C3bi receptors, respectively) enhance phagocytosis. CR1 also controls the metabolism of C3b to C3dg by factor I and thus may protect host cell surface against complement damage.

Immunoglobulin bridges the gap between microbe and host cell by binding microbe to its Fab or antigen-binding site and its Fc portion to the Fc receptor on the host cell. Many Fc receptors for immunoglobulins (FcγR) are now known; among the earliest described are the high-avidity Fc receptors found in monocytes (FcγRI, FcγR$_{p72}$, and CD64) enhanced by γ-interferon (IFN-γ) and are important for phagocytosis, antigen capture for presentation to T cells, antibody-dependent cell-mediated cytotoxicity,[45] and release of cytokines and reactive oxygen products. A low-avidity Fc receptor (FcγRII, FcγR$_{p40}$, or CD32) is found on neutrophils, monocytes, macrophages, dendritic cells, some endothelial cells, and platelets. This receptor is considered important for endocytosis, cytotoxicity, and immunomodulation. FcγRIIIa, FcγR$_{p50-70}$, or CDI6a is found in neutrophil natural killer cells and monocytes, and some T cells probably are involved in antibody-dependent cell-mediated cytotoxicity and cytokine production. These receptors represent just a sampling of the increasing number of cell surface antigens in the immunoglobulin supergene family.

Development of monoclonal antibodies to leukocyte antigens also has allowed the identification of a family of leukocyte adherence glycoproteins. Examples include CD11a (formerly called "receptor for leukocyte function-associated antigen-1"), CD11b (formerly called "MO-l," "Mac-l," or "CR3", and CD11c (formerly called "p150/95"). All three proteins promote cell adhesion and appear to be part of a family of adherence-mediating receptor proteins that include fibronectin receptors and perhaps others with which they share substantial J3-chain sequence homology and the capacity to recognize the RGD sequence (Arg-Gly-Asp) for binding. In addition, all can directly bind both lipopolysaccharide- and non–lipopolysaccharide-containing microbes independent of antibody or complement. Thus these proteins may be part of an important defense system in neonates before development of acquired immunity.

Receptors may detach from the cell surface and solubilize in plasma. Soluble receptors may modify cell function by acting as sponges that divert ligands away from cells. The most recently characterized example of this phenomenon is the TNF receptor–associated periodic syndrome,[16] in which the periodic fever and inflammatory manifestations are the result of failure of TNF receptors from detaching from the cell anchor because of a missense mutation in the gene encoding the 55-kd TNF receptor. The defect affects normal cleavage at the extracellular disulfide subdomains of the receptor, leading to diminished shedding.

A move is under way to rename all leukocyte surface antigens using the "CD" nomenclature. With redesignations of previously described receptors and discovery of new ones, the number of CD-designated molecules is now up to 247 and increasing.*

Signal Transduction   Signal transduction begins once the ligand binds to the cell receptor. Although evidence is incomplete, signal transduction and intracellular events resulting from cellular activation of neutrophils, monocytes, and lymphocytes appear to follow a similar basic mechanistic pattern. Briefly, the pattern involves conversion of cell surface signals into chemical energy, which is further translated to mechanical action or function. Activation begins with interaction of the signal (ligand or activator molecule) with a specific cell surface receptor, activating a membrane phospholipase C, which hydrolyzes phosphatidylinositol 4,5-bisphosphate into two secondary messengers, diacylglycerol and inositol 1,4,5-triphosphate. Diacylglycerol activates protein kinase C, which phosphorylates a Na^+-H^+ pump that raises intracellular pH. High intracellular pH activates phosphorylation reactions of pH-sensitive proteins, and phosphorylation reactions in turn provide the energy needed to translate signals to action or function. The other second messenger, 1,4,5-inositol triphosphate, releases Ca^{++} from Ca^{++} stores. A complex of free Ca^{++} ions, calmodulin, and a kinase is formed, which similarly leads to phosphorylation of other proteins and generates energy to convert signal to function.

Cellular Myoskeleton   Myoskeletal elements in the presence of energy provided by phosphorylation reactions are the "hardware" that converts the signal, such as a chemotactic molecule, into mechanical responses for directed locomotion, engulfment (phagocytosis and pinocytosis), degranulation or exocytosis, and secretion. As such, these element play important roles in cellular function.

The myoskeletal elements of leukocytes are composed of two major filamentous cytoplasmic structures, microtubules and microfilaments. Microtubules are hollow filaments made up of polymers of the protein tubulin. The interaction of microtubules with membranes apparently controls the movement, distribution, and traffic of membrane transport proteins, lysosomal granules, and cell surface receptors. These effects suggest their importance as regulators in the movement of substances through the cell membrane and in membrane-membrane or membrane-substrate interactions in cell adherence and locomotion. The effects of microtubule disturbance on cell function are shown in Chédiak-Higashi cells and cells treated with the antitubulin drug colchicine.[35]

Microfilaments are smaller in diameter than microtubules and made up of actin polymers. These structures are arranged randomly or oriented in subplasmalemmal (subcortical) bundles. At present, cell-substrate contact is believed to activate actin-binding protein and myosin, which gel and contract the actin filaments. The impor-

---

*Readers are referred to Sundy et al.[51]; for the latest updates, consult Protein Reviews On the Web (PROW)[37] (available from: http://www.ncbi.nlm.nih.gov/prow).

tance of microfilaments has been demonstrated for cell locomotion, phagocytosis, and degranulation. Cells treated with low concentrations of cytochalasin B, which dissolves actin gels, show defects in all functional parameters. Cells from a child with abnormal leukocytic actin also showed profound functional abnormalities.[5]

Phagocytes As the names implies, *phagocytes* are cells that have the ability to engulf particles. In general, these cells include the polymorphonuclear granulocytes (neutrophils and eosinophils), the monocytes of the blood, and at the tissue level the macrophages. To facilitate engulfment, phagocytes must be brought in close proximity to their target particles. This movement requires leukocytic mobilization, a phenomenon that involves two events: adherence to endothelial surfaces and locomotion. Adherence to endothelial cells allows phagocytes to gain a foothold on the vascular endothelium, an important prerequisite for the mobilization of leukocytes into extravascular sites. Adherence to endothelial cells also is important because the phagocyte moves by "pulling itself ahead," which requires firm anchoring of a part of the cell. Cell adhesion glycoprotein receptors play an important role in the regulation of cell adherence. Patients with glycoprotein receptor deficiency have recurrent infections at an early age, delayed separation of the umbilical cord and wound healing, early onset of severe periodontitis, defective inflammatory responses, and impaired neutrophil and monocyte adherence, aggregation, and chemotaxis.[1]

Cell locomotion is either random or chemotactic. Random locomotion is similar to the movements of a person who is blind left in the middle of an open field with no signals to which to respond. The probability of moving in one direction would be equal to the probability of going in any other direction. Chemotaxis is the unidirectional response to a concentration gradient of a chemical attractant. This response is similar to a person who is blind going toward the direction of a sound. Random locomotion is nonstimulated or stimulated (chemokinetic, a multidirectional response to the presence of a chemical substance). Endogenous chemotactic factors are derived from various sources including the complement system, from which is derived the chemotactic fragment of C5, and from various cells (cytokines) such as macrophages, lymphocytes, and granulocytes. The humoral regulation of leukocyte locomotion has been studied more extensively than regulators of other leukocyte functions such as phagocytosis. These regulators include the anaphylatoxin inactivator (carboxypeptidase N), the chemotactic factor inactivator, and the cell-directed inhibitor of leukotaxis.

The anaphylatoxin inactivator (carboxypeptidase N) is present in normal serum or plasma. This factor regulates C5a anaphylatoxin and chemotactic factor by splitting the C-terminal arginine of the molecule to produce C5a des Arg, completely abolishing anaphylatoxin activity and reducing chemotactic activity to approximately 10% of original C5a potency.[23] Plasma anaphylatoxin inactivator activity is elevated in Hodgkin's disease, pregnancy, cystic

fibrosis, and chronic lung diseases; low levels are observed in chronic liver disease (because it is derived from the liver) in the presence of intravascular complement activation such as during hemodialysis, during cardiopulmonary bypass, and in trauma.[28] A familial carboxypeptidase N deficiency has been described in a patient with long-standing angioedema.

The chemotactic factor inactivator is another regulator present in normal human serum.[28,58] Chemotactic factor inactivator acts directly on chemotactic factors to inactive them. Two types of inactivators have been identified, both of which are heat labile and nondialyzable. Elevations of serum chemotactic factor inactivator have been associated with chemotactic defects and have been observed in patients with Hodgkin's disease, cirrhosis, sarcoidosis, lepromatous leprosy, hairy cell leukemia, and systemic lupus erythematosus. The cell-directed inhibitor of leukotaxis, which is present in normal serum, is another regulator of cell locomotion.[28] This inactivator acts directly on polymorphonuclear cells and monocytes to inhibit locomotion and phagocytosis. Immunoglobulins are responsible for much of the cell-directed inhibitor activity in normal serum and partly may explain the immunosuppressive effects of high-dose intravenous IgG. Elevations of cell-directed inhibitor in serum have been associated with abnormal leukocyte locomotion and observed in patients with cirrhosis and cancer and some with recalcitrant periodontitis. A low molecular weight cell-directed inhibitor specific against monocytes has been described in patients with cancer.[47] The material is lower in molecular weight, dialyzable, and inactive against polymorphonuclear cells, and it does not inhibit phagocytosis. In disease states, abnormally high serum heavy molecular weight cell-directed inhibitor activity may result from aggregated, complexed, or transformed immunoglobulins.

Phagocytosis is initiated by attachment of a particle to the surface of the phagocyte, followed by invagination of that portion of the cell membrane, formation of a vacuole, and entrapment of the particle in the vacuole. Several enhancers of phagocytosis have been described: the opsonins (immunoglobulins and complement products), which coat the target particles to render them palatable to the phagocyte, and tuftsin, which acts directly on the cell to stimulate its phagocytic activity.[34] The heat-stable specific opsonin is a specific antibody acting alone or with complement activated by the classic pathway. The heat-labile opsonin includes the complement activation products C3b and C5b, which are generated through activation of the classic and the alternative complement pathways. Opsonins enhance phagocytosis by acting as ligands that attach to the bacterial surface antigen through the $F(ab)_2$ portion of the IgG or IgM molecule and specific receptor sites on the phagocyte cell surface through its Fc portion. Opsonic deficiencies have been described in newborns, in sickle cell disease, and in deficiency states of the C3 and C5 components of complement. Tuftsin, a phagocytosis-enhancing material present in normal serum, is a tetrapeptide that acts directly on the cell to stimulate phagocytosis of opsonized bacteria. Two types of tuftsin disorders have been described in the literature: one is congenital and caused by the presence of an abnormal (mutant) peptide that competitively inhibits normal tuftsin; the other is a deficiency state observed in patients who have undergone splenectomy because of the lack of a tuftsin-releasing enzyme derived from the spleen.

Once a microbe is phagocytized, a series of events occurring within the neutrophil leads to the eventual killing and digestion of the microbe. First, the phagosomal membrane fuses with the lysosomal granule membrane to form a phagolysosome, resulting in discharge of the lysosomal granule contents into the phagocytic vacuole. This action is followed by a burst of metabolic activity leading to killing and digestion of the microbe. Two microbicidal mechanisms exist: the oxygen-dependent system and the oxygen-independent system. The former consists of myeloperoxidase and its cofactors (halides, thiocyanate, thyroxine, and triiodothyronine), hydrogen peroxide, superoxide anions, hydroxyl radicals, and singlet oxygen. This system, by a series of powerful oxidation-reduction reactions, is assumed to destroy phagocytized microbes. The oxygen-independent system includes low pH and a variety of catalytic and noncatalytic proteins, including antimicrobial peptides. Some factors are microbicidal or microbistatic, and some potentiate the effects of other more potent microbicides. Acid-sensitive organisms may be killed by the low pH achieved in the phagocyte vacuole. Lysozyme may potentiate the lytic action of other microbicidal factors on the bacterial cell wall. Lactoferrin binds iron and deprives the organism of an essential nutrient in addition to its antimicrobial peptide moiety. The cationic proteins may interfere with microbial viability by punching holes through microbial membrane (defensins and bacterial/permeability-increasing protein), similar to that produced by the C5b-9 membrane attack complex of complement and cytotoxic T cells, or by inhibiting microbial metabolism and protein synthesis (defensins and cathepsin G).

Unlike the PMNs (Figure 1-5), the mononuclear phagocytes the mononuclear phagocytes (monocytes and macrophages) move and respond to chemotactic stimuli more slowly, and they appear in the later phase of the inflammatory reaction, when certain microbes may have escaped or resisted neutrophil activity. Consequently, monocytes and macrophages are critical elements in the defense against intracellular microorganisms. In addition, they "clean up the battlefield" by removing the debris of dead cells remaining from the preceding acute inflammatory process. Also, unlike the neutrophils, the mononuclear phagocytes usually do not die after ingestion and digestion of bacteria. Their survival is due partly to their ability to synthesize new phospholipid, replenishing the phospholipid lost in the cell membrane during phagocytic activity. Myeloperoxidase does not appear to be an important bacterial-killing substance in the mature mononuclear phagocyte, which contains little or none of this enzyme.

The killing activity of mononuclear phagocytes may be

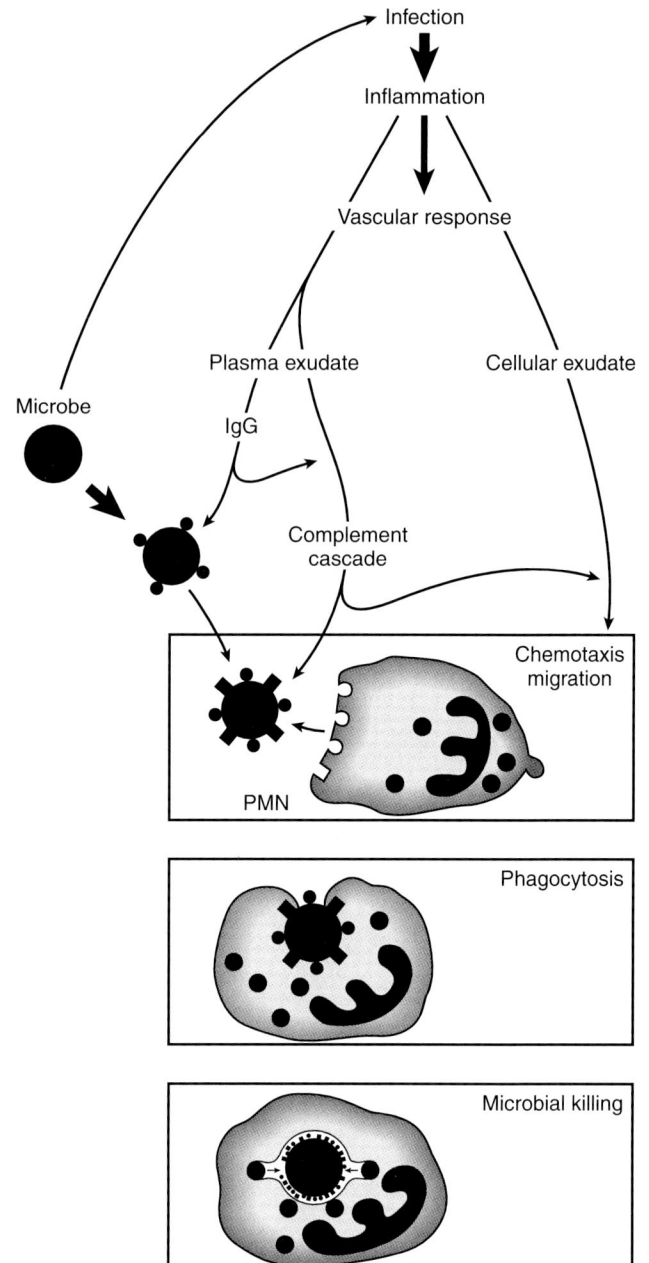

Figure 1-5 Polymorphonuclear leukocytic reactions after microbial invasion, terminating in microbial digestion and killing.

activated by products of lymphocytes formerly known collectively as "macrophage-activating factors" but now known to be many distinct factors, including IFN-γ, GM-CSF, IL-3, and IL-4. In addition to the phagocytic and scavenger activities of mononuclear phagocytes, other important functions have been assigned to these cells. For example, as the primary antigen-processing or antigen-presenting cells, they have essential immunoregulatory function on T lymphocytes, T-cell–B-cell collaboration in response to thymus-dependent antigen, and antigen presentation to B cells. Recognition of antigen by the immune system involves this important activity of the macrophage. This process involves several steps that begin with the

TABLE **1-3**

Differential Characteristics of B and T Lymphocytes

Characteristics	B Lymphocytes	T Lymphocytes
Differentiation of precursor cells	Bursa of Fabricius in birds or the equivalent in humans (fetal liver, bone marrow, or gut lymphoid tissue)	Thymus
Location	Predominates in bone marrow and in germinal centers and medullary cords of lymph nodes	Predominates in thymus, blood, thoracic duct lymph, spleen, and deep cortex of lymph nodes
Surface markers		
Rosette with sheep erythrocytes (CD2)	No	Yes
Fc receptors	Yes	No (activated cell may develop Fc receptors)
CR2 (C3dg receptor)	Yes	No
Responses to mitogens	Proliferate with pokeweed mitogen in the presence of helper T cells	Proliferate with phytohemagglutinin, concanavalin A, and pokeweed mitogens
Functions	Mainly antibody production	Mainly cell-mediated immunity or delayed hypersensitivity

binding of antigen to a mannose receptor or major histocompatibility complex (MHC) molecule on the surface of the macrophage, the antigen-presenting cell. This binding is followed by cell-cell contact between the antigen-bearing presenter macrophage and a T cell, for example, through cell adhesion receptor proteins on the T-cell surface and their specific ligands on the macrophage surface. Thus T-cell receptors CD11a and CD2 may bind to the macrophage ligand proteins intercellular adhesion molecule-I (ICAM-I) and LFA-3. Recognition of the antigen then proceeds with the involvement of another set of receptor-ligand interaction. The antigen bound to the MHC protein (antigen-MHC complex) on the macrophage surface interacts with the T-cell receptor (TCR-CD3 complex). Helper T cells possess the TCR-$\alpha\beta$-CD4 receptor, which specifically interacts with antigen bound to the MHC class II molecule; cytotoxic T cells have the TCR-$\gamma\delta$-CD8 receptor, which interacts with antigen on the MHC class I molecule.

In addition to the antigen-processing mechanism that requires cell-cell contact, mononuclear phagocytes may communicate with other cells by secretion of soluble substances (monokines), important inflammatory mediators.

Lymphocytes Host versus microbe interactions primarily involve nonspecific responses. In immunoglobulin responses, microbial antigen is recognized as foreign and specific antibodies recognize and bind it. Such recognition of a foreign antigen as "nonself" involves immunological memory and specificity that resides in lymphocytes. Antigens derived from microbes bind to cell surface receptors on macrophages, processed and presented to specific antigen-reactive lymphocytes through specific receptor-ligand interactions. If the antigen is recognized as foreign, the specific reactive lymphocytes respond by transformation and proliferation into more of the similarly specific

reactive cells, increasing the number of cells that can react against the antigen. Unlike the phagocytic cells, lymphocytes do not function by engulfment and digestion of particles but mainly by secretion of effector substances called *lymphokines*. The lymphocyte immune system consists of two distinct types of cells: the B cells, so called because their development requires processing by the bursa of Fabricius in birds or its equivalent in mammals, and the T cells, which require processing by the thymus. Although morphologically indistinguishable, the B and T cells differ considerably in their locations in various anatomical sites, responses to different mitogens, production of lymphokines, kinetics, function, and development (Table 1-3).

The most important difference between B and T cells is function. B cells are responsible primarily for the antibody-dependent reactions, whereas T cells are responsible for the so-called cell-mediated immunity (CMI). In both instances the reactions are mediated through production and release of lymphokines. B cells synthesize and release mainly immunoglobulins; T cells produce an array of substances with various functions. Of the nonimmunoglobulin lymphokines, one of the earliest described is IL-2, which is required for proliferation of certain subpopulations of lymphocytes, in particular CD4+ helper T cells, CD8+ suppressor and cytotoxic T cells, and natural killer cells; various chemotactic factors; and the migration inhibitory factor. Small numbers of lymphocytes can produce migration inhibitory factor in sufficient quantity to inhibit great numbers of macrophages; thus blast transformation is not necessary for its expression. The migration inhibitory effect of migration inhibitory factor may result from its ability to increase macrophage adherence, and most likely it functions by promoting mononuclear phagocyte accumulation at sites of T-cell–mediated inflammation.

Some lymphokines that have not been fully defined chemically are named mostly according to their observed in vitro effects. In general, these effects can be grouped into three kinds of activities: regulation of inflammatory reactions (migration inhibitory factor and chemotactic lymphokines), inhibition or killing of target cells (interferon and cytotoxic factors), and stimulation of cell proliferation (growth and other mitogenic factors).

Although distinct, B and T cells are derived from a common uncommitted lymphocyte precursor, and their functional differences are narrow. Under certain conditions B cells also can produce nonimmunoglobulin lymphokines such as migration inhibitory factor, macrophage chemotactic factor, and interferon. The mechanisms involved in the commitment process or the signals that initiate the development of the uncommitted cells into B or T cells are beginning to be defined. During their development, these cells acquire or lose certain surface receptors and antigenic characteristics as they differentiate further into the various subsets of B- and T-cell populations. In the thymus, cells acquire some or all other surface antigens, and further differentiation is manifested by a loss of some of these antigens, the progessive expression of new surface antigens, and activation of the γ, β, or α genes. For example, the earliest thymocytes express the CD2 surface antigen followed by TCR-$\gamma\delta$-CD3 receptor protein. As the cells mature further, they acquire the TCR-$\alpha\beta$-CD3 receptor, CD4, CD5, and CD8 markers. Differentiation then diverges into two distinct lineages: to helper-inducer cells, which are CD4$^+$, CD8$^-$, or to suppressor or killer cells, which are CD4$^-$, CD8$^+$. A direct route apparently also occurs in which the T cells acquire only CD4 or CD8 along with other surface antigens. (The genetic control of lymphocyte differentiation and macrophage–B-cell–T-cell interactions is discussed in greater detail in several reviews by Reinherz and Schlossman,[40] Waldmann et al.,[55] and Gallin et al.[15])

CD4$^+$ T helper cells differentiate further into two distinct subsets, Th1 and Th2, which produce a distinct array of cytokines. The Th1 subset produces cytokines, mainly IL-2, IFN-γ, and TNF-α, associated with phagocyte-dependent responses, whereas the Th2 subset produces cytokines IL-4, IL-5, IL-6, IL-9, IL-10, and IL-13, associated with phagocyte-independent responses. A Th0 subset also has been designated for T helper cells that produce cytokines of both Th1 and Th2 subclasses. Although this subset differentiation is clear in the murine model, it is not as clear in humans; however, Th1 and Th2 clones specific for a particular antigen have been identified. Studies have identified IL-12 and IL-4 as driving the development of Th1 and Th2.[14b] In humans, IL-12 has been shown to shift Th0/Th2 cells to the Th1 profile. Furthermore, antibodies that block IL-12 also switch the response back to Th0/Th2. IL-12 not only induces IFN-γ production by T lymphocytes but also blocks the development of IL-4–producing Th2 cells. Interestingly, IFN-γ appears to upregulate IL-12 receptor (β chain) expression on T cells, which may help to initiate their susceptibility to IL-12.

CD4$^+$ T lymphocytes stimulated with purified protein derivative generally have a Th1 cytokine response. How-

ever, addition of exogenous IL-4 shifts the response to Th0 (IFN-γ/IL-2) and Th2 (IL-4, IL-5, or both). Early production of IL-4 is key to drive the response in a Th2 direction. FcϵR1$^+$ cells may produce the IL-4 early. Hormones such as glucocorticoids, androgen steroids, and calcitriol also may regulate Th1 and Th2 cytokine secretion.

Many examples exist of the possible roles of Th1/Th2 cells in human diseases.[42] Th1-type cytotoxic activity and delayed-type hypersensitivity may play a role in transplant rejection. For example, rejected allografts had IL-2 and IFN-γ protein expression. Th2 clones have been isolated from allergy sufferers, and Th2 cytokines were detected in bronchial biopsy specimens of patients with asthma. Th1 cytokines IFN-γ and TNF-α have been associated with pathogenesis of multiple sclerosis.

T cells have key roles in CMI. Unlike antibody-dependent or humoral immunity, which can be defined and quantitated more clearly, CMI is much more complex. Transfer of immunity from a reactive donor to a nonreactive recipient can be made by cells or extracts of such cells but not serum. The best-known reaction to demonstrate CMI is the cutaneous delayed hypersensitivity reaction (DHR), such as occurs after intradermal tuberculin injection into a previously sensitized individual. Typically, the reaction develops slowly, not reaching its peak until 24 to 72 hours later with the development of erythema and indurated swelling at the site of injection. Histologically, a transient neutrophilic response is noted in the early lesion, followed by a change to mononuclear phagocytes, lymphocytes, and basophils. Fibrin is seen commonly and believed to be responsible for the induration because it can be suppressed effectively with anticoagulants.[8] Systemic injection of tuberculin into a sensitized animal produces a generalized reaction characterized by fever, lymphopenia, and shock and a DHR around tuberculous lesions.

In addition to cutaneous DHR, CMI is involved in the protection against infectious agents (mainly intracellular microbes), graft rejection, and tumor cell proliferation. In these instances, killer T cells are of primary importance. Moreover, CMI is involved in autoimmune disorders. Animal and human models of autoimmune disease show the presence of a defective suppressor cell network. Whether this defect is primary, thus allowing the expression of certain immunological mechanisms (the "forbidden clones") that otherwise would have been suppressed, or secondary to chronic stimulation from a real or perceived foreign antigen is unknown.

The mechanisms involved in CMI are complex. In general, the mechanisms include an afferent limb that involves mainly antigen processing by the macrophages; a central position occupied by the CD4$^+$ T lymphocytes or macrophages, which interpret and translate the afferent signals; and the efferent pathway, which involves the execution of effector functions by a constellation of cells and factors directly responsible for the expression of the inflammatory reaction such as DHR. The central importance of CD4$^+$ T cells in host immune response against infections and surveillance and defense against neoplasms is illustrated best in acquired immunodeficiency syndrome, in which the causative virus, the human immunodeficiency virus, specifically attacks and kills CD4$^+$ T cells. In full-blown disease, patients have recurrent or frequent infections produced by unusual organisms and from uncommon neoplastic diseases.[49]

The inability of a previously sensitized individual to express DHR is called *anergy,* and such individuals can be assumed to have one or more abnormalities in the afferent, central, or efferent limb of CMI. Anergy may result from defective antigen processing by macrophages, abnormal lymphocyte function, or a disorder in effector functions. In most instances, it may result from a combination of several abnormalities. For example, in Hodgkin's disease and sarcoidosis, anergy may result from increased serum CFI activity and defective lymphocytes. By inactivating chemotactic factors, CFI could render defective the chemotactic response to the antigen (afferent limb) and the phagocytic release of phlogistic lysosomal granule contents (efferent limb).

Despite increasing sophistication of testing for CMI, skin testing for DHR is still the most practical and clinically useful single test. Before a failure of response to skin test antigens can be interpreted as anergy, however, two issues should be considered. First, has the subject been previously sensitized to the specific antigens used? Testing with a battery of three to four antigens (*Candida,* mumps, trichophyton, and tetanus toxoid) usually answers this question. Although actual reported percentages vary, generally most normal individuals react (induration $\geq$ 5 mm) to at least one of three antigens. If anergy is still questioned after multiple skin tests have been performed, the patient can be sensitized with a specific antigen with subsequent retesting; a variety of vaccines have been used for this purpose, including tetanus toxoid. The second consideration is whether the test was performed correctly. Among the more common problems in skin testing are improper route of administration (e.g., subcutaneous instead of intradermal), errors in interpreting reactions, and high variability in interpretation of reactions. Reactions to mumps antigen and tuberculin antigen in individuals who have had previous skin testing peak earlier (24 to 36 hours); hence, reading at 48 to 72 hours may miss the maximum reaction.

Although measurement of induration has become the standard means of assessment of cutaneous DHRs, several objections to this method exist. One is the difficulty of accurate measurement of the indurated area. Another objection is that the induration does not result primarily from inflammatory cell infiltration but from fibrin deposition; thus anticoagulants suppress the induration, although they have no effect on mononuclear cell infiltration.[8] Therefore the absence of induration does not necessarily indicate the absence of CMI or anergy. For this reason a tuberculin reaction without palpable induration but with significant erythema in a patient who has received anticoagulant must not be interpreted as negative.[27]

EFFECTS OF INFECTION ON THE HOST

NONSPECIFIC EFFECTS OF INFECTION

When the host encounters potentially injurious agents, an intricate series of reactions is triggered for protection against injury. These reactions initially are nonspecific and known collectively as *inflammation,* or the *inflammatory reaction* (Figure 1-6). The acute response consists of the release of mediators, vascular changes (vasospasm, vasodilation, and increased vasopermeability), and exudation of cells, mainly the polymorphonuclear leukocytes. When the reaction continues, the subacute inflammatory reaction begins, with the appearance of mononuclear cells (monocytes and lymphocytes) and the subsequent formation of granulation tissue. If inflammation still fails to restore homeostasis, the chronic inflammatory response ensues, which is characterized by further exudation of lymphocytes, monocytes, and plasma cells.

Plasma-Derived Mediators of Inflammation　Mediators of inflammation have been variously classified. For example, they have been classified according to their time of appearance during inflammation; thus the term *immediators* is used for those that appear early (histamine, serotonin, slow-reacting substance A, kinins, and the lipid-derived mediators) and *intermediators* for those that appear later (complement and lysosomal enzymes).[59] A more useful method involves their function as linkages of key systems that help manifest the inflammatory reaction.

Mediators are derived from plasma substrates or directly from cells. Mediators acting in groups to serve a common general function compose systems. The coagulation, fibrinolytic, kinin, and complement systems are examples (Figure 1-7). Hageman factor (factor XII) is the central component (the hub) interconnecting the first three systems, and plasmin is the key component linking these systems to complement. Numerous hubs and linkages exist because most mediators are multifunctional, and as their functional characteristics are understood, they too become hubs. For example, thrombin is a hub for fibrin clot formation, and recently activated protein C is another hub for fibrinolysis. These soluble mediator systems work with cells (endothelial cells, granulocytes, monocytes and macrophages, and lymphocytes) to link inflammation and coagulation, but the steps that result in expression of inflammatory and coagulation responses also trigger regulatory negative feedback loops. Thus proinflammatory factors often initiate "on demand" antiinflammatory factors, and coagulation triggers anticoagulation (fibrinolysis). The result is a complex protective network with a goal of returning to a balanced state.

Kinin System　In addition to activating proenzymes of the coagulation and fibrinolytic systems, the activation of

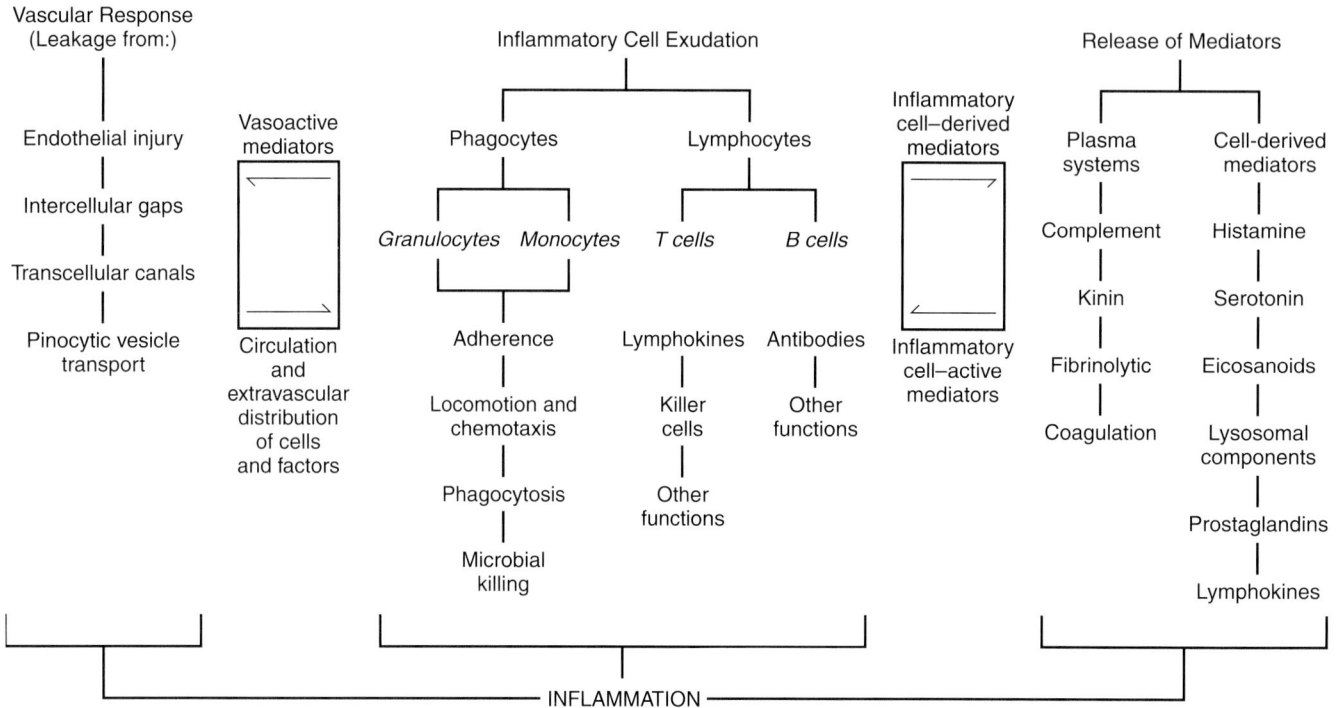

Figure 1-6 The various mechanisms involved in the production of inflammation in response to injury or infection. Connections among the vascular response, inflammatory cell exudation, and release of mediators indicate their close interdependence and interactions.

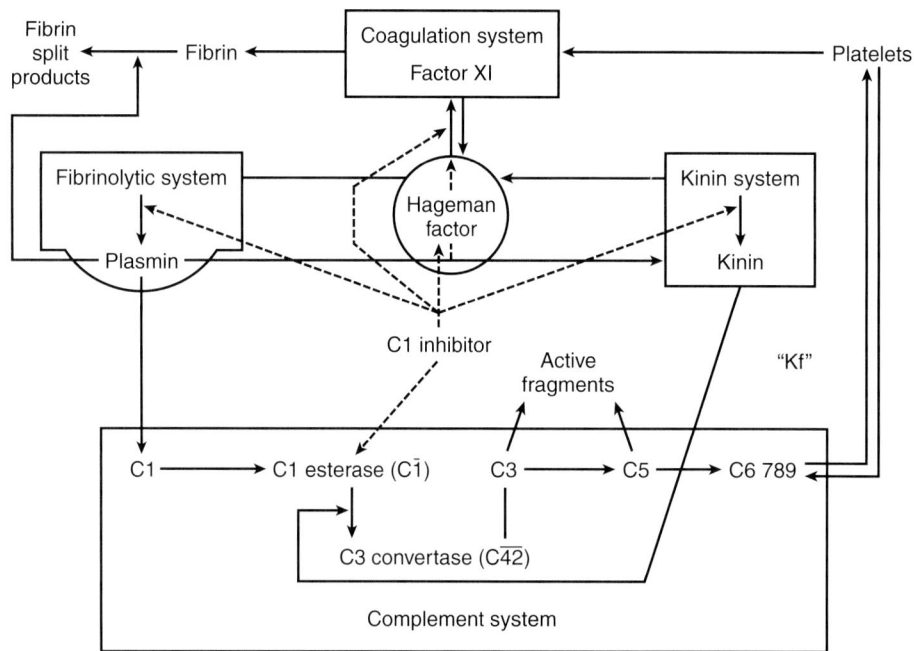

Figure 1-7 Relationships among the coagulation, fibrinolytic, kinin, and complement systems. Hageman factor is the hub that links the first three systems. Plasmin and to some extent, "Kf" fragment of the kinin-generating system provide the connection to complement. An additional link is present between the complement system and coagulation cascade through the platelet intermediary. A negative link of all four systems exists with the presence of C1 inhibitor (see text). ---▸, Inhibition; ——▸, stimulation.

factor XII to XIIa results in a cascade that leads to the formation of bradykinin. Factor XIIa converts prekallikrein to kallikrein, which is a cleaving enzyme of its plasma substrate, kininogen, the precursor of the active nonapeptide bradykinin. Positive and negative feedback loops modulate the system. For example, kininogen may act as a nonenzymatic cofactor that enhances activation of XII and the formation of kallikrein. Bradykinin, the major active end product of kinin system generation, is a potent vasodilatory, vasopermeable, and pain-inducing factor in vivo and elicits slow contractions of certain smooth muscles in vitro.[41a] Ascertainment of its exact role in inflammation is difficult, but studies in rats suggest its importance in the causation of the edema that occurs early in inflammation. Evidence exists that bradykinin also enhances the synthesis and release of prostaglandins through its activating effect on phospholipase A_2, an enzyme involved in releasing arachidonate for biosyntheses of lipid-derived mediators, prostaglandins, leukotrienes, and lipoxins.

The kinin system is regulated by inactivators (kininases) and inhibitors that are present in plasma and tissues. Two kininases are known to rapidly destroy bradykinin: kininase I, or carboxypeptidase, which is identical to the C3 and C5a inactivator; and kininase II, or phenylalanine arginine carboxydipeptidase, which splits the carboxyterminal dipeptide of bradykinin and is identical to the angiotensin I converting enzyme. Additional less well-defined cell-derived kininases for leukokinin and C-kinin also exist. The inhibitors of the kinin-forming system include kallikrein antagonist, the C1 esterase inhibitor (which also inhibits the esterase, chemotactic, and kinin-generating activities of kallikrein), and α_2-macroglobulin (which inhibits the chemotactic and kininogenase activities of kallikrein).

Coagulation and Fibrinolytic Systems Coagulation may be initiated by the intrinsic or extrinsic pathways. The intrinsic pathway is triggered by the activation of XII to XIIa and through a series of reactions and activations called the *intrinsic coagulation cascade,* eventually resulting in the formation of thrombin. Thrombin formation also results from activation of tissue factor that in turn activates VII to VIIa and initiates a cascade by the extrinsic pathway (so called because tissue factor is on the endothelial cell surface and extrinsic to plasma). Thrombin then acts on fibrinogen to form fibrin, the major component of the fibrin clot.

In turn, the persistence of the clot is modulated by the fibrinolytic system, which is triggered simultaneously during the initiation of coagulation by the action of XIIa on plasminogen activator. The latter acts on plasminogen to produce plasmin, and plasmin is the principal fibrin clot-lysing factor. Fibrinolysis also is triggered by binding of thrombin to thrombomodulin on the endothelial cell surface. The resulting thrombin-thrombomodulin complex activates the protein C system, which in turn activates plasmin formation indirectly by inhibiting plasminogen activator inhibitor-1.

Linking Inflammation, Coagulation, and Fibrinolysis
Each plasma-derived system does not function as a totally independent unit but rather interrelates with the various other systems, including the inflammatory cells and cell-derived mediators. Factor XII provides the common link among the coagulation, fibrinolytic, and kinin systems because XIIa activates the initiating proenzymes for these systems (Figure 1-7). The link between these systems and the complement system is then provided by plasmin through its activity on C1 and its ability to release the inflammatory fragments of C3. An additional link is provided by Kf, which enhances the formation of C3 convertase, the activating enzyme for C3. Direct links of the complement system to the coagulation system also exist because the terminal sequence of complement activity can be initiated and enhanced by platelets. Reciprocal modulation of platelet and clotting effects in the rabbit also have been shown by the enhancement of platelet clot-promoting factors by C6 and modulation of platelet membrane function by C5-9 membrane attack complex. Finally, a common modulating factor for all four systems is present because the inhibitor for activated C1 inhibits factor XII and the fibrinolytic system through its inhibitory effect on plasmin, the coagulation system through its inhibitory effect on the activation of clotting factor, and the kinin system through its inhibitory effect on kallikrein.[11a] Although factor XII seemingly plays a central role in these interrelated phenomena in vitro, patients with a deficiency of this factor have no demonstrable defect in the inflammatory response and no bleeding tendencies, despite abnormal in vitro coagulation. Thus other pathways of activation, such as the extrinsic coagulation pathway, may operate to bypass factor XII steps in vivo if factor XII is unavailable.

In addition to its procoagulant effects and activation of the fibrinolytic pathway, thrombin also has proinflammatory effects (endothelial cell P-selectin expression and platelet-activating factor synthesis and enhancement of prostacyclin, phagocytic adherence, and chemotactic response), and cell growth–promoting effects for wound healing (fibroblast mitogenic effect, enhanced platelet-derived growth factor, and TGF-β). Thrombin is inhibited by forming a complex with antithrombin. Therefore thrombin occupies a central role in the inflammation, coagulation and anticoagulation, wound-healing axis. Activated protein C, an on-demand product of thrombin formation, also occupies a central role in modulating inflammatory, coagulant, and fibrinolytic responses to systemic infection through its multiple actions, including (1) antithrombin effect by inactivating factors VIIa and Va, (2) fibrinolytic effect by inhibiting plasminogen-activator inhibitor-1, (3) antiinflammatory effect by inhibiting syntheses of inflammatory cytokines (TNF-α, IL-1, and IL-6) by monocytes and selectin-mediated leukocyte binding to endothelial cells.[3]

Products of fibrinogen and fibrin have inflammatory effects. For example, fibrinopeptides released by the action of thrombin on fibrinogen enhance capillary permeability, chemotactically attract leukocytes, and potentiate the smooth muscle effect of bradykinin. Fibrin fragments, released on proteolysis of fibrin by plasmin, are chemotactic for leukocytes and enhance vascular permeability.

Hemostasis requires a base on which these critical reactions can occur, and the endothelial cell provides this base.[10,15] Under normal conditions the endothelial cell provides a nonthrombotic and noninflammatory medium with expression of antithrombin activity such as heparan sulfate proteoglycan (required for antithrombin III activity); profibrinolytic activity such as thrombomodulin and receptors for activated protein C, plasminogen, and tissue plasminogen activator; and potent inhibitors of platelet activation such as prostacyclin and CD39/ectoADPase. On endothelial cell stimulation such as with TNF-α or microbial toxins, antithrombotic activities are reduced and converted to a prothrombotic and proinflammatory phenotype with expression of inflammatory cytokines and chemokines, leukocyte adhesion molecules, and procoagulant factors such as platelet growth and activating factors, plasminogen-activator inhibitor-1, and von Willebrand factor.

Cell-Derived Mediators of Inflammation The mediators previously discussed generally are derived from plasma. Various inflammatory mediators are derived directly from cells. These mediators include vasoactive amines (histamine and serotonin), eicosanoids (prostaglandins, leukotrienes, and lipoxins), lysosomal components, and cytokines. These substances are released by cell lysis or active secretion. Cell lysis can occur for a variety of reasons, for instance, as a result of exposure to physical and chemical agents or through the cytotoxic activities of complement and lysosomal enzymes. Cytotoxic release is associated with cell death and liberation of its cytoplasmic and granular constituents. Secretion, on the other hand, involves the active release of mediators from intracellular granules and is not associated with cell disruption and death. In the case of lysosomal granule contents, secretion is preceded by movement of granules toward the plasma membrane, fusion of the granule membrane with the plasma membrane, and discharge of granule contents extracellularly. Although the precise mechanisms are not understood fully, lysosomal enzyme release from granules involves similar signal transduction mechanisms and the activities of serine esterase, cyclic nucleotides (wherein increase of cyclic adenosine monophosphate [cAMP] inhibits release and increase of cyclic guanosine monophosphate [cGMP] increases the release response), adenosine triphosphate, microfilaments (which apparently control movement of granules), microtubules (which presumably direct the traffic of moving granules), and the divalent cations Mg^{++} and Ca^{++}. These mechanisms are relatively well studied in the neutrophil, but they are less clear in other cells. In platelets, secretion may be facilitated by a network of intracellular canalicular systems that connects with the exterior. However, the exact role of these canals is only assumed.

Histamine is a potent vasoactive amine that is distributed widely in mammalian tissues. The two types of histamine-containing cells are the circulating histamine-containing cells (basophils, platelets, and eosinophils) that are found in blood and the fixed histamine-containing cells (mast cells and other fixed cells in the gastrointestinal mucosa and elsewhere). On its release, histamine is rapidly bound to tissues and the remainder is inactivated quickly by diamine oxidase (histaminase) and N-methyltransferase. Normally, histamine is not detectable in tissue fluids and plasma, but during anaphylaxis, histamine may be found transiently at sites of local injury, in plasma, and in urine. Although histamine is considered an important mediator for immediate hypersensitivity reactions (such as in asthma), the inability of antihistaminic drugs to abort the anaphylactic response in humans and the short duration of its biological activities suggest the operation of other mediators.

Two types of histamine receptors are recognized: H_1 and H_2. Type 1 (H_1) receptors mediate the vascular and smooth muscle effects of histamine and are blocked by the conventional antihistamines (e.g., diphenhydramine). H_1 blockers resemble histamine chemically with a charged ammonium group on their side chains. This group is believed to be the recognition unit for the H_1 receptor. Conversely, type 2 (H_2) receptors mediate histamine action on the gastric parietal cell, guinea pig atrium, rat uterus, polymorphonuclear leukocytes, and lymphocytes and are not blocked by classic antihistamines (H_1 blockers). Rather, they are blocked by the thiourea derivatives (burimamide and metiamide) and the cyanoguanidine derivative (cimetidine) of histamine; these drugs are categorized as *H_2 blockers*. The H_2 blockers resemble histamine by possessing an imidazole ring, the recognition determinant for the H_2 receptor. The discovery of the H_2 receptor–blocker drugs has clarified some controversies surrounding histamine for many years, particularly its activity on gastric acid secretion. The use of these probes may uncover more unsuspected modulating effects of histamine on inflammatory cells.

The inflammatory effects of histamine include dilation and increased permeability of small blood vessels, contraction of smooth muscles of the gastrointestinal tract and bronchi, and modulation of various inflammatory cells. The third effect involves chemotactic attraction of eosinophils, inhibition of neutrophil locomotion, inhibition of release of lysosomal enzymes, reduction of antibody-forming leukocytes, and inhibition of cell-mediated immune responses such as cutaneous DHR, thymidine uptake, migration-inhibitory factor production, and cytolytic activity of T cells. Most effects are mediated through the induction of increased intracellular cAMP levels in leukocytes by histamine. The strategic location of mast cells around blood vessels in connective tissues, the rapid inactivation of histamine by potent enzymes on its release from cells, and the recently observed inhibitory effects of histamine on a variety of leukocytic functions indicate that histamine is designed mainly to initiate a quick and transient vascular response and, with the possible exception of eosinophil mobilization, abrogate the cellular reactions that follow.[14a,23a]

Serotonin (5-hydroxytryptamine) is another vasoactive amine whose precise role in human inflammation is less clear than that of histamine. Serotonin is found in mast cells of rats and mice and the platelets of most mammalian species. Some effects resemble those of histamine; it induces smooth muscle contractions, vascular dilation, and vascular permeability. These effects, however, vary considerably among mammalian species. Serotonin induces an intracellular accumulation of cGMP in monocytes, which is associated with enhanced chemotactic response. The same effect, however, has not been shown in neutrophils. Whether serotonin itself produces other effects attributed to cGMP and other agents that increase cGMP levels has not been studied. In the past few years, interest has focused more on the effects of serotonin as a neurotransmitter in brain function (thermoregulation, pituitary hormone release, behavior, sleep, and pain responsiveness) than as a mediator of inflammatory response.

Arachidonic Acid Metabolites Considerable knowledge now exists of lipid-derived mediators, receptors and enzymes involved, and biosynthetic pathways.[15] Arachidonic acid, a component of cell membrane phospholipid released by the action of phospholipase A, is an important precursor of a group of mediators that possess a variety of functions and are known collectively as *eicosanoids*. Arachidonic acid is metabolized by enzymatic oxidation reactions into two biosynthetic pathways: the cyclooxygenase (COX) pathway, resulting in the formation of prostaglandins (including prostacyclin) and thromboxanes, and the lipoxygenase (LO) pathway, with the production of leukotrienes and lipoxins. At least two COX isozymes exist: COX-1, which is constitutive and responsible for the basal COX activity, and COX-2, which is the inducible isoform (except in the brain and kidney where it is constitutively expressed) at sites of injury and inflammation. The discovery of COX-2 has led to the finding and eventual marketing of specific COX-2 inhibitor antiinflammatory agents with reduced gastrointestinal and renal adverse effects.

Prostaglandins (and the intermediate endoperoxides, prostaglandin G$_2$ [PGG$_2$] and prostaglandin H$_2$ [PGH$_2$]) are derivatives of a 20-carbon prostanoic acid containing a cyclopentane ring produced by a bond between C8 and C12. The name originated from the mistaken belief that the active compound in fresh human semen inducing rhythmic contractions in human myometrium was produced in the prostate gland; seminal prostaglandin actually is derived from the seminal vesicles, not the prostate.[13] Prostaglandins do not exist preformed in tissue but are synthesized locally from available substrates such as cell membrane phospholipids to exert local effects. Prostaglandins are inactivated by prostaglandin dehydrogenase, which prevents their accumulation in tissue sites and their overflow into the systemic circulation. The effects of prostaglandins are mediated by specific receptors (one sub-

type each for PGD$_2$, PGF$_{2\alpha}$, PGI$_2$, and thromboxane A$_2$ and four for PGE$_2$) followed by signal transduction and changes in intracellular calcium, cGMP, and cAMP.

With regard to the effect of these products on inflammation, products of the cyclooxygenase pathway generally do not have direct potent edema- or pain-producing effects, but most potentiate the effects of other direct mediators such as bradykinin and histamine, perhaps by means of vasodilator activity. The stable prostaglandins are potent vasodilators, whereas the intermediate endoperoxides (PGG$_2$ and PGH$_2$) are not, and thromboxane A$_2$ is a potent vasoconstrictor. Prostaglandins are involved in fever production. The fever-producing effect of endogenous pyrogens (IL-1, TNF-α, IFN-α, and IL-6) occurs through induction of local prostaglandin production, which stimulates increased firing by temperature-sensitive neurons and raises the set-point of the thermoregulatory center.[16] Their effects on inflammatory cells are quite complex and at times paradoxical. For example, PGE in pharmacological doses produces vasodilation and increased vascular permeability, both of which are proinflammatory responses, whereas its ability to augment intracellular accumulation of cAMP depresses leukocytic activity and is antiinflammatory. PGF stimulates vasoconstriction and inhibits the PGE-induced microvascular effect, both of which are antiinflammatory; it also increases cellular cGMP, which is proinflammatory. The effect of PGE on cAMP, however, is different at low concentrations because low-dose PGE lowers cAMP cellular levels and enhances histamine release from the human lung. This dose-related activity may have some regulatory function and may operate in vivo, as evidenced by cAMP levels varying with time in acute and chronic experimental inflammation in animals. These changes consist of an initial decrease in cAMP, which coincides with an early low PGE concentration, followed by an increase in cAMP that may exceed resting levels.

Another regulatory mechanism that may operate in prostaglandins in vivo is the relative concentrations of PGE and PGF. In the reversed passive Arthus reaction in the pleural cavity, Capasso et al[6] noted an initial predominance of PGE$_2$ for as long as 6 hours during the stage of increased vascular permeability. This predominance was followed by an increase in PGF$_{2\alpha}$ levels, which exceeded PGE$_2$ levels after the initial 6 hours, at which time vascular permeability was waning. Thus prostaglandins may control inflammation by their unique dose effects on cyclic nucleotides and changes in the relative concentrations of PGE and PGF. From these findings, the role of prostaglandin in inflammation has been speculated by Dun et al.[12] Cell membrane phospholipids released during tissue injury or immunological reactions are hydrolyzed into a 20-carbon unsaturated fat by lysosomal phospholipases (with the potentiating effect of bradykinin). Prostaglandins then are formed from this substrate in the presence of prostaglandin synthetase. PGE indirectly increases vascular permeability through its potentiating effect on histamine and bradykinin, and the initial low concentration lowers intracellular cAMP, which results in stimulation of mediator release, lysosomal enzyme release, and leukocytic mobilization. Initially, more PGE than PGF is formed, which favors continuation of increased vascular permeability; at high doses, PGE may have direct vascular permeability effects and at this time PGF concentration may yet be insufficient to counteract PGE. As the PGE concentration reaches pharmacological levels, cellular cAMP increases, stopping mediator and lysosomal enzyme release and slowing phagocytic mobilization. In the later stages of inflammation, PGF levels may exceed PGE levels, which is believed to be caused by preferential PGF synthesis through the endoperoxide intermediate PGG_2. PGF stimulates vasoconstriction and allows subsidence of the erythema and fluid exudation induced by PGE. PGF also stimulates cGMP cellular accumulation, resulting in persistence of inflammation and perhaps initiation of a more chronic inflammatory process (enhancement of monocyte and lymphocyte functions).

The leukotrienes are divided into two groups (with leukotriene A_4 [LTA_4] as a common precursor): the dihydroxy acids, LTB_4, its isomers, and metabolites; and the cysteinyl or sulfidopeptide leukotrienes, LTC_4, LTD_4, and LTE_4 (formerly called the "slow-reacting substances"). LTB_4 differs from the other leukotrienes structurally and in its biological activity; it is a potent chemotactic attractant of neutrophils and eosinophils and stimulates immunoglobulin production by B lymphocytes. The cysteinyl leukotrienes, on the other hand, have no chemotactic activity but possess potent smooth muscle–contracting activity, resulting in bronchoconstriction and vasoconstriction. LTE_4 is only one tenth as potent as LTC_4 and LTD_4 on bronchial smooth muscles, but its duration of action is more prolonged. Speculation exists that LTE_4 may be involved in the prolonged bronchoconstriction of asthma.[26c] LTF_4 is relatively new and not well characterized. Consistent with their smooth muscle–contracting activity, both LTC_4 and LTD_4 also are potent vasoconstrictors of several vascular beds, such as the coronary, femoral, carotid, and renal beds. Leukotrienes may play a role in vasospastic conditions such as in Prinzmetal's angina and pulmonary hypertension and fetal circulation during hypoxemia. In addition to their bronchoconstricting and vasoconstricting effects, the cysteinyl leukotrienes may increase mucous secretion and have a modest vasopermeability effect that is enhanced by PGE_2 in experimental animals.[26c] LTB_4 also produces erythema and wheals when injected into human skin. The reaction is enhanced when LTB_4 is coadministered with prostaglandins. Several therapeutic products based on 5-lipoxygenase inhibition (zileuton [Zyflo]) or cysteinyl leukotriene receptor blockade (zafirlukast [Accolate] and montelukast [Singulair]) are clinically available for the treatment of asthma.

Lipoxins are products of 15-lipoxygenase and 5-lipoxygenase interaction through transcellular routes, by leukocytic 5-lipoxygenase and platelet 12-lipoxygenase interaction, or by the aspirin triggered 15-epi-lipoxin synthesis. Lipoxins have counterregulatory effects that may provide a more balanced lipid-derived mediator response.

Lysosomal Granule Contents   In addition to subserving the microbicidal and digestive functions of PMNs intracellularly, under certain conditions, lysosomal contents are discharged outside the cell. This extracellular release may have some useful functions, such as destruction of nonphagocytosable antigens, regulation of PMNs and other inflammatory cells, and control of the evolution of the inflammatory response.

Most known lysosomal factors are proteolytic enzymes, each with a pH requirement for optimal activity. Acid proteases, for example, are most active in acidic pH environments and probably are most useful inside an active phagolysosome in which their pH requirements may be met, but they are of doubtful significance extracellularly. Neutral proteases are most active at higher pH levels. Like acid proteases, they possess digesting capacity for renal basement membrane and vascular wall elastin in vitro. In addition, neutral proteases possess collagenase activity. When released extracellularly, proteolytic enzymes, particularly the neutral proteases, may digest foreign proteins but, in the process, also may digest normal host tissues, resulting in injury. If injected, these enzymes produce local Arthus-like lesions.

In addition to their direct digesting effect, lysosomal products may influence leukocytic function indirectly by their effects on inflammatory mediators. Lysosomal fractions of PMNs contain a C5-cleaving enzyme that generates chemotactic activity.[57] This enzyme activity is segregated in the "specific" or "secondary" granules of PMNs.[61] Conversely, chemotactic factor inactivator activity also is released from phagocytosing PMNs. The C5 chemotactic fragment inactivator is located in the azurophil, or primary, granules. Because specific granules tend to release early and more easily than azurophil granules, this segregation of prochemotactic and antichemotactic activities in distinct granules is consistent with the need for neutrophil accumulation initially and inhibition of further neutrophil migration in the later stages of inflammation. Another neutrophil-derived factor that may be important in modulating the later phase of inflammation is the neutrophil-immobilizing factor.

Other products of lysosomal granules have no known enzymatic activity; these include cationic proteins, histamine, and endogenous pyrogen. In addition to their well-known microbicidal activity, cationic proteins induce histamine release from mast cells, directly enhance capillary permeability, and possess chemotactic activity for monocytes and macrophages. Cationic proteins also have coagulant and anticoagulant activities, antiheparin activity, and pyrogenic activity. The pyrogenic activity in leukocytes is believed to be predominantly granular, but this is questionable. Histamine is found in PMN lysosomal granules and released extracellularly together with other lysosomal products during phagocytosis of opsonized staphylococci.

Cytokines   Phagocytes and lymphocytes may be considered as mobile or transportable endocrine glands. Both cells secrete small protein mediators that allow the host cells to communicate with one another. These proteins are called by the general term *cytokines,* the more specific terms *monokines* when produced by monocytes and macrophages, and *lymphokines* when derived from lymphocytes; they also called *chemokines* if they are chemotactic. Their effectiveness at very low concentrations and production by cells that are mobile or capable of being transported through the circulation suggest that they are designed for short-range, local communication or effects. When released in excess, these mediators may lose any semblance of their original protective function and produce profound systemic effects that may lead to discomfort, injury, or death of the host. Thus considerable effort is being exerted to discover ways to modify or nullify their inappropriate effects in these situations.

An increasing number of cytokines have now been described.[51] One of the first to be characterized was IL-l. On stimulation with antigen or pyrogens, mononuclear phagocytes synthesize and release this monokine, which has a range of biological activities. In the past these activities were not known to be derived from a single substance and thus IL-l is identical to several previously described factors: endogenous pyrogen (the fever-producing mediator), leukocytic endogenous mediator (the acute-phase reaction mediator), lymphocyte-activating factor (the potentiating factor of lymphocyte responses), and mononuclear cell factor (an inducer of PGE and collagenase synthesis by synovial cells). IL-l is an important mediator of host responses to infection and responsible for several aspects of acute-phase reaction.[16] Sequenced IL-l precursor contains 270 amino acids.[2] Another monokine of interest is TNF (or cachectin]; its widespread physiological effects resemble and overlap with those observed with IL-l.[59] TNF and IL-l are produced primarily by mononuclear phagocytes (monocytes and macrophages). In addition to interferon-α and IL-6, they induce fever and are endogenous pyrogens. Both induce production of acute-phase proteins, play important roles in recruiting inflammatory cells and the profound systemic changes in endotoxic shock, and induce synthesis of other cytokines. Some similarities in vivo can be explained by the apparent ability of TNF to induce the synthesis of IL-l and other cytokines. After bacterial challenge or endotoxemia the increase in serum concentration of TNF occurs before that of IL-l and anti-TNF inhibits 95% of the IL-l response.

The two types of TNF, TNF-α and TNF-β, have been cloned; they have similar specific receptors and similar effects. TNF-β has 30% homology with TNF-α, but unlike TNF-α, which is produced mainly by mononuclear phagocytes, TNF-β is produced primarily by T lymphocytes. TNF and other cytokines, particularly IL-l, play important roles in endotoxin shock.[59] Injection of recombinant TNF in experimental animals mimics the hematologic, metabolic, and lethal consequences of endotoxemia, and antibody to TNF protects animals against these effects.[7,48] Cytokines appear to possess multiple functions that interrelate. The precise cause-and-effect relationships of many cytokines and their apparent functions have not been determined;

therefore a fully coherent picture of the immune communication network they serve is not possible.

VASCULAR COMPONENT

The vascular system provides ready access by which cells and mediators produced elsewhere are brought to distant sites to participate in inflammatory reactions. The vessels that compose the microcirculation are dynamic and respond with changes in flow and permeability governed mainly by structural and functional changes of the endothelial lining cells. Although vascular leakage and exudation depend mainly on permeability, they are influenced in part by blood flow, as shown by marked diminution of edema and Arthus reaction in hypovolemic animals. Increased permeability can occur either directly by injury to the vessel wall or through the effects of chemical mediators. In the latter case the postcapillary venules are the most sensitive and most responsive part of the vasculature. The various mechanisms of vascular leakage include endothelial injury, formation of intercellular gaps by endothelial cell contraction (such as that occurring in the venules on exposure to histamine or histamine-like mediators) or "unzipping" of the endothelial cell junctions (as in mild injuries produced by heat, turpentine, or nitrogen mustard), leakage through transcellular endothelial cell canals,[43] and increased active transport by the pinocytic vesicles. Transudates resulting from arteriolar vasodilation and possibly from the increased secretion by connective tissue cells (e.g., exposure to toxins) also may contribute to inflammatory exudate formation. Three types of kinetic patterns of vascular leakage are described.[43] The first is immediate-transient leakage, which occurs in the venules beginning soon after injury and lasts only about 15 to 30 minutes. This leakage can be caused by histamine and other chemical mediators. The second type is immediate-prolonged leakage, which is characterized by its prompt appearance, more prolonged duration, and involvement of all vessels. This type of leakage occurs as a result of severe direct injury such as burns. The third type is delayed-prolonged leakage, which is believed to be a mild version of immediate-prolonged leakage. Delayed-prolonged leakage results from mild direct injury, involves all vessels, and is preceded by an immediate-transient type of leakage.

Considerable, albeit incomplete, knowledge of the function of endothelial cells and its role in the inflammatory response now exists. In addition to the structural changes in response to the microenvironment that are important to the flow of fluids and cells, the endothelial cell has many other critically important functions in clotting and inflammation. These include expression or elaboration of many factors such as (1) adhesion molecules that control leukocyte adherence; (2) cytokines such as IL-1, IL-6, IL-8, and macrophage inflammatory protein 1; (3) growth factors such as platelet-derived growth factor, CSFs, and TGF-β; (4) vasoactive and antithrombotic mediators such as nitric oxide, prostacyclin, and other eicosanoids; and (5) coagulation mediators such as tissue factor, tissue plasminogen activator, plasminogen-activator inhibitor-1, receptors for thrombomodulin, annexin, and activated protein C.[10,15] The endothelial cell is another critical link of the inflammatory, coagulation, and fibrinolytic responses.

Specific Effects of Infection   In addition to inducing the stereotypical nonspecific inflammatory reaction, infections can induce more specific effects on the host. Pathogens can produce tissue injury directly by invasion of host tissues and release of toxic products or indirectly by inducing an "altered" host inflammatory response. Practically every host cell and function or mediator involved in acute inflammation is a potential target for the microbe or its products.

Microbes can invade host cells directly and produce injury. An example is *Rickettsia rickettsii,* the agent of Rocky Mountain spotted fever, which invades vascular endothelial cells, injures the endothelium, triggers platelet and leukocyte adherence, and activates complement, kinin production, coagulation, and fibrinolysis. The result is vasculitis and, in severe cases, disseminated intravascular coagulation. In the later stages of this infection, immune complex–associated injury may be the major factor for the persistence of vasculitis. Viral agents that invade cells are another example of direct injury caused by microbes. The agents produce injury by altering host cell metabolism. Products derived from infectious agents may enhance microbial virulence by their direct injurious effects on tissues, enhancement of microbial invasiveness, or neutralization of host defenses. Examples of toxic effects that are directly harmful to the host include the strychninelike effects of tetanospasmin, the water and ion transport effects of enterotoxins, and the neuronal effects of botulinum toxin. Products that produce not only direct tissue damage but also enhance microbial invasiveness are hyaluronidase, which digests the ground substance of connective tissues; streptokinase, which lyses fibrin; and collagenase and elastase, which digest connective tissue proteins. Other products are poorly defined and have been given names that connote their effects, such as *leukocidin* (for leukocyte "-cidal" effect) and *aggressin,* which increases the aggressiveness of tissue injury by staphylococci. Numerous bacterial factors may interfere with host humoral defenses, immune responses, and phagocytic function, including many surface factors of microorganisms, lipid-specific enzymes and toxins, and complement-inactivating enzymes. Microbial synergism, whereby one infection promotes a second infection by a different microbe, has been observed frequently. Although these microbes appear to be nonspecific inhibitors of host defenses, the exact mechanisms involved are not clear.

BACTERIAL TOXINS

Endotoxin   Gram-negative bacteria have a unique cell wall composition. The outer portion consists of a layer of lipopolysaccharide (endotoxin). This layer has three distinct regions: the polysaccharide side chain region that confers the O-antigenic specificity on the organism, the lipid portion (lipid A) that confers the biological properties of endotoxin, and a core region that consists of carbohydrate (heptose, glucose, galactose, glucosamine, and 2-keto-3-deoxyoctonic acid).[41]

Endotoxin has many in vitro effects. It activates phagocytes, endothelial cells, Hageman factor, and the complement system by means of the alternative pathway. Thus it can trigger the coagulation, fibrinolytic, kinin-generating, and complement cascades. Although endotoxin induces release of mediators from rabbit platelets, probably with the help of complement, it does not appear to do so with human platelets. In neutrophils, endotoxin enhances the release of hydrolytic lysosomal enzymes, and in phagocytosing neutrophils it releases neutrophil-immobilizing factor. Endotoxin also increases neutrophil adherence and results in a transient leukopenia that may be caused at least in part by an expanded marginated pool.

In vivo, endotoxin produces a variety of biological effects. When given intravenously to experimental animals or humans, it initiates a febrile response with a latent period of 15 minutes in rabbits and 90 minutes in humans.[32a] (The difference probably is the result of the small dose relative to weight used in humans.) The febrile response is mediated through the release of endogenous pyrogen (IL-l, TNF-α, IFN-γ, and IL-6) from mononuclear phagocytes. Repeated injections of endotoxin induce tolerance that lasts for only a few days; this tolerance is nonimmunologically mediated. In high doses, endotoxin is lethal in many animals. When two doses are given at 18- to 24-hour intervals in rabbits, a local Shwartzman reaction results (if the initial dose is given intradermally and the second dose is given intravenously). The local reaction is characterized by hemorrhagic necrosis at the site of the intradermal injection. A generalized Sanarelli-Shwartzman reaction occurs if both doses are given intravenously. This reaction is characterized by bilateral renal cortical necrosis. The reactions require neutrophils and are inhibited by heparin administration. In primates, endotoxin produces a gradual development of hypotension without the hepatosplanchnic pooling of blood observed in dogs.

Recent studies have shown that lipopolysaccharide or endotoxin binds to a circulating serum transfer protein called *lipopolysaccharide-binding protein* (LBP).[45a] The lipopolysaccharide-LBP complex then binds to the CD14 receptor on the surface of the macrophage, initiating its activation and inducing synthesis of TNF, IL-l, and other cytokines. These macrophage-derived proteins, particularly TNF, are considered the major factors responsible for the adverse metabolic and hemodynamic changes in endotoxemia and sepsis. Several lines of evidence convincingly link TNF to the pathophysiological events that occur during endotoxemia.[7,48] First, an increase in serum TNF occurs coincident with the onset of chills, fever, and tachycardia after endotoxin injection into human volunteers. High serum TNF concentration in sepsis correlates with poor outcome. Many of the harmful effects of endotoxin, including hypotension and shock, multiple organ damage, and severe vascular leak syndrome, have been duplicated in experimental animals by infusion of recombinant human TNF. Finally, anti-TNF antibodies appear to reduce the harmful changes that follow endotoxin or live bacterial challenge in experimental animals, but studies in humans have not confirmed this reduction.[21]

Streptococcal and Staphylococcal Superantigens

Gram-positive bacteria now are a relatively more common cause of sepsis in many hospitals. Because these organisms do not contain endotoxin, the mechanism by which they produce sepsis and septic shock is not well understood. Streptococcal and staphylococcal exotoxins are responsible for streptococcal and staphylococcal toxic shock syndromes. These exotoxins act as superantigens by virtue of their ability to interact with the variable β domains on T lymphocytes, providing a more direct route to macrophage stimulation, production of inflammatory monokines, and toxic shock. The pyrogenic exotoxins of group A *Streptococcus* and the enterotoxins of *Staphylococcus* organisms are structurally related superantigens with highly conserved molecular domains that could be developed as potential vaccines. Evidence suggests that intravenous IgG, perhaps because it contains antibodies to the superantigens, is a useful therapeutic modality for streptococcal toxic shock syndrome.[24]

Peptidoglycan is a component of the bacterial cell wall of both gram-positive and gram-negative bacteria that consists of repeating units of neuraminic acid-*N*-acetyl glucosamine molecules with varying interpeptide bridges. Some parts of the peptidoglycan and lipid A molecules resemble each other, and peptidoglycan-like lipid A binds to CD14, has pyrogenic and cytotoxic activities, and can induce release of TNF-α and septic shock.[21]

Bacterial or prokaryotic deoxyribonucleic acid (DNA) differs from mammalian or eukaryotic DNA mainly by its unmethylated cytidine-guanidine (CpG) and also may be a molecular pattern recognized by the pattern recognition receptors of the host. Bacterial DNA can stimulate the release of TNF and cause septic shock in experimental animals and therefore may be a significant inflammatory mediator in gram-positive and gram-negative bacteria.[21] Although peptidoglycan and bacterial DNA can mediate inflammatory response and septic shock, their main significance could be their additive or synergistic effects on endotoxin and bacterial superantigens.

Sepsis and Systemic Inflammatory Response Syndrome

The term *sepsis* and associated complications have undergone yet another redefinition[4] (Box 1-1). Uniformity of definition is advantageous because it allows comparison of studies. The term *systemic inflammatory response syndrome* was proposed for when criteria for manifestations (temperature, heart rate, respiratory rate, and white blood cell count) are fulfilled and no infectious cause is found to explain the manifestations. *Sepsis* is used if there is an infectious cause is documented and the manifestations are changes from the patient's baseline and do not result from

---

BOX 1-1

Definition of Sepsis Terminologies

Systemic inflammatory response syndrome (SIRS) is response to any or a combination of severe clinical insults manifested by two or more of the following conditions:
1. Temperature >38° C or <36° C
2. Heart rate >90 beats/min
3. Respiratory rate >20 breaths/min or Paco$_2$ <32 mm Hg
4. White blood cell count >12,000/mm^3, <4000/mm^3, or >10% immature neutrophils (bands)

Sepsis is systemic inflammatory response, as similarly defined for SIRS, to a documented infection.

Severe sepsis occurs with associated hypotension, *hypoperfusion,* or *organ dysfunction. Sepsis-induced hypotension* is defined as systolic blood pressure <90 mm Hg or reduction of ≥40 mm Hg from baseline in the absence of other causes for hypotension. Observed abnormalities related to hypoperfusion include but are not limited to lactic acidosis, oliguria, and an acute change in mental status. Organ dysfunction is the presence of altered organ function in an acutely ill patient such that homeostasis cannot be maintained without intervention.

Septic shock is severe sepsis in which hypotension and hypoperfusion abnormalities persist despite adequate fluid resuscitation. Patients receiving inotropic or vasopressor agents who are no longer hypotensive by the time they manifest hypoperfusion abnormalities and organ dysfunction are still considered to have septic shock.

Data from Bone RC, Balk RA, Cerra FB, et al: American College of Chest Physicians/Society of Critical Care Medicine Consensus Conference: definitions for sepsis and organ failure and guidelines for the use of innovative therapies in sepsis, *Chest* 101:1644, 1992.

---

other known causes. Sepsis may progress as a continuum from the less severe sepsis to septic shock to multiple organ dysfunction syndrome.

Although infections caused by nonbacterial pathogens such as viruses, rickettsial organisms, and fungi occasionally are complicated by hypotension, the infectious agents most commonly responsible for shock are bacteria. McCabe and Jackson[29] observed hypotension in approximately 40% of their patients with gram-negative bacteremia. A decrease in arterial blood pressure is a usual finding in shock, but the most consistent event that defines the shock syndrome is ineffective tissue perfusion resulting in inadequate tissue oxygenation, decreased oxygen consumption, a shift to anaerobic metabolism, and accumulation of lactic acid in the blood. A more easily determined expression of ineffective tissue perfusion is oliguria and a change in mental status.

The pathophysiological process of sepsis is complex and involves the initiation of the inflammatory process by infection resulting in release of inflammatory mediators, loss of physiological balance between proinflammatory and antiinflammatory mediators and procoagulants and anticoagulants, oxidative damage, intravascular coagulation and endothelial injury tissue damage organ dysfunction, and death. Although other mediators of the kinin and complement systems are activated, inflammatory cytokines such as TNF-α, IL-1, IL-6 and IL-8 and the endothelial cell may play leading roles in producing the severe and life-threatening effects of sepsis. TNF in particular induces fever, release of other cytokines, and production of acute-phase proteins; recruits inflammatory cells; and stimulates expression of tissue factor on monocytes and endothelial cells. TNF induces the profound systemic changes in endotoxic shock. Recently, understanding of the linkage among inflammation, coagulation, and fibrinolysis during sepsis through the thrombin and APC systems has been enhanced.[52] TNF and other inflammatory cytokines increase expression of tissue factor on the surfaces of monocytes and endothelial cells, triggering the coagulation cascade by the extrinsic coagulation pathway and leading to activation of factor VII. Briefly, tissue factor activation is followed by a series of other activating steps that results in the formation of thrombin and fibrin clot. Aside from its procoagulant effects, thrombin also affects inflammation, fibrinolysis, and wound healing. Binding of thrombin by antithrombin III inhibits its clot-forming activity. Binding with thrombomodulin results in activation of protein C anticoagulant system. In turn, activated protein C occupies a central role in modulating the coagulant effects of thrombin with its antithrombin effect by inactivating factors VIIa and Va and fibrinolytic effect by inhibiting plasminogen-activator inhibitor-1. Activated protein C may terminate the vicious cycle induced by the initiating inflammatory reaction mediated by cytokines through its antiinflammatory effects because it inhibits syntheses of inflammatory cytokines (TNF-α, IL-1, and IL-6) by monocytes and inhibits selectin-mediated leukocyte binding to endothelial cells.[3]

The inflammatory and coagulation systems generally are balanced responses. In the presence of severe infection, however, this balance may be lost, resulting in excessive and self-propagating inflammatory and procoagulant effects. Because of the complexity of the networks involved and the presence of multiple positive- and negative-feedback loops and amplification systems, determination of which step or switch should be turned off to restore balance has been difficult. The inflammatory, antiinflammatory, coagulation, and fibrinolytic systems are linked intimately, and mediators involved have multiple effects.[39] For example, thrombin affects on all systems, as does activated protein C. Under normal or low-stress conditions, thrombin is a potent procoagulant, yet when infused in an animal model of sepsis, it becomes primarily an anticoagulant and blocks the lethality of the *Escherichia coli* sepsis.[52] This action is caused by an apparent switch in the direction of reactions favoring the thrombomodulin–acitvated protein C system. The processes that determine the direction of reactions still are not understood clearly, but most likely the direction is influenced mainly by availability of substrates,

kinetics of reactions, and activity of inhibitors. Much of the research in the treatment of severe sepsis has been almost purely trial and error. Many early treatment studies have ended in blind alleys but contributed immensely to the understanding of the pathophysiological process and relative importance of the various factors involved.[52]

Despite significant improvements in antibiotic treatments and critical care, mortality rates from sepsis remain high, with estimates ranging from 20% to 50%. Treatments that do not improve survival include high-dose steroids, antithrombin III, E5, a murine monoclonal antiendotoxin antibody, murine monoclonal anti-TNF antibody, and tissue factor pathway inhibitor.[14] Bernard et al.[3] recently reported the results of a randomized, double-blind, placebo-controlled, multicenter phase 3 trial using the recombinant human activated protein C (drotrecogin-alfa) in the treatment of sepsis and found significant reduction of mortality (30.8% placebo vs. 24.7% treatment, $P = .005$), 19.4% reduction of relative risk of death, and 6.1% reduction of absolute risk of death. Although murine monoclonal anti-TNF antibody was not found to be useful, murine monoclonal Fab$_2$ fragment yielded positive results (4% reduction of absolute risk of death) in a prospectively defined subgroup with high IL-6 levels (>1000 pg/mL), and a polyclonal murine monoclonal antibody fragment significantly improved ventilator-free and organ failure-free days.[14] Although these treatments resulted in insignificant or significant but relatively meager results, present understanding of the pathogenesis of sepsis suggests that restoration of balance in severe sepsis involves deactivation of many switches; thus further inroads in treatment require a combination of modalities.

Fever and Endogenous Pyrogens   Another fairly consistent, nonspecific reaction to infection is the development of fever. Cooper et al.[9] hypothesized that fever occurs as a result of an upward resetting of the host's "thermostat" and its consequent effects on the thermal reflex arc. This reflex arc consists of an afferent limb, which carries sensory input from thermal sensors scattered in the skin and other areas, such as the central nervous system, abdomen, and spinal cord; the thermostat, primarily localized in the hypothalamus, which processes and interprets the sensory thermal input; and the efferent pathway, which carries the integrated messages from the thermostat to the effector organs that then should respond appropriately (i.e., peripheral vasoconstriction and shivering if the body temperature is lower than the thermostat set-point, or vasodilation and sweating if the body temperature is higher). The events that accompany fever in infections support this concept. In the presence of microbial toxins, mononuclear phagocytes are stimulated to elaborate and release endogenous pyrogens (IL-1, TNF, IFN-γ, and IL-6), one or all of which then can induce local production of PGE$_2$ in the thermoregulatory center, which results in increased firing by temperature-sensitive neurons and an increase in the thermostat set-point. The body temperature becomes hypothermic relative to the elevated set-point, and the effector mechanisms are activated to raise the body temperature. This activity leads to vasoconstriction to conserve body heat; the individual feels cold, starts to shiver, and performs maneuvers designed to increase body heat. As the body temperature increases and reaches the thermostat setting, the individual becomes warm and equithermic with the high set-point and the feeling of coldness disappears and shivering stops. This equalization of the body temperature with the high thermostat set-point is known as *fever*. When the release of pyrogens ends, after a diminution or elimination of microbial toxins, the thermostat resets back to the lower (normal) set-point, the body temperature becomes hyperthermic relative to the new set-point, and the thermal reflexes activate the effector systems to lower the temperature. Peripheral vasodilation now occurs, and the individual feels warm, perspires, and performs actions to lower the temperature. These cycles are most evident in the malarial paroxysm, which typically consists of the cold, febrile, and sweating stages.

Studies in animals and human subjects have clarified some mediators involved in the production of fever.[26d] The first of these mediators are the endogenous pyrogens, which are produced by mononuclear phagocytes that include the circulating monocytes and fixed tissue macrophages. Other cells, such as keratinocytes, Langerhans' cells, corneal epithelial cells, gingival exudate cells, astrocytes and glial cells, renal mesangial cells, and renal cell carcinoma cells, also produce IL-1 and perhaps other pyrogens.

The biochemical events that lead to the production of fever in the presence of IL-l are not well understood, but prostaglandins, cyclic nucleotides, and monoamine neurotransmitters may be involved. IL-1 increases firing from temperature-sensitive neurons in the hypothalamus, which is responsible for the resetting of the hypothalamic thermostat. Evidence also suggests that IL-1 activity is mediated through induction of local prostaglandin synthesis in the hypothalamus. This finding is based on the thermogenic effects of prostaglandin when it is injected into IL-1–sensitive sites in the hypothalamus, inhibition of IL-1–induced fever by inhibitors of prostaglandin synthesis, and accumulation of prostaglandins in cerebrospinal fluid during endotoxin- or IL-1–induced fever. However, the significance of prostaglandin fever has been questioned.[11] If prostaglandins are significant, their action may be mediated by their effects on cyclic nucleotides. The induction of fever by cAMP injection into the anterior hypothalamus of the rabbit supports this view. Finally, the use of monoamine-depleting drugs has shown the importance of serotonin and norepinephrine in the maintenance of body temperature, but the mechanism by which monoamine neurotransmitters relate to IL-1, prostaglandins, and cyclic nucleotides is unknown. Whether fever is harmful or beneficial to the infected human host is not clear. Kluger et al.[26] showed that elevated temperature increased survival in infected lizards, and they postulate that a beneficial effect may extend to higher animals and humans.

WOUND HEALING

Immediately after injury, concomitant with the unleashing of factors to prevent infection, the host also begins the process of healing. The components of wound healing include coagulation and inflammation, fibroplasia, matrix repair, angiogenesis, epithelialization, and contraction. The precise process and regulators involved in wound healing are not fully understood, but more components are being defined. Various cells are involved in the process, and platelets, neutrophils, macrophages, fibroblasts, endothelial cells, keratinocytes, and epithelial cells play crucial roles. The role of lymphocytes is less clear, but they appear to increase collagen deposition and granulation strength.[15,36,46]

Platelet activation and clotting occur immediately after injury to stop the bleeding and provide a base on which cells crucial to wound healing migrate and serve their functions. Simultaneously, endothelial cells are activated by the injury, and together with platelets, initiate the inflammatory response by sending chemical signals that attract phagocytic cells to the site. In addition, endothelial cells that grow into the matrix provide the early beginnings of angiogenesis. PMNs, mainly neutrophils, respond to the chemical signals of injury and arrive within hours (peak within 24 to 48 hours) and then begin to clear fibrin debris and release proinflammatory cytokines that attract more cells to the site and induce keratinocyte growth factors and matrix metalloproteinases. Blood monocytes are transformed into macrophages and follow the neutrophils (peak within 5 to 7 days) to the wound. These cells are crucial in most if not all stages of wound healing after coagulation. Macrophages are important in completion of neutrophil-initiated matrix debridement and remodeling with their ability to orchestrate opposing factors, such as secretion of proteases, inhibition of metalloproteinases, and synthesis of extracellular matrix while they stimulate fibroblasts and other cells to proliferate and then inhibit tissue growth when healing is complete. Macrophages also clear the way for new vessel growth. Within 10 to 14 days, fibroblasts become the predominant cells in the wound. These cells proliferate under the influence of macrophages and secrete matrix to form granulation tissue and eventually the scar.

Epithelialization occurs simultaneously with the dermal repair process. The most important cells in this phase are the keratinocytes. These cells migrate and proliferate to regenerate the lost epithelial cover of the wound. Proliferation of the epithelial cells is controlled by many factors, including TGF-β, platelet-derived growth factor, fibroblast growth factors, and the keratinocyte growth factors 1 and 2, which were shown recently to increase the proliferation of keratinocytes at wound edges.[46] Some well-studied wound repair factors include TGF-β, platelet-derived growth factor, and platelet-activating factor. Local application of these factors to wounds enhances tissue repair, probably by attracting macrophages and fibroblasts into the area and modulating keratinocytes (Table 1-4). Other factors also affect wound healing: IL-2 enhances wound breaking strength, IFN-γ decreases collagen synthesis,

TABLE 1-4

Some Cytokines Involved in Wound Healing

| | | | LOCAL APPLICATION ENHANCES TISSUE REPAIR | | | |
| | | | ABNORMAL TISSUE REPAIR | | | |
Cytokine	Source	Normal Tissue Repair	Steroid Induced	Doxorubicin Induced	Total Body Irradiation	Megavolt EB
TGF-β	Macrophages platelets	Yes	Yes	Yes	Yes	Yes
PDGF	Platelets, fibroblasts	Yes	No	—	No	Yes
PAF	Cell membranes of inflammatory cells	Yes	—	—	—	—

EB, Electrical burn; *TGF-β,* transforming growth factor-β; *PDGF,* platelet-derived growth factor; *PAF,* platelet-activating factor; —, no data available.

monocyte chemotactic protein-1 promotes collagen deposition by fibroblasts, and GM-CSFs promote faster wound healing.

MECHANISMS OF IMMUNOLOGICAL INJURY

Although the immune response exists as a host-protective mechanism, its effects are not always beneficial. These harmful reactions are termed *hypersensitivity,* or *allergic reactions,* to distinguish them from the protective immune reactions generally called *immunity.* Immunological injuries can be classified as immediate or delayed depending on the latent period of the reactions and the cells involved. Immediate hypersensitivity reactions can be mediator or nonmediator determined depending on whether the manifestations of the reaction are produced with or without the intervention of mediators. The more commonly used classification of Gell and Coombs[17] groups the mechanisms of immunological injury into type I (reagin-dependent anaphylactic), type II (cytotoxic antibody), type III (immune complex toxic), and type IV (CMI or DHR) reactions. One or more of these reactions can be involved in any hypersensitivity disease process and overlapping can occur. One example is anaphylaxis produced by cytotoxic antibody reaction. Of the first three types, type III reaction is the most frequent of immunological injury associated with infections.

TYPE I REACTION

The type I reaction is initiated by antigen bridging of adjacent membrane-bound IgE (reaginic) antibody molecules present on the surface of mediator cells. This process results in the release of various mediators. The cells involved are mast cells and basophils, which can release the following preformed mediators: histamine, heparin, eosinophil chemotactic factor of anaphylaxis, neutrophil chemotactic factor, and kallikrein. The cells also synthesize and release peptidolipid leukotrienes and platelet-activating factor. The biological effects of these factors presumably are responsible for allergic manifestations. The preferential distribution of mast cells in the skin, res-

piratory tract, and gastrointestinal tract makes these organs vulnerable; consequently, they become the area of expression for immediate hypersensitivity reactions. The frequency of asthma, hay fever, allergic diarrhea, and some forms of urticaria reflects these unique mast cell locations. Generalized anaphylaxis can be produced by intravenous infusion of an allergen in an appropriately sensitized host. Anaphylactic shock after intravenous injection of penicillin in a few individuals who are penicillin sensitive is an example.

With the possible exception of metazoan infections in which hyperimmunoglobulinemia E and eosinophilia are observed, the role of type I reactions in infection-associated immunological injury is limited. However, evidence indicates that the type I reaction plays a cooperative role in localizing circulating immune complexes in the kidney.[7a]

TYPE II REACTION

The type II reaction requires antibody with specificity against tissue antigen. Antibody binds with antigen, which is a component of the host cells. The antigen-antibody complex formed can lead to tissue damage by activation of complement, with generation of cytolytic activity, induction of influx of PMNs resulting in the extracellular release of lysosomal contents or attachment to macrophages, in the presence of "killer T cells," causing toxic changes (antibody-dependent cell-mediated cytotoxicity reactions). Cytotoxic reactions are presumed to be the mechanism of glomerular injury in Goodpasture's syndrome. Whether this mechanism is involved in other diseases such as rheumatic fever is not known. Other than the antigen being part of the host in type II reactions, type II and type III reactions are similar.

TYPE III REACTION

These events that accompany immune complex injury include interaction of antibody and antigen, deposition of immune complexes in tissues, activation of complement, accumulation of leukocytes, and production of tissue damage.[9a,26b] Binding of antigen to antibody is primarily a protective mechanism, but under certain conditions such as in persistent antigenemia the complexes cannot be rapidly and adequately cleared, resulting in their deposition in tissues and consequent tissue damage. Type III reactions often involve the action of complement-fixing antibodies. Because nonsoluble immune complexes are cleared easily and more rapidly, only soluble complexes are thought to be responsible for tissue injury. Studies of combining ratios of antigen to antibody have shown that the greatest number of soluble complexes occurs in the zone of antigen excess; thus the greatest danger to immune complex injury exists in the presence of persistent antigenemia. Deposition of complexes in the blood vessel basement membrane appears to depend to some extent on trapping, which is influenced by the size of the immune complexes and activity of vascular permeability factors. Studies of serum sickness in animals have shown that a sedimentation coefficient of greater than 19S is required of immune complexes for deposition in blood vessel walls. This deposition can be reduced and tissue damage prevented by administration of antagonists to histamine and serotonin. Therefore speculation exists that the vasoactive amines, by producing intercellular gaps between endothelial cells, expose the basement membrane and allow deposition of circulating complexes.

Complement and neutrophils are important in the production of immune complex injury, as shown by inhibition of immune complex injury (particularly vasculitis) in experimental animals depleted of complement or neutrophils. Both IgG and IgM complexes fix complement mainly through the classic pathway, whereas IgA and IgE do not. Aggregated IgA and IgE also may fix complement by the alternative pathway, but their importance in immune complex injury is not clear. Complement activation releases various mediators with diverse activities, including cytolytic, opsonizing, phagocytosis-enhancing, and perhaps more important in immune complex injury, chemotactic activities. The chemotactic factors released at the site of complex deposition attract neutrophil accumulation. If these complexes are tightly bound to the tissues, they may become nonphagocytosable; consequently, PMNs may release their lysosomal contents extracellularly. These lysosomal contents include tissue-digesting proteases, which are directly damaging to tissues; permeability factors, which permit more deposition of complexes; and chemotactic factors, which enhance further neutrophil accumulation.

A growing list of infectious diseases is believed to be associated with immune complex injury. These infectious diseases include the nephritides of subacute bacterial endocarditis, shunt infections, poststreptococcal infections, infectious mononucleosis, pneumococcal otitis, syphilis, babesiosis, and typhoid fever; the skin rash, arthritis, and arteritis of hepatitis B virus infection; disseminated gonococcal infection; Rocky Mountain spotted fever; and other infections in humans and experimental animals associated with persistent antigenemia.

TYPE IV REACTION

Type IV reactions are mediated by the action of T cells that, for reasons still mostly unclear, fail to recognize host antigens as "self" and react against them, with resulting host injury. Examples of type IV reactions are contact hypersensitivity and autoimmune disorders. In the former, the actual target is a low molecular weight foreign material, which is bound to a host carrier protein in the skin. The low molecular weight substance itself is nonimmunogenic but acts as a hapten and, in the presence of a carrier protein, becomes immunogenic. With the hapten the host carrier protein is mistaken as "nonself" and the host T cells may respond against it, resulting in a lesion that resembles a typical cutaneous DHR. In autoimmune diseases, any host tissue can be the antigen. In systemic lupus erythematosus, for example, the host fails to recognize and mounts an attack against its own nuclear DNA, which results in production of antinuclear antibodies and, consequently, damage in potentially every host organ. Studies in animals have uncovered some information that may be relevant to the causation and treatment of autoimmune diseases. These studies were performed in New Zealand black (NZB) mice and New Zealand black/white (NZB/W) hybrid mice. These animals are unique in that with aging, they spontaneously develop an autoimmune disorder resembling systemic lupus erythematosus in humans. These studies showed that the autoimmune phenomenon in adult NZB/W mice is related to a reduction of suppressor cell activity, that suppressor cell activity is mediated through secretion of a "soluble immune response suppressor," and that replacement of the soluble suppressor (by injection three times weekly) can prevent development of autoimmune disease and prolong the survival of NZB/W mice.[26a] These studies provide evidence that suppressor cell activity is necessary to prevent the development and expression of forbidden clones with specificity against self antigens. Regardless of the cause of autoimmune diseases, disorders of the immune system usually resolve as a regulatory gene problem with variable environmental influence.

SUMMARY

The host defense system consists of three major components: local, humoral, and cellular defenses. However, these components do not have boundaries, overlap extensively, and interact closely to provide a unified protection for the host. Infectious agents initiate in the host a series of reactions that are collectively called the *inflammatory reaction*. This response results in the generation and release of mediators, microvascular changes, and mobilization and activation of leukocytes, all designed to eliminate the infectious pathogen and repair tissue injury. Therefore these reactions are primarily protective. In addition to initiating the inflammatory reaction, infectious agents or their products also produce myriad effects on the host. These effects include direct injury to the host cells, enhancement of the parasite's invasiveness, and amplification of these effects by neutralization of host defenses. Other products may trigger systemic effects, some beneficial or benign (e.g., fever), others inappropriate and harmful (e.g., endotoxic shock). Finally, in certain abnormal situations, host defenses may fail to limit collateral damage or recognize self and produce harmful immunological effects such as in hypersensitivity (allergic) and autoimmune diseases. The latter represent imperfections in nature's otherwise flawless design of the host immune system.

REFERENCES

1. Anderson DC, Schmalsteig FC, Finegold MJ, et al: The severe and moderate phenotypes of heritable Mac-l, LFA-l deficiency: the quantitative definition and relation to leukocyte dysfunction and clinical features, *J Infect Dis* 152:668, 1985.
2. Auron PE, Webb AC, Rosenwasser LJ, et al: Nucleotide sequence of human monocyte interleukin-l precursor cDNA, *Proc Natl Acad Sci USA* 81:7907, 1984.
3. Bernard GR, Vincent J, Laterre P, et al: Efficacy and safety of recombinant human activated protein C for severe sepsis, *N Engl J Med* 344:699, 2001.
4. Bone RC, Balk RA, Cerra FB, et al: American College of Chest Physicians/Society of Critical Care Medicine Consensus Conference: definitions for sepsis and organ failure and guidelines for the use of innovative therapies in sepsis, *Chest* 101:1644, 1992.
5. Boxer LA, Hedley-Whyte ET, Stossel TP: Neutrophil actin dysfunction and abnormal neutrophil behavior, *N Engl J Med* 291:1093, 1974.
6. Capasso F, Dunn C, Yamamoto S, et al: Pharmacological mediators of various immunological and nonimmunological inflammatory reactions produced in the pleural cavity, *Agents Actions* 5:528, 1975.
7. Cerami A: Inflammatory cytokines, *Clin Immunol Immunopathol* 62:S3, 1992.
7a. Chen XM, Tanaka T, Kobayashi Y, et al: Experimental glomerulonephritis induced by immune complexes of monoclonal antibodies produced by immunoglobulin class-switch variants, *Lab Invest* 57:665, 1987.
8. Cohen S: The role of cell-mediated immunity in the induction of inflammatory responses, *Am J Pathol* 88:502, 1977.
9. Cooper KE, Cranston WI, Snell ES: Temperature regulation during fever in man, *Clin Sci* 27:593, 1964.
9a. Cooper NR: The biology of the complement system. In Gallin JI, Snyderman R, editors: *Inflammation: basic principles and clinical correlates,* New York, 1999, Lippincott Williams & Wilkins.
10. Cotran RS, Biscoe DM: Endothelial cells in inflammation. In Kelley W, Ruddy S, Harris E, editors: *Textbook of rheumatology,* Philadelphia, 1997, WB Saunders.
11. Cranston WI, Duff GW, Hellon RF, et al: Is brain prostaglandin synthesis essential in fever? In *Drugs, biogenic amines and body temperature,* Proceedings of the Third International Symposium on the Pharmacology of Temperature Regulations, Basel, 1977, S Karger.
11a. de Agostini A, Lijnen HR, Pixby RA, et al: Inactivation of factor XII active fragment in normal plasma: predominant role of C1-inhibitor, *J Clin Invest* 73:1542, 1984.
12. Dun CJ, Willoughby DA, Giroud JP, et al: An appraisal of the interrelationships between prostaglandins and cyclic nucleotides in inflammation, *Biomedicine* 24:214, 1976.
13. Eliasson R, Mossberg B, Cammer P, et al: The immotile-cilia syndrome: a congenital ciliary abnormality as an etiologic factor in chronic airway infections and male sterility, *N Engl J Med* 297:1, 1977.
14. Ely EW Jr: New evolutions in the understanding and managing patients with sepsis. Available from: http://id.medscape.com/Medscape/CriticalCare/TreatmentUpdate/2000
14a. Falus A: Histamine modulates the acute phase response at multiple points, *Immunol Today* 15:59, 1994.
14b. Fitch FW, McKisic MD, Lancki DW, et al: Differential regulation of murine T lymphocyte subsets, *Annu Rev Immunol* 11:29, 1993.
15. Gallin JI, Snyderman R, editors: *Inflammation: basic principles and clinical correlates,* New York, 1999, Lippincott Williams & Wilkins.
16. Galon J, Aksentijevich I, McDermott MF, et al: TNFRSF1A mutations and autoinflammatory syndromes, *Curr Opin Immunol* 12:479, 2000.
17. Gell PGH, Coombs RRA: *Clinical aspects of immunology,* ed 2, Philadelphia, 1968, FA Davis.
18. Hancock REW, Chapple DS: Peptide antibiotics, *Antimicrob Agents Chemother* 43:1317, 1999.
19. Hemerhorst EJ, Hodgson R, van't Hof W, et al: The effects of histatin-derived basic antimicrobial peptides on oral biofilms, *J Dent Res* 78:1245, 1999.
20. Heiner DC: Significance of immunoglobulin G (IgG) subclasses, *Am J Med* 76:1, 1984.
21. Horn DL, Morrison DC, Opal SM, et al: What are the microbial components implicated in the pathogenesis of sepsis? *Clin Infect Dis* 31:851, 2000.
22. Houten SM, Wanders, RJ, Waterham HR: Biochemical and genetic aspects of mevalonate kinase and its deficiency, *Biochim Biophys Acta* 1529:19, 2000.
23. Hugli TE, Morgan EC: Mechanism of leukocyte regulation by complement-derived factors, *Contemp Topics Immunobiol* 14:109, 1984.
23a. Jutel M, Watanabe T, Klunker S, et al: Histamine regulates T-cell and antibody responses by differential expression of H_1 and H_2 receptors, *Nature* 413:420, 2001.
24. Kaul R, McGeer A, Norrby-Teglund A, et al: Intravenous immunoglobulin therapy for streptococcal toxic shock syndrome: a comparative observational study, the Canadian Streptococcal Study Group, *Clin Infect Dis* 28:800, 1999.
25. Klebanoff SJ, Smith D: Peroxidase-mediated antimicrobial activity of rat uterine fluid, *Gynecol Invest* 1:21, 1970.
26. Kluger MJ: The evolution and adaptive value of fever, *Am Sci* 66:38, 1978.
26a. Krakauer RS, Strober W, Waldman TA: Loss of suppressor T cells in the pathogenesis of the autoimmunity of NZB/W mice, *Arthritis Rheum* 21:S185, 1978.
26b. Leber P, McCluskey R: Immune complex disease. In Zweifach B, Grant L, McCluskey R, editors: *The inflammatory process,* vol 3, New York, 1974, Academic Press.
26c. Leff AR: Regulation of leukotrienes in the management of asthma: biology and clinical therapy, *Annu Rev Med* 52:1, 2001.
26d. Mackowiak PA, editor: Fever: basic mechanisms and management, Philadelphia, 1997, Lippincott-Raven.
27. Maderazo EG: Interpreting tuberculosis skin tests, *Lancet* 348:832, 1996.

28. Maderazo EG, Woronick CL, Ward PA: Inhibitors of chemotaxis, *Methods Enzymol* 162:223, 1988.

29. McCabe WR, Jackson GG: Gram-negative bacteremia. II. Clinical, laboratory, and therapeutic observations, *Arch Intern Med* 110:856, 1962.

30. McKay IA, Leigh IM: Epidermal cytokines and their roles in cutaneous wound healing, *Br J Dermatol* 124:513, 1991.

31. Moll GN, Konings WN, Driessen AJ: Bacteriocins: mechanism of membrane insertion and pore formation, *Antonie Van Leeuwenhoek* 76:185, 1999.

32. Mooney JK, Mooney JS, Hinman F: The antibacterial effect of the bladder surface: an electron microscopic study, *J Urol* 115:381, 1976.

32a. Morrison DC, Ulevitch RJ: The effects of bacterial endotoxins on host mediation systems, *Am J Pathol* 93:526, 1978.

33. Muller-Eberhard HJ: Complement: chemistry and pathways. In Gallin JI, Goldstein IM, Snyderman R, editors: *Inflammation: principles and clinical correlates,* New York, 1988, Raven Press.

34. Najjar VA: Defective phagocytosis due to deficiencies involving the tetrapeptide tuftsin, *J Pediatr* 89:1121,1975.

35. Oliver JM: Impaired microtubule function correctable by cyclic GMP and cholinergic agonists in the Chédiak-Higashi syndrome, *Am J Pathol* 85:395, 1976.

36. Proceedings of the National Institutes of Health Conference on Advances in Understanding Trauma and Burn Injury, Session IV: Wound healing, Washington, DC, June 21-23, 1990, *J Trauma* 30(suppl):SI16, 1990.

37. Protein Reviews On the Web (PROW). Available from: http://www.ncbi.nlm.nih.gov/prow

38. Putnam FW, editor: *The plasma proteins: structure, function and genetic control,* vol 3, ed 2, New York, 1977, Academic Press.

39. Ratnoff OD: A tangled web: the interdependence of mechanisms of blood clotting, fibrinolysis, immunity, and inflammation, *Thromb Diath Haemorrh* 45(suppl):109, 1971.

40. Reinherz EL, Schlossman SF: Regulation of the immune response-inducer and suppressor T-lymphocyte subsets in human beings, *N Engl J Med* 303:1153, 1980.

41. Rietschel ET, Brade H: Bacterial endotoxins, *Sci Am* 267:54, 1992.

41a. Regoli D, Barabe J: Pharmacology of bradykinin and related kinins, *Pharmacol Rev* 32:1, 1980.

42. Romagnani S: Cytokines and the Th1/Th2 paradigm. In Blackwill F, editor: *The cytokine network,* Chicago, 2000, Oxford University Press.

43. Ryan GB, Majno G: Acute inflammation: a review, *Am J Pathol* 86:183, 1977.

44. Schenkein HA, Genco RJ: Gingival fluid and serum in periodontal disease, *J Periodontol* 48:772, 1977.

45. Schreiber AD, Rossman MD, Levinson AI: The immunobiology of human Fcγ receptors on hematopoietic cells and tissue macrophages, *Clin Immunol Immunopathol* 62:S62, 1992.

45a. Schumann RR, Leong SR, Flaggs GW, et al: Structure and function of lipopolysaccharide binding protein, *Science* 164:777, 1990.

46. Singer AJ, Clark RAF: Cutaneous wound healing, *N Engl J Med* 341:738, 1999.

47. Snyderman R, Pike MC: An inhibitor of macrophage chemotaxis produced by neoplasms, *Science* 192:370, 1976.

48. Spooner CE: The role of tumor necrosis factor in sepsis, *Clin Immunol Immunopathol* 62:SII, 1992.

49. Streicher HZ, Reitz MS Jr, Gallo R: Human immunodeficiency virus. In Mandell GL, Bennett JE, Dolin R, editors: *Principles and practice of infectious diseases,* Philadelphia, 2000, Churchill Livingstone.

50. Sturgess JM, Chao J, Wong J, et al: Cilia with defective radial spokes: a cause of human respiratory disease, *N Engl J Med* 300:53, 1979.

51. Sundy JS, Patel DD, Haynes BF: Cytokines in normal and pathologic inflammatory responses. In Gallin JI, Snyderman R, editors: *Inflammation: basic principles and clinical correlates,* New York, 1999, Lippincott Williams & Wilkins.

52. Taylor FB Jr, Chang A, Hinshaw LB, et al: A model for thrombin protection against endotoxin, *Thromb Res* 36:177, 1984.

53. Tsai H, Bobek LA: Human salivary histatins: promising antifungal therapeutic agents, *Crit Rev Oral Biol Med* 9:480, 1998.

54. van Wetering S, Sterk PJ, Rabe KF, et al: Defensins: key players or bystanders in infection, injury, and repair in the lung? *J Allergy Clin Immunol* 104:1131, 1999.

55. Waldmann TA, Blaese RM, Broder S, et al: Disorders of suppressor immunoregulatory cells in the pathogenesis of immunodeficiency and autoimmunity, *Ann Intern Med* 88:226, 1978.

56. Walport MJ: Complement, *N Engl J Med* 344:1058, 2001.

57. Ward PA, Hill JH: Biologic role of complement-derived leukotactic activity extractable from lesions of immunologic vasculitis, *J Immunol* 108:1137, 1972.

58. Ward PA: Leukotaxis and leukotactic disorders: a review, *Am J Pathol* 77:520, 1974.

59. Weissmann G, editor: *Mediators of inflammation,* New York, 1974, Plenum.

60. Williams RC, Gibbons RJ: Inhibition of bacterial adherence by secretory immunoglobulin A: a mechanism of antigen disposal, *Science* 177:697, 1972.

61. Wright DG, Gallin JI: Mechanisms of modulation of the inflammatory response: generation and inactivation of C5a by products stored in the granules of human neutrophils. In Gallin JI, Quie PG, editors: *Leukocyte chemotaxis: methods, physiology, and clinical implications,* New York, 1978, Raven Press.

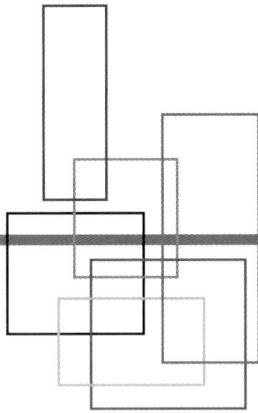

Microbiology of the Orofacial Region

George S. Schuster

The microbial residents of the oral cavity constitute one of the most varied and numerous floras in the human body. More than 500 bacterial taxa are found in the oral cavity, of which approximately 22 predominant ones have been identified. In addition, several fungal species, two or more protozoal genera, and likely many viruses are normal residents. Numerous microorganisms also have been detected but not definitely characterized or classified. The variation relates to the many microenvironments in the oral cavity, such as the various surfaces of the teeth, gingival sulcus, tongue, and buccal mucosa. Each has a unique set of conditions that permits the organisms to establish residency and thrive, including receptors for selective adherence, appropriate nutrients and oxygen tension, or simply physical protection from unfavorable conditions. Although the subtypes and proportions of organisms differ among individuals, the general patterns of the indigenous microfloras are similar in healthy individuals. However, changes in systemic disease patterns and concurrent use of medications result in the presence of unusual organisms as part of the "normal" flora and an increase in disease caused by normal organisms that usually are considered to have low pathogenicity. Generally, in the orofacial region, most bacterially mediated conditions involve disturbances of the normal flora or displacement of normal organisms to abnormal sites. However, as discussed later in this chapter, oral microorganisms also have been linked to systemic diseases. For these reasons, an understanding of the nature of the oral flora and its dynamics is important in orofacial infections.

ACQUISITION AND VARIATION

During birth and immediately thereafter the neonate contacts the microbial inhabitants of the immediate environment. Nevertheless, the oral cavity is considered sterile at birth. The numbers of detectable organisms in the oral cavity increase rapidly beginning about 8 hours after birth. The early flora varies and is relatively simple, but it includes streptococci, lactobacilli, staphylococci, *Veillonella, Neisseria,* and coliform organisms. Streptococci generally are the dominant forms (reportedly up to 80% of the recoverable forms) in neonates. These particularly include *Streptococcus salivarius, S. oralis,* and *S. mitis,* and the group B streptococci.[7,14] Yeasts also are present soon after birth and are found in as many as 44% of infants tested by about 6 months after birth. *Candida albicans* and *C. parapsilosis* appear to be the dominant species.[33,42] *Streptococcus sanguis (sanguinius)* has a median age of colonization of about 9 months. This correlates with the time of tooth emergence.[11] Anaerobic bacteria also establish themselves early. By 2 months of age, *Veillonella* spp., *Actinomyces* spp., and *Prevotella melaninogenica* were present in more than 10% of the population tested, whereas by 6 months of age, *Fusobacterium nucleatum,* nonpigmented *Prevotella* spp., *Porphyromonas catoniae,* and *Leptotrichia* spp. were present. By 12 months of age, *Capnocytophaga* spp., other fusobacteria, and corroding rods were present. *Prevotella intermedia* and *Clostridium, Eubacterium,* and *Selenomonas* spp. also were present by 12 months of age, although with lesser frequency.[38,45] In young children with primary dentition a variety of microorganisms may be found, including species of *Streptococcus, Peptostreptococcus, Bacteroides, Prevotella, Porphyromonas, Selenomonas, Capnocytophaga, Campylobacter, Fusobacterium,* and *Gemella.* The predominant type varies with the intraoral location. The patterns in children with mixed dentition are similar to those associated with primary dentition, but a greater variety of species representing the various genera are present.[39,40] Changes in the microbiota are associated with various disease states, including caries and periodontal disease. As teeth are lost, spirochetes, some streptococcal strains, and lactobacilli are reduced, often to undetectable levels, as are periodontal pathogens such as *Actinobacillus actinomycetemcomitans* and *Porphyromonas gingivalis.* In edentulous individuals without artificial dentures, some species of streptococci, spirochetes, and yeasts are reduced or virtually eliminated, although they return to near-preextraction levels after placement of dentures.[18,44,66] In general, the factors that influence development of the flora include frequency of introduction, nutritional and physiochemical conditions at the time of introduction, and the nature of any existing microbiota. The environment of the neonate tends to favor oxygen-tolerant organisms, but as sites with more anaerobic conditions appear, the number of anaerobes increases. Furthermore, aerobes may scavenge oxygen, facilitating growth of anaerobes. Similarly, organisms that adhere to hard tissues become established later than those that favor soft tissues. These various factors and microbial interactions are important in the development and regulation of the flora throughout life.[47]

REGULATING FACTORS

Once established, the oral microbial flora remains relatively constant. As indicated, with the eruption or loss of teeth, the microenvironments associated with these structures appear or disappear and the organisms associated with them change, either in number or proportion. Similarly, as disease appears or disappears, the associated flora changes. With the appearance of caries and periodontal disease, the microorganisms associated with them change the number and proportion of the flora. Alterations in the flora also may occur with physiological changes such as pregnancy. The hormonal changes associated with pregnancy may affect not only tissue cytokines but also the growth of certain microbial species. Various disease conditions, drugs, and even aging can change the flora by altering the flow rate and composition of saliva and levels and activity of defense components such as immunoglobulins.[26,46,48,54]

SALIVA

Saliva is probably one of the most important regulators of the oral microbiota. Not only does it vary with age and disease state, but the flow rate and composition demonstrate diurnal variations, which in turn affect numbers and composition of the flora. Salivary flow is greatest during waking hours due to repeated stimulation, and the composition varies with secretion. Thus osmolarity increases with secretion, as do the bicarbonate levels and pH, whereas ammonia, urea, and the antimicrobial thiocyanate concentration vary inversely with the flow rate. Other flow-dependent components, components that remain constant, and dietary factors affect the number and proportion of the organisms present. Xerostomia caused by drugs, local conditions such as salivary gland disease and irradiation, and systemic diseases such as human immunodeficiency virus (HIV) infection can profoundly affect the flora and diseases that result from the oral flora.[54]

Saliva, with its complex composition, serves as an environment for the oral microorganisms; thus its fluctuations help regulate the microbiota (Table 2-1). Mineral and ionic content affects the buffering capacity, pH, and Eh and regulates enzyme activity. The gaseous environment regulates the survival and growth of various organisms. The Eh de-

TABLE 2-1

Factors Regulating the Oral Flora

Factor or Component	Role
Salivary Factors	
Ion content: Na, K, Cl, SO_4, Mg, Mn, Ca, Cl, PO_4	Maintain ionic strength and osmotic balance, buffering capacity
CO_2, bicarbonate, flow rate	Maintain buffering capacity
Bicarbonate/CO_2 ratio	Determines pH
Oxidation-reduction potential	Determines which types of organisms (aerobes, facultative, anaerobes) will grow
CO_2, O_2	Act as growth regulators and regulate pH, Eh, buffering capacity
Organic components: vitamins, amino acids, proteins, carbohydrates, glycoproteins	Influence adherence, aggregation, viscosity
Host Diet	
Carbohydrate, proteins, lipids	Affect growth of organisms, proportions of acidogenic and nonacidogenic organisms

From Schuster GS: Oral flora and pathogenic organisms, *Infect Dis Clin North Am* 13:757, 1999.

termines whether anaerobes, aerobes, or facultative organisms predominate. pH is a key factor in the establishment and maintenance of the flora, and even transient changes may affect the presence (or detectability) of an organism. Plaque, with its generally acidic pH, may be a natural reservoir for *Helicobacter pylori,* serving as a source for reinfection of the gut. However, *H. pylori* may be transient and associated with gastric reflux.[48]

The organic components include proteins, amino acids, vitamins, and carbohydrates derived from plasma, salivary gland secretions, microbial metabolic or breakdown products, and the host diet. They serve directly as microbial nutrients, facilitating growth of some organisms while inhibiting others. The free amino acid content varies in amount and composition. Alanine, serine, and glycine are regularly present, whereas others may or may not be present. The amino acids serve as nutrients for the bacteria, and those in saliva may provide adequate nutrition for growth of some organisms. Some proteins have enzymatic activity, providing nutrients such as sugars for organisms or inhibiting organisms (e.g., lactoperoxidase). Glycoproteins are major components of saliva. They impart viscosity and influence adherence and aggregation of the organisms. Others influence the organisms' ability to adhere to surfaces or other bacteria. Immunoglobulins (Igs) are an important group of glycoproteins that serve a defensive role. Studies have shown that in healthy human beings the salivary flow rate, protein content, and Ig levels remain unchanged with age but opsonic activity decreases significantly, possibly affecting an individual's ability to handle abnormal bacteria.[26] The salivary carbohydrates that produce the greatest effects on the oral microbiota are those derived from the host diet because the amounts secreted in the saliva are low and probably insufficient to sustain optimal microbial growth.

HOST DIET

Microorganisms require an adequate nutrient supply for growth and survival, and the availability of this supply helps determine their ecological niche. Although many organisms use the end products of metabolism of other organisms, much nutrition is derived from the host diet (see Table 2-1). Nevertheless, with the notable exceptions of dietary carbohydrates and certain streptococci, reliable evidence of a direct relationship between specific dietary substances and the ecology of individual microorganisms is scarce.

A significant number of oral microorganisms use dietary carbohydrates as a major energy source. Thus large amounts of refined sugar favor microorganisms that ferment carbohydrates. The best known example is the major increase in oral streptococci when the host diet is high in sucrose. Many oral species are able to persist because they can convert host-derived carbohydrate into storage forms to be used when dietary carbohydrates are unavailable.

The effects of dietary proteins on the oral flora are largely unknown. The slow rate of protein breakdown, especially as a result of short exposure to weakly proteolytic salivary enzymes, suggests that dietary protein does not provide a significant source of amino acids to the organisms. However, a high-protein diet, especially if coupled with a reduction in carbohydrates, results in a reduction of the acidogenic flora. A similar situation occurs with dietary lipids.

The physical consistency of the diet affects the retention of organisms in some sites, particularly supragingival areas. Nevertheless, retention of foods at various sites can influence local microbial growth. Consistency also can affect the saliva. Liquid diets can cause a significant reduction in volume and total protein content of parotid secretions, which in turn can affect the principal salivary bicarbonate buffer system.

RETENTION OF THE MICROBIAL FLORA

To become or remain a member of the oral microbial flora, the organism must have a mechanism to localize and remain at a site. As with other sites, oral organisms have specific and nonspecific mechanisms for localizing or remaining in a favorable environment. Nonspecific retention involves physical entrapment, usually in a favorable site such as occurs with nonadherent bacteria that reside in pits, fissures, or carious lesions of teeth, soft tissue sites such as the gingival sulcus, or breaks in the tissues.

Specific interactions and selective adherence also occur.

These may be metabolic, as when growth of *Veillonella* strains is facilitated in the presence of streptococci.[30] Selective adherence between microorganisms and among groups of microorganisms likely accounts for more retention of normal organisms and pathogens than does physical entrapment. The organisms have different attachment abilities and the strength of the attachment varies, with the result that some organisms can displace others, or in other circumstances successors cannot displace predecessors but readily occupy a niche when it becomes vacant. These various phenomena may result in coaggregation pairs or even multigeneric aggregations that produce a resident flora at a particular locale.[43] Often these interactions involve fimbriae. Such attachment patterns can affect disease production by the organisms. Thus selective attachment of the periodontal pathogen *P. gingivalis* to various host proteins occurs while the organism stimulates cytokine production and bone resorption; *S. sanguis* antagonism and delayed attachment of *S. mutans*[11] also occurs in addition to localization of *Actinobacillus actinomycetemcomitans* to periodontal sites through binding to tissue cells. Fimbriae of *P. intermedia* induce hemagglutination reactions, whereas those of *Prevotella loescheii* have been found to cause coaggregation with other bacteria (i.e., *Actinomyces viscosus* and *S. sanguis*). Similarly, a fimbria-mediated coaggregation occurs between the oral anaerobes *Treponema medium* and *P. gingivalis*.[16,32,65] Some adherences relate to the presence of specific tissue cell receptors (e.g., the attachment, through lipoteichoic acid, of group A streptococci to mucosal epithelial cells) and the affinity of *C. albicans* for distinct subpopulations of oral epithelial cells.[3,57] These mechanisms help establish the retention patterns and thus the resident microflora at a site and facilitate the persistence of pathogens, if only for a brief time. The importance of the organism-tissue interactions in pathogenesis can be illustrated by the often-seen phenomenon of overgrowth by oral *Candida* spp. when an individual is treated with certain antibiotic agents. When agents reduce the number of bacteria, yeast takes over the poorly populated site and produces a candidal infection. When antibiotic use is discontinued, the normal bacterial flora reasserts itself. A similar situation occurs when antibiotic agents selectively reduce the gram-positive bacterial population, resulting in an overgrowth of gram-negative bacteria.

MICROORGANISMS

As noted earlier, the oral microbiota is complex and, although relatively stable, does fluctuate with age, disease conditions, and preferred site of residence. Thus the presence of a particular organism at a site of infection must be viewed in the context of the aforementioned conditions. For example, in debilitated or compromised patients the flora varies and unusual organisms may be present as pathogens or members of the flora. The best studied example of this phenomenon is the changes in the periodontal flora associated with the development of acquired immunodeficiency syndrome.[5,12,23]

The classification and nomenclature of the oral micro-biotica are in a state of flux, especially from the perspective of relationships based on genetic information, which is a practical method. Although organisms are generally grouped as aerobes, facultatives, microaerophils, and obligate anaerobes, a spectrum of optimal living conditions exists. For example, organisms may grow in the presence of small amounts of oxygen, survive but not grow at these low levels, or actually be killed by these levels. Thus the groupings based on environment are somewhat arbitrary. Classification by schemes other than genetics shows similar problems.

The following sections discuss the major groups of microorganisms in the oral cavity. Some organisms have not been cultured or characterized. The major genera are included, and where appropriate, specific species are described.

STREPTOCOCCI

Facultative streptococci form the most numerous group of organisms in the oral cavity. Although the actual percentages vary among sites, the streptococci represent approximately one half of the viable counts from saliva and the dorsum of the tongue and one fourth the counts from plaque and gingival sulcus. The most abundant oral streptococci are members of the viridans group, which have been classified by several schemes (Table 2-2).[8,60,67] Viridans streptococci lack many features that distinguish other major streptococcal pathogens. The hemolytic characteristics are important parameters for the classification of streptococci. Indeed, the original basis for the category viridans streptococci was their α-hemolysis. However, according to recent schemes some streptococci that are α-, β-, or γ-hemolytic sometimes may be included with the viridans streptococci.[60]

TABLE 2-2

Major Aerobic and Facultative Bacterial Genera and Species of the Head and Neck Region

Current Name	Locale	Comments
Gram-Positive Cocci		
Staphylococcus aureus	Oral cavity, pharynx	
Staphylococcus epidermidis	Oral cavity, pharynx, skin	
Staphylococcus asaccharolyticus	Oral cavity	Formerly *Peptococcus asaccharolyticus*
Stomatococcus mucilaginosus		Common finding in cases of pericoronitis
Streptococci		"Viridans" streptococci
Mitis group		
Streptococcus mitis	Oral cavity, oropharynx	
Streptococcus oralis	Oral cavity, oropharynx	
Streptococcus parasanguis (parasanguinius)	Throat	
Streptococcus gordonii	Oral cavity, oropharynx	
Streptococcus sanguis (sanguinius)	Oral cavity	
Streptococcus crista	Oral cavity, throat	
Streptococcus pneumoniae	Upper respiratory tract	Causative agent for pneumonia
Salivarius group		"Viridans" streptococci
Salivarius salivarius	Oral cavity, especially saliva and tongue	
Salivarius vestibularis	Oral cavity, especially vestibular mucosa	
Anginosus group		"Viridans" streptococci
Anginosus aginosus	Oral cavity, upper respiratory tract, vagina	
Anginosus constellatus	Oral cavity, upper respiratory tract	
Anginosus intermedius	Oral cavity, upper respiratory tract	
		"Viridans" streptococci
Anginosus mutans	Dental plaque, carious teeth	
Anginosus sobrinus	Tooth surface, carious teeth	
Anginosus cricetus	Oral cavity of rodents, occasionally humans	
Anginosus rattus	Oral cavity of rats, occasionally humans	
Gemella morbillorum	Association with the periodontium	Previous classification with streptococci
Streptococcus pyogenes	Throat, oropharynx, oral cavity (transient)	Lancefield group A, β-hemolytic
Group B	Oropharynx of neonates (common)	
Group D:		
Enterococcus spp.	Oral cavity and intestine	Possible problem in endodontic infections
Enterococcus faecium		
Enterococcus faecalis		

Data from Bruckner DA, Colonna P, Bearson BL: Nomenclature for aerobic and facultative bacteria, *Clin Infect Dis* 29:713, 1999; Whiley RA, Beighton D: Current classification of the oral streptococci, *Oral Microbiol Immunol* 13:195, 1998. *Continued*

TABLE 2-2

Major Aerobic and Facultative Bacterial Genera and Species of the Head and Neck Region—cont'd

Current Name	Locale	Comments
Gram-Negative Cocci		
Neisseria spp.	Orapharynx and mouth	Generally minor component in mouth and major component of oropharynx
Neisseria subflava		
Neisseria sicca		
Gram-Positive Rods		
Bacterionema matruchotii	Oral cavity, especially dental plaque	
Rothia dentocariosa	Oral cavity, throat, dental calculus	Possible appearance as coccoid, diphtheroid, or bacillary form
Diphtheroids	Tongue, gingival sulcus, plaque	Poor characterization, rods and filaments, some belonging to *Corynebacterium* or *Propionobacterium* genera but not assigned to any species
Lactobacillus spp.	Various areas of the oral cavity, especially carious teeth	Multiple species
Gram-Negative Rods and Coccobacilli		
Moraxella catarrhalis	Oropharynx	Formerly *Branhamella catarrhalis* and *Neisseria catarrhalis*
Actinobacillus actinomycetemcomitans	Gingival sulcus	Producer of potent leukotoxin, association with various forms of periodontal disease
Campylobacter spp.	Gingival sulcus	
Capnocytophaga spp.	Gingival sulcus	CO_2 necessary
Eikenella corrodens	Gingival sulcus	Common association with pericoronitis and osteomyelitis
Helicobacter pylori	Plaque (possibly transient)	Association with recurrent aphthous ulcers

Data from Bruckner DA, Colonna P, Bearson BL: Nomenclature for aerobic and facultative bacteria, *Clin Infect Dis* 29:713, 1999; Whiley RA, Beighton D: Current classification of the oral streptococci, *Oral Microbiol Immunol* 13:195, 1998.

Viridans streptococci prevent colonization of the oral cavity by being more aggressive than other organisms. They compete for mucosal adherence sites and produce bacteriocins that exert a bactericidal effect on some competitors. Viridans streptococci are usually of low virulence but cause serious infections when the oral mucosa is disrupted, the host's defense mechanisms are compromised, or a combination of these conditions occurs. Little is known about the pathogenic mechanisms of viridans streptococci. They may produce some exotoxins and lytic enzymes, activate complement, induce production of cytokines, or perform a number of these actions.

Oral streptococci may account for a major proportion of the organisms associated with bacterial endocarditis, especially in individuals with prosthetic valves. The most common isolates are *S. mitis*, *S. oralis*, *S. sanguis*, and *S. gordonii*. *S. anginosus*, *S. constellatus*, and *S. intermedius* often are isolated from purulent infections, especially deep-seated abscesses. Streptococci of the "mutans" group tend to colonize on teeth and are associated with dental caries.

In addition to their roles in abscesses and endocarditis in otherwise healthy persons, oral streptococci are important in infections of individuals who are immunocompromised and neutropenic. Oral mucositis, often related to cancer chemotherapy, may predispose patients to such infections. The initial feature of *S. viridans* sepsis is fever that may persist for several days, even after cultivable organisms are cleared from the blood. Most patients recover, although fulminant septic shock may occur.[60]

OTHER GRAM-POSITIVE COCCI

Enterococci may frequently be found in the oral cavity, although they do not compose a large percentage of the flora (see Table 2-2). However, when present in infections, they may be persistent and difficult to eliminate. The genus *Peptostreptococcus* contains obligately anaerobic, gram-positive cocci that are found in varying but low percentages at different sites in the oral cavity, although they may represent a significant proportion of the subgingival flora in advanced periodontal disease. They also have been found in odontogenic and soft tissue abscesses. This genus is poorly classified but includes many species previously classified in the genus *Peptococcus* (see Table 2-2).

Facultative, catalase-positive, gram-positive organisms classified as staphylococci are present in nearly every mouth, albeit not in large numbers. *S. aureus* is present intraorally in about half the population, including in the saliva, although the number of organisms is not large. They are more likely to be present and in larger numbers in the nose and throat, and often are components of mixed infections of the orofacial region.

GRAM-POSITIVE RODS AND FILAMENTS

Gram-positive rod-shaped and filamentous bacteria are present in the oral cavity (Table 2-3). Although organisms typically have this characteristic morphological pattern, they may be somewhat pleomorphic, with various lengths and widths. *Actinomyces* spp. are some of the more common gram-positive filamentous and rod-shaped bacteria in the oral cavity. This genus also includes some of the more common and persistent pathogens of the head and neck region. They are primarily anaerobes, although some are facultative. The more frequently found oral species include *A. israelii, A. viscosus, A. naeslundii,* and *A. odontolyticus.* The latter organism may be isolated from deep dentinal caries, as well as other sites in the oral cavity. The normal habitat of *A. naeslundii* includes the tonsillar crypts and dental calculus. Human infections with this organism have been reported, but its exact role is not proved. *A. viscosus,* isolated from the oral cavity of humans and rodents, produces a viscous sediment in culture. It produces transmissible periodontal disease in hamsters, is found in dental calculus and root surface caries in humans, and has been isolated from human abscesses. *A. israelii* species are usually isolated from cases of human actinomycosis. Such infections are usually of endogenous origin, since dental calculus and tonsillar crypts are their normal habitat.

The genus *Rothia* contains one species, *R. dentocariosa* (see Table 2-2). It has a branching, filamentous shape but also may appear as coccoid, bacillary, and diphtheroid forms. *Rothia* is anaerobic, but some strains grow under aerobic conditions. A few natural infections have been reported in humans.

Eubacterium spp. are anaerobic, pleomorphic, gram-positive, rod-shaped or filamentous bacteria found at various sites in the oral cavity (see Table 2-3). They have been found in plaque *(E. saburreum),* calculus, carious dentin, and necrotic pulp. *E. lentum (Eggerthella lenta)* in particular has been related to percussion pain in endodontic infections.[35] Other species isolated from periodontal pockets include *E. timidum, E. brachy,* and *E. nodatum,* whereas *E. combesii* has been seen in many endodontic lesions.

The bacterial flora of the oral cavity includes a large number of pleomorphic gram-positive rods and filaments grouped under the general term *diphtheroid* (see Table 2-3). This categorization is based on morphological characteristics, and the organism's true classifications are not known. Organisms may be isolated from the dorsum of the tongue, gingival sulcus, and plaque. Some strains are aerobic, some facultative, and some obligate anaerobes. They appear club shaped and in angular arrangements in clusters and branched forms. Some belong to the genus *Corynebacterium* and others to *Propionibacterium,* although they are not assigned to any species. Diphtheroids are abundant in the oral cavity, but their roles in disease are not known.

Lactobacilli are characteristic oral bacteria. They are probably present soon after birth. *Lactobacillus* counts vary widely in adults but constitute only a small proportion of the total viable count of oral microorganisms. They are usually not pathogenic, although fair correlation exists between their presence and caries activity (see Table 2-2).

GRAM-NEGATIVE COCCI

Veillonellae are anaerobic, gram-negative cocci that are among the more numerous of the oral bacteria, composing 5% to 10% of the organisms of the tongue and saliva. They are among the first colonizers of the oral cavity. Of the seven recognized species, *V. parvula, V. atypica,* and *V. dispar* are found in the oral cavity and in the respiratory and intestinal tracts. They contain endotoxin that is pyrogenic. They also may participate as components of polymicrobial infections, often in individuals who are debilitated.[37]

Gram-negative, facultative cocci designated as *Neisseria* have been found in the oral cavity and nasopharynx of humans. *N. sicca* is the major species (see Table 2-2), although it may be a type of *N. subflava.* This organism can produce inflammation of the oral mucosa and may produce lesions resembling oral gonorrhea.

GRAM-NEGATIVE RODS AND FILAMENTS

Many gram-negative, anaerobic, microaerophilic, or facultative rods and filaments are located in the oral cavity (see Tables 2-2 and 2-3). In the healthy mouth these may constitute nearly 25% of the flora, but the proportions double with the development of gingivitis or periodontitis. The more common organisms include species of *Prevotella, Porphyromonas, Selenomonas, Bacteroides, Fusobacterium, Campylobacter, Actinobacillus,* and *Capnocytophaga.*[51,58,64] Similarly, some of the same organisms and different species of the same genera are associated with endodontic infections.[20,28,35,56,68] However, they and similar species do cause infectious disease or tissue damage at other sites. Fusobacteria have been isolated from infections of the respiratory tract, pleural cavity, oral cavity (in addition to sites of periodontitis), and trauma sites such as bite wounds. *Eikenella corrodens* has been found in human infections of the respiratory and intestinal tracts, brain abscesses, and infections of the oral cavity and associated with infective endocarditis[13] (see Table 2-2). *Porphyromonas* and *Prevotella* spp. have been isolated from abscesses, pulmonary and ear infections, wound infections, peritonitis, and sinusitis[6,15,27] (see Table 2-3). Most infections are polymicrobial, involving various combinations of gram-negative and gram-positive cocci and gram-negative rods. Pathogen(s) isolated from such infections or the proportions of such pathogens

TABLE 2-3

Major Anaerobic Bacterial Genera and Species of the Head and Neck Region (except spirochetes)

Current Name	Locale	Comments
Gram-Negative Rods		
Bacteroides spp.	Periodontium	Relation to *Porphyromonas* spp.
Bacteroides forsythus		
Bacteroides distasonis		Relation to *Porphyromonas* spp.
Bacteroides ureolyticus		Relation to *Campylobacter* organisms
Fusobacterium spp.	Periodontium	Several subspecies
Fusobacterium nucleatum		
Fusobacterium periodonticum		Relation to *F. nucleatum*
Porphyromonas spp.	Periodontium	
Porphyromonas gingivalis		
Porphyromonas asaccharolyticus	Periodontium	
Porphyromonas endodontalis	Oral cavity	Usual isolation from endodontic lesions
Prevotella spp.		
Prevotella intermedia	Most in periodontium and peri-	
Prevotella buccalis	odontal lesions, some in en-	
Prevotella dentalis	dodontic lesions	
Prevotella denticola		
Prevotella heparinolytica		
Prevotella loescheii		
Prevotella melaninogenica		
Prevotella nigrescens		Endodontic lesions (common)
Prevotella oralis		
Prevotella oris		
Prevotella tannerae		Endodontic and periodontic lesions
Centipeda periodontii	Periodontal tissue	Relation to *Selenomonas* spp.
Leptotrichia buccalis	Oral mucosa	
Selenomonas spp.		
Selenomonas noxia	Periodontal tissue	Early adult periodontitis (often)
Selenomonas sputigena		
Gram-Negative Cocci		
Veillonella spp.	Tongue and saliva	Total 5% to 10% of cultivable organisms on tongue and in saliva
Veillonella atypica		
Veillonella dispar		
Veillonella parvula		
Gram-Positive Rods		
Actinomyces spp.	Dental plaque, calculus	
Actinomyces meyeri		
Actinomyces naeslundii		
Actinomyces odontolyticus		
Actinomyces viscosus		
Bifidobacterium dentium	Dental plaque	
Eggerthella lenta	Endodontic lesions, gingival tissues	Previously *Eubacterium lentum*
Eubacterium spp.	Gingival tissues and areas	
Eubacterium combesii	Gingival areas	
Eubacterium contortum		
Eubacterium moniliforme		
Eubacterium nitrogenes		
Eubacterium saburreum		
Eubacterium tenue		
Gram-Positive Cocci		
Peptococcus niger	Subgingival areas	
Peptostreptococcus spp.	Subgingival areas	Many species formerly classified as *Peptococcus*
Peptostreptococcus anaerobius		
Peptostreptococcus asaccharolyticus		
Peptostreptococcus magnus		
Peptostreptococcus micros		

Data from Jousimies-Somer H, Summanen P: Microbiology terminology update: clinically significant anaerobic gram-positive and gram-negative bacteria (excluding spirochetes), *Clin Infect Dis* 29:724, 1999; Tanner ACR, Taubman MA: Microbiota of initial periodontitis in adults, *Anaerobe* 5:229, 1999.

may vary depending on the stage of the infection. As conditions within the lesion change because of environment, microbial metabolism (e.g., oxygen scavenging by aerobes), or treatment, the organisms present or dominant at one stage may decrease or even disappear at a later stage while others become dominant.

SPIROCHETES

The basic structure of a spirochete is a helical cylinder consisting of cytoplasm enclosed in a membrane and surrounded by a thin layer of peptidoglycan that allows the organism to flex. Spirochetes also have one or more fibrils that are likely associated with motility. Spirochetes vary in length, thickness, and number and amplitude of spirals.

Of the four genera in the family Spirochaetaceae, only two, *Treponema* and *Borrelia,* appear to be pathogenic for humans. Members of the genus *Treponema* usually produce local tissue lesions. Included are the agents that cause syphilis, yaws, and pinta and the oral spirochetes. Organisms in the genus *Borrelia* include the causative agents for Lyme disease and relapsing fever in humans.

Spirochetes commonly inhabit the oral cavity and can invade connective tissue or intact epithelium in diseased sites (Table 2-4). Most spirochetes likely belong to the genus *Treponema.* Seven *Treponema* species have been cultured: *denticola, pectinovorum, socranskii, vincentii, maltophilum, medium,* and *amylovorum.* Some others have been cultivated but not named, and numerous uncultivated species exist.[22] Treponemes are best observed with dark-field or phase-contrast microscopy because of their size and resistance to staining. Where cultivable, they are slow growing and require anaerobic conditions and the medium generally requires enrichment with blood, serum, or ascites fluid. Spirochetes almost always are present in the oral cavity of healthy adults and find conditions in periodontal pockets quite favorable.

The pathogenicity of the oral spirochetes is not clear because separation of their effects from those of other bacteria with which they often are found, especially the fusiforms, is difficult; the two types frequently are found together in lesions. A variety of potential virulence factors have been identified, including cytotoxic factors, proteases, hemolysins, and immunomodulatory mechanisms.[24] Pure cultures of oral spirochetes do not cause characteristic, transferable infections as occurs when mixed populations of spirochetes and other oral bacteria are inoculated. Lesions seen include acute necrotizing ulcerative gingivitis, lesions of the upper respiratory tract, and noma, a spreading, gangrenous stomatitis that may develop in children with poor nutrition or debilitating disease.

MYCOPLASMA

Mycoplasma are small bacteria that lack a rigid cell wall, causing them to appear mainly as cocci or coccoid forms. Most are facultative anaerobes, although they tend to grow better under aerobic conditions. Although the most common human infection is pneumonia, caused by *Mycoplasma pneumoniae,* other species are found in the oral cavity, including *M. salivarium* and *M. penetrans* (Table 2-5). Of particular interest is *M. penetrans,* which has been shown to augment the cytotoxicity of HIV.[12,29]

FUNGI AND YEASTS

C. albicans is the most common oral yeast. Its reported incidence in the oral cavity of healthy individuals varies from 10% to 80%. In addition to *C. albicans,* other species of *Candida* have been isolated from significant numbers of individuals, including *C. dubliniensis, parapsilosis, krusei, famata, guillermondii,* and *zeylanoides.* The predominant species and strains appear to vary as a function of host age.[42] Not surprisingly, an increased incidence of fungal infections with

TABLE 2-4

Major Species of Oral Spirochetes

Current Name	Locale	Comments
Treponema spp.	Periodontal	
Treponema medium	tissues,	
Treponema denticola	especially	
Treponema maltophilum	in various	
Treponema amylovorum	forms of	
Treponema socranskii	periodontal	
sp Smibert-2	disease	
sp Smibert-3		
sp Smibert-5		
Treponema pectiovorum		
Treponema vincentii		
Uncultivated		At least 47 as
Treponema spp.		yet uncultivated species

Data from Dewhirst FE, Tamer MA, Ericson RE, et al: The diversity of periodontal spirochetes by 16S rRNA analysis, *Oral Microbiol Immunol* 15:196, 2000.

TABLE 2-5

Mycoplasma Species Associated with the Head and Neck Region

Current Name	Locale	Comments
Mycoplasma (no Gram stain reaction)		
Mycoplasma spp.	Periodontal	Some species appear
Mycoplasma hominis	tissues	to increase in individuals who are
Mycoplasma orale		viduals who are
Mycoplasma penetrans		HIV positive
Mycoplasma salivarium		
Mycoplasma bucalle		

Candida spp. has been noted in patients who are immunocompromised. Colonization rates increase with severity of illness, and in such individuals, systemic infections have become increasingly important in causing morbidity and mortality. Some species have greater resistance to antifungal agents, especially the azole antifungals.[25,33,34] Species of *Penicillium, Geotrichum, Hormodentrum, Aspergillus, Hemispora,* and *Scopulariopsis* also have been isolated from the oral environment, including from normal individuals. These groups may be considered normal inhabitants.

Candida spp. may play a symbiotic or an opportunistic role with bacteria in the oral ecology. For example, *Candida* spp. may cause oral lesions in adults and children, particularly if the bacterial flora is disturbed. In turn, oral bacteria may inhibit or limit the attachment or growth of oral yeast (see Chapter 11).

VIRUSES

With the exceptions of herpes simplex virus and cytomegalovirus, viruses appear to be oral transients. Herpes simplex virus infection is present in a large proportion of the population, often in a latent form. Its characteristic recurrence and the persistence of significant antibody titers indicate that it persists throughout life, in either its latent form in the trigeminal ganglion or the infectious stage in the oral cavity during acute episodes. Virus may be recovered from the saliva or an individual up to 2 months after recovery from an acute exacerbation of disease and from that of a small percentage of adults who do not display symptoms.[63]

Cytomegaloviruses infect a variety of tissues, including salivary glands. They also have been detected in deep periodontal pockets of adults and children, suggesting an ability to replicate in periodontal tissues.[15] Infections in children can be asymptomatic or may produce jaundice, enteritis, and central nervous system disturbances. If a child's mother was infected during pregnancy, this may be manifest as congenital defects. In adults, infection may be asymptomatic or produce a mononucleosis-like illness. Because the virus has been recovered from tissues such as adenoids of apparently healthy persons, the virus is likely present in the saliva of healthy carriers who are asymptomatic (see Chapter 11).

HOST-MICROBIAL INTERACTIONS

PARASITISM

The initial contact between a host and a microorganism usually results in a transient relationship in which the organism is quickly eliminated by host defenses or establishes a temporary residency followed by later elimination from the host. These responses occur whether the organism is relatively benign or a potential pathogen. If the organisms find the host suitable for growth, they may cause an infection. The host may eliminate the organism, or the host may die. In either instance the organism is an unsuccessful parasite. Alternatively, the host may neither eliminate the organism nor die, but rather adapt to the organism, in which case a carrier state occurs; the organism survives, often retaining its virulence, but the host no longer manifests the disease. On the other hand, the organism may adapt, losing its virulence for that host, a situation known as *attenuation.* In either type of adaptation the organism has established a state of successful parasitism. In some instances organisms may be successful parasites as long as they remain in their accustomed locations. However, the adaptation, host or microbial, may break down or the organism may acquire pathogenic potential through mutation or transfer of genetic information from a pathogenic strain of organism, in which case it produces infectious disease.

Another and perhaps more common form of parasitism occurs, namely that of *aberrant parasitism.* In this relationship the organism moves from its usual site to an unaccustomed site where it behaves as a pathogen. An example is the movement of normal, "harmless" inhabitants of the oral cavity into the deeper tissues, resulting in a soft tissue or bone infection.

In addition to infections caused by indigenous organisms or invasion by exogenous ones, infections can be superimposed on a disease that has already affected a patient. Superimposed infections result from activities or disease processes that disrupt the balance of the flora, such as the use of antibiotics, from clinical disorders that increase susceptibility to indigenous or exogenous parasites (e.g., immunosuppression caused by HIV infection), or use of chemotherapeutic agents. In the one instance, drugs may eradicate or suppress susceptible organisms, resulting in overgrowth by resistant forms. The most common example is a patient treated with broad-spectrum antibiotics. Suppression or eradication of groups of bacteria results in a loss of interactions or factors that maintain the stability of the resident microflora and facilitates the rapid multiplication of drug-resistant, potential pathogens. However, simple suppression is not the entire cause for diseases. Although suppression is a universal reaction, the superimposed diseases develop in some individuals only. Factors involved include age, presence of chronic disease, type of antibiotic agent, and duration of exposure. The most notable example is the overgrowth by *Candida* spp. after tetracycline therapy or overgrowth by gram-negative bacteria after penicillin therapy.

Superinfections also may be related to the presence of clinical conditions, infectious or noninfectious, that increase susceptibility to exogenous or endogenous organisms. Superinfection may occur when the natural defenses are compromised. For example, catheters provide pathways to the deeper tissues or circulation. Surgical procedures or injections also provide such routes because they disrupt the mucocutaneous barriers. Use of antibiotics to help control the disease-related infections may actually further exacerbate the problem at another site.

The importance of the various mechanisms that regulate the flora, thus controlling superimposed infections, is exemplified by patients who are immunosuppressed through treatment or disease. These individuals are particularly susceptible to infections by a variety of organisms that are opportunistic or considered minimally pathogenic or nonpathogenic. Viridans streptococci are a particular cause of sepsis or pneumonia in the patient with neutropenia.[60] Individuals who are HIV seropositive with periodontitis harbor a range of exogenous pathogens rarely associated with common types of periodontitis. The lack of adequate immune effector and regulatory cells in these individuals may explain the increase in opportunistic pathogens and the rapid progression of the periodontal disease. This may be compounded by altered levels of cytokines such as interleukin (IL)-1β, IL-6, and tumor necrosis factor α in the gingival crevicular fluid of patients who are HIV positive.[2,5,53] Multiple factors increase the risk of infection from indigenous and exogenous organisms, but the basic problem is a breakdown in the regulation of host-parasite interactions.

PATHOGENICITY AND VIRULENCE

Although pathogens, pathogenicity, and virulence typically have been defined in terms of the organisms and based on the recognition that host response is a key factor in infectious disease, recent modifications of these definitions have been suggested. Thus the definition of a *pathogen* has been expanded from that of a microbe capable of causing a disease to encompass host damage by mechanisms related to the presence or activity of the organism, but not a direct result of the organism's action (e.g., an immunopathological response). *Pathogenicity* is defined as the capacity of a microbe to cause damage in a host. *Virulence* is now recognized as a more relative term—the relative capacity of a microbe to cause damage in a host. Similarly, a *virulence factor* relates to the ability to damage the host as opposed to simply being a microbial component.[10] In keeping with the relationships between the organism and the host, other factors must be considered. The organisms must be able to enter the host, multiply, resist host defenses, and damage the host. Although each step is complex, all these processes must occur to produce an infectious disease.

Role of Attachment   Many infections begin on the mucous membranes such as those of the oral cavity despite various defense mechanisms. To initiate an infection, an organism must be able to adhere to the mucosal surface and resist elimination by various mechanical means, compete for space and nutrients, resist antagonisms by other organisms and host defenses, and penetrate the epithelium to infect the deeper tissues. Adherence may be directly to the mucosa or other organisms, either of the same genus and species or different ones. The physicochemical properties of the specific surface sites or structures on bacteria and tissue cell surfaces apparently account for the interactions that result in adherence and are likely important in the disease process. Importance of the

cell surface is exemplified by adherence of *C. albicans*. Distinct subpopulations of epithelial cells have different affinities for attachment.[57] Importance of the microbial surface is exemplified by rheumatic fever. Although group A streptococci associated with rheumatic fever may adhere to buccal mucosal and pharyngeal epithelial cells through mechanisms involving M protein and lipoteichoic acid fimbriae, in the case of *Streptococcus pyogenes*–induced skin infections, the mechanisms are not M-protein mediated and are unknown.[19]

Many bacteria possess fibrils that mediate adherence to cells and other bacteria and thus affect their ability to produce disease. In the case of pathogenic neisseriae, adhesions and fimbriae mediate the organism's interaction with cell receptors. These interactions allow colonization of the mucosa, stimulate signaling cascades and pathways that are essential for cellular entry and intracellular accommodation of the organisms, and lead to induction of cytokine release, priming the immune response.[50]

The fimbriae of various oral streptococci that colonize surfaces in the oral cavity play important roles in adherence and coaggregation. These determine whether the organisms adhere to soft tissues, tooth structure, other bacteria, and so on.[16,32] Similarly, adherence factors associated with periodontal pathogens may contribute to other forms of disease caused by these same organisms. In the case of *P. gingivalis*, adherence is associated with fimbriae, as are other biological activities including immunogenicity, stimulation of cytokine production, and promotion of bone resorption. Proteases may enhance binding by degrading host proteins, which can expose cryptic receptors for microorganisms.[31,32]

A. actinomycetemcomitans also can adhere to and interact with oral structures. This involves fimbriae, microbial vesicles, and amorphous proteinaceous material. The vesicles may serve as a delivery mechanism for the leukotoxin that destroys polymorphonuclear leukocytes and macrophages. The adherence and delivery mechanisms may facilitate invasion by the organism and its ability to produce a local or systemic disease. Fimbriae of various *Prevotella* species induce hemagglutination and coaggregation with other bacteria.[32,49,61]

BACTERIAL TOXINS AND VIRULENCE FACTORS

Microorganisms produce a variety of toxins and virulence factors, including endotoxins, exotoxins, and enzymes, and structural factors important for pathogenicity, such as the adhesins discussed previously. Endotoxins are important in the pathogenesis of gram-negative bacteria. They can produce effects such as leukopenia, increased capillary permeability, pyrexia, shock, and death. Endotoxins also may contribute to the pathogenesis of systemic diseases associated with various oral diseases. Endotoxin damage is more likely when invasion of tissues and the circulation occurs. Although the majority of endotoxin release occurs when the organisms undergo lysis, some may be released from cells during active growth, usually in vesicles. The potency of various endotoxins varies with the source, although this does not necessarily relate to the severity of the infection. Toxicity derives from actions on host cell membranes, immune responses induced by the endotoxin, and activation of complement by the alternative pathway. The importance of these agents is now being more fully appreciated as the varied activities of immune response–related tissue reactions (i.e., related to cytokines) become better understood.

Exotoxins are potent toxins produced by and released from both gram-positive and gram-negative bacteria during growth. In contrast to endotoxins, they tend to be rather specific in their sites and modes of action and tend to act at a site distant from that of production. Several have been associated with orofacial infections. Strains of *S. aureus* have been isolated from the oral cavity of individuals who were dehydrated and had severe oral mucositis. These strains produced toxic shock syndrome toxin I and enterotoxin D.[1] Others have been associated with chronic orofacial pain.[9] Cases of orofacial and cervical necrotizing fasciitis have been reported as a result of group A streptococci. The disease is manifest as a rapidly invasive necrotizing infection that displays myositis and necrosis of tissues and overwhelming sepsis, requiring surgical debridement, fasciotomy, or amputation.[41,62]

Enzymes capable of damaging the host by cytolysis or destruction of other tissue components are well recognized as contributing to disease processes. Some staphylococci produce coagulase that may help establish a localized infection. Coagulase also may result in production of a fibrin coat that helps the organisms resist phagocytosis or produce a clot around the infection that keeps phagocytes from the site. The metalloproteinases produced by some oral bacteria such as *Prevotella* spp. may be potent factors in the pathogenesis of infections by digesting connective tissues. Enzymes such as hyaluronidase, proteases, and lipases produced by various bacteria such as streptococci and staphylococci contribute to the disease process by digesting extracellular matrices.

HOST RESISTANCE

Host defenses are generally divided into innate and acquired defenses. Innate defenses are those present at birth. These include mechanical barriers, secretions, the resident microbial flora, and inflammatory responses. The role of the resident flora in protecting the host against exogenous microorganisms has already been discussed. Mechanical barriers include the intact skin and mucosa and the entrapping and washing actions of the secretions and cilia. Saliva washes many organisms out of the oral cavity into the alimentary canal, where they are destroyed by the low gastric pH and enzymes. Mucous secretions trap organisms and the organisms are destroyed by enzymes or other antimicrobial substances if swallowed or eliminated if washed up and out by the cilia. If organisms enter the deeper tissues, they elicit an inflammatory response that involves phagocytosis, actions of cytokines, and activities of the immune response. All these responses interact to protect the host against pathogens.

The acquired defenses, unlike the innate defenses, usually are specific for the organisms. The immune responses tend to be divided into those that are antibody mediated and those that are cell mediated, although this distinction is no longer clear. The immune responses can provide a variety of protections for the host, including toxin neutralization, opsonization, bacteriolysis, inhibition of attachment, enhancement of chemotaxis, and localization of the organisms to prevent spread of the infection. At the same time, these responses may facilitate tissue damage, since immunopathological effects are a significant component of some diseases.

Relationships between Oral Infections and Systemic Diseases   Although the oral microbiota is generally confined to the oral cavity and contiguous structures, evidence is increasing that it does participate in various systemic diseases. This appears especially true of the periodontopathic organisms because periodontal disease permits the organisms to enter deeper tissues and perhaps become systemic. A particular association between periodontal pathogens such as *P. gingivalis* and atherosclerosis has been suggested. The possible mechanisms include direct effects of the organisms on atheroma formation, indirect or host-mediated effects triggered by infections, common predispositions for periodontal disease and atherosclerosis, and common risk factors such as lifestyle. Of importance to the current discussion is the direct relationship between the periodontal bacteria and atheroma formation. *P. gingivalis* has been found in carotid and coronary atheromas. The organism can invade and proliferate in heart and coronary artery endothelial cells in vitro, and along with *S. sanguis,* it may induce platelet aggregation thought to be associated with thrombus formation. In addition, in a nonhuman primate model, a number of host factors related to atherosclerosis have been shown to significantly increase during gingivitis and periodontitis. Changes in serum lipid levels, especially cholesterol, triglycerides, low-density lipoprotein, high-density lipoprotein, and lipoproteins such as apoprotein A-I were noted during periodontitis. Some of these were exacerbated when the fat content of the diet was increased.[17,21,23,55,59] As has been well recognized, oral microorganisms can enter the deeper tissues after damage to the oral mucosa through trauma, surgery, or disease-related destruction, contributing to systemic disease processes. One commonly cited model is infective endocarditis. Glucans synthesized by oral streptococci from dietary sucrose have been suggested to enhance adherence to fibrin-platelet clots. In addition, oral organisms can enter the circulation and lodge on prosthetic heart valves and joints, producing severe systemic and local problems.[36,49,52] These results further emphasize the importance of the oral microbial flora, its pathogenic mechanisms, and its relationships to local and systemic diseases.

REFERENCES

1. Bagg J, Sweeney MP, Wood KH, et al: Possible role of *Staphylococcus aureus* in severe oral mucositis among elderly dehydrated patients, *Microb Ecol Health Dis* 8:51, 1995.

2. Baqui AA, Meiller TF, Jabra-Rizk, et al: Enhanced interleukin 1 beta, interleukin 6 and tumor necrosis factor alpha in gingival crevicular fluid from periodontal pockets of patients infected with human immunodeficiency virus 1, *Oral Microbiol Immunol* 15:67, 2000.

3. Beachey EH, Courtney HS: Bacterial adherence: the attachment of group A streptococci to mucosal surfaces, *Rev Infect Dis* 9(suppl 5):S475, 1987.

4. Birek C, Grandhi R, McNeill K, et al: Detection of *Helicobacter pylori* in oral aphthous ulcers, *J Oral Pathol Med* 28:197, 1999.

5. Brady LJ, Walker C, Oxford GE, et al: Oral diseases, mycology and periodontal microbiology of HIV-infected women, *Oral Microbiol Immunol* 11:371, 1996.

6. Brook I: *Prevotella* and *Porphyromonas* infections in children, *J Med Microbiol* 42:340, 1995.

7. Broughton RA, Baker CJ: Role of adherence in the pathogenesis of neonatal group B streptococcal infection, *Infect Immun* 39:837, 1983.

8. Bruckner DA, Colonna P, Bearson BL: Nomenclature for aerobic and facultative bacteria, *Clin Infect Dis* 29:713, 1999.

9. Butt HL, Dunstan RH, McGregor NR, et al: An association of membrane-damaging toxins from coagulase-negative staphylococci and chronic orofacial muscle pain, *J Med Microbiol* 47:577, 1998.

10. Casadeval A, Pirofski L-A: Host-pathogen interactions: redefining the basic concepts of virulence and pathogenicity, *Infect Immun* 67:3703, 1999.

11. Caulfield PW, Dasanayake AP, Li Y., et al: Natural history of *Streptococcus sanguinis* in the oral cavity of infants: evidence for a discrete window of infectivity, *Infect Immun* 68:4018, 2000.

12. Chattin BR, Ishihara K, Okuda K, et al: Specific microbial colonizations in the periodontal sites of HIV-infected subjects, *Microbiol Immunol* 43:847, 1999.

13. Chen CKC, Wilson ME: *Eikenella corrodens* in human oral and non-oral infections: a review, *J Periodontol* 63:941, 1992.

14. Cole MF, Bryan S, Evans MK, et al: Humoral immunity to commensal oral bacteria in human infants: salivary secretory immunoglobulin A antibodies reactive with *Streptococcus mitis* biovar 1, *Streptococcus oralis, Streptococcus mutans*, and *Enterococcus faecalis* during the first two years of life, *Infect Immun* 67:1878, 1999.

15. Contreras A, Slots J: Active cytomegalovirus infection in human periodontitis, *Oral Microbiol Immunol* 13:225, 1998.

16. Crowley PJ, Fischlschweiger W, Coleman SE, et al: Intergeneric bacterial coaggregations involving mutans streptococci and oral actinomyces, *Infect Immun* 55:2695, 1987.

17. Cutler CW, Shinedling EA, Nunn M, et al: Association between periodontitis and hyperlipidemia: cause or effect? *J Periodontol* 70:1429, 1999.

18. Danser MM, van Winklehoff AJ, van der Velden U: Periodontal bacteria colonizing oral mucous membranes in edentulous patients wearing dental implants, *J Periodontol* 68:209, 1997.

19. Darmstadt GL, Mentele L, Podbielski A, et al: Role of group A streptococcal virulence factors in adherence to keratinocytes, *Infect Immun* 68:1215, 2000.

20. Debelian GJ, Olsen I, Tronstad L: Distinction of *Prevotella intermedia* and *Prevotella nigrescens* from endodontic bacteremia through their fatty acid contents, *Anaerobe* 3:61, 1997.

21. Deshpande RG, Khan MB, Genco CA: Invasion of aortic and heart endothelial cells by *Porphyromonas gingivalis, Infect Immun* 66:5337, 1998.

22. Dewhirst FE, Tamer MA, Ericson RE, et al: The diversity of periodontal spirochetes by 16S rRNA analysis, *Oral Microbiol Immunol* 15:196, 2000.

23. Ebersole JL, Capelli D, Mott G, et al: Systemic manifestations of periodontitis in the non-human primate, *J Periodontal Res* 34:358, 1999.

24. Fenno CJ, McBride BC: Virulence factors of oral treponemes, *Anaerobe* 4:1, 1998.

25. Fidel PE, Vazquez JA, Sobel JD: *Candida glabrata*: review of epidemiology, pathogenesis, and clinical disease with comparison to *C. albicans, Clin Microbiol Rev* 12:80, 1999.

26. Ganguly R, Stablein J, Lockey RF, et al: Defective antimicrobial functions of oral secretions in the elderly, *J Infect Dis* 153:163, 1986.

27. Goldstein EJC: Clinical anaerobic infections, *Anaerobe* 5:347, 1999.

28. Gomes B, Drucker DD, Lilley JD: Endodontic microflora of different teeth in the same mouth, *Anaerobe* 5:241, 1999.

29. Grau O, Slizewicz B, Tuppin P, et al: Association of *Mycoplasma penetrans* with human immunodeficiency virus infection, *J Infect Dis* 172:672, 1995.

30. Gutierrez de Ferro MI, Ruiz de Valladares, RE, Benito de Cardenas IL: Physiological aspects and conservation of a *Veillonella* strain isolated from the oral cavity: interaction with streptococci, *Anaerobe* 5:255, 1999.

31. Hamada S, Fujiwara T, Morishima S, et al: Molecular and immunological characterization of the fimbriae of *Porphyromonas gingivalis, Microbiol Immunol* 38:921, 1994.

32. Hamada S, Amamo A, Kimura S, et al: The importance of fimbriae in the virulence and ecology of some oral bacteria, *Oral Microbiol Immunol* 13:129, 1998.

33. Hannula JJ, Saarela M, Jousimies-Somer H, et al: Age-related acquisition of oral and nasopharyngeal yeast species and stability of colonization in young children, *Oral Microbiol Immunol* 14:176, 1999.

34. Hannula J, Saarela M, Dogan B, et al: Comparison of virulence factors of oral *Candida dubliniensis* and *Candida albicans* in healthy people and patients with chronic candidosis, *Oral Microbiol Immunol* 15:238, 2000.

35. Hashioka K, Yamasaki M, Nakane A, et al: The relationship between clinical symptoms and anaerobic bacteria from infected root canals, *J Endodont* 18:558, 1992.

36. Herzberg MC, Meyer MW: Effects of oral flora on platelets: possible consequences in cardiovascular disease, *J Periodontol* 67:1138, 1996.

37. Jousimies-Somer H, Summanen P: Microbiology terminology update: clinically significant anaerobic gram-positive and gram-negative bacteria (excluding spirochetes), *Clin Infect Dis* 29:724, 1999.

38. Jousimies-Somer HR, Bryk A, Asikainen S, et al: Oral colonization of infants with *Veillonella* species, *Anaerobe* 5:251, 1999.

39. Kamma JJ, Diamanti-Kapioti A, Nakou M, et al: Profile of subgingival microbiota in children with primary dentition, *J Periodontal Res* 35:33, 2000.

40. Kamma JJ, Diamanti-Kipioti A, Nakou M, et al: Profile of subgingival microbiota in children with mixed dentition, *Oral Microbiol Immunol* 15:103, 2000.

41. Kantu S, Har-El G: Cervical necrotizing fasciitis, *Ann Otol Rhinol Laryngol* 106:965, 1997.

42. Kleinegger CL, Lockhart SR, Vargas K: Frequency, intensity, species, and strains of oral *Candida* vary as a function of host age, *J Clin Microbiol* 34:2246, 1996.

43. Kolenbrander PE, Anderson RA: Multigeneric aggregations among oral bacteria: a network of independent cell-to-cell interactions, *J Bacteriol* 168:851, 1986.

44. Kononen E, Asikainen S, Kononen M, et al: Are certain oral pathogens part of normal oral flora in denture-wearing edentulous subjects? *Oral Microbiol Immunol* 6:119, 1991.

45. Kononen E, Kanervo A, Takala A, et al: Establishment of oral anaerobes during the first year of life, *J Dent Res* 78:1634, 1999.

46. Kornman KS, Loesche WJ: The subgingival microbial flora during pregnancy, *J Periodontal Res* 15: 111, 1980.

47. Kroes I, Lepp PW, Relman DA: Bacterial diversity within the human subgingival crevice, *Proc Natl Acad Sci U S A* 96:14547, 1999.

48. Madinier IM, Fosse TM, Monteil RA: Oral carriage of *Helicobacter pylori:* a review, *J Periodontol* 68:2, 1997.

49. Meyer DH, Fives-Taylor PM: Oral pathogens: from dental plaque to cardiac disease, *Curr Opin Microbiol* 1:88, 1998.

50. Meyer TF: Pathogenic neisseriae: complexity of pathogen-host cell interplay, *Clin Infect Dis* 28:433, 1999.

51. Moreno M, Romero P, Nieves B, et al: Microbiological characteristics of adult periodontitis associated with anaerobic bacteria, *Anaerobe* 5:261, 1999.

52. Munro CL, Macrina FL: Sucrose-derived exopolysaccharides of *Streptococcus mutans* V403 contribute to infectivity in endocarditis, *Mol Microbiol* 8:133, 1993.

53. Nakou M, Kamma J, Garganglianos P, et al: Periodontal microflora of HIV infected patients with periodontitis, *Anaerobe* 3:97, 1997.

54. Phelan JA: Oral manifestations of human immunodeficiency virus infection, *Med Clin North Am* 81:511, 1997.

55. Progulske-Fox A, Kazarov E, Dorn B, et al: *Porphyromonas gingivalis* virulence factors and invasion of the cardiovascular system, *J Periodontal Res* 34:393, 1999.

56. Roques CG, El kaddouri S, Barthet P, et al: *Fusobacterium nucleatum* involvement in adult periodontitis and possible modification of strain classification, *J Periodontol* 71:1144, 2000.

57. Sandin RL, Rogers AL, Fernandez MI, et al: Variations in affinity to *Candida albicans* in vitro among human buccal epithelial cells, *J Med Microbiol* 24:151, 1987.

58. Sawada S, Kokeguchi S, Nishimura F, et al: Phylogenetic characterization of *Centipeda periodontii, Selenomonas sputigena,* and *Selenomonas* species by 16S rRNA gene sequence analysis, *Microbios* 98:133, 1999.

59. Scannapieco FA, Genco RJ: Association of periodontal infections with atherosclerotic and pulmonary diseases, *J Periodontal Res* 34:340, 1999.

60. Shenep JL: Viridans-group streptococcal infections in immunocompromised hosts, *Int J Antimicrob Agents* 14:129, 2000.

61. Siqueira JF, Magalhaes FAC, Lima KC, et al: Pathogenicity of facultative and obligate anaerobic bacteria in monoculture and combined with either *Prevotella intermedia* or *Prevotella nigrescens, Oral Microbiol Immunol* 13:368, 1998.

62. Stevens DL: The flesh-eating bacterium: what's next? *J Infect Dis* 179(suppl 2):S366, 1999.

63. Tanner A, Maiden MF, Macuch PJ, et al: Microbiota of health, gingivitis, and initial periodontitis, *J Clin Periodontol* 25:85, 1998.

64. Tanner ACR, Taubman MA: Microbiota of initial periodontitis in adults, *Anaerobe* 5:229, 1999.

65. Umemoto T, Yoshimura F, Kureshiro H, et al: Fimbria-mediated co-aggregation between human oral anaerobes *Treponema medium* and *Porphyromonas gingivalis, Microbiol Immunol* 43:837, 1999.

66. Van der Weijden GA, Van der Velden U: Fluctuations of the microbiota of the tongue in humans, *J Clin Periodontol* 18:286, 1991.

67. Whiley RA, Beighton D: Current classification of the oral streptococci, *Oral Microbiol Immunol* 13:195, 1998.

68. Xia T, Bumgartner JC, David LL: Isolation and identification of *Prevotella tannerae* from endodontic infections, *Oral Microbiol Immunol* 15:273, 2000.

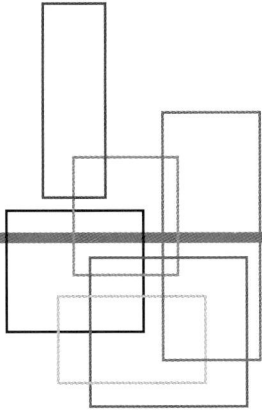

Laboratory Microbiological Diagnostic Techniques

Yvette S. McCarter

The isolation, identification, and susceptibility testing of microorganisms associated with infection are important components in determination of the diagnosis and appropriate therapy for many infectious diseases. This testing usually is accomplished by microscopic examination and culture of specimens representative of the site of infection. The infectious diseases associated with the oral and maxillofacial region have unique microbiological features because of the abundance and variety of microorganisms in this region. Culture detection of a specific organism or the determination of an organism's significance from culture often is complicated. The normal flora of the oral cavity consists of up to 10^{11} bacteria per gram of tissue, with anaerobic bacteria composing the majority of the flora present.[40] In some individuals this represents more than 300 species of bacteria.[19] Because of the large numbers of flora, the risk of specimen contamination with bacteria unrelated to infection is increased. Thus the careful collection of appropriate specimens is extremely important in the accurate diagnosis of infections from this region.

In general, the role of the microbiology laboratory is to aid the clinician in the diagnosis of infectious diseases. Although cultures may require several days to several weeks for completion depending on the organism, the results of rapid tests such as the Gram stain and noncultural methods are available to guide the initiation of therapy. The performance of susceptibility testing, when appropriate, also provides guidelines for the judicious use of antimicrobial agents. Reliance on microbiological techniques will likely increase because of the emergence of new pathogens, reemergence of old pathogens, and substantial increase in antimicrobial resistance. For clinicians to make optimal use of the microbiology laboratory, an understanding of the contemporary principles and practices of microbiology diagnostic techniques is critical. This chapter provides information regarding appropriate specimen collection and transportation, direct methods of specimen examination, and methods used for organism isolation, identification, and antimicrobial susceptibility testing. Exposure to these microbiological techniques allows the clinician to maximize the information gained by laboratory examination.

SPECIMEN ACQUISITION AND TRANSPORT

The results obtained from microbiological examination and culture depend on the care observed in specimen collection.[44] Because the optimal site and time of collection have an important influence on the usefulness of microbiology results, specimens should always be collected from a site representative of infection.[4] Improper collection techniques or collection from an inappropriate site results in a specimen of little clinical value and may produce misleading results (Box 3-1). Collection of a quality specimen from the oral or maxillofacial region is often a challenge because of the presence of indigenous oral flora and/or cutaneous flora. Therefore adherence to appropriate specimen collection guidelines is of the utmost importance.

Although the collection of an appropriate specimen is the first step in the achievement of quality, clinically relevant microbiological results, proper collection should be followed by appropriate transportation to the laboratory. All specimens for microbiological examination and culture should be transported to the laboratory promptly because they are subject to deterioration and overgrowth during transit. Extremes of temperature, delay, dehydration, and the presence of nutrients in body fluids result in the death of more fastidious organisms and overgrowth of rapidly growing but less important organisms, thus producing misleading reports. The optimum time for specimen transport to the laboratory is less than 2 hours.[27,28] This transport time may be possible in a hospital setting, but longer transport times almost always occur when specimens are collected in the office setting and transported to a distant laboratory site. Thus appropriate transport devices specific

General Guidelines for Specimen Collection

1. When possible, collect specimen before administration of antimicrobial therapy.
2. Minimize contamination of the specimen with indigenous flora so that specimen is representative of the site of infection.
3. Collect an appropriate amount of specimen for the test or tests required. This will minimize false-negative results.
4. Use appropriate collection devices.
5. Submit specimens submitted in sturdy, sterile leakproof containers to minimize the potential safety hazards. Use containers that promote survival of suspected organisms.
6. Label the specimen container with the patient's name, identification number (if appropriate), specific source, and date and time of collection.
7. Identify the specimen source as specifically as possible to ensure proper processing by the microbiology laboratory.
8. Submit specimens in a protective plastic bag in accordance with universal precautions.

Data from Miller JM, Holmes HT: Specimen collection transport, and storage. In Murray PR, Baron EJ, Pfaller MA, et al, editors: *Manual of clinical microbiology,* ed 7, Washington, 1999, American Society for Microbiology Press; National Committee for Clinical Laboratory Standards: *Protection of laboratory workers from infectious disease transmitted by blood, body fluids and tissue;* approved standard M29-A2, Wayne, Pa, 1991, The Committee; and Shea YR: Specimen collection and transport. In Isenberg HD, editor: *Clinical microbiology procedures handbook,* Washington, 1992, American Society for Microbiology Press.

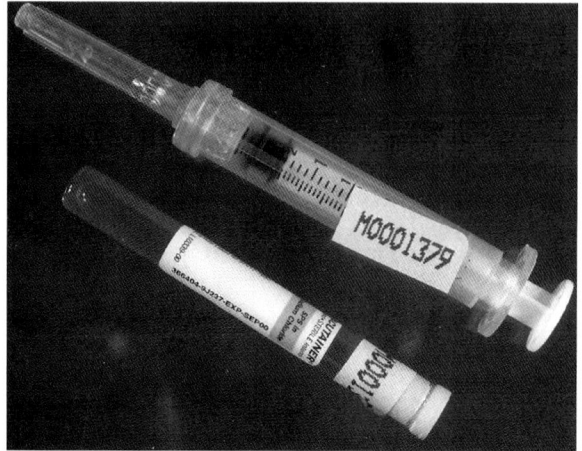

Figure 3-1 Material may be aspirated into a syringe but should be transferred into a sterile, appropriately labeled transport tube containing sodium polyanethol sulfonate anticoagulant before transport. Submission in a syringe may result in leakage and unnecessary potential for needle stick exposures.

for the test and organism suspected should be used. Specimens should also be held and transported at a temperature optimum for organism recovery. Specimens for viral or *Chlamydia* culture should be transported refrigerated or on ice; all others should be transported at room temperature.

ASPIRATES

The collection of oral and maxillofacial specimens by aspiration is useful because of the potential to minimize or prevent contamination with indigenous oral flora. The aspiration of material is always preferable to collection with a swab because swabs collect a relatively small amount of specimen, are readily contaminated, and needlessly subject the specimen to an oxygen-containing environment. Aspiration provides the most reliable information of the organisms associated with maxillary sinusitis, and aspiration of tissues such as lymph nodes provides optimal specimens to establish a specific cause of infection.[5,38]

Optimally, collection of aspirate specimens in head and neck infections should use an extraoral approach to eliminate contamination with oral flora.[40] The site should be cleansed with germicidal soap, alcohol, povidone-iodine,

or a combination of these cleansers to remove cutaneous flora. If an intraoral approach must be used, preparation of the site with a compound such as chlorhexidine minimizes contamination with oral flora. The injection of local anesthetics into the infected site should be avoided whenever possible because of the inhibitory effect of anesthetic agents on bacteria.[22]

Specimen collection is accomplished using a needle and syringe. Depending on the sampling area (tissue vs. abscess), injection of a small amount (0.5 to 1 mL) of nonbacteriostatic, sterile saline solution into the site and respiration may be necessary. Collection of specimens from fistulas and sinus tracts is performed after careful superficial cleaning of the stoma and introduction of a plastic catheter deep enough to obtain a representative specimen. Although this method was advocated in the past, needles should not be recapped or placed in a rubber stopper before specimen submission because this process provides an unnecessary opportunity for needle stick exposures. In addition, if a small amount of specimen is present, especially in the needle, it may be subject to drying and unnecessary exposure to oxygen, resulting in loss of viability or misleading culture results (Figure 3-1). Aspirate specimens should be transferred to a sterile tube, preferably a tube containing sodium polyanethol sulfonate (SPS) anticoagulant or an anaerobic transport vial before transport to the laboratory. Anticoagulants other than SPS should not be used because of their inhibitory effect on bacteria. If a small amount of specimen is obtained, a small amount of nonbacteriostatic saline solution or broth should be drawn into the syringe with the contents then expelled into an appropriate transport tube.

TISSUE AND BONE

Tissue is the optimal specimen for microbiological examination and culture providing it is collected such that nor-

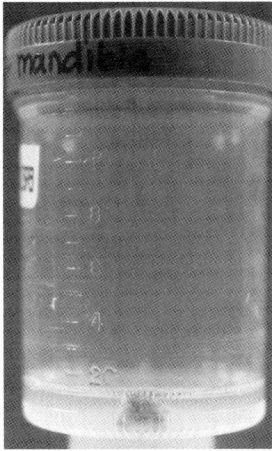

Figure 3-2 Optimally, tissue should be placed in a sterile screw-top cup for transport to the laboratory. A small amount of saline solution is added to prevent desiccation. The container should be labeled with the type of specimen and a patient identifier.

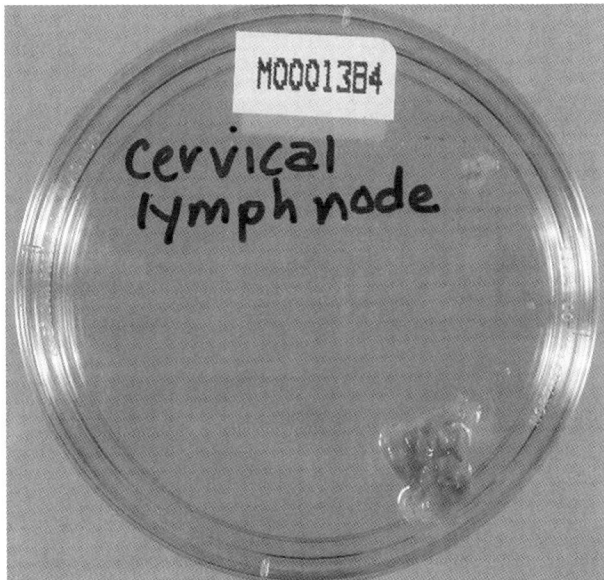

Figure 3-3 Tissue received in a sterile Petri dish is also optimal for microbiological examination. A small amount of saline solution is added to prevent desiccation. This method is used frequently for specimens that are hand carried to the laboratory.

mal flora is minimized or eliminated. Most tissue and bone specimens are collected aseptically during surgical procedures. These specimens should be submitted for both microbiological and histological examination. However, specimens for microbiological examination should not be submitted in formalin. Tissue specimens should be submitted to the microbiology laboratory in a sterile, screw-topped container or Petri dish with a small amount of nonbacteriostatic saline solution to prevent desiccation (Figures 3-2 and 3-3). Although advocated by some, the use of saline solution–moistened gauze is not advisable because the specimen may become lost in the fibers. Speci-

mens should not be submitted in an open container because of the likelihood of desiccation and contamination during transport. The use of an anaerobic transport medium is not required because tissue provides its own reduced conditions for protection of anaerobic organisms during transport. Transport time of these specimens should not exceed 15 minutes.[18,28]

Although surgical biopsy is the standard for tissue diagnosis, recent reports have promoted the use of fine-needle aspiration biopsy as an adjunct to open excision. Fine-needle aspiration offers advantages over surgical biopsy in terms of cost, convenience, lack of complications, and rapidity with which preliminary results can be obtained.[10,43] Fine-needle aspiration has proved useful in obtaining adequate microbiological samples for the diagnosis of soft tissue infections, infected surgical wounds, and chronic osteomyelitis caused by bacteria, fungi, mycobacteria, and viruses.[15,22]

SUPERFICIAL SITES

The use of swabs is the least desirable method of collecting and transporting material. Cells, bacteria, and especially fungal hyphae are trapped among the fibers and may not be recoverable for direct examination or culture. The use of swabs to collect specimens from sites that contain large amounts of indigenous flora is of no clinical value. This includes the use of nasal, pharyngeal, and nasopharyngeal cultures in lieu of an aspirate to establish the cause of maxillary sinusitis.[11,52] Swab specimens are also less satisfactory for the recovery of anaerobic organisms because swabs collect a small sample, are easily contaminated, and subject anaerobes to undue oxygen exposure.[3] In some instances, the collection of specimens using swabs may be necessary. In this case the site should be adequately cleansed and a specimen should be obtained from deep within the lesion, minimizing and preferably avoiding contact with indigenous flora. Swab specimens have been useful in the diagnosis of pharyngitis caused by *Streptococcus pyogenes*, *Corynebacterium diphtheriae*, and *Neisseria gonorrhoeae*. In addition, swabs may be used for the collection of oral specimens for the diagnosis of *Candida* and herpes simplex virus infection.

The appropriate swab should be chosen for specimen collection. Cotton swabs and swabs with wooden shafts should not be used because of the presence of antibacterial fatty acids and antiviral properties. The use of Dacron and rayon swabs with plastic or wire shafts is preferred. Calcium alginate swabs may be used to collect specimens for *Chlamydia* culture. Dry swabs are unacceptable for microbiological examination. Swabs should always be submitted in a transport medium that provides an environment for organism survival with minimal organism multiplication or death (Figure 3-4). Most transport devices contain liquid or semisolid Stuarts or Amies medium. Historically, a specialized anaerobic transport medium has been encouraged for swab specimens from the oral and maxillofacial region; however, swab transport devices containing semisolid

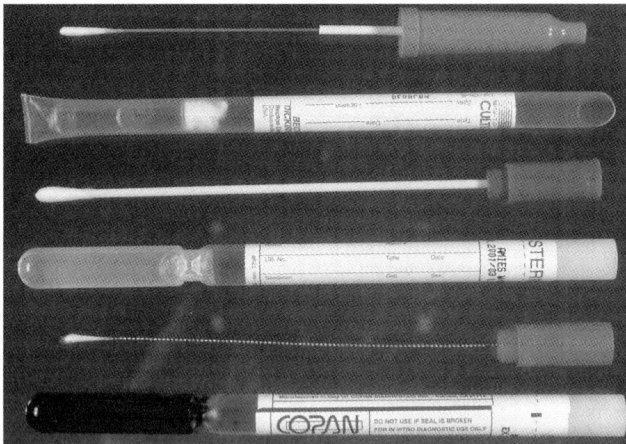

Figure 3-4 Commercially prepared swab transport kits. The top kit provides a small, tipped swab on a rigid wire shaft and a transport sleeve containing liquid transport medium. After placement of the swab into the transport sleeve, the liquid-containing ampule must be crushed to saturate the swab. The middle kit provides a plastic-shafted Dacron swab and a transport sleeve containing semisolid medium. Note the pinching of the sleeve above the medium, which promotes an atmosphere favorable for the preservation of anaerobic bacteria. The bottom kit provides a small, tipped swab on a flexible wire shaft and a transport sleeve containing semisolid medium with charcoal. This collection is often is used to obtain nasopharyngeal specimens for *B. pertussis.*

medium are of equivalent use for the preservation of anaerobes.[8] Commercially available transport media for viruses, *Chlamydia,* and *Mycoplasma* also are available. As with other specimens for microbiological examination, swab specimens should be transported to the laboratory as quickly as possible, preferably within 2 hours of collection.

COLLECTION OF SPECIMENS FOR OTHER DIAGNOSTIC TESTS AND CULTURES

The diagnostic evaluation of patients with oral and facial infections may include the collection of blood specimens for serum chemistry studies, complete blood cell counts, and urine samples for urinalysis as appropriate.[18] The presence of abnormal serum chemistry findings and leukocytosis often provides useful information regarding the presence of acute or chronic infection. In addition to the collection of specimens for nonmicrobiological analysis, the collection of blood for cultures is indicated in all serious infections of the head and neck when clinical sepsis is present. Blood cultures are also useful in the determination of the causative agent or agents of osteomyelitis and can provide a bacteriological diagnosis of infection in the oral and facial region in cases in which a diagnosis might not have been possible otherwise or specimens collected from these infections demonstrate a mixture of organisms.[24]

As with the collection of other specimens for microbiological examination, the appropriate collection of blood for culture is paramount for the production of clinically useful results. Cultures are easily contaminated during collection by organisms present on the skin. Thus proper skin preparation is essential, preferably with a bactericidal agent such as povidone-iodine, and alcohol before specimen collection. Other factors such as the volume of blood cultured and the number and timing of cultures also affect blood culture yield. The volume of blood obtained per culture sampling is the most important factor in organism recovery because the concentration of organisms in most cases of bacteremia, especially in adults, is low. The magnitude of bacteremia in children is often higher than in adults; therefore the collection of smaller volumes is acceptable. The recommended volume of blood for culture is 10 to 30 mL per venipuncture in adults and 1 to 5 mL per venipuncture in children. Studies have shown that two or three blood cultures, with appropriate amounts of blood, are sufficient for detection of almost all bacteremic episodes.[12] The collection of a single sample for blood culture should be avoided because a single collection may miss an intermittent bacteremia and the interpretation of the clinical significance of some organisms such as coagulase-negative staphylococci, viridans streptococci, and *Corynebacterium* spp. isolated from a single blood culture can be problematic. The dissemination of organisms into the blood actually occurs before the presence of chills or fever. Therefore, blood ideally should be collected in the hour before the chill or fever spike. Because this is not realistic and because bacteria are rapidly cleared from the blood, blood should be collected as quickly as possible after the chill or fever spike. Because specimens should be collected before the start of antimicrobial therapy, the separation of venipunctures by an arbitrary time is not recommended. The simultaneous collection of two or three 20- to 30-mL specimens by separate venipuncture should be performed.[12] Blood may be collected by syringe with immediate transfer into culture medium or a transfer set that allows direct inoculation of the blood culture bottles. The collection of specimens involving an intermediate collection tube containing SPS is discouraged. The increased final concentration of SPS in the blood culture medium is inhibitory to certain organisms, and the additional step of transfer of blood from the intermediate collection tube to the blood culture bottle provides additional opportunity for culture contamination and exposure to bloodborne pathogens.

Blood culture systems have improved significantly since the modern two-bottle system was first described in 1951. Blood culture bottles contain a defined amount of an appropriate nutrient broth medium to promote the growth of aerobic, facultatively anaerobic, and anaerobic organisms. When an appropriate volume of blood is added to the broth medium, a 1:5 to 1:10 blood/broth ratio is achieved. This dilution minimizes the effects of microbial inhibitors present in blood and dilutes any antimicrobial agents to subinhibitory levels. The presence of the recommended concentration of SPS in the blood culture bottles inhibits serum bactericidal activity and phagocytosis and inactivates complement. The use of commercial automated blood culture systems is preferred by most laboratories because of their ease of use and rapid detection of positive cultures. More recently developed continuous monitoring systems automatically detect organism growth by means of colorimetric, fluorometric, or pressure sensors and monitor the bottles for growth frequently (every 10 to 30 minutes). Cultures are incubated for 5 days; however, the majority of pathogens are isolated within the first 48 hours of incubation. This includes organisms of the HACEK group *(Haemophilus aphrophilus, Actinobacillus actinomycetemcomitans, Cardiobacterium hominis, Eikenella corrodens,* and *Kingella kingae)* that were previously considered causes of culture-negative endocarditis. The isolation of more fastidious organisms such as *Brucella* spp. may require an extended incubation time. After detection of a positive blood culture result, a Gram stain is performed and an aliquot of the culture medium is removed from the bottle and placed on the appropriate solid growth medium. The performance of Gram stains after negative blood culture results is not routine. The isolation of microorganisms from blood cultures should be interpreted in the context of other clinical findings. Organisms that may be considered contaminants such as coagulase-negative staphylococci, *Corynebacterium,* and *Propionibacterium* spp. may be significant in certain patient populations, especially those patients with indwelling prosthetic devices.

DIRECT METHODS OF SPECIMEN EXAMINATION

The initial step in the processing of most clinical material is microscopic examination of the specimen. Much information can be obtained from smear preparations. A Gram-stained direct smear provides the clinician with rapid information regarding the quality of the specimen and the bacterial morphotypes present. Similarly, fungal stains, wet preparations, and acid-fast stains provide rapid evidence of fungal and mycobacterial infection, respectively. The commercial availability of monoclonal antibody reagents allows the microbiology laboratory to offer rapid fluorescent antibody tests for the detection of bacteria such as *Legionella pneumophila* and *Bordetella pertussis* and viruses such as herpes simplex, varicella zoster, adenovirus, influenza, and parainfluenza. In addition to staining techniques, direct detection of microbial antigens or nucleic acids provides rapid evidence of the causative agents of disease and may be the most reliable detection method for microorganisms that do not grow well in culture.

STAINING METHODS

Gram Stain

Preparation and Staining   Care should be taken to prepare a smear that is representative of the specimen and not too thick (Box 3-2). Thick smears are often uninterpretable and material has a tendency to wash off the slide during staining.

BOX 3-2

Preparation and Staining of Gram-Stained Direct Smears

Preparation
1. Examine the material. Select portions of the specimen representative of exudate. Avoid saliva or saline solution (if used to prevent desiccation).
2. The material must be thin enough to produce a monolayer of organisms and cells. Emulsify thick specimens in saline solution before smear preparation.
3. Keep glass slides in an alcohol container or clean them with alcohol before use to obtain the best results.
4. Smear the specimen in a circular area in the center of the slide and allow to air dry.
   a. Roll swabs gently on the slide to prevent destruction of cellular material.
   b. Concentrate fluids by centrifugation before smear preparation. Place a drop of sediment on the slide.
   c. Gently touch tissue specimens to several areas of the slide.

Staining
1. Methanol-fix slides to minimize loss of material during the staining process.
2. Flood the slide with an alcoholic solution of crystal violet (Hucker's solution recommended for general use) for 5 to 10 seconds.
3. Rinse the slide briefly with tap water.
4. Flood the slide with Gram's iodine (a mixture of iodine and potassium iodide) for 5 to 10 seconds. This results in fixation of crystal violet to proteins in the bacterial cell wall.
5. Rinse the slide briefly with tap water.
6. Wash the slide briefly with a solution of equal parts of acetone and alcohol (vol/vol). This organic solvent removes the outer lipid layer from some bacteria.
7. Rinse the slide briefly with tap water.
8. Flood the slide with safranin counterstain for 5 to 10 seconds.
9. Rinse the slide with tap water and allow to dry. Use paper towels to blot slides dry if needed.

Methanol is the preferred method of specimen fixation before staining because heat fixation may distort the morphological appearance of cells and bacteria.[3] Proper performance of the Gram stain does not rely on the timing of the steps performed. Rather, the most common errors in Gram stain performance center on the decolorization step. The use of a 50% mixture of acetone and alcohol provides an optimal decolorizing solution. The use of acetone causes excessively rapid decolorization; similarly, alcohol alone provides inappropriately slow decolorization.

Examination and Interpretation   The preparation, examination, and staining of smears may be performed in the office setting and laboratory. Gram stains should only be performed by clinicians who are skilled in the technique and examine and interpret smears frequently enough to remain proficient. Clinicians who are inexperienced in smear interpretation should submit specimens to the laboratory so that another smear can be prepared and interpreted.

Examination of Gram-stained smears in the office or laboratory setting requires a suitable compound microscope with a good 10× and 100× objective. In addition, the illumination must be moderately dense for oil immersion use to permit adequate resolution of bacteria. The microscope should be kept clean and covered when not in use and should be serviced regularly. Before specimen examination, a drop of immersion oil is placed on the slide. The slide is then examined using the low-power (10×) objective to determine the relative numbers of squamous epithelial cells and neutrophils. An abundance of squamous cells in the absence of neutrophils suggests superficial material unrelated to infection (Plate 1). Bacteria observed in these specimens represent indigenous flora of the mouth or skin and are not related to infection (Plate 2). Specimens of this type should be re-collected avoiding sources of contamination. An abundance of neutrophils suggests an inflammatory exudate indicative of a site of infection (Plates 3 and 4). After the assessment of specimen quality, the 100× objective is used to assess the bacterial morphotypes present. The Gram stain differentiates bacteria based on their ability (gram-positive) or inability (gram-negative) to retain the crystal violet dye and their size and shape (rod shaped vs. cocci). Of the gram-positive organisms, micrococci, staphylococci, and streptococci appear as spherical gram-positive organisms (Box 3-3). Micrococci and staphylococci are often arranged in tetrads (groups of four) or appear as irregular grapelike clusters (Plate 5). Streptococci are often arranged in pairs or chains (Plate 6). *Streptococcus pneumoniae* displays a characteristic lancet-shaped cocci most often in pairs (Plate 7). Members of the genera *Bacillus* and *Clostridium* appear as large gram-positive rods often with squared-off ends (Plate 8). Although vacuoles may be present, spores are rarely seen in clinical specimens. Other gram-positive rods display morphological features varying from small and uniform to pleomorphic and branching (Plates 9 and 10).

Gram-negative cocci occur singly *(Veillonella)* or in pairs *(Neisseria, Moraxella, Acinetobacter)*. The gram-negative rods constitute a large number of pathogenic species but can be subdivided into four categories. The largest gram-negative rods are represented by the family Enterobacteriaceae. These enteric bacteria often display bipolar staining with intensification of safranin staining at the poles of the cell with a less intense staining in the center of the cell (Plate 11). Gram-negative rods with a thinner, more uniform staining appearance are often of the genus *Pseudomonas* or a related genera (Plate 12). Small, coccobacillary gram-negative rods represent *Bacteroides, Haemophilus,* and related genera (Plate 13). Long, filamentous and pleomorphic forms may be seen depending on the specimen type. The final group of Gram-negative rods are those that display curved or spiral-shaped morphological findings.

The Gram stain is particularly helpful in providing presumptive evidence of the presence of anaerobes because many anaerobic organisms display distinctive features on microscopic examination.[3] The presence of small, faint-staining gram-negative rods is often indicative of organisms such as *Bacteroides, Fusobacterium, Prevotella,* and *Porphyromonas.*

Long, thin gram-negative rods with pointed ends are suggestive of *Fusobacterium nucleatum,* and large box car–shaped gram-positive rods are suggestive of *Clostridium* from appropriate specimens. The characteristic pattern of fusiform bacteria and spirochetes in cases of Vincent's angina or gingivitis makes the Gram stain more diagnostic than culture in this situation (Plate 14).

Brown-Brenn Tissue Gram Stain   The Brown-Brenn Gram stain method is used exclusively on histological sections of tissue to demonstrate the same gram-positive and gram-negative characteristics shown with the Gram method. The identification of gram-negative organisms is often difficult in these preparations because of their confusion with tissue artifacts.

Fungal Stains   All specimens of sufficient quantity should be examined microscopically if fungi are suspected. Fungal elements including yeast, pseudohyphae, and true hyphae may be visualized using a 10% potassium hydroxide preparation or any of the following stains: calcofluor white, periodic acid–Schiff (PAS), and methenamine silver. Calcofluor white, a fluorescent brightener used in the textile industry, binds to cellulose and chitin in fungal cell walls and fluoresces when exposed to ultraviolet light. Calcofluor is a nonspecific stain and relies on the microscopist's expertise to identify fungal morphological features. PAS stain is used by both microbiologists and pathologists to demonstrate fungi in clinical specimens and histological sections. In addition to staining the carbohydrate component of the fungal cell wall, PAS stains mucins, glycogen, basement membrane, and fibrin.[9] Therefore PAS-positive structures must display fungal morphological characteristics (Plate 15). The use of methenamine silver stain is reserved primarily for histological specimens. This stain produces an intense black staining of the cell walls of fungi (Plate 16).

Acid-Fast Stains   Acid-fast smears play an important role in the early diagnosis of mycobacterial infection because of the relatively slow growth rate of mycobacteria in culture. Acid-fast organisms are difficult to stain because of the high lipid content of their cell walls. Acid-fast stains take advantage of mycobacteria's retention of basic fuchsin dyes or fluorochrome stains after decolorization with an acid-alcohol solution.

The Ziehl-Neelsen and Kinyoun carbol-fuschin methods and the fluorochrome dyes, rhodamine and auramine, are used to demonstrate mycobacteria in clinical specimens and histological sections. The stains use phenol to allow penetration of the primary stain. The older Ziehl-Neelsen method requires heat because of the lower concentration of phenol present in the stain. The Kinyoun modification uses a higher concentration of both carbol-fuschin and

BOX 3-3

Categories of Bacterial Identification Based on Gram Stain Reaction and Morphology

Positive	Negative	Positive	Negative
Cocci	**Cocci**	*Propionibacterium*	*Curved or spiral*
Singly or in clumps	*Spherical or kidney bean–shaped*	*Rothia*	*Arcobacter*
Aerococcus	Acidaminococcus	*Tsukamurella*	*Campylobacter*
Alloiococcus	Megasphaera	*Turicella*	*Helicobacter*
Gemella	Veillonella	**Branching**	*Pectobacterium*
Helcococcus	**Pairs**	*Actinomadura*	*Vibrio*
Micrococcus	Acinetobacter	*Actinomyces*	*Nonspecific morphology*
Pediococcus	Moraxella	*Nocardia*	*Actinobacillus*
Peptostreptococcus	Neisseria	*Nocardiopsis*	*Aeromonas*
Staphylococcus		*Streptomyces*	*Anaerobiospirillum*
Stomatococcus	**Rods**		*Anaerorhabdus*
Pairs and chains	*Large, possible display of bipolar*		*Bilophila*
Abiotrophia	*staining*		*Capnocytophaga*
Enterococcus	Enterobacteriaceae		*Cardiobacterium*
Globicatella	*Thin, uniform*		*Catonella*
Lactococcus	Alcaligenes		*Centipeda*
Peptostreptococcus	Burkholderia		*Chromobacterium*
Streptococcus	Legionella		*Chryseobacterium*
	Pseudomonas		*Chryseomonas*
Rods	Stenotrophomonas		*Desulfomonas*
Large, uniform size	*Coccobacillary*		*Desulfovibrio*
Bacillus	Bacteroides		*Dialister*
Clostridium	Bartonella		*Dichelobacter*
Small, uniform size	Bordetella		*Empedobacter*
Erysipelothrix	Brucella		*Fibrobacter*
Eubacterium	Eikenella		*Flavimonas*
Kurthia	Francisella		*Johnsonella*
Lactobacillus	Haemophilus		*Leptotrichia*
Listeria	Kingella		*Megamonas*
Rhodococcus	Pasteurella		*Methylobacterium*
Irregular, pleomorphic	Porphyromonas		*Mitsuokella*
Arcanobacterium	Prevotella		*Myroides*
Arthrobacter			*Plesiomonas*
Aureobacterium			*Rikenella*
Bifidobacterium			*Roseomonas*
Brevibacterium			*Ruminobacter*
Cellulomonas			*Sebaldella*
Corynebacterium			*Selenomonas*
Dermabacter			*Shewanella*
Dermatophilus			*Sphingobacterium*
Eubacterium			*Sphingomonas*
Gardnerella			*Tissierella*
Gordona			*Weeksella*
Microbacterium			
Oerskovia			

phenol and does not require heating. After decolorization with an acid alcohol solution, smears are counterstained to highlight stained organisms. Carbol-fuchsin–based stains usually are counterstained with methylene blue, whereas rhodamine-auramine–stained smears are counterstained with potassium permanganate. Acid-fast organisms stain red with carbol-fuchsin procedures (Plate 17) and acid-fast organisms fluoresce yellow to orange with fluorochrome procedures (Plate 18). The use of rhodamine-auramine stains for primary specimen smears is preferred over carbol-fuchsin methods because of its increased sensitivity.[48] Although organisms such as *Nocardia* display acid-fast properties, the acid-alcohol decolorizer used for staining of mycobacteria is inappropriate for the demonstration of acid fastness in *Nocardia*. Instead, a weak acid solution (usually 1% sulfuric acid) is used as the decolorizing agent. This "modified Kinyoun" method also stains other organisms with acid-fast properties such as *Rhodococcus, Tsukamurella,* and *Gordona.*

Wet Preparations and Dark-Field Microscopy   Wet preparations may be prepared from exudates, scrapings, fluids, and tissue. The addition of 10% potassium hydroxide to the specimen dissolves mucous and cellular material, thus facilitating visualization of fungal structures. After the addition of potassium hydroxide, the slide is held at room temperature for 5 to 30 minutes to allow digestion to occur. Fungi remain undamaged because of the presence of chitin in their cell walls. This method is particularly useful for identification of patients with mucocutaneous candidiasis (Plate 19). Examination of wet preparations demonstrates budding yeast, pseudohyphae, or both, which is suggestive of *Candida,* round budding yeast suggestive of *Cryptococcus,* or the presence of true hyphae. Broad aseptate hyphae are suggestive of a zygomycete, whereas septate hyphae with dichotomous branching may indicate the presence of *Aspergillus* spp. Finer-branching filaments suggest the presence of *Actinomyces* or *Nocardia* spp. The use of a stain such as calcofluor white enhances the recognition of fungal structures. In unstained preparations, fungal structures may be enhanced by the use of a phase-contrast microscope. Phase-contrast microscopy also may prove useful in the evaluation of oral samples for the relative number of bacterial morphotypes and organism motility.

Dark-field microscopy is a modification of the wet preparation in which the specimen is examined using a microscope with a dark-field condenser. This condenser improves the resolving power of the microscope by blocking light from the center of the condenser and allowing light to reach the object from the periphery of the objective. Thus organisms with very small diameters (0.1 to 0.15 μm) can be observed. Direct examination of specimens by dark-field microscopy is most frequently used for the detection of *Treponema pallidum* in suspected syphilitic lesions. Exudates from specimens collected from mucosal and skin lesions of primary, secondary, and early congenital syphilis are most useful because they tend to contain large numbers of treponemes. Lesions should be carefully cleaned with soap and water. The lesion should be abraded with dry gauze to express serosanguinous fluid from the base of the lesion. Gross bleeding should be prevented. The specimen is placed on a glass slide, a cover slip is added, and the specimen is examined immediately. The demonstration of tightly coiled spirochetes composed of 6 to 14 spirals ranging in length from 6 to 20 μm with characteristic "corkscrew" motility is suggestive of *T. pallidum.* Characteristic motility must be present, so specimens should be examined immediately. Extended transport times, which leads to drying or cooling of the slide, result in death and distortion of the organism. Because of the presence of saprophytic spirochetes in the oropharynx, the evaluation of potential syphilitic lesions in this region by dark-field microscopy is not recommended.

Fluorescent Antibody Stains   Immunofluorescence is the oldest and one of the most widely used techniques for the rapid detection of certain bacterial, fungal, parasitic, and viral pathogens from direct clinical specimens.[23,25,53] This test uses a fluorescent molecule, most commonly fluorescein isothiocyanate, conjugated to a monoclonal antibody that is directed against an organism or antigen. The formation of the resulting antibody and antigen complex is visualized by fluorescence microscopy. The advantage associated with use of immunofluorescence techniques is that both the quality of the specimen and the morphology or staining pattern of the organism or cell can be assessed. The disadvantage of the immunofluorescent assay is its subjectivity of interpretation. The use of immunofluorescence has proved useful in the direct detection of bacteria such as *L. pneumophila, B. pertussis, Rickettsia, T. pallidum,* and *Chlamydia trachomatis.* Parasites such as *Giardia lamblia* and *Cryptosporidium parvum* and fungi such as *Pneumocystis carinii* also are detectable using immunofluorescence.

Viral culture does not provide information rapidly enough to influence initial treatment. The use of immunofluorescence has greatly reduced the time required for diagnosis of many viral pathogens. Immunofluorescence may be used to demonstrate the presence of influenza viruses, parainfluenza viruses, adenovirus, and respiratory syncytial virus (RSV) from respiratory specimens, herpes simplex virus, varicella zoster virus in cutaneous and mucocutaneous lesions, and rabies virus in tissue (Plate 20). In the case of RSV infection, direct detection is superior to detection in culture. Recent advances in immunofluorescence include the development of bivalent and dichromatic reagents.[21] These reagents can detect more than one virus simultaneously in direct specimens. The continued development of improved monoclonal antibodies likely will increase the number of pathogens detectable with this method.

DIRECT DETECTION OF MICROBIAL ANTIGENS AND NUCLEIC ACIDS

Advances in immunological and molecular techniques have provided clinicians with a variety of assays to diagnose infectious diseases more rapidly and accurately. These assays also provide the ability to detect microorganisms that grow slowly in culture or not at all. These techniques include latex agglutination, immunoassays, deoxyribonucleic acid (DNA) probes, and most recently, nucleic acid amplification. Latex agglutination uses a stable colloid (polystyrene latex particles) coated with antibody specific for a microbial pathogen. When the clinical specimen is mixed with the suspension, antibody-coated latex particles bind to the antigen of interest, resulting in agglutination. This method has been used to detect common causes of bacterial meningitis including *Haemophilus influenzae* type b, *S. pneumoniae, Neisseria meningitidis,* and group B streptococcus. This test is most useful in cases of partially treated meningitis when cultures may be sterile. These tests do not detect other causes of meningitis such as *Listeria monocyto-*

genes, Citrobacter koseri, or organisms most frequently associated with shunt infections. Latex agglutination is also useful for the detection of cryptococcal antigen in patients with active nonmeningeal and meningeal cryptococcosis.

Other assays, including fluorescence, optical, and enzyme-linked immunoassays, are assuming an increasingly prominent role in the laboratory and the office practice setting. These tests use an antibody bound to a solid phase that captures the microbial antigen and a second antibody conjugated to an enzyme or a fluorescent substrate that is used to detect the presence of the antigen of interest. The most recent development of the optical immunoassay uses antibody bound to a molecular thin film (silicon wafer). After the addition of substrate, the presence of antigen is detected as a color change caused by increased thickness of the molecular thin film. Immunoassays have been widely used for the detection of group A streptococcus in throat specimens, RSV and influenza virus in respiratory specimens, and rotavirus and *Clostridium difficile* in stool specimens.

The birth of molecular biology and the availability of nucleic acid probes and nucleic acid amplification has significantly affected the ability of the laboratory to provide more rapid and accurate diagnosis of infectious diseases.[47] Nucleic acid probes use pieces of DNA or ribonucleic acid (RNA) that are labeled with a radioactive, a chemiluminescent, or an affinity tag. These probes bind to complementary nucleic acid sequences in the target organism. This reaction is very specific because the probes used are unique to a given organism. In addition, the molecular targets of the probes are often present in many copies, thus enhancing the detection of fewer organisms in clinical specimens. Nucleic acid probes are commercially available for the detection of *N. gonorrhoeae, Chlamydia trachomatis,* and human papilloma virus from genital specimens and group A streptococcus from throat specimens. Probes have been developed in the research setting for anaerobic organisms.[3] The development of commercial sources for these probes will enable the rapid detection of these important head and neck pathogens directly from patient specimens.

Several nucleic acid amplification strategies have been developed including polymerase chain reaction (PCR), ligase chain reaction, and the Q beta replicase system; PCR is the most widely used. With PCR a small amount of nucleic acid present in the target organism is amplified repeatedly. Each PCR cycle involves three basic steps: (1) denaturation of target DNA into single strands, (2) binding of single-stranded DNA primers to the single DNA strands near the target nucleic acid sequence, and (3) extension (replication) of the target genetic material. After each cycle the target sequence is doubled so that after 30 cycles of replication the target sequence has been amplified more than a million-fold. This amplification allows for the detection of the equivalent of close to a single virion or bacterium present in clinical samples. Few infectious agents exist for which PCR assays have not been described. Commercial PCR and ligase chain reaction assays are available for the direct detection of *Mycobacterium tuberculosis, N. gonorrhoeae, C. trachomatis,* human immunodeficiency virus (HIV), hepatitis C virus, hep-

atitis B virus, cytomegalovirus, enterovirus, and human T-cell lymphotrophic virus.[46] Many laboratories offer in-house–developed PCR assays for detection of a wide variety of microorganisms, including *Borrelia burgdorferi, Bartonella hensellae, Bordetella pertussis, Ehrlichia* spp., *Tropheryma whippelii, Mycobacterium genavense,* varicella zoster virus, herpes simplex virus, and JC polyoma virus. The availability of PCR assays to detect more microbial pathogens will only increase in the future. Amplification-based techniques also can produce quantitative results of the amount of microbe present. These results are of particular value in HIV and hepatitic C infection for monitoring of disease progression and response to therapy. Special attention should be used in the interpretation of molecular diagnostic results because they can detect nucleic acids in nonviable organisms. In addition, the presence of nucleic acid of a specific organism does not necessarily imply infection by that organism, especially in nonsterile specimens.

SPECIMEN PROCESSING, ISOLATION, AND IDENTIFICATION OF MICROORGANISMS

Although direct methods of examination provide rapid results of the presence or absence of microorganisms, the isolation and identification of viable organisms is still considered the "gold standard" for the diagnosis of most pathogens. Culturing offers the advantages of providing an exact organism identification, and the ability to perform antimicrobial susceptibility testing on the isolate. Although viruses and *Chlamydia* spp. require the use of living tissue cells for growth, the isolation of most organisms (bacteria, fungi, and mycobacteria) is accomplished using synthetic or semisynthetic media. Once the specimen reaches the laboratory, a determination is made regarding the need for specimen pretreatment. In general, fluid specimens, with the exception of urine, are concentrated by centrifugation before processing and tissue samples are homogenized to release organisms present. Homogenization should be performed carefully especially if fungi are suspected because fungal hyphae may be destroyed if homogenization is too intense.

BACTERIA

A combination of enriched, selective, and differential media is used for the isolation and presumptive identification of bacteria from clinical samples. The basic components of these media include digests of casein or plant and animal proteins and salts to provide an isotonic and buffered environment. Agar is added to solidify the media, or the media may be used in a liquid state. The addition of blood, carbohydrates, or other factors to the media enhances the growth of some bacteria (enriched media) and provides an environment in which the growth or metabolic characteristics of certain organisms can be differentiated from others (differential media). The addition of dyes and antibiotics to media provides inhibitory properties that permit the selective detection of certain pathogens (selective media). Enriched media such as sheep blood and chocolate agar provide the nutrients necessary to cultivate a wide variety of bacteria. The growth of more fastidious bacteria such as some *Neisseria* and *Haemophilus* spp. is enhanced by the free hemoglobin present in chocolate agar. Sheep blood agar also enables the distinction of the various types of hemolysis produced by streptococci. The omission of blood and addition of dyes or bile salts produce media inhibitory to gram-positive cocci. The addition of antibiotics such as colistin and nalidixic acid and kanamycin and vancomycin produces media that favor the growth of gram-positive and anaerobic gram-negative organisms, respectively. Differential media such as MacConkey and eosin–methylene blue agar are used extensively because of their ability to differentiate gram-negative rods based on carbohydrate fermentation. The use of selective and nonselective media increases the yield of cultures for both aerobic and anaerobic organisms and permits enhanced isolation and recognition of colonies.[14,27]

The selection of media used for primary isolation is based on the source of the specimen and types of organisms anticipated from the site. The results of direct microscopic examination may provide additional clues. For example, anaerobic organisms often display distinctive morphological characteristics on Gram staining. In this case, media should be added to enable the recovery of these organisms. After inoculation, the specimen is spread or "streaked" across the surface of the agar. This can be performed with a sterile inoculating loop or automated plater. As the inoculum passes over the agar, bacteria are deposited, and after incubation, each develops into a colony visible to the naked eye.

Most organisms grow best when they are incubated at 35° to 37° C. In addition, growth is enhanced in an atmosphere of increased humidity. Although many organisms grow in the presence of an ambient environment, the growth of other organisms requires specialized atmospheric conditions for growth. An enhanced CO_2 environment permits the growth of all aerobic organisms and stimulates the growth of certain bacteria such as *Haemophilus* and *Neisseria*. Some streptococci and bacteria such as *Campylobacter* grow preferentially in an atmosphere of reduced oxygen tension (no more than 6% O_2). These organisms are designated as microaerophilic. Culture for anaerobic bacteria is performed in an anaerobic environment (85% N_2, 10% H_2, 5% CO_2). This environment is essential because most obligately anaerobic bacteria lack the enzyme peroxidase. Peroxides are formed in the presence of oxygen. Thus without peroxidases these organisms are killed in the presence of oxygen. Anaerobic media contain reducing agents such as cysteine and should be prereduced before inoculation. If specimen inoculation cannot be performed in an anaerobic chamber or a glove box, specimens may be held in a holding system that is flushed free of oxygen by a nonoxygen gas (e.g., N_2) before placement in an anaerobic environment.

After incubation, the initial interpretation of growth on primary media by the microbiology laboratory provides the clinician with a preliminary identification of the clinically significant organisms present. Colonies present may be presumptively identified by gross colonial morphology, Gram stain morphology, and spot biochemical tests applied directly to the plate. Further identification of organisms to the genus and species level requires characterization of their biochemical and often immunological characteristics. Most laboratories use methods such as latex agglutination and rapid identification systems that rely on the detection of preformed enzymes, and growth in and utilization of a variety of substrates. These systems can provide identifications in as little as 10 minutes. In addition, the development of automated systems for identification has reduced the time necessary for the complete identification of both gram-positive and gram-negative organisms to as little as 4 hours in some cases. These include biochemical systems for the identification of aerobic organisms and systems that base identification on the determination of cellular fatty acid patterns.[14]

The identification of organisms in pure culture is relatively straightforward; however, the appropriate evaluation and identification of organisms in a mixed culture presents a greater challenge. The possibility that a culture contains bacteria representing indigenous or colonizing flora complicates evaluation. In most cases these organisms are reported as "normal flora" or "mixed flora" from that site (Box 3-4). Organism identification that exceeds diagnostic and therapeutic needs is of minimal clinical value.[4]

Historically, laboratories spent substantial time and resources identifying organisms of questionable significance in mixed cultures. The complete identification of more than three potential pathogens from a mixed culture usually is not clinically essential. An aid to the interpretation of mixed cultures is the correlation of the culture results with the bacteria observed in the direct specimen Gram stain. Organisms that were observed in the direct Gram stain and grow in culture are likely more relevant than those organisms that grow only in culture. Establishing an open line of communication between the clinician and the microbiology laboratory is imperative. Consultation with the clinical microbiologist regarding the results of direct smears and cultures provides the opportunity for dialogue with the clinician regarding the significance of organisms isolated and the need for complete identification and susceptibility testing.

MYCOBACTERIA

The recovery of mycobacteria from clinical specimens requires proper specimen processing. Because mycobacteria grow slowly (with a doubling time of up to 20 hours) and require lengthy periods of incubation, nonmycobacterial species may overgrow cultures from nonsterile sites. Thus specimens from nonsterile body sites are digested to free mycobacteria from mucus and cells, and decontaminated to reduce or eliminate contaminating bacteria. In addition,

BOX 3-4

Common Commensal Organisms of the Oral and Maxillofacial Region

Oropharynx	Nose (nares)
Actinomyces	Coagulase-negative
Bacteroides	*Staphylococcus*
Bifidobacterium	*Corynebacterium*
Candida	*Haemophilus influenzae*
Capnocytophaga	*Moraxella catarrhalis*
Clostridium	*Neisseria**
Coagulase-negative	*Propionibacterium*
Staphylococcus	*Streptococcus pneumoniae*
Corynebacterium	**Nasopharynx and**
Eikenella corrodens	**Sinuses**
Entamoeba gingivalis	Coagulase-negative
Enterobacteriaceae	*Staphylococcus*
Enterococcus	*Corynebacterium*
Eubacterium	Enterobacteriaceae
Fusobacterium	*Haemophilus influenzae*
Haemophilus	*Haemophilus parainfluenzae*
Lactobacillus	*Moraxella catarrhalis*
Micrococcus	*Neisseria**
Moraxella	*Streptococcus* spp.
Mycoplasma	(viridans group)
Neisseria	**Skin**
Nocardia	*Acinetobacter*
Oral spirochetes	*Aerococcus*
Peptostreptococcus	*Candida*
Porphyromonas	*Clostridium*
Prevotella	*Corynebacterium*
Propionibacterium	*Micrococcus*
S. aureus	Nonpathogenic *Neissera* spp.
Streptococcus anginosus group†	*Peptostreptococcus*
Streptococcus mitis group‡	*Propionibacterium*
Streptococcus mutans group§	*Staphylococcus*
S. pneumoniae	*Streptococcus* (viridans group)
Streptococcus salivarius	
Streptococcus vestibularis	
Stomatococcus	
Trichomonas tenax	
Veillonella	

*Neisseria spp. other than *N. gonorrhoeae.*
†Anginosus group: *Streptococcus anginosus, S. constellatus,* and *S. intermedius.*
‡Mitis group: *S. mitis, S. sanguis, S. parasanguis, S. gordonii, S. crista,* and *S. oralis.*
§Mutans group: *S. mutans, S. sobrinus, S. cricetus, S. rattus, S. downei,* and *S. macacae.*

all specimens also should be concentrated by centrifugation to maximize the yield of mycobacteria. The presence of a high lipid content in the cell wall of mycobacteria necessitates the use of specialized media for recovery of these organisms. Media used include egg-based and agar-based solid media and liquid media culture systems. Antimicrobial agents may be added to the media to inhibit the growth of contaminating bacteria, and supplements such as hemin may be added to support the growth of more fastidious mycobacteria. Although egg-based media support the growth of most mycobacteria, agar-based media often are preferred because of the ease with which early growth can be detected. The necessity for the rapid detection of mycobacteria, especially *M. tuberculosis,* has led to the recommendation by the Centers for Disease Control and Prevention that broth-based automated culture systems be used for the primary isolation of mycobacteria.[6] The use of these liquid-based systems has decreased the time to detection of mycobacteria from 6 to 8 weeks to as little as 7 to 14 days depending on the amount of organism present in the specimen. The medium is incubated at 35° to 37° C for 6 to 8 weeks to ensure optimal recovery of mycobacteria. The incubation of solid medium occurs in an enhanced-CO_2 atmosphere.

Historically, the identification of mycobacteria required the use of biochemical tests that were slow and limited. Newer laboratory methods for the identification of mycobacteria include the use of the compound *p*-nitro-α-acetylamino-β-hydroxypropiophenone, nucleic acid probes, and analysis of mycobacterial fatty acids by chromatography.[7] These methods have greatly reduced the time necessary to speciate mycobacteria.

FUNGI

Although fungi may be isolated on routine bacteriological media, the recovery of fungi is optimized by the use of appropriate fungal media. Both selective and nonselective media are available. Selective medium contains antibiotics to inhibit the growth of contaminating bacteria. It also may contain compounds such as cyclohexamide to inhibit the growth of saprophytic fungi. The recovery of dimorphic fungi *(Sporothrix, Coccidioides, Blastomyces, Histoplasma,* and *Paracoccidioides)* is enhanced by the addition of blood to the media. Both tubed media (slants) and plates are available for fungal culture. Tubed media often are used in the office setting to culture specimens, particularly hair, skin, and nail samples. Similar to bacterial culture, the processing of specimens onto various fungal media depends on the fungi suspected and the body site cultured. The addition of selective media is necessary for the culture of specimens likely to be contaminated with bacteria.

The methods used to identify fungi vary depending on whether the isolate is a unicellular yeast or multicellular mold. Commercial yeast identification systems rely on the detection of preformed enzymes, substrate assimilation, or cellular fatty acids for organism identification.[16] These tests require as little as 1 to 2 hours or as long as 72 hours to perform. Rapid enzymatic and morphological tests also are available for the identification of specific organisms such as *Candida albicans* and *Cryptococcus neoformans.* The identification of filamentous fungi (molds) is most commonly based on colony characteristics, growth characteristics, nutritional requirements, enzymatic properties, and the microscopic morphological characteristics of the mold's reproductive structures. In addition, rapid nucleic acid probes are available for the confirmatory identification of *Histoplasma capsulatum, Coccidioides immitis,* and *Blastomyces dermatitidis.*

VIRUSES AND *CHLAMYDIA* SPECIES

Viruses and *Chlamydia* are obligate intracellular organisms and require living cells for growth and reproduction. The isolation and identification of these organisms is more difficult than those previously discussed because of their small size, growth requirements, and greater lability. Viruses can be cultivated in cell cultures, embryonated eggs, and laboratory animals; however, cell cultures are the only host system used routinely for isolation. Cell cultures are composed of monolayers of cells grown in a glass tube. A combination of cell culture types must be used to maximize the recovery of viruses. After a period of specimen adsorption onto the monolayers, cell culture tubes are incubated at 35° to 37° C for up to 4 weeks. Cultures are observed periodically for evidence of viral replication in the form of cellular cytopathic effects (CPE). These morphological cellular changes are often characteristic for a given virus and aid in identification. Viral isolates are definitively identified by various techniques, including immunofluorescence, enzyme immunoassay, acid lability, hemagglutination inhibition, and neutralization. Because of the time required to recover most viruses in culture, rapid culture techniques including centrifugation-enhanced cultures, pre-CPE detection, and genetically modified cell lines are used by many laboratories.[25] Centrifugation-enhanced cultures increase cell culture sensitivity to viral infection and permit detection of virus in 18 to 48 hours. This method is used for the detection of herpes simplex, varicella zoster virus, cytomegalovirus, and respiratory viruses such as adenovirus, influenza virus, parainfluenza virus, and RSV. The earlier detection of these viruses is accomplished by their pre-CPE detection using immunofluorescence. The specific detection of herpes simplex virus has been enhanced by the use of genetically modified cell lines. These cell lines have been engineered to express the enzyme β-galactosidase when infected with the virus. Enzyme detection using a specific substrate is performed 16 to 24 hours after infection.

ANTIMICROBIAL SUSCEPTIBILITY TESTING

EMPIRICAL THERAPY

The choice of the appropriate antimicrobial agent for treatment of an infection depends on several important factors. First, antimicrobial therapy must be directed as specifically as possible against the infecting organisms. Therefore before the isolation of these organisms, the clinician must consider the organisms likely to be found at the site of infection. Second, an antimicrobial agent must be

chosen that will exhibit appropriate pharmacological properties and activity against the target organisms. In the absence of specific susceptibility data on an individual isolate, an institutional susceptibility profile indicating the susceptibility of commonly isolated pathogens to commonly used antimicrobials is useful when empirical therapy is initiated (Table 3-1). Third, host factors such as age, renal and hepatic function, site of infection, and previous adverse drug reactions must be evaluated for their influence on the choice of antimicrobial used.[29] The most important host factor to be considered is the site of infection, which influences not only the choice of an agent but also the dose and route of administration. The effectiveness of antimicrobial therapy depends on delivery of an adequate concentration of antibiotic to the site of infection. Material should be collected for direct smear and culture from the site of infection before the administration of antimicrobial agents because culture specimens collected subsequently may yield false-negative results because of suppression of microbial growth. In addition to the factors considered previously, the results of direct methods of specimen examination provide important information that may influence the choice of an antimicrobial agent. The use of empirical therapy often accompanies but should not serve as a replacement for necessary surgical therapy.[41] Surgical intervention often augments empirical therapy because the drainage of abscess cavities and the removal of necrotic tissue and sequestra (bone and teeth) are necessary for effective action of the antimicrobial at the site of infection.

RATIONALE FOR SUSCEPTIBILITY TESTING

Although treatment of infection often begins before the availability of susceptibility results, the microbiology laboratory has an important role in the selection and use of antimicrobial agents by clinicians. The goal of susceptibility testing is to predict the likely outcome of treating a specific organism with a particular antimicrobial agent.[20] Susceptibility testing of organisms with a predictable susceptibility pattern is unnecessary. For example, susceptibility testing is not necessary with penicillin against group A streptococcus, erythromycin against *Legionella,* and penicillin against *N. meningitidis* in the United States because of the predictable susceptibility of these organisms to these agents. Antimicrobial susceptibility testing is most important and should be routinely performed with species that do not display predictable susceptibility results. These include members of the Enterobacteriaceae family, *Pseudomonas, Staphylococcus, and Enterococcus* spp., and *S. pneumoniae.* In addition, the increase in the incidence of antimicrobial resistance in *H. influenzae* and *N. gonorrhoeae* has increased requests for susceptibility testing of these organisms. Susceptibility testing should never be performed on organisms unrelated to infection or those representing indigenous flora. In addition, susceptibility testing should never be performed directly on patient specimens because of the potential presence of mixed cultures and the lack of a standardized test inoculum.

TABLE 3-1

Percent Susceptibility of Commonly Isolated Bacteria to Commonly Used Antimicrobial Agents*

					AEROBIC BACTERIA							
Organism	AMP	CFZ	CIP	COT	GEN	PIM	PIP	TAX	TOB	TAZ	UNA	ZOS
Acinetobacter baumanii	—†	—	83	89	85	81	75	62	88	88	92	100
Alcaligenes xylosoxidans	—	—	19	89	1	11	79	—	1	60	67	82
Burkholderia cepacia	—	—	28	72	3	19	22	—	6	34	—	50
Citrobacter freundii	—	—	91	82	92	97	66	71	90	72	58	89
Citrobacter koseri	—	—	99	99	99	100	42	99	100	100	94	100
Enterobacter aerogenes	—	—	96	99	99	100	72	79	99	74	52	80
Enterobacter cloacae	—	—	83	84	86	85	51	53	89	55	20	61
Escherichia coli	66	94	97	87	98	100	68	99	98	99	70	98
Klebsiella oxytoca	—	47	97	94	96	99	64	99	96	96	70	94
Klebsiella pneumoniae	—	94	95	90	94	97	71	95	94	97	84	96
Morganella morganii	—	—	93	90	93	100	68	77	99	80	—	95
Proteus mirabilis	90	94	96	94	96	100	92	99	97	100	90	100
Proteus vulgaris	—	—	96	100	93	89	54	75	93	93	81	100
Pseudomonas aeruginosa	—	—	72	—	70	78	89	—	90	84	—	90
Serratia marcescens	—	—	84	97	97	98	83	78	94	85	—	76
Stenotrophomonas maltophilia	—	—	33	99	29	14	22	—	27	50	—	—

	AMP	CFZ	CLI	COT	ERY	OXA	PEN	VAN
Staphylococcus aureus	—	58	68	77	49	58	—	100
Staphylococcus, not *aureus*	—	37	65	66	34	37	—	100
Streptococcus pneumoniae	—	—	—	—	—	—	73	100
Enterococcus	87	—	—	—	—	—	—	87

		ANAEROBIC BACTERIA‡			
	CLI	MET	PIP	TRO	UNA
Bacteroides fragilis	90	100	92	100	99
Bacteroides fragilis group§	84	100	91	100	99
Prevotella species	100	100	100	100	100
Fusobacterium species	93	100	100	100	96

AMP, Ampicillin; *CFZ,* cefazolin; *CIP,* ciprofloxacin; *COT,* cotrimoxazole (trimethoprim/sulfamethoxazole); *GEN,* gentamicin; *PIM,* cefepime; *PIP,* piperacillin; *TAX,* cefotaxime; *TOB,* tobramycin; *TAZ,* ceftazidime; *UNA,* ampicillin/sulbactam; *ZOS,* piperacillin/tazobactam; *CLI,* clindamycin; *ERY,* erythromycin; *OXA,* oxacillin; *PEN,* penicillin; *VAN,* vancomycin; *MET,* metronidazole; *TRO,* trovafloxacin.

*Based on testing at Hartford Hospital, Hartford, Conn, October 1999 to October 2000.

†Indicates drug is not useful or not first line choice.

‡Based on data from references 1, 2, 35, 45, and 51.

§*B. thetaiotao micron, B. distasonis, B. vulgatus, B. ovatus, B. uniformis, B. fragilis, B. caccae, B. merdae, B. stercoris,* and *B. eggerthii.*

The selection of antimicrobials to test and report should be appropriate for the organism isolated, site of infection, and clinical setting (inpatient vs. outpatient) to which the results will be reported. The panel of antimicrobial agents tested and reported often is determined by a team of microbiology, infectious disease, and pharmacy personnel. Laboratories most frequently test antimicrobial agents that are part of an institution's formulary or used routinely in the outpatient environment. The organism to be tested also determines the type and number of antimicrobial agents that will be tested and reported. The National Committee for Clinical Laboratory Standards publishes a list of antimicrobials appropriate for testing of the Enterobacteriaceae, *Pseudomonas* spp. and other nonglucose fermenters, staphylococci, enterococci, streptococci, *H. influenzae,* and *N. gonorrhoeae.*[30,32] Most laboratories use the list as a guide for determining routinely tested antimicrobials. Finally, the availability of the antimicrobial agent in the appropriate form affects its ability to be tested.

Antimicrobial susceptibility results most often are reported using the following interpretations: susceptible, intermediate, and resistant. Susceptibility indicates that the organism is susceptible to a given antimicrobial at the appropriate dosage for that type of infection. The intermediate susceptibility category includes isolates with testing results that approach usually attainable levels in blood and tissue, but with response rates that may be lower than for susceptible isolates. The antimicrobial agent still may be used to treat infections in body sites where the drug is physiologically concentrated (e.g., urine) or in cases when a higher dose of drug can be used. Resistant isolates are not inhibited by clinically achievable blood or tissue levels of an antimicrobial agent. As indicated, the choice of antimicrobials to report on a given organism depends on the species isolated and the site of the infection (Table 3-2). In addition, many new antimicrobials are similar to one another and older

agents (e.g., azithromycin, clarithromycin, erythromycin); thus the testing and reporting of one drug (erythromycin) from each group is usually sufficient. The limited number of antimicrobials reported is intended to discourage the use of inappropriate antibiotics and combinations of antibiotics and encourage the use of the antibiotic with the narrowest spectrum, lowest toxicity, and lowest cost. Selective reporting may take several forms, including cascade reporting and

TABLE 3-2

Antimicrobial Agents Commonly Reported against Selected Organisms

Enterobacteriaceae	Pseudomonas aeruginosa and Other Nonfermenting Gram-Negative Rods	Staphylococcus	Enterococcus
Primary Antimicrobials to Be Tested and Reported Routinely			
Ampicillin	Ceftazidime	Oxacillin	Penicillin or ampicillin
Cefazolin	Gentamicin		
Cephalothin	Mezlocillin or ticarcillin		
Gentamicin	Piperacillin		
Secondary Antimicrobials Tested Routinely but Reported Selectively			
Amikacin	Amikacin	Azithromycin or	Vancomycin
Amoxicillin/clavulanic acid	Cefepime	clarithromycin or	
or ampicillin/sulbactam	Cefoperazone	erythromycin	
Piperacillin/tazobactam	Aztreonam	Clindamycin	
Ticarcillin/clavulanic acid	Ciprofloxacin	Trimethoprim/	
Cefamandole or cefonicid	Imipenem or meropenem	sulfamethoxazole	
or cefuroxime	Ticarcillin/clavulanic acid	Vancomycin	
Cefepime	Tobramycin		
Cefmetazole	Trimethoprim/		
Cefoperazone	sulfamethoxazole		
Cefotetan			
Cefoxitin			
Cefotaxime or ceftizoxime			
or cefuroxime			
Ciprofloxacin or levofloxacin			
Imipenem or meropenem			
Mezlocillin or piperacillin			
Ticarcillin			
Trimethoprim/			
sulfamethoxazole			
Supplemental Antimicrobials Tested but Not Reported except under Special Circumstances			
Aztreonam	Cefotaxime or ceftriaxone	Chloramphenicol	Chloramphenicol
Ceftazidime	Chloramphenicol	Ciprofloxacin or levofloxacin	Erythromycin
Chloramphenicol		Gentamicin	Rifampin
Tetracycline		Rifampin	Tetracycline*
Tobramycin		Tetracycline	Gentamicin (screen for
			high-level
			resistance only)
Antimicrobials Used Primarily for Treating Urinary Tract Infections and Not Reported on Organisms Recovered From Other Sites of Infection			
Carbenicillin	Carbenicillin	Lomefloxacin or norfloxacin	Ciprofloxacin
Lomefloxacin or norfloxacin	Ceftizoxime	Nitrofurantoin	Levofloxacin
or ofloxacin	Levofloxacin or lomefloxacin		Norfloxacin
Loracarbef	or norfloxacin or ofloxacin		Nitrofurantoin
Nitrofurantoin	Tetracycline		Tetracycline

*Data from ancomycin-resistant strains of *Enterococcus* only.

reporting based on body site (Box 3-5). The selective reporting of antibiotic susceptibilities helps prevent the indiscriminate use of antimicrobial agents and the development of antibiotic resistance and minimizes the risk of misleading a clinician by reporting erroneous information.

SUSCEPTIBILITY TESTING METHODS

Aerobic Bacteria   The procedures used to determine antimicrobial susceptibility can be divided into two categories: quantitative and qualitative tests. As the name implies, quantitative tests produce numerical results in the form of a minimum inhibitory concentration (MIC). This indicates the minimum concentration of antibiotic necessary to inhibit the growth of the organism. Conversely, qualitative tests produce results solely in the form of susceptibility categories: susceptible, intermediate, and resistant. All susceptibility testing methods are highly standardized to ensure consistent results.

Dilution susceptibility testing methods are used to determine quantitative results. These tests may be performed in either agar (agar dilution) or broth (broth dilution) and may be totally manual or completely automated. Twofold serial dilutions of antibiotics are prepared and inoculated with a standardized suspension of the test organism. After incubation the lowest concentration of antibiotic that inhibits visible growth is considered the MIC (Figure 3-5). The MIC must then be correlated with the achievable serum level for that antibiotic depending on the frequency and route of administration to determine antimicrobial effectiveness. A fourfold margin is necessary to ensure successful therapy. This interpretation may present a challenge to clinicians; therefore most laboratories translate the significance of the MIC value into the more familiar susceptible, intermediate, and resistant categories. Dilution methods offer flexibility in that both nonfastidious and fastidious bacteria may be tested. In addition, broth dilution methods are highly amenable to automation.

Qualitative susceptibility results are determined with the disk diffusion procedure. The test is performed by application of a standardized suspension of test organism to the surface of an agar plate. Antibiotic-containing disks are then placed on the inoculated surface. After incubation the zone of growth inhibition around the disk is measured (Figure 3-6). The zone size is then compared with interpretive criteria published by the National Committee for Clinical Laboratory Standards.[32] These criteria have been established after large-scale testing and correlation of disk diffusion zone diameters with MIC breakpoints for susceptibility and resistance for a given microorganism and antibiotic combination. Disk diffusion testing is inexpensive, highly reproducible, and capable of testing a large number of antimicrobials at one time. In addition, the ability to perform disk diffusion susceptibility testing of newer antimicrobial agents usually precedes the availability of these antimicrobials in commercial dilution panels. Disk diffusion, however, is not appropriate for the testing of some fastidious organisms and has experienced difficulty in the detection of some methicillin-resistant *S. aureus* and vancomycin-resistant *Enterococcus* isolates.

A recently developed gradient diffusion (also referred to as *E test*) method incorporates the principles of disk diffusion testing and produces a quantitative result (Figure 3-7). Test organisms are inoculated to an agar surface in

---

BOX 3-5

Selective Reporting of Antimicrobial Agents

Cascade Reporting
Enterobacteriaceae
   Report second-generation cephalosporins only if first-generation cephalosporins resistant.
   Report third-generation cephalosporins only if second-generation cephalosporins resistant. Report tobramycin or amikacin only if gentamicin resistant.
Pseudomonas
   Report tobramycin or amikacin only if gentamicin resistant.
Staphylococcus
   Report vancomycin only if methicillin (oxacillin) resistant.
Enterococcus
   Report vancomycin only if ampicillin resistant.

Reporting According to Body Site
For isolates from cerebrospinal fluid, report the susceptibilities of antimicrobials that cross the blood-brain barrier.
   For isolates from urine, report the susceptibilities of antimicrobials that are used exclusively in the treatment of urinary tract infection.

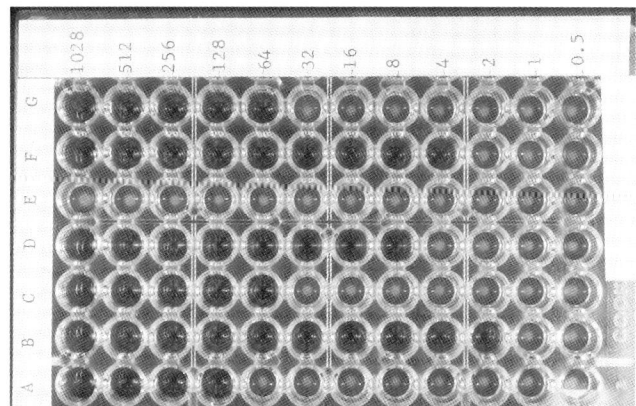

Figure 3-5 Broth dilution susceptibility testing using a microdilution plate; this method permits the simultaneous antimicrobial susceptibility testing of a single organism to seven antimicrobial agents *(rows A through G)*. After inoculation of a standardized organism suspension into a plate containing serial twofold dilutions of antimicrobials (1028 µg/mL through 0.5 µg/mL), the MIC is interpreted as the lowest concentration of antibiotic that inhibits organism growth. The MICs for this organism are as follows: antibiotic A, 128 µg/mL; antibiotic B, 2 µg/mL; antibiotic C, 64 µg/mL, antibiotic D, 8 µg/mL; antibiotic E, >1028 µg/mL; antibiotic F, 4 µg/mL; and antibiotic G, 64 µg/mL.

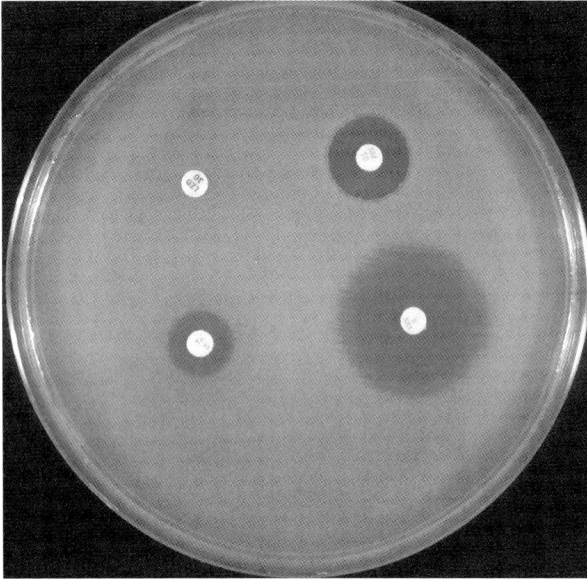

Figure 3-6 Qualitative susceptibility testing using the disk diffusion procedure. Antibiotic-containing disks are placed on the agar surface after inoculation with a standardized organism suspension. The diameter of the zone of growth inhibition is measured and compared with established guidelines to determine the organism's susceptibility to the antimicrobial agents tested.

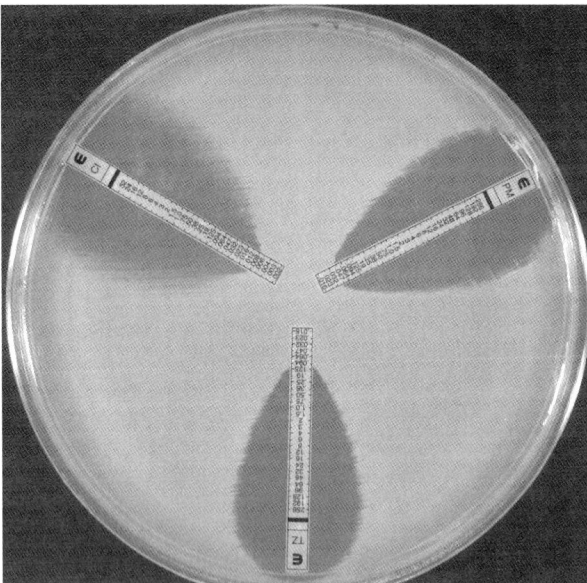

Figure 3-8 Interpretation of susceptibility test performed using the E test method. The MIC is read as the point on the scale where the ellipse of organism growth intersects the plastic strip. The MIC of this organism to ceftazidime is 0.094 µg/mL.

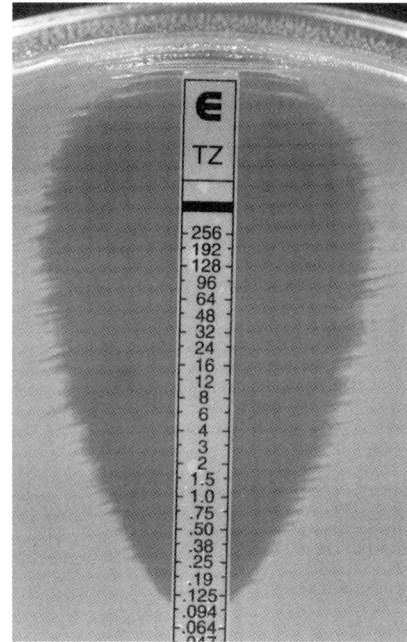

Figure 3-7 Quantitative susceptibility testing using the gradient diffusion (E test) method. Agar plates are inoculated in the same process as for disk diffusion susceptibility testing. A plastic antimicrobial-impregnated strip is placed on the inoculated surface. Subsequent MIC values are read from the top surface of the strip.

the same method as for disk diffusion testing. However, instead of antibiotic-containing disks, a plastic strip with a continuous gradient of antibiotic on one side and an MIC scale on the other is placed on the inoculated plate.[26] After incubation the MIC is interpreted as the point on

the scale where the ellipse of organism growth intersects the test strip (Figure 3-8). This method offers the simplicity of disk diffusion testing and the flexibility of dilution methods because fastidious organisms can be tested. However, the E test method is more expensive than disk diffusion and has not been mechanized to the level of disk diffusion testing.

Anaerobic Bacteria   The routine susceptibility testing of anaerobic bacteria is controversial. Because most anaerobic infections involve mixed organisms and the time required for the laboratory to isolate and identify anaerobic bacteria is longer, the empirical therapy of these infections is necessary. Some have advocated therapy choices based on the use of published antibiograms. However, geographical variations in susceptibility patterns and increasing resistance encountered among some species, particularly the *Bacteroides fragilis* group, has led to the recommendation that at least periodic susceptibility testing of anaerobic bacteria is appropriate.[13,50] The testing of individual patient isolates may be necessary in cases of life-threatening infection, relapse, or failure of therapy and prolonged therapy. The only currently approved methods for determination of susceptibility of anaerobic bacteria are broth and agar dilution.[31] The E test method has been used by some laboratories because of its convenience and ease of use. Recent studies have demonstrated a good correlation of results obtained by E test and approved methods.[26,37,39] The continued emergence of more resistant organisms may necessitate routine susceptibility testing in the future.

Fungi With the increase in the number and complexity of fungal infections and an increase in resistance to commonly used antifungal agents, the laboratory now plays an important role in the selection and monitoring of antifungal therapy. Susceptibility testing of fungi is performed for many of the same reasons as bacterial susceptibility testing. However, evidence supporting the correlation of antifungal susceptibility testing results and clinical efficacy has been lacking. The development of a standardized method for the performance of fungal susceptibility testing has improved test reproducibility and provided interpretive breakpoints for some agents.[34,36] The approved standardized method is broth dilution; however, agar dilution, disk diffusion, and E test methodologies have been used to determine antifungal susceptibilities. Although the principle of broth dilution testing is similar to the testing of bacteria, actual test performance and interpretation are more laborious and complicated. Testing of yeast isolates, particularly *Candida* spp., is routinely performed in some large hospital and reference laboratories, whereas testing of filamentous fungi (*Aspergillus* spp., zygomycetes, *Pseudallescheria boydii,* and others) is limited to a few reference centers.

Mycobacteria Mycobacteria represent a diverse group of organisms that display differing roles in the cause of human disease. Thus mycobacteria, like bacteria, differ in the antimicrobial agents used to treat them. Historically, the need for susceptibility testing of mycobacteria was limited to *M. tuberculosis* and testing was indicated only in instances of relapse or high levels of resistance in the community. With the resurgence of tuberculosis, especially multidrug-resistant tuberculosis, the Centers for Disease Control and Prevention has recommended the routine testing of all *M. tuberculosis* isolates.[48] The emergence of nontuberculosis mycobacteria, including *M. avium* complex, *M. kansasii,* and rapidly growing mycobacteria as pathogens, has increased the need to perform testing on these isolates under certain circumstances, including relapse and intractable infection. Rapidly growing mycobacteria (*M. fortuitum, M. chelonae,* and *M. abscessus*) are not treated with the same types of drugs used to treat other mycobacterial infections. Thus susceptibility testing of significant isolates provides important information for appropriate antimicrobial therapy.

Because of the media and growth requirements of mycobacteria, susceptibility testing of these organisms is conducted differently than that for other bacteria or fungi. Historically, susceptibility was performed by the indirect proportion method.[17] In this method a suspension of *M. tuberculosis* organisms is inoculated onto agar medium containing empirical concentrations of antimycobacterial agents and agar that contains no drugs. After a 3-week incubation period the percentage of resistant organisms is reported based on the comparison between growth on drug-containing and drug-free media. More recently, commercial liquid-based systems used for the isolation of mycobacteria also have been used for an-

timycobacterial susceptibility testing. With these systems, organism suspensions are added to drug-containing and drug-free liquid vials and growth is monitored by the automated system. The advantage of these systems is the rapidity with which results are produced (5 days). Susceptibility testing methods used for nontuberculosis mycobacteria have included broth and agar dilution, automated liquid-based systems, agar disk elution, and disk diffusion.

Viruses Bacterial resistance to antimicrobial agents is well known. In contrast, the resistance of viruses to specific antiviral agents is a relatively recent phenomenon. Resistance is rarely demonstrated in individuals who are immunocompetent. Rather, resistance most frequently develops in patients who are immunocompromised (those with HIV, transplant recipients, and patients with cancer) after lengthy antiviral therapy. Although antiviral susceptibility testing is not the norm, testing may be indicated to determine whether resistance has emerged during therapy and to evaluate the potential use of alternative agents. Testing most frequently has been performed on isolates of herpes simplex virus, cytomegalovirus, and varicella-zoster virus. The recent development of assays for the evaluation of HIV susceptibility has enabled clinicians to tailor antiretroviral regimens.

Antiviral susceptibility testing assays measure the inhibitory effects of agents on the entire virus population (phenotypic assays), whereas others are designed to detect specific genetic mutations resulting in resistance (genotypic assays). To date, antiviral susceptibility testing remains unstandardized, and because of other variables affecting clinical response, some patients may not respond to therapy despite in vitro susceptibility. Future efforts have been aimed at addressing sources of testing variability and developing testing interpretive guidelines.

Molecular Methods The development and routine use of molecular technology in the laboratory has extended into its use for the detection of antimicrobial resistance genes. This testing is based on the supposition that the detection of a gene mediating resistance equates to resistance. Although molecular susceptibility testing likely will not replace routine testing methods in the near future, the detection of resistance genes is particularly helpful in instances in which routine susceptibility results are near the breakpoint between susceptibility and resistance (e.g., methicillin resistance in *S. aureus*) and those in which the detection of resistance genes directly in clinical samples could guide early therapy (e.g., resistance in *M. tuberculosis*).[47,49] The detection of mutations affecting resistance also is possible in cytomegalovirus, influenza virus, and HIV. The one drawback of this method is that only one resistance gene may be detected at a time. The development of commercially available assays will enable laboratories to provide more rapid susceptibility information. Future endeavors may enable the simultaneous detection of multiple resistance determinants.

SUMMARY

Knowledge regarding the pathogenesis of infections in the oral and facial region continues to increase. Diagnosis of infections from this region may be complicated by the complexity of the flora present. However, the accurate diagnosis of infections from these sites is crucial for the administration of appropriate therapy. The first step in an accurate diagnosis is adherence to appropriate collection and transport protocols. The availability of direct methods of specimen examination provides clinicians with rapid results on which to base empirical therapy decisions. The ability of clinicians to evaluate Gram-stained smears and perform rapid tests for microbial antigens enables them to make immediate decisions regarding patient care.

The laboratory isolation, definitive identification, and antimicrobial susceptibility testing of microorganisms serves an important role in the diagnosis and appropriate treatment of infectious diseases. The development of rapid methods for microbial identification and susceptibility testing has enabled the laboratory to provide complete culture results more quickly than in the past. The use of molecular techniques now permits the identification of organisms and the detection of resistance traits at the genetic level. The automation of these techniques will likely increase the use and significance of these tests. An increased emphasis on communication and cooperation between the clinician and the microbiology laboratory is necessary to produce the maximal benefit from laboratory results and minimize the production of potentially misleading information. Thus the consultative role of the clinical microbiologist will likely increase in an effort to ensure the clinical relevance of microbiology laboratory results.

REFERENCES

1. Aldridge KE, Gelfand M, Reller LB, et al: A five-year multicenter study of the susceptibility of the *Bacteroides fragilis* group isolates to cephalosporins, cephamins, penicillins, clindamycin, and metronidazole in the United States, *Diagn Microbiol Infect Dis* 18:235, 1994.
2. Aldridge KE, Johnson WD: A comparison of susceptibility results of the *Bacteroides fragilis* group and other anaerobes by traditional MIC results and statistical methods, *J Antimicrob Chemother* 39:319, 1997.
3. Allen SD, Siders JA, Marier LM: Current issues and problems in dealing with anaerobes in the clinical laboratory, *Clin Lab Med* 15:333, 1995.
4. Bartlett RC: Making optimum use of the microbiology laboratory. I. Use of the laboratory, *JAMA* 247:857, 1982.
5. Brook I: The swollen neck: cervical lymphadenitis, parotitis, thyroiditis, and infected cysts, *Infect Dis Clin North Am* 2:221, 1988.
6. Centers for Disease Control and Prevention: CDC guidelines for tuberculosis control in healthcare facilities, *MMWR Morb Mortal Wkly Rep* 43:24, 1994.
7. Christie JD, Callihan DR: The laboratory diagnosis of mycobacterial diseases: challenges and common sense, *Clin Lab Med* 15:279, 1995.
8. Citron DM, Warren YA, Hudspeth MK, et al: Survival of aerobic and anaerobic bacteria in purulent clinical specimens maintained in the Copan Venturi Transystem and Becton Dickinson Port-a-Cul transport systems, *J Clin Microbiol* 38:892, 2000.
9. Cleveland DB, Miller AS: Diagnostic laboratory aids in oral and maxillofacial surgical pathology, *Oral Maxillofac Surg Clin North Am* 6:377, 1994.
10. Davidson D, Platt J, Nelson C: Fine needle aspiration biopsy: what good is it? In Worthington P, Evans JR, editors: *Controversies in oral and maxillofacial surgery*, Philadelphia, 1994, WB Saunders.
11. Doern GV: Laboratory diagnosis of infectious diseases. In Gwaltney JM, Grandis JR, Sugar AM, editors: *Infectious diseases and antimicrobial therapy of the ears, nose and throat*, Philadelphia, 1997, WB Saunders.
12. Dunne WM Jr, Nolte FS, Wilson ML: Blood cultures III. In Hindler JA, editor: *Cumulative techniques and procedures in clinical microbiology*, Washington, 1997, American Society for Microbiology Press.
13. Finegold SM: Perspective on susceptibility testing of anaerobic bacteria, *Clin Infect Dis* 25(suppl 2):S251, 1997.
14. Finegold SM, Jousimies-Somer HR, Wexler HM: Current perspectives on anaerobic infections: diagnostic approaches, *Infect Dis Clin North Am* 7:257, 1993.
15. Gerbino G, Bernardi M, Secco F, et al: Diagnosis of actinomycosis by fine-needle aspiration, *Oral Surg Oral Med Oral Pathol* 81:381, 1996.
16. Hazen KC: Methods for fungal identification in the clinical mycology laboratory, *Clin Microbiol Newslett* 18:137, 1996.
17. Heifets LB: Drug susceptibility testing, *Clin Lab Med* 16:641, 1996.
18. Horswell BB: Infections. In Kwon PH, Laskin DM, editors: *Clinician's manual of oral and maxillofacial surgery*, ed 2, Chicago, 1997, Quintessence.
19. Jenkinson, HF, Dymock D: The microbiology of periodontal disease, *Dent Update* 26:191, 1999.
20. Jorgensen JH: Antimicrobial susceptibility testing of bacteria that grow aerobically, *Infect Dis Clin North Am* 7:393, 1993.
21. Landry ML, Ferguson D: SimulFluor respiratory screen for rapid detection of multiple respiratory viruses in clinical specimens by immunofluorescence staining, *J Clin Microbiol* 38:708, 2000.
22. Lee PC, Turnidge J, McDonald PJ: Fine-needle aspiration biopsy in diagnosis of soft tissue infections, *J Clin Microbiol* 22:80, 1985.
23. Long EG, Christie JD: The diagnosis of old and new gastrointestinal parasites, *Clin Lab Med* 15:307, 1995.
24. Mader JT, Calhoun J: Osteomyelitis. In Mandell GL, Bennett JE, Dolin R, editors: *Principles and practice of infectious diseases*, ed 4, New York, 1995, Churchill Livingstone.
25. Mann LM, Woods GL: Rapid diagnosis of viral pathogens, *Clin Lab Med* 15:389, 1995.
26. Massey VE, Lannigan R, Hussain Z: Evaluation of susceptibility of anaerobic organisms by the E test and the reference agar dilution method, *Clin Infect Dis* 20(suppl 2):S337, 1995.
27. Miller CH: Isolation and systematic examination of pathogenic microorganisms. In Schuster GS, editor: *Oral microbiology and infectious disease*, Philadelphia, 1990, BC Decker.
28. Miller JM, Holmes HT: Specimen collection transport, and storage. In Murray PR, Baron EJ, Pfaller MA, et al, editors: *Manual of clinical microbiology*, ed 7, Washington, 1999, American Society for Microbiology Press.

29. Moellering RC Jr: Principles of anti-infective therapy. In Mandell GE, Douglas RG Jr, Bennett JE, editors: *Anti-infective therapy,* New York, 1985, John Wiley & Sons.

30. National Committee for Clinical Laboratory Standards: *Methods for dilution antimicrobial susceptibility tests for bacteria that grow aerobically;* approved standard M7-A5, Wayne, Pa, 2000, The Committee.

31. National Committee for Clinical Laboratory Standards: *Methods for antimicrobial susceptibility testing of anaerobic bacteria;* approved standard M11-A4, Wayne, Pa, 1997, The Committee.

32. National Committee for Clinical Laboratory Standards: *Performance standards for antimicrobial disk susceptibility tests;* approved standard M2-A7, Wayne, Pa, 2000, The Committee.

33. National Committee for Clinical Laboratory Standards: *Protection of laboratory workers from infectious disease transmitted by blood, body fluids and tissue;* approved standard M29-A2, Wayne, Pa, 1991, The Committee.

34. National Committee for Clinical Laboratory Standards: *Reference method for broth dilution antifungal susceptibility testing of yeasts;* approved standard M27-A, Wayne, Pa, 1997, The Committee.

35. Pankuch GA, Jacobs MR, Appelbaum PC: Susceptibilities of 428 Gram-positive and -negative anaerobic bacteria to Bay y3118 compared with their susceptibilities to ciprofloxacin, clindamycin, metronidazole, piperacillin, piperacillin-tazobactam, and cefoxitin, *Antimicrob Agents Chemother* 37:1649, 1993.

36. Pfaller MA, Rinaldi MG: Antifungal susceptibility testing: current state of technology, limitations and standardization, *Infect Dis Clin North Am* 7:435, 1993.

37. Poulet PP, Duffant D, Lodter JP: Evaluation of the E test for determining the in-vitro susceptibilities of *Prevotella intermedia* isolates to metronidazole, *J Antimicrob Chemother* 43:610, 1999.

38. Rafetto LK: Clinical examination of the maxillary sinus, *Oral Maxillofac Surg Clin North Am* 11:35, 1999.

39. Rosenblatt JE, Gustafson DR: Evaluation of the E test for susceptibility testing of anaerobic bacteria, *Diagn Microbiol Infect Dis* 22:279, 1995.

40. Salit IE: Diagnostic approaches to head and neck infections, *Infect Dis Clin North Am* 2:35, 1988.

41. Sandor GKB, Low DE, Judd PL, et al: Antimicrobial treatment options in the management of odontogenic infections, *J Can Dent Assoc* 84:508, 1998.

42. Shea YR: Specimen collection and transport. In Isenberg HD, editor: *Clinical microbiology procedures handbook,* Washington, 1992, American Society for Microbiology Press.

43. Silverman JF, Gay RM: Fine-needle aspiration and surgical pathology of infectious lesions: morphologic features and the role of the clinical microbiology laboratory for rapid diagnosis, *Clin Lab Med* 15:251, 1995.

44. Slack RCB: Use of the laboratory. In Greenwood D, editor: *Antimicrobial chemotherapy,* ed 3, New York, 1995, Oxford University Press.

45. Spangler SK, Jacobs MR, Appelbaum PC: Susceptibility of anaerobic bacteria to trovafloxacin: comparison with other quinolones and non-quinolone antibiotics, *Infect Dis Clin Pract* 5(3 suppl):S101, 1996.

46. Tang Y-W, Persing DH: Molecular detection and identification of microorganisms. In Murray PR, Baron EJ, Pfaller MA, et al, editors: *Manual of clinical microbiology,* ed 7, Washington, 1999, American Society for Microbiology Press.

47. Tenover FC: DNA hybridization techniques and their application to the diagnosis of infectious diseases, *Infect Dis Clin North Am* 7:171, 1993.

48. Tenover FC, Crawford JT, Huebner RE, et al: The resurgence of tuberculosis: is your laboratory ready? *J Clin Microbiol* 31:767, 1993.

49. Tenover FC, Rasheed JK: Genetic methods for detecting antibacterial and antiviral resistance genes. In Murray PR, Baron EJ, Pfaller MA, et al, editors: *Manual of clinical microbiology,* ed 7, Washington, 1999, American Society for Microbiology Press.

50. Wexler HM, Finegold SM: Current susceptibility patterns of anaerobic bacteria, *Yonsei Med J* 39:495, 1998.

51. Wexler HM, Molitoris E, Finegold SM: In vitro activities of three of the newer quinolones against anaerobic bacteria, *Antimicrob Agents Chemother* 36:239, 1992.

52. Weymouth LA: Microbiology of the maxillary sinus, *Oral Maxillofac Surg Clin North Am* 11:21, 1999.

53. Winn WC Jr, Keathley JD: Direct immunofluorescence identification of bacteria in clinical specimens. In Coonrod JD, Kunz LJ, Ferraro MJ, editors: *The direct detection of microorganisms in clinical specimens,* New York, 1983, Academic Press.

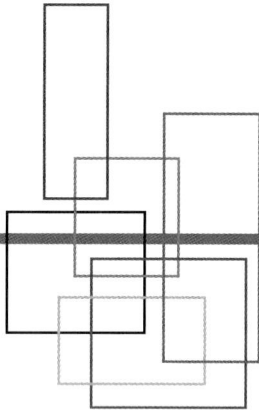

Diagnostic Imaging of Maxillofacial and Fascial Space Infections

Angelo M. DelBalso
Richard E. Hall

Diagnostic imaging has assumed a central role in the management of patients with deep-seated head and neck infections. Information gained from various diagnostic studies, especially computed tomography (CT), is essential in accurately delineating the anatomical extent of the process, demonstrating surgically drainable abscesses and fluid collections, and demonstrating and assessing associated complications. In addition, CT-guided needle aspiration of fluid collections can be used to obtain material for microbial analysis. This chapter examines the role of diagnostic imaging in the treatment of patients with head and neck infections.

IMAGING MODALITIES

The modern diagnostic armamentarium contains a number of different imaging modalities that can be used in the assessment of head and neck pathological conditions.

PLAIN FILM EXAMINATION

Diagnostic imaging of maxillofacial and fascial space disorders often starts with some form of a plain film study. Panoramic radiographs are commonly obtained if the inflammatory process involves the oral or paraoral region to rule out pathological conditions of odontogenic origin and demonstrate the extent of the process.[67] Anteroposterior and lateral views of the cervical soft tissues are especially important if patency of the airway is a concern (Figure 4-1); these views are especially indicated in the treatment of inflammatory or infectious processes involving the submandibular, parapharyngeal, or retropharyngeal spaces that can cause airway compromise.

COMPUTED TOMOGRAPHY

CT has become the most widely used and readily available advanced imaging modality for the evaluation of head and

neck infections. In contrast to plain film radiographs in which information is directly recorded on film, CT images are computer generated. In CT, digitized data are obtained by the rotation of an x-ray source and detector array about a structure in either the axial or the direct coronal plane. These detectors measure the intensity of a fine beam of radiation passing through the object. This information is then sent to a computer, which determines the physical densities of many small volumes of tissue making up the larger structure through a series of complex mathematical equations. These small volumes, or voxels, are assigned a numerical value relative to water. These numerical values, or CT numbers, are expressed in Hounsfield units (HU). Examples of commonly cited CT numbers include air (-1000 HU), fat (-80 to -100 HU), water (0 HU), blood (60 to 110 HU), and bone (1000 HU). The final CT image is composed of many two-dimensional picture elements, or pixels. Each pixel corresponds to the average density of one voxel. The final CT image is displayed using a gray scale, with the more negative numbers appearing toward the black end of the scale, and the more positive numbers appearing toward the white end of the gray scale.

Terms often used in the CT display of images are the *window level* and the *window width*.[21] The lowest value of the CT number range being displayed is determined by the window level, whereas the window width, or range of numbers displayed, determines the contrast (degree of difference in brightness or darkness) being displayed. A number of techniques are available to enhance the diagnostic yield of a CT study. These include imaging at a level and window width combination in order to emphasize bone or soft tissue, reformatting in different planes, and using iodinated contrast media. Iodinated contrast medium administered intravenously before and/or during the study can greatly enhance the diagnostic yield of a study by demonstrating the location of normal vascular structures and enhancing pathological processes or structures such as abscess walls. Major advantages of CT in the evaluation of head and neck fascial

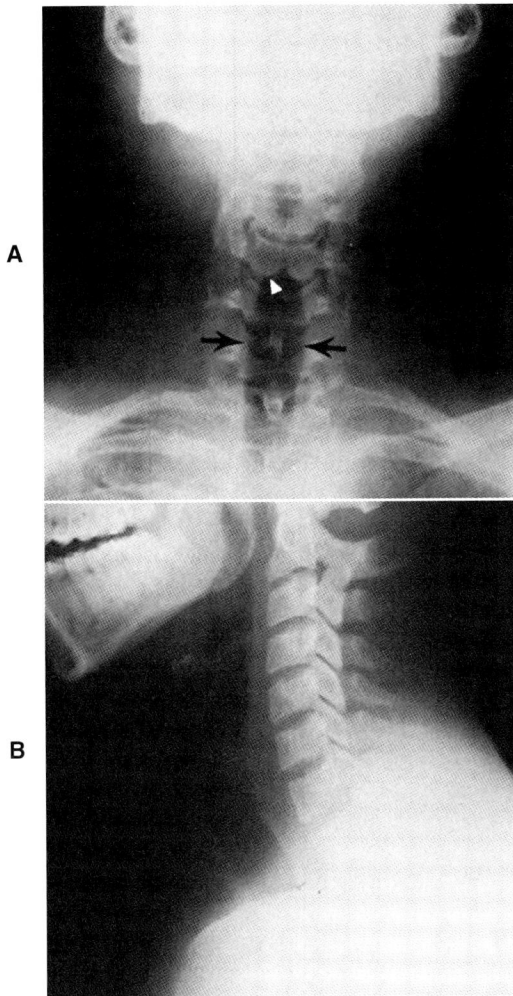

Figure 4-1 A, Anteroposterior view of the normal cervical airway. The normal cervical airway *(arrows)* should appear symmetrical over the middle third of the cervical spine. It should have distinct shoulders in the proximal segment of the trachea *(arrowhead).* **B,** Lateral view of cervical airway. In the adult the width of the prevertebral soft tissue at the C3 level should not exceed 7 mm or 20 mm at the C7 level.

space infections include (1) CT's ability to readily assess the integrity of cortical bone, (2) the short times required for CT examination, (3) the ready availability of CT scanners, and (4) the relatively low cost of a CT study compared with magnetic resonance imaging (MRI) studies. Major advancements in CT technology have included the development of the helical, or spiral, CT scanner and the multidetector CT scanner. These advancements have greatly reduced the time needed to scan a given area. Scans that formerly took several minutes to perform can now be performed in less than a minute. This is especially important for patients who have limited ability to remain still because of the discomfort associated with various inflammatory processes.

MAGNETIC RESONANCE IMAGING

MRI does not involve the use of ionizing radiation to generate images but instead relies on a combination of a magnetic field and radiofrequency energy. In an MRI system the patient is placed in a strong magnetic field and the hydrogen atoms are allowed to align in the direction of the field. This alignment is then altered by pulsing radiofrequency energy in the form of a radio wave perpendicular to the magnetic field. This typically results in a 180-degree shift in the orientation of some of the hydrogen nuclei such that the bulk magnetization, or average of all proton magnetic moments, is rotated away from the direction of the magnetic field, typically by 90 degrees. Cessation of the radio wave results in a return of the bulk magnetization toward the original field direction. Emission of radiofrequency energy from these protons as they return toward the equilibrium state is detected and used to generate diagnostic images. A major advantage of MRI over CT is its ability to generate images in not only the axial planes but also the direct coronal and sagittal planes.

MRI images are described in terms of being either *T1-* or *T2-weighted* images. T1 refers to a rate constant at which magnetic polarization or relaxation occurs about the longitudinal or Z axis. Stated more simply, T1 measures the rate at which tissue becomes magnetized. The T2 constant is the rate at which spins become disorganized as a result of local inhomogeneities in the field. When different imaging parameters are varied, the images that are obtained emphasize T1 or T2 characteristics of a group of tissues in an imaging plane. T1 images provide good anatomical detail, whereas T2 images are very sensitive in detecting disease processes.

The final image generated in an MRI system is governed by the hydrogen atom density and T1 and T2 time constants. Descriptions of a tissue or lesion often refer to *signal intensity,* or *brightness,* on a given weighted sequence. Fat and highly proteinaceous tissues characteristically produce high signal intensity on T1-weighted images. Inflammatory processes, tumors, and fluid collections usually have low signal intensity on T1-weighted sequences and high signal intensity on T2 sequences reflecting their increased water content (Figure 4-2). Structures appearing dark on T1 and T2 images include rapidly flowing blood, dense calcification, and organized fibrous tissue.

The use of intravenous MRI contrast agents can demonstrate the vascularity of a lesion, which can be important in neoplastic and inflammatory lesions. The most widely used MRI contrast agent is gadolinium–diethylenetriamine pentaacetic acid (DPTA). In contrast to the iodinated contrast agents used in CT scanning, the intravenous contrast agents used in MRI scanning are safer, with adverse reactions occurring only rarely.

NUCLEAR MEDICINE

Although CT and MRI provide excellent anatomical information about the tissues under study, one major drawback is their inability to provide significant physiological information about these tissues. In contrast, radionuclide imaging can provide excellent information about various physiological and pathological processes. This capability can result in earlier detection before morphological changes become evident.

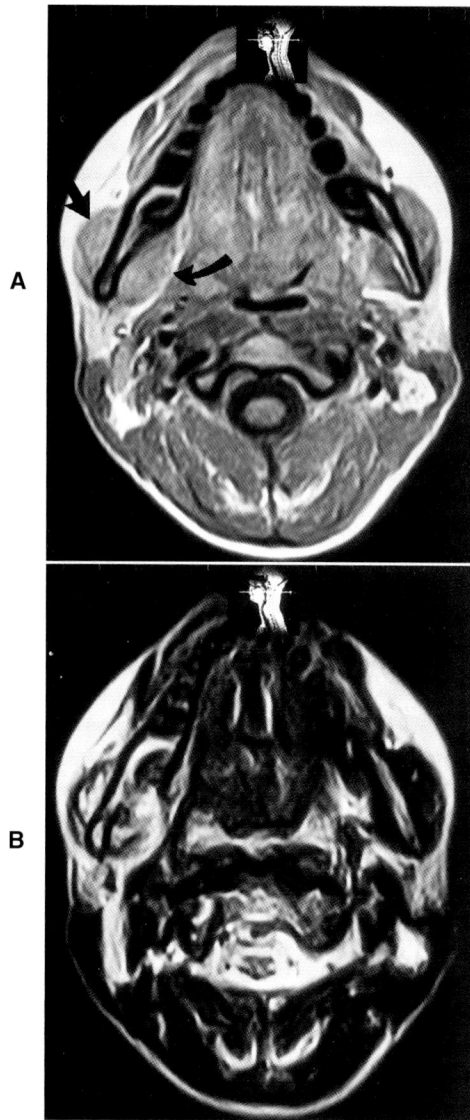

Figure 4-2 MRI scan of masticator space cellulitis resulting from a mandibular molar periapical abscess. Axial T1- and T2-weighted images through masticator space and floor of mouth. On the T1 sequence the right masseter *(straight arrow)* and medial pterygoid *(curved arrows)* muscles appear increased in size and demonstrate decreased signal intensity **(A).** Decreased signal intensity of the marrow within the mandible reflective of marrow edema. On the T2-weighted sequence, increased signal intensity is seen within muscles and mandibular marrow indicating edema. Contrast with normal-appearing structure on the right **(B).**

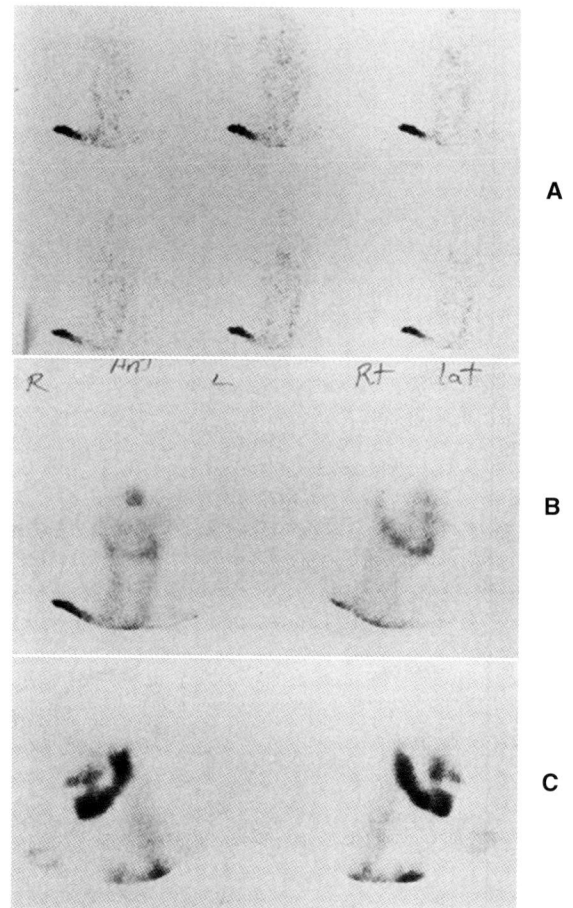

Figure 4-3 Radionuclide bone scan in a patient with chronic osteomyelitis of the premaxilla and mandible. **A,** Initial flow phase taken immediately after the injection of ^{99m}Tc-labeled methylene diphosphonate demonstrates flow in the vessels of the head and neck; however, no accumulation of activity in the mandible exists to suggest an osteomyelitis. Static images obtained immediately after **(B)** and at 5 hours after **(C)** the injection demonstrate progressive uptake of the radiopharmaceutical in the mandible and premaxilla. The overall pattern is consistent with chronic osteomyelitis.

Radionuclide imaging involves the use of radiopharmaceuticals, consisting of an organic substance specific for a given tissue or structure and a nonspecific radionuclide label, usually ^{99m}Tc. This intermediate, metastable radionuclide is formed during the decay of ^{99}Mo to ^{99}Tc. It has a half-life of 6.3 hours and undergoes isomeric transformation to ^{99}Tc by releasing a gamma photon. In radionuclide imaging, the number and distribution of gamma rays emitted from the radionuclide in the patient during a set period are detected by a gamma camera and depicted in the final image. Radionuclide images are often referred to as *dynamic,* or *static,* images. Dynamic images or flow studies are obtained during and/or immediately after injection and are intended to demonstrate blood flow to an area, an organ or lesion's vascularity, or both (Figure 4-3). Static images are obtained after injection or after an appropriate period for uptake to occur; these images are intended to visualize a specific organ or structure or to better delineate a physiological or pathological process.

Radionuclide bone scanning is particularly useful in the evaluation of inflammatory and neoplastic conditions involving the osseous maxillofacial structures.[21,80,92,93] These studies demonstrate osseous involvement before changes are evident on standard plain films. In conventional radiography, approximately 60% of the mineral content of a pathologically involved segment of bone must be lost before the pathological changes become evident. Radiopharmaceuticals commonly used in bone scanning are ^{99m}Tc-phosphate compounds such as polyphosphate, pyrophosphonate, hydroxyethylene diphosphonate (HEDP), and methylene diphosphonate (MDP). Although the exact mechanisms underlying the uptake of the phosphate by bone are not fully understood, adsorption to the hydroxyapatite surface is believed to play an important role. Factors influencing the uptake of radiopharmaceuticals by bone include regional blood flow, bone formation rate, and extraction efficiency. Common indications for radionuclide bone scan include demonstration of primary or secondary malignancies, metabolic and dysplastic bone disorders, and differentiation between cellulitis and osteomyelitis. Differentiating between cellulitis and osteomyelitis is especially important clinically and is readily accomplished using a three- or four-phase radionuclide bone scan. Sequential images of the area under study are obtained during injection, resulting in a radionuclide arteriogram (Figure 4-3, *A*), followed by an immediate static or blood pool image.[94] The arteriogram images obtained during phase 1 of the study demonstrate increased vascularity in osteomyelitis or cellulitis. The blood pool images demonstrate increased soft tissue uptake in cellulitis and in involved soft tissue overlying a focus of osteomyelitis. The second phase of the study is obtained approximately 2 hours after injection and demonstrates increased osseous uptake in osteomyelitis (Figure 4-3, *B*). The third phase is performed approximately 5 hours after injection (Figure 4-3, *C*). In patients with osteomyelitis a continued increase in the activity of the pharmaceutical in the involved bone relative to surrounding normal bone should occur compared with the ratio at 2 hours. Images also can be obtained at 24 hours after injection; these images constitute the fourth phase of the study and should demonstrate increased accumulation of radiopharmaceutical in areas involved by osteomyelitis. These later images sometimes are referred to as the fourth phase of the bone scan.

In addition to technetium-containing radiopharmaceuticals, other agents used in the evaluation of acute or chronic osteomyelitis include ^{67}Ga citrate and ^{111}In-labeled leukocytes.[80,94] Gallium scanning is useful in the detection of a number of neoplastic and inflammatory conditions, particularly salivary abnormalities because increased salivary gland uptake can occur in malignant salivary tumors, lymphoma, acute and chronic inflammation, postirradiation sialadenitis, abscesses, and active sarcoidosis. Patients with active sarcoidosis frequently demonstrate increased uptake by the parotid and lacrimal glands. Gallium scanning involves the intravenous administration of 3 to 5 mCi of ^{67}Ga citrate and imaged obtained at 6, 24, 48, and 72 hours after administration. Although gallium scanning is an extremely useful imaging tool, it cannot totally differentiate between an inflammatory and a neoplastic process, and false-negative results can occur with an encapsulated, inactive abscess.

Tagging of white blood cells (WBCs) with ^{111}In allows for the early localizing of acute inflammatory processes. WBC tagging is achieved by isolation and in vitro labeling of WBCs from a venous sample. The labeled WBCs are then injected back into the patient and imaging is performed at 3 and 24 hours after injection.

ULTRASONOGRAPHY

Ultrasonography has been used as a diagnostic tool in other areas of the body; however, it has not been used ex-

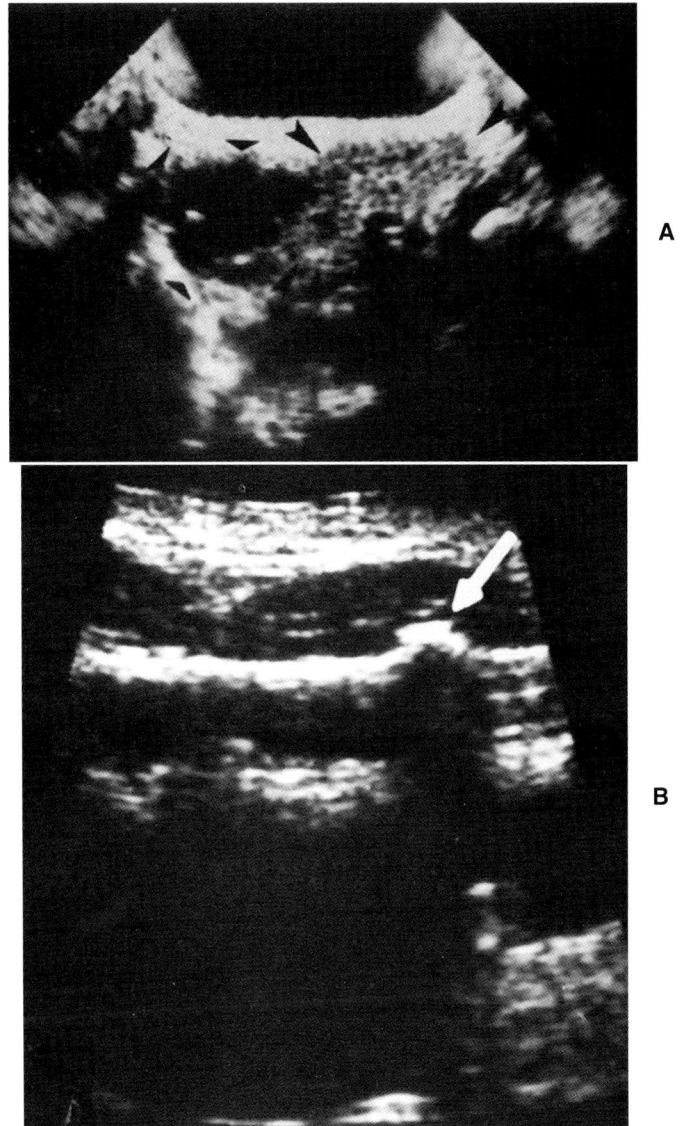

Figure 4-4 A, Ultrasound of submandibular region demonstrating a branchial cleft cyst. A sonolucent area devoid of internal echoes *(arrowheads)* is noted. Acoustic enhancement, typical of cysts, is represented by the echogenic area beneath the cyst. The normal, echogenic submandibular gland is demonstrated *(long arrowheads)*. **B,** Ultrasound examination of the right parotid demonstrating an echogenic shadowing sialolith in the hilus of the right parotid *(arrow)*. (From DelBalso AM, editor: *Maxillofacial imaging,* Philadelphia, 1990, WB Saunders.)

tensively in the evaluation of inflammatory lesions involving the head and neck.[54,62] One major limitation of ultrasound is its inability to penetrate osseous structures such as the maxilla and mandible. Consequently, its use is restricted to areas of the maxillofacial region where the sound wave does not have to penetrate bone (e.g., superficial lobe of parotid, lower maxillofacial region [submandibular triangle and neck]). Ultrasound is useful in differentiating between solid and cystic masses and in demonstrating the relationship of these masses to various structures (Figure 4-4). An echomorphological classification of soft tissue head and neck swelling, consisting of edema, infiltrate, preabscess, and echo-poor and echo-free abscess, has been reported.[104] Ultrasound is useful in the evaluation of sialoliths in patients with acute obstructive sialoadenitis or in whom contrast sialography was contraindicated because of a known history of iodine allergy. In these cases, the sialolith appears as a focal echogenic density exhibiting acoustic shadowing[22] (Figure 4-4, *B*).

MAXILLOFACIAL AND FASCIAL SPACE ANATOMY

MIDFACE AND PARANASAL SINUSES

The paired maxillae are the keystones of the maxillofacial skeleton. Located within each maxilla is a pyramidal air-filled space commonly known as the "maxillary sinus" (Figures 4-5 through 4-7).[125] The lateral wall of the maxilla, or infratemporal surface, separates the infratemporal fossa from the maxillary sinus; the medial wall of the maxilla, or nasal surface, forms a significant portion of the lateral wall of the nasal cavity. The superior, or orbital surface, of the maxillary bone forms the greatest portion of the floor of the orbit (roof of the sinus), separating the maxillary sinus from the orbit. Superomedially, the ethmomaxillary plate separates the maxillary sinus from the ethmoid air cells (Figure 4-8). The anterior wall of the maxilla provides contour to the midface and separates the maxillary sinus from the adjacent subcutaneous tissues of the face. The posterior wall of the sinus separates the maxillary sinus from the pterygopalatine fossa space. The maxillary sinuses drain into the middle meatus, in close proximity to the ducts draining the frontal sinuses and anterior ethmoid air cells. This close proximity of draining ostia is one pathway of spread of infection from one sinus to another.[26] Each maxillary sinus may have three extensions or recesses extending into adjacent structures. The alveolar recess is a

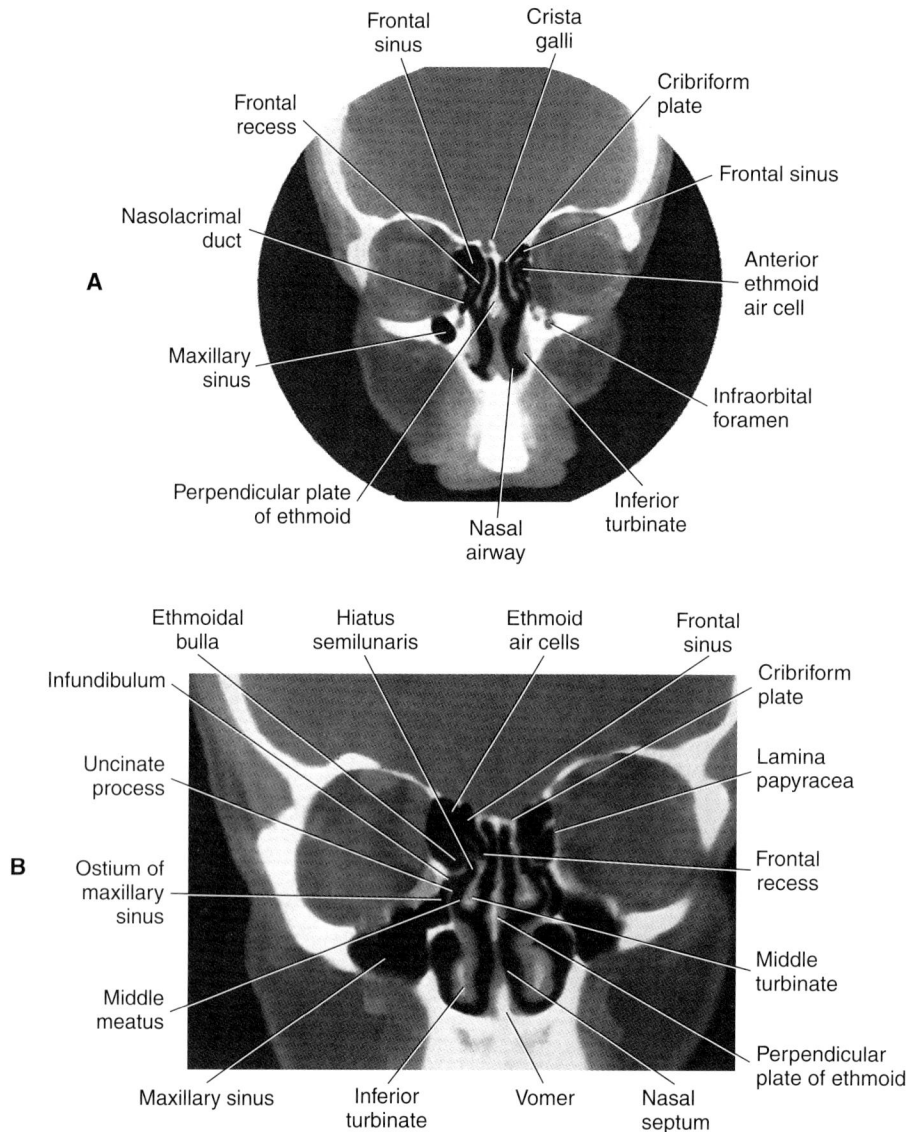

Figure 4-5 Coronal CT anatomy of paranasal sinuses. CT sections through the anterior face **(A),** osteomeatal unit **(B).** (From DelBalso AM, editor: *Maxillofacial imaging,* Philadelphia, 1990, WB Saunders.) (*A to E, G,* and *H* from DelBalso AM, editor: *Maxillofacial imaging,* Philadelphia, 1990, WB Saunders.)

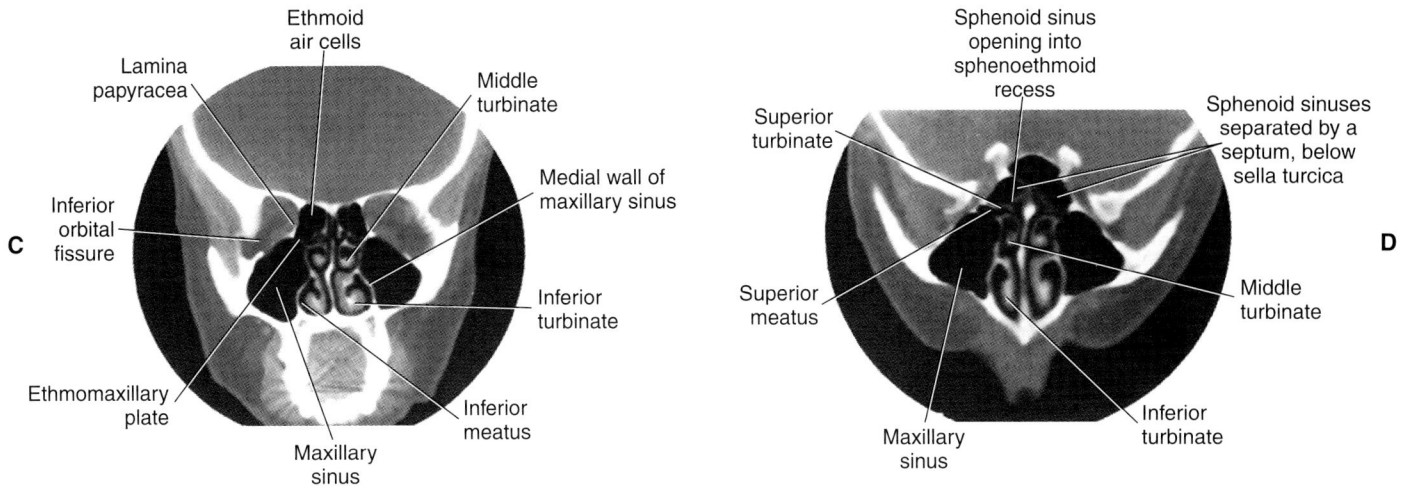

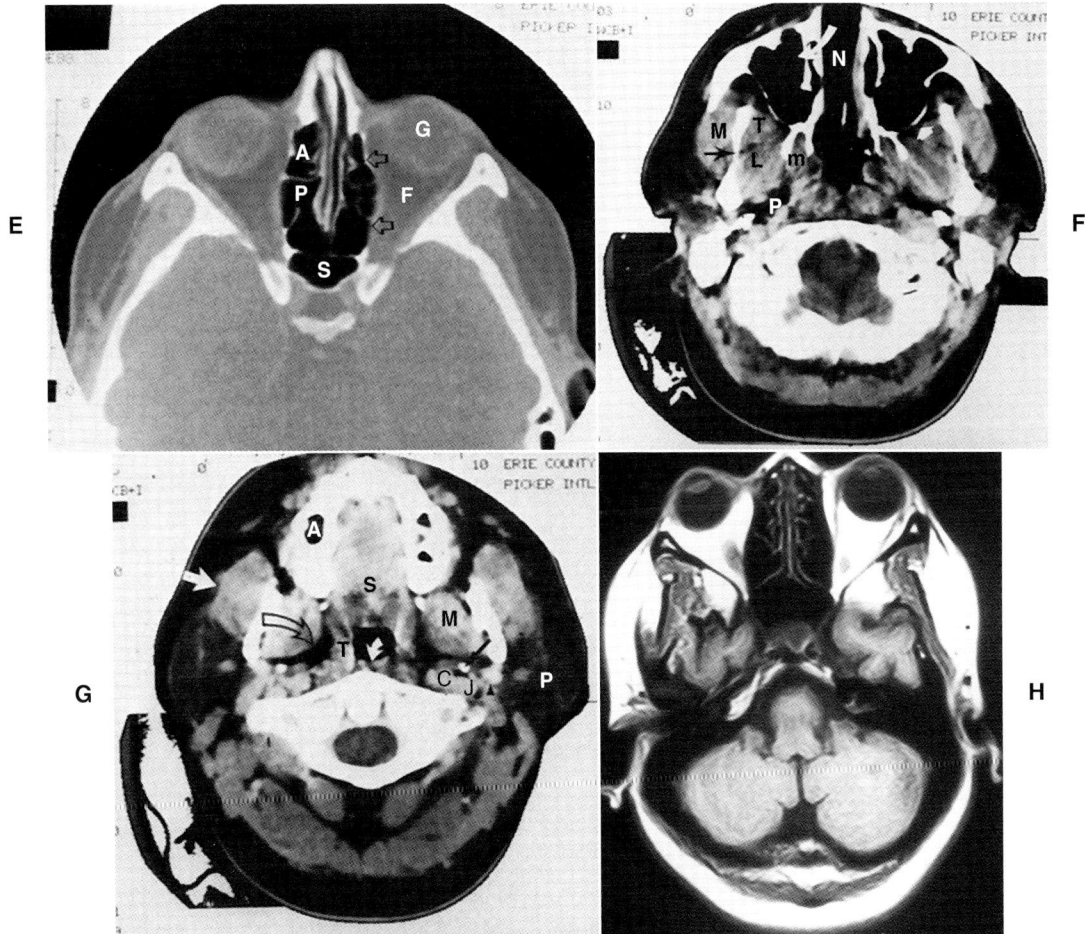

Figure 4-5, cont'd Posterior maxillary sinuses and ethmoid air cells **(C),** and posterior maxillary and sphenoid sinuses **(D).** Axial anatomy of maxillofacial and upper cervical regions. The following contrast-enhanced and T1-weighed axial images demonstrate the normal anatomy of the maxillofacial region. **E,** Axial CT section through ethmoid air cells and orbit. The anterior *(A)* and posterior *(P)* ethmoid air cells, sphenoid sinus *(S),* lamina papyracea *(open arrows),* globe *(G),* and intraconal fat *(F)* are identified. **F,** Axial T1-weighted MRI section through ethmoid sinuses and orbits. The orbital fat demonstrates high signal intensity, whereas the pneumatized ethmoid sinuses are devoid of signal intensity. The maxillary sinus *(curved white arrow),* nasal airway *(N),* retroantral fat pad *(arrowhead),* lateral *(L)* and medial *(m)* pterygoid muscles, masseter muscle *(M),* proximal ramus of mandible *(black straight arrow),* temporalis muscle *(T),* and parapharyngeal space *(P)* are identified. **G,** Axial CT image through maxillary sinus and nasopharynx. The alveolar recess of the maxillary sinus *(A)* masseter muscle *(large white arrow),* parotid gland *(P),* retromandibular vein *(small black arrowhead),* medial pterygoid muscle *(M),* ramus of mandible *(R),* parapharyngeal space *(curved open arrow),* styloid process *(small black arrow),* carotid artery *(C),* jugular vein *(J),* tonsillar pillars *(T),* and prevertebral soft tissues *(small curved white arrow)* are identified. **H,** Contrast-enhanced axial CT section through oral cavity at level of soft palate *(S).*

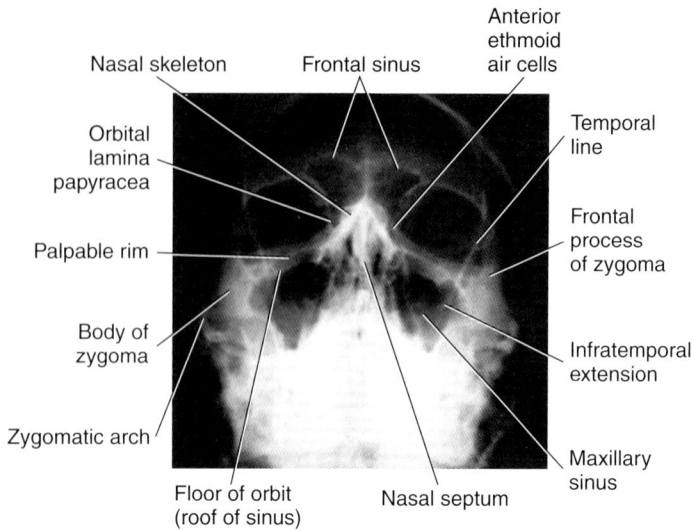

Figure 4-6 Waters' view of paranasal sinuses demonstrating the frontal, ethmoid, and maxillary sinuses and adjacent structures. (From DelBalso AM, editor: *Maxillofacial imaging*, Philadelphia, 1990, WB Saunders.)

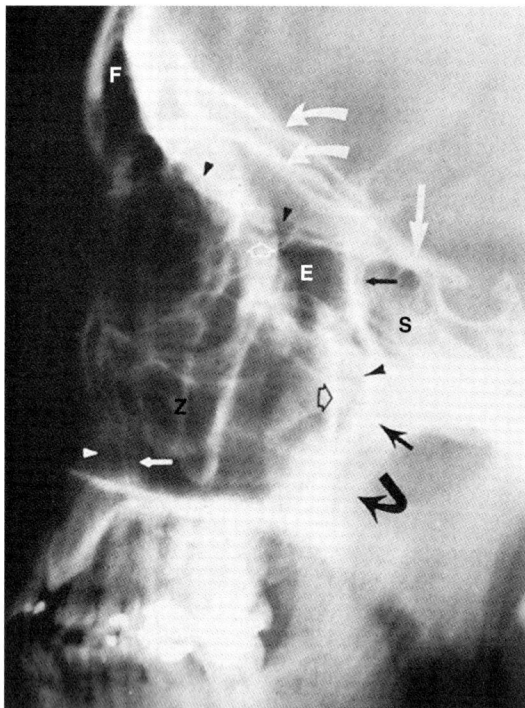

Figure 4-7 Lateral view of the paranasal sinuses demonstrating their relationship to adjacent anatomical structures: frontal sinus *(F)*, ethmoid sinus *(E)*, sphenoid sinus *(S)*, ethmoid-sphenoid septum *(small black arrow)*, planum sphenoidale *(large white arrow)*, cerebral surface of the roof of the ethmoid *(black arrowheads)*, cribriform plate of the ethmoid *(open white arrowhead)*, orbital roofs *(curved white arrows)*, posterior wall of the maxillary sinus *(open black arrowhead)*, pterygopalatine fossa *(large black arrowhead)*, pterygoid plates *(large black arrows)*, zygomatic recess of the maxillary sinus *(Z)*, anteromedial extent of the maxillary sinuses *(small white arrowhead)*, parallel lines representing anterolateral extent of the maxillary sinus *(small white arrow)*, and simulated "mass" produced by the confluence of the posterior turbinates and coronoid processes *(curved black arrow)*. (From DelBalso AM, editor: *Maxillofacial imaging*, Philadelphia, 1990, WB Saunders.)

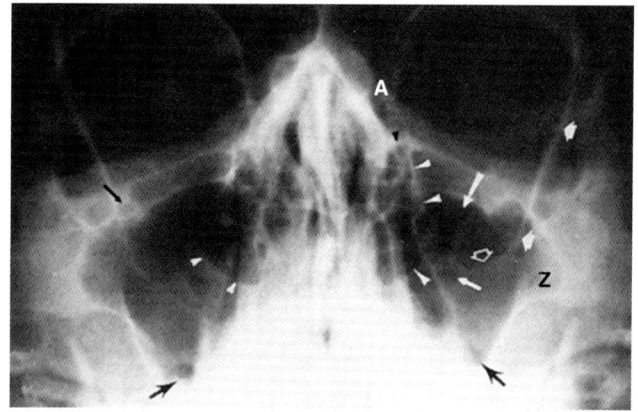

Figure 4-8 Coned-down Waters' view of maxillary sinuses demonstrating structures commonly superimposed over the maxillary sinuses. These include infraorbital foramen *(small black arrow)*, superior orbital fissure *(large white arrow)*, foramen rotundum *(small white arrow)*, foramen ovale *(large black arrow)*, lateral extension of sphenoid sinus *(small white arrowhead)*, ethmomaxillary plate *(black arrowhead)*, posterior ethmoid air cells *(large white arrowheads)*, infratemporal extension *(open arrowheads)* of temporal line *(solid white arrowhead)*, zygomatic recess *(Z)*, and anterior ethmoid air cells *(A)*. (From DelBalso AM, editor: *Maxillofacial imaging*, Philadelphia, 1990, WB Saunders.)

ventral extension into the alveolar ridge, the orbital recess represents the apical most portion of the sinus, and the zygomatic recess represents pneumatization of the medial segment of the zygoma. The alveolar recess is often intimately related to the roots of the maxillary molars.* This close proximity allows for the extension of odontogenic infections from the molars to the sinus. Approximately 10% to 15% of bacterial sinusitis infections involving the maxillary sinus are of odontogenic origin. Once an infection of odontogenic or other origin has involved the sinus, it can extend through the sinus to involve any structure bordering the sinus.

The ethmoid bone lies deep to the maxilla. It is an important anatomical bridge between the paired maxillae and base of the skull (Figure 4-9). The ethmoid bone is composed of bilateral, pyramidal-shaped bodies termed the *labyrinth*, each containing 5 to 18 individual air cells.[15,75,83] These air cells are often collectively referred to as an *ethmoid sinus* and are divided into anterior, middle, and posterior groups. Each group has a different drainage pattern. The ethmoid air cells are separated from the maxillary sinuses by the ethmomaxillary plate and from the sphenoid sinuses by the ethmosphenoid septum (Figure 4-10).[83] The lateral portion of each ethmoid labyrinth forms a large segment of the medial orbital wall. This segment of the ethmoid is known as the orbital plate of the ethmoid bone, or *lamina papyracea*. The lamina papyracea is a relatively thin bone that can readily allow the extension of ethmoid sinusitis to the orbit.

Paranasal sinuses are also located in the frontal and sphenoid bones. The frontal sinuses are paired, often

*References 3, 43, 101, 102, 107, 124, 129.

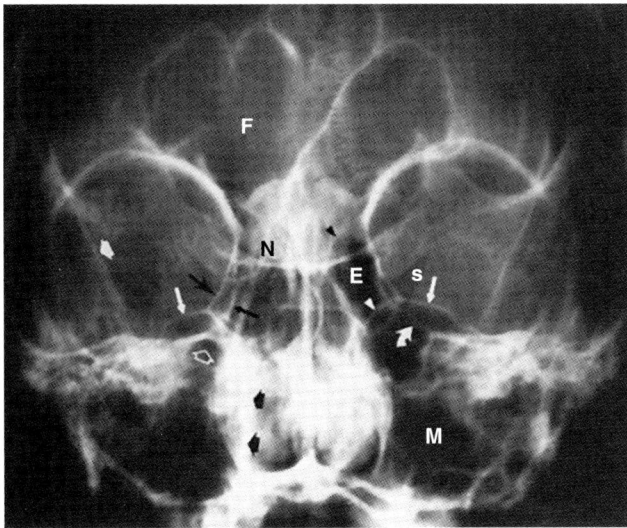

Figure 4-9 Caldwell's view. Posterior roof of the maxillary sinus *(small white arrow)*, anterior roof of the maxillary sinus *(curved white arrow)*, maxillary sinus *(M)*, ethmomaxillary plate *(white arrowhead)*, anterior *(small black arrow)* and posterior segment of the lamina papyracea *(large black arrow)*, superior orbital fissures *(S)*, roof of the ethmoid sinus *(small black arrowhead)*, ethmoid sinus *(E)*, temporal line or linea innominata *(solid white arrowhead)*, superior recess of nasal cavity *(N)*, medial wall of the maxillary sinuses, *(solid black arrowheads)*, foramen rotundum *(open white arrowhead)*, and frontal sinus *(F)* are demonstrated. (From DelBalso AM, editor: *Maxillofacial imaging*, Philadelphia, 1990, WB Saunders.)

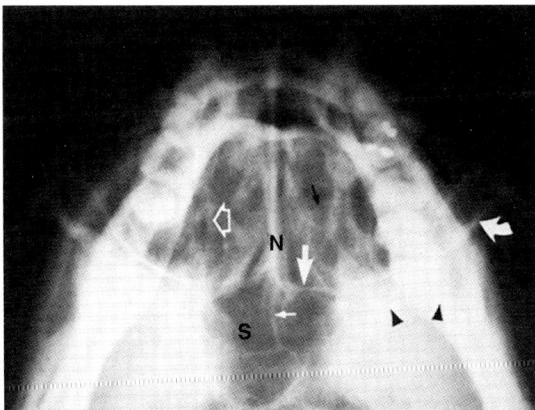

Figure 4-10 Submentovertex (base) view of the paranasal sinuses demonstrating the relationship of the paranasal sinuses to adjacent structures. The antral *(large black arrow)*, orbital *(curved white arrow)*, and cranial *(solid black arrowhead)* lines; medial wall of the maxillary sinus *(open white arrowhead)*; nasal septum *(N)*; sphenoid sinus *(S)*; intrasphenoid septum separating the sphenoid sinuses *(small white arrow)*; ethmoid-sphenoid septum *(large white arrow)*; and ethmoid air cells *(small black arrow)* are indicated. (From DelBalso AM, editor: *Maxillofacial imaging*, Philadelphia, 1990, WB Saunders.)

asymmetrically developed air spaces located entirely within the frontal bone. They demonstrate the greatest amount of variation in development, ranging from complete agenesis to massive pneumatization of the frontal bone. The paired sphenoid sinuses are located within the sphenoid

bone below the sella turcica. The midline sphenoid sinuses are intimately related to a number of important structures, including the orbit, pituitary, optic chiasm, cavernous sinus, and internal carotid arteries.

Like the frontal sinus, the sphenoid sinuses can demonstrate variable degrees of pneumatization. The two often asymmetrical sinuses are separated by an intrasinus septum and infrequently communicate. The septum is usually located in the midline anteriorly and usually deviates to one side posteriorly (see Figure 4-10).

An important functional entity is the ostiomeatal complex, which is a functional entity composed of the middle turbinate and meatus, ethmoid bulla, hiatus semilunaris, uncinate process, ostium of the maxillary sinus, and infundibulum (see Figure 4-5). The ostia of all paranasal sinuses, except for the posterior ethmoid air cells and sphenoid sinuses, open into the complex. The middle meatus is located between the middle inferior turbinates on the lateral wall of the nasal cavity. Located in the cephalad segment of the middle meatus is the ethmoid bulla. The ethmoid bulla receives drainage from the middle ethmoid air cells by means of ostia located on or above the bulla. Located immediately below the ethmoid bulla is a groove known as the *hiatus semilunaris*. Inferiorly, the *hiatus semilunaris* is delineated by a ridge known as the *uncinate process*. The anterior ethmoid air cells can drain directly into the anterior segment of the hiatus semilunaris known as the *ethmoid infundibulum* or into the frontonasal duct. The frontonasal duct, which drains the frontal sinus, may drain in front of, above, or directly into the ethmoid infundibulum. The ostium of the maxillary sinus is located posterior to the ethmoid infundibulum. In the ostiomeatal complex the draining ostia are in close proximity, which allows for the rapid spread of infection from one sinus to another. In addition, anatomical abnormalities of one or more components of the ostiomeatal complex can impair sinus ventilation, drainage, or both, thereby facilitating the development of a sinusitis.

DIAGNOSTIC IMAGING OF THE MIDFACE AND PARANASAL SINUSES

Plain Film Studies Diagnostic imaging of inflammatory processes involving the midface usually starts with plain film study, which generally consists of a facial bone or paranasal sinuses series. Essential views that must be included in any study of the midface and paranasal sinuses are the Waters, Caldwell, and lateral views. Additional views such as a posteroanterior or submentovertex (SMV) view also may be needed to evaluate the patient fully. The Waters, Caldwell, lateral, and SMV views are intended to demonstrate inflammatory processes involving the paranasal sinuses.

The Waters view provides optimal visualization of anterior facial structures free of superimposed posterior structures such as the petrous ridge of the temporal bone (see Figures 4-6 and 4-8). Particularly useful in the evaluation of the maxillary sinuses, this view provides optimal visualization of the lateral and medial walls of the maxillary sinus, inferior orbital (palpable orbital) rim, and floor of the orbit (roof of the sinus). The Waters view also demonstrates the anterior portion of the medial wall of the orbit free from superimposed posterior segments.[86] An important structure often identified on the Waters and Caldwell views is the ethmomaxillary plate, a bony plate separating the ethmoid air cells and maxillary sinus (see Figure 4-9). Destruction of this plate indicates a neoplastic or an aggressive inflammatory process. The alveolar recess, a normal extension of the maxillary sinus, often is intimately related to the roots of the maxillary molars. This close relationship can result in the spread of odontogenic infections to the maxillary sinuses. Although not considered the primary view for the evaluation of the ethmoid and frontal sinuses, the Waters view can provide information concerning their status because it is the only view that projects the anterior and posterior ethmoid cells independent of each other.[86] The anterior ethmoid air cells are projected superiorly into the medial aspect of the orbit, and the posterior air cells are projected over the medial aspect of the maxillary sinus.

The Caldwell view provides optimal visualization of midline and posterior facial structures such as the orbits, the ethmoid and frontal sinuses, and nasal fossae (see Figure 4-9). The lower half of the maxillary sinus is not well visualized on the Caldwell view because of the superimposed petrous ridges of the temporal bone. The orbital floor or roof of the sinus is represented by two lines: a superior line representing the posterior roof and an inferior line representing the anterior roof. This projection can provide a good overview of the relative lucency or opacity of the entire ethmoid sinus complex. However, individual assessment of groups of ethmoid air cells is impossible because of the superimposition of anterior and posterior air cells. The laminae papyraceae and ethmomaxillary plate are well demonstrated on this projection. The laminae papyraceae are visualized as two lines: a more medially located line representing the anterior segment and a more laterally located line representing the posterior segment. The ethmomaxillary plate is visualized as is the osseous septum separating the maxillary and ethmoid sinuses. The Caldwell view provides the best demonstration of the frontal sinuses, which often demonstrate the greatest degree of anatomical variation of the paranasal sinuses.

The lateral view in a facial bone series is usually an upright, left lateral view; in cases with right-sided symptoms, a right lateral view should be obtained instead (see Figure 4-7). Cross-table lateral views of the facial bones can be obtained in patients who are debilitated, those in whom acute sphenoid sinusitis is suspected and those in whom a definite air-fluid level cannot be demonstrated on upright lateral views. On the lateral view the respective sinuses are superimposed. However, the lateral view can provide important information concerning the various sinuses. This view often best demonstrates the presence of an air-fluid level in the maxillary sinuses and sphenoid sinuses. The anterior and posterior walls of the frontal sinuses are well demonstrated on the lateral view, making it an essential

view in the evaluation of destructive lesions that expand or erode the sinus walls (e.g., mucocele, osteomas). In addition, the lateral view is useful in differentiating between decreased translucency of the frontal sinuses as a result of sinus wall thickening or sinusitis. The lateral view also demonstrates the sphenoid sinuses and their relationships to the sella turcica and planum sphenoidale. Opacification of the sphenoid sinus can occur as a result of sphenoid sinusitis, mucocele formation, superior extension of a nasopharyngeal tumor, or inferior extension of a pituitary tumor.

The SMV view can be useful in assessing inflammatory processes involving the midface because it demonstrates the boundaries of the ethmoid, maxillary, and sphenoid sinuses, ethmosphenoid septa, and secondary septae between individual ethmoid air cells (see Figure 4-10). Three lines that should be noted on the SMV view are the antral, orbital, and middle cranial fossa lines. The antral line is shaped like an S or reverse S and defines the lateral and posterolateral walls of the maxillary sinus. The orbital line appears as a straight line superimposed over the orbital line and defines the lateral wall of the orbit. The C-shaped middle cranial fossa line is located slightly posterior to the antral and orbital lines and defines the anterior extent of the middle cranial fossa. The SMV is the only sinus projection demonstrating the sphenoid sinuses as separate structures, thereby pathological conditions noted on the lateral view can be localized and defined.

Computed Tomography and Magnetic Resonance Imaging   CT is the preferred imaging modality for the evaluation of inflammatory processes of the paranasal sinuses. CT allows ready demonstration of important soft tissue and osseous components of the paranasal sinuses and surrounding structures. Images obtained using bone windows can provide detailed anatomical information about the status of the ostiomeatal complex and underlying osseous structures. In addition, CT studies are readily performed and not subject to artifacts that can result from the dessication of sinus secretions that occurs in long-standing chronic sinusitis.

MRI is especially useful in the evaluation of sinonasal neoplasms because direct images can be obtained in planes other than the axial plane and MRI has superior soft tissue resolution. Contrast-enhanced MRI examinations are especially useful in demonstrating early tumor extension.

CT studies for the evaluation of infections involving the paranasal sinuses, midface, or both regions should be performed in the axial and direct coronal planes. The coronal sections must provide optimal demonstration of the ostiomeatal complex. Direct coronal images are also important when volume averaging may be occurring in segments of bone parallel to the CT scan plane, resulting in suboptimal demonstration of an area (e.g., the floor of the orbit). The scans should include all paranasal sinuses and adjacent structures. All axial and direct coronal sections should be imaged using bone and soft tissue win-

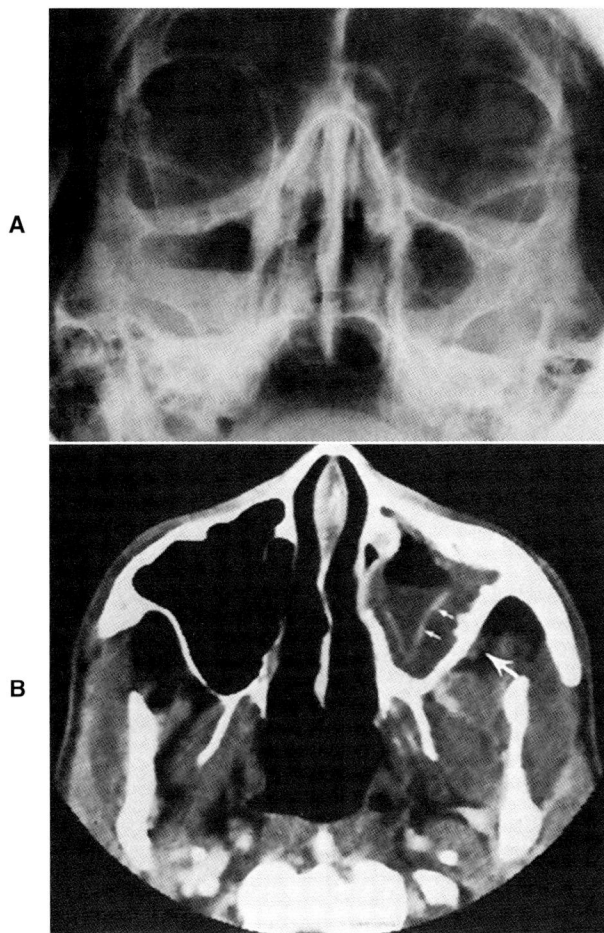

Figure 4-11 Acute sinusitis. **A,** Waters' view demonstrating air-fluid levels in both maxillary sinuses in a patient with acute bacterial sinusitis. Chronic mucosal thickening in the lateral aspect of the left maxillary sinus also is present. **B,** Contrast-enhanced axial computed tomographic section through the maxillary sinuses demonstrating bone and soft tissue changes associated with chronic and acute left maxillary sinusitis. Chronic changes include mucosal thickening and hyperostotic changes of the sinus walls. Extension of the inflammatory process into the retroantral fat pad *(arrow)* is noted. Acute changes consist of an air-fluid level in the sinus and mucosal enhancement *(small arrows).* (From DelBalso AM, editor: *Maxillofacial imaging,* Philadelphia, 1990, WB Saunders.)

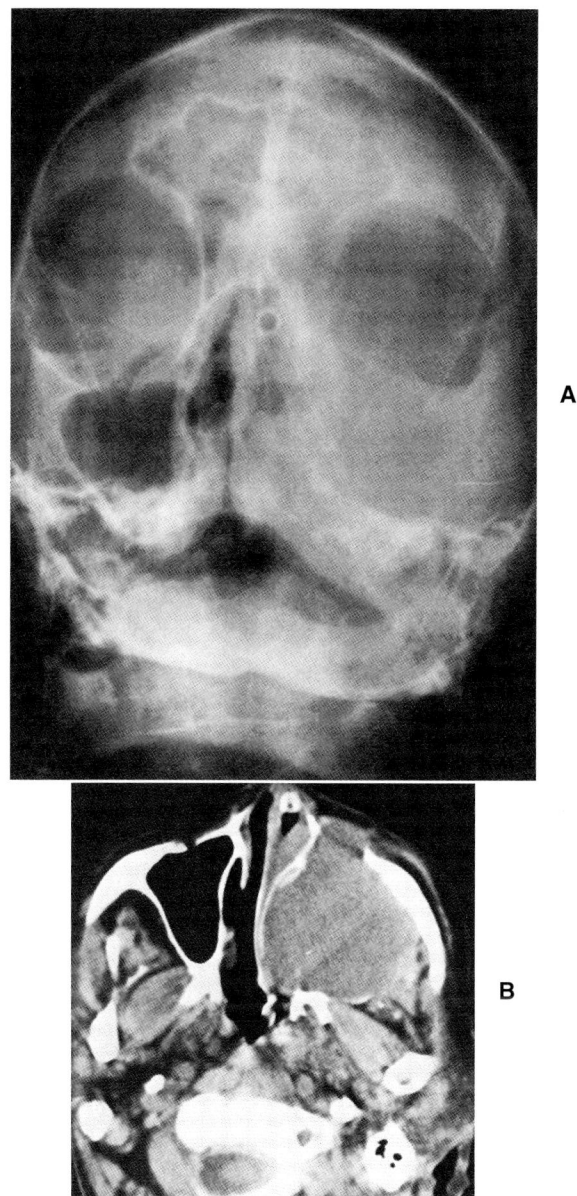

Figure 4-12 Left maxillary sinus mucocele. **A,** Waters' view demonstrating opacification of the left maxillary sinus and absence of the lateral and medial walls suggestive of a neoplastic process. **B,** Axial CT section through maxillary sinuses demonstrates an expansile soft tissue mass involving the left maxillary sinus with pressure atrophy of the sinus walls. (From DelBalso AM, editor: *Maxillofacial imaging,* Philadelphia, 1990, WB Saunders.)

dows. In addition, lung windows may be useful in evaluating the various air-containing components of the ostiomeatal complex.

Important abnormalities to be noted in the evaluation of the paranasal sinuses include opacification, presence of air-fluid levels (Figure 4-11), mucosal thickening and enhancement, soft tissue masses, hyperostotic changes, and bone displacement or destruction (Figure 4-12). In the evaluation of pathological processes involving the maxillary sinuses, involvement of adjacent structures should be noted. An important fat pad to be evaluated on axial CT sections is the retroantral fat pad, located adjacent to the lateral wall of the sinus (see Figures 4-5, *G,* and 4-11, *B*). Loss of this fat pad can occur as a result of the transmural extension of an inflammatory

or a neoplastic process involving the sinus. The ethmomaxillary plate is another important osseous structure to be identified and evaluated on direct coronal CT sections. The ethmomaxillary plate separates the maxillary sinus from the adjacent ethmoid air cells (see Figures 4-8 and 4-9). Destruction of this plate of bone occurs with aggressive inflammatory and neoplastic processes involving both the maxillary and the adjacent ethmoid sinus.

Soft tissue abnormalities to be noted on CT examinations of the paranasal sinuses and midface include orbital

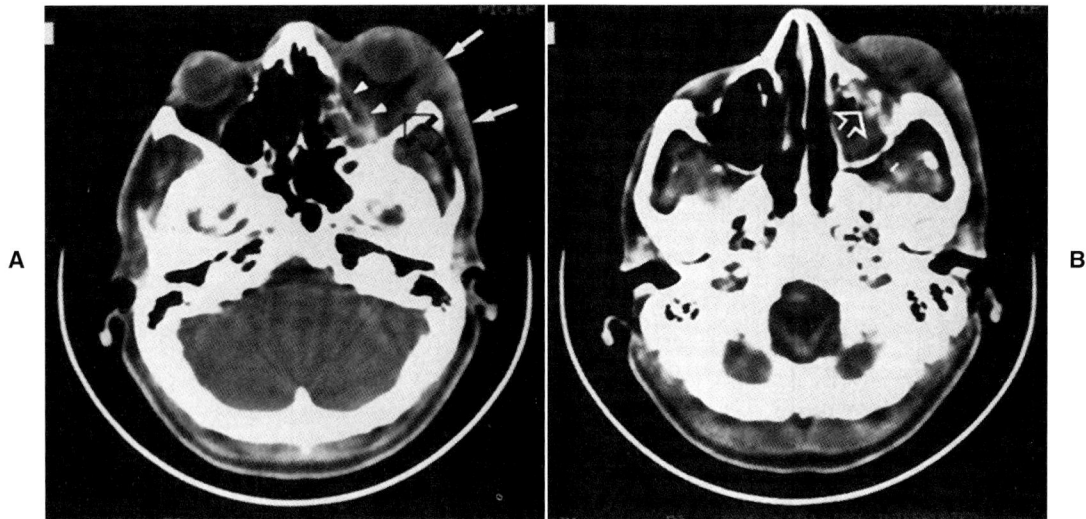

Figure 4-13 Development of an acute left pansinusitis with involvement of the left orbit 2 weeks after the extraction of a left maxillary molar. **A,** Axial CT section through the orbit demonstrates opacification of the left ethmoid air cells, thickening, and displacement of the medial orbital tissues caused by a subperiosteal abscess *(arrowhead),* and increased density of the orbital fat and thickening of the lateral rectus muscle *(open arrow)* reflecting the development of orbital cellulitis of the soft tissues of the left side of the face are also demonstrated *(white arrow).* **B,** Osteomyelitis of the orbital floor is evident on this section through the superior maxillary sinus *(white arrow).* (From DelBalso AM, editor: *Maxillofacial imaging,* Philadelphia, 1990, WB Saunders.)

involvement (Figure 4-13), bone destruction (Figure 4-14), thickening and ill definition of muscles (myositis), ill definition or loss of fascial planes (fasciitis), edema of overlying skin and subcutaneous tissues (cellulitis), mass effect, fluid collections with or without peripheral contrast enhancement, and adenopathy.

The evaluation of the paranasal sinuses must also include a thorough evaluation of the ostiomeatal complex (see Figure 4-5, *B*). This complex is a particularly important area because the draining ostia of all of the paranasal sinuses except for the posterior ethmoid and sphenoid sinuses are in close proximity. Anatomical abnormalities of one or more components of the ostiomeatal complex can impair sinus ventilation, drainage, or both, thereby facilitating the development of a sinusitis. In addition, the close proximity of the draining ostia allows for the rapid spread of infection from one sinus to another. Abnormalities commonly encountered on coronal images of the ostiomeatal complex include prominent pneumatization of the middle turbinate (concha bullosa), paradoxically curved turbinate, uncinate bulla, medially curved uncinate process, septal deviation, and oversized ethmoid bulla. Pathological abnormalities that can be seen in this area include chronic mucosal thickening in any segment of the osteomeatal complex, nasal polyps, and rarely, nasal neoplasms.

PARANASAL SINUS PATHOLOGY

Inflammatory Disorders   Inflammatory disorders represent the most common pathological conditions in-

volving the midface and paranasal sinuses. Inflammatory disorders involving the paranasal sinuses may be divided into three general categories based on the underlying cause: infectious, noninfectious, and granulomatous disorders.*

INFECTIOUS SINUSITIS

The paranasal sinuses can be affected by a number of infectious agents, including viruses, bacteria, and fungi. Infectious processes involving the paranasal sinuses are often classified according to duration or clinical course of the disease, with acute lasting days or weeks, subacute lasting weeks, and chronic lasting weeks to months. The radiographic manifestations of these diverse entities cover a limited spectrum of radiographic findings.

Acute Infectious Sinusitis   Acute sinusitis most often follows an upper respiratory tract infection; however, it may occur after trauma, excessive drying, allergic edema with occlusion of draining ostia, nasal obstruction, or the introduction of foreign bodies.† Acute sinusitis is most often viral, occurring in conjunction with a viral nasal infection. The radiographic findings in acute viral sinusitis vary, ranging from clear sinuses, to a slight increased thickness of the mucoperiosteum, to generalized increased radiographic density. These findings are a reflection of mucosal edema

---

*References 1, 17, 35, 37, 43, 60, 70, 101, 102, 106, 122, 124, 129.
†References 1, 3, 46, 106, 107, 116.

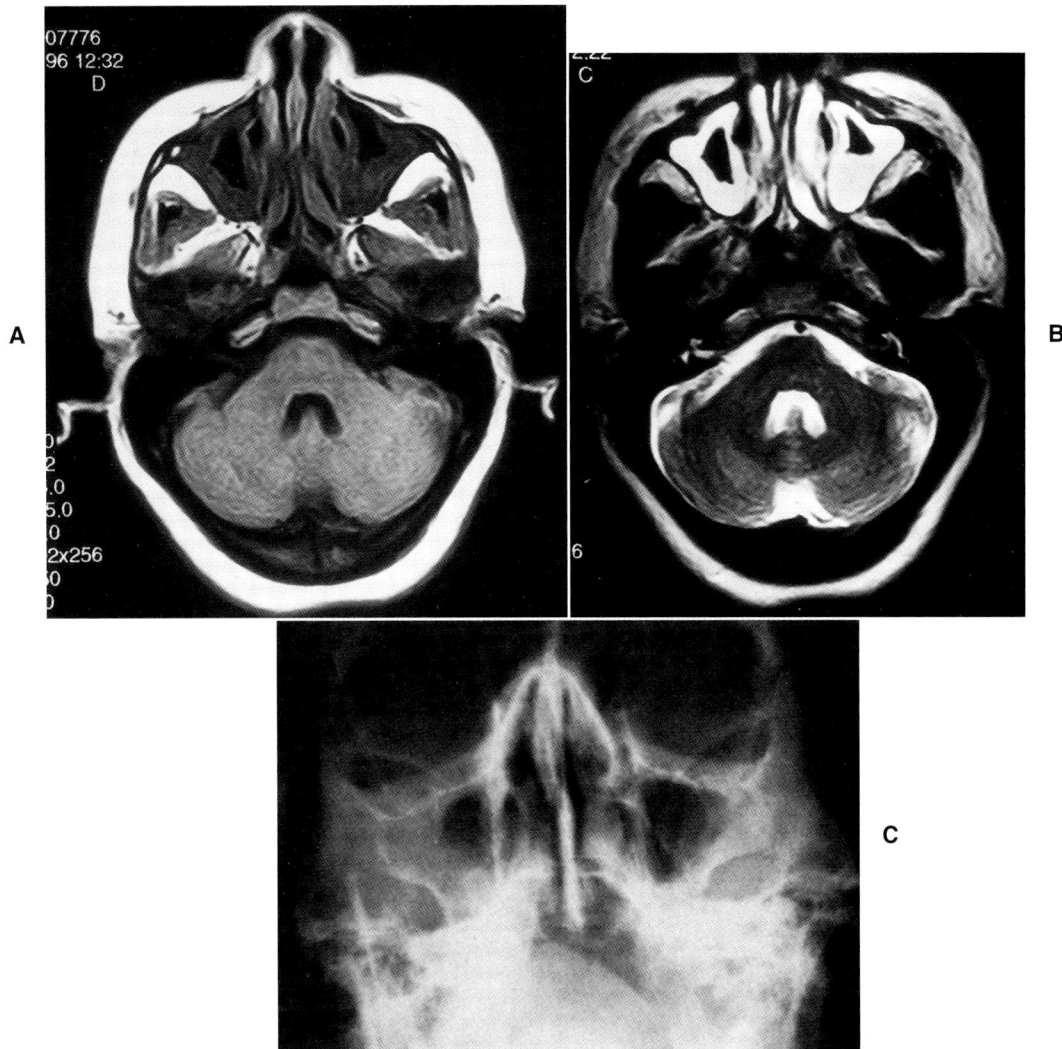

Figure 4-14 A and **B,** MRI scan of chronic sinusitis. **A,** T1- and **B,** T2-weighted axial sections through maxillary sinuses demonstrating chronic mucosal thickening. On the T1-weighted sequence the mucosal changes are of low signal intensity, whereas on the T2-weighted sequences, they are of high intensity. A small air-fluid level is noted on the T2 sequence that is not readily apparent on the T1 sequences. **C,** Waters' view demonstrating chronic mucosal changes in both maxillary sinuses.

caused by vasodilation and increased production of mucus by the goblet cells and mucosal glands.

In the evaluation of a sinus demonstrating increased radiographic density, correlation of the radiographic and clinical findings is important because a number of pathological processes can begin with a similar radiographic appearance. In addition to mucosal edema, increased radiographic density can result from chronic mucosal changes caused by chronic sinusitis, previous trauma, and prior surgical procedures. Other factors that can result in an apparent increased radiographic density of a sinus include hypoplasia of the sinus with or without variations in the thickness of the osseous walls of the sinus.

Acute bacterial sinusitis results from secondary bacterial infection of the obstructed sinus by bacteria normally found in the nasal airway and oral cavity. The two bacteria most frequently involved in acute bacterial sinusitis are *Haemophilus influenzae* and *Streptococcus pneumoniae.* Other less commonly involved bacteria include *Staphylococcus epidermidis, Streptococcus viridans, Branhamella catarrhalis,* and the diphtheroids.[3,17,43,101,102] Approximately 10% to 15% of maxillary sinus pathological conditions are dental in origin and often are associated with abscessed molars and premolars, the roots of which are closely related to the floor of the maxillary sinus.* Acute sinusitis also may occur after violation of the sinus and the introduction of oral bacteria during dental surgical procedures (see Figure 4-13). Improper closure of a communication can result in an oral-antral fistula and chronic sinusitis. Purulent mucosal discharge results in purulent exudate fluid accumulating in

---

*References 1, 3, 102, 103, 124, 129, 130.

the sinus, causing an air-fluid level[17,70,106,122,130] (see Figure 4-11). The radiographic findings in acute bacterial sinusitis vary and range from a generalized increased density reflective of mucosa edema, to an air-fluid level caused by a buildup of purulent material, to a complete opacification of the sinus caused by the presence of a large amount of purulent material and mucosal edema. In bacterial sinusitis the air-fluid level, if present, is limited to one or two sinuses. Although the air-fluid level is most often the result of acute bacterial sinusitis, it also can result from recent antral lavage, recent trauma, or blood dyscrasia with bleeding into the sinus, stressing the need to always correlate radiographic findings with clinical history. CT examinations demonstrate air-fluid levels in the dependent portion of involved sinuses (see Figure 4-11, *B*). On MRI examination the appearance of an uncomplicated acute sinusitis reflects the underlying pathological condition. Inflamed, edematous mucosa and free fluid typically demonstrate low signal intensity on T1-weighted and increased signal intensity on T2-weighted sequences[43,66,111,122] (see Figure 4-14).

Acute Noninfectious Sinusitis   Allergic rhinitis and sinusitis are noninfectious, inflammatory processes affecting approximately 10% of the population.[1,43,116] These two conditions represent the most common acute, noninfectious processes invading the sinonasal tract.[3,106] The seasonal conditions are the result of immunoglobulin E reagin–antibody reactions. In allergic sinusitis the mucoperiosteum associated primarily with the maxillary sinuses becomes hyperplastic and grossly edematous. Similar changes often occur in the mucosa lining the ethmoid, frontal, and sphenoid sinuses. This thickening is often uniform and symmetrical, although the formation of localized polypoid masses often occurs. The radiographic findings in allergic sinusitis mirror these various mucosal changes. In addition to generalized or local mucosal thickening, radiographic studies demonstrate edema of the turbinates. Air-fluid levels are not associated with acute allergic sinusitis and, when present, indicate the presence of bacterial superinfection.[106]

Acute sinusitis, regardless of the cause, may evolve into a chronic sinusitis. Factors that may facilitate this evolution include impaired drainage and aeration of the involved sinus, persistent infection, loss of cilia, and mucosal changes.[1,3] Inadequate sinus drainage and aeration may result from mechanical factors such as a deviated septum, nasal polyps, adenoid hypertrophy, nasopharyngeal tumors, and edematous mucosa in the region of the draining ostia. Inadequate sinus drainage can result in the accumulation within the sinus of a medium favorable to bacterial growth, whereas impaired aeration may facilitate the growth of the pathogenic anaerobic and microaerophilic bacteria. Inadequate treatment of an acute bacterial sinusitis may result in a chronic, smoldering infection that can involve the adjacent bone. Mucosal changes, often irreversible in nature, may result from chemical injuries or through an allergic mechanism. Chemical injuries may result in a loss of ciliated epithelium, thereby impairing normal sinus toilet and destroying the regenerative capacity of the mucosa. Allergies may promote the development of chronic sinusitis by causing mucosal edema and hypersecretion; both impair normal sinus drainage and facilitate the growth of bacteria. Grossly and radiographically, chronic sinusitis is characterized by irreversible mucosal hyperplasia and thickening that often results in mucosal folds or pseudopolyps[97,106,119,129,130] (see Figure 4-11). In addition to involving the mucosa, the inflammatory process can extend to the underlying bone, resulting in hyperostotic changes, the hallmark of chronic sinusitis.

Acute bacterial infections may occur in patients with chronic sinusitis. Radiographically, an air-fluid level and mucosal thickening in the involved sinus may be noted. CT studies demonstrate contrast enhancement of the inflamed mucosa, mucosal thickening, and an air-fluid level.

On MRI examination the thickened edematous mucosa typically demonstrates low signal intensity on T1-weighted and increased signal intensity on T2-weighted sequences similar to that seen in acute sinusitis (Figure 4-14). However, the appearance of entrapped secretions can vary depending on the degree of hydration. On T1- and T2-weighted sequences, the signal intensities decrease as the secretions become more concentrated. Signal voids on T1 and T2 sequences are noted when the secretions are dried and solid.[111]

Complications of Sinusitis   The development of chronic sinusitis represents one complication associated with acute or recurrent episodes of sinusitis. In addition, a number of other complications are associated with acute and chronic sinusitis. These complications can be divided into two main groups: those limited solely to the sinus and those involving adjacent structures. The first group of complications includes formation of hypertrophic polyps, mucosal cysts, and mucoceles. The second group results from extension of the inflammatory process to adjacent structures and includes a number of inflammatory nasal, orbital, and intracranial lesions or osteomyelitis of the sinus walls.

Mucous Retention Cysts   The most common local complication of sinusitis is the formation of mucous retention cysts, occurring in approximately 10% of the population.[7,70,106,119,128] These cysts result from blockage of the ducts draining seromucous glands followed by cystic expansion. The lesions occur most often in the maxillary sinus and range from less than 1 cm to large lesions filling nearly all the sinus. In contrast to mucoceles that mold the sinus walls, mucous retention cysts adhere to the sinus cavity without causing any bone expansion. Radiographically, these lesions usually appear as rounded, soft tissue densities within the involved sinus (Figure 4-15). A lesion of dental origin that at times can have an initial radiographic appearance identical to that of a retention cyst is a periapical dental lesion involving one of the maxillary molars. These cystic lesions are the result of inflammatory processes occurring at the apex of a nonvital tooth. They can either directly involve the maxillary sinus or be located

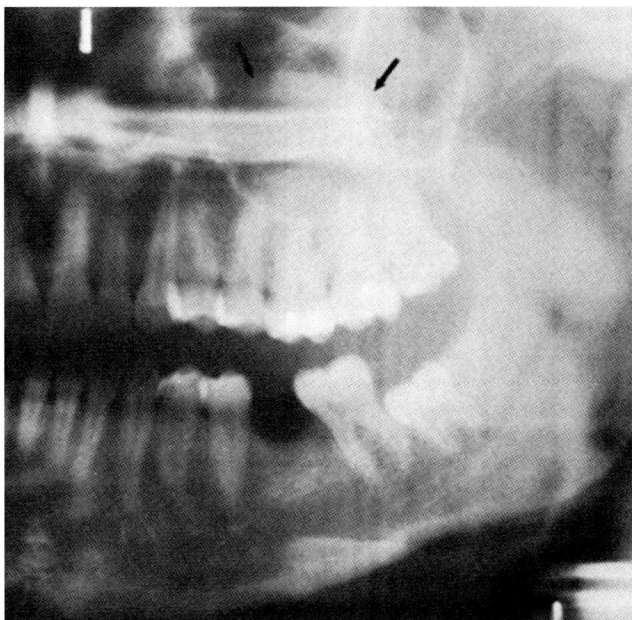

Figure 4-15 Mucous retention cysts. Panoramic view of mandible demonstrating a mucous retention cyst in the left maxillary sinus *(arrows)*.

within the adjacent alveolar bone and projected over the sinus, thereby simulating pathological findings of sinus origin. In these cases, correlation with the vitality of adjacent teeth is required to distinguish between lesions of sinus and dental origin. On MRI examinations these lesions typically demonstrate low to intermediate signal intensity on T1 and high signal intensity on T2 sequences.

Mucocele   The most significant local complication of sinusitis is the formation of a mucocele. Mucoceles are true cystic lesions lined by the sinus mucosa. Mucoceles result from obstruction of the draining ostia followed by the continued secretion of fluid in the obstructed sinus or air cell.* Ostial obstruction is usually the result of inflammatory or allergic processes, although it also can result from neoplastic, postsurgical, or traumatic factors.[106,112,119] As a result of the continued fluid secretion into the obstructed sinus or air cell, a buildup of fluid results in pressure atrophy, osseous remodeling, and bowing of the sinus walls (see Figure 4-12). The expansile character of mucoceles underlies their clinical presentation. Mucoceles occur most commonly in the frontal sinus and ethmoid air cells.[106,107] Frontal mucoceles constitute approximately two thirds of all mucoceles, whereas ethmoid mucoceles constitute approximately 25% to 30%.[7,106,109] Ethmoid sinus mucoceles more often involve the anterior ethmoid air cells; however, they also can originate in the posterior ethmoid air cells and expand into the adjacent sphenoid sinus.[109,122] These mucoceles are sometimes referred to as *sphenoethmoid mucoceles*. Maxillary sinus mucoceles are uncommon and constitute approximately 5% to 10% of all mucoceles.[106] On rare occa-

sions, mucoceles occur in the sphenoid sinus and within septated compartments in the maxillary sinus.[38,84,109,112] They also may occur in the maxillary sinuses after Caldwell-Luc procedures. Mucoceles can become infected and are then termed *pyoceles*. Certain radiographic characteristics are common to all mucoceles on plain film and CT studies. In addition, some radiographic findings are related to the local effects of the mucocele. Common plain film and CT findings include the presence of an expansile mass causing displacement or bowing of the sinus or air cell walls. Axial CT sections through all noninfected mucoceles typically demonstrate a well-circumscribed, nonenhancing soft tissue mass. Peripheral macroscopic calcification is evident in approximately 5% of mucoceles.[129] The presence of rim enhancement or increased density of the soft tissue mass suggests the presence of infection and are more accurately diagnosed as a pyocele.

Plain film findings associated with frontal mucoceles include clouding of the involved sinus, erosion of the intrasinus septae, the presence of a smooth wall sinus cavity, and ill definition or loss of the mucoperiosteal line.[106] Axial CT sections through frontal sinus mucoceles also may demonstrate intracranial and intraorbital extension, proptosis, sutural diastasis, and supraorbital soft tissue masses.

Ethmoid mucoceles are best diagnosed on CT studies and demonstrate a nonenhancing, expansile, soft tissue mass causing bowing of the walls of air cells. Ethmoid mucoceles originating in the posterior ethmoid sinuses (sphenoethmoid mucoceles) may demonstrate significant involvement and expansion of the adjacent sphenoid sinus. In addition, axial CT scans also demonstrate orbital and nasal involvement. Maxillary sinus mucoceles often initially display plain film findings suggestive of a malignancy. These findings include opacification of the involved sinus and often loss or apparent destruction of the sinus walls (see Figure 4-12). CT studies show a well-circumscribed mass filling the sinus with bowing or atrophy of the sinus. On MRI examination the appearance of mucoceles can vary depending on the degree of hydration of mucoid material present. Uncomplicated mucoceles demonstrate low signal intensity on T1 and high signal intensity on T2 sequences. However, depending on the degree of hydration present, mucoceles also may demonstrate increased signal intensity on T1 and T2 sequences or an absence of signal intensity on the sequences.[111]

Sphenoid sinus mucoceles on plain film and CT studies demonstrate opacification of the sinus and expansion and thinning of the sinus walls.[84] Intracranial extension and anterior extension also can occur. Intracranial extension can result in sellar or parasellar masses on CT studies.[84,106] Anterior extension into the posterior ethmoid air cells also can occur, often resulting in bone destruction indistinguishable from that caused by a malignancy.[106]

Orbital and Extrasinus Complications of Sinusitis   If improperly treated or unresponsive to appropriate therapy, acute sinusitis and, more rarely, chronic sinusitis can

---

*References 7, 97, 106, 119, 129, 130.

involve the adjacent orbit and structures.* Acute orbital complications include cellulitis or abscess formation, subperiosteal abscess formation and superior orbital fissure syndrome, and osteomyelitis of the osseous walls (see Figure 4-13). Orbital complications usually are the result of an isolated ethmoiditis, ethmoiditis and sinusitis involving the adjacent frontal or maxillary sinuses, or both. Improperly treated intracranial extension of an acute sinusitis is associated with significant morbidity and mortality rates. Intracranial extension can occur along anatomical pathways including perineural by means of a retrograde thrombophlebitis or through direct spread from an involved sinus bordering the cranial fossa or hematogenous routes. Intracranial complications include purulent meningitis, acute subdural or epidural empyemas, brain abscesses, and cavernous sinus thrombosis. Osteomyelitis of the wall of an involved sinus also can occur. This usually is found in the frontal sinus, although it also can occur in the maxillary sinus, usually after dental extractions. An unusual complication of osteomyelitis of the frontal sinus in the pediatric age group is extension of the inflammatory process into the cranium and the development of a superficial subgaleal abscess without evidence of bone destruction, resulting in a clinical entity known as a *Pott's puffy tumor*.[1,39,97,106] Radiographic findings associated with osteomyelitis are evident 7 to 14 days and include loss of the sharp outline of the sinus margin and a patchy "motheaten" appearance of involved bone resulting from localized decalcification.[97] These areas subsequently may develop sclerotic changes, focal sequestration, or both. CT provides optimal demonstration of sequestrae that may not be readily seen on plain films (see Chapter 14).

Fungal Sinusitis   The two major fungal infections involving the paranasal sinuses are aspergillosis (caused by genus *Aspergillus*) and mucormycosis (caused by genera *Rhizopus, Mucor,* and *Absidia*). Aspergillosis is the most common fungal infection of the paranasal sinuses.[53,95] Aspergilli are ubiquitous saprophytic molds that occasionally become pathogenic in humans. Aspergillosis of the paranasal sinuses can occur in a number of distinct forms. In the otherwise healthy person, it may be found as a chronic, noninvasive form of sinusitis, usually limited to a single maxillary sinus.[8,14,72,77,121] The radiographic findings associated with this form of aspergillosis are nonspecific. In the early phases a soft tissue mass representing a mass of mycelia may be noted, whereas in later phases, a homogeneous opacification of the involved sinus may be found.[8,61,64,122] In approximately half the advanced cases, dense concretions accumulate within the sinus; such findings are considered pathognomonic of aspergillosis. These radiodensities are composed primarily of tertiary calcium phosphate (apatite) and smaller quantities of calcium sulfide and heavy metal salts.[61,117] These materials are deposited in necrotic areas of the mycelium, usually in the center of the mass filling the sinus, and are readily detected on plain film and CT studies.[61] CT sections also demonstrate thickening of the osseous sinus walls and low-density areas within the soft tissue mass filling the sinus.[65] *Aspergillus* infection also may be found initially as a fungus ball (aspergilloma) in the involved sinus, which can radiographically simulate a neoplasm. In patients who are debilitated or immunocompromised, *Aspergillus* infection may be first seen as a fulminating infection with rapid destruction of the nasal cavity and involved paranasal sinuses.[18,76,77] Extensive and rapid bone destruction suggestive of a malignancy can be seen in such cases.

Mucormycosis represents the most fatal, acute, opportunistic fungal infection. It is caused by fungi belonging to the Mucoraceae family, which includes species of the genera *Rhizopus, Mucor,* and *Absidia.** The fungi in mucormycosis invade the arterial wall and produce an arteritis followed by vascular thrombosis and infarction of the surrounding tissue. Rhinocerebral mucormycosis starts with nasal involvement, followed by extension into the paranasal sinuses and orbits and intracranial effects. Fungal dissemination usually occurs through vascular channels.[31] Intracranial extension can result in either infarction or abscess formation.[14,31,33] Plain film and CT findings associated with mucormycosis include nodular thickening of the mucoperiosteum lining the maxillary sinus, usually without air-fluid levels; clouding of the ethmoid sinuses; and multiple focal areas of bone destruction.[14,17,33]

CT plays an important role in known or suspected *Mucor* infections. Gamba et al.[33] described a number of CT findings in patients with mucormycosis. The initial clinical findings of craniofacial mucormycosis reflect the structures involved.[10] Initial involvement of the sinonasal tract is reflected by a nonspecific mucosal thickening, often without air-fluid levels. Involvement of the deep soft tissues of the infratemporal and pterygopalatine fossae results in the loss of the retroantral fat pad and the various fat planes separating the muscles of mastication. Orbital involvement can result in preseptal edema, ptosis, infiltration of fat in the orbital apex, subperiosteal abscess formation, and changes in the orbital musculature. Intracranial extension usually involves the cerebellum and brain parenchyma at the base of the brain, resulting in either focal abscesses, areas of infarction, or both features. Bone destruction, when present, occurs late in the disease process (see Chapter 11).

Granulomatous Disease   The granulomatous diseases affecting the nose and paranasal sinuses represent a heterogenous group of pathological entities characterized by the formation of soft tissue granulomata that often exhibit similar clinical and radiographic findings.[62] The gross destruction noted on clinical examination is often indistinguishable from that of neoplastic processes. The granulomatous diseases involving the nose and paranasal sinuses include a number of infectious diseases: tuberculosis, leprosy, syphilis, yaws, autoimmune diseases such as Wegener's granulomatosis, idiopathic midline granuloma,

---

*References 1, 3, 39, 43, 97, 106, 122, 128, 129.

*References 10, 14, 17, 31, 33, 102.

sarcoidosis and foreign body–induced granulomata resulting from long-term exposure to beryllium and chromate salts.[62,106,129] The radiographic and CT findings in these different entities are similar. Initial CT examination demonstrates nasal soft tissue nodules and thickening. Subsequent involvement of the paranasal sinuses can occur. In the later phases of the disease process, bone destruction and soft tissue masses suggestive of a neoplastic process are present.

FASCIAL SPACES

The fascial spaces of the head and neck represent major pathways for the spread of deep infections. Failure to recognize and appropriately treat a fascial space infection can result in death from airway obstruction or mediastinitis. Diagnostic imaging is important in the evaluation of fascial space infections.

ANATOMY

The soft tissues of the head and neck can be divided into a series of spaces. Some spaces are normal anatomical spaces containing various structures (e.g., masticator space), whereas others are potential spaces, identifiable only when involved by a pathological process (e.g., retropharyngeal space). Important anatomical connections exist between these various actual and potential spaces that can allow for the rapid dissemination of infections throughout the head and neck and even into the mediastinum.

Conceptually, the fascial planes of the head and neck may be visualized as a series of "conduits."* The outer envelope, which surrounds the neck and head, is composed of the skin and superficial fascia (subcutaneous tissues). Two features of the superficial fascia are that (1) it contains the muscles of facial expression, including the platysma, and (2) by virtue of its superficial location, it is readily evaluated on clinical examination and usually does not necessitate diagnostic imaging of pathological processes.

Anatomically the deep neck can be divided into a superficial investing layer, middle or pretracheal layer, and deep or prevertebral layer. These spaces are major pathways for the spread of inflammatory processes and must be thoroughly evaluated in any imaging study. The investing layer is the most superficial layer and surrounds the entire neck. It is attached posteriorly to the spinous processes and ligamentum nuchae and anteriorly to the chin, body of the hyoid bone, and manubrium sterni. Superiorly, the superficial layer is attached to the external occipital protuberance and nuchal line, tip of the mastoid process, lower border of the zygomatic arch, and lower border of mandible between the angle and the chin. Inferiorly, it is attached to the sternum, clavicle, and acromion of the scapula.[9] In the neck the investing fascia splits to enclose the trapezius, sternocleidomastoid, and infrahyoid musculature (omohyoid, sternohyoid, sternothyroid, and thyrohyoid). In the maxillofacial region the investing layer

*References 46, 50, 51, 69, 96, 118.

splits to form the submandibular, sublingual, masticator, and parotid spaces (Figure 4-16).

The middle layer of the deep cervical fascia extends from the skull base to the pericardium through the carotid sheath. It is divided into a muscular and visceral division. The muscular division surrounds strap muscles and the adventitia of the great vessels; the visceral division surrounds the constrictor muscles of the pharynx and esophagus, and forms the buccopharyngeal fascia and anterior wall of the retropharyngeal space. The larynx, trachea, and thyroid gland also are enveloped by the middle layer of deep cervical fascia.

The deep layer of the deep cervical fascia is composed of the prevertebral and alar divisions. The alar division forms the posterior border of the retropharyngeal space and surrounds the deep neck muscles. The alar division also contributes to the carotid sheath and fuses with the middle layer of the deep cervical fascia at the approximate level of T1 to T2. The prevertebral division is attached to the anterior aspects of the vertebral bodies and extends laterally to the transverse processes of the vertebrae. An important potential space for the spread of head and neck infections to the mediastinum is the potential space between the alar and prevertebral division of the deep layer of the deep cervical fascia known as the "danger space." This potential space is bounded laterally by the fusion of the alar and prevertebral divisions of the deep cervical fascia with the transverse processes of the vertebrae. The danger space extends from the base of the skull to the level of the diaphragm (see Chapter 8).

DIAGNOSTIC IMAGING

Plain Film   Diagnostic imaging of a patient with a known or suspected fascial space infection often starts with a plain film study of the pharyngeal and cervical airway. This study usually consists of anteroposterior and lateral views of the airway taken with a lesser degree of penetration than comparable views of the cervical spine (Figure 4-17, see Figure 14-1). Plain film findings associated with acute fascial space infections include thickening of the retropharyngeal soft tissues, distortion with or without displacement of the pharyngeal air column caused by soft tissue edema or abscess formation, soft tissue gas, and radiodense foreign bodies. In addition, plain films obtained using standard techniques for osseous tissues may demonstrate osteomyelitis of the mandible or cervical spine and radiodense sialoliths. The lateral view of the cervical airway is especially important in the evaluation of retropharyngeal, parapharyngeal, and submandibular space infections. In such studies, evaluation of not only the gross patency of the airway but also the width of the prevertebral soft tissues is important. In the adult with the neck in the neutral position, the thickness of prevertebral soft tissues should not exceed 10 mm at the C1 level, 7 mm at the C3 level, and 20 mm at the C7 level.[59] In school-aged children the normal maximum width of the retropharyngeal tissues at C2 should not exceed 6 mm and 15 mm at C6.[47] These measurements represent the maximum width of normal

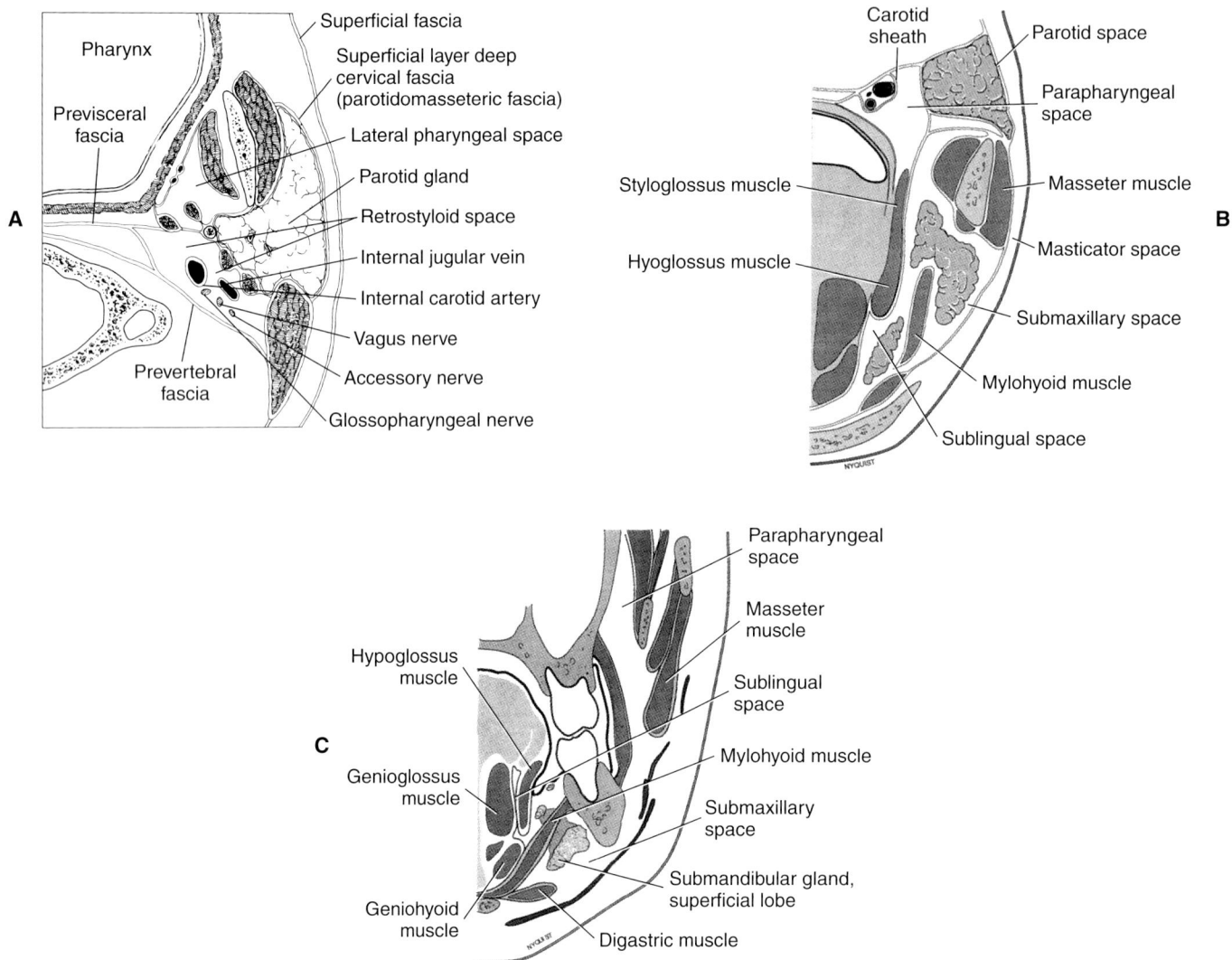

Figure 4-16 A, Cross-section of cervical fascia, potential anatomical spaces, and proximate vital structures at the level of the oropharynx. The parapharyngeal space is referred to as the *lateral pharyngeal space.* (From Hatton MH, Hall RE, DelBalso AM: Radiology of head and neck deep space infections: the clinician's perspective. In DelBalso AM, editor: *Maxillofacial imaging,* Philadelphia, 1990, WB Saunders.) The relationship of the various fascial spaces at the level of the midoral cavity in the axial plane **(B)** and coronal plane at the level of the posterior oral cavity **(C).**

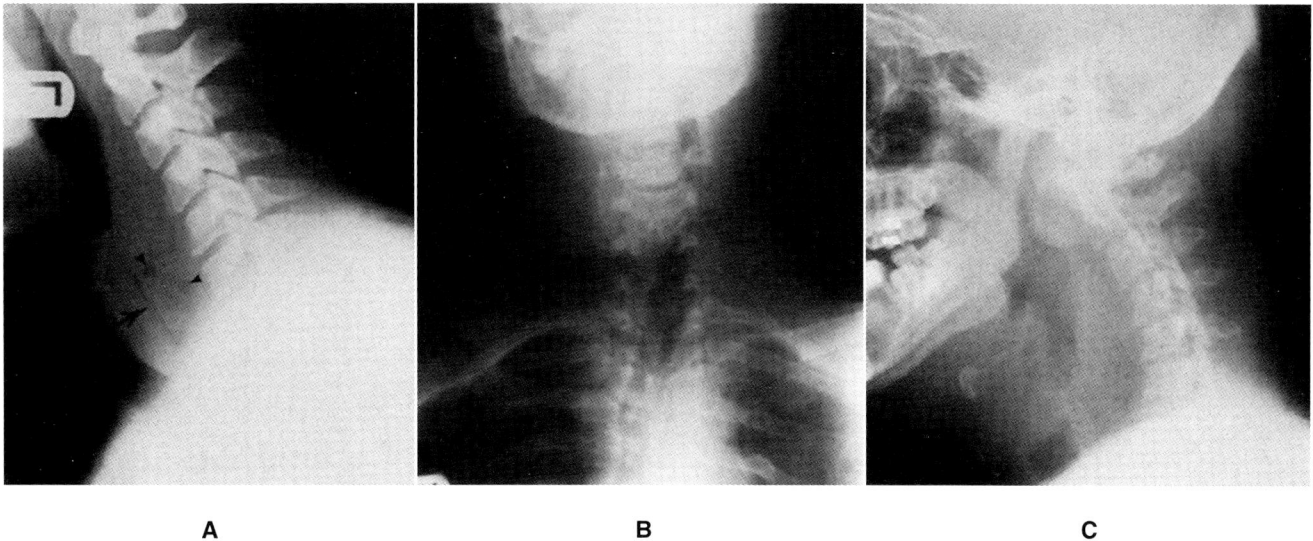

A   B   C

Figure 4-17 A, Lateral view of neck with soft tissue detail demonstrating a retropharyngeal abscess after ingestion of a foreign body 5 days earlier. Marked thickening of the prevertebral soft tissues with anterior displacement of the hypopharyngeal, laryngeal, and tracheal airways is present. Air is present with the retrolaryngeal and retrotracheal soft tissues *(arrowheads).* A plastic foreign body *(large arrow)* was removed endoscopically. Anteroposterior and lateral views of airway demonstrating airway displacement caused by diffuse fasciitis and abscess formation in the left submandibular, parapharyngeal, and retropharyngeal spaces. **B,** Anteroposterior view of the neck demonstrates a marked displacement of the cervical airway to the left. **C,** Lateral view of the cervical airway demonstrates a marked increased in the width of the prevertebral soft tissues in the middle and lower neck. (Case courtesy Y. Barodawala, Buffalo, New York.)

tissues; the average values for the population from which these values were derived are less. Because retropharyngeal or parapharyngeal space infections may occur with measurements within normal limits, clinicians should always look for other signs of infection on the lateral view such as focal increases in soft tissue thickness, soft tissue emphysema, foreign bodies, and localized deviations of the airway. In addition, the anteroposterior view of the airway should be examined for signs of pathological conditions. On the normal, properly positioned anteroposterior view of the airway, the air column should appear symmetrical over the middle third of the cervical spine (see Figure 4-1, *A*). Displacement of the pharyngeal or tracheal airway reflects involvement of the parapharyngeal, retropharyngeal, or pretracheal spaces. An important area to evaluate is the subglottic region of the trachea; a distinct shoulder should be evident in the subglottic segment. A concentric narrowing of this area resulting in an inverted V appearance is seen in patients with croup.

Computed Tomography CT is probably the most widely used advanced imaging modality in the evaluation of deep fascial infections.* It can provide important information concerning the extent of soft tissue involvement, including demonstration of the full extent of the inflammatory process and its probable epicenter, differentiation between myositis-fasciitis and abscess forma-

tion, accurate demonstration of the status of the airway, and involvement of various groups of lymph nodes. The differentiation between myositis-fasciitis and abscess is especially important clinically because abscesses require prompt surgical intervention to establish good drainage, whereas cellulitis may respond solely to appropriate antibiotics. CT also can provide important information concerning the status of adjacent osseous structures and may demonstrate early periosteal reactions associated with osteomyelitis.

Contrast-enhanced axial CT sections should be performed in the axial plane in 5-mm increments through all the involved fascial spaces and the major lymph node chains receiving drainage from involved regions of the head and neck. In cases of mediastinal involvement the full extent of mediastinal involvement must be demonstrated.

CT findings associated with fascial space involvement include myositis and fasciitis (Figure 4-18), airway deformity, inflammatory masses, fluid collections and abscesses, and osteomyelitis of involved bone. A variety of interventional procedures can be performed using CT guidance. Fine-needle aspiration of fluid collections to obtain material for microbial analysis is routinely performed. In addition, abscess drainage and drain placement can be readily performed under CT guidance.

Although MRI has been used extensively in the evaluation of conditions in the head and neck, it has not been used extensively in the evaluation of deep fascial space infections. Major advantages of MRI include the ability to

*References 4, 29, 49, 52, 82, 99.

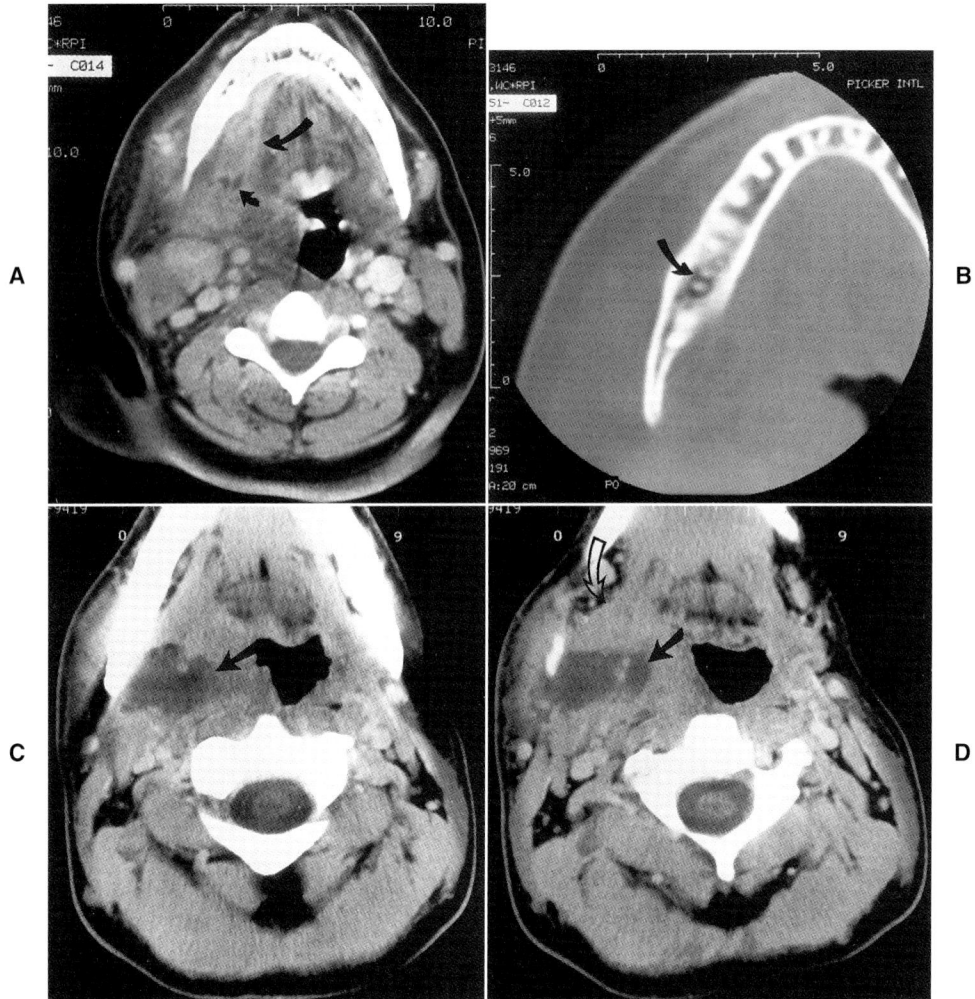

Figure 4-18 Submandibular space abscess. Myositis and fasciitis of right submandibular space caused by extension of a dental abscess involving the right second molar. **A,** Contrast-enhanced axial CT section through floor of mouth demonstrating a diffuse myositis and fasciitis involving the right submandibular and lower portion of right masticator space. Low-density areas representing early abscess formation are noted *(small curved arrow).* **B,** Axial CT section of mandible with bone windows demonstrates a periapical abscess around the apices of mandibular second molar *(curved arrow).* This case demonstrates the need to always obtain appropriate bone windows when evaluating fascial space infections of possible odontogenic origin. **C** and **D,** Contrast-enhanced axial CT sections through the deep and superficial segments of the right submandibular space demonstrating an abscess involving the deep and superficial portions of the right submandibular space. The normal-appearing superficial segment of the submandibular gland *(open curved arrow)* is displaced anteriorly by the abscess *(straight arrow).* Deformity of the right half of the airway is present.

obtain direct images in not only the axial plane but also the coronal and sagittal planes. Images are less susceptible to artifacts caused by dental restorations, and the intravenous contrast material used in MRI studies is less toxic than the iodinated contrast used in CT scanning.[49] The ability to image in the sagittal and parasagittal planes is especially useful in the demonstration of retropharyngeal and superior mediastinal involvement in the region of the thoracic inlet, an area that is sometimes difficult to image on routine axial CT examinations because of artifacts from adjacent bones. However, MRI does have a number of major disadvantages in the evaluation of head and neck infections, including length of imaging time and the similar appearances of abscesses and cellulitis on T2-weighted im-

ages, making differentiation between the two difficult at times.[49,74] In addition, mural enhancement by an abscess wall may be isointense with respect to surrounding fat after gadolinium administration, resulting in limited detection or delineation of the abscess. The cutaneous manifestations also may not be obvious on MRI if imaging parameters are not monitored.[49] In addition, MRI examinations are more expensive than standard CT examinations and may not be available in an emergency.

MRI findings associated with myositis and fasciitis include an apparent increase in the size of the involved muscles or tissue planes associated with a variable low signal intensity on T1-weighted and increased signal intensity on T2-weighted sequences (Figure 4-19, see

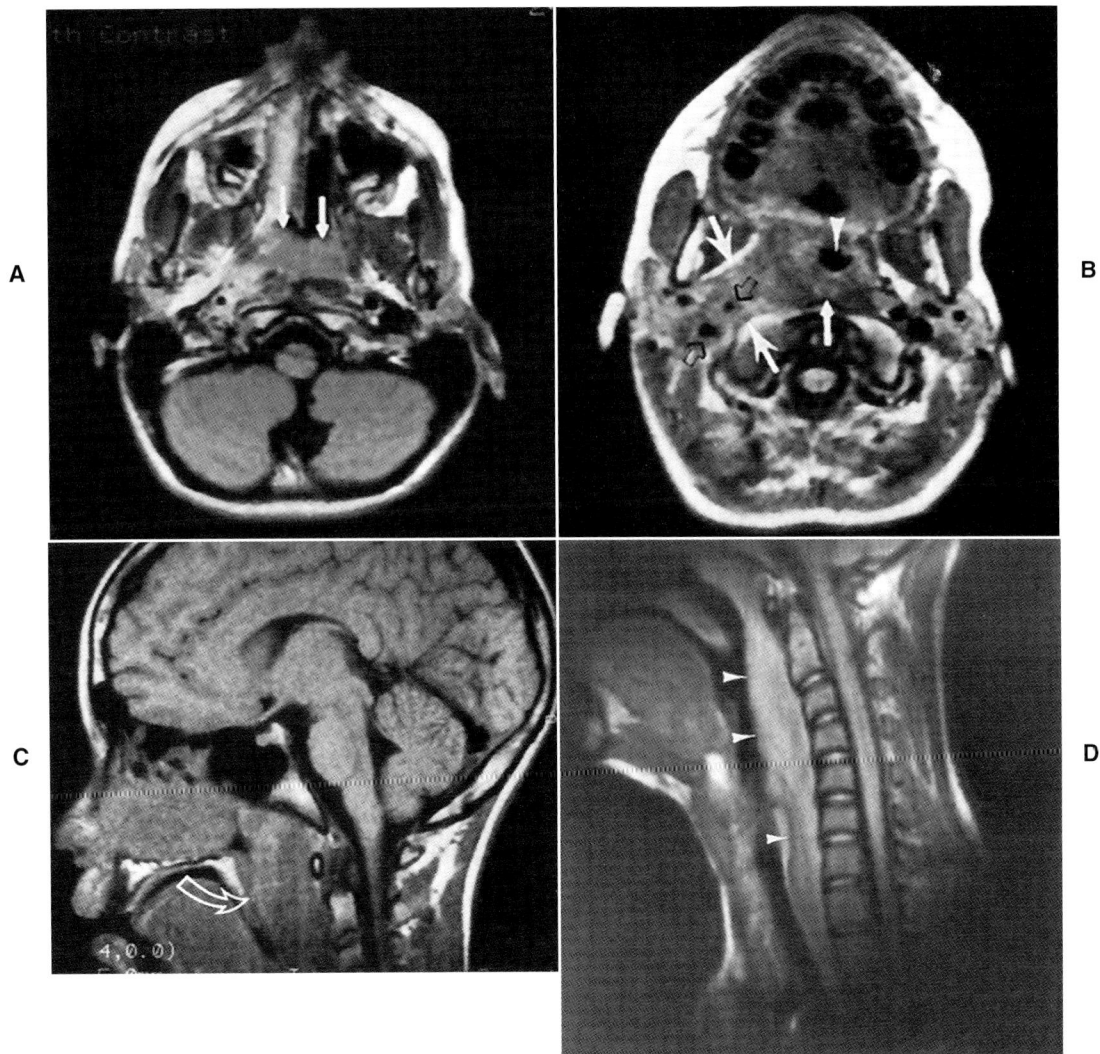

Figure 4-19 MRI scan of a right parapharyngeal and retropharyngeal fasciitis. **A** and **B,** Axial T1-weighted image through the nasopharynx and oral pharynx after gadolinium administration demonstrates thickening of the retropharyngeal and nasopharyngeal soft tissues (**A** and **B,** *small arrows*), and extension of the inflammatory process into the retrostyloid compartment of right parapharyngeal space (**B,** *large arrows*). Enhancement of the inflammatory process involving the parapharyngeal space and extension of the inflammatory process around the carotid and jugular vessels is noted. These vessels appear as areas devoid of signal (flow voids). Displacement of the airway to the left *(arrowhead)* is noted. **C** and **D,** Inflammatory processes involving the nasopharyngeal soft tissues (**C,** *open arrow*) and prevertebral tissues (**D,** *arrowheads*) are evident on sagittal images through the nasopharynx and cervical region. (Case courtesy Lindell Gentry, Madison, Wisconsin.)

Figure 4-2). Enhancement of the inflammatory process occurs on T1-weighted sequences after gadolinium administration.[74,120,126] Abscesses demonstrate similar signal characteristics and mass effect. Abscess walls may be distinguishable on T2-weighted or T1-weighted sequences after gadolinium administration. Demonstration of the abscess wall may not be always possible because the increased signal intensity of the cellulitis surrounding an abscess may be similar to that of the abscess wall on T2-weighted sequences. Similarly, mural enhancement after gadolinium enhancement may result in the mural ring becoming isointense with the surrounding fat. Marrow space involvement by an inflammatory process results in a decrease in the normally high signal intensity of the marrow seen on T1-weighted sequences and an increase in the signal intensity of the marrow on T2-weighted sequences.

FASCIAL SPACES

Submandibular Fascial Space   The submandibular fascial space is formed by the investing layer splitting above the hyoid bone to enclose the submandibular gland; superiorly, this layer of fascia is attached to the mentum and anterior body of the mandible.[9,46,100] The investing layer ascends to cover the superficial surfaces of the muscles constituting the floor of the mouth (mylohyoid and digastrics). The submandibular fascial spaces are considered anterior extensions of the parapharyngeal space and are divided into the upper sublingual and lower submandibular spaces by the mylohyoid muscle (Figure 4-20, see Figure 4-16); these two spaces communicate freely around the posterior border of the mylohyoid muscle. The sublingual space is located between the mylohyoid muscle inferiorly and laterally, and the genioglossus and hyoglossus-styloglossus muscle complexes medially.[9,100,105] Major components of the sublingual space include the geniohyoid and genioglossus muscle, the hyoglossus-styloglossus muscle complex, the sublingual gland, deep portion of the submandibular gland and duct, the lingual nerve and artery, and the twelfth (hypoglossal) nerve. The styloglossus muscle arises from the tip of the styloid process and passes downward and forward between the middle and superior pharyngeal constrictor muscles. As the styloglossus muscle passes between the constrictor muscles, it creates a potential communication between the submandibular and parapharyngeal spaces known as the *buccopharyngeal gap*. This gap is a potential pathway for the spread of infection between these two respective spaces. The submaxillary space is located below the level of the mylohyoid muscle and contains the superficial lobe of the submandibular gland, submandibular and submental lymph nodes, and anterior belly of the digastric muscle. The fascial attachments to the anterior belly of the digastric muscle subdivide the submandibular space into the central submental and lateral submandibular space.[105] No major anatomical barriers exist between the two submental and submandibular spaces proper; consequently, infections can extend readily across the midline (see Chapters 8 and 9).

An understanding of the basic axial and coronal cross-sectional anatomy is essential in the evaluation of inflammatory processes involving the submandibular space and its various divisions. The submandibular gland is located within the submandibular space. CT sections show that it normally has a CT density comparable with that of adjacent muscle. On axial CT sections through the submandibular space proper, the superficial lobe of the submandibular gland appears as a well-defined, soft tissue density usually surrounded by a fat plane (see Figure 4-20). Loss of this soft tissue plane is associated with extension of a neoplastic or an inflammatory process involving either the gland or the structures bordering the gland. Although it does not contain any intraglandular lymph nodes, the submandibular gland is closely related to a number of small submandibular lymph nodes. These lymph nodes should have a homogenous, nonenhancing appearance and never exceed 1.5 cm in diameter.[90,92,108] The deep lobe of the submandibular gland is not well demonstrated on axial CT sections because its CT density is close to that of the adjacent soft tissues of the floor of the mouth; however, it can be identified on direct coronal CT sections.

On MRI sections through the submandibular space, the muscles are of low signal intensity on T1 and T2 sequences, whereas fat within the fascial spaces demonstrates high signal intensity on T1-weighted sequences. The submandibular and sublingual glands demonstrate intermediate signal intensity on T1-weighted and relatively high signal intensity on T2-weighted sequences. The superficial lobes of the submandibular gland are readily identified because they are surrounded by high signal intensity fat immediately anteriorly. The deep lobe of the submandibular gland can be identified between the mylohyoid and styloglossus and hyoglossus muscles.

In addition to the submandibular glands, several muscles should be identified in the evaluation of the submandibular region on CT and MRI studies because these define not only the space but also the major subdivisions of the space.[24,58,68,105] These muscles include the mylohyoid and genioglossus muscles, and the anterior belly of the digastric muscle (see Figure 4-20). The mylohyoid is a fan-shaped muscle arising from the mylohyoid ridge on the medial aspect of the mandible and, along with the paired genioglossus muscles, is readily identifiable on axial and direct coronal scans. On axial CT sections through its origin the mylohyoid appears as a band of soft tissue density adjacent to the medial aspect of the mandible; on direct coronal scans, it appears as a muscular sling extending between the medial aspects of both hemimandibles. The genioglossus muscles appear as two paramedian muscular bands separated by a low-density vertical cleft or midline lingual septum. These muscles originate from the genial tubercles on the internal aspect of the anterior mandibular midline and pass superiorly into the substance of the tongue. The sublingual space appears as a low-density area between the paramidline genioglossus muscle medially and the mylohyoid muscle and medial surface of the mandible laterally. Its roof is formed by the mucosa of the

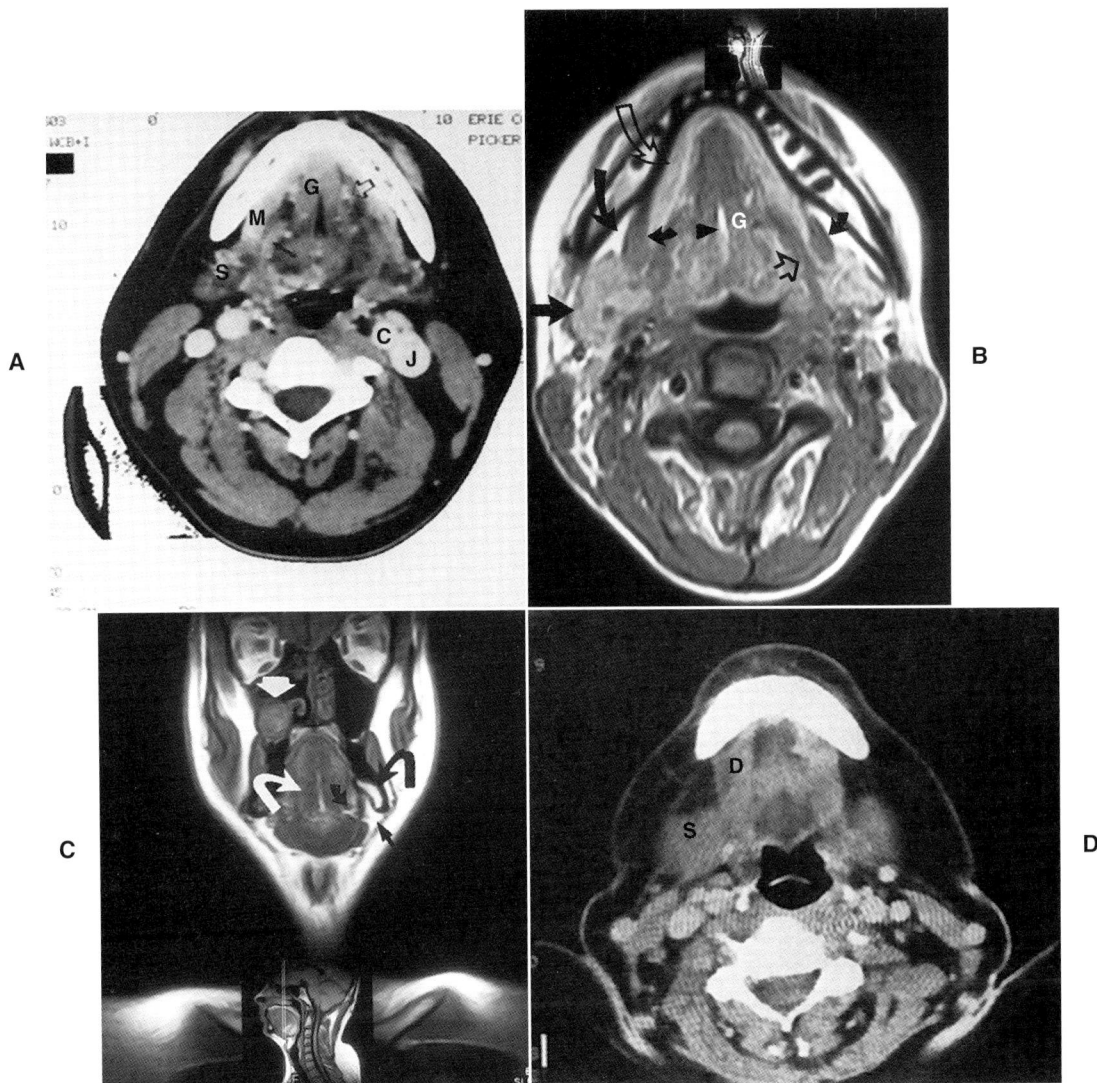

Figure 4-20 A, Contrast-enhanced axial CT section through submandibular space. The paired midline genioglossus muscles *(G),* curvilinear hyoglossus-styloglossus muscle complex *(arrows),* mylohyoid muscle *(M)* arising from the mylohyoid ridge, and superficial lobe of the submandibular gland *(S)* in the submandibular space are indicated. The low-density sublingual space with its enhancing lingual vessels *(open arrow),* carotid artery *(C),* and jugular vein *(J)* are indicated. **B,** T1-weighted axial section through submandibular space. The normal submandibular gland *(short straight arrow),* fat anterior to gland *(curved arrow),* mylohyoid muscle *(short curved arrow),* styloglossus and hypoglossal muscles *(open arrowhead),* sublingual gland *(open curved arrow),* genioglossus muscle *(G),* and lingual septum *(solid arrowhead)* are indicated. The deep lobe of the submandibular gland is located between the mylohyoid and styloglossus/hypoglossal muscles. **C,** T1-weighted coronal MRI section through anterior maxillofacial region demonstrating the high signal intensity of fat in the left submandibular space *(short straight arrow)* and sublingual spaces *(short curved arrow)* and midline genioglossus muscles *(curved white arrow)* are noted. The band of low signal intensity between the submandibular and sublingual spaces is the mylohyoid muscle. High signal intensity is noted in the normal marrow of the left hemimandible. An odontogenic keratocyst also is present in the right maxillary sinus *(white arrowhead).* **D,** Axial CT section through hypopharynx. The anterior belly of the digastric muscle *(D)* and superficial lobe of the submandibular gland *(S)* are identified.   *Continued*

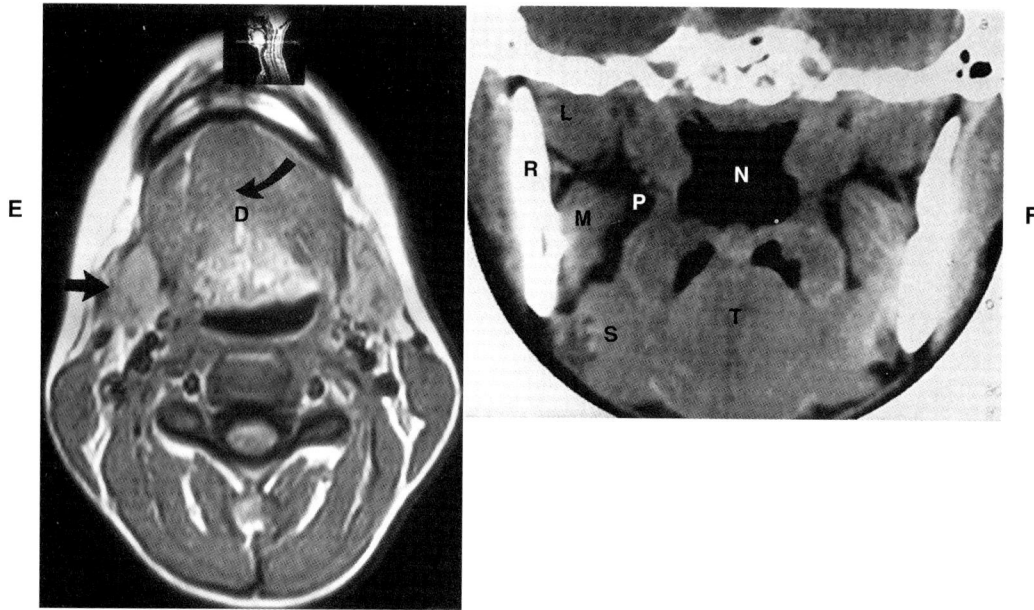

Figure 4-20, cont'd E, T1-weighted axial section through hypopharynx. The superficial lobe of the submandibular gland, anterior belly of the digastic muscle *(D)*, and geniohyoid muscles *(curved arrow)* are indicated. **F,** Direct coronal CT section through nasopharynx. The lateral *(L)* and medial *(M)* pterygoid muscles, nasal airway *(N)*, parapharyngeal space *(P)*, ramus of the mandible *(R)*, tongue, and submandibular gland *(S)* are indicated.

floor of the mouth. Important landmarks useful in the identification of this space are the lingual blood vessels, which enhance after intravenous contrast injection, and the hyoglossus-styloglossus muscle complex, which appears as a thin, curvilinear muscle complex medially. On successively lower axial scans a low-density area is noted between the mandible and mylohyoid muscle, representing the submandibular space. Lower scans demonstrate the superficial lobe of the submandibular gland and submandibular nodes. On direct coronal scans, the submandibular space is readily apparent between the medial aspect of the mandible and mylohyoid muscle. The anterior belly of the digastric extends downward and backward from the digastric fossa on the inferior border of the chin to the greater horn of the hyoid bone and divides the submandibular space into the central submental and lateral submandibular space proper. On axial CT sections through the inferior mandible the anterior belly of the digastric muscle can be identified in the digastric fossa located on the undersurface of the anterior mandible. On axial CT sections below the level of the mandible the paired anterior bellies of the digastric are noted below the subcutaneous tissues of the neck, extending between the anterior mandible and greater horn of hyoid bone. Infections involving the submandibular space often are the result of dental infections, adenitis in the sublingual or submandibular lymph nodes, penetrating trauma, or sialoadenitis.[37,46] Odontogenic infections initially involving the sublingual space usually are associated with the premolars, whereas infections involving the submandibular space are associated with the molars (see Figure 4-18).

One potentially fatal infection involving the submandibular space is Ludwig's angina.[37,46,79,127] Ludwig's angina is a brawny, hard cellulitis of the entire submandibular fascial space bilaterally. It usually results from a dental infection or suppurative nodes in the submandibular space; however, it also may occur as a result of acute sialoadenitis. This cellulitis, often associated with phlegmon formation, can extend into the mediastinum by way of the parapharyngeal and retropharyngeal spaces. Involvement of these spaces can result in airway embarrassment and death, whereas involvement of the superior mediastinum can result in mediastinitis.[50,52,96,127] Plain film findings include soft tissue swelling of the floor of the mouth and suprahyoid neck and airway deformity (see Figure 4-17). CT findings include cellulitis of the soft tissues of the submandibular and sublingual spaces (Figure 4-21, see Figure 4-18), abscess formation, and fluid collections. Extension into the parapharyngeal, retropharyngeal, or both spaces or the mediastinum can result in cellulitis with or without abscess formation in these spaces. Airway displacement or deformity invariably accompanies involvement of these anatomical spaces.

Space of the Body of the Mandible and Osteomyelitis of the Jaws   The space of the body of the mandible is formed by the upward extension of the superficial layer of the deep cervical fascia as it splits to enclose the buccal and lingual aspect of the mandible.[46,100] The space is continuous with the mandibular periosteum. Infections of the space of the body of the mandible are primarily acute or chronic osteomyelitis of the mandible. Acute osteomyelitis

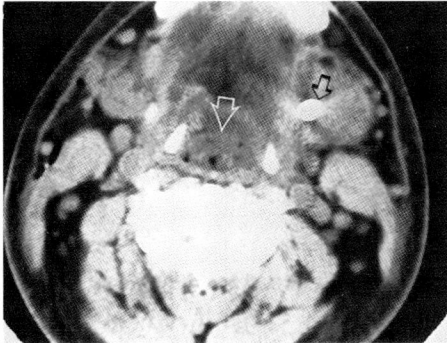

Figure 4-21 Left submandibular sialadenitis with cellulitis of floor of mouth *(open white arrow)*. Axial CT section through floor of mouth demonstrating a sialolith in the proximal portion of the left submandibular duct *(open black arrow)*. The left submandibular gland is enlarged, with diffuse myositis and fasciitis of the floor of the mouth. The inflammatory response has extended to the hypopharynx, resulting in narrowing of the hypopharyngeal airway.

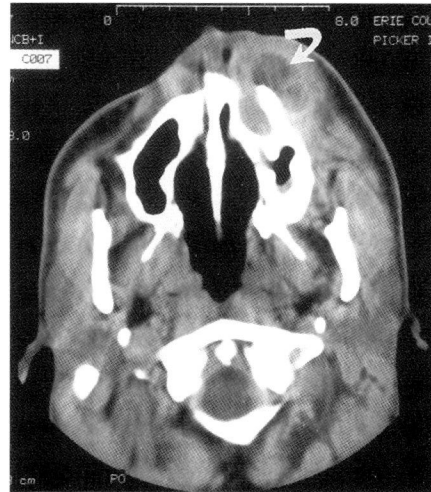

Figure 4-22 Acute osteomyelitis arising in a preexisting periapical lesion. Contrast-enhanced axial CT section through maxilla demonstrating a large intraosseous periapical abscess with cortical breakthrough and extension into overlying soft tissues. The walls of the abscess demonstrate peripheral enhancement *(curved white arrow)*. The initial lesion in this patient was a long-standing periapical lesion that became acutely infected.

of both the mandible and the maxillary alveolar ridges most often occurs as a result of the contiguous spread of an odontogenic infection originating in the tooth-bearing regions of the involved jaw to the adjacent spongiosa. Other less common causes of acute osteomyelitis include a surgical procedure (e.g., extraction, apical curettage), passage of bacteria through the periodontal ligament, the hematogenous dissemination of bacteria from a distant site, or osseous involvement by a soft tissue infection. Acute osteomyelitis of odontogenic origin results from either the direct extension of an acute pulpal infection without the formation of a granuloma or the acute exacerbation of a chronic periapical lesion (Figure 4-22). Extension of the inflammatory process throughout the marrow cavity can result in a fulminating acute osteomyelitis involving a large segment of the involved bone. Transcortical extension of the inflammatory process can result in cortical destruction, fistula formation, and periosteal reaction. Extension into the soft tissues bordering the bone may result in myositis, fasciitis, cellulitis, and abscess formation (see Figures 4-2, 4-18, and 4-22).

Initial radiographic findings in acute osteomyelitis arising de novo are typically absent for the first 7 to 14 days except for a possible widening of the periodontal space around the root apex or generalized osteoporosis around the apex of an involved tooth (Figure 4-23). Definitive plain film findings usually become evident between 7 and 14 days. Findings include poor definition of trabeculae, single or multiple ill-defined radiolucent areas, and loss of the lamina dura between the lucent lesion and tooth apex. Acute osteomyelitis also may develop in a preexisting chronic periapical lesion. In these cases the progressive loss of discrete margination of the lesion initially may be noted

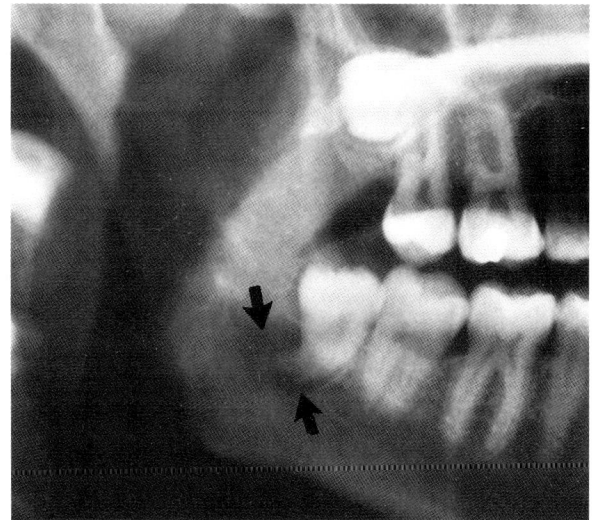

Figure 4-23 A periapical abscess *(arrows)*. This is the same case as in Figure 4-2.

on plain films, followed by loss of trabeculation in the adjacent bone as the process extends into the area. Extension of the infection into adjacent soft tissues and fascial spaces is common and often the initial clinical symptom for which a CT study is indicated, and should be ordered immediately. CT studies of these patients should be performed with intravenous contrast unless otherwise contraindicated. CT sections should be imaged using soft tissue and bone windows. Information gained can have a definite effect on patient management. Images obtained using soft tissue windows with contrast are useful in demonstrating the extent of soft tissue abscesses, whereas images obtained using bone windows may demonstrate a periapical abscess that may not be apparent on plain films or CT images obtained with soft tissue windows (see Figure 4-18, *B*). Surgical drainage of osseous and soft tissue abscesses often is central to effective treatment of such patients.

CT findings in these patients may include periosteal reactions, myositis, fasciitis, cellulitis, abscess formation, and sinus tracts. Osseous changes may include localized osseous breakdown resulting from abscess formation, sequestrae, and periosteal new bone formation. MRI is useful in assessing patients with acute osteomyelitis. On MRI examination, inflammatory changes involving the marrow and soft tissues demonstrate decreased signal on T1-weighted sequences, intermediate signal intensity on proton density sequences, and high signal intensity on T2-weighted sequences (see Figure 4-2).

Chronic osteomyelitis may result from an acute osteomyelitis that was inadequately treated or a low-grade inflammatory process that never evoked an acute phase. Chronic osteomyelitis is essentially a persistent infection of bone, often with abscess formation. The radiographic appearances are variable, ranging from a single radiolucent area representing an abscess to a "moth-eaten" appearance consisting of multiple areas of bone destruction separated by normal-appearing bone.[35,67,95] Often sclerotic changes are evident around the abscess. Sequestrae, foci of increased density representing dead bone, become more apparent as the surrounding bone becomes osteoporotic. These changes are best demonstrated on CT examination (Figure 4-24). CT sections may demonstrate a prominent involucrum or fistulous communication, which might not be apparent on plain films.

Masticator Space   The *masticator space,* as it name implies, contains the muscles of mastication; these are the

masseter, lateral, and medial pterygoids and insertion of the temporalis muscle (Figures 4-25 and 4-26; see Figures 4-5, 4-16, and 4-20).[20,46,55] It also contains the ramus and posterior portion of the body of the mandible and branches of the mandibular division of the trigeminal nerve. These branches include the masticator, buccal, lin-

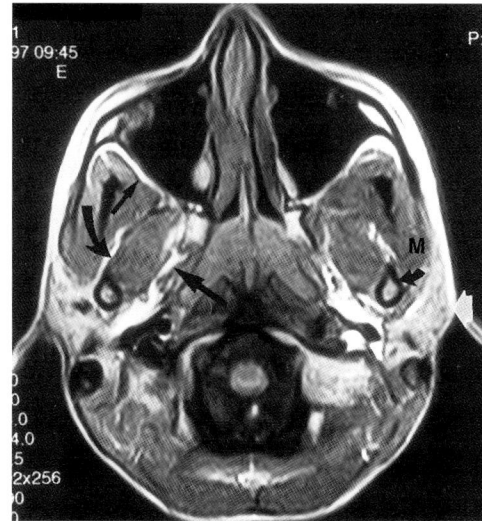

Figure 4-25 Axial T1-weighted magnetic resonance image section at level of zygomas demonstrating the lateral pterygoid muscle *(large curved arrow),* masseter muscle *(M),* condylar neck of mandible *(short curved arrow),* and parotid gland *(white arrowhead).* These muscles are noted to be of low signal intensity. The normal-appearing parotid gland is of intermediate signal intensity, whereas the retroantral fat pads *(small straight arrow)* and parapharyngeal spaces *(large straight arrow)* demonstrate high signal intensity reflecting their high fat content.

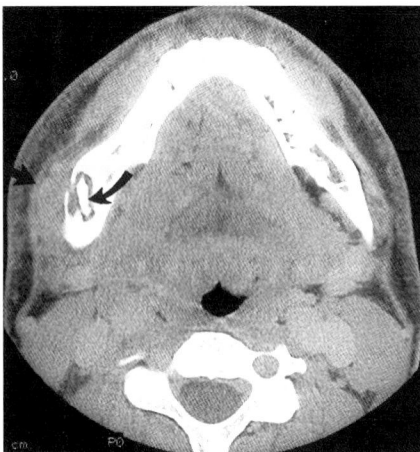

Figure 4-24 Chronic osteomyelitis. Axial CT section through maxilla demonstrating chronic osteomyelitis after third molar extraction. An involucrum is demonstrated within the bone *(curved arrow).* Cortical breakthrough and extension of the inflammatory process into adjacent masseter muscle has resulted in myositis of the muscle *(straight arrow).*

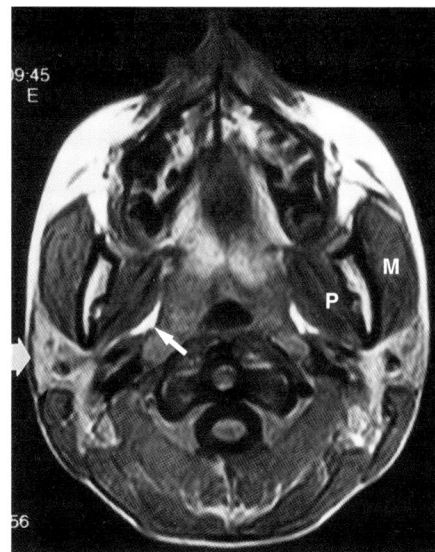

Figure 4-26 Axial magnetic resonance image section through oral cavity at level of soft palate. The masseter *(M),* medial pterygoid *(P),* parapharyngeal space *(straight arrow),* and parotid gland *(white arrowhead)* are indicated.

gual, and inferior alveolar nerves. The masticator space is divided into a lateral and medial compartment by the ramus of mandible. The masticator space is formed by a splitting of the investing fascia into superficial and deep layers that define the lateral and medial extent of the space. The superficial layer lies along the lateral surfaces of the masseter and lower half of the temporalis muscles. Superiorly, the superficial layer fuses with the periosteum of the zygoma and temporalis fascia. The deep layer passes along the medial surface of the pterygoid muscles before attaching to the base of the skull superiorly. The masticator space borders on a number of other spaces. Posteriorly, it borders on the parotid space, medially on the parapharyngeal space, and inferiorly on the submandibular and sublingual spaces. Potential communications exist among these respective spaces, thereby allowing for the spread of infections and neoplasms. The ramus of the mandible and the overlying masseter muscle are readily identified on frontal views of the skull and facial bones. However, the medial portion of the masticator space is not well demonstrated on routine plain film examination.

Axial CT and direct coronal CT sections through the masticator space demonstrate the ramus of the mandible dividing the masticator space into its lateral and medial segments (Figure 4-27; see Figures 4-5, 4-20, and 4-26). The masseter muscle is noted throughout the lateral compartment. In the upper half of the medial compartment, the horizontally oriented lateral pterygoid muscle is readily identified extending between the lateral pterygoid plate and temporo-

mandibular joint. In the lower half of the medial compartment the obliquely oriented medial pterygoid muscle, extending between the medial pterygoid plate and angle of the mandible, is well demonstrated. The lower half of the temporalis muscle and its attachment to the coronoid process is demonstrated on axial and coronal sections through the lower portion of the infratemporal fossa and coronoid process.

Primary infections of the masticator space are usually of odontogenic origin.[45,46] Uncommon primary causes of masticator space infections include iatrogenic introduction of bacteria during local anesthesia administration and penetrating trauma. More commonly, the masticator is secondarily involved by infections affecting the adjacent parapharyngeal or parotid spaces.

Plain film findings associated with masticator space infections include soft tissue swelling over the lateral aspect of the ramus and, rarely, osteomyelitis of the ramus of the mandible. CT findings associated with masticator space infections include myositis and fasciitis of involved muscles and fascial planes (Figure 4-28), fluid collections, abscess formation, periosteal reactions, and rarely, osteomyelitis of the ramus. MRI findings include decreased signal intensity on T1-weighted and increased signal intensity on T2-weighted sequences of the involved bone marrow and surrounding soft tissues.

Parotid Space   Posterior to the masticator space, the superficial layer of the deep cervical fascia splits to form the parotid space. The parotid space contains the parotid gland and lymph nodes (see Figures 4-5, 4-16, and 4-25). Inferiorly, it is separated from the submandibular space by

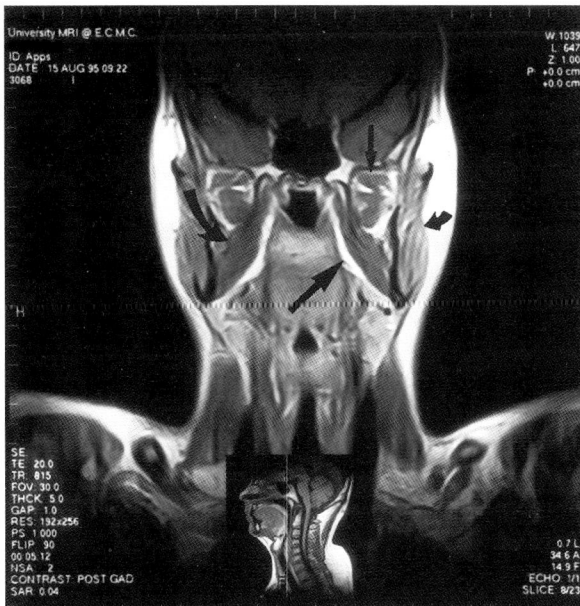

Figure 4-27 T1-weighted coronal image through nasopharynx. The parapharyngeal spaces demonstrate high signal intensity reflecting its high fat content *(large straight arrow)* . The lateral *(small straight arrow)* and medial pterygoid *(large curved arrow)* and masseter muscles *(short curved arrow)* are noted.

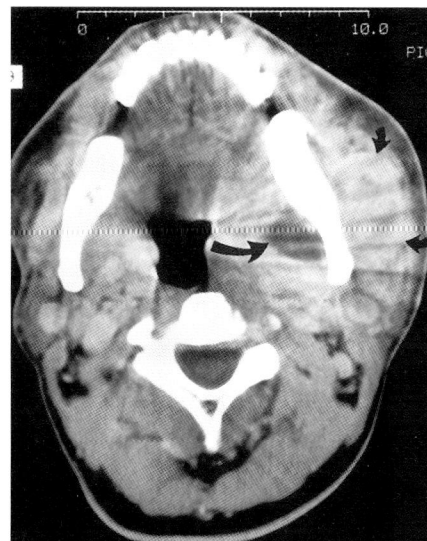

Figure 4-28 Masticator space abscess. Contrast-enhanced axial CT section through oral cavity demonstrating an abscess in the medial compartment of the left masticator space *(large curved arrow)*. A generalized edema of the visualized portion of the left masseter and generalized contrast enhancement of the lateral compartment and surrounding tissues reflect the inflammatory process *(short curved arrows)*.

the stylomandibular ligament. Communications do exist between the two spaces through anterior branches of the posterior facial vein.

The parotid gland is readily identified on axial and direct coronal CT sections posterior to the masseter muscle. On axial sections the parotid gland has a triangular shape, with a relatively low CT number on nonenhanced scans (−10 to 10 HU) reflecting its high fat and fluid content.[12,22,88,89] In addition to the glandular tissues, the parotid gland also contains a number of intraparotid lymph nodes, the facial nerve, the retromandibular vein, and the external carotid artery. The facial nerve divides the parotid into superficial (lateral) and deep (medial) lobes and can be laterally displaced by pathological processes involving the deep lobe or adjacent parapharyngeal space. Although the facial nerve cannot be identified on direct axial scans, its location can be approximated by the readily identifiable retromandibular vein. The facial nerve lies lateral to the retromandibular vein, and lateral displacement of the retromandibular vein is indicative of a pathological condition arising in the deep lobe.

On MRI examinations the signal intensity of the normal parotid gland is greater than that of muscle but lower than that of fat in the subcutaneous tissues or parapharyngeal space on T1-and T2-weighted sequences (see Figure 4-25). On T2-weighted images the parotid gland's signal intensity is greater than that of adjacent muscle but lower than that of fat. Areas devoid of signal are noted within the parotid gland representing the retromandibular vein and external carotid artery. The facial nerve is an important structure that can be identified on T1-weighted images, appearing as a curvilinear density of relatively low signal intensity. The high signal intensity of fat within the parapharyngeal space adjacent to the deep lobe of the parotid and in the subcutaneous tissue around the superficial lobe is identified readily on T1-weighted images.

The parotid gland is surrounded by and contains a number of lymph nodes. These nodes normally appear as focal areas of increased density on non–contrast-enhanced CT sections and filling defects on contrast-enhanced CT studies[12,13,22,56] (see Chapter 12).

Parapharyngeal and Retropharyngeal Spaces   Two major pathways for the spread of head and neck infections are the parapharyngeal and retropharyngeal spaces.[23,103,109,125] These spaces form a "ring" around the pharynx and together form a pathway for the spread of maxillofacial infections into the neck and mediastinum. The parapharyngeal space is a fat-filled space extending from the base of skull to the hyoid bone, separating the muscles of mastication from the muscles of deglutition; the space is well demonstrated on routine axial and coronal CT and MRI sections (see Figures 4-5; 4-20, *F;* 4-25, and 4-27). The parapharyngeal space is bounded anteriorly by the pterygomandibular raphe, laterally by the parotid and masticator spaces, medially by the pharyngeal wall, and posteriorly by the styloid muscle and carotid sheath. Its lateral wall is formed by the ascending ramus of the mandible, insertion

of the medial pterygoid muscle, and medial surface of the deep lobe the parotid. Its medial wall is formed by the palatal muscles at the level of the nasopharynx and the pharyngeal constrictors at the level of the oropharynx. The parapharyngeal spaces communicate directly with the submandibular space anteroinferiorly and the retromandibular space posteriorly.

On MRI studies the parapharyngeal space exhibits a high signal intensity on T1 sequences, reflecting its high fat content. On axial sections through the superior nasopharynx the parapharyngeal space appears as a cleft between the pharyngeal and pterygoid muscles. At the level of the midnasopharynx through lower oropharynx, the parapharyngeal space assumes a triangular shape. Inferiorly, the space is limited by the sheath of the submandibular gland and appears as a fat space medial to the submandibular gland and anterior to the carotid artery and jugular vein.

Parapharyngeal space infections represent extensions of infections that occur in structures bordering on it or through anatomical pathways communicating with the space. Infections that most commonly involve the parapharyngeal space include those of dental, tonsil, mastoid, and salivary origin.

Plain film findings associated with parapharyngeal space infections consist primarily of soft tissue swelling and airway displacement with or without distortion (see Figure 4-17). CT findings associated with parapharyngeal infections include fasciitis of the space and edema (myositis) of muscles bordering it, fluid collections, and abscess formation (Figure 4-29).

The retropharyngeal space is a potential midline space between the pharyngobasilar fascia, which attaches to the pharyngeal constrictors to the base of the skull, and prevertebral fascia.[23,118] It is bounded laterally by the alar fascia of the deep layer of deep cervical fascia. The retropharyngeal space extends from the skull base to the approximate

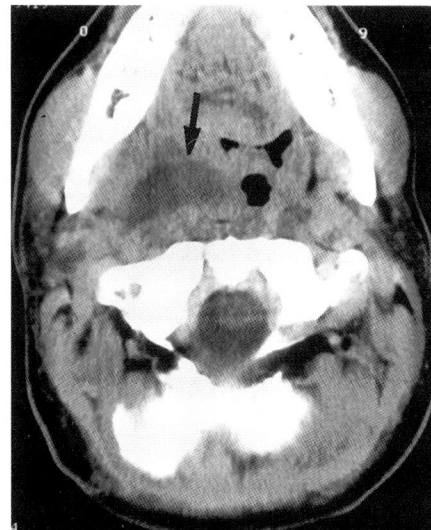

Figure 4-29 Contrast-enhanced axial CT sections through floor of mouth demonstrating a right parapharyngeal abscess *(arrow).* Mass effect is noted on the airway.

level of T2. No midline attachments are present in the retropharyngeal space, thereby permitting unimpeded inferior extension of inflammatory and neoplastic processes into the mediastinum. Infections of the retropharyngeal spaces usually represent extension of infections in spaces communicating with the retropharyngeal space; however, primary infections may occur after penetrating trauma. Danger space infections result from the extension of infections involving adjacent regions such as the retropharyngeal, parapharyngeal, and prevertebral spaces.

The normal retropharyngeal space is a potential space and, in the absence of pathological conditions, is not usually identifiable on plain films or CT studies. Plain film findings associated with retropharyngeal space infections include widening of the prevertebral soft tissues, air within the retropharyngeal soft tissues, airway distortion with or without displacement, and the presence of radiodense foreign bodies. CT findings may demonstrate the findings noted for plain films and cellulitis of the tissue bordering the space, fluid collection in the space, and abscess formation (Figure 4-30). MRI is particularly useful for the as-

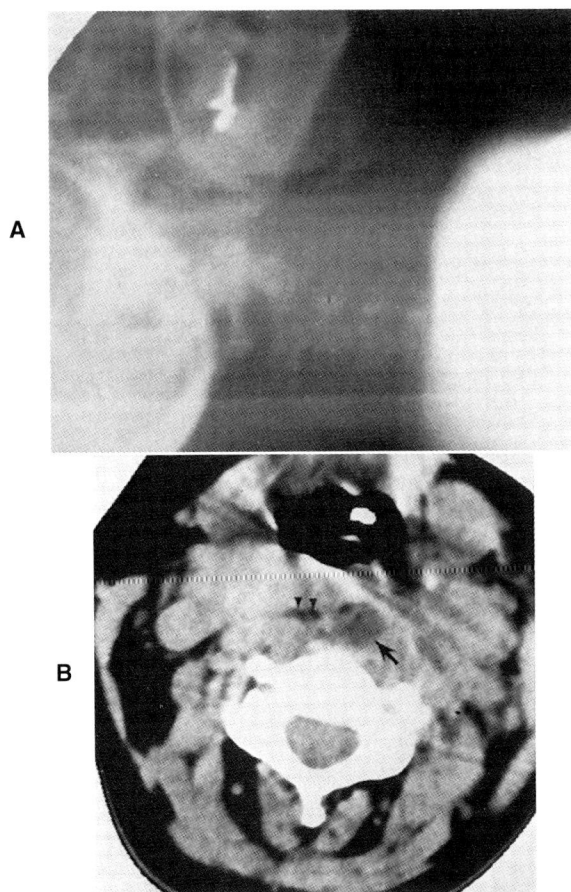

Figure 4-30 Retropharyngeal space abscess. **A,** Lateral view of the neck from a CT pilot image demonstrating thickening of the prevertebral soft tissues and anterior displacement of the airway. **B,** Axial CT section through the hypopharynx demonstrating a low-density fluid collection *(arrow)* representing a retropharyngeal abscess. Focal collection of air is present in the retropharyngeal space *(arrowheads).* (From DelBalso AM, editor: *Maxillofacial imaging,* Philadelphia, 1990, WB Saunders.)

sessment of retropharyngeal space involvement because it permits direct sagittal and parasagittal views, thereby allowing ready identification of the inferior extent of the inflammatory process (see Figure 4-19).

Pretracheal Space The pretracheal space is a potential space located between the pretracheal fascia and esophagus. The pretracheal space represents an important pathway for the spread of head and neck infections into the superior mediastinum. In the absence of a pathological process this potential space is not identifiable on routine plain film or CT studies. In the presence of infection, CT findings similar to those noted for infections involving other fascial spaces may be evident.

LYMPH NODE EVALUATION

Evaluation of any inflammatory process involving the maxillofacial region also must include evaluation for draining lymphatics; these include the parotid, submandibular, submental, internal jugular, retropharyngeal, spinal accessory, transverse cervical, and anterior cervical nodes (Figure 4-31).[56,90,91,105,108] These cervical lymph nodes have been organized into seven levels for the purpose of describing the spread of neoplastic processes. Level I includes the submandibular and submental lymph nodes; level II includes the upper cervical chain nodes; level III consists of the middle deep cervical chain; level IV consists of the lower deep cervical nodes; level V consists of the spinal accessory and transverse cervical chain nodes; level VI nodes consists of the pretracheal, paratracheal, and prelaryngeal nodes; and level VII consists of the upper mediastinal nodes (see Chapter 9).

The parotid lymph nodes are divided into two groups, superficial and deep. The superficial, or extraglandular, group receives drainage from the scalp above the parotid, the lateral portion of the eyelid, auricle, and external auditory canal; and the posterior portion of the cheek, buccal mucosa, and parotid gland.[56,108] The deep lymph nodes are located within the substance of the gland and receive drainage from the deep portion of the face, including the oropharynx and nasopharynx, and the middle ear. Efferent drainage is to the internal jugular chain.

The submandibular gland, although not containing any intraglandular lymphatics, is closely related to a number of small lymph nodes located on the anterior aspect of the submandibular gland and the lateral aspect of the anterior belly of the digastric muscle between its insertion and the angle of the mandible (see Figure 4-31, *B*). These nodes are collectively referred to as the *submandibular nodes* and receive drainage from the submental and sublingual lymph nodes, lateral segment of the lower lip, all the upper lip and external nose, the submandibular and sublingual glands, and the anterior two thirds of the tongue. Efferent drainage is to the internal jugular chain through lymphatics located along the anterior facial vein and artery.

The submental lymph nodes are a group of nodes located between the anterior bellies of the digastric muscles,

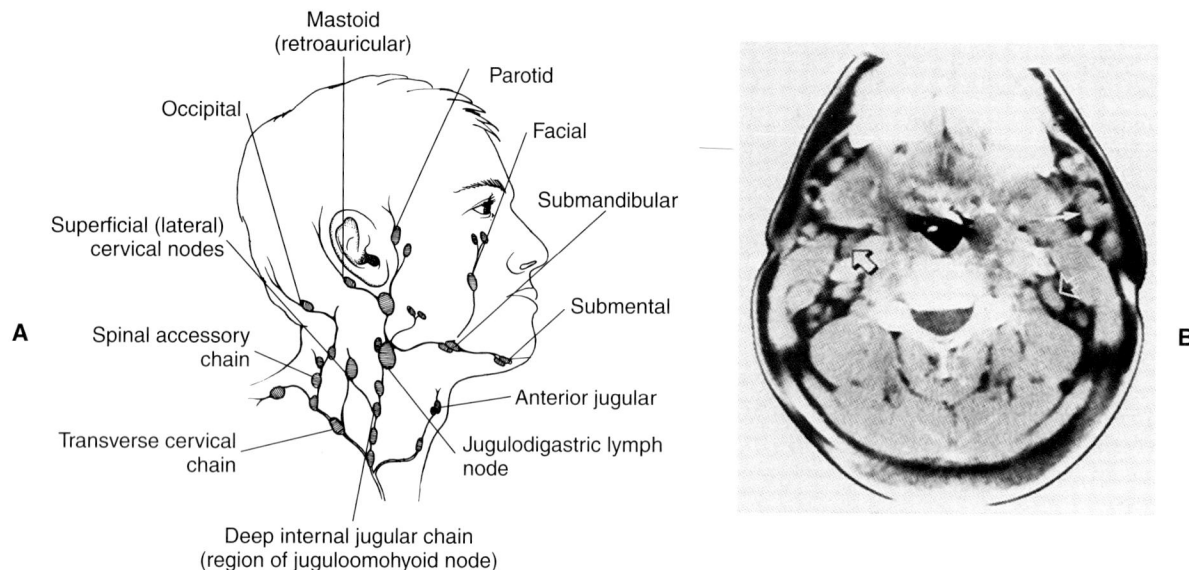

Figure 4-31 A, The major lymphatics of maxillofacial and upper cervical regions. **B,** Contrast-enhanced axial CT section through lower maxillofacial region demonstrating left spinal accessory *(open white arrowhead),* submandibular nodes *(white arrow),* and right internal jugular node *(open black arrow).* (From DelBalso AM, editor: *Maxillofacial imaging,* Philadelphia, 1990, WB Saunders.)

superficial to the mylohyoid muscle. Consisting of up to eight nodes, the submental lymph nodes receive drainage from the chin, lower lip, cheeks, anterior gingiva, floor of mouth, and tip of tongue. Efferent drainage is to the ipsilateral or contralateral submandibular lymph nodes and rarely directly to the internal jugular chain.

The anterior jugular chain is located in the superficial fascia of the neck and receives afferent drainage from the skin and anterior portion of the neck. Efferent drainage on the right is to the lowest internal jugular chain or highest intrathoracic node and on the left is into the thoracic duct or anterior mediastinal lymph nodes.[56] The superficial cervical nodes are superficial to the sternocleidomastoid muscle along the course of the external jugular vein. Afferent drainage is from the superficial tissues of the preauricular and postauricular scalp and overlying skin.[56] Efferent drainage is to the deep internal jugular or transverse cervical chain.

The retropharyngeal lymph nodes consist of a bilateral median and lateral group. In adults these nodes are often not identifiable except when involved by pathological conditions.[105] The median group is located along the midline; the lateral group is located along the lateral border of the longus capitis muscle, medial to the carotid artery. These lymph nodes receive afferent drainage from the nasal fossae, sinuses, nasopharynx and oropharynx, palate, and middle ear. Efferent drainage is to the internal jugular chain.

The deep lymphatics of the neck can be divided into three major groups: the internal jugular, spinal accessory, and transcervical lymph nodes. The internal jugular nodes

lie anterolateral to the internal jugular vein, beneath the sternocleidomastoid muscle (see Figure 4-31, *B*). They receive efferent drainage from the parotid, submental, submandibular, retropharyngeal, and anterior cervical lymph nodes.[56] Two important nodes in this chain are the jugulodigastric and juguloomohyoid lymph nodes. These two lymph nodes are larger than the other nodes in the chain and often enlarge in response to infection or neoplasms in one of the regions from which they receive drainage. The jugulodigastric lymph node is located below the posterior belly of the digastric muscle at the level of the hyoid bone and receives drainage from the posterior third of the tongue and palatine tonsils. The juguloomohyoid lymph node is located either at or above the level at which the middle tendon of the omohyoid crosses the internal jugular vein. It receives direct or indirect afferent drainage from the entire tongue. Indirect drainage occurs through the submental, submandibular, and upper deep cervical nodes.

The spinal accessory lymph nodes are located in the posterior triangle of the neck, along the course of the spinal accessory nerve. These nodes receive afferent drainage from various lymphatics located in the occipital region and lateral neck; efferent drainage is primarily to the transverse cervical nodes. The transverse cervical lymph nodes are located along the course of the transverse cervical artery. They receive drainage from the spinal accessory lymph nodes and the skin of the anterolateral neck and upper anterolateral chest wall. Efferent drainage is similar to that described for the internal jugular nodes.

The CT findings in inflammatory and neoplastic disease cover a wide spectrum of changes, often of similar appearances, stressing the need to correlate clinical and imaging findings. A number of diagnostic criteria have been established to evaluate the lymphatics of the head and neck; these criteria consider size, number, appearance, and enhancement patterns. With the exceptions of the submandibular and jugulodigastric nodes, any node larger than 1 cm is considered abnormal.[56,73,91,108] The upper limit of normal for the submandibular and jugulodigastric lymph nodes is 1.5 cm. The presence of a low-density area (10 to 18 HU) representing central necrosis is abnormal regardless of size or pattern of peripheral enhancement. Central necrosis may occur in metastatic, inflammatory, and lymphomatous nodes.[90,91,108] Peripheral enhancement may occur in inflammatory and neoplastic lymph nodes; inflammatory lymph nodes often exhibit a thick, irregular zone of peripheral enhancement around a necrotic center and most often are seen in tuberculosis.[90,91] Metastatic lymph nodes often demonstrate peripheral enhancement that is of uniform thickness and density. Lymphomatous nodes often are found as smooth, bulky nodes with peripheral enhancement. Inflammatory and neoplastic lymph nodes can exhibit loss of the adjacent fascial planes; however, the degree of obliteration associated with inflammatory lymph nodes is usually more extensive than that associated with metastatic disease.

ORBITAL INFLAMMATORY PROCESSES

CT represents the most commonly used imaging modality in the evaluation of orbital inflammatory processes.[44,71,78] CT scanning of the orbit is ideally performed ideally using slice thicknesses of 3 to 5 mm in the axial and direct coronal planes. At times, imaging in the direct coronal plane may be impossible because patients must maintain their heads in an extended position while the scan is performed; in patients with cervical spine problems, especially the elderly, this position often is difficult or impossible to attain. In addition, the presence of metallic dental restorations may result in nondiagnostic images. Multiplanar reformatted images in the coronal and parasagittal planes can be obtained using data obtained in thin-slice axial scans. The generation of reformatted images requires special software normally present on most CT scanners. Intravenous contrast, although not essential in defining normal orbital anatomy, may afford better definition of a pathological process, especially abscesses. MRI has been reported useful in the evaluation of orbital inflammatory processes and in the differentiation of pseudotumors from other inflammatory processes involving the orbit (see Chapter 15).

The majority of inflammatory processes involving the orbit are infectious in origin, usually resulting from inadequately treated acute or chronic sinusitis. However, they also may occur as a result of infections elsewhere in the maxillofacial region. Orbital complications often are the first manifestation of an ethmoiditis and occur most often in children.[1,36] Bacteria most commonly isolated from orbital infections are *Staphylococcus, Streptococcus, Pneumo-*

coccus, Pseudomonas, Neisseria, Haemophilus, and *Mycobacterium*.[71,78] Viral infections are usually secondary herpes simplex or herpes zoster virus.[72] Opportunistic fungal or parasitic infections can develop in patients who are immunocompromised including those with poorly controlled diabetes.[72]

Acute orbital complications resulting from an extension of sinusitis include cellulitis, orbital abscess formation, subperiosteal abscess formation (see Figure 4-13), superior orbital fissure syndrome, orbital apex syndrome, and osteomyelitis of the osseous walls. The mildest complication is reactionary edema of eyelid and orbital contents that occurs as a result of the close proximity of the orbit to the involved sinus. This complication (preseptal edema) is not associated with bacterial invasion of the orbit. Opacification of the involved sinus is noted on plain film studies. CT studies show inflammatory changes in the involved sinus and soft tissue and periorbital edema, but osseous destruction is absent.[39,72,106]

Bacterial invasion of the orbit results initially in a cellulitis. CT findings are similar to those described for reactionary edema. Orbital cellulitis may be complicated by the formation of an orbital or a subperiosteal abscess with or without osteomyelitis of the orbital wall. Clinically, patients are first seen with varying degrees of proptosis, ophthalmoplegia, and visual impairment. Plain film findings demonstrate opacification of involved sinuses. CT studies, in addition to the findings noted for orbital inflammation, also demonstrate sinus opacification, proptosis, orbital mass with or without abscess, and subperiosteal abscess. Osteomyelitis with breakdown of the orbital wall can occur in untreated or rapidly fulminating infections. Posterior and superior extension of the abscess can result in cavernous sinus thrombosis. On MRI examinations, orbital cellulitis can result in a decrease in the normally high signal intensity of orbital fat seen on T1-weighted sequences.[6] These changes are believed to reflect an increase in the free water content.

ORBITAL PSEUDOTUMORS

Orbital pseudotumors (idiopathic orbital inflammatory syndrome) represent a group of orbital inflammatory disorders involving one or more tissues of the orbit except the eye.[19] Orbital pseudotumors are believed to be of immunological origin; however, no local or identifiable cause can be identified.[19,78,81] Clinically, these patients usually have proptosis as a result of inflammatory infiltration of one or more tissues. Orbital pseudotumors can occur at any age. CT plays a central role in the diagnostic imaging of orbital pseudotumors. A number of systems have been proposed for classifying orbital pseudotumors; however, one of the easiest to understand and apply is that proposed by Nugent et al.[81] These investigators proposed a classification of orbital pseudotumors based on anatomical location and radiographic features as determined by CT. According to this system, orbital pseudotumors are classified as lacrimal, anterior, posterior, diffuse, or myositic. Lacrimal pseudotumors involve the lacrimal glands and are located in the superolateral aspect of the orbit. Inferomedial displacement is present in these cases. Anterior pseudotumors are located on the posterior aspect of the globe, resulting in thickening of the posterior sclera. These lesions also extend posteriorly at variable distances along the optic nerve. Posterior pseudotumors are located in the apical portion of the orbit and result in poor definition of the extraocular muscles and optic nerve. Diffuse pseudotumors involve the entire orbit and extend from the orbital apex to the posterior margin of the globe. Myositic pseudotumors involve the extraocular muscle or muscles, resulting in diffuse enlargement of the muscle. Orbital pseudotumors can present as masses that are isointense to orbital muscles on T1 sequences and isointense or minimally hyperintense to orbital fat on T2 sequences.[6]

DIAGNOSTIC IMAGING OF SALIVARY INFLAMMATORY DISORDERS

Inflammatory disorders of the major salivary glands or sialoadenitis may be classified as acute or chronic (see Chapter 12). Acute sialoadenitis may be further subdivided into obstructive or nonobstructive causes. Obstructive sialoadenitis is the result of sialoliths (ductal stones) with or without strictures, whereas nonobstructive sialoadenitis is most commonly the result of infectious agents such as bacteria and viruses. Obstructive and nonobstructive sialoadenitis often are interrelated with respect to causative factors and clinical presentation; ductal damage (stricture) and intraductal debris from bacterial sialoadenitis may be predisposing factors in the development of a sialolith, whereas a sialolith, strictures, or both may result in a ductal obstruction facilitating a superimposed bacterial infection.

Clinically, patients with acute obstructive sialoadenitis often report colicky pain and glandular or periglandular swelling associated with meals. Acute obstructive sialoadenitis in the absence of an accompanying acute bacterial infection is readily evaluated using CT. Thin axial CT sections through the suspect gland and its duct demonstrate not only the offending stone but also inflammatory changes involving the gland and periglandular tissues (Figure 4-32).

Acute nonobstructive sialadenitis is usually related to several viral or bacterial pathogens. Mumps is the most common form of viral parotitis, the diagnosis of which is based largely on clinical and serological findings, with no indication for additional imaging studies. However, diagnostic imaging can play an important role in the evaluation of patients with acute pyogenic or suppurative sialadenitis. Suppurative parotitis, the most common form of acute pyogenic sialadenitis, can occur at any age and is characterized by diffuse swelling of the gland and adjacent soft tissue.[22] Suppurative parotitis usually occurs in patients who are immunocompromised or debilitated and results from an ascending retrograde infection. Bacteria frequently responsible for this condition include *Staphylococcus aureus, S. viridans,* and pneumococci. Bacterial sialadenitis also can occur in obstructed glands, especially the submandibular gland.

CT scanning before and after the administration of intravenous contrast is the imaging study of choice in these patients. The CT findings in nonobstructive sialadenitis are variable and range from generalized increases in the size and CT density of the gland, to ill-defined areas of increased density representing inflammatory masses on non–contrast-enhanced studies, to abscess formation with a low-density central region and peripheral mural en-

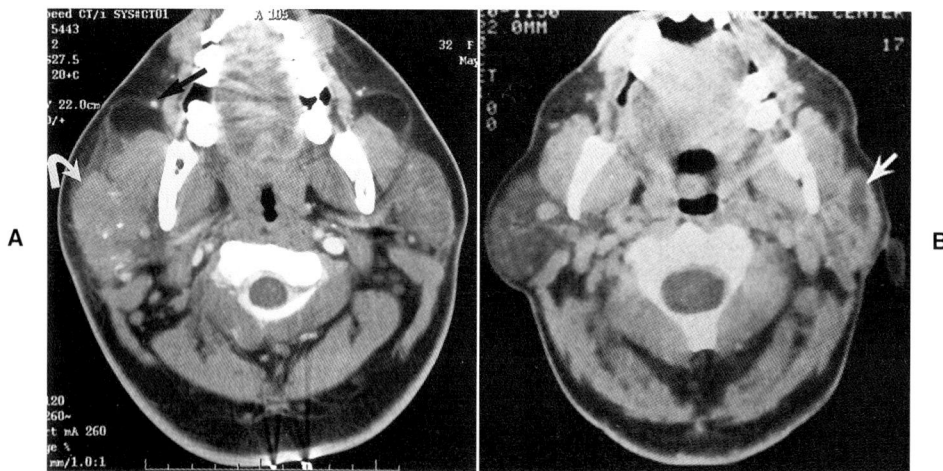

Figure 4-32 A, Non-contrast-enhanced axial CT section through parotid glands demonstrating obstructive parotitis on the left caused by a stone in the distal parotid duct *(straight arrow).* A similar nonobstructing duct is present on the left. Multiple intraglandular stones are noted in the right parotid gland. Generalized edema of the gland has resulted in an overall increase in its CT density. Extension of the inflammatory process into the surrounding tissues has resulted in loss of sharp marginations of the gland and extension of the inflammatory process into the adjacent subcutaneous tissues *(curved white arrow).* **B,** Contrast-enhanced axial CT section through the parotid glands demonstrating an abscess in the superficial lobe the left parotid *(arrow).* A generalized increased density of the remainder of the gland is noted, reflecting inflammatory changes.

hancement on contrast-enhanced studies (see Figure 4-32, *B*). In some instances the inflammatory masses or abscesses may be indistinguishable from neoplasms without an adequate clinical history. CT sections also may demonstrate sialoliths in those cases with an associated ductal obstruction. Extension of the inflammatory process beyond the gland into adjacent soft tissue results in a loss or ill definition of adjacent soft tissue planes.

MRI can be used in the evaluation of acute and chronic inflammatory processes. Acute inflammation of the parotid can result in increased signal intensity on T2-weighted sequences and contrast enhancement on T1-weighted sequences. Chronic inflammation can result in shrinkage of the gland and hypointensity on T1 and T2 sequences.[63]

Chronic recurrent sialoadenitis is characterized by recurrent episodes of pain and swelling, often associated with glandular swelling.[27] As the name implies, this condition is characterized by a recurrent cycle of ascending glandular infections followed by scarring or stricture of the major ducts. Often an acute obstructive or a nonobstructive bacterial sialoadenitis may occur in these glands. Chronic recurrent sialadenitis can be evaluated with sialography. In such patients, sialography is primarily intended to assess the status of the ductal system; demonstrate the presence, location, or both of strictures that may predispose or impede the movement of a stone; and differentiate between obstructive sialoadenitis and other forms of sialoadenitis that can result in salivary enlargement. These may be mistaken for obstructive sialoadenitis[34,85-89,109] and include chronic recurrent sialoadenitis, sialosis, and autoimmune sialoadenitis.* The sialographic hallmark of chronic recurrent sialadenitis is ductal scarring or stricture formation with focal areas of dilation involving the primary ducts. Information provided by a contrast sialogram can play an important role in determining whether gland removal is warranted.

Autoimmune sialoadenitis is used to describe a group of salivary gland disorders resulting from underlying autoimmune processes such as Sjögren's syndrome and Mikulicz's disease.† These conditions are characterized by salivary gland enlargement, diffuse lymphocytic infiltration, and the formation of benign lymphoepithelial lesions. In contrast to chronic recurrent sialadenitis, in which extensive involvement of the primary ducts occurs, the sialographic findings in autoimmune sialadenitis are related to the rupture of weakened secondary ducts, especially early in the disease process, and is referred to as *pseudosialectasis*.[110,111] Later sialographic changes include cavity formation and the significant glandular destruction as a result of cavitation caused by abscess formation.[110,111]

Sialosis or benign parotid hypertrophy is a noninflammatory, nonneoplastic bilateral enlargement of the parotid glands of unknown origin. The sialographic findings in sialosis reflect the underlying pathological process. Sialosis exclusively involves the underlying parenchyma while spar-

ing the ductal system. Sialography may demonstrate a splaying of the major ductal system as a result of parenchymal edema; however, no morphological changes occur in the ducts.

CT should be considered in patients in whom a strong clinical indication for an obstructive and a pyogenic sialadenitis is evident. In these instances, non–contrast-enhanced axial sections may demonstrate the presence of the sialolith, ductal dilation, and signs of pyogenic sialadenitis.

PEDIATRIC MAXILLOFACIAL INFECTIONS

The radiographic manifestations of pediatric maxillofacial odontogenic and nonodontogenic infections are very similar if not identical to those described for the same disease processes in adults (see Chapter 21).

TYPES OF PEDIATRIC MAXILLOFACIAL INFECTIONS

Periorbital and Orbital Infections   Periorbital and orbital involvement occur fairly commonly as a complication of the spread of infections originating in the maxillary dentition and paranasal sinuses or a result of trauma to the area. Periorbital or preseptal involvement tends to occur in a younger age group (younger than 5 years of age), whereas postseptal involvement tends to occur in older children.[25,39,57] Although plain films may be helpful in documenting the cause of infection in certain circumstances (e.g., presence of a foreign body, dental infections, sinusitis), specific radiographic findings are difficult to delineate, particularly if only the preseptal area is involved (Figure 4-33). Consequently, CT scanning is considered the radiographic study of choice.[39,42] Indeed, a CT classification of

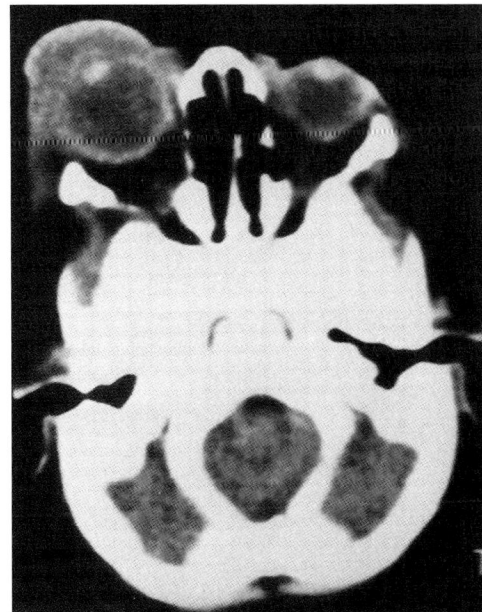

Figure 4-33 Preseptal cellulitis. Axial CT section through the orbits of a 1-year-old child demonstrating proptosis and preseptal cellulitis of the right orbit. (From DelBalso AM, editor: *Maxillofacial imaging,* Philadelphia, 1990, WB Saunders.)

---

*References 22, 27, 34, 40, 41, 93, 109.
†References 2, 7, 30, 110, 111, 123.

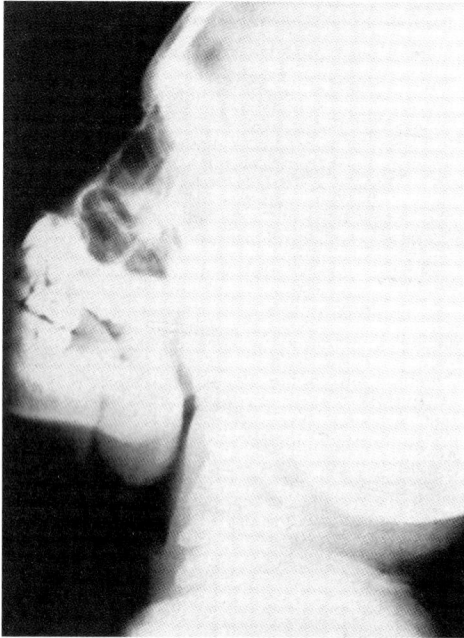

Figure 4-34 Lateral view of neck with soft tissue detail demonstrating marked tonsillar enlargement resulting from abscess formation in the orbit. (From DelBalso AM, editor: *Maxillofacial imaging,* Philadelphia, 1990, WB Saunders.)

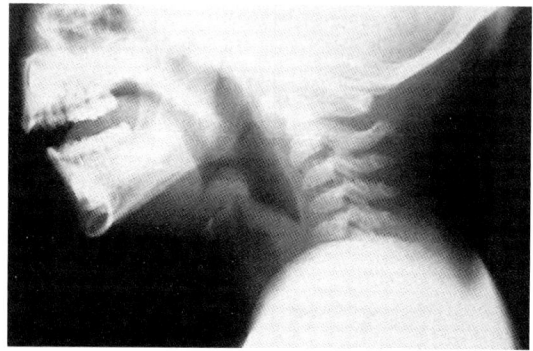

Figure 4-35 Epiglottitis. Lateral view of cervical airway in a 3-year-old boy demonstrating thickening and smoothness of the epiglottis and aryepiglottic folds. (From DelBalso AM, editor: *Maxillofacial imaging,* Philadelphia, 1990, WB Saunders.)

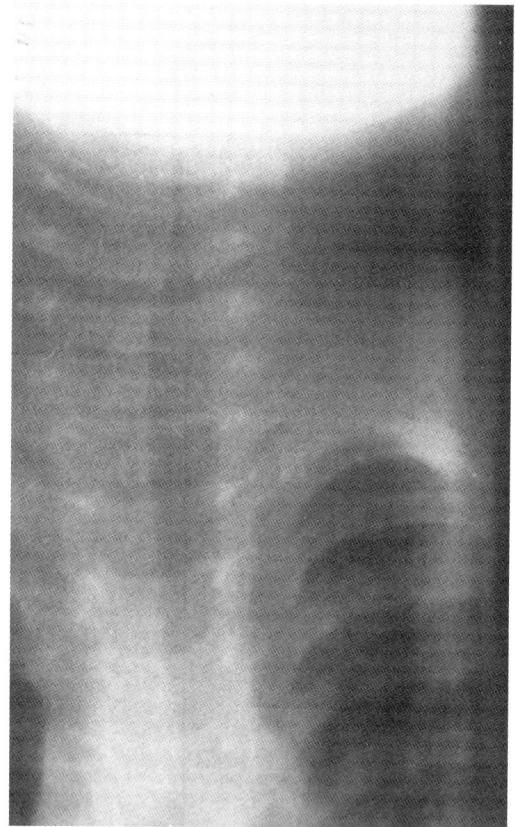

Figure 4-36 Croup. Anteroposterior view of airway demonstrating symmetrical narrowing of the subglottic airway for several centimeters below the vocal cords. (From DelBalso AM, editor: *Maxillofacial imaging,* Philadelphia, 1990, WB Saunders.)

orbital involvement by infectious processes has been delineated to assist in diagnosis and treatment planning by assessing radiographic features associated with the preseptal region, orbital involvement, and complication with or without local extension.[16,43,98]

Tonsillar and Peritonsillar Infections   Radiographic changes in the tonsillar and peritonsillar region can be produced by hypertrophy, allergic reactions, infections, and neoplasms. Although these changes can be identified on plain films, MRI, and CT, a plain lateral neck film is often the view obtained initially to assess the degree of soft tissue enlargement and upper airway and nasopharyngeal patency[5] (Figure 4-34). In the assessment of adenoidal hypertrophy, a ratio of adenoidal mass to nasopharynx may be obtained to determine whether adenoidectomy is necessary.[11,32,48] However, a radiograph should not supplant an adequate examination of the airway, and radiography is probably no better in gauging airway patency than a thorough physical examination.[11,28,32] In addition, poor patient cooperation or poor positioning on the table may give the radiographic appearance of adenoid hypertrophy and airway obstruction; again, radiographic findings must be correlated with the physical examination. Although an anteroposterior plain film may be of little use in the determination of adenoid hypertrophy, it can be of great help in the evaluation of tonsillar hypertrophy, particularly if a small amount of barium is used to coat the tonsils to delineate the location of the inferior pole.[11] Lateral plain films of the neck cannot be used to determine the impingement of tonsillar hypertrophy on airway patency.

Occasionally, plain films may be of benefit in assessment of a mass effect or the presence of gas in the tissues as the result of an infection, but these features are more readily demonstrated on axial or coronal CT projections. The diagnostic capabilities of this study can be enhanced further by the coincident use of intravascular contrast.

Epiglottitis   Epiglottitis is an acute, bacterial inflammation or infection of the epiglottis, usually caused by

H. influenzae. In the pediatric population, epiglottitis usually begins abruptly with a severe pharyngitis, high fever, and an inability to handle saliva. Its rapid progression leading to dysphagia and upper airway obstruction makes it a pediatric medical emergency. Radiographically, the epiglottis and the aryepiglottic folds are edematous and swollen with smooth borders optimally seen on a lateral neck film (Figure 4-35). The epiglottis looks like a thumb projecting into and compromising the hypopharynx; indeed, this feature is referred to as the "thumb sign." Placement of a patient in the supine position to obtain lateral or anteroposterior neck films may lead to acute airway obstruction. In addition, the time expended in obtaining the radiographs may delay the establishment of an adequate airway; consequently, these films should never be performed unless the means to establish and maintain an airway are at hand. Finally, epiglottitis is occasionally accompanied by a bacterial pneumonia, which is evident on appropriate chest radiographs.

Croup As opposed to epiglottitis, croup, or laryngotracheobronchitis, is a viral infection characterized by inspiratory stridor, hoarseness, and a distinctive barking cough. Croup usually is caused by parainfluenza or respiratory syncytial virus. In this disease the diagnostic radiograph is the plain anteroposterior or posteroanterior projection, which demonstrates a distinctive subglottic narrowing resulting from mucosal and submucosal edema, giving the appearance of a church steeple (steeple sign) or a wine bottle (bottle sign) (Figure 4-36).

REFERENCES

1. Adams GL, Boles LR, Paparella MM: *Boies' fundamental of otolaryngology,* ed 5, Philadelphia, 1978, WB Saunders.
2. Alarcon-Segovia D, Ibanez G, Valezquez-Forero F, et al: Sjögren's syndrome in systemic lupus erythematosus: clinical and subclinical manifestations, *Ann Intern Med* 81:577, 1974.
3. Alberti PW: Inflammatory disease of the maxillary sinus and its complications, *Otolaryngol Clin North Am* 9:153, 1976.
4. Ariji E, Moriguchi S, Kuroki T, et al: Computed tomography of maxillofacial infection, *Dento-Maxillo-Facial Rad* 20:147, 1991.
5. Assael LA, McGarvy LL: Use of soft tissue radiographs for assessing impending airway obstruction in head and neck infections: report of a case, *J Oral Maxillofac Surg* 44:398, 1986.
6. Atlase SW: Orbit. In Stark DS, Bradley WG, editors: *Magnetic resonance imaging,* vol 3, ed 3, St Louis, 1999, Mosby.
7. Batsakis JG: Cysts, sinuses and "coeles." In Batsakis JG, editor: *Tumors of the head and neck,* ed 2, Baltimore, 1984, Williams & Wilkins.
8. Beck-Mannagetta J, Necek D: Radiologic findings in aspergillosis of the maxillary sinus, *Oral Surg* 62:345, 1986.
9. Berkovitz BKK, Moxhax BJ: *Textbook of head and neck anatomy,* Chicago, 1988, Year Book Medical.
10. Blitzer A, Lawson W, Meyers BR, et al: Patient survival factors in paranasal sinus mucormycosis, *Laryngoscope* 90:635, 1980.
11. Brodsky L: Modern assessment of tonsils and adenoids, *Pediatr Clin North Am* 36:1551, 1989.
12. Bryan RN, Miller RH, Ferreyro RI, et al: Computed tomography of the major salivary glands, *AJR Am J Roentgenol* 139:547, 1982.
13. Carter BL, Karmody CS, Blickman JR, et al: Computed tomography and sialography. I. Normal anatomy, *J Comput Assist Tomogr* 5:42, 1981.
14. Centeno RS, Bentson JR, Mancuso AA: CT scanning in rhinocerebral mucormycosis and aspergillosis, *Radiology* 140:383, 1981.
15. Chakeres DW: Computed tomography of the ethmoid sinuses, *Otolaryngol Clin North Am* 18:29, 1985.
16. Chandler JR, Lagenbrunner DS, Stevens EF: The pathogenesis of the orbital complications of acute sinusitis, *Laryngoscope* 92:1414, 1970.
17. Chapnik JS, Bach MC: Bacterial and fungal infections of the maxillary sinus, *Otolaryngol Clin North Am* 9:43, 1976.
18. Colman MF: Invasive aspergillus of the head and neck, *Laryngoscope* 95:898, 1985 (abstract).
19. Curtin HD: Pseudotumor, *Radiol Clin North Am* 25:583, 1987.
20. Curtin HD: Separation of the masticator space from the parapharyngeal space, *Radiology* 163:195, 1987.
21. DelBalso AM: Advances in maxillofacial imaging. In Myers HW, editor: *New biotechnology in oral research,* Basel, 1989, Karger.
22. DelBalso AM, Ellis GE, Hartman KS, et al: Diagnostic imaging of the salivary glands and periglandular regions. In DelBalso AM, editor: *Maxillofacial imaging,* Philadelphia, 1990, WB Saunders.
23. DelBalso AM, Pruet CW, Heffner DK, et al: The parapharyngeal and retropharyngeal spaces. In DelBalso AM, editor: *Maxillofacial imaging,* Philadelphia, 1990, WB Saunders.
24. Dillon WP: The pharynx and oral cavity. In Som PM, Bergeron RT, editors: *Head and neck imaging,* ed 2, St Louis, 1990, Mosby.
25. Dolan KD: The ethmoid sinus: plain film and tomographic radiology, *Otolaryngol Clin North Am* 18:15, 1985.
26. Eichel B: Ethmoiditis: pathophysiology and medical management, *Otolaryngol Clin North Am* 18:43, 1985.
27. Eisenbud L, Cranin N: The role of sialography in the diagnosis and therapy of chronic obstructive sialadenitis, *Oral Surg* 16:1181, 1961.
28. Elwany S: The adenoidal-nasopharyngeal ratio (A-N ratio): its validity in selecting children for adenoidectomy, *J Laryngol Otol* 101:569, 1987.
29. Endicott JN, Nelson RJ, Saraceno CA: Diagnosis and management decisions in infections of the deep fascial spaces of the head and neck utilizing computerized tomography, *Laryngoscope* 92:630, 1982.
30. Ericson S: The parotid gland in patients with and without rheumatoid arthritis: a sialographic and physiologic study, *Acta Radiol Diagn (Stockh)* 275(suppl):1, 1968.
31. Finn DG, Farmer JC: Chronic mucormycosis, *Laryngoscope* 92:761, 1982.
32. Fusioka M, Young W, Giradany B: Radiographic examination of adenoidal size in children: adenoid-nasal pharyngeal ratio, *AJR Am J Roentgenol* 133:401, 1979.
33. Gamba JL, Woodruff WW, Djang WT, et al: Craniofacial mucormycosis: assessment with CT, *Radiology* 160:207, 1986.
34. Gates GA: Sialography and scanning of the salivary glands, *Otolaryngol Clin North Am* 10:379, 1977.

35. Goaz PW, White SC: Infection and inflammation of the jaws and facial bones. In Goaz PW, White SC, editors: *Oral radiology: principles and interpretation,* St Louis, 1987, Mosby.

36. Goldberg MH, Eichel B: Ethmoiditis: pathophysiology and medical management, *Otolaryngol Clin North Am* 18:43, 1985.

37. Goldberg MH, Topazian RG: Odontogenic infections and deep fascial space infections of dental origin. In Topazian RG, Goldberg MH, editors: *Oral and maxillofacial infections,* ed 2, Philadelphia, 1987, WB Saunders.

38. Gore RM, Weinberg PE, Kwang SK, et al: Sphenoid sinus mucoceles presenting as intracranial masses on computed tomography, *Surg Neurol* 13:375, 1980.

39. Greiner FG: Pediatric maxillofacial imaging. In DelBalso AM, editor: *Maxillofacial imaging,* Philadelphia, 1990, WB Saunders.

40. Greyson ND, Noyek AM: Radionuclide salivary scanning, *J Otolaryngol* 11:3, 1982.

41. Grove AS, DiChiro G: Salivary gland and technetium 99m pertechnetate, *Am J Roentgenol Radium Ther Nucl Med* 102:109, 1968.

42. Gutowski WM, Mulberry PE, Hengerer AS, et al: The role of CT scans in managing the orbital complications of ethmoiditis, *Int J Pediatr Otorhinolaryngol* 15:117, 1988.

43. Hall RE, DelBalso AM, Carter LC: Radiography of the sinonasal tract. In DelBalso AM, editor: *Maxillofacial imaging,* Philadelphia, 1990, WB Saunders.

44. Hammerschlag SB, Hesselink JR, Weber AL: *Computed tomography of the eye and orbit,* Norwalk, Conn, 1983, Appleton-Century-Crofts.

45. Hardin CW, Harnsberger HR, Osborn AE: Infection and tumor of the masticator space, *Radiology* 157:413, 1987.

46. Hatton MN, Hall RE, DelBalso AM: Radiology of head and neck deep space infections: the clinician's perspective. In DelBalso AM, editor: *Maxillofacial imaging,* Philadelphia, 1990, WB Saunders.

47. Haug RH, Wible RT, Lieberman J: Measurement standards for the prevertebral region in the lateral soft-tissue radiograph of the neck, *J Oral Maxillofac Surg* 49:1149, 1991.

48. Hibbert J, Whitehouse GH: The assessment of adenoidal size by radiographic means, *Clin Otolaryngol* 3:43, 1978.

49. Holliday RA, Pendergast NC: Imaging inflammatory processes of the oral cavity and suprahyoid neck, *Oral Maxillofacial Surg Clin North Am* 4:215, 1992.

50. Hollinshead WH: *Anatomy for surgeons, the head and neck,* ed 2, vol 1, New York, 1968, Harper & Row.

51. Hollinshead WH: Fascia and fascial spaces of the head and neck. In Hollinshead WH, editor: *Anatomy for surgeons: the head and neck,* Philadelphia, 1982, JB Lippincott.

52. Holt GR, McManus K, Newman RK, et al: Computerized tomography in the diagnosis of deep-neck infections, *Arch Otolaryngol* 108:693, 1982.

53. Hora JF: Primary aspergillosis of the paranasal sinuses and associated areas, *Laryngoscope* 75:768, 1964.

54. Ishikawa H, Ischii Y, Ono T: Evaluation of gray scale ultrasonography in the investigation of oral and neck mass lesions, *J Oral Maxillofac Surg* 41:775, 1983.

55. Jarenwattananon A, Gentry L: Magnetic resonance imaging of the upper maxillofacial region. In DelBalso AM, editor: *Maxillofacial imaging,* Philadelphia, 1990, WB Saunders.

56. Jinkins JR: Computed tomography of the cranio-cervical lymphatic system: anatomical and functional considerations, *Neuroradiology* 29:317, 1987.

57. Kaban LB: Infections of the maxillofacial region. In Kaban LB, editor: *Pediatric oral and maxillofacial surgery,* Philadelphia, 1990, WB Saunders.

58. Kassel EE: Radiographic evaluation of the floor of the mouth and tongue base. In DelBalso AM, editor: *Maxillofacial imaging,* Philadelphia, 1990, WB Saunders.

59. Keat TE: *Atlas of roentgenographic measurements,* ed 6, St Louis, 1990, Mosby.

60. King WP: Allergic disorders in the otolaryngologic practice, *Otolaryngol Clin North Am* 18:677, 1985.

61. Kopp W, Fotter R, Steiner H, et al: Aspergillosis of the paranasal sinuses, *Radiology* 156:715, 1985.

62. Kornblut AD: Granulomatous inflammations of the nose and para-nasal sinuses, *Otolaryngol Clin North Am* 15:529, 1982.

63. Kramer LA, Mafee Mahmoud: Salivary glands. In Stark DS, Bradley WG, editor: *Magnetic resonance imaging,* vol 3, ed 3, St Louis, 1999, Mosby.

64. Kristensen S: Fungal infection of the maxillary sinus, *Rhinology* 22:281, 1984.

65. Kumazawa H, Zehm S, Nakamura A: CT findings of aspergillosis in the paranasal sinuses, *Arch Otorhinolaryngol* 244:77, 1987.

66. Lam EWN, Hannam AG, Wood WW, et al: Imaging of orofacial tissues by magnetic resonance, *Oral Surg* 68:2, 1988.

67. Langland O, Langlais R, McDavid WD, et al: *Principles and practice of panoramic radiology,* Philadelphia, 1989, Lea & Febiger.

68. Larson SG: The base of the tongue. In Carter BL, editor: *Computed tomography of the head and neck,* New York, 1985, Churchill Livingstone.

69. Last RJ: *Anatomy: regional, and applied,* New York, 1978, Churchill Livingstone.

70. Lee KJ: The nose and sinuses. In Lee KJ, editor: *Essential otolaryngology. Head and neck surgery,* ed 3, New Hyde Park, NY, 1983, Medical Examination Publishing.

71. Logalbo FA: Computed tomography of the orbit. In DelBalso AM, editor: *Maxillofacial imaging,* Philadelphia, 1990, WB Saunders.

72. Mafee MF, Schatz. CJ: The orbit. In Som PM, Bergeron RT, editors: *Head and neck imaging,* ed 2, St Louis, 1990, Mosby.

73. Mancuso A, Maceri D, Rice D, et al: CT of cervical lymph node cancer, *AJR Am J Roentgenol* 136:381, 1981.

74. Matt BH, Lusk RP: Delineation of a deep neck abscess with magnetic resonance imaging, *Ann Otol Rhinol Laryngol* 96:615, 1987.

75. Mattox DE, Delaney RG: Anatomy of the ethmoid sinus, *Otolaryngol Clin North Am* 18:3, 1985.

76. McGill TJ, Simpson G, Healy GB: Fulminant aspergillosis of the nose and paranasal sinuses: a new clinical entity, *Laryngoscope* 90:748, 1980.

77. McGuirt WF, Harrill JA: Paranasal sinus aspergillosis, *Laryngoscope* 89:1563, 1979.

78. Momose KJ: Orbital pathology. In Taveras JM, Ferrucci JT, editors: *Radiology,* vol 3, New York, 1993, JB Lippincott.

79. Nguyen VD, Potter JL, Hersh-Schick MR: Ludwig angina: an uncommon and potentially lethal neck infection, *AJNR Am J Neuroradiol* 12:215, 1991.

80. Noyek AM, Kirsch JC, Greyson ND, et al: The clinical significance of radionuclide bone and gallium scanning in osteomyelitis of the head and neck, *Laryngoscope* 94(pt 2 suppl 34):1, 1984.

81. Nugent RA, Rootman J, Robertson WD: Acute orbital pseudotumor: classification and CT features, *AJR Am J Roentgenol* 137:957, 1981.

82. Nyberg DE, Jeffrey RB, Brant-Zawadzki M, et al: Computed tomography of cervical infection, *J Comput Assist Tomogr* 9:288, 1985.

83. O'Rahilly R: Nose and paranasal sinuses. In Gardner E, Gray DJ, O'Rahilly R, editors: *Anatomy,* ed 2, Philadelphia, 1967, WB Saunders.

84. Osborn AG, Johnson L, Roberts TS: Sphenoidal mucoceles with intracranial extension, *J Comput Assist Tomogr* 3:335, 1979.

85. Potter GD: Sialography and the salivary glands, *Otolaryngol Clin North Am* 6:509, 1977.

86. Potter GD, Gold RP: Radiographic analysis of the skull, *Med Rad Photogr* 5:2, 1975.

87. Rabinov K: Sialography, *Contemp Diagn Radiol* 4:1, 1981.

88. Rabinov K, Kell T, Gordon PH: CT of the salivary glands, *Radiol Clin North Am* 22:145, 1984.

89. Rabinov K, Weber AL: *Radiology of the salivary glands,* Boston, 1985, GC Hall Medical.

90. Reede DL, Bergeron RT, Osborn AG: CT of the soft tissues of the neck. In Bergeron RT, Osborn AG, Som PM, editors: *Head and neck imaging excluding the brain,* St Louis, 1984, Mosby.

91. Reede DL, Bergeron RT, Whelan MA, et al: Computed tomography of cervical lymph nodes, *Radiographics* 3:339, 1983.

92. Reiskin AB: Diagnostic imaging and other techniques. In Topazian RG, Goldberg MH, editors: *Oral and maxillofacial infections,* Philadelphia, 1987, WB Saunders.

93. Reiskin AB, Lurie AG: Special radiographic techniques. In Goaz PW, White SC, editors: *Oral radiology principles and interpretation,* St Louis, 1987, Mosby.

94. Resnick D, Niwayama G: Osteomyelitis, septic arthritis, and soft tissue infections: mechanisms and situations. In Resnick D, editor: *Bone and joint imaging,* Philadelphia, 1989, WB Saunders.

95. Robb PJ: Aspergillosis of the paranasal sinuses: a case report and historical perspective, *J Laryngol Otol* 100:1071, 1986.

96. Rubin M, Cozzi GM: Fatal necrotizing mediastinitis as a complication of an odontogenic infection, *J Oral Maxillofac Surg* 45:529, 1987.

97. Samuel E, Lloyd GA: *Clinical radiology of the ear, nose and throat,* Philadelphia, 1978, WB Saunders.

98. Schramm VL, Curtain H, Kennerdell J: Evaluation of orbital cellulitis and the results of treatment, *Laryngoscope* 92:732, 1982.

99. Schwimmer AM, Roth SE, Morrison SN: The use of computerized tomography in the diagnosis of temporal and infratemporal spaces abscesses, *Oral Surg* 66:17, 1988.

100. Scott JH, Dixon AD: The circumoral spaces. In Scott JH, Dixon AD, editors: *Anatomy for students of dentistry,* ed 3, Baltimore, 1972, Williams & Wilkins.

101. Shafer WG, Hine MK, Levy BM: Bacterial, viral and mycotic infections. In Shafer WG, Hine MK, Levy BM, editors: *A textbook of oral pathology,* ed 4, Philadelphia, 1983, WB Saunders.

102. Shafer WG, Hine MK, Levy BM: Spread of oral infections. In Shafer WG, Hine MK, Levy, BM, editors: *A textbook of oral pathology,* ed 4, Philadelphia, 1983, WB Saunders.

103. Sicher H: The propagation of dental infections. In Sicher H, editor: *Oral anatomy,* St Louis, 1965, Mosby.

104. Siegert R: Ultrasonography of inflammatory tissue swellings of the head and neck, *J Oral Maxillofac Surg* 45:842, 1987.

105. Smoker WRK, Harnsberger HR, Reede DL, et al: The neck. In Som PM, Bergeron RT, editors: *Head and neck imaging,* ed 2, St Louis, 1990.

106. Som PM: The paranasal sinuses. In Bergeron RT, Osborn, AG, Som PM, editors: *Head and neck imaging excluding the brain,* St Louis, 1984, Mosby.

107. Som PM: Paranasal sinuses and pterygopalatine fossa. In Carter BL, editor: *Computed tomography of the head and neck,* New York, 1985, Churchill Livingstone.

108. Som PM: Lymph nodes of the neck, *Radiology* 165:593, 1987.

109. Som PM: Parapharyngeal space. In Som PM, Bergeron RT, editor: *Head and neck imaging,* ed 2, St Louis, 1990, Mosby.

110. Som PM, Biller HF, Shugar JMA, et al: Manifestations of parotid gland enlargement: radiographic, pathologic, and clinical correlations. Part II. The diseases of the Mikulicz syndrome, *Radiology* 141:421, 1981.

111. Som PM, Curtain HD: Sinuses. In Stark DS, Bradley WG, editors: *Magnetic resonance imaging,* vol III, St Louis, 1999, Mosby.

112. Som PM, Sacher M, Lanzieri CF, et al: The hidden antral compartment, *Radiology* 152:463, 1984.

113. Som PM, Sanders DP: The salivary glands. In Bergeron RT, Osborn AG, Som PM, editors: *Head and neck imaging excluding the brain,* St Louis, 1984, Mosby.

114. Som PM, Shugar JM: Antral mucoceles: a new look, *J Comput Assist Tomogr* 4:484, 1980.

115. Som PM, Shugar JM, Train JS, et al: Manifestations of parotid gland enlargement: radiographic, pathologic, and clinical manifestations. Part I. The autoimmune pseudosialectasis, *Radiology* 141:415, 1981.

116. Stahl RH: Allergic disorders of the nose and paranasal sinuses, *Otolaryngol Clin North Am* 7:703, 1974.

117. Stammberger H, Jakse R, Beaufort F: Aspergillosis of the paranasal sinuses: x-ray diagnosis, histopathology, and clinical aspects, *Ann Otol Rhinol Laryngol* 93:251, 1984.

118. Stiernberg CM: Deep-neck space infections, *Arch Otolaryngol Head Neck Surg* 112:1274, 1986.

119. van Nostrand AWP, Goodman WS: Pathologic aspects of mucosal lesions of the maxillary sinus, *Otolaryngol Clin North Am* 9:21, 1976.

120. Wall SD, Fisher MR, Amparo EG, et al: Magnetic resonance imaging in the evaluation of abscesses, *AJR Am J Roentgenol* 144:1217, 1985.

121. Warder FR, Chikes PG, Hudson WR: Aspergillosis of the paranasal sinuses, *Arch Otolaryngol* 101:683, 1975.

122. Weber AL: Inflammatory diseases of the paranasal sinuses and mucoceles, *Otolaryngol Clin North Am* 21:421, 1988.

123. Whaley K, Blair S, Low PS, et al: Sialographic abnormalities in Sjögren's syndrome, rheumatoid arthritis, and other arthritides and connective tissue disease: clinical and radiological investigation using hydrostatic sialography, *Clin Radiol* 23:474, 1972.

124. Williams P: Diseases of the maxillary sinus of dental origin. In Kruger GO, editor: *Textbook of oral surgery,* ed 3, St Louis, 1968, Mosby.

125. Wong YK, Novotony GM: Retropharyngeal space: review of anatomy, pathology, and clinical presentation, *J Otolaryngol* 7:528, 1978.

126. Yucel EK, Carter BL: Neck, oropharynx, and nasopharynx in clinical magnetic resonance. In Runge VM: *Clinical magnetic resonance imaging*, Philadelphia, 1991, JB Lippincott.

127. Zachariades N, Mezitis M, Stavrinidis P, et al: Mediastinitis, thoracic empyema, and pericarditis as complications of a dental abscess: report of a case, *J Oral Maxillofac Surg* 46:493, 1988.

128. Zizmor J, Noyek AM: Cyst, benign tumors, and malignant tumors of the paranasal sinuses, *Otolaryngol Clin North Am* 6:487, 1973.

129. Zizmor J, Noyek AM: Inflammatory diseases of the paranasal sinuses, *Otolaryngol Clin North Am* 6:459, 1973.

130. Zizmor J, Noyek AM: The radiologic diagnosis of maxillary sinus disease, *Otolaryngol Clin North Am* 9:93, 1976.

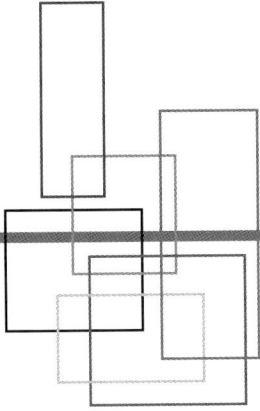

Principles of Surgical and Antimicrobial Infection Management

Larry J. Peterson

PRINCIPLES OF THERAPY

PRESENCE OF INFECTION

In most clinical situations it is easy to determine whether a patient has an infection. Locally, the classic signs and symptoms of pain, swelling, surface erythema, pus formation, and limitation of motion are present. Systemically, fever, lymphadenopathy, malaise, a toxic appearance, and an elevated white blood cell count are found.

However, frequently a patient reports some, but not all, of the signs of infection. Such a situation occurs when the patient has a painful tooth but has no swelling, trismus, elevated temperature, or other signs of infection. In this situation an inflammatory process such as pulpitis, rather than an infectious one, is probably the cause of the pain and antibiotic therapy is inappropriate.

Another example of a noninfectious condition occurs in the patient who has had third molar removal 2 days before being seen with persistent pain and swelling, but who does not have an elevated temperature, foul mouth odor, or malaise. Assessment of the character of the swelling, the presence of surface erythema, and the severity of pain may help in the diagnosis of infection. In most of these situations, the pain and swelling are the result of surgery, not of infection.

Diagnostic difficulty also may be encountered in the patient who has had a major maxillofacial procedure performed while under general anesthesia. During the second and third days after surgery, swelling and pain are commonly significant. Similarly, an elevated temperature and white blood cell count is not uncommon. Thus many of the signs of infection are present, but in fact, the more likely cause of these clinical findings is a combination of factors. Surgical insult causes pain and swelling and an elevation in neutrophils; and prolonged general anesthesia with insufficient postoperative pulmonary care often results in temperature elevation because of atelectasis. Clinical judgment is important in making the diagnosis, and the clinician should weigh all

information available before making the diagnosis of infection.[2]

Thus whenever the diagnosis is infection, the clinician's judgment should be based on a logical process of elimination. Although recognition of the signs and symptoms of infection is important, other disease conditions with some of the same signs and symptoms must be excluded as possible causes of the patient's discomfort.

STATE OF HOST DEFENSES

Host defense mechanisms are the most important factor in the final outcome of a bacterial insult. The inflammatory response, with its migration of white blood cells and the production of antibodies, provides most of this protection. If this mechanism or the other host defenses are impaired, infection may result from an otherwise minor bacterial exposure. Thus when considering prophylactic therapy for infection, the surgeon must evaluate the general state of the host defense mechanisms. (Extensive discussions of host defenses and the compromised host are presented in Chapters 1 and 24.)

Understanding that infections are ultimately cured by the host, not by antibiotics, is critical. Antibiotics help in situations in which the host has been overwhelmed by bacteria or when especially virulent bacteria are involved. In addition, when a patient's defenses are impaired, antibiotics play a more important role in the control of infection. Certain patient population groups are more susceptible to infection caused by depressed defenses. For discussion purposes, the causes of depressed defenses can be divided into four categories: physiological, disease-related, defective immune system–related, and drug suppression–related.

The physiological depression of host defenses relates primarily to the patient's inability to deliver the defending agents, such as white blood cells, antibodies, and complement, to the site of bacterial invasion. Shock, disturbances in circulation caused by advanced age or obesity, and fluid imbalances are examples of this type of depressed defenses.

Several diseases and disease states may inhibit host defenses. Malnutrition syndrome, often as a result of alcoholism, is an important example. Patients with cancer and leukemias also are more likely to become infected. Although diabetes is a predisposing factor to infection in the extremities, it is not an important contributing factor in the orofacial region, except in patients with poorly controlled diabetes.

Defective immune systems may be the result of congenital defects such as agammaglobulinemia, diseases such as multiple myeloma, and total-body radiation therapy. Patients with these conditions may be unable to fight successfully against the invading bacteria. Children who have had splenectomy are more susceptible to pneumonia caused by *Streptococcus pneumoniae.*

Finally, a variety of therapeutic drugs may suppress the patient's ability to handle infectious insults. Two groups of drugs are important in this regard. First is the cytotoxic drug group, used primarily for the treatment of a variety of malignancies. As documentation of their effectiveness increases, new and more potent cytotoxic drugs are being developed. Patients may have increased susceptibility to infections for up to 1 year after a course of cancericidal therapy.

The other group of drugs affecting host defenses is given to intentionally depress the immune system. These immunosuppressive drugs, such as glucocorticoids, azathioprine, and cyclosporine, are used in a variety of clinical situations such as organ transplantation. Steroid and azathioprine immunosuppressive therapy depresses T- and B-cell lymphocytes. When these drugs are used, there is a substantial increase in the incidence of severe infection. Cyclosporine depresses the T cells preferentially, leaving the B cells unaffected to continue their antibacterial activity. Aggressive antibiotic therapy must be considered in treating established infections in patients in any of these categories.

When surgery is anticipated in any compromised host, antibiotic prophylaxis of wound infection must be strongly considered.[29] The principles of wound infection prevention are discussed in Chapter 25. Even minor procedures in some patients with depressed host defenses may result in an overwhelming infection.

SURGICAL DRAINAGE AND INCISION

It is an established principle of treatment of deep tissue infections that surgical drainage must be achieved.[30] The objective in most situations is to drain pus from tissue spaces and to insert drains so that more pus does not accumulate in these spaces. This procedure removes the infected pus and relieves tissue pressure. In many odontogenic infections, surgical drainage can be accomplished by extraction of the affected tooth (or by opening, cleaning, and treating the pulp chamber). Removal of the tooth also serves to eliminate the bacteria's portal of entry (ie, the necrotic pulp) to deeper tissues. In some odontogenic infections

opening the pulp chamber or removal of the tooth is not possible or does not provide adequate drainage. In these situations intraoral or extraoral incisions must be made (see Chapter 8).

Surgical incision also plays an important role in the patient with cellulitis without pus formation. In patients with indurated swelling, incision through the tissues allows for faster resolution of the infection. In some situations, in fact, performance of this procedure is essential to achieve a cure. The purpose of this procedure is to release the pressure that has built up in the tissues, thereby increasing vascular flow. If unrelieved, this pressure substantially reduces the vascularity of the tissue and prevents the host defense substances from reaching areas where they are needed.

In most patients with moderate to severe cellulitis, incision and exploration of the spaces involved almost always reveal small areas of abscess formation. The clinical presentation in these situations is induration without fluctuation. Yet, when adequate incision and exploration are performed, areas of abscess formation are usually found. In some patients, these abscess pockets may be surprisingly large. Therefore consideration of early incision and drainage is prudent in the patient with rapidly progressing cellulitis or moderately advanced cellulitis. In summary, surgical intervention is necessary in both chronic abscesses with pus formation and acute indurated cellulitis. Many infections demonstrate abscess formation and indurated cellulitis. In such situations, incision and drainage of the abscess result in reduction of pressure in the area of cellulitis. Surgical drainage and incision may also obviate the use of an antibiotic or may increase the effectiveness of an antibiotic as the vascular flow is restored.

THE DECISION TO USE ANTIBIOTIC THERAPY

When the clinician is treating a patient with a possible infection, each of the factors in the previous section must be weighed carefully. Only then can an appropriate decision be made about whether antibiotic therapy is necessary.[23,31] The decision of when to treat a patient with antibiotics should be easy: give antibiotics to cure an existing infection. However, this easy step becomes difficult in critically evaluating the risk/benefit ratio of drug administration. This section discusses the principles that serve as guidelines in treatment decisions for antibiotic management of infections.

Truly, we live in the "antibiotic era." Beginning with the early work of Sir Alexander Fleming in 1929, when penicillin became the first "miracle drug," innumerable lives have been saved from such scourges as pneumococcal pneumonia, wound sepsis, and bacteremias.[13] Dentists benefited greatly from the discovery of penicillin because most odontogenic infections are caused by penicillin-sensitive microorganisms.

It soon became evident, however, that antibiotic usage had considerable risks.[16,25] First, allergy to penicillin was noted rather early. Second, a variety of toxic and idiosyncratic reactions emerged, ranging from simple nausea to fatal aplastic anemia. Selective organ and nerve damage was also observed. Third, superinfection by normally non-pathogenic bacterial inhabitants of the skin, the mucosal surfaces, and the gastrointestinal tract resulted from the death of susceptible bacteria. Finally, the development of antibiotic resistance was noted. Penicillinase-producing staphylococci were described early and became a major problem as the widespread use of penicillin resulted in recognition of "new" diseases caused by antibiotic-resistant species.

The problem of resistant bacteria is an ecological one. The microbiological environment has been polluted with bacteria that are resistant to many antibiotics. This alteration in antibiotic sensitivity is now the expected result of antibiotic administration. The risk to the individual patient from a single prescription of penicillin is small, but altered bacterial flora represent a present and future risk to the community in general. Community risk must somehow be balanced against individual benefit.

As these problems of antibiotic usage became apparent and their seriousness became clear, the need was evident that steps should be taken to decrease the inappropriate use of antibiotics.[34] This effort continues through individual hospital guidelines and through the periodic and regular review of antibiotic use in hospitals, as now required by the Joint Commission on Accreditation of Healthcare Organizations.

Despite the problems associated with antibiotic use, antibiotics are an essential weapon against infection. The treatment of odontogenic infections involves a complex series of diagnostic and therapeutic maneuvers, including determining the severity of infection, evaluating the patient's host defenses, treating the infection surgically, and prescribing the appropriate antibiotic. This section discusses the principles of antibiotic use. A set of guidelines for therapeutic and prophylactic use of antibiotics is also presented.[31,35] Information relating to specific antibiotic pharmacology appears in Chapter 6.

In some patients in whom an infection exists antibiotic therapy may not be indicated because the host normal immune defenses will be responsible for curing the infection. Therefore minor infections in patients with intact host defenses may not require antibiotic therapy. Even some moderately severe infections can be treated without antibiotics if surgical drainage, especially removal of the source of the infection, can be achieved. For example, routine extraction of an infected tooth does not typically require antibiotic therapy even when a limited periapical infection exists. Conversely, minor infections in patients with depressed host defenses must be treated aggressively, that is, medically with bactericidal drugs and surgically as early as possible. Also, an antibiotic may be required in treating minor infections that do not lend themselves to surgical intervention, such as a diseased tooth that must be retained but does not drain when the pulp chamber is opened.

Wise use of anitbiotics requires the clinician to take the stance that positive indications must be present before antibiotic drugs are prescribed. The clinician should not assume that antibiotics must be given in all instances of infection.

PRINCIPLES FOR CHOOSING THE APPROPRIATE ANTIBIOTIC

Once the decision has been made to use antibiotics as an adjunct to treating an infection, the antibiotic should be properly selected. The following guidelines are useful in making this decision.

IDENTIFICATION OF THE CAUSATIVE ORGANISM

The identity of a pathogen may be determined scientifically either in the laboratory, where the organism can be isolated from pus, blood, or tissue, or empirically based on knowledge of the pathogenesis and clinical presentation of specific infections. Antibiotic therapy is then either initial or definitive, depending on whether the organism is even identified precisely.

Initial empirical therapy may be instituted with a fair degree of reliability if the following criteria are met: the site and features of the infection have been well defined, the circumstances leading to the infection are well known; and the organism or organisms that most commonly cause such infections are well known.

The microbiology of odontogenic infections has been very clearly defined in recent years.* The use of improved aseptic, anaerobic techniques for obtaining culture specimens, as well as the use of standard anaerobic culture and identification techniques, has resulted in a clear, consistent picture of the usual causative bacteria (Box 5-1).

Several factors regarding the type of bacteria (aerobic vs. anaerobic) and their specific identification are important to the clinician. The typical odontogenic infection is caused by a mixture of aerobic and anaerobic bacteria; approximately 70% of these infections are caused by this mixed flora. Infections caused by aerobic bacteria only are much less common, accounting for approximately 5%. Similarly, pure anaerobic infections are seen in only approximately 25% of odontogenic infections. These data are derived from aspirates of pus, usually taken percutaneously, and cultured using sophisticated methodology.

Although clinical correlation of these results is not absolutely proved, enough information is available to suggest that the bacteria found in the well-circumscribed chronic nonadvancing abscess are almost always anaerobic bacteria only. In a similar finding, those few studies that report microbiology of cellulitis-type infections, that do not have abscess formation, show almost exclusively aerobic bacteria. Therefore it appears that early infections that present as a cellulitis without abscess formation are most likely caused

*References 1, 3, 5, 10, 11, 15, 17, 18, 19, 20, 22.

BOX 5-1

Bacteria Responsible for Odontogenic Infections

Aerobic Bacteria	Frequency	Anaerobic Bacteria	Frequency
Gram-positive cocci		**Gram-positive cocci**	
Streptococcus		*Streptococcus*	Common
Viridans	Very common		
β-Hemolytic	Unusual		
Group D	Rare		
Staphylococcus	Rare		
Gram-negative bacilli		**Gram-negative bacilli**	
Haemophilus influenzae	Rare	*Porphyromonas (Bacteroides)*	Rare
Escherichia coli	Rare	*Prevotella (Bacteroides)*	Very common
Klebsiella	Rare	*Fusobacterium*	Common
Eikenella corrodens	Unusual	*Bacteroides fragilis*	Rare

by aerobic bacteria. As the infection becomes more severe, the microbiology becomes a mixed flora of aerobic and anaerobic bacteria. If the infection process becomes contained and controlled by the body's host defenses, the aerobic bacteria are no longer able to survive in the hypoxic, acidotic environment, and only anaerobic bacteria are found.

The aerobic bacteria found in odontogenic infections are primarily gram-positive cocci, most of which are of the viridans type of streptococci. These streptococcal species are typical oral flora and include *Streptococcus milleri, S. sanguis, S. salivarius,* and *S. mutans.* These oral streptococci, also known as α-hemolytic cocci, account for approximately 85% of the aerobic bacteria found in odontogenic infections. Also seen are occasional isolates of *S. pyogenes,* a few staphylococci, and a variety of other bacteria that appear to play no pathogenic role. In summary, the aerobic component of the mixed aerobic-anaerobic bacteria causing odontogenic infections consists overwhelmingly of α-hemolytic streptococci, all of which are susceptible to penicillin and other antibiotics with an antimicrobial spectrum similar to that of penicillin.

The number of anaerobic bacteria found in the typical odontogenic infection is greater than the number of aerobic bacteria. There are two major groups of anaerobic bacteria: anaerobic gram-positive cocci and anaerobic gram-negative rods. The two main groups of gram-positive cocci are anaerobic streptococci and peptostreptococci. Anaerobic gram-positive cocci are found in approximately one third of odontogenic infections and account for approximately 30% of the anaerobic bacteria isolated from these infections. Their antibiotic susceptibility is similar to that of aerobic streptococci; that is, they are universally sensitive to penicillin and to other antibiotics with a penicillin-like antimicrobial spectrum.

Anaerobic gram-negative rods account for approximately 50% of the anaerobic bacteria isolated from odontogenic infections. The two important genera of anaerobic gram-negative rods are *Bacteroides* and *Fusobacterium.*

Recent investigations have led to the differentiation of the many species and subspecies that exist in the genus previously known as *Bacteroides.* There have been two main groups of *Bacteroides;* the first is the oropharyngeal group, which is found in the mouth and contributes to odontogenic infections. The other group, the enteric *Bacteroides,* is found in the gut. The gut species include *B. fragilis, vulgatis, distasonis, thetaiota omicron,* and *ovatus.* These are usually known as the fragilis group. They are rarely seen in the oral cavity and generally do not cause odontogenic infections.

Oropharyngeal *Bacteroides* has been reclassified into two separate genera: *Porphyromonas* and *Prevotella.* The *Porphyromonas* group currently includes three species: *P. asaccharolyticus, gingivalis,* and *endodontalis.* The *Prevotella* group includes *P. melaninogenica, buccae, intermedia, oralis, loeschii, ruminicola,* and *denticola.* The gram-negative anaerobic rod most commonly isolated from odontogenic infections is *Prevotella. Porphyromonas* are rarely identified in these infections, even though *P. gingivalis* is a common causative organism found in periodontitis. *Prevotella* organisms have a natural resistance to penicillin; between 40% and 80% are resistant.

The third important group of anaerobic gram-negative rods is the genus *Fusobacterium.* As with the *Prevotella* spp., *Fusobacterium* organisms are quite pathogenic and can destroy tissue through production of proteolytic enzymes and endotoxins. *Fusobacterium* organisms are usually sensitive to penicillin and penicillin-like drugs, but they are frequently resistant to erythromycin. In fact, approximately 50% of *Fusobacterium* organisms isolated from odontogenic infections are resistant to erythromycin. *Fusobacterium* also seems to be associated with the most severe type of odontogenic infection. The specific combination of *Fusobacterium* and *S. milleri* has been noted by several investigators as common in severe infections that have descended into the lateral and retropharyngeal spaces and into the mediastinum.

In summary, anaerobic bacteria play an important role in the origin of odontogenic infection. Anaerobic gram-

Bactericidal and Bacteriostatic Antibiotics

Bactericidal Antibiotics	Bacteriostatic Antibiotics
Penicillin(s)	Tetracyclines
Cephalosporin(s)	Erythromycin
Aminoglycosides	Clarithromycin
Vancomycin	Arithromycin
Metronidazole	Clindamycin
Imipenem	Sulfa
Fluoroquinalones	

positive cocci are seen in approximately one third of all odontogenic infections, and gram-negative rods are seen in approximately 50% of odontogenic infections. The main species of the gram-positive cocci are *Streptococcus intermedius* and *Peptostreptococcus* spp. The main gram-negative rods are *Prevotella* and *Fusobacterium*. The *Fusobacterium* spp. appear to be the most virulent, and when found in conjunction with *S. milleri*, are associated with the most aggressive odontogenic infections (Box 5-2).

The pathobiology of mixed odontogenic infections is relatively clear.[40] Entrance to the underlying tissue is gained primarily by the aerobic bacteria. During this time the infection is established and a cellulitis develops. The cellulitis process, if left untreated, produces a hypoxic-acidotic condition in the tissue that allows the proliferation and ingrowth of anaerobic bacteria. The anaerobic bacteria then produce a variety of proteolytic enzymes, endotoxins, and exotoxins, which results in a significant amount of tissue destruction. This tissue destruction, combined with the ingress of large numbers of white blood cells, results in the formation of an abscess cavity and pus. If the infection becomes well-circumscribed and walled off by the host body's defenses, the aerobic bacteria disappear from the infection and it is populated by only anaerobic bacteria. Therefore this model of infection substantiates the critical observation that the early cellulitis is the result primarily of *Streptococcus,* the typical moderate to severe infection is caused by a combination of aerobic and anaerobic bacteria, and the well-circumscribed chronic abscess is caused primarily by anaerobic bacteria alone.

These facts have major clinical implications. The antibiotic that is useful for odontogenic infections must be effective against *Streptococcus* and anaerobes. In the cellulitis type infection, antistreptococcal activity is more important. In the later-stage, chronic abscess situation, antianaerobic activity is the major antibiotic goal.

This information is so clearly defined at this time that routine cultures for mild and moderate odontogenic infections are not necessary. At the time of surgical treatment, a smear of the pus should be made on a glass slide for future Gram staining should additional information be required (see Chapter 3).

Several clinical situations indicate obtaining cultures. If a patient seen with an infection has compromised host defenses and will require aggressive, unerring treatment, major efforts should be made to obtain culture material. Other situations in which cultures should be performed include the following: (1) if the patient has received appropriate treatment for 3 days without improvement, (2) if the infection is a postoperative wound infection, (3) if the infection is recurrent, (4) if actinomycosis is suspected, or (5) if osteomyelitis is present. In these situations deviation from the normal bacterial pattern is likely. More precise information about the bacteria must be available for definitive treatment.

Empirical antibiotic choices can be made in a variety of other situations in which the microbiological patterns are well established.

DETERMINATION OF ANTIBIOTIC SENSITIVITY

In the treatment of an infection that has not responded to initial antibiotic therapy or a postoperative wound infection, the causative agent must be precisely identified, and the antibiotic sensitivity must also be determined. The results of these studies provide the information needed to prescribe the most appropriate antibiotic.

Most odontogenic infections are caused by organisms such as streptococci that do not vary much in their antibiotic sensitivity patterns. Viridans streptococci that have been exposed to β-lactam antibiotics may become quite resistant in a short time (2 to 4 days).[9] Resistant viridans streptococcal organisms may cause serious infections in certain patients. However, a few others are caused by organisms of unexpected resistance and sensitivity. For example, *Staphylococcus* infections must be treated with antibiotic susceptibility information on hand. Penicillin G has been the drug of choice in past years, but because of the predominance of penicillinase-producing strains, both in *S. aureus* and *S. epidermidis* species, penicillin G can be used only if sensitivity studies support its effectiveness. Instead, penicillinase-resistant penicillins should be used. Also of importance is the increasing incidence of resistance to penicillinase-resistant drugs, which currently is high enough to warrant antibiotic routine susceptibility testing for staphylococcal infections.

Several other subtle susceptibility differences are important. Penicillin is excellent for treatment of *Streptococcus* infection and is good to excellent for the major anaerobes of odontogenic infections. Erythromycin is effective against *Streptococcus, Peptostreptococcus,* and *Prevotella* but is ineffective against *Fusobacterium*. Clindamycin is good for *Streptococcus* and for the five major anaerobic groups. Cephalexin is only moderately active against *Streptococcus* (approximately 10% of strains are resistant, 70% are intermediately sensitive, and 20% are sensitive) and is good to very good against the five groups of anaerobes. Metronidazole has no activity against *Streptococcus* but has excellent activity against the five anaerobic groups.

USE OF A SPECIFIC, NARROW-SPECTRUM ANTIBIOTIC

When considering which antibiotic to use, a choice of four or five drugs may exist. Selection should be based on consideration of several factors.[31,37] First, the antibiotic with the narrowest antibacterial spectrum should be chosen. For example, if the organism is a *Streptococcus* sensitive to penicillin, a cephalosporin, and a tetracycline, penicillin should be used because it has the narrowest spectrum. The other two have broad antibacterial activity against a variety of gram-negative organisms, and their use leads to development of resistant organisms.

The opportunity for development of resistant strains is presented each time bacteria are exposed to antibiotics. Thus when a broad-spectrum antibiotic is used, many different bacteria also present in the body are exposed to the antibiotic. However, if a narrow-spectrum antibiotic is used, fewer organisms have the opportunity to become resistant because they are not even partially sensitive. Thus for a given streptococcal infection, penicillin would result in less exposure of the host flora to antibiotics than would a broader-spectrum cephalosporin.[27]

The use of narrow-spectrum antibiotics also minimizes the risk of superinfections. When large numbers of normal host flora are eliminated, overgrowth of resistant organisms occurs, and this may result in clinical infection in some patients, ranging from moniliasis to gram-negative pneumonias. Use of narrow-spectrum antibiotics allows larger proportions of the host flora to be maintained, thereby reducing superinfections to a minimum.

USE OF THE LEAST TOXIC ANTIBIOTIC

Another principle in the choice of an antibiotic is selection of the least toxic drug from among those that are effective. Antibiotics are used to kill living bacteria, but some antibiotics also can kill or injure human cells. Thus they can be highly toxic. At times these drugs must be used, but in other clinical situations, less toxic drugs that are equally effective may be used. For example, the bacteria that cause odontogenic infections are usually sensitive to penicillin and to chloramphenicol. In fact, chloramphenicol may be somewhat more effective in 2% to 3% of these infections. However, it is a toxic drug with the potential for causing severe bone marrow depression. Even though treatment may fail slightly more often with penicillin than with chloramphenicol, penicillin is preferable because of its lower toxicity. However, treatment failure with penicillin would result in a more prolonged treatment period because of the need to switch drugs. The clinician should continuously be alert for signs of toxicity and also instruct the patient to look for and report them as well.

PATIENT DRUG HISTORY

Knowledge of the patient's drug reaction history is critical. Two items must be reviewed: previous allergic reactions and previous toxic reactions.

Because penicillin is so widely used and because the allergy rate to penicillin is approximately 5%, most clinicians routinely obtain a history of previous allergies, especially to antibiotics. When actually treating a patient with an infection, antibiotic allergy must be carefully checked from a reliable source and recorded.

A recurring and important question about penicillin-allergic patients is whether the cephalosporin antibiotics can be used safely. Patients who are allergic to penicillin tend to have more allergies than patients who are not allergic to penicillin. Although it is unlikely that there is actual cross-sensitivity between the penicillins and cephalosporins, it is well documented that coincident allergies to cephalosporins and penicillins do exist. Therefore the usual recommendation is that if the patient had a documented anaphylactic (type I) allergic reaction to penicillin, a cephalosporin should be avoided unless deemed absolutely essential, and then only after preparations have been made to treat a severe reaction. Conversely, if the patient had a less severe reaction to the penicillin antibiotic, the cephalosporins can more than likely be used safely. The patient should be observed for approximately 30 minutes after the cephalosporin has been administered for any signs of emerging allergic reactions.

Patients with a history of previous major toxic or minor side effects from an antibiotic are likely to experience the same problem again. Attempts should be made to identify the drug and the precise reaction. An alternative drug should be used if possible.

Potential interactions with other drugs that the patient is taking also must be considered. Antibiotics may prolong, enhance, or interfere with the other medications that the patient is taking.

USE OF A BACTERICIDAL RATHER THAN A BACTERIOSTATIC DRUG

Whether an antibiotic is bactericidal or bacteriostatic is a property of the antibiotic and depends primarily on its mechanism of activity against bacteria. Although there is slight variation in the effect of a specific antibiotic against different bacteria, each antibiotic is usually classified as either bacteriostatic or bactericidal (see Box 5-2). Antibiotics are used as an adjunct to combat infection inasmuch as cure of the infection is the result of the host defense mechanisms. Antibiotic therapy reduces the bacterial challenge and allows host defenses to complete the treatment. Bacteriostatic antibiotics exert their influence by inhibiting growth and reproduction of the bacteria, usually by inhibiting protein synthesis. Because growth is slowed, the host defenses can now eliminate a static population of bacteria and cure the infection. If the host defense system is compromised, the use of an antibiotic that can kill the bacteria (bactericidal) becomes critical. The two major mechanisms of antibiotic killing are interference with cell wall synthesis and nucleic acid synthesis.

The advantages of the bactericidal antibiotic are (1) less reliance on host resistance, (2) killing of the bacteria by the antibiotic itself, (3) faster results than with bacteriostatic drugs, and (4) greater flexibility with dosage intervals. Bactericidal drugs exert their influence after they are incorporated into the bacterial cell and the cell eventually dies. Bacteriostatic drugs, on the other hand, exert their influence only when present in the patient's tissues. The bacteria resume their normal growth after the drug is eliminated. Therefore it is important that bacteriostatic drugs be given (taken) according to a rigorous time schedule. Bactericidal rather than bacteriostatic antibiotics should be used for patients who are pathologically or therapeutically immunosuppressed (see Box 5-2). The action of bactericidal antibiotics results in death of the invading microorganisms, whereas the bacteriostatic antibiotics merely retard growth of the bacteria. When bacteriostatic antibiotics are used, the host defenses must play a more important role in the eradication of the bacteria. For example, the bactericidal drugs such as penicillin or a cephalosporin should be used in immunodeficient patients instead of the bacteriostatic drugs erythromycin or clindamycin for the treatment of bacteria susceptible to all four agents.

USE OF THE ANTIBIOTIC WITH A PROVEN HISTORY OF SUCCESS

The best evaluation of the efficacy of a drug in a particular situation is the critical observation of its clinical effectiveness over a prolonged period. This observation helps in the assessment of the frequency of treatment success and failure, the frequency of adverse reactions, and the frequency of side effects. By such observations, a few drugs deservedly become standards for use and should not be disregarded for an unproved drug without good reason.

The treatment of oral infections is an almost classic example of this principle. Since its initial availability penicillin has been used for oral infections, and it has been very effective with a low incidence of adverse reactions. As new drugs were developed and new bacteria were identified, the role of penicillin as the drug of choice was repeatedly challenged. The tetracyclines, erythromycin, lincomycin, and clindamycin all have been claimed to be superior. However, the historically proven overall performance of penicillin has not been surpassed in the treatment of most odontogenic infections.

Enthusiasm for the use of the most recently developed antimicrobials is also valid. Most clinicians have a desire to be current in their treatment of patients. However, when a new drug is released for general use, there is often haste to use it, despite a lack of good reasons to abandon the old drug. When new antibiotics are available, subtle toxicities not seen in the investigational phase of the drug become evident, inasmuch as it may take as long as 4 or 5 years for enough clinical experience to be gained before these problems become clearly defined.

In addition, initially sensitive bacteria become more resistant to the antibiotic being used with increasing exposure. This development of resistance to an antibiotic may be slowed by limiting its use, or it may be hastened by its wide use. If the wide use is the result of special benefits of the drug, development of rapid resistance must be accepted. However, if the wide use is not consistent with the prudent choice of drugs, the resistance that develops must be viewed as a loss.

Newer antibiotics should be used only when they offer clear advantages over older ones. They may be effective for bacteria against which no other antibiotic is effective, as was the case when methicillin became available for penicillinase-producing staphylococci. In such a situation, that antibiotic must be reserved for those patients with infections caused by bacteria that have a proven sensitivity to that antibiotic. In addition, a new antibiotic may be more active at lower concentrations (thus reducing cost and dose-related toxicity reactions), it may be less toxic, or it may have less bothersome side effects than the older antibiotic. Finally, the new antibiotic may be less expensive, although this is rarely the case. For these reasons, the surgeon may elect to use a new antibiotic but should use it with caution and with good cause.

COST OF THE ANTIBIOTIC

It is difficult to place a price tag on health, but the surgeon should consider the cost of the antibiotic prescribed. In some situations, the more expensive antibiotic is the drug of choice. In other situations, there may be a substantial difference in price for drugs of equal efficacy. For example, the price of penicillin V differs dramatically from the prices of cephalexin and clindamycin. When expensive drugs are to be prescribed, the patient should be told of the drug costs before visiting the pharmacist. This helps prevent angry feelings from the patient.

In addition to the actual cost of the drug, the administration costs must be considered. Most parenteral antibiotics given in the hospital are administered intravenously. They are prepared in the hospital pharmacy as a single-dose piggyback administration set. If the cost for each set is $25, the daily administration costs for a drug given every 4 hours would be 6 × $25, or $150. This cost is added to the drug expense. The use of a drug with a long half-life but more expensive itself on a per-gram basis may be less expensive when all costs are included.

ENCOURAGE PATIENT COMPLIANCE

It is clear that patients often, if not usually, fail to take the medication in the way in which it was prescribed. In fact, Socrates in 400 BC cautioned physicians to be aware that patients will lie about taking the medications prescribed.[33]

Hard data exist from many studies that demonstrate that patient compliance decreases with increasing number of pills per day.[32] When the prescription is for once-daily administration, patient compliance is approximately 80%. However, when it is necessary to take the pill twice daily, compliance decreases to 69% and drops even further to 35% for four times daily. Therefore if there is a choice, the clinician should prescribe antibiotics that can be given the fewest times daily to improve patient compliance.

It is also clear that patients stop taking their antibiotics after the acute symptoms have subsided and rarely take their drugs as prescribed after 5 or 6 days. Despite what the prescription says, it appears quite clear that patients rarely take antimicrobial agents as prescribed longer than 3 or 4 days. Therefore the antibiotic that would have the highest compliance would be the drug that could be given once a day for 4 or 5 days.

PRINCIPLES OF ANTIBIOTIC ADMINISTRATION

Once it has been established that the patient has an infection that requires antibiotic therapy, and the kind of antibiotic has been chosen, it must be administered properly. This involves consideration of dosage, route of administration, and combination therapy.

PROPER DOSE

The goal of any drug therapy should be to prescribe or administer sufficient amounts to achieve the desired therapeutic effect but not enough to cause injury to the host.

The laboratory plays an important role in helping the clinician to calculate the proper dosage. When sensitivity testing by the disk diffusion method is used, the amount of antibacterial activity in the zone surrounding the disk is comparable to that present in the normal patient's plasma after a standard dose of the antibiotic. The laboratory can supply even more specific information by determining the minimum inhibitory concentration (MIC) of an antibiotic for a specific bacterium (see Chapter 3). The MIC of the usual antibiotics for most common bacteria has been established. For therapeutic purposes the peak concentration of the antibiotic at the site of infection should be three to four times the MIC. Therefore the dosage prescribed must be capable of establishing a concentration of antibiotic that is three to four times the MIC.

The blood levels of various antibiotics, as well as their dosages and routes of administration, have been established. Given the MIC for an antibiotic and the specific organism to be treated, the dose of that antibiotic that should be given to achieve three to four times the MIC can be determined. For example, if a patient is infected with a penicillinase-producing *Staphylococcus,* the MIC will be about 6.0 μg/mL for cephalexin, thus requiring a plasma level about three times 6.0, or 18.0 μg/mL. Five hundred milligrams of cephalexin given orally yields a plasma level of 17 μg/mL; that is, a therapeutic level based on the favorable therapeutic responses of patients receiving these drugs. The usual recommended dose of an antibiotic is usually sufficient to provide a threefold MIC concentration against the common susceptible organisms.

Therapeutic levels greater than three to four times the MIC generally do not improve the therapeutic results. Administration of doses above that level increases the likelihood of toxicity and is wasteful. This issue is critical with some antibiotics. For example, gentamicin is usually effective in concentrations of 4 to 6 μg/mL, but the incidence of nephrotoxicity increases dramatically if the plasma level reaches 10 μg/mL. It is clear that with gentamicin and all antibiotics plasma concentrations greater than three to four times the MIC are potentially hazardous and add unnecessarily to the cost of treatment.

Increased doses may be justified when the site of infection may be isolated from the blood supply, as in abscess formation or in nonvital tissue. These high plasma concentrations may allow a greater amount of antibiotic to reach the sealed-off bacteria by simple diffusion. In such cases, early surgical intervention must also be considered. Actinomycosis and osteomyelitis are examples in which such problems may occur.

Another important point is that sufficient antibiotic must be given to reach therapeutic levels, because subtherapeutic levels may mask the infection and suppress the clinical manifestations without actually killing the invading microbes. Furthermore, subtherapeutic doses may cause a recurrence of the infection once the drug is discontinued. Underdosing commonly occurs when the clinician uses a drug of great potential toxicity and fears a toxic reaction. This problem can be avoided by use of a less toxic drug, if available, or by regular measurement of plasma antibiotic levels. Recently it has become recommended practice to monitor aminoglycoside plasma levels to ensure that therapeutic levels of the antibiotic have been achieved and that toxic levels are avoided.

PROPER TIME INTERVAL

The frequency of dosing is also of importance in administration of antibiotics. Just as there is a usual recommended dose of each antibiotic, there is a usual recommended dosage interval. Knowledge of the pharmacokinetics of the drug is important. Each antibiotic has an established plasma half-life ($t_{1/2}$), during which one half of the absorbed dose is excreted. This time interval has been established for various antibiotics. The usual dosage interval for the therapeutic use of antibiotics is four times the $t_{1/2}$. At five times the $t_{1/2}$, 95% of the drug has been excreted. For example, the $t_{1/2}$ for cefazolin is almost 2 hours. Thus the interval between doses should be 8 hours.

Because most antibiotics are eliminated by the kidneys, the patient with preexisting renal disease and subsequent decreased clearance may require longer intervals between doses if overdosing is to be avoided, for if the usual dosage schedule is maintained, excessive plasma levels and a resultant increase in toxicity reactions occur. To prevent excessive plasma levels, an alternative technique is to decrease the dose and maintain the same interval between doses. However, because therapeutic response depends primarily on a high peak level, most clinicians prefer to increase the interval between doses. Not all antibiotics must be modified by the same amount. A consultation with a specialist in infectious diseases is useful when treating such patients.

Special monitoring of plasma antibiotic concentrations also must be considered. An alternative treatment plan would be to use an antibiotic that is excreted by the liver, such as erythromycin.

PROPER ROUTE OF ADMINISTRATION

In some infections, only parenteral administration produces the necessary serum level of antibiotic. For example, the maximum peak plasma level of penicillin V that can be reached by using the oral route is 2 g. This dose gives a plasma level of almost 4 µg/mL. Some bacteria are not susceptible at that level, but they are quite susceptible to the concentrations of penicillin achievable by parenteral routes of administration. The oral route also results in the most variable absorption. Most antibiotics should be taken in the fasting state (30 minutes before or 2 hours after a meal) for maximum absorption.

When long-term parenteral administration is necessary, repeated intramuscular injections are poorly accepted by patients. In such situations, use of the intravenous route should be considered. If intravenous fluid therapy is not being used, a heparin well or lock facilitates administration of the drug.

CONSISTENCY IN ROUTE OF ADMINISTRATION

When treating a serious, established infection, parenteral antibiotic therapy is frequently the method of choice. After an initial response has been achieved, immediate discontinuation of the parenteral route and oral administration of the drug is tempting. When this is done, the infection may recur because blood levels of the drug are higher when it is given parenterally than when it is given orally. Maintenance of peak blood levels of antibiotic for an adequate period is important to achieve maximum tissue penetration and effective bacterial killing. Bacteria usually are not eradicated until the antibiotic has been given for 5 or 6 days. Thus, recurrence of the infection is more likely by switching from the parenteral to the oral route on the second or third day of antibiotic therapy. After the fifth day of parenteral administration, the blood levels achievable with oral administration are usually sufficient. If the infection is mild enough not to require parenteral therapy initially, the blood levels achievable with oral therapy are sufficient.

COMBINATION ANTIBIOTIC THERAPY

In addition to treating infections with the most specific antibiotics possible and avoiding broad-spectrum antibiotics, combination drug therapy should also be avoided when not specifically indicated. The usual result of combination therapy is a broad-spectrum exposure that leads to depression of the normal host flora and increased opportunity for resistant bacteria to emerge. For routine infections, the disadvantages of combination therapy outweigh the advantages.

However, there are several situations in which the use of antibiotic combinations clearly is indicated. The first occurs when it is necessary to increase the antibacterial spectrum in the patient with life-threatening sepsis of unknown cause. Here, the bactericidal drugs that cover the broadest spectrum of organisms are frequently indicated.

The second situation occurs when increased bactericidal effect against a specific organism is desired (e.g., treatment of infections caused by enterococcus [group D *Streptococcus*], which usually must be treated by a penicillin and an aminoglycoside).

The third situation in which combined therapy is desirable is in the prevention of the rapid emergence of resistant bacteria. The primary example of this situation is the use of multiple drugs for the treatment of tuberculosis. However, combined therapy generally should be avoided in the absence of specific indications.

A fourth situation in which combined antibiotic therapy may be useful is in the empiric treatment of certain odontogenic infections. If the patient has a severe cellulitis/abscess type of infection that is rapidly progressing posteriorly around the lateral and retropharyngeal spaces, bactericidal activity against *Streptococcus* and the oral anaerobes is important. Because a significant component of *Prevotella* may be resistant to penicillin, a rational approach to antibiotic management in such patients would be to prescribe parenteral penicillin G and parenteral metronidazole. This combination therapy provides rapid bactericidal activity against both streptococci and anaerobes.

PATIENT MONITORING

Once the antibiotic administration has been initiated, the patient's response must be carefully observed. Issues such as adjunctive surgery, fluid balance, and nutritional support are critical. Monitoring related specifically to the antibiotic therapy should be directed at the response to treatment and at the development of adverse reactions.

RESPONSE TO TREATMENT

Patients rarely have a noticeable response to antibiotic therapy for the first 24 to 48 hours unless surgery to accomplish drainage is also performed. Most commonly, the response begins by the second day and initially is a subjective sense of feeling better. This state is difficult to define precisely, other than to note that it is an improvement. Thereafter objective signs of improvement occur, including a decrease in temperature, swelling, and pain, and a lessening of trismus.

At that time a decision must be made about the duration of antibiotic therapy.[26] Ideally, antibiotics should be given until all offending bacteria have been eradicated. If this goal is not achieved, infection may recur. Eradication of the infection generally is reached by the third day after the patient becomes relatively asymptomatic, that is, when there is no temperature and little or no swelling, pain, or drainage. In an uncomplicated odontogenic infection, improvement would be expected to begin by the second day of therapy and marked resolution by the third day. Allowing an additional 2 days results in a 5-day course of antibiotics. Occasionally resolution may take longer than 4 days, so a 7-day course of antibiotics is necessary. By observing the patient's progress closely, the clinician can individualize the treatment for the proper duration of therapy.[21]

Occasionally the patient's condition does not improve or may in fact deteriorate after the initial course of antibiotic therapy. The clinician should resist the temptation to change antibiotics in the first day or two inasmuch as it takes several days to actually determine whether an antibiotic will be effective. If no improvement is noted by the end of the second day or on the third day, the patient must be carefully reevaluated. Special attention should be given to determining the need for additional surgical intervention for drainage of pus, release of pressure, or removal of nonvital tissue or a foreign body. Other possible sites of infection also should be examined, and for the hospitalized patient, portals of entry such as intravenous and Foley catheters should be examined as possible sites of infection. The state of the host's defenses must be reassessed, and supportive therapy must be given whenever possible. Adequate hydration and nutritional support are also essential.

If the initial antibiotic therapy has failed, the choice of antibiotic should be reevaluated. Several questions should be considered. (1) Have the route of administration and the dose of the antibiotic been adequate to deliver effective amounts to the site of infection? (2) Is the patient taking the antibiotic as prescribed? (3) Have the physician's orders on the chart been understood and carried out? (4) Finally, was the initial choice of antibiotic correct? If a culture was performed initially, reevaluation of the sensitivity report may be necessary. If no cultures were performed initially, repeated efforts should be directed toward this goal. A second empirical choice should be avoided if at all possible because the likelihood of success is substantially less. Consultation with other clinicians and laboratory personnel may be of value in evaluating the patient's condition (Box 5-3).

Occasionally a patient with a maxillofacial infection responds to therapy quite adequately, but when the culture

and sensitivity report is received, it states that the bacteria present are resistant to the antibiotic being used for initial empirical therapy. In this situation, the combination of surgical and antibiotic treatment and natural host defenses has resulted in resolution of the infection. The antibiotic may or may not have played an important role. Certainly, in vivo activity is not always the same as in vitro activity as reported by the laboratory. The antibiotic that was clinically effective for the patient should be continued despite contradictory laboratory data.

Conversely, empirical therapy may not have resulted in resolution, even though the culture and sensitivity reports support the use of the drug chosen empirically. In this case, other factors may be important. These include the virulence of the bacteria involved and the severity and location of the infection, as well as the dose and route of administration of the drug.

DEVELOPMENT OF ADVERSE REACTIONS

Adverse reactions occur all too commonly. An estimated 15% to 20% of hospitalized patients receiving antibiotics experience an adverse reaction.[8] Hypersensitivity reactions occur with all antibiotics; penicillins and cephalosporins have the highest incidence of reactions. These reactions may include accelerated anaphylactic (type I) reactions or less severe reactions associated with edema, urticaria, and itching, or they may be delayed reactions, presenting only as a low-grade temperature elevation. Diagnosis of anaphylactic reactions is not difficult, but treatment must be rapid and deliberate.

The less severe reaction that develops as a rash or urticaria may begin immediately or many hours after exposure (types II and III). Thus when giving an antibiotic prescription to an outpatient, the surgeon should describe the signs and symptoms of allergy and instruct the patient to call if any of these develop. When a reaction is reported, the patient must be examined carefully and provided with the indicated treatment. Additionally, if an allergic reaction actually occurred, the patient should know the name of the drug and the kind of reaction that occurred and should be advised to relate this information to the physician during future treatment. A written statement for the patient's future use may be indicated if the allergic reaction has been severe.

Diagnosis of delayed hypersensitivity reactions may be difficult. These type IV reactions are mediated by T lymphocytes rather than by antibodies. Only if the clinician is alert to such problems is he or she in a position to make the diagnosis. The most common sign is a persistent, low-grade temperature. In a typical situation, the patient no longer has swelling, pain, trismus, or drainage but continues to have a mild temperature elevation despite a normal pulse. The white blood cell count is decreased from its elevated levels to a nearly normal number, but the differential count usually shows an increased number of eosinophils. If the patient has been receiving long-term antibiotic therapy, the diagnosis of drug hypersensitivity

BOX 5-3

Causes of Failure in Treatment of Infection

Inadequate surgical treatment
Depressed host defenses
Presence of foreign body
Antibiotic problems
   Drug not reaching infection
   Dose not adequate
   Wrong bacterial diagnosis
   Wrong antibiotic

must be considered. The temperature elevation resolves 24 to 48 hours after the drug is withdrawn.

Antibiotics frequently cause bothersome side effects that are often unique to the drug, such as gastrointestinal distress. These reactions are usually not dose related. If the patient complains, the clinician must be able to differentiate the bothersome side effects from potentially serious toxic reactions.

Although toxic reactions are seen rather often with antibiotic use, primary care clinicians rarely encounter toxicity problems with the commonly used penicillin, a drug with an extremely low toxicity potential. However, surgeons who use a greater variety of antibiotics encounter various manifestations of toxicity. Most of these are dose related, and many are reversible if the diagnosis is made early and the therapy discontinued. Early diagnosis requires the clinician to be familiar with the toxic effects associated with the prescribed antibiotic. Informing the patient of the possible early signs of toxicity also helps in the early diagnosis and prevention of permanent damage. Of course, avoidance of excessive doses is important to prevent toxicity. Therapeutic levels must be reached, but the higher the level, the more likely a toxic reaction. Factors that alter drug metabolism also should be noted, and because most antibiotics are eliminated by the kidneys or liver, the function of these organs should be specifically checked. Information regarding the toxicity potential of the various antibiotics is readily available in package inserts and standard textbooks.

One toxic reaction that should be discussed specifically is antibiotic-associated colitis (AAC). AAC was originally associated with clindamycin therapy but has now been recognized to be caused by almost every antibiotic, with the exception of the aminoglycosides.[4] The three most common drugs that lead to AAC are clindamycin, ampicillin/amoxicillin, and the cephalosporins. Each of these antibiotic groups causes about one third of the reported cases of AAC. The pseudomembranous colitis is caused by toxins from *Clostridium difficile*. Patients receiving antibiotics that alter colonic flora may have an overgrowth of *C. difficile*, which leads to AAC. The clinical features of AAC are profuse watery diarrhea that may be bloody, cramping abdominal pain, fever, and leukocytosis. The population most readily affected by AAC are patients who are severely medically compromised, are usually inpatients, are frequently elderly, and are more frequently female. Treatment involves discontinuation of the causative antibiotic, restoration of fluid and electrolyte balance, and administration of anti-clostridia antibiotics. The usual choice is oral vancomycin but metronidazole also may be used.

SUPERINFECTION AND RECURRENT INFECTION

During antibiotic treatment of an infection normal host bacteria that are susceptible to the drug are eliminated or dramatically reduced. In the normal state, these bacteria live in peaceful coexistence with the host and by their phys-

ical presence prevent bacteria capable of producing disease from growing in large numbers. Thus the normal flora acts as a defense mechanism against infection, but when the indigenous flora is altered or eliminated by an antibiotic, the pathogenic bacteria resistant to the antibiotic may cause a secondary infection, or superinfection.

A common secondary infection is the overgrowth of *Candida* in the oral cavity or vagina. Candidiasis (thrush) is primarily the result of the use of penicillin, which eliminates the gram-positive cocci, and it occurs most commonly after relatively high-dose, long-term penicillin therapy. Patients treated for osteomyelitis or actinomycosis with penicillin are susceptible to thrush for this reason. When it occurs, thrush should be treated with antifungal agents such as clotrimazole.

Hospitalized patients have a rather high incidence of secondary infections. Approximately 3 of every 100 patients admitted to a hospital in the United States develop a secondary infection. Such infection is related to several factors, but perhaps the most important is the high percentage of patients who receive broad-spectrum antibiotics. Secondary pneumonia caused by gram-negative organisms that are resistant to common antibiotics occurs frequently, causing great expense, considerable morbidity, and death. The use of broad-spectrum antibiotics results in decreased normal host flora, permitting invasion of antibiotic-resistant bacteria.

Facial surgeons occasionally face recurrent infection when treating patients with odontogenic infections. The evaluation of the patient should not end after the patient is "cured." An occasional infectious situation may be masked or put into a remissive state by antibiotic therapy, only to recur when antibiotic therapy is stopped. Although recurrent infections are unusual after odontogenic infections, the patient must be observed for several weeks after the clinical signs of infection subside to ensure that it does not recur. Some infections, such as osteomyelitis and actinomycosis, require more careful and longer follow-up. Because nonvital bone provides a barrier to antibiotic effectiveness and is a potential focus of bacteria, recurrences of the infection are possible weeks after antibiotic therapy has been stopped. In such situations, reculture and reinstitution of antibiotic therapy with consideration of additional surgical intervention must be done. Similarly, actinomycosis may recur months after therapy has stopped. Careful long-term follow-up is therefore necessary in osteomyelitis and actinomycosis.

THERAPEUTIC USES OF ANTIBIOTICS IN MAXILLOFACIAL SURGERY

Surgeons frequently must use antibiotics in the treatment of their patients. Consideration of the previously discussed principles allows them to select those situations in which antibiotic therapy is indicated and those in which it is not. As a general guideline, antibiotic therapy should be reserved for those patients with clearly established infections who have systemic manifestations of infection, that is, fever, malaise, swelling, and pain. Such patients should also be treated surgically as early as possible.

Abscess   Acute dentoalveolar cellulitis and abscess usually require antibiotic therapy. Penicillin is usually the drug of choice. Adjunctive treatment should include endodontic therapy, or extraction of the causative tooth and surgical drainage of any areas of pus accumulation. The patient must be monitored carefully to determine the response to this therapy. Conversely, many chronic dentoalveolar abscesses need no antibiotic therapy. The patient often has no temperature, little induration, and little malaise. Treatment may be entirely surgical without antibiotic therapy (see Chapter 7).

Pericoronitis   Acute pericoronitis, if severe, may require antibiotic therapy. Most patients seek treatment when pain and intraoral swelling begin. The bacteria responsible for pericoronitis are all anaerobic bacteria,[28] including gram-positive cocci *(Peptostreptococcus)* and gram-negative rods *(Prevotella)*. Debridement by irrigation and possible extraction of the offending or opposing tooth usually are sufficient therapy. Many patients can be treated without antibiotics. Occasionally, however, a patient has a clearly established infection with temperature elevation and sufficient trismus to prevent adequate local therapy. In such cases, antibiotics may be necessary for several days before surgery can be performed. Again, penicillin is the drug of choice.

Osteomyelitis   A third indication for antibiotics in maxillofacial surgical patients is the presence of osteomyelitis. Although infection of the jaws usually requires surgical intervention, antibiotic therapy also is essential for successful treatment. Special care must be taken to identify the causative organisms, using anaerobic and aerobic cultures of tissue removed at surgery, if necessary. Osteomyelitis must be treated with antibiotics for a much longer period than soft tissue infections. Specific management of osteomyelitis is discussed in detail in Chapter 10.

Fractures   A final therapeutic use of antibiotics is in the management of compound maxillofacial fractures.[39] All compound fractures may be assumed to be contaminated, if not frankly infected. All fractures through tooth-bearing alveolar bone should be considered compound because they communicate with the oral cavity through the socket. Antibiotics must be given in therapeutic doses as soon as possible and continued until the active fracture treatment is completed, whether it be closed reduction with arch bars or open reduction with rigid fixation; then the antibiotic should be discontinued. Once a patient is discharged from the hospital, it is highly unlikely that he or she will continue to take antibiotics. Administration of the antibiotic should begin as early as possible after diagnosis to diminish the chance of a clinical infection. As with all infections, adjunctive treatment is essential, and in the case of fractures, early reduction and fixation decrease morbidity from infection. Penicillin is the drug of choice for facial fractures.

If cerebrospinal fluid leaks are present or if other major extrafacial trauma exists, other antibiotics may be chosen. This decision should be made in consultation with the other members of the trauma team, especially the neurosurgeon. At one time, antibiotics given to trauma patients were considered prophylactic, but as understanding of the behavior of bacteria in the presence of prophylactic antibiotics has increased, it has become clear that in the trauma patient antibiotics are, in fact, therapeutic. Therefore the patient who has sustained a facial fracture must be given antibiotics according to the therapeutic principles presented in this section, not according to prophylactic guidelines (see Chapter 17).

Soft Tissue Wounds   The need for antibiotics in the treatment of soft tissue wounds has been less well-defined.[36] Antibiotics are of no benefit if a facial wound can be cleaned, debrided of nonvital tissue and other debris, and closed adequately in a reasonable time. Even through-and-through wounds of the lips and cheeks may be treated without antibiotic support if adequate soft tissue debridement is performed. Antibiotics may be of some benefit in several other situations. If a wound has been open for 6 hours or more, it should be considered infected, and if primary closure is elected, a delayed primary closure is the method of choice. If the delayed technique cannot be used, antibiotic support is helpful.

Wounds caused by animal and human bites should be considered special situations.[7,14,24] The principal management of these wounds is thorough debridement and excision of all nonvital tissue. As a general rule, the wound should be closed primarily after thorough debridement except for bite wounds of the hand. These should be managed by delayed primary closure. The bacteria isolated from animal bites include *Staphylococcus, Streptococcus, Bacteroides,* and *Fusobacterium* spp. and *Pasteurella multocida.* The microbiology of human bite wounds is the same except that *P. multocida* is not seen. Instead, the gram-negative aerobic rod *Eikenella corrodens* is frequently isolated. Recent controlled studies have indicated that primary closure after thorough debridement of devitalized-compromised tissue, copious irrigations with saline solution, and primary closure without the use of antibiotics result in infection rates that are as low as if antibiotics were used. When antibiotics are indicated, the drug of choice is amoxicillin with clavulanic acid, as it is effective against essentially all of the usual bacteria, including *P. multocida* and *E. corrodens*[38] (see Chapter 17).

Miscellaneous   Anaerobic bacteria are the causative agents in some odontogenic infections.[6,12] Of the anaerobes found in the mouth, only *Prevotella* is resistant to penicillin at about a 50% level. Only rarely does *B. fragilis* cause infections in the oral cavity, and because it is resistant to penicillin, the drug of choice remains clindamycin.

Of interest is the increasing use of metronidazole for the treatment of anaerobic infections. This drug has been used in the past for the treatment of infections caused by *Trichomonas* but recently has been used in the treatment of anaerobic infections. It has no effect on aerobic facultative organisms, however. The toxicity of metronidazole is quite low and it can be administered orally, which is the usual route, or parenterally.

Penicillinase-resistant antibiotics are almost always required with staphylococcal infections. Although several such antibiotics exist, one or two should be selected as drugs for routine use. This allows the surgeon to become familiar with doses, dosage intervals, side effects, and toxicities. Oxacillin is recommended for parenteral use and dicloxacillin for oral use. These choices are based primarily on favorable pharmacokinetic patterns.

REFERENCES

1. Aderhold L, Knothe H, Frenkel G: The bacteriology of dentogenous pyogenic infections, *Oral Surg* 52:583, 1981.
2. Altemeier WA: *Manual on control of infection in surgical patients,* Philadelphia, 1984, Lippincott Williams & Wilkins.
3. Baker PJ, Evans RT, Slots J, et al: Antibiotic susceptibility of anaerobic bacteria from the human oral cavity, *J Dent Res* 64:1233, 1985.
4. Bartlett JG: Antimicrobial agents implicated in *Clostridium difficile* toxin-associated diarrhea or colitis, *Johns Hopkins Med J* 149:6, 1981.
5. Bartlett JG, O'Keefe P: The bacteriology of perimandibular space infections, *J Oral Surg* 37:407, 1979.
6. Brook I: Aerobic and anaerobic bacterial flora of normal maxillary sinuses, *Laryngoscope* 91:372, 1981.
7. Brook I: Human and animal infections, *J Fam Pract* 28:713, 1989.
8. Caldwell JR, Cluff LE: Adverse reactions to antimicrobial agents, *JAMA* 230:77, 1974.
9. Carratalá VJ, Alcaide F, Fernández-Sevilla A, et al: Bacteremia due to viridans streptococci that are highly resistant to penicillin: increase among neutropenic patients with cancer, *Clin Infect Dis* 20:1169, 1995.
10. Chow AW, Roser SM, Brady FA: Orofacial odontogenic infections, *Ann Intern Med* 88:392, 1978.
11. Dornbusch K: Antibiotic susceptibility in oral bacteria, *Swed Dent J* 4:9, 1980.
12. Edson RS, Rosenblatt JE, Lee DR, et al: Recent experience with antimicrobial susceptibility of anaerobic bacteria, *Mayo Clin Proc* 57:737, 1982.
13. Fleming A: On the antibacterial action of cultures of a penicillium, with special reference to their use in the isolation of H. influenzae, *Br J Exp Pathol* 10:226, 1929.
14. Guy RJ, Zook EG: Successful treatment of acute head and neck dog bite wounds with antibiotics, *Ann Plast Surg* 17:45, 1986.
15. Heimdahl A, Yon Konow L, Satoh T, et al: Clinical appearance of orofacial infections of odontogenic origin in relation to microbiological findings, *J Clin Microbiol* 22:299, 1985.
16. Jackson GG: Perspective from a quarter century of antibiotic usage, *JAMA* 227:634, 1974.
17. Konow LY, Nord CE, Nordenram A: Anaerobic bacteria in dentoalveolar infections, *Int J Oral Surg* 10:313, 1981.
18. Labriola JD, Mascaro J, Alpert B: The microbiologic flora of orofacial abscesses, *J Oral Maxillofac Surg* 41:711, 1983.
19. Lewis MAO, Carmichael F, MacFarlane TW, et al: A randomized trial of co-amoxiclav (Augmentin) versus penicillin V in the treatment of acute dentoalveolar abscess, *Br Dent J* 175:169, 1993.
20. Lewis MAO, MacFarlane TW, McGown DA: Quantitative bacteriology of acute dentoalveolar abscesses, *J Med Microbiol* 21:101, 1986.
21. Lewis MAO, McGowan DA, MacFarlane TW: Short-course, high-dosage amoxycillin in the treatment of acute dentoalveolar abscess, *Br Dent J* 161:299, 1986.
22. Lewis MAO, Parkhurst CL, Douglas CW, et al: Prevalence of penicillin resistant bacteria in acute suppurative oral infection, *J Antimicrobial Chem* 35:785, 1995.
23. Ma MY, Rho JP: Considerations in antimicrobial prescribing, *Med Clin North Am* 79:537, 1995.
24. Maimaris C, Quinton DN: Dog-bite lacerations: a controlled trial of primary wound closure, *Arch Emerg Med* 5:156, 1988.
25. Maki DG, Schuna AA: A study of antimicrobial misuse in a university hospital, *Am J Med Sci* 275:271, 1978.
26. Martin MV, Longman LP, Hill JB, et al: Acute dentoalveolar infections: an investigation of the duration of antibiotic therapy, *Br Dent J* 183:135, 1997.
27. Paterson SA, Curzon MEJ: The effect of amoxycillin versus penicillin V in the treatment of acutely abscessed primary teeth, *Br Dent J* 174:443, 1993.
28. Peltroche-Llacsahuanga H, Reichhart E, Schmitt W, et al: Investigation of infectious organism causing pericoronitis of the mandibular third molar, *J Oral Maxillofac Surg* 58:611, 2000.
29. Peterson LJ: Antibiotic prophylaxis against wound infections in oral and maxillofacial surgery, *J Oral Maxillofac Surg* 48:617, 1990.
30. Peterson LJ: Microbiology of head and neck infections, *Oral Maxillofac Surg Clin North Am* 3:255, 1991.
31. Polk R: Optimal use of modern antibiotics: emerging trends, *Clin Infect Dis* 29:264, 1999.
32. Raz R, Elchanan G, Colodner R, et al: Penicillin V twice daily vs four times daily in the treatment of streptococcal pharyngitis, *Infect Dis Clin Pract* 4:50, 1995.
33. Sclar DA, Tartaglione TA, Fine MJ: Overview of issues related to medical compliance with implications for the outpatient management of infectious disease, *Infect Agents Dis* 3:266, 1994.
34. Simmons HE, Stolley PD: This is medical progress? Trends and consequences of antibiotic use in the United States, *JAMA* 227:1023, 1974.
35. Thompson RL, Wright AJ: General principles of antibiotic therapy, *Mayo Clin Proc* 73:995, 1998.
36. Uman SJ, Kunin CM: Needle aspiration in the diagnosis of soft tissue infections, *Arch Intern Med* 135:959, 1975.
37. Veterans Administration Ad Hoc Interdisciplinary Advisory Committee on Antimicrobial Drug Usage: Guidelines for peer review, *JAMA* 237:1001, 1977.
38. Weber DJ, Tolkoff-Rubin NE, Rubin RH: Amoxicillin and potassium clavulanate: an antibiotic combination, *Pharmacotherapy* 4:122, 1984.
39. Zallen RD, Curry JT: A study of antibiotic usage in compound mandibular fractures, *J Oral Surg* 33:431, 1975.
40. Zalelnik DF, Kasper DL: The role of anaerobic bacteria in abscess formation, *Annu Rev Med* 33:217, 1982.

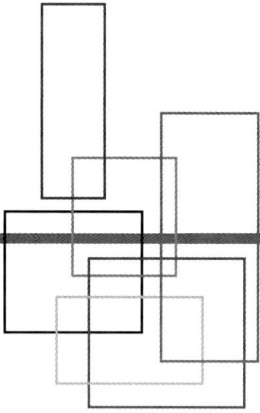

Antimicrobial Pharmacology for Maxillofacial Infections

James R. Hupp

This chapter focuses on the pharmacology, spectrum, and clinical uses of antimicrobial drugs in the management of infections of the head and neck (see Chapter 5). Not all antibiotics available in the United States are discussed; rather the coverage is limited to the major drugs frequently used for infections of the maxillofacial region (Tables 6-1 and 6-2, Box 6-1). Comprehensive infectious disease textbooks or *Mosby's Drug Consult** provide more complete information about specific antibiotics.

Most infections in the maxillofacial region resolve without the use of antimicrobial drugs because the host defenses are potent in the head and neck given the region's abundant vascularity (see Chapter 1). Even when the body cannot completely manage a facial infection, surgical intervention can provide the needed assistance by removing the nidus of infection, facilitating drainage of accumulated products of inflammation, or both. Antibiotics serve an adjunctive role in the management of most infections. However, they also help prevent infections after contamination occurs or abort a developing infection if administered early in the course of an infection. Antibiotics should not be used as a substitute for needed surgical treatment, nutritional support, or other basic therapies.

β-LACTAMS

Antibiotics of the β-lactam class remain the mainstay for prevention and treatment of most bacterial infections of the head and neck because of their effectiveness and relative safety.[27] Their name refers to a β-lactam ring common to these agents. These antibiotics inhibit replication of susceptible bacteria by interfering with cell wall cross-linking and kill them by activation of murein hydrolases that break down cell walls.[36] A variety of side chains confer differences in absorption, spectrum, and metabolism. Resistance to the β-lactam antibiotics occurs when bacteria can

synthesize β-lactamase, which breaks the β-lactam ring and neutralizes the antibiotic[43] (Figure 6-1). Many bacteria produce specific penicillinases, that is, β-lactamases that destroy only penicillin. In addition, some bacteria develop altered permeability to penicillins in their cell walls by changes in penicillin-binding proteins.[63] Five general categories of β-lactams exist[10]: penicillins, cephalosporins, monobactams, carbapenems, and combination drugs that are formulated with β-lactamase inhibitors.

PENICILLINS

The penicillins are a diverse group of β-lactam antibiotics that vary considerably in their spectrum (Figure 6-2 and Table 6-3). Because oral aerobes and anaerobes dominate the flora of the maxillofacial region, only some penicillins are useful: natural penicillins, aminopenicillins, and penicillinase-resistant penicillins such as oxacillin and methicillin. The other major group of penicillins is termed *extended-spectrum penicillins* and includes ticarcillin, mezlocillin, and piperacillin. The spectrum of these drugs extends to *Pseudomonas aeruginosa,* but their effectiveness for oral aerobes is limited.[36]

Although penicillins generally are well distributed after administration, they do not enter the cerebrospinal fluid (CSF) well. Concentrations in the CSF typically are less than 1% of serum values; with inflammation this concentration increases to only 5%.[61]

The principal contraindication to use of penicillins for treatment of susceptible bacteria is hypersensitivity. The incidence of allergy to penicillins ranges from 1% to 10% among various populations.[61] Most hypersensitivity cases are limited to dermatological reactions (2% to 3%), but anaphylactic responses to penicillin are not unusual, occurring in 0.004% to 0.015% of patients.[32,36] This incidence represents 75% of fatal anaphylactic reactions in the United States each year.[53] Cephalosporins and other β-lactams can be used safely in patients who are penicillin allergic even though cross-reactivity occurs in approximately 10% of

---

Mosby's drug consult, St Louis, 2002, Mosby (in press).

TABLE 6-1

Antibiotics of Choice for Specific Pathogens

Pathogen	First-Choice Antibiotic	Alternative Antibiotic
Actinomyces	Penicillin G	Minocycline Clindamycin
Bacteroides fragilis (enteral)	Metronidazole	Clindamycin Cefoxitin Chloramphenicol
Clostridium	Penicillin G	Cephalosporin Clindamycin Tetracycline
Escherichia coli (nosocomial)	Cefotaxime Ceftizoxime Ceftriaxone	Cefamandole TMP/SMX
E. coli (urinary)	TMP/SMX	Ampicillin
Eikenella corrodens	Ampicillin	Erythromycin Tetracycline
Fusobacterium	Penicillin	Metronidazole Clindamycin
Haemophilus influenzae	TMP/SMX	Amoxicillin Cefaclor Cefaroxime Chloramphenicol
Klebsiella pneumoniae	Cefotaxime Ceftizoxime	Aminoglycoside Cephalosporin TMP/SMX
Mycoplasma pneumoniae	Erythromycin	Clarithromycin
Neisseria gonorrhoeae	Ceftriaxone	Spectinomycin Ciprofloxacin
Peptostreptococcus	Penicillin G	Clindamycin Metronidazole
Prevotella (oropharyngeal)	Penicillin G	Metronidazole Clindamycin Cefoxitin Tetracycline
Proteus (indole-positive)	Cefotaxime Ceftizoxime	Cefoxitin TMP/SMX
Proteus mirabilis	Ampicillin	Aminoglycoside Cephalosporin
Pseudomonas aeruginosa	Gentamicin + ticarcillin	Imipenem and aminoglycoside
Salmonella	Ceftriaxone	TMP/SMX Ampicillin
Serratia	Cefotaxime Ceftizoxime	Aminoglycoside
Shigella	Ciprofloxacin	TMP/SMX Ampicillin
Staphylococcus aureus	PRP	Cephalosporin Vancomycin Amoxicillin/clavulanic acid
Staphylococcus epidermidis	PRP	Cephalosporin Vancomycin Amoxicillin/clavulanic acid
Streptococcus (enterococci)	Ampicillin + aminoglycoside	Erythromycin
Streptococcus pneumoniae	Penicillin G	Erythromycin Cephalosporin
Streptococcus pyogenes	Penicillin	Erythromycin Cephalosporin Clarithromycin
α-Hemolytic streptococci	Penicillin	Erythromycin Cephalosporin Clarithromycin

Modified from Topazian RG, Goldberg MH: *Oral and maxillofacial infections*, ed 3, Philadelphia, 1994, WB Saunders.
TMP/SMX, Trimethoprim-sulfamethoxazole; *PRP*, penicillinase-resistant penicillin.

TABLE 6-2

Pharmacology of Commonly Used Antibiotics

Drug	Route of Administration	Usual Adult Dosage	Special Features	$t_{1/2}$ (hr)	Peak Serum Level (μg/mL) and Dose	Major Adverse Effects
Penicillin G	IM, IV	600,000-1,200,000 U q4h	—	0.5	7.0 (600,000 U)	Allergy
Penicillin V	PO	500 mg qid	—	1.0	2.0 (250 mg PO)	Allergy
Oxacillin	IM, IV	500-1000 mg q4-6h	Penicillinase-resistant	0.5	11.0 (500 mg IM)	Allergy
Dicloxacillin	PO	250-500 mg q6h	Penicillinase-resistant	0.5	14.0 (500 mg PO)	Allergy
Ampicillin	PO, IM	250-500 mg q6h	Useful against *Proteus* (indole-negative)	0.7	2.4 (250 mg PO)	Allergy
Amoxicillin	PO	250-500 mg q6-8h	—	1.0	4.7 (250 mg PO)	Allergy
Cefazolin	IM, IV	250-1000 mg q8h	Excellent pharmacokinetics	1.8	38 (500 mg IM)	Allergy
Cefalexin	PO	500-1000 mg q6h	Oral cephalosporin	0.7	8 (250 mg PO)	Allergy
Cefoxitin	IM, IV	500-2000 mg q6h	Useful for anaerobes	0.7	24 (1000 mg IM)	Allergy
Cefaclor	PO	250-1000 mg q6h	Oral cephalosporin	0.7	18 (500 mg PO)	Allergy
Erythromycin	PO, IV	500 mg q6h	For mild gram-positive infections	1.5	1.0 (250 mg PO)	GI upset
Clindamycin	PO, IM, IV	150-450 mg q6h	Anaerobic antibiotic	4	2.5 (150 mg PO)	Diarrhea (20%)
Metronidazole	PO	1000 mg, then 250-500 mg tid	Anaerobic antibiotic	8	11.5 (500 mg PO)	Nausea
Vancomycin	IV (PO)	500 mg q6h	For severe gram-positive infections (PO for *Clostridium difficile*)	6	30 (500 mg IV)	Phlebitis
Tetracycline	PO, IV	500 q6h	—	—	3 (250 mg PO)	GI upset
Doxycycline	PO, IV	100 mg q12h × 2, then 50 mg bid	—	18.5	2.4 (100 mg PO)	GI upset
Chloramphenicol	PO, IV	250-750 mg q6h PO 15-20 mg/kg q6h IV	—	2.5	4 (500 mg PO)	Aplastic anemia
Trimethoprim-sulfamethoxazole	PO	(400 mg SMX and 80 mg TMP/tab) 1 tab bid	Broad-spectrum, bactericidal oral antibiotic	10 10	TMP 2 SMX 60 (1 tab)	Allergy to SMX
Ciprofloxacin	PO	250 mg q12h	Broad-spectrum, bactericidal oral antibiotic	3.3	1.5 (250 mg PO)	Secondary infection

Modified from Topazian RG, Goldberg MH: *Oral and maxillofacial infections,* ed 3, Philadelphia, 1994, WB Saunders.
GI, Gastrointestinal; *SMX,* sulfamethoxazole; *TMP,* trimethoprim.

BOX 6-1

Antimicrobial Spectrum of Common Antibiotics

Amoxicillin/Clavulanic Acid
As amoxicillin
Haemophilus influenzae
Escherichia coli
Proteus
Klebsiella
Staphylococcus aureus
Staphylococcus epidermidis
Enterococci
Anaerobes
Gonococci

Ampicillin and Amoxicillin
As penicillin
E. coli
H. influenzae
Proteus mirabilis

Cefaclor
As cephalexin
H. influenzae

Cefazolin
Streptococcus
Staphylococcus
E. coli
P. mirabilis
Klebsiella

Cefoxitin
As cefazolin
Enterobacter
Bacteroides fragilis
Oral anaerobes

Cephalexin
Streptococcus (except group D)
Staphylococcus (including penicillinase-producing)
E. coli
Proteus mirabilis
Klebsiella

Clindamycin
Streptococcus
Staphylococcus
Actinomyces
Anaerobes
B. fragilis

Chloramphenicol
Oral anaerobes
B. fragilis
Streptococcus
Staphylococcus
H. influenzae
E. coli
Shigella
Salmonella
Rickettsia

Erythromycin + Clarithromycin
Streptococcus
Staphylococcus
Mycoplasma
H. influenzae
Legionella
Oral anaerobes

Metronidazole
Only anaerobic bacteria

Oxacillin and Dicloxacillin
For treatment of penicillinase-
producing *Staphylococcus*

Penicillin G and Penicillin V
Streptococcus (except group D)
Staphylococcus (non-
penicillinase-producing)
Treponema
Neisseria
Actinomyces
Oral anaerobes

Tetracyclines
Streptococcus
Staphylococcus
Bacteroides
Mycoplasma
E. coli
H. influenzae
Shigella

Vancomycin
Streptococcus (including group D)
Staphylococcus (including
penicillinase-producing)
Clostridia

Modified from Topazian RG, Goldberg MH: *Oral and maxillofacial infections,* ed 3, Philadelphia, 1994, WB Saunders.

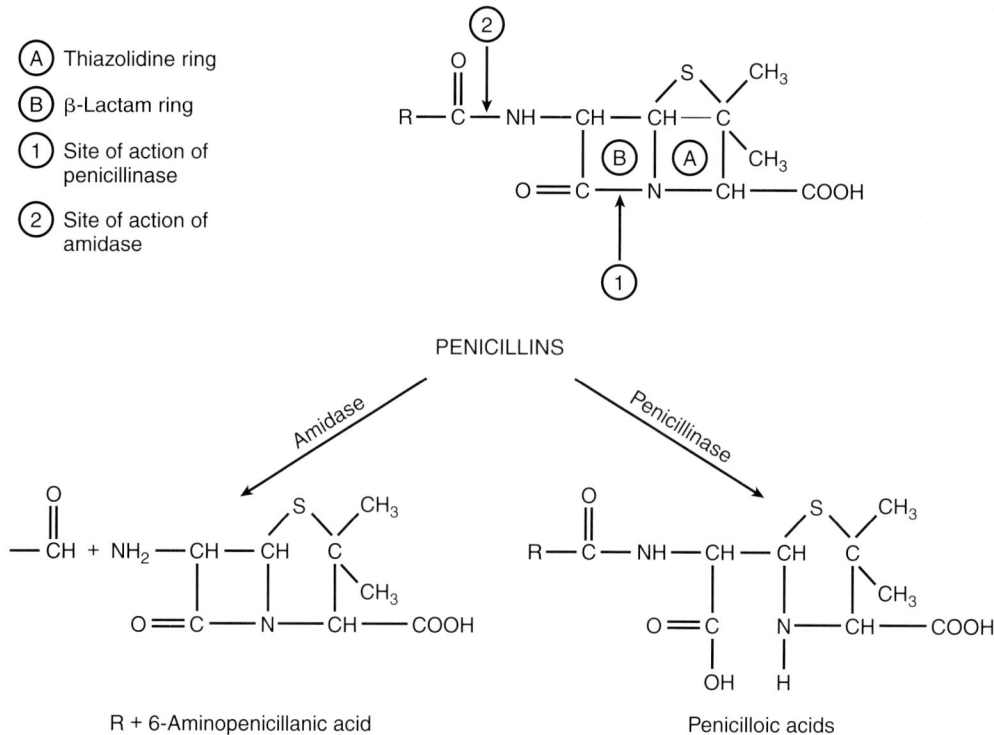

Figure 6-1 Destruction of the penicillins by penicillinase and amidase. *A*, Thiazolidine ring; *B*, β-lactam ring; *1*, site of action of penicillinase; *2*, site of action of amidase. (From Hardman JG, Limbird LE, editors: *Goodman and Gilman's the pharmacologic basis of therapeutics*, New York, 1996, McGraw-Hill.)

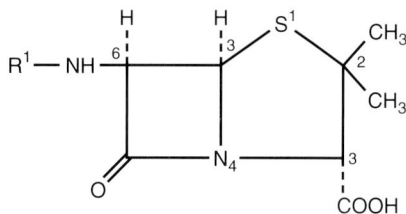

Figure 6-2 Basic penicillin structure. Substitutions at the R[1] site create the extended-spectrum penicillins. (From Johnson JT, Yu VL: *Infectious diseases and antimicrobial therapy of the ears, nose and throat*, Philadelphia, 1997, WB Saunders.)

them.[62] Clinical prudence dictates avoidance of all β-lactam antibiotics in any patient with a history of anaphylaxis or other serious reaction to any β-lactam antibiotic. Only 70% of patients who died of anaphylaxis after taking a penicillin had a history of ever receiving a penicillin.[58] Most cases of penicillin-induced anaphylaxis occur during or after intravenous administration.

The main natural penicillins are penicillin G and penicillin V. Penicillin G is a salt with either sodium or potassium. The K+ salt contains 1.7 mEq of potassium per unit. Because it is acid labile, penicillin G usually is given parenterally. The typical adult dose is 2 to 5 million units administered intramuscularly. Procaine penicillin G is a longer-acting formulation used to achieve adequate serum

levels for 8 to 12 hours; levels remain effective for 1 to 2 days when the drug is administered intramuscularly. Penicillin G benzathine produces an even longer duration of serum levels with the drug detectable for 1 to 3 weeks. Penicillin V is acid stable and administered orally. The typical adult dosage is 500 mg four times a day. Peak levels of penicillin V are achieved within 30 to 45 minutes, and most of the drug disappears in the serum by 6 hours after administration (Table 6-4). The spectrum of natural penicillins includes most gram-positive aerobes and most anaerobes (see Table 6-3). Notable bacteria that commonly are resistant to natural penicillins include *Staphylococcus aureus*, *Bacteroides fragilis*, and *Haemophilus influenzae*.

When a gram-negative bacteria is the likely cause of an oral or a facial infection, ampicillin and amoxicillin are reasonable alternatives. Ampicillin is absorbed poorly from the gastrointestinal tract and therefore typically is administered parenterally. Amoxicillin, in contrast, is very well absorbed by the enteral route. Both drugs are susceptible to β-lactamases. They are available in formulations with β-lactamase inhibitors using sulbactam (for ampicillin) (Unasyn) or clavulanic acid (for amoxicillin) (Augmentin) to overcome β-lactamases, thus improving their ability to eradicate bacteria such as *S. aureus* and *H. influenzae*.[58]

Although extended-spectrum penicillins such as mezlocillin (Mezlin), nafcillin (Nafcil), piperacillin (Pipracil), and ticarcillin (Timentin) exist, they have lost much of their efficacy against gram-positive organisms as they gained

TABLE 6-3

Penicillin Classes

Class	Examples	Useful Spectrum
Natural penicillins	Penicillin G Penicillin V	*Streptococcus* spp.* Enterococci* *Listeria* *Neisseria meningitidis** Anaerobes (not *Bacteroides fragilis* or some *Prevotella* spp.) Spirochetes *Actinomyces*
Penicillinase-resistant	Methicillin, nafcillin Oxacillin Dicloxacillin	*Staphylococcus aureus*† *Stapylococcus epidermidis*†
Aminopenicillins	Ampicillin Amoxicillin Bacampicillin	Extension of penicillin spectrum to Enterobacteriaceae, (*Escherichia coli*,‡ *Proteus mirabilis*,‡ *Salmonella*,‡ *Shigella*‡), *Haemophilus influenzae*,‡ and *Helicobacter pylori*§
Extended-spectrum	Piperacillin Ticarcillin Mezlocillin	Extension of ampicillin spectrum to *Pseudomonas aeruginosa*, Enterobacteriaceae, and *B. fragilis* group‖
β-lactamase inhibitor combinations	Amoxicillin-clavulanate Ampicillin-sulbactam	Extension of ampicillin spectrum to β-lactamase–producing strains of *H. influenzae, Moraxella (Branhamella) catarrhalis, S. aureus*, Enterobacteriaceae, *Neisseria*, and *Bacteroides*
	Ticarcillin-clavulanate Piperacillin-tazobactam	Extension of ticarcillin-piperacillin spectrum to β-lactamase–producing strains of *H. influenzae, M. catarrhalis, S. aureus*, Enterobacteriaceae, *Neisseria*, and *Bacteroides*¶

Modified from Johnson JT, Yu VL: *Infectious diseases and antimicrobial therapy of the ears, nose and throat,* Philadelphia, 1997, WB Saunders.
*Except for penicillin-resistant isolates.
†Except for methicillin-resistant isolates.
‡Except for β-lactamase–producing isolates.
§In combination with bismuth salt and metronidazole.
‖Except for some β-lactamase–producing isolates. Piperacillin is the most potent agent of this class against *P. aeruginosa*.
¶Except for chromosomally and some plasmid-encoded β-lactamases. The currently recommended dose of piperacillin-tazobactam may be inadequate to treat *P. aeruginosa*.

TABLE 6-4

Pharmacology of Selected Penicillins

Antibiotic	Usual Adult Dose	Peak Serum Levels (µg/mL)
Penicillin G	20 million units continuous infusion over 24h (high dose)	20 (3 million units IV)
Procaine penicillin G	300,000-600,000 units IM q12h	
Benzathine penicillin G	1.2-2.4 million units q15-20d	
Penicillin V	125-500 mg PO q6h	2.1-2.8 (250 mg PO)
Nafcillin	1-2 g IV q4h	40 (500 mg IV)
Cloxacillin	250-500 mg PO q6h	7.7 (500 mg PO)
Dicloxacillin	125-500 mg PO q6h	10-18 (500 mg PO)
Oxacillin	500 mg PO q6h	2.6-3.9 (500 mg PO)
Ampicillin	40-50 mg/kg IV q6h	3-6 (500 mg PO)
Amoxicillin	250 mg PO q6h	5.5-11 (500 mg PO)
Bacampicillin	400 mg PO q12h	5.8-8.3 (400 mg PO)
Piperacillin	3-4 g IV q4-6h	389-484 (2 g IV)
Ticarcillin	3 g IV q3-6h	200-218 (2 g IV)
Mezlocillin	3 g IV q4h	161-364 (2 g IV)
Carbenicillin indanyl	382-764 mg PO q6h	6.8-17 (764 mg PO)
Amoxicillin-clavulanate	250-500 mg PO q6h	3.7-4.8 (250 mg PO)
Ampicillin-sulbactam	1.5-3 g IV/IM q6h	40-71 (1.5 g IV)

Modified from Johnson JT, Yu VL: *Infectious diseases and antimicrobial therapy of the ears, nose and throat,* Philadelphia, 1997, WB Saunders.

strength against gram-negative bacteria. This property limits their benefits for typical head or neck infections.[58]

CEPHALOSPORINS

Cephalosporins are another important group of β-lactam antibiotics (Figure 6-3). Fortunately, they are less susceptible to β-lactamases compared with natural penicillins. Like penicillin, the first-generation cephalosporins and to a lesser degree the second-generation ones, cephalosporins provide good coverage against the oral flora.[37] Generations of cephalosporins generally relate to their respective spectrums (Table 6-5). The first-generation agents have the greatest gram-positive activity, but as the generation numbers increase, the gram-positive coverage decreases somewhat while effectiveness for gram-negative bacteria increases.[47] A similar trend occurs for anaerobes, in which the earlier the generation, the better the killing power. As the generation increases,

---

TABLE 6-5

Cephalosporin Generations

Examples	Useful Spectrum
First Generation	
Cefazolin	Is active against streptococci*
Cephradine	Is active against *Staphylococcus aureus*†
Cephalexin	Is not active against enterococci, *Listeria,* or MRSA
Cefadroxil	
Cephapirin	
Second Generation	
Cefuroxime	Expands first-generation spectrum to include greater gram-negative activity (*Haemophilus influenzae,* including ampicillin-resistant strains, and *Escherichia coli, Neisseria, Klebsiella, Acinetobacter, Enterobacter,*
Cefaclor	
Cefonicid	*Citrobacter, Proteus, Providencia,* and *Moraxella* [*Branhamella*] *catarrhalis*)
Cefpodoxime	Is not as active against gram-positive organisms as first generation; not active against enterococci,
Cefprozil	*Listeria,* MRSA, or *Pseudomonas*
Cefoxitin	Has spectrum similar to that of cefuroxime, but also active against *Bacteroides fragilis, Bacteroides* spp.,
Cefotetan	and other anaerobes
Cefmetazole	
Third Generation	
Cefotaxime	Achieves therapeutic concentrations in CSF, unlike first and second generations
Ceftriaxone	Is less active than first generation against gram-positive bacteria;‡ less active than cefoxitin or cefotetan
Ceftazidime	against anaerobes
Cefixime	Has expanded gram-negative spectrum§ compared with first and second generations, including
Cefoperazone	*Citrobacter, E. coli, Klebsiella, Enterobacter, Pseudomonas aeruginosa,*‖ *Proteus, Morganella, Providencia, Serratia,*
Ceftibuten	*Neisseria gonorrhoeae*
Ceftizoxime	Is not active against enterococci, *Listeria,* or MRSA
Cefditoren	Is more effective than oral third-generation antibiotics (cefixime, cefpodoxime), which lack useful
Cefdinir	activity against most strains of *Enterobacter* and *Pseudomonas* and have limited antianaerobic activity
Fourth Generation	
Cefepime	Compares with that of third generation but more resistant to some extended-spectrum β-lactamases

Modified from Johnson JT, Yu VL: *Infectious diseases and antimicrobial therapy of the ears, nose and throat,* Philadelphia, 1997, WB Saunders.
CSF, Cerebrospinal fluid; *MRSA,* methicillin-resistant *S. aureus.*
*Except for penicillin-resistant strains.
†Except for methicillin-resistant strains.
‡Cefotaxime is most active in class against *S. aureus* and *Streptococcus pyogenes.*
§Resistance to cephalosporins may be rapidly induced during therapy by de-repression of bacterial chromosomal β-lactamases, which destroy the cephalosporins, especially in the case of *Enterobacter* spp. and *Citrobacter freundii.*
‖Ceftazidime and cefoperazone only.

Figure 6-3 Basic cephalosporin structure. Substitutions at positions 1, R^1, R^2, and C^7 create the therapeutically important classes. (From Johnson JT, Yu VL: *Infectious diseases and antimicrobial therapy of the ears, nose and throat,* Philadelphia, 1997, WB Saunders.)

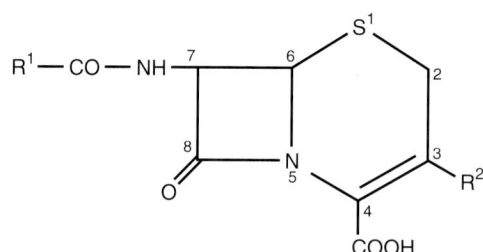

so too does the resistance to β-lactamases. The anti–*B. fragilis* activity of second-generation cephalosporins can be useful in head and neck infections caused by that organism.

The first-generation cephalosporins commonly used for maxillofacial infections and prophylaxis are cephalexin (Keflex) and cephradine (Cefadyl) for oral use and cefazolin (Ancef, Kefzol) for parenteral administration. Cefuroxime (Ceftin, Zinacef), a second-generation drug, is useful for sinusitis[58] but has been shown to be no more efficacious than traditional drugs.[58a] A newer, third-generation cepha-

TABLE 6-6

Pharmacology of Selected Cephalosporins

Cephalosporin	Usual Adult Dosage
First Generation	
Parenteral	
Cefazolin (Ancef, Kefzol)	0.5-1.5 g IV/IM q6-8h
Cephapirin (Cefadyl)	0.5-2 g IV/IM q4-6h
Cephradine (Velosef)	0.5-2 g IV/IM q4-6h
Oral	
Cephalexin (Keflex, Keftab, Biocef)	0.25-1 g PO q6h
Cephradine (Velosef, Anspor)	0.25-1 g PO q6h
Cefadroxil (Duricef, Ultracef)	1-2 g PO q12-24h
Second Generation	
Parenteral	
Cefamandole (Mandol)	0.5-2 g IV/IM q4-6h
Cefonicid (Monocid)	0.5-2 g IV/IM q24h
Cefuroxime (Kefurox, Zenacef)	0.75-1.5 g IV/IM q6-8h
Parenteral, antianaerobic	
Cefoxitin (Mefoxin)	1-2 g IV/IM q6h
Cefotetan (Cefotan)	1-2 g IV/IM q12h
Cefmetazole (Zefazone)	2 g IV q6-12h
Oral	
Cefaclor (Ceclor)	0.25-0.5 g PO q8h
Cefuroxime axetil (Ceftin)	0.25-0.5 g PO q12h
Cefprozil (Cefzil)	0.25-0.5 g PO q12-24h
Loracarbef (Lorabid)	0.2-0.4 g PO q12h
Third Generation	
Parenteral	
Cefotaxime (Claforan)	1-2 g IV/IM q4-8h
Ceftizoxime (Cefizox)	1-4 g IV/IM q8-12h
Ceftriaxone (Rocephin)	0.5-2 g IV/IM q12-24h
*Parenteral, anti-*Pseudomonas	
Cefoperazone (Cefobid)	2-4 g IV/IM q8-12h
Ceftazidime (Fortaz, Tazidime, Tazicef)	0.5-2 g IV/IM q8-12h
Oral	
Cefixime (Suprax)	0.2 g PO q12h
Cefpodoxime proxetil (Vantin)	0.2-0.4 g PO q12h
Cefditoren (Spectracef)	0.2-0.4 g PO q12h
Cefdinir (Omnicef)	0.6 g PO q24h
Fourth Generation	
Cefepime (Maxipime)	1-2 g IV q12h

Modified from Johnson JT, Yu VL: *Infectious diseases and antimicrobial therapy of the ears, nose and throat,* Philadelphia, 1997, WB Saunders.

losporin available in an oral form, cefditoren pivoxil (Spectracef), appears promising for serious sinus and skin infections[42] (Table 6-6).

MONOBACTAMS

Monobactams are a class of β-lactam antibiotics with bactericidal action similar to other drugs in their class. Only one monobactam, aztreonam (Azactam), is approved for use in the United States. Like other monobactams, aztreonam has no activity against gram-positive organisms,[33] which limits its use for head or neck infections. It can be useful for *Pseudomonas* and *Proteus* infections.[55]

Aztreonam does not cross-react with other β-lactams and has a low incidence of toxicity.[70] The usual dosage is 1 to 2 g every 8 hours.

CARBAPENEMS

Another group of β-lactam antibiotics is the carbapenems. These agents function like other β-lactam antibiotics by binding to penicillin-binding proteins and inhibiting cell wall synthesis. Their spectrum of activity is extremely broad, in part because of their stability in β-lactamases.[17] They are used to treat *P. aeruginosa* infections resistant to other antimicrobials.[29,44] The two carbapenems available for use in the United States are imipenem and meropenem. These drugs are not absorbed from the enteral route and so are administered parenterally.[54]

Imipenem by itself is toxic to and inactivated by the kidneys. However, when the drug is combined with cilastatin, an inhibitor of dehydropeptidase I, the nephrotoxicity from and inactivation of imipenem by the kidneys is blocked.[30] Imipenem/cilastatin (Primaxin) in a 1:1 combination is available for use when other more narrow-spectrum drugs are ineffective or cannot be used. The usual dosage is 0.5 to 1 g every 6 to 8 hours. Meropenem (Merrem) is the other carbapenem available for use; the dosage is 0.5 to 1 g every 8 hours.[18,76]

TETRACYCLINES, VANCOMYCIN, AND CHLORAMPHENICOL

TETRACYCLINES

Tetracyclines provide adequate antibacterial action, but the rapid appearance of resistance has limited their utility. These drugs function by reversibly binding to the 30S ribosomal subunit blocking the binding of aminoacyl-transfer ribonucleic acid, thus inhibiting bacterial protein synthesis. Although tetracyclines are used clinically, other than for use in lower molar osteitis sicca (dry socket) prevention, acne therapy, and management of periodontal disease, these drugs rarely are used for maxillofacial region infections.[68]

Side effects of tetracyclines include gastrointestinal disturbance, discoloration of bone and teeth, and growth disturbance of teeth. The effects on teeth contraindicate their use in pregnant patients and children.[61] Tetracyclines should be used with caution in conjunction with phenytoin, carbamazepine, and oral anticoagulants and in patients with renal insufficiency.

VANCOMYCIN

Vancomycin (Vancocin) is a relatively toxic antibiotic used primarily for treatment of methicillin-resistant staphylococci, although resistance to vancomycin by methicillin-resistant staphylococci and enterococci is developing in some hospitals.[27,41] Its acts by inhibiting peptidoglycan synthesis.[52] Vancomycin enters many tissue and fluid compartments but does not enter the vitreous humor and CSF in amounts adequate for therapeutic needs.[14]

Vancomycin is administered intravenously but requires a very slow infusion. Otherwise, patients may experience unpleasant symptoms, including flushing, pruritus, dyspnea, muscle spasms, and chest pain. Blood pressure also may decrease. This reaction to infusion of vancomycin is called "red man syndrome" and seems preventable by administering the infusion over at least 1 hour.[14,56,75]

Other toxic effects of vancomycin include nephrotoxicity, particularly when the drug is used with other potentially nephrotoxic drugs.[20] Ototoxicity also is considered by many as a risk of vancomycin therapy, particularly when plasma levels exceed 40 µg/mL. However, this risk is controversial because some believe the ear damage is related to other ototoxic drugs used concurrently with vancomycin.[9,19] Monitoring of serum levels is prudent, with targeted peak levels of 30 to 40 µg/mL and trough values of 5 to 15 µg/mL.

Vancomycin dosage in patients with normal renal function is 2 g per day, given as two 1-g infusions or 500-mg infusions every 6 hours. Dosage in patients with renal compromise varies based on creatinine clearance values.

CHLORAMPHENICOL

Chloramphenicol (Chloromycetin) is a now rarely used antibiotic that inhibits bacterial protein synthesis by binding to the 50S ribosomal subunit; thus it is a bacteriostatic agent. Because of its broad spectrum, it is potentially useful for treatment of ampicillin-resistant *H. influenzae* and anaerobic bacteria. It penetrates the central nervous system well and thus is a good agent for brain abscesses and meningitis.[23] However, its rare side effect of aplastic anemia greatly limits its use to only those situations in which less toxic antibiotics cannot be used or are ineffective. The drug more commonly causes dose-related reversible bone marrow suppression. In neonates the inability to conjugate chloramphenicol can lead to the so-called gray baby syndrome with cyanosis and circulatory collapse.[7] The usual dosage of chloramphenicol for older children and adults is 50 mg/kg per day divided in four doses. Serum levels and complete blood cell counts should be monitored.

MACROLIDES

Macrolide antibiotics frequently are useful for maxillofacial infections. This group shares a common structure of macro-

TABLE 6-7

Dosages for Macrolides

Drug	Adult (> age 12 years)	Child (≤12 years)
Azithromycin	250-500 mg/d	5-10 mg/kg daily
Clarithromycin*	250-500 mg q12h	15 mg/kg day 2 times daily
Dirithromycin	250-500 mg/d	NA
Erythromycin base	250-1000 mg q6h	30-50 mg/kg day 4 times daily

Modified from Johnson JT, Yu VL: *Infectious diseases and antimicrobial therapy for the ears, nose and throat,* Philadelphia, 1997, WB Saunders.
Administer all macrolides at least 1 hour before or 2 hours after meals.
*Dosage modification is required for severe renal failure.

cyclic lactam rings linked with amino sugars. These antimicrobials are bacteriostatic in that they interfere with protein synthesis by attaching to the 50S procaryotic ribosomal subunits. Although it does not kill the organism, this interference with protein manufacture neutralizes the bacteria.[49] Resistance to macrolide antibiotics may occur by receptor site alteration or bacterial modification of the antibiotic. Gram-negative bacteria can resist macrolides inherently because of their outer cell membranes. In addition, methicillin-resistant *S. aureus* infections are macrolide resistant.[51]

Erythromycin is the best known macrolide. Its gram-positive antibacterial properties are similar to those of penicillin, but erythromycin is not as effective as penicillin against anaerobes. Esters of erythromycin help overcome the native drug's poor bioavailability and its tendency to cause gastrointestinal upset. For serious oral and facial infections, other agents typically are preferred over erythromycin, even in cases of penicillin allergy. Erythromycin still is used often for legionellosis and *Mycoplasma pneumoniae* infections[51] (Table 6-7).

Clindamycin (Cleocin) is a lincoamide antibiotic that has reemerged as a commonly used drug for serious odontogenic infections including osteomyelitis. Poorly founded fear of pseudomembranous colitis limited this agent's use for many years, but a more scientifically based examination of antibiotic-related colitis failed to confirm any special danger from clindamycin compared with other antibiotics in individuals who are immunocompetent.[22,39]

Clindamycin is well absorbed orally but also is available as a parenteral drug. It readily enters hard and soft tissues because of its relatively small molecular size but does not pass through inflamed meninges.[22] Its spectrum includes aerobic gram-positive bacteria and facultative and strict anaerobic bacteria. The usual adult dosage is 150 to 450 mg every 6 hours orally or 300 to 900 mg every 8 hours parenterally. The pediatric dosage is 10 to 20 mg/kg per day in three to four divided doses (Box 6-2).

Azithromycin (Zithromax) is a macrolide with broad-spectrum coverage including gram-positive and gram-negative aerobes and strict anaerobes, including *Acti-*

Pediatric Dosages of Commonly Used Antibiotics

Amoxicilllin—25 mg/kg/day PO in 3 doses
Ampicillin—100 mg/kg/day PO, IM, or IV in 4 doses
Cephalothin—80-160 mg/kg/day IM or IV in 6 doses
Cephalexin—25-50 mg/kg/day PO in 4 doses
Chloramphenicol—75-100 mg/kg/day IV in 4 doses
Clindamycin—10-20 mg/kg/day PO, IM, or IV in 3-4 doses
Cloxacillin—50-100 mg/kg/day PO in 4 doses
Dicloxacillin—12.5-50 mg/kg/day PO in 4-6 doses
Doxycycline—5.0 mg/kg/day PO in 2 doses
Erythromycin—40 mg/kg/day PO in 4 doses
Metronidazole—30-40 mg/kg/day PO
Minocycline—4.0 mg first day, then 4.0 mg/kg/day in 2 doses
Penicillin G—100,000 U/kg/day IM or IV in 3 doses
Penicillin V—50 mg/kg/day PO in 3-4 doses
Vancomycin—50 mg/kg/day IV in 4 doses

Modified from Topazian RG, Goldberg MH: *Oral and maxillofacial infections,* ed 3, Philadelphia, 1994, WB Saunders.

nobacillus actinomycetemcomitans and *Porphyromonas gingivalis.*[45] Its oral absorption is better than that of erythromycin and it penetrates tissue well. In fact, even when measured blood levels are relatively low, tissue levels are 10 times higher and the levels in saliva, bone, and the gingiva can be 100 times higher. Azithromycin has a low incidence of side effects and is well tolerated in all age groups.[27]

Azithromycin is available in 250-mg capsules and tablets, 600-mg tablets, various strengths for oral suspension, and a form for intravenous infusion. The drug's long half-life allows once-a-day enteral doses of 500 mg initially and 250 mg thereafter. The capsular form of the drug should be given at least 1 hour before or after meals, and the suspension should be given at least 2 hours before or after food intake.[61] Tablets may be taken at any time (see Table 6-7).

Clarithromycin (Biaxin) is a macrolide available in many formulations. It is used frequently in combination with other drugs for treatment of *Helicobacter pylori* infections causing duodenal ulceration. It also is active against *Bacteroides* spp. and *Prevotella melaninogenica*. Its half-life allows dosage of 250 to 500 mg two times daily[11] (see Table 6-7).

A final group of macrolides is the aminoglycosides. These drugs are useful for many gram-negative bacteria but they rarely are used for head or neck infections because of their limited coverage for gram-positive or anaerobic bacteria.

NITROIMIDAZOLES

Metronidazole (Flagyl) belongs to the nitroimidazole class of antibiotics. These agents stimulate the production of toxic metabolites able to kill susceptible bacteria. Metro-

nidazole is effective only against strict anaerobic bacteria including those in the oral cavity.[60] This drug can be a useful adjunct to antibiotics with an aerobic spectrum in treatment of a mixed aerobic and anaerobic infection or for empirical treatment of stubborn odontogenic infections. Metronidazole is administered orally (500 mg every 8 hours). Its major adverse effect is a disulfiram-type reaction caused by the collection of acetaldehyde with the consumption of ethanol by patients taking metronidazole. It also can increase the action of anticoagulants. Patients may report nausea, headache, metallic taste, or anorexia while taking metronidazole. This drug should not be used in pregnant patients.[8]

QUINOLONES

The quinolones generally are effective for gram-positive and gram-negative aerobes, including *P. aeruginosa,* but are not useful for strict anaerobes.[4] These agents interfere with a bacterial enzyme critical for deoxyribonucleic acid transcription.[31,46] Quinolones are useful when susceptible bacteria such as *Streptococcus pneumoniae* are known as the cause of infection but should not be considered as a sole drug for empirical treatment when anaerobes may be present.[15] Ciprofloxacin (Cipro) is the most commonly used drug when quinolones are used for head and neck infections. Oral absorption ranges between 50% and 90%. Ciprofloxacin passes into most fluid compartments and crosses the placental barrier.[72] Cipro is effective particularly in the treatment of malignant otitis externa.[13] Side effects include gastrointestinal upset, photosensitivity, xerostomia, and central nervous system symptoms such as insomnia, headache and dizziness. Electrocardiographic changes also may occur.[2] The usual adult dosage is 500 to 750 mg orally every 12 hours (Table 6-8).

Moxifloxacin (Avelox), a third-generation quinolone, provides good coverage against oral streptococci and anaerobes and has proven efficacy for acute sinusitis.[15] It is well absorbed orally and not affected by concurrent food intake. Tissue levels commonly increase above plasma levels; the drug also appears in saliva and nasal secretions. Adverse effects are rare and typically consist of gastrointestinal disturbance.[72] Safety in children and pregnant patients is not yet established. The usual dosage is one 400-mg tablet daily (see Table 6-8).

ANTIFUNGAL AGENTS

Four types of antifungal agents are available for management of fungal infections of the head and neck: amphotericin B, flucytosine, the azole drugs, and topical antifungal agents. Amphotericin B and flucytosine typically are reserved for life-threatening infections or infections that cannot be resolved with azole drugs. These restrictions are based on amphotericin B's adverse effects on the kidneys and flucytosine's bone marrow–suppressive effects.

Amphotericin B (Fungizone) has a broad spectrum of antifungal activity including *Candida* spp., dermatophytes,

TABLE 6-8

Dosage of Quinolones in Patients with Normal and Impaired Renal Function

Quinolone	DOSAGE WITH NORMAL RENAL FUNCTION		DOSAGE WITH IMPAIRED RENAL FUNCTION WITH GFR (mL/mm)	
	Oral	Intravenous	10-50	<10
Ciprofloxacin (Cipro)	250-750 mg q12h	200-400 mg q12h	1 × dose q18h	1 × dose q24h
Ofloxacin (Floxin)	200-400 mg q12h	200-400 mg q12h	1 × dose q24h	½ × dose q24h
Lomefloxacin (Maxaquin)	400 mg q24 h	No IV form	½ × dose q24h	½ × dose q24h
Moxifloxacin (Avelox)	400 mg q24h	No IV form	None	None
Trovafloxacin (Trovan)*	200 mg q24h	300 mg q24h	None	None

Modified from Johnson JT, Yu VL: *Infectious diseases and antimicrobial therapy of the ears, nose and throat,* Philadelphia, 1997, WB Saunders.
GFR, Glomerular filtration rate.
*Adjust dosage downward in patients with hepatic compromise.

filamentous fungilike *Aspergillus, Rhizopus* and *Mucor* spp., and dimorphic endemic mycoses.[34] It is the treatment of choice for life-threatening mycotic infections.[46] In the head and neck, amphotericin B is used most commonly for severe sinusitis, cavernous sinus thrombosis, orbital apex syndrome, and otitis externa caused by fungal organisms.[25] Flucytosine typically is given in conjunction with amphotericin B for cryptococcal meningitis and serious candidal infections.[50,67]

The amphotericin B dosing regimen is complex, and assistance from an infectious disease specialist or others with regular experience using this drug may be indicated. The drug is given intravenously, and titration from a low to therapeutic dose is performed over several days while renal function is monitored. Patients frequently experience nausea and vomiting, rigors, and fever during administration. Veins used for infusion are irritated and phlebitis is common. Anemia occurs while the drug is in use but reverses once the drug is discontinued. Different forms of amphotericin B are available (Abelcet, Amphotec, AmBisome) and were created to reduce the toxic side effects. These new formulations use lipid complexes or lipid encapsulation to diminish the toxicity of the parent compound.[3,67]

Flucytosine (Ancobon) is available as 250- and 500-mg-capsules; the drug is administered every 6 to 12 hours to a total of 100 mg/kg daily. If the creatinine clearance decreases to critical levels, the total daily dose should be reduced with guidance from infectious disease physicians. The bone marrow suppression caused by flucytosine usually reverses once the drug is discontinued. Side effects include nausea, vomiting, hepatotoxicity, and rashes. Peak and trough blood levels should be monitored.[71]

Five azole drugs commonly are used for fungal infections of the head and neck. These include clotrimazole, used as a topical agent for fungal infections; fluconazole; itraconazole; ketoconazole; and miconazole (Table 6-9).

Fluconazole (Diflucan) is the most versatile of the azole antifungal drugs. It is available in oral and intravenous formulations and does not require the action of gastric acid or absorption. It is not highly protein bound, allowing wide distribution among body compartments.[6] Its long serum half-life allows once-daily dosing of 100 mg for minor infections and up to 400 to 800 mg daily for serious infections.[48,73]

Itraconazole (Sporanox) is available only as a 100-mg capsule, and doses greater than 200 mg do not appear to increase serum levels. Thus it must be given in separate doses if used for a severe infection requiring a daily dose of 400 mg. For less serious infections a total daily dose of 100 to 200 mg usually is adequate.[28] Itraconazole is not well distributed to areas such as the CSF, eye, and urine.[16,48,73] Intravenous itraconazole offers a less toxic alternative for patients with deep fungal infections who are unable to take amphotericin B.[65]

Ketoconazole (Nizoral) is available in 200-mg tablets that, similar to itraconazole capsules, require gastric acid for absorption. This requirement may affect absorption in elderly patients and others with low gastric acidity.[35] Like itraconazole, ketoconazole poorly penetrates into the CSF, eye, urine, and saliva because of a high degree of protein binding. As with fluconazole, once-daily dosing is possible; the dose ranges from 200 to 800 mg depending on the severity of the fungal disease.[69,73]

The azoles' spectrum of coverage varies to some degree among the various agents.[64] All have good activity against *Candida* spp. and *Coccidioides immitis.* Itraconazole and ketoconazole are best for dimorphic endemic mycoses. The only azole active against *Aspergillus* is itraconazole.[12] None of the azoles are useful for *Mucor* or *Rhizopus* organisms.

The most frequent use of azoles is management of mucocutaneous candidiasis.[5] Fluconazole is more effective than ketoconazole or clotrimazole troches for thrush in patients who are human immunodeficiency virus positive. For minor infections a 100-mg daily dose is sufficient.

Common side effects of ketoconazole are decreased libido and gynecomastia, particularly at higher doses.[34] Adrenal suppression also has been reported.[38] Other side effects include fatigue, rash, and nausea. Hepatitis is a rare complication of ketoconazole use.

TABLE 6-9

Clinically Important Features of the Pharmacology of Azoles

Feature	Ketoconazole	Itraconazole	Fluconazole
Formulation	200-mg tablets	100-mg capsules	50-, 100-, 150-, 200-mg tablets 2 mg/mL IV solution 50-mg or 200-mg/5 mL suspension
Absorption	Requires acid; decreased with antacids, omeprazole, histamine$_2$ blockers, sucralfate	Requires acid; decreased with blockers, omeprazole, histamine$_2$ blockers, (?) sucralfate	Excellent; not affected by antacids, omeprazole, histamine$_2$ blockers, sucralfate
Distribution	Minimal in CSF, eye, and other sites	Minimal in CSF, eye, and other sites	Excellent in CSF, eye, and other sites
Protein binding	High (~99%)	High (~99%)	Low (~10%)
Metabolism	Almost entirely hepatic	Almost entirely hepatic	Minimal hepatic metabolism
Excretion in urine	Little unchanged drug in urine	Little unchanged drug in urine	>80% excreted by kidneys
Reduction of dose in renal failure	Not necessary	Not necessary	20-50 mL/min: ↓ by 50% <20 mL/min: ↓ by 75% Hemodialysis: administer dose after dialysis
Dosing regimen	Once-daily dosing	Once daily for 200 mg; twice daily if higher dose required	Once-daily dosing
Usual daily dose	200-800 mg	100-400 mg	100-800 mg

From Johnson JT, Yu VL: *Infectious diseases and antimicrobial therapy of the ears, nose and throat,* Philadelphia, 1997, WB Saunders.
CSF, Cerebrospinal fluid.

Side effects of itraconazole are less severe than those of ketoconazole, and those of fluconazole are even more minor. Itraconazole side effects include nausea, fatigue, rash, and hepatitis. Azoles have some important drug interactions with terfenadine (Seldane) and loratadine (Claritin). Levels of these drugs tend to increase in patients concurrently taking azole agents.[34]

Two useful antifungals that are not used systemically are nystatin and clotrimazole. Nystatin (Micostatin) is a polyene antifungal similar in structure to amphotericin B, whereas clotrimazole is an azole.[66] Both agents are helpful as topical therapy for mild to moderate mucocutaneous candidiasis. Nystatin is available as a suspension (100,000 units/mL) and pastilles (200,000 units each). The suspension is administered in a swish-and-swallow format four times a day and also can be used for soaking dental prostheses. The pastilles should be dissolved in the mouth until gone and are taken one or two at a time four to five times a day for 10 to 14 days. Nystatin is nontoxic and usually effective during use, but relapses after therapy are common.[24]

Clotrimazole (Mycelex) troches contain 10 mg of active drug and are used for oral thrush. The troches contain sugar and so may promote caries if used excessively, but they otherwise are nontoxic. Like nystatin pastilles, clotrimazole troches must be dissolved in the mouth completely because any swallowed troche has no benefit. Some clinicians have used clotrimazole prophylactically, but a reliable protocol is not yet established.[57] The typical dosage is four to five troches per day for 10 to 14 days for treatment of oral candidiasis.

ANTIVIRAL AGENTS

Most viral infections are self-limiting and antiviral agents are unnecessary. However, oral and facial surgeons often treat patients with recurrent herpes simplex virus infections that affect the oral and perioral tissues. These infections sometimes are severe, or patients are bothered by frequent recurrences or fear spreading the virus to others.[40] In these circumstances, some clinicians prescribe antiviral agents to speed the resolution of lesions or prevent outbreaks of herpetic lesions.[21,24,59,74]

Two agents in regular use for management of oral herpes simplex are acyclovir (Zovirax) and valacyclovir (Valtrex). Both are acyclic analogues of guanine deoxyribase; valcyclovir is a prodrug of acyclovir.[1] Both agents inhibit herpes simplex virus replication. The drugs also have activity against varicella zoster, Epstein-Barr virus, human herpesvirus 6, and cytomegalovirus. Viruses in their latent stage are not affected, and therefore these antiviral agents do not eradicate viruses.

Because these drugs are highly selective for viral deoxyribonucleic acid, they do not harm human cells. Their low protein binding improves distribution to the CSF, saliva, and other fluid compartments. Oral absorption is low and therefore the intravenous form of these drugs is necessary for serious infections. The toxicity of these agents is low, although reversible encephalopathy or nephropathy occurs rarely.[1]

Primary or recurrent orolabial herpes is managed with oral acyclovir (200 to 400 mg five times a day). Topical acyclovir decreases viral shedding but does not significantly hasten the resolution of herpetic lesions. Prophylactic use of acyclovir frequently prevents outbreaks but is not curative. Resistance to the drug does occur, and a dose of 400 mg twice a day reduces recurrences by approximately 50%. Suppression of herpes during periods of therapeutic immunosuppression is achieved using intravenous acyclovir (250 mg/m^2 over 8 hours).[26]

REFERENCES

1. Acosta EP, Fletcher C: Valacyclovir, *Ann Pharmacother* 31:185, 1997.
2. Ball P: Quinolone-induced QT interval prolongation: a not-so-unexpected class effect, *J Antimicrob Chemother* 45:557, 2000.
3. Bishara J, Weinberg M, Lin AY, et al: Amphotericin B—not so terrible, *Ann Pharmacother* 35:308, 2001.
4. Blondeau JM, Yaschck Y, Suter M, et al: In vitro susceptibility of 1982 respiratory tract pathogens and 1921 urinary tract pathogens against 19 antimicrobial agents: a Canadian multicentre study, *J Antimicrob Chemother* 43(suppl A):3, 1999.
5. Bodey GP: Azole antifungal agents, *Clin Infect Dis* 14(suppl 1):S161, 1992.
6. Brammer KW, Farrow PR, Faulkner JW: Pharmacokinetics and tissue penetration of fluconazole in humans, *Rev Infect Dis* 12(suppl 2):S318, 1990.
7. Brook I: Chloramphenicol. In Johnson JT, Yu VL, editors: *Infectious diseases and antimicrobial therapy of the ears, nose and throat,* Philadelphia, 1997, WB Saunders.
8. Brook I: Metronidazole. In Johnson JT, Yu VL, editors: *Infectious diseases and antimicrobial therapy of the ears, nose and throat,* Philadelphia, 1997, WB Saunders.
9. Brummett RE: Ototoxicity of vancomycin and analogs, *Otolaryngol Clin North Am* 26:821, 1993.
10. Bush K, Jacoby GA, Mederiros AA: A functional classification scheme for beta-lactamases and its correlation with molecular structure, *Antimicrob Agents Chemother* 39:1211, 1995.
11. Carbon C, Rubinstein E: Macrolides, lincosamides and streptogramins. In Armstrong D, Cohen J, editors: *Infectious diseases,* St Louis, 1999, Mosby.
12. Como JA, Dismukes WE: Oral azole drugs as systemic antifungal therapy, *N Engl J Med* 330:263, 1994.
13. Cooper MA, Andrews JM, Wise R: Ciprofloxacin resistance developing during treatment of malignant otitis externa, *J Antimicrob Chemother* 32:163, 1993.
14. Cooper GL, Given DB: *Vancomycin: a comprehensive review of 30 years of clinical experience,* New York, 1986, Park Row.
15. Cubbon MD, Masterton RG: New quinolones: a fresh answer to the pneumococcus, *J Antimicrob Chemother* 46:869, 2000.
16. DeBaule K, van Gestel J: Pharmacology of itraconazole, *Drugs* 61(suppl 1):27, 2001.
17. Edwards JR: Meropenem: a microbiological overview, *J Antimicrob Chemother* 36(suppl A):1, 1995.
18. Edwards JR, Betts MJ: Carbapenems: the pinnacle of the beta-lactams antibiotics or room for improvement? *J Antimicrob Chemother* 45:1, 2000.
19. Eliopoulous GM: Vancomycin. In Johnson JT, Yu VL, editors: *Infectious diseases and antimicrobial therapy of the ears, nose and throat,* Philadelphia, 1997, WB Saunders.
20. Eng RH, Wynn L, Smith SM, et al: Effect of intravenous vancomycin on renal function, *Chemotherapy* 35:320, 1989.
21. Esmann J: The many challenges of facial herpes simplex virus infection, *J Antimicrob Chemother* 47(suppl T1):17, 2001.
22. Falagae ME, Gorbach SL: Clindamycin and metronidazole, *Med Clin North Am* 79:845, 1995.
23. Feder HM Jr, Osier C, Maderazo EG: Chloramphenicol: a review of its use in clinical practice, *Rev Infect Dis* 3:479, 1981.
24. Fleischman J: Topical and systemic antifungal and antiviral agents. In Newman MG, van Winkelhoff AJ, editors: *Antibiotic and antimicrobial use in dental practice,* ed 2, Chicago, 2001, Quintessence.
25. Gallis HW, Drew RH, Pickard WW: Amphotericin B: 30 years of clinical experience, *Rev Infect Dis* 12:308, 1990.
26. Gnann JW Jr: Antiviral agents. In Armstrong D, Cohen J, editors: *Infectious diseases,* St Louis, 1999, Mosby.
27. Goldberg M: Antibiotics: old friends and new acquaintances, *Oral Maxillofac Surg Clin North Am* 13:15, 2001.
28. Grant SM, Clissold SP: Itraconazole, *Drugs* 37:310, 1989.
29. Hamilton-Miller JM: Beta-lactams: variations on a chemical theme, with some surprising biologic results, *J Antimicrob Chemother* 44:729, 1999.
30. Hellinger WC, Brewer NS: Imipenem, *Mayo Clin Proc* 66:1074, 1991.
31. Hooper DC: Quinolone mode of action, *Drugs* 49(suppl 2):10, 1995.
32. Idose O, Guthe T, Wilcox RR, et al: Nature and extent of penicillin side-reactions with particular reference to fatalities from anaphylactic shock, *Bull World Health Organ* 38:159, 1968.
33. Johnson CC: Susceptibility of anaerobic bacteria to beta-lactam antibiotics in the United States, *Clin Infect Dis* 16(suppl 4):371, 1993.
34. Kauffman CA: Antifungal agents. In Johnson JT, Yu VL, editors: *Infectious diseases and antimicrobial therapy of the ears, nose and throat,* Philadelphia, 1997, WB Saunders.
35. Kauffman CA: Fungal infections in older adults, *Clin Infect Dis* 33:550, 2001.
36. Kendler JS, Hartman BJ: Beta-lactam antibiotics. In Armstrong D, Cohen J, editors: *Infectious diseases,* St Louis, 1999, Mosby.
37. Kessler RE, Fung-Tome J: Susceptibility of bacterial isolates to beta-lactam antibiotics from U.S. clinical trials over a 5-year period, *Am J Med* 100(suppl 6A):135, 1996.
38. Khosla S, Wolfson JS, Demerjian Z, et al: Adrenal crisis in the setting of high-dose ketoconazole therapy, *Arch Intern Med* 149:802, 1989.
39. Knopp FC, Owens M, Crocker IC: *Clostridium difficile:* clinical disease and diagnosis, *Clin Microbiol Rev* 6:251, 1993.
40. Koelle DM, Wald A: Herpes simplex virus: the importance of asymptomatic shedding, *J Antimicrob Chemother* 45(suppl T3):1, 2000.
41. Kollef M, Niederman M: Antimicrobial resistance in the ICU: the time for action is now, *Crit Care Med* 29(4 suppl):N63, 2001.
42. Kuti JL, Quintiliani R: Cefditoren pivoxil, *Formul* 36:265, 2001.
43. Livermore DM: Beta-lactamases in laboratory and clinical resistance, *Clin Microbiol Rev* 8:557, 1995.
44. Livermore DM: Of *Pseudomonas,* porins, pumps, and carbapenems, *J Antimicrob Chemother* 47:247, 2001.

45. Lo Bue AM, Sammartino R, Chisari G, et al: Efficacy of azithromycin compared with spiramycin in the treatment of odontogenic infections, *J Antimicrob Chemother* 31(suppl 3):119, 1993.

46. Lortholary O, Denning DW, Dupont B: Endemic mycoses: a treatment update, *J Antimicrob Chemother* 43:321, 1999.

47. Marshall WF, Blair JE: The cephalosporins, *Mayo Clin Proc* 74:187, 1999.

48. Martin MV: The use of fluconazole and itraconazole in the treatment of *Candida albicans* infections: a review, *J Antimicrob Chemother* 44:429, 1999.

49. Mazzei T, Mini E, Novelli A, et al: Chemistry and mode of action of macrolides, *J Antimicrob Chemother* 31(suppl C):1, 1993.

50. Medoff G, Kobayashi GS: Strategies in the treatment of systemic fungal infections, *N Engl J Med* 302:145, 1980.

51. Mulazimoglu L, Young LS: Macrolides. In Johnson JT, Yu VL, editors: *Infectious diseases and antimicrobial therapy of the ears, nose and throat*, Philadelphia, 1997, WB Saunders.

52. Nagarajan R: Antibacterial activities and modes of action of vancomycin and related glycopeptides, *Antimicrob Agents Chemother* 35:605, 1991.

53. Neugut AI, Ghatak AT, Miller RL: Anaphylaxis in the United States, *Arch Intern Med* 161:15, 2001.

54. Norrby SR: Carbapenems, *Med Clin North Am* 79:745, 1995.

55. Norrby SR: Monobactams. In Johnson JT, Yu VL, editors: *Infectious diseases and antimicrobial therapy of the ears, nose and throat*, Philadelphia, 1997, WB Saunders.

56. O'Sullivan TL, Ruffing MJ, Lamp KC, et al: Prospective evaluation of red man syndrome in patients receiving vancomycin, *J Infect Dis* 168:773, 1993.

57. Owens NJ, Nightingale CH, Schweizer RT, et al: Prophylaxis of oral candidiasis with clotrimazole troches, *Arch Intern Med* 144:290, 1984.

58. Petri WA Jr, Mandell GL: Beta-lactam antibiotics. In Johnson JT, Yu VL, editors: *Infectious diseases and antimicrobial therapy of the ears, nose and throat*, Philadelphia, 1997, Saunders.

58a. Piccirillo JF, Mager DE, Frisse ME, et al: Impact of first-line vs second-line antibiotics for the treatment of acute uncomplicated sinusitis, *JAMA* 286:1849, 2001.

59. Rooney JF, Straus SE, Mannix ML, et al: Oral acyclovir to suppress frequently recurrent herpes labialis, *Ann Intern Med* 118:268, 1993.

60. Rosenblatt JE, Edson RS: Metronidazole, *Mayo Clin Proc* 62:1013, 1987.

61. Sanz M, Herrera D: Individual drugs. In Newman MG, van Winkelhoff AJ, editors: *Antibiotic and antimicrobial use in dental practice*, ed 2, Chicago, 2001, Quintessence.

62. Saxon A, Beal NG, Rohr AS, et al: Immediate hypersensitivity reactions to beta-lactam antibiotics, *Ann Intern Med* 107:204, 1987.

63. Schmitz F, Fluit AC : Mechanisms of resistance. In Armstrong D, Cohen J, editors: *Infectious diseases*, St Louis, 1999, Mosby.

64. Sheehan DJ, Hitchcock CA, Sibley CM: Current and emerging azole antifungal agents, *Clin Microbiol Rev* 12:40, 1999.

65. Slain D, Rogers PD, Cleary JD, et al: Intravenous itraconazole, *Ann Pharmacother* 35:721, 2001.

66. Speed B: A review of antifungal agents, *Aust Fam Physician* 25:717, 1996.

67. Terrell CL, Hughes CE: Antifungal agents used for deep-seated mycotic infections, *Mayo Clin Proc* 67:69, 1992.

68. Threlkeld SC, Tierney MR: The tetracyclines. In Johnson JT, Yu VL, editors: *Infectious diseases and antimicrobial therapy of the ears, nose and throat*, Philadelphia, WB Saunders, 1997.

69. van Tyle JH: Ketoconazole, *Pharmacotherapy* 4:343, 1984.

70. Vega JM, Blanca M, Garcia JJ, et al: Tolerance of aztreonam in patients allergic to beta-lactam antibiotics, *Allergy* 46:196, 1999.

71. Vermes A, Guchelaar H-J, Dankert J: Flucytosine: a review of its pharmacology, clinical indications, pharmacokinetics, toxicity and drug interactions, *J Antimicrob Chemother* 46:171, 2000.

72. Walker RC, Wright AJ: The fluoroquinolones, *Mayo Clin Proc* 66:1249, 1991.

73. White MH: Antifungal agents. In Armstrong D, Cohen J, editors: *Infectious diseases*, St Louis, 1999, Mosby.

74. Whitley RJ, Gnann JW: Acyclovir: a decade later, *N Engl J Med* 327:782, 1992.

75. Wilhelm MP: Vancomycin, *Mayo Clin Proc* 66:1165, 1991.

76. Wiseman LR, Wagstaff AJ, Brogden RN, et al: Meropenem: a review of its antibacterial activity, pharmacokinetic properties, and clinical efficacy, *Drugs* 50:73, 1995.

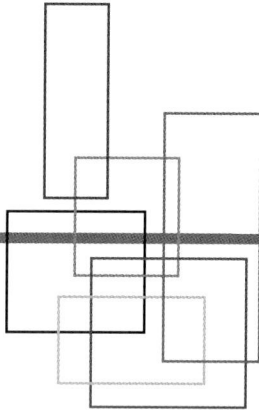

Periodontal and Pulpal Infections

Clarence L. Trummel
Ali Behnia

PERIODONTAL INFECTIONS

The soft and hard tissues that invest and support the teeth are the target of a diverse group of complex and often interrelated diseases. Some diseases are primary (i.e., arising in and largely limited to the periodontal tissues) and others are secondary (i.e., manifestations of systemic disorders). In addition, systemic conditions can modify the presentation and course of primary periodontal diseases. Recent findings suggest that the reverse also may be true: primary periodontal disease of a destructive nature may modulate systemic diseases such as atherosclerosis.[6] Because periodontal diseases, particularly those of bacterial origin, are ubiquitous, may reflect serious systemic problems, and often are first observed in an acute phase, clinicians who treat such patients initially should be familiar with the causes of these diseases and their management.

CLASSIFICATION OF PERIODONTAL DISEASES

As knowledge of their causes and pathogenesis expands, the classification of diseases of the periodontium improves.[2,128] However, to date no universally accepted system exists. A modification of a recent classification system of periodontal disorders and conditions was adopted by the American Academy of Periodontology[4] (Box 7-1). The diseases affecting periodontal tissues are classified according to characteristic pathological features or origin. This system divides periodontal diseases into gingival diseases, several categories of destructive periodontal diseases (periodontitis), necrotizing periodontal diseases, acute infections of the periodontium (abscesses), and periodontitis associated with endodontic lesions.

Of all diseases affecting the periodontium, the most prevalent and clinically important are those caused by oral bacteria that colonize the dentogingival crevice, gingivitis and periodontitis, in acute and chronic forms. Because

inflammation is a feature of periodontal diseases caused by bacteria, this group is frequently referred to as *inflammatory periodontal disease* or more simply as *periodontal disease*. The latter term, although inherently nonspecific, is used widely by clinicians. Based on the present knowledge of the essential causative role of bacteria in inflammatory periodontal disease, more appropriate terms might be *infectious periodontal diseases* or *periodontal infections. Pyorrhea alveolaris,* a term used more than 100 years ago to describe destructive inflammatory periodontal disease, reflected an emerging perception of the nature of the disease.[130]

Although inflammatory periodontal diseases of bacterial origin are diverse, they can be classified as *acute* or *chronic*. The term *acute* does not connote a purely acute inflammatory process occurring abruptly in a previously healthy site because most "acute" periodontal diseases represent an exacerbation of a chronic process. This chapter focuses on the diseases that constitute the acute group: abscesses, acute necrotizing ulcerative gingivitis-periodontitis (ANUGP), pericoronitis, and periodontal diseases associated with human immunodeficiency virus (HIV) infection.

FUNCTIONAL ASPECTS OF THE PERIODONTIUM

In the context of infectious periodontal diseases, some important functional properties of the periodontium are noteworthy. The most obvious is the structural support provided by the alveolar bone that allows the tooth to withstand the enormous and repetitive forces of mastication. Related to this is the suspensory action of the periodontal ligament through which these forces are transmitted to and dispersed within alveolar bone. A less appreciated but no less important function of the periodontium is the role of the gingiva in protecting alveolar bone from infection. Bone ordinarily is a highly protected tissue; with the exception of the oral cavity, it is well sequestered from the external environment by an intact cutaneous or mucosal barrier. Serious infections of bone of-

BOX 7-1

Classification of Periodontal Diseases and Conditions

I. Gingival Diseases
  A. Dental plaque-induced gingival diseases*
    1. Gingivitis associated with dental plaque only
      a. without other local contributing factors
      b. with local contributing factors (See VIII A)
    2. Gingival diseases modified by systemic factors
      a. associated with the endocrine system
        1) puberty-associated gingivitis
        2) menstrual cycle-associated gingivitis
        3) pregnancy-associated
          a) gingivitis
          b) pyogenic granuloma
        4) diabetes mellitus-associated gingivitis
      b. associated with blood dyscrasias
        1) leukemia-associated gingivitis
        2) other
    3. Gingival diseases modified by medications
      a. drug-influenced gingival diseases
        1) drug-influenced gingival enlargements
        2) drug-influenced gingivitis
          a) oral contraceptive-associated gingivitis
          b) other
    4. Gingival diseases modified by malnutrition
      a. ascorbic acid-deficiency gingivitis
      b. other
  B. Non-plaque-induced gingival lesions
    1. Gingival diseases of specific bacterial origin
      a. *Neisseria gonorrhoeae*-associated lesions
      b. *Treponema pallidum*-associated lesions
      c. streptococcal species-associated lesions
      d. other
    2. Gingival diseases of viral origin
      a. herpesvirus infections
        1) primary herpetic gingivostomatitis
        2) recurrent oral herpes
        3) varicella-zoster infections
      b. other
    3. Gingival diseases of fungal origin
      a. *Candida*-species infections
        1) generalized gingival candidosis
      b. linear gingival erythema
      c. histoplasmosis
      d. other
    4. Gingival lesions of genetic origin
      a. hereditary gingival fibromatosis
      b. other
    5. Gingival manifestations of systemic conditions
      a. mucocutaneous disorders
        1) lichen planus
        2) pemphigoid
        3) pemphigus vulgaris
        4) erythema multiforme
        5) lupus erythematosus
        6) drug-induced
        7) other
      b. allergic reactions
        1) dental restorative materials
          a) mercury
          b) nickel
          c) acrylic
          d) other
        2) reactions attributable to
          a) toothpastes/dentifrices
          b) mouthrinses/mouthwashes
          c) chewing gum additives
          d) foods and additives
        3) other
    6. Tramatic lesions (factitious, iatrogenic, accidental)
      a. chemical injury
      b. physical injury
      c. thermal injury
    7. Foreign body reactions
    8. Not otherwise specified (NOS)
II. Chronic Periodontitis†
  A. Localized
  B. Generalized
III. Aggressive Periodontitis†
  A. Localized
  B. Generalized
IV. Periodontitis as a Manifestation of Systemic Diseases
  A. Associated with hematological disorders
    1. Acquired neutropenia
    2. Leukemias
    3. Other
  B. Associated with genetic disorders
    1. Familial and cyclic neutropenia
    2. Down syndrome
    3. Leukocyte adhesion deficiency syndromes
    4. Papillon-Lefèvre syndrome
    5. Chediak-Higashi syndrome
    6. Histiocytosis syndromes
    7. Glycogen storage disease
    8. Infantile genetic agranulocytosis
    9. Cohen syndrome
    10. Ehlers-Danlos syndrome (Types IV and VIII)
    11. Hypophosphatasia
    12. Other
  C. Not otherwise specified (NOS)
V. Necrotizing Periodontal Diseases
  A. Necrotizing ulcerative gingivitis (NUG)
  B. Necrotizing ulcerative periodontitis (NUP)

From Armitage GC: Development of a classification system for periodontal diseases and conditions, *Ann Periodontol* 4:1, 1999.
*Can occur on a periodontium with no attachment loss or on a periodontium with attachment loss that is not progressing.
†Can be further classified on the basis of extent and severity. As a general guide, extent can be characterized as Localized = ≤30% of sites involved and Generalized = > 30% of sites involved. Severity can be characterized on the basis of the amount of clinical attachment loss (CAL) as follows: Slight = 1 or 2 mm CAL, Moderate = 3 or 4 mm CAL, and Severe = ≥5 CAL.   *Continued*

BOX 7-1

Classification of Periodontal Diseases and Conditions—cont'd

VI. Abscesses of the Periodontium
   A. Gingival abscess
   B. Periodontal abscess
   C. Pericoronal abscess
VII. Periodontitis Associated With Endodontic Lesions
   A. Combined periodontic-endodontic lesions
VIII. Developmental or Acquired Deformities and Conditions
   A. Localized tooth-related factors that modify or predispose to plaque-induced gingival diseases/periodontitis
     1. Tooth anatomic factors
     2. Dental restorations/appliances
     3. Root fractures
     4. Cervical root resorption and cemental tears
   B. Mucogingival deformities and conditions around teeth
     1. Gingival/soft tissue recession
       a. facial or lingual surfaces
       b. interproximal (papillary)

     2. Lack of keratinized gingiva
     3. Decreased vestibular depth
     4. Aberrant frenum/muscle position
     5. Gingival excess
       a. pseudopocket
       b. inconsistent gingival margin
       c. excessive gingival display
       d. gingival enlargement (See I.A.3. and I.B.4.)
     6. Abnormal color
   C. Mucogingival deformities and conditions on edentulous ridges
     1. Vertical and/or horizontal ridge deficiency
     2. Lack of gingiva/keratinized tissue
     3. Gingival/soft tissue enlargement
     4. Aberrant frenum/muscle position
     5. Decreased vestibular depth
     6. Abnormal color
   D. Occlusal trauma
     1. Primary occlusal trauma
     2. Secondary occlusal trauma

From Armitage GC: Development of a classification system for periodontal diseases and conditions, *Ann Periodontol* 4:1, 1999.

ten follow wounds such as compound fractures that breach this barrier and contaminate bone. Yet teeth obviously transgress this barrier, with roots intimately embedded in bone and crowns projecting into a body cavity with a multitude of bacterial and other pathogens. The solution to this unique, constant, and potentially dangerous threat to the skeleton is the gingival epithelial attachment. With inflammatory and immune mechanisms in the subjacent connective tissue, the epithelial attachment usually effectively limits the invasion of oral bacteria into alveolar bone or the host beyond. Although the chronic accumulation of bacteria at the dentogingival crevice can and often does lead to local disease and destruction of tooth-supporting bone and periodontal ligament, development of serious or disseminated infection from this localized infectious process is uncommon.

CHRONIC INFLAMMATORY PERIODONTAL DISEASES: GINGIVITIS AND PERIODONTITIS

CLINICAL FEATURES

Chronic inflammatory periodontal disease generally is a painless, asymptomatic, and slowly progressive disorder that begins as inflammation of the marginal gingiva in response to microbial colonization of the adjacent tooth surface. If this inflammatory response persists (i.e., becomes chronic), it likely will extend into deeper periodontal tissues and eventually result in progressive destruction of the periodontal ligament and adjacent alveolar bone, apical migration of the epithelial attachment and pocket formation, and possibly the ultimate loss of the affected tooth.[170] The disease can be subdivided clinically into chronic gingivitis

(inflammation only) and periodontitis (inflammation and loss of connective tissue attachment and bone) (Figure 7-1). Although distinction between these two conditions is important, it often is difficult given the present means of determining gingival inflammation and attachment loss.

Gingival inflammation commonly is assessed on the basis of visual signs (erythema and edema) and the tendency of the gingiva to bleed on sulcular probing.[45,94] Loss of connective tissue attachment and bone is measured primarily by determination of the attachment level relative to the cementoenamel junction using a probe[110] and secondarily by analysis of radiographs.[13] Because the presence and severity of periodontitis often is poorly correlated with the severity of marginal gingival inflammation, especially when the latter is assessed by purely visual criteria, a diagnosis of periodontitis must be based on measurement of attachment levels by probing. Like gingival inflammation, three other features traditionally associated with chronic inflammatory periodontal disease—pockets, purulent exudation, and mobility—must be interpreted cautiously in evaluation of the periodontium. Pockets may result from inflammatory or hyperplastic enlargement of the gingiva in the absence of attachment loss; conversely, attachment loss can occur with little or no pocket formation.[15] Although pus may be a prominent feature, it may not reflect the severity or even presence of periodontitis.[15] Similarly the presence or absence of mobility is not an infallible measure of the extent of attachment loss.

Gingivitis and periodontitis collectively compose the predominant pathological processes that affect the periodontium. Although the transition from gingivitis to periodontitis is not well understood, chronic gingival inflammation historically has been considered an early

HEALTH   GINGIVITIS   PERIODONTITIS

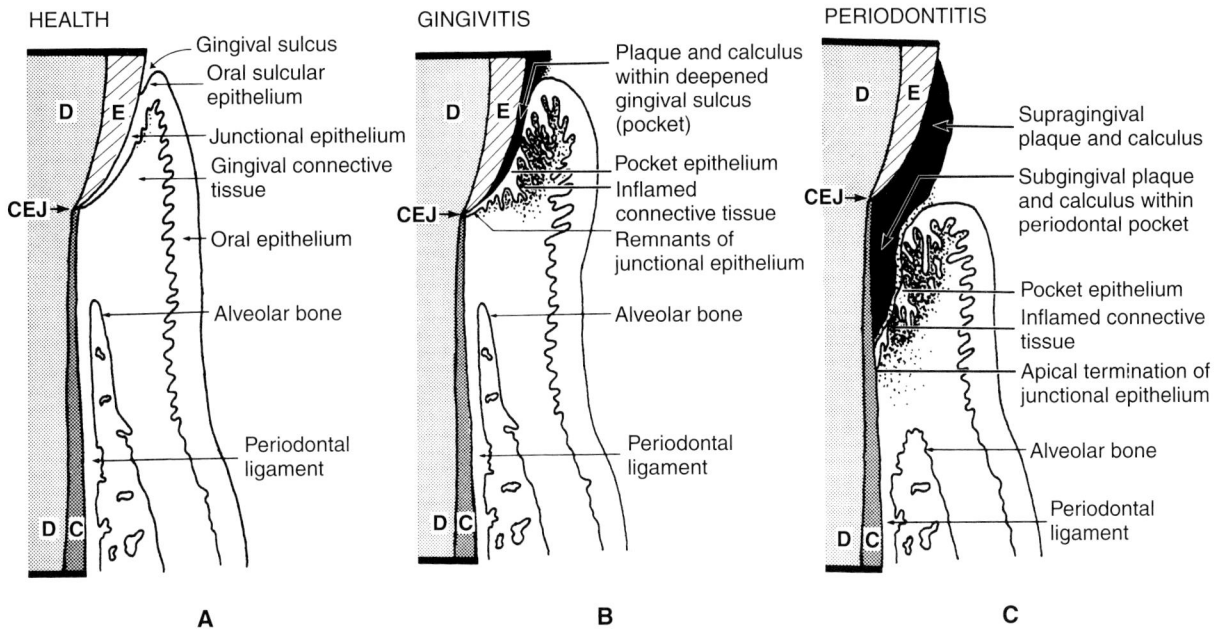

A   B   C

Figure 7-1   Essential features of the periodontium in health, gingivitis, and periodontitis. **A,** Healthy periodontium. The gingival sulcus is shallow (0 to 0.2 mm). The apical termination of the junctional epithelium is at the cementoenamel junction *(CEJ)*. The junctional epithelium is attached to enamel *(E)* by hemidesmosomes. Very few, if any, inflammatory cells are present in the gingival connective tissue. *D,* Dentin; *C,* cementum. **B,** Gingivitis. The gingival margin is enlarged (edematous). Gingival sulcus has deepened as a result of disruption of the epithelial attachment by dental plaque (i.e., hemidesmosomes of junctional epithelia have been disrupted). Some or all of the junctional epithelium has been transformed into pocket epithelium. Gingival connective tissue is infiltrated heavily with inflammatory cells. Proliferation of pocket epithelium into inflamed connective tissue is a prominent feature. No apical migration of the junctional epithelium or resorption of alveolar bone has occurred. The apical termination of junctional epithelium is still at the CEJ. *D,* Dentin; *C,* cementum; *E,* enamel. **C,** Periodontitis. Major features include apical migration of the junctional epithelium from the CEJ, bone loss, and recession of the gingival margin (not always observed). Most of the histopathological features of gingivitis, such as heavily inflamed connective tissue and proliferation of pocket epithelium, are present. *D,* Dentin; *C,* cementum; *E,* enamel. (From Armitage GC: *The biologic basis of periodontal maintenance therapy,* Berkeley, Calif, 1980, Praxis.)

phase of periodontitis (i.e., an inevitable continuum from gingivitis to periodontitis exists) (Figure 7-2). An alternative concept assumes that chronic gingivitis, although it may predispose the patient to development of pathological conditions affecting deeper periodontal structures, is a separate disease entity that may convert to periodontitis.[38,119] Not all gingivitis progresses to periodontitis, but periodontitis always is preceded and accompanied by gingivitis. A complex interplay between factors such as the duration and severity of gingival inflammation, the virulence of the associated microbial flora, and the effectiveness of the host's resistance likely determines if and when the transition to periodontitis occurs. Nonetheless, clinical management of chronic inflammatory periodontal disease presumes that gingivitis progresses to periodontitis because those sites with gingivitis that will *not* progress cannot be determined a priori.

The onset of gingivitis in previously healthy gingiva is difficult to determine clinically. Even gingiva with all of the characteristic visual and physical signs of health usually shows histological evidence of mild inflammation.[118] However, at some point the inflammatory process sufficiently intensifies to produce the classic clinical features of gingivitis: erythema, edematous enlargement, a tendency for crevicular

bleeding after gentle insertion of a blunt probe, and the presence of an inflammatory exudate. Based on the severity of these changes, gingivitis often is roughly classified as mild, moderate, or severe. Mild gingivitis exhibits the first recognizable signs of inflammation: slight erythema and enlargement of the papilla and gingival margin, some loss of gingival stippling (if previously present), and minimal bleeding on probing. Moderate gingivitis simply represents a more overt and extended expression of these changes. Finally, severe gingivitis is identified by markedly intense gingival erythema (blue to fiery red) and enlargement, complete loss of stippling, and profuse bleeding on probing. Frank ulceration, especially interdentally, bleeding induced by mastication or mild digital compression of the gingiva, or spontaneous bleeding also may be present.

A usual consequence of increasingly severe gingivitis is the development of progressively deeper pockets. Because such pockets are caused by gingival enlargement rather than attachment loss, they are referred to as *gingival pockets* or *pseudopockets*. Pseudopockets initially are the result of edema and inflammatory cell infiltration, but fibrous hyperplasia may become the major contributor in longstanding gingivitis.[14]

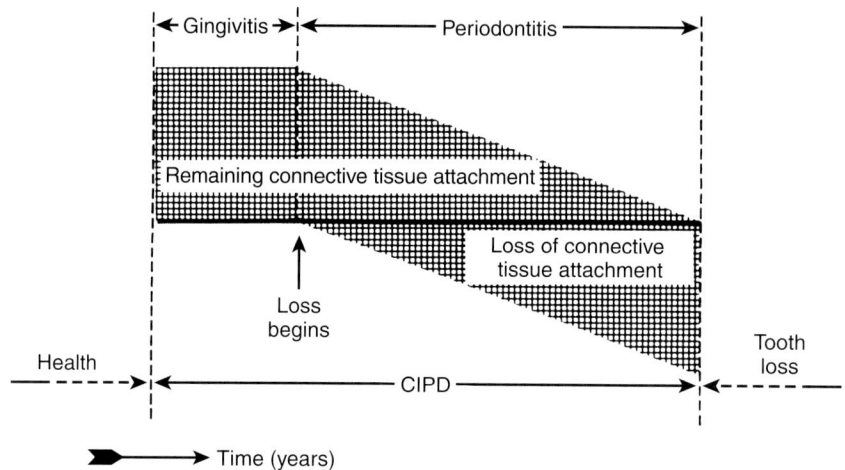

Figure 7-2 Spectrum of chronic inflammatory periodontal disease *(CIPD)*. Gingivitis and periodontitis are stages of CIPD and are distinguished by attachment loss. The transition from gingivitis to periodontitis involves apical migration of the junctional epithelium from the cementoenamel junction. The rate of attachment loss probably is not constant as shown. (From Armitage GC: *The biologic basis of periodontal maintenance therapy,* Berkeley, Calif, 1980, Praxis.)

Gingivitis in an individual who is systemically healthy is often termed *simple gingivitis.* It is perhaps the most ubiquitous of all human diseases.[158] The rapid onset and ultimate intensity of gingivitis are a function of a complex interplay between the quantity and quality (virulence) of the bacterial challenge and the individual's defense mechanisms. Alteration of the balance between these two opposing forces, particularly by perturbation of the latter, can affect the expression of gingivitis significantly. The importance of the host response often is illustrated dramatically in conditions such as neutropenia, HIV infection, leukemia, type I diabetes mellitus, malnutrition, and immunosuppressive chemotherapy in which resistance to infection is impaired. Individuals so affected typically have more severe gingivitis than would be expected for a given level of plaque. The acute occurrence of severe gingivitis in an individual with previously healthy or only mildly inflamed gingiva may indicate the onset or worsening of systemic disease and should trigger periodontal and medical evaluation.

Certain hormonal conditions also can exacerbate gingival inflammation. Although the mechanisms are poorly understood, physiological alterations in the levels of sex steroids during puberty and pregnancy worsen the severity and prevalence of preexisting gingivitis.[65,81] After puberty or parturition, gingival inflammation decreases even though plaque levels may remain unchanged. Localized granulomatous gingival enlargement (pyogenic granuloma) also may occur during pregnancy, especially when gingival inflammation is severe. These masses often resolve spontaneously after the pregnancy.

On the basis of clinical characteristics and the age group, several forms of periodontitis are recognized. The most common is chronic periodontitis with onset in early adulthood and rather slow but relatively continuous progression thereafter.[79,164] Chronic periodontitis frequently does not manifest clinically (or is diagnosed) until well into the third or fourth decade of life. Although the number and pattern of affected teeth varies, posterior teeth and proximal surfaces are affected more frequently than are anterior teeth and facial or lingual surfaces, respectively. The marginal gingiva may exhibit notable visual signs of inflammation (red to red-blue color and enlargement) or may appear relatively normal. Periodontal pockets usually are present and bleed on gentle probing; a watery or frankly purulent exudate also may be present. Radiographs reveal highly variable patterns of bone loss on affected teeth ranging from generalized and uniform (horizontal) to highly localized (vertical or angular). Clinical experience and epidemiological data support the concept that the severity of attachment loss in adult periodontitis generally is correlated with the abundance of soft and hard microbial deposits on supragingival and subgingival surfaces.[79] Although adult periodontitis usually is independent of systemic factors, its clinical appearance may be altered dramatically and the rate of connective tissue destruction increased by coexistent diseases such as diabetes,[1,51] neutropenia, leukemia,[115,121,176] and HIV infection.

Other forms of periodontitis represent assorted and less common variants of the disease that most frequently affect children and young adults. In the classification scheme used in this text, these forms are considered collectively as aggressive periodontitis[119] (Box 7-1). Several clinically distinct forms of aggressive periodontitis are recognized, including prepubertal periodontitis, juvenile periodontitis, and rapidly progressive periodontitis. Whether these conditions represent biologically unique subsets of aggressive periodontitis or simply age-dependent expressions of this disease is unknown.

Prepubertal Periodontitis Prepubertal periodontitis is a relatively rare entity that occurs in children as young as 4 years.[117] The disease may be localized or generalized and affect the deciduous or mixed dentition or both. The generalized form is characterized by severe inflammation and rapid progression that frequently leads to tooth loss. Although the number of reported cases is limited, most patients with generalized prepubertal periodontitis have leukocyte function abnormalities or other systemic conditions associated with reduced resistance to infection (e.g., neutropenia). Prepubertal periodontitis affecting the deciduous dentition may predispose patients to localized juvenile periodontitis but this suggestion has not been well documented.[168]

Juvenile Periodontitis   Juvenile periodontitis, formerly known as periodontosis, has a circumpubertal onset, usually between the ages of 10 and 15 years. The most widely recognized form, localized juvenile periodontitis, affects only incisors and first molars. Estimates of the prevalence of localized juvenile periodontitis in the United States vary; two recent studies found the disease in approximately 0.5% of 12- to 17-year-old adolescents with a higher prevalence in certain minority groups.[78,109] In typical localized juvenile periodontitis, modest levels of bacterial plaque and gingival inflammation are present but rapid progression of attachment and angular bone loss on the affected teeth occurs. Although localized juvenile periodontitis once was considered a degenerative, noninflammatory disease[41]—hence the term *periodontosis*—clinical, histological, and microbiological studies confirm its infectious-inflammatory nature.[178] A generalized form of juvenile periodontitis has been described but may be the more frequently termed *rapidly progressive periodontitis.*

Rapidly Progressive Periodontitis   As the name implies, *rapidly progressive periodontitis* is a rapidly destructive form of periodontitis that usually affects much or all of the dentition. Although it can occur at any age after puberty, onset typically occurs in the late second or third decade of life.[116] Severe florid gingival inflammation and rapid progression of attachment loss, frequently culminating in tooth loss, is common. Although juvenile and rapidly progressive periodontitis sometimes occur in association with systemic conditions that impair immune or inflammatory function (Plate 21), most affected individuals appear healthy. However, the majority of patients exhibit measurable defects in neutrophil or monocyte function.[128] The importance of these defects to the occurrence or progression of periodontitis is unknown.

EPIDEMIOLOGY

Inflammatory diseases of the periodontium are one of the longest recognized and most common conditions of humans. Alveolar bone destruction consistent with periodontitis has been observed in fossil remains of Neanderthal man, and detailed descriptions of periodontal disease and its treatment in Chinese and Egyptian writings predate this text by more than 4000 years.[35] Epidemiological surveys suggest that essentially all adult populations experience some form of inflammatory periodontal disease.[16,158]

Interpretation of studies of the distribution and frequency of periodontal disease is complicated by several issues. One is the various indices used for measurement of disease. Objective laboratory tests and clinical "gold standards" for assessment of the various forms of gingivitis and periodontitis do not exist.[43] Consequently, investigators used numerous, disparate, and often deficient indices to assess presence and severity of disease. Another issue is the assumption in many earlier studies that all inflamma-

tory periodontal disease is a single entity. The validity of this assumption is in doubt. Finally, epidemiological surveys frequently reported data from populations with divergent racial, cultural, socioeconomic, and geographical backgrounds.

Despite these problems the results of epidemiological surveys generally have been uniform with respect to the universality of periodontal disease and the strong positive correlation among inflammatory periodontal disease, age, and microbial plaque.[92,126,132,138] Accumulation of microbial deposits on the teeth is related directly to the presence and severity of periodontal disease and, conversely, controlled removal of plaque results in resolution of gingivitis and marked improvement in measures of periodontitis.[5,74,88]

Gingivitis affects the majority of young children and its prevalence is estimated at 60% to 80% in adolescence, declining somewhat thereafter. Estimates of gingivitis in adults range from approximately 40% to 100%.[158] Although periodontitis in young children is uncommon, numerous studies show that periodontal pocket formation and loss of attachment and alveolar bone often occurs before age 20.[79,133] With increasing age the prevalence of periodontitis increases almost linearly, and in U.S. adults older than 65 years of age, periodontitis may account for approximately 30% of missing teeth.[10] A recent survey of employed persons in the United States found that nearly half of 18- to 19-year-olds had one or more sites with at least a 2-mm loss of attachment.[96] This study also showed that the proportion of individuals with attachment loss had increased nearly 90% by age 65. Approximately one fourth of these individuals had attachment loss of 4 mm or more at one or more sites. Despite its widespread prevalence in older adults the severity of periodontitis has decreased slightly in recent years.[12,24]

The association of periodontal disease with gender, race, and social and demographic factors is less clear. In Western cultures, females have a lower severity of disease than males. Increased levels of education, income, and socioeconomic status have been associated with a lower incidence and less severe disease. In the United States a higher prevalence and greater severity of periodontal disease exist in black individuals compared with white individuals. The correlation for all these factors is weak and often lost entirely when groups are stratified based on measures of oral hygiene.[126,167]

The natural history of periodontal disease in adults was described recently in longitudinal studies of populations in Norway and Sri Lanka.[76,77] The two groups had major racial, geographical, cultural, socioeconomic, and educational differences and represented extremes with respect to dental care. The predominant diseases reported in both populations were gingivitis and periodontitis. Destruction of supporting structures associated with chronic periodontitis was continuous and progressed at a relatively constant rate in both groups. However, annual rates of periodontal attachment loss were significantly different, averaging 0.09 mm in the Norwegian population and 0.25 mm in Sri Lankans. Within the Sri Lankan population the rate of attachment loss varied; three subpopulations were identified: a rapidly progressive group (8% of subjects; 13-mm average attachment loss by age 45); a moderately progressive group (81% of subjects; 7-mm average attachment loss); and a group with essentially no progression of disease beyond chronic gingivitis (11% of subjects). These differences are notable because all subjects had similarly high levels of plaque, calculus, and gingival inflammation over the same period.

ETIOLOGY OF PERIODONTITIS

Plaque Factors   *Dental plaque,* a general term for a complex tooth-adherent mass composed principally of microorganisms and their products, is the primary cause of gingivitis and periodontitis. The evidence implicating the plaque microflora is the subject of numerous reviews[61,100,147,155] and includes epidemiological observations,* experimental induction of the disease process in a previously healthy periodontium solely by allowing the accumulation of bacteria,[82,161] and reversal of the inflammatory periodontal lesion by either mechanical removal[5] or chemical inhibition[75] of plaque.

Previous theories proposed that all plaque was similar qualitatively and disease was presumed to result when an adequate mass of plaque was present for a sufficient period. This view was articulated more than 100 years ago by the dentist-microbiologist, W.D. Miller,[97] who stated, ". . . Pyorrhea alveolaris is not caused by any specific bacterium which occurs in every case . . . , but various bacteria may participate in it." Several studies during the past two decades using improved techniques for sampling, anaerobic culture, and identification of organisms in subgingival plaque provided substantial evidence for a very different point of view, namely, that microbial specificity operates in inflammatory periodontal diseases.[148,155,156] Currently various stages and forms of inflammatory periodontal disease are acknowledged as related to qualitatively different plaque microfloras. Moreover, only a few[5,7] of the more than 350 bacterial species found in plaque appear to be associated with inflammatory periodontal disease.[101]

Although the origin of the pathogenic species for all forms of inflammatory periodontal disease has not been determined conclusively, most forms represent opportunistic infections: the responsible organisms are part of the indigenous oral flora.[33,160] Infection results from the creation of favorable ecological niches, alteration of host defenses, or other disturbances that allow pathogenic species to colonize and propagate. Once established in sufficient numbers these "disease-associated" floras can cause disease. Although the subgingival floras typically linked to various forms of inflammatory periodontal diseases vary considerably, all are characterized by the dominance of gram-negative, anaerobic, motile bacteria.†

The scanty subgingival plaque in individuals with clinically healthy gingiva is composed largely of gram-positive,

facultatively anaerobic, nonmotile bacteria (85%). Most of these organisms are streptococci, followed by species of *Actinomyces,* especially *Actinomyces viscosus* and *Actinomyces naeslundii,* and *Rothia dentocariosa.*[146] The small proportion of gram-negative organisms usually consist of *Fusobacterium, Capnocytophaga,* and saccharolytic *Bacteroides* spp. On microscopic examination, spirochetes and other motile forms are present but rarely constitute more than 5% of the total flora.

Individuals in initially perfect periodontal health consistently develop gingivitis within 1 to 3 weeks after all methods of plaque control are withdrawn.[82] The onset of gingivitis is associated with a marked increase in the mass of plaque at the gingival margin and a striking shift in the composition of the plaque microflora.[86,151] The proportion of streptococci decreases and the proportion of *Actinomyces* spp. increases sharply. The proportion of gram-negative and anaerobic forms also increases; in long-standing gingivitis these organisms may account for 40% or more of the total cultivable flora. Spirochetes and other motile organisms also increase to as much as 20% of the flora.

Periodontitis is associated with further qualitative shifts in the subgingival flora. In adult periodontitis, high proportions of anaerobes (90%), gram-negative organisms (75%), and motile forms, largely spirochetes (30%), are present.[84,153] The specific bacteria composing such floras can vary considerably between patients with clinically similar disease; even in a single patient with periodontitis the bacterial populations may vary in similar pockets. Thus association of a unique set of specific organisms with given stages or forms of periodontitis is impossible.[92,102,129] Nonetheless, greater numbers of a few species usually are found in the subgingival microflora of periodontitis. In particular, three organisms are strongly associated with periodontitis on the basis of their high occurrence and proportions in active periodontitis lesions and their well-known virulence properties: *Porphyromonas gingivalis, Bacteroides forsythus,* and *Actinobacillus actinomycetemcomitans.*[48,150,154] The first two organisms are associated especially with chronic periodontitis[18] and aggressive periodontitis[177]; the latter is associated with localized juvenile periodontitis.[178,179] Other bacteria also related to periodontitis are *Prevotella intermedia, Fusobacterium nucleatum, Wolinella recta, Eikenella corrodens,* and species of *Capnocytophaga, Eubacterium,* and *Treponema* (Box 7-2).

Nonplaque Factors   Epidemiological and experimental studies have not identified any local or systemic factors, independent of bacteria, that initiate gingivitis or periodontitis. However, several factors may modify the progress of the disease once established. One factor is calculus, once believed to be a major cause of inflammatory periodontal disease. Now the role of calculus is viewed as one of "nurturing" by providing a highly receptive substrate for the development and retention of a mature plaque.[79] Similarly, other local factors such as defective restorations or prostheses that intrude into the gingival crevice or crowded or malposed teeth may interfere with the patient's ability to remove plaque or provide an environment favoring the es-

---

*References 5, 74, 88, 92, 126, 132, 138.
†References 66, 85, 100, 150, 153, 159.

Bacterial Species Associated with Periodontal Health and Diseases

Healthy gingiva	Porphyromonas* gingivalis
Streptococcus mutans and other species	Bacteroides forsythus
Actinomyces viscosus and other species	Actinobacillus actinomycetemcomitans
Rothia dentocariosa	Prevotella* intermedia
Veillonella species	Fusobacterium spp.
Prevotella* intermedia	Wolinella recta
Gingivitis	Eikenella corrodens
Actinomyces viscosus and other species	Peptostreptococcus micros
Streptococcus spp.	Eubacterium spp.
Prevotella* intermedia	Treponema spp.
Veillonella parvula	Juvenile periodontitis
Fusobacterium spp.	Actinobacillus actinomycetemcomitans
Treponema spp.	Porphyromonas* gingivalis
Chronic periodontitis and rapidly progressive periodontitis	Prevotella* intermedia
	Eikenella corrodens

*Formerly *Bacteroides.*

tablishment of a more pathogenic flora.[69] Systemic conditions such as hormonal changes associated with puberty and pregnancy,[81] deficits in neutrophil number or function, and impairment of immunological responses may facilitate increased severity of gingivitis and periodontitis by altering the microbial flora, depressing host defense mechanisms, or both.[19-21,32,106] Evidence suggests that smoking has a negative effect on the periodontium, particularly in the presence of inflammatory disease.[136] Although smokers of any age have an increased risk of periodontitis, this effect is much greater for young individuals. Smokers as a group have greater bone loss than age- and plaque-matched nonsmokers[9,162] and have a poorer response to surgical periodontal therapy.[8] Several studies showed that half of the observed periodontitis in smokers younger than 33 years of age is smoking related with the odds ratio for smoking and the presence of periodontitis greater than 14.[70,139] The association of smoking with ANUGP is well established.[37]

Despite claims of the need for various vitamins (e.g., ascorbic acid), minerals (e.g., calcium), and other dietary factors for good periodontal health, little evidence exists that nutritional deficiencies except extreme ones act as initiating or modifying factors in inflammatory periodontal disease. Metabolic bone disease, most commonly osteoporosis, has been suggested as a contributor to alveolar bone loss in periodontitis. This assertion has not been substantiated experimentally, and evidence in animals and humans shows that loss of tooth-supporting bone in inflammatory periodontal disease is unrelated to systemic bone mass.[25]

The contribution of occlusal loading and stress to the progression of periodontal disease remains controversial. Studies in humans, primates, and dogs have demonstrated consistently that excessive occlusal forces alone do not ini-

tiate gingivitis or periodontitis or convert an established gingivitis to periodontitis.[18] Superimposition of occlusal trauma on experimentally induced periodontitis accelerated the rate of periodontal attachment loss in dogs[71] and was associated with reduction of bone regeneration after resolution of periodontitis in monkeys.[125]

PATHOGENESIS OF PERIODONTITIS

Sufficient bacterial colonization (plaque formation) of the tooth surface adjacent to the gingival margin initiates an inflammatory lesion in the gingival tissue. This lesion, if sufficiently severe and persistent, likely leads to irreversible loss of the connective tissue attachment and supporting alveolar bone. However, beyond acceptance of plaque bacteria as the principal causative agent in gingivitis and periodontitis and despite much research, neither specific causal organisms nor related pathogenic pathways have been defined clearly. Considerable progress has led to understanding the fundamental pathogenesis of inflammatory periodontal disease, and well-supported concepts of disease initiation and progression are emerging.

Whether bacterial invasion of tissues is an important aspect of the pathogenesis of chronic inflammatory periodontal disease is not established. For the most part, subgingival bacteria are confined to the periodontal pocket, attached to the root surface as a biofilm (plaque), free-living in the pocket fluid, or attached to pocket epithelium. Although single organisms or small colonies of bacteria, including *A. actinomycetemcomitans,* have been demonstrated in pocket epithelium and gingival connective tissue and on the surface of alveolar bone in advanced periodontitis,[29,134,135,137] overt tissue invasion by bacteria is not a feature of chronic forms of gingivitis and periodontitis. Therefore the inflammatory lesion and possibly the tissue destruction associated with periodontitis result from cellular components or metabolic products derived from the microbial mass within the sulcus or periodontal pocket.[32] In acute forms of disease, such as ANUGP or abscesses, bacterial penetration into periodontal tissues is essential to the disease and its manifestations.

Several substances that can mediate disease, either alone or in concert with others, have been identified in bacteria associated with inflammatory periodontal diseases.[149] Moreover, the ability of these substances, such as endotoxin, to penetrate sulcular epithelium and enter the adjacent connective tissue has been demonstrated. These substances may act by either direct or indirect mechanisms. Direct mechanisms are those in which a bacterial substance directly injures or destroys periodontal tissues. Examples of these are toxic metabolites, such as hydrogen sulfide, histolytic enzymes, such as collagenase, and substances that impair host defenses, such as *A. actinomycetemcomitans* leukotoxin. Indirect mechanisms are those in which bacterial factors trigger biochemical or cellular events in the host which in turn lead to tissue destruction. The production of collagenase by macrophages stimulated by bacterial endotoxin, and bone resorption stimulated by products of activated mononuclear cells such as interleukin-1 and prostaglandin E_2 are examples of indirect mechanisms. Recent reviews detail the complex interplay between bacterial virulent factors and host responses that leads to this uniquely destructive disease.*

The histopathological events that occur after microbial colonization of tooth surfaces adjacent to healthy gingiva and during the progression from gingivitis to periodontitis have been divided into four general and overlapping stages: initial, early, established, and advanced.[118,119] The initial stage consists of vasculitis concomitant with increased migration of neutrophils into the connective tissue immediately subjacent to the junctional epithelium. Alterations in the junctional epithelium and some loss of perivascular collagen may be observed. The early stage, beginning approximately 4 to 7 days after plaque accumulation, is characterized by migration of neutrophils through the epithelium into the sulcus and the appearance in connective tissue of an inflammatory cell infiltrate consisting primarily of lymphocytes. Continuing collagen destruction and proliferation of basal junctional epithelial cells occur. Over the ensuing weeks, plasma cells increase and in the established stage dominate the inflammatory cell infiltrate. The area of infiltrated connective tissue continues to increase in size, lateral proliferation and apical migration of the junctional epithelium are apparent, and the continued outpouring of neutrophils into the sulcus continues. The established lesion is compatible with a clinical diagnosis of chronic gingivitis and may persist without further involvement of deeper supporting structures. However, under conditions or influences that are not well understood the established lesion may progress to the advanced lesion, with loss of collagen fibers attached to cementum, apical migration of epithelium along the root surface, destruction of alveolar bone, and subsequent pocket formation. This stage represents the initiation of periodontitis, which leads to destruction of the periodontal ligament and alveolar bone if it persists.[103]

Once periodontitis ensues, its rate of progression—slow or rapid—is a function of the particular form of disease. Regardless of the rate, presumed to be continuous, attachment loss is constant. This assumption is based on substantial epidemiological evidence demonstrating increasing loss of attachment with age.[103] However, recent studies with attachment loss in sites with periodontitis closely monitored at frequent intervals indicate that tissue destruction proceeds episodically.[40,47,49] This finding has engendered a concept that the course of periodontitis is cyclical: variably long periods of quiescence marked by acute bursts of net connective tissue destruction.[143,157] Moreover, these bursts of destructive activity apparently occur independently of other periodontitis sites in the same mouth. The events that cause a stable inflammatory lesion to become acutely destructive are unclear; such exacerbations may result from abrupt shifts to a more pathogenic flora. Efforts to identify biochemical markers in gingival crevicular fluid or other parameters that predict or reflect disease activity at sites of periodontitis have been unsuccessful.

Although the effect of systemic disorders on the expression of periodontitis is appreciated, data from the past decade suggest that the opposite relationship also exists: periodontitis may predispose an individual to a variety of systemic conditions and disorders. One of these is preterm low birth weight, a condition with major medical and public health consequences. Several studies have shown that women with periodontitis have a significantly increased risk of delivering a preterm low birth weight infant.[57,114,171] In one study the odds ratio for preterm very low birth weight and periodontitis was 7.5 after adjusting for other low birth weight risk factors such as age, race, number of births, use of tobacco or alcohol, level of prenatal care, and bacteriuria.[114] Although the association of periodontitis and preterm low birth weight does not prove causality, the release of prostaglandins and proinflammatory cytokines from chronic periodontal infection and the effects of these substances on the fetal-placental unit has been proposed as a plausible biological mechanism.[172]

Several studies have noted that association of cardiovascular disease and periodontitis.[93] A large prospective study of male subjects extended over 18 years. During this period, nearly 20% of the subjects developed coronary heart disease (CHD), including angina pectoris, nonfatal myocardial infarction, and CHD-related death. The risk of these events was related to the periodontal status at baseline. After adjusting for other known CHD risks, subjects with pockets of more than 3 mm on more than half the teeth had a twofold increase risk of CHD and those with pockets of more than 3 mm on all teeth had a threefold increase of CHD.[6] An increased risk of stroke also was associated with more severe periodontitis in this study. Other studies have confirmed the association of atherosclerotic disease and periodontitis with adjusted odds ratios ranging from 1.2 to 2.0.[93]

The mechanisms by which periodontitis could be related to atherosclerotic disorders such as CHD and stroke are unknown. As an infection, periodontitis likely results in episodic bacteremias and chronic systemic dissemination of products of gram-negative periodontal pathogens such as lipopolysaccharide. Either or both of these events could trigger vascular consequences, such as an influx of monocytes and macrophages into vessel walls, or release of proinflammatory cytokines that may be atherogenic and alter coagulability.[6,113]

Although most evidence supports an association between periodontitis and CHD, a conclusion of direct or indirect links between the two diseases is premature. One large cross-sectional study reported no increased risk of CHD in patients with periodontitis,[53] and another showed that subjects with definitive elimination of all periodontal infection through extraction of all teeth did not have a lower risk of CHD over time than subjects with periodontitis.[52]

TREATMENT

Treatment of infection depends on control of the causative organism. Because chronic inflammatory periodontal disease is a consequence of the bacterial flora that colonizes the

*References 22, 23, 31, 55, 131, 144.

dentogingival area, treatment of gingivitis and periodontitis requires control of this flora. The means of control is of little importance provided the level of control is sufficient and sustained. In the case of gingivitis, suppression of bacterial plaque adjacent to the gingiva by physical or chemical means resolves inflammation and the tissue returns to its previously intact state (i.e., the disease is reversible).[82]

The same treatment principle is used for periodontitis—suppression of plaque bacteria reverses the inflammatory lesion—but two factors complicate the outcome. First, control of the disease-associated bacteria is generally more difficult in periodontitis than in gingivitis because of pocket formation and subgingival colonization of the root surface. The affected area is relatively inaccessible, and the subgingival microflora increases in mass and proportion of anaerobic, gram-negative species with known virulence properties.[149] Second, unlike gingivitis, periodontitis leads to irreversible loss of connective tissue attachment, which usually creates a periodontal pocket. These anatomical defects tend to persist even after resolution of inflammation and are highly prone to reinfection and exacerbation of disease.

Although the essential causative role of plaque bacteria in chronic inflammatory periodontal disease has been validated only in recent times, the importance of antiinfective measures in the treatment of chronic inflammatory periodontal disease has been recognized and practiced for more than a century. These measures have been and remain largely mechanical in nature: regular removal of supragingival plaque by simple cleaning techniques performed by the patient, debridement of root surfaces and subgingival spaces by scaling and root planing, and surgical reduction of pockets to facilitate plaque removal by patient and therapist and thereby lower the risk of reinfection.[170] The mundane nature of these mechanical strategies does not diminish their biological rationale or fundamental therapeutic importance. Resolution of gingivitis and arrest of periodontitis through mechanical control of the periodontal microflora is clinically and scientifically irrefutable.[5,74,88]

In practice, however, antiinfective therapy of chronic inflammatory periodontal disease based on mechanical techniques is not always successful. Frequent and thorough removal of supragingival plaque from the dentogingival interface is necessary to prevent or resolve gingivitis. Although the frequency of removal in each case depends on the particular oral microflora and host resistance, a study in healthy young adults suggest that plaque removal at intervals no greater than 48 hours is necessary to maintain gingival health.[68] Furthermore, consistent control of supragingival plaque may be important in delaying the reestablishment of a pathogenic subgingival flora in previously treated periodontal pockets.[64] Although techniques for self-removal of plaque are relatively simple and straightforward, many patients do not clean their teeth sufficiently well or frequently enough to prevent plaque-induced inflammation. Such failure often results from lack of motivation, stemming in part from the deceptively benign, asymptomatic nature of chronic inflammatory periodontal disease throughout much of its course. Another factor is the level of dexterity required for the self-removal of plaque, especially in patients with crowded teeth, restorations with plaque-retentive margins and contours, open furcations, or large areas of exposed root surfaces.

The conventional treatment of periodontitis relies on thorough removal of hard and soft bacterial deposits from subgingival surfaces by mechanical debridement. The ability of even highly-skilled and experienced clinicians to accomplish this task declines as access to subgingival surfaces decreases; factors such as attachment loss and pocket depth, posterior teeth, proximal surfaces, large restorations, and exposed furcations contribute to lack of access. The difficulty of definitive removal of all bacterial debris from root surfaces in periodontitis is lessened but not completely alleviated even when surgical access to these surfaces is obtained.[11] The persistence of inflammation after root surface debridement in sites with periodontitis is caused in large part by incomplete debridement and persistence of a sufficient mass of subgingival bacteria at these sites.

Various surgical techniques have been advocated and used to manage periodontitis. Resective procedures such as gingivectomy to remove soft tissue pockets or apically positioned flaps with osseous recontouring to remove intrabony pockets were widely used in the past. These procedures were aimed at pocket reduction and creation of normal gingival architecture to facilitate removal of plaque by both patient and therapist. Although useful, these procedures are not without problems. For example, anatomical considerations may prevent complete elimination of pockets by surgical resection. Even if pockets can be eliminated the resultant exposure of roots may create cosmetic problems, increase susceptibility to root caries, or cause protracted thermal hypersensitivity. Some patients never are sufficiently skillful in effectively cleaning surgically exposed root surfaces or over time may lose their motivation to do so; in either case, plaque accumulates, disease recurs, and the benefit of surgery is lost. Furthermore, longitudinal studies have demonstrated that regular subgingival debridement by scaling and root planing is as effective in arresting the progression of periodontitis as various surgical techniques.[63,122] These observations have led to a decline in the use of surgical procedures for the sole objective of pocket elimination. Other procedures, such as the modified Widman flap to gain access to root surfaces for debridement, have been emphasized. Although not the primary purpose, some pocket reduction resulting from tissue removal and resolution of inflammation usually follows surgical access procedures. Although the established place of surgical procedures in the management of periodontitis is unquestioned, they are not inherently curative but adjunctive to the primary therapeutic goal of bacterial control.

Given the nature of chronic inflammatory periodontal disease, the use of chemical agents to control the periodontal microflora has been an area of keen interest in periodontics. Initial efforts were directed at finding topically effective agents for control of supragingival plaque. Numerous products were promoted but none were useful. As antibiotics were introduced in the 1950s, several, including penicillin, were evaluated as topical antiplaque agents. Although some agents showed modest activity, they were considered unacceptable because of their low substantivity, side effects, and the potential for hypersensitivity reactions.

The first well-tolerated antibacterial agent with clinically significant antiplaque effects—chlorhexidine—was introduced in Europe in 1970 as a 0.2% oral rinse.[80] It was approved for use in the United States in 1986 as a 0.12% oral rinse (chlorhexidine gluconate [Peridex]). This agent, applied twice daily, strongly inhibits supragingival plaque formation and significantly retards gingivitis by 50% to 80%.[67] Because agents applied as a rinse poorly penetrate subgingival areas, chlorhexidine rinse has little effect on subgingival plaque and therefore cannot be used alone in the treatment of periodontitis. Experience and specific studies indicate that long-term application of chlorhexidine does not affect oral microbial ecology and does not lead to development of resistant strains.[141,142] Although the long-term safety of chlorhexidine oral rinse is established,[140-142] some problems limit its long-term use. These include dental staining (reversible), bitter taste, transient disturbance of taste, and cost.

Chlorhexidine oral rinse may be useful in a variety of clinical situations ranging from transient postsurgical situations in which mechanical cleaning cannot be performed to long-term plaque control in individuals with physical impairments (Box 7-3). Several over-the-counter antiplaque-antigingivitis rinses also are available, including mixtures of phenolic oils (e.g., Listerine), sanguinaria extracts, mixtures of surfactant/detergents, and quaternary ammonium compounds. Although these products have fewer side effects, they are inferior to chlorhexidine in antiplaque-antigingivitis activity. Further research may yield new agents with greater efficacy and fewer side effects.

Coinciding with advances in periodontal microbiology over the past quarter century has been a surge of interest in systemic antibacterial therapy in the management of periodontitis. The object of chemotherapy is to reduce or eliminate subgingival organisms that are presumed pathogens. Because thorough debridement of the subgingival root surface and pocket is almost impossible by mechanical means, the rationale for the adjunctive use of a systemically delivered antibacterial agent seems sound. This approach was evaluated initially in localized juvenile periodontitis. Although these studies generally had few subjects, were not well controlled, and used varied drug dosages and regimens, the results suggested that tetracycline modestly enhanced the clinical improvement (reduction in pocket depth, gain in attachment level, bleeding on probing) obtained by scaling and root planing.[152]

Systemic antimicrobial therapy also has been studied extensively in adult periodontitis and rapidly progressive periodontitis. A variety of agents, singly and combined, have been tested, including penicillin, ampicillin, amoxicillin, tetracycline, doxycycline, minocycline, clindamycin, spiramycin, cephalexin, and metronidazole. Although some studies suggest that a particular antimicrobial may improve the outcome of mechanical therapy, overall the available evidence does not support adjunctive antimicrobial use in adult periodontitis.[152,165] Because most cases of uncomplicated adult periodontitis respond readily to mechanical therapy, the benefit does not seem to justify the risk. In cases of rapidly progressive periodontitis, evidence of the utility of antibacterial agents is more compelling.[152] Further research is needed to define the most efficacious agent or agents and regimen for use in these cases.

One problem with systemic chemotherapy is achievement of effective drug levels in the fluid phase of the pocket. Another is that systemic administration exposes a large mass of nontarget tissue to the drug; only a small fraction of the dose enters gingival tissue and ultimately the pocket. Both problems may be circumvented by delivery of the drug directly into the pocket. This approach in the form of subgingival irrigation has been used for many years. Unfortunately, drug solutions delivered by irrigation are rapidly "washed out," or cleared, from the pocket and maximum concentrations prevail only briefly and quickly decline. Therefore efforts to suppress subgingival bacteria by pocket irrigation with antibacterial agents are largely unsuccessful. Several systems for the controlled release of drugs delivered into a pocket have been developed and introduced clinically to overcome this problem. One system uses tetracycline physically incorporated into a monolithic synthetic fiber of ethylene vinyl acetate (Actisite). The fiber is packed into a periodontal pocket and the tetracycline is released slowly into the fluid phase over a 10- to 14-day period. Very high concentrations of tetracycline are obtained, resulting in marked suppression of the pocket microflora, including putative pathogens, and significant clinical improvement.[39,50]

BOX 7-3

Clinical Applications of Chlorhexidine Oral Rinse

Adjunctive supragingival plaque control
For management of recurrent or persistent gingivitis
After oral/periodontal surgery
After crown preparation and during wearing of provisional restorations
In patients with physical mental handicaps
Treatment of oral and mucosal infections
For rampant caries
For gingivitis in patients who are immunocompromised (e.g., HIV infection)
For prevention and control of mild candidiasis in patients who are immunocompromised
For aphthous ulcers
Adjunctive control of bacterial recolonization
In association with treatment of periodontitis
In association with controlled-release antibiotic treatment of subgingival bacteria

Adapted from Korman KS: Topical antimicrobial agents: individual drugs. In Newman MG, Kornman KK, editors: *Antibiotic/antimicrobial use in dental practice,* Chicago, 1990, Quintessence.

Two other systems for sustained intrapocket delivery of antibiotics are available. One is a gel of poly(DL-lactide) containing doxycycline (Atridox).[30] The gel is injected into the pocket where it solidifies and slowly releases the drug into ambient fluid as it bioresorbs over 7 days. Another product consists of bioresorbable microspheres composed of a polymer, poly(glycolide-co-DL-lactide), and contains minocycline (Arestin). The gel microspheres are introduced into the pocket space by syringe and slowly release the drug. All three current systems for intrapocket delivery—fiber, gel, and microspheres—when combined with mechanical debridement of the pocket have similar efficacy as measured by reduction of probing pocket depth and bleeding on probing.[46] The latter two devices offer the advantage of being bioresorbable. All are approved for use as an adjunct to scaling and root planing in patients with chronic periodontitis. They are neither approved nor recommended for treatment of acute periodontal abscesses.

ACUTE PERIODONTAL DISEASES

The most common inflammatory periodontal diseases, gingivitis and periodontitis, essentially are chronic throughout their course. Although their occurrence is less common, acute infectious diseases of the periodontium are not rare and, in some cases, may be increasing (e.g., periodontal diseases associated with HIV infection). In the usual pathological sense, these diseases are not strictly acute because they usually are superimposed on a chronic inflammatory process. Gingivitis and periodontitis seem to be prerequisites for most acute periodontal diseases. Acute periodontal diseases develop rapidly, often are aggressively destructive, and cause considerable pain and disability. Their management is based on the same principle applicable to any acute infection—suppression of the causative organisms—and most respond to standard antiinfective measures. The clinician must understand that recurrence of the acute problem is likely unless the underlying chronic disease is addressed.

ABSCESSES

The periodontal abscess probably is the most common acute periodontal infection. In its simplest form this infection represents an acute exacerbation of the chronic lesion of periodontitis; this is reflected in the usual definition of a *periodontal abscess:* an acute, destructive inflammatory lesion in the periodontium resulting in localized accumulation of pus in the gingival wall of a periodontal pocket.[15] The periodontal tissues also may be involved secondarily by abscesses arising from an acute or long-standing pulpal-periapical infection. From a diagnostic and treatment standpoint the most complicated periodontal abscess is one in which both periodontitis and an infected pulp or periapical lesion are present before abscess formation. The term *gingival abscess* has been used to describe a periodontal abscess occurring in the absence of a periodontal pocket and therefore confined to the marginal gingiva. Gingival abscesses frequently are the result of sub-

gingival impaction of rigid fragments of food debris or foreign material and are much less uncommon than periodontal abscesses.

Clinical Features and Diagnosis A periodontal abscess often presents all or most of the signs of acute local inflammation and infection: abrupt onset, gingival or mucosal swelling or both, intense erythema of the affected tissue, and pain. Of these, pain is noted first and foremost by the patient, who is frequently unaware of other signs. Pain may range from mild tenderness of the involved soft tissues and the affected tooth or its neighbors to percussion, palpation, or occlusion to severe, spontaneous throbbing radiating from the site. The patient may note that the offending tooth is mobile, "high" on occlusion, or both. The affected tissues are deep blue to bright red (Plate 22). Swelling may affect only a limited area of gingiva or may extend into the alveolar mucosa and vestibule and may be visible or palpable extraorally. Submandibular and sublingual lymph nodes may be palpable and variably tender. If lymphadenopathy is present, body temperature may be elevated slightly. Depending on the stage of the abscess the swollen area may be firm or fluctuant, with rupture and spontaneous drainage apparently imminent. More advanced lesions may have one or more fistulous tracts opening into the gingiva or mucosa. Gentle digital pressure over the swollen area usually elicits variable amounts of a purulent and sometimes bloody exudate from the sulcus, or fistula if present. Gentle probing of the involved periodontal pocket also usually causes extrusion of pus after withdrawal of the probe. Radiographs may reveal bone loss consistent with the presence and severity of periodontitis as determined by probing or may reveal little if the abscess is located on the facial or lingual aspect of the tooth.

Patients frequently are seen with an asymptomatic fistula in the gingiva draining a periodontal pocket. On the reasonable presumption that such lesions were once acute abscesses, they are often referred to as *chronic abscesses.* The patient usually recalls one or more cycles of acute swelling and gingival tenderness at the site followed by remission.

As in most diseases, appropriate treatment of a periodontal abscess depends on correct diagnosis. Because the typical findings are not unique to an uncomplicated periodontal abscess (i.e., an abscess arising solely from periodontitis), accurate diagnosis of abscesses involving the periodontium requires careful and complete clinical and radiographic assessment (Figure 7-3). First, the status of the periodontal attachment must be determined by probing. Attachment loss and a pocket must be present for a periodontal abscess to exist. If the abscess is confined to the marginal gingiva or a papilla without loss of attachment, then the lesion likely is a gingival abscess. A pericoronal abscess represents a form of gingival abscess. Next, the status of the pulp must be determined to rule out pulpal and associated periapical lesions as the source of infection. The presence of deep carious lesions or large or defective restorations or crowns should be considered, although such findings alone are not indicative of pulpal-periapical disease. If the tooth has either an intact (i.e., vital) pulp or a filled root canal and

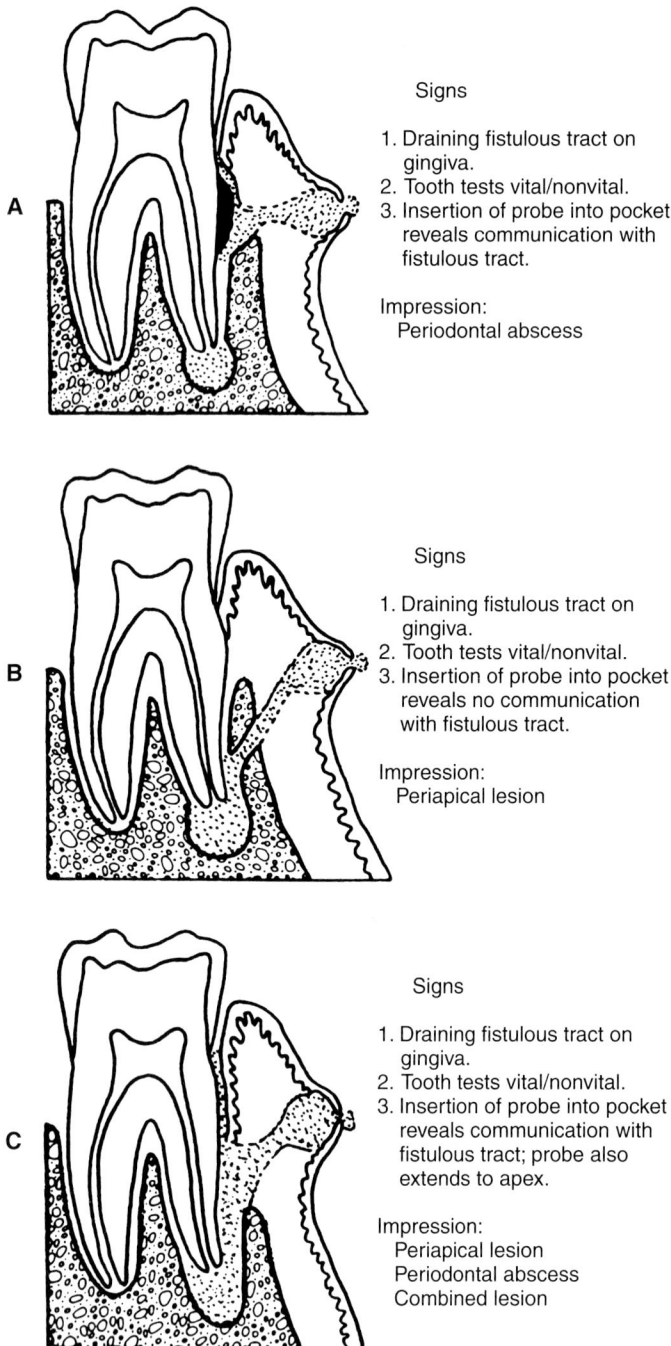

Signs

1. Draining fistulous tract on gingiva.
2. Tooth tests vital/nonvital.
3. Insertion of probe into pocket reveals communication with fistulous tract.

Impression:
   Periodontal abscess

Signs

1. Draining fistulous tract on gingiva.
2. Tooth tests vital/nonvital.
3. Insertion of probe into pocket reveals no communication with fistulous tract.

Impression:
   Periapical lesion

Signs

1. Draining fistulous tract on gingiva.
2. Tooth tests vital/nonvital.
3. Insertion of probe into pocket reveals communication with fistulous tract; probe also extends to apex.

Impression:
   Periapical lesion
   Periodontal abscess
   Combined lesion

Figure 7-3 Distinguishing features of abscesses involving the periodontium. **A,** Periodontal abscess. **B,** Pulpal-periapical abscess. **C,** Combined periodontal-periapical abscess. Periodontal probing and assessment of pulpal status are critical in differentiating these three possibilities. (From Armitage GC: *The biologic basis of periodontal maintenance therapy,* Berkeley, Calif, 1980, Praxis.)

no evidence of periapical disease, then a diagnosis of a periodontal abscess is rational. Unfortunately, diagnostic decisions frequently are equivocal because of the difficulty in assessing pulpal and associated periapical pathological conditions. In an early periapical abscess, tests of pulpal vitality may be indeterminate, particularly in teeth with multiple canals, and radiographs may not reveal apical lesions.

Another complicating factor in diagnosis is an incomplete fracture of the root, usually running in a vertical direction. Such fractures may occur in vital teeth but most often are found in endodontically treated teeth, especially those with restorative posts or pins. Fractures may be difficult or impossible to detect but must be considered when an abscess apparently is associated with an endodontically treated tooth. A finding suggestive of vertical root fracture is attachment loss that extends far apically but is extremely limited in a horizontal direction.

The nature of the pain experience often is helpful in distinguishing between a pulpal-periapical and a periodontal abscess. Acute pulpal-periapical infections typically manifest in severe, sharp pain of an intermittent and spontaneous nature. Sensitivity to heat or cold is common and may be severe and persist long after removal of the stimulus. In contrast, pain associated with a periodontal abscess usually is not severe or spontaneous and is dull and throbbing. Thermal sensitivity is not common.

Etiology   In histopathological terms a periodontal abscess is like an abscess elsewhere in the body: pyogenic bacteria locally invade the gingival connective tissue adjacent to the pocket wall. An intense but circumscribed suppurative inflammatory lesion results. The ensuing accumulation of pus ultimately seeks drainage through the pocket orifice or by formation of a fistulous tract through the pocket wall into the gingiva or mucosa. Although infection is highly localized, rapid and often extensive destruction of periodontal attachment and adjacent bone occurs.

The critical events that convert a chronic inflammatory lesion of periodontitis into an acute abscess are not understood. The balance between host defenses and the bacteria flora of the pocket is tipped abruptly and markedly in favor of the flora, allowing sufficient numbers of organisms to invade and propagate in gingival connective tissue. One possibility is that continuous drainage of a periodontal pocket is impaired by any measure that reduces gingival inflammation in the coronal aspect of the pocket but leaves the bacterial mass in the apical portion of the pocket largely untouched. Such measures include improved plaque removal by the patient and superficial or incomplete scaling by a dental professional. The reduced drainage of the products of a chronic inflammatory process could create an environment that promotes a dramatic increase in the total pocket microbiota, allows more virulent organisms to dominate the flora, or both. The frequent clinical observation that patients with untreated periodontitis often are seen with periodontal abscesses a few days after dental "prophylaxis" supports this concept. Such patients also can develop abscesses shortly after initiation of rigorous home care programs but before thorough subgingival debridement. Another factor contributing to acute exacerbation and abscess formation in periodontitis is systemic disease (e.g., type I diabetes mellitus or chemotherapy) that impairs resistance to infection.[115,121,176] Although a single abscess in a patient with periodontitis is not itself a reason to refer a patient for medical evaluation, multiple periodontal abscesses that occur simultaneously or repeated abscesses are cause for concern regarding systemic health. Periodontal abscesses that occur after systemic antibiotic therapy also have been reported[163] and presumably are related to alteration of the subgingival microflora.

The microbiology of acute periodontal abscesses has been studied to a limited extent. Before current techniques for anaerobic sampling and culture were available, several investigators reported that *Streptococcus viridans* and *Staphylococcus albus* most commonly were associated with abscesses, followed by nonhemolytic streptococci, *Neisseria, Escherichia coli,* and diphtheroids. These findings prompted the conclusion that periodontal abscesses were "mixed infections," with streptococci representing key organisms.[90,95,99] More recently, Newman and Sims,[111] by sampling bacteria at the most apical portion of pockets associated with acute abscesses and using more rigorous techniques for culturing oxygen-sensitive organisms, found a predominantly gram-negative (66%) and anaerobic (65%) flora, in contrast to the heavily gram-positive (71%) and facultative (78%) flora found at the gingival crevice sites. The gram-negative organisms most commonly detected in the apical ("abscess") flora were *Prevotella melaninogenica* subspp., *Fusobacterium* spp., and *Capnocytophaga. Porphyromonas gingivalis* was found in virtually all acute periodontal abscesses in two recent studies.[163] In one study, *F. nucleatum* and *Streptococcus intermedius* were detected in more than 60% of abscess sites.[163] Thus the organisms that seem to be associated most closely with periodontitis—gram-negative and anaerobic—also may be associated closely with the periodontal abscess. The conclusion that periodontal abscesses are not microbiologically distinct from the chronic periodontitis that precedes them is reasonable given current knowledge.

Treatment   Prompt treatment of a periodontal abscess is important to relieve symptoms and minimize tissue destruction and attachment loss. As with all pyogenic infections the step in achieving these goals, especially the former, is to establish drainage. Drainage leads to an immediate reduction of swelling and internal tissue pressure, resulting in almost immediate pain relief. If the tooth is extruded, drainage also allows it to return to a more normal position, thus lessening occlusal loading and tenderness.

Drainage can be achieved either through the pocket by means of the sulcus, by incision through the external surface of the abscess into the pus cavity, or both. The former pathway often is realized during assessment of the lesion by probing. If considerable pus is evacuated by probing, further drainage through the sulcus by purposeful instrumentation is indicated. Instrumentation is done with appropriate periodontal scalers and curettes after anesthesia is obtained. The objective is twofold: enlargement of the opening to promote drainage and debridement of the root surface. The latter usually is incomplete because of the inevitable heavy bleeding, enlarged edematous gingiva, and

often deep and tortuous pocket. However, any reduction of the bacterial load on the root surface and within the pocket contributes to resolution of the acute infection. Firm digital pressure over the most fluctuant part of the abscess during instrumentation of the pocket may aid in the evacuation of pus. Vigorous rinsing with warm water or saline solution at frequent intervals for several days may promote further drainage and reduce tenderness.

Traditional incision and drainage also is highly effective in evacuating the suppurative content of a periodontal abscess, particularly if the abscess is just starting to "point" or spontaneously open a fistula. Incision may be least effective in the early stage of abscess formation because location of the pus cavity is more difficult. A disadvantage of the incision approach is the tendency of the incision to close; if the suppurative process is not well resolved, premature closure may lead to exacerbation of the acute phase of infection. If prolonged drainage through an incision is important, a drain should be placed in the incision to maintain patency. Another disadvantage of incision for drainage of an acute periodontal abscess is that debridement of the pocket still is required. For these reasons, attempted drainage through the pocket during the process of pocket and root debridement is the most rational first approach. If this strategy does not appear to fully "deflate" the abscess, incision should be done.

Although the treatment of acute periodontal abscesses by systemic antimicrobials alone usually alleviates symptoms and leads to transient resolution of the infection, the basic cause remains and recurrence is highly likely. Consequently, such therapy is not justified. However, the routine use of antibacterial chemotherapy as an adjunct to drainage and debridement in the management of periodontal abscesses has been advocated.[28] Although this approach is still favored by some clinicians, the large majority of periodontal abscesses resolve promptly and without complication after drainage of the exudate and debridement of the pocket without chemotherapy. Therefore systemic antibacterial therapy currently is reserved for specific situations. These include patients with multiple abscesses occurring simultaneously and patients who are febrile or with acute periodontal infections which do not appear to be localizing but rather are spreading diffusely (i.e., developing cellulitis). Use of adjunctive antimicrobials in patients with systemic conditions that may reduce resistance to infection and who have a history of past infections may be prudent.

Culture and sensitivity testing of organisms involved in a periodontal abscess before using an antimicrobial drug is not feasible for several reasons. First, a periodontal abscess is an acute problem that requires immediate treatment. Second, obtaining a "clean" bacterial sample for culture is difficult. Consequently, if use of an antibiotic is deemed appropriate in managing a particular case, it is selected purely on empirical grounds. Penicillin, 500 mg qid (with erythromycin as an alternative) commonly is used despite evidence that many bacteria isolated from deep pockets and abscesses are resistant to this agent.[36] On the basis of its greater activity against gram-negative bacteria frequently found in periodontitis and ability to accumulate in gingival crevicular fluid, tetracycline (250 mg qid) has been advocated.[62] Although the acute phase is likely to resolve within a few days, antibiotic therapy should be continued for 7 to 10 days.

The decision to use antimicrobial chemotherapy in the management of a periodontal abscess must be made in terms of a cost-benefit evaluation. As an adjunct to mechanical therapy the benefit may be small or nonexistent, but the cost may be considerable both financially and in terms of morbidity. Recent evidence supports a common clinical observation that systemic antimicrobial therapy in patients with untreated periodontitis may dispose patients to acute periodontal abscess by altering the subgingival microflora,[163] a risk that should be considered carefully.

Marked improvement in symptoms and signs should occur within 12 to 24 hours of drainage and debridement. The patient should be monitored carefully to ensure this outcome. After 1 to 2 weeks the patient should be reexamined and definitive periodontal therapy planned. Therapy can range from scaling and root planing by a closed or open approach or pocket reduction surgery with or without osseous recontouring. Many clinicians believe that periodontal attachment and bone destroyed by acute infection is more amenable to repair than that lost in chronic periodontitis.[108] Although this belief is unsubstantiated by experimental evidence, regenerative rather than resective procedures, promptly applied, are preferred in the definitive management of postabscess defects.

The previously described treatment presumes a diagnosis of uncomplicated periodontal abscess (i.e., no pulpal-periapical contribution to the lesion). If the infection represents a periapical abscess that has affected a previously intact periodontium, treatment must be directed specifically at the primary disease in the pulp or periapical area. However, if concomitant pulpal-periapical and primary periodontitis lesions exist that physically communicate and are acutely infected, management is more complicated. If the affected tooth is salvageable, endodontic treatment and periodontal abscess therapy must be instituted without delay. Infection in the periodontal pocket of such combined lesions does not resolve well or at all until pulpal infection is cleared.[9]

ACUTE NECROTIZING ULCERATIVE GINGIVITIS-PERIODONTITIS

ANUGP is perhaps the most interesting and distinct of all inflammatory periodontal diseases. ANUGP was first described several centuries ago and since then has intrigued clinicians and researchers. Given its high incidence in certain subsets of the population and discovery of spirochetes in its lesions, AGUNP once was considered a highly contagious disease of a quasi-venereal nature.[143] It has been known by more than a dozen names, including Vincent's infection, Vincent's ulceromembranous gingivostomatitis, fusospirochetal stomatitis, putrid sore mouth, Gilmer's disease, diphtheroid angina, trench mouth, necrotizing gingivitis, necrotic ulcerative gingivitis, and acute ulcerative gingivitis.[3] The most widely used current designation is *acute necrotizing ulcerative gingivitis* (ANUG). When the clinical features of ANUG are considered, most notably its destructive aspect, the effects obviously are not limited to the gingiva. Hence, the term *acute necrotizing ulcerative gingivitis-periodontitis*, although more cumbersome, better describes this infectious disease.

Clinical Features and Diagnosis   ANUGP most commonly occurs in patients with poor oral hygiene, calculus, and chronic gingivitis. Patients with ANUGP typically are seen initially with these conditions. The distribution of lesions varies: one, several, or many sites may be infected, with anterior sites more frequently involved than posterior.

Like periodontal abscesses, ANUGP has an abrupt onset. Although occasional patients report prodromal symptoms consisting of vague gingival itching or burning, most cases begin acutely with gingival pain with or without bleeding. The pain may begin as tenderness in the marginal and papillary gingiva but spontaneous gingival aching or burning pain is common as the disease worsens. In contrast to common gingivitis, which usually is not painful to touch, the affected gingiva in ANUGP is exquisitely tender to probing or other gentle manipulation. Patients with ANUGP may report gingival pain on mastication. Gingival bleeding often is marked and may occur spontaneously or with only slight provocation.

The gingival lesion in ANUGP is highly characteristic, consistent with its name. The gingival surface, which appears as a grey-white "membrane" or layer of debris, is necrotic. This membrane is removed easily by mild abrasion such as eating or toothbrushing and therefore may not be present at initial examination. Beneath the membrane is an ulcerated surface that tends to bleed copiously when disturbed. Considerable erythema and edema of the adjacent gingival tissue is present, and the ulcer often is bordered by a narrow, bright red zone. The infection typically affects the tips of papillae first (Plate 23) and then extends to the entire interdental gingiva and, in more severe cases, the facial and lingual gingiva (Plate 24). One or several sites of infection may occur; anterior sites are affected more frequently than posterior sites. Without intervention the disease may progress rapidly and cause marked loss of interdental tissue. The resultant soft tissue defect is craterlike and classically described as a "punched-out" papilla. Necrosis of the gingival margin can create a notched or ragged contour.

In addition to pain, bleeding, and gingival necrosis, other signs and symptoms associated with ANUGP include lymphadenopathy, increased salivation, general malaise, and fever. In older literature reports, fever was commonly cited. However, subsequent extensive investigation has refuted this finding; temperature elevation, if any, is slight and in some patients temperature may be slightly below normal.[37] Another putative classic feature of ANUGP is a foul oral odor ("fetor oris"). However, severe halitosis is not unique to this form of periodontal disease.[37]

The course of ANUGP varies. If treated promptly and appropriately the disease can be resolved with few or no tissue defects. If untreated, ANUGP often cycles through periods of spontaneous remission and exacerbation. In these cycles the acute signs and symptoms diminish and the lesion reverts to chronic gingivitis. Some clinicians refer to this quiescent phase as *subacute* or *latent ANUGP,* but because the ulcerations disappear *gingivitis* is a more appropriate term. The loss and altered contour of gingival tissue usually remain after remission. After a variable period, acute relapse to full-blown ANUGP generally occurs. Tissue destruction progresses with each cycle. Destruction is not limited to gingiva but quickly can affect the periodontal attachment and bone (i.e., ANUG becomes ANUGP).[91] Destruction is severe particularly in interproximal areas; over time the interdental gingival and bony septum may be lost completely. Although the disease may occur in patients with periodontitis, ANUGP itself leads to minimal pocket formation. The necrotizing process destroys the attachment, adjacent alveolar bone, and overlying gingiva. Large amounts of plaque and calculus accumulate on root surfaces exposed by ANUGP and considerable oral debris accumulates in interproximal craters. Effective oral hygiene is difficult because of tenderness and altered gingival contours.

The pattern of cyclic recurrences of ANUGP may be altered dramatically in individuals with impaired host responses (e.g., HIV infection) or those who are otherwise severely debilitated by disease or malnutrition. In these individuals the disease may not include cycles of spontaneous remission but follows a relatively steady progression, causing severe lesions and loss of affected teeth. Moreover, the infection can spread well beyond the periodontium and alveolar process, invading the palate, nose, and face (see Chapter 6). Dissemination and tissue destruction to this degree is termed *noma* (cancrum oris), a poorly understood fusospirochetal orofacial infection that can occur in the absence of ANUGP.[27,58,123] The relationship between these two similar but yet different diseases remains obscure.

In patients first seen with ANUGP the clinician should be aware that the current episode may not be the first occurrence of the disease. Severe lesions, if present, may represent numerous previous episodes of necrosis and tissue destruction. This possibility should be considered in taking the history to obtain the most accurate description of disease progression.

Etiology The microbial cause of ANUGP infection has been known for many years, and early microscopic studies pointed to its fusospirochetal nature. More recent investigations have confirmed the specific role of microorganisms, particularly spirochetes.[72,73,83] The simplest and most illustrative demonstration of the microbial basis of ANUGP may be its dramatic resolution after either mechanical or chemical suppression of tooth-adherent bacterial debris.

Bacterial invasion of gingival tissue is a characteristic and well-studied histological feature of ANUGP. Fusiform bacteria and medium and large spirochetes are found deep into connective tissue, even beyond the zone of frank ulceration. Definitive information pertaining to the particular organisms involved and their interrelationships is limited because obtaining representative samples and culturing of spirochetes is difficult. Currently the primary pathogens recognized in ANUGP are spirochetes (*Treponema vincentii* and others) and *Fusobacterium* spp. The ubiquitous *Prevotella intermedia* and other gram-negative rods also have been reported.[87] The ability of this combination of organisms to cause ulceration appears to be unique among oral bacteria. The dramatic resolution of ANUGP after a short course of systemic antimicrobial therapy supports the notion that bacterial invasion of tissue by these bacteria is a critical mechanism in the pathogenesis of this disease.

ANUGP, like other inflammatory periodontal diseases, may be an opportunistic infection. Although it usually is preceded by well-established gingivitis, most people with poor plaque control and gingivitis do not develop ANUGP. Such individuals may harbor ANUGP-associated bacteria in the oral flora.[59] These observations indicate that other causative factors allow this unique fusospirochetal gingival infection to occur. Numerous possibilities have been proposed. A clear predisposition to ANUGP exists in patients with impaired resistance to infection as a result of disease or general debilitation. Severe ANUGP or an ANUGP-like syndrome is common in patients with HIV infection.[124,174,175]

Another factor that has received much attention is psychological or emotional stress. ANUGP frequently occurs in young individuals (age 17 to 35 years) who are in apparent good physical health. However, these individuals often experience emotionally trying or anxiety-producing life events or situations; such individuals also are sleep deprived and have poor dietary habits.[34,37] Thus psychological stress, through its impairment of host immune or other defensive functions, may predispose patients to ANUGP. A strong association between heavy cigarette smoking and ANUGP has been well established.[34,37] Smoke, either directly or through products taken up in blood, may affect gingiva by impairing resistance to the organisms associated with ANUGP. Although the association between factors such as emotional stress and smoking with ANUGP is clear, many individuals under great emotional strain smoke heavily or have reduced host defenses but never develop ANUGP. Therefore a complex set of circumstances is necessary for development of this infection.

Treatment In the absence of systemic complications, routine antiinfective measures yield a dramatic "cure" of the signs and symptoms of ANUGP. These measures are mechanical debridement of involved teeth, systemic antimicrobial therapy, or both. Diminution of pain sometimes occurs within hours, especially if palliative measures such as nonsteroidal antiinflammatory analgesics and frequent oral lavage with warm saline solution also are used. Most symptoms resolve within 24 hours with distinct improvement in clinical signs. Healing of ulcerated areas is apparent after 3 days.

Mechanical debridement is accomplished easily with periodontal scalers. Although affected tissue is exquisitely painful, soft debris and readily accessible calculus often can be removed without anesthesia. Avoidance of anesthesia at the initial visit may be prudent given the usual level of distress in patients with full-blown ANUGP. Copious bleeding results from even the mildest tissue manipulation. Frequent and abundant irrigation with saline solution improves visibility in the operative area and aids removal of loosely attached debris. Depending on the extent of debridement, additional appointments at daily intervals may be needed to remove all plaque and calculus.

Because of the somewhat more gentle action and the irrigant effect, some clinicians advocate use of ultrasonic scalers for initial debridement in ANUGP. Because of the abundant and contaminated aerosol generated by these instruments this practice is not recommended.

The analgesics and oral lavage are helpful in the initial treatment of ANUGP. Because pain improves dramatically after debridement, analgesics may not be needed for an extended period. However, if the initial pain is severe or the infection widespread, a nonsteroidal antiinflammatory analgesic should be prescribed in full doses. Vigorous rinsing with warm saline solution at frequent intervals provides symptomatic relief and removes loose debris. Although mechanical plaque control is important, initially it may be difficult or impossible. Use of 0.4% chlorhexidine oral rinse is helpful until mechanical cleaning is possible. The alcohol content of the commercially available preparation may cause considerable burning if applied to the acute lesions. This problem ceases after a few days of healing.

Although a short course of an antimicrobial agent, such as penicillin, without other treatment reduces the signs and symptoms of ANUGP, the use of antimicrobials alone is poor therapy because it does not address fully the underlying causes. An antimicrobial may be indicated in the relatively uncommon ANUGP cases with fever or affected lymph nodes and no apparent systemic disease, or in more generalized or severe cases in which at least partial debridement of all sites cannot be accomplished at the first visit. Given the aggressive course of ANUGP in patients with impaired defenses, administration of an appropriate antimicrobial agent with local mechanical therapy is important. The most widely used agent is penicillin (500 mg qid). The drug should be continued for at least a week, although dramatic improvement may occur early in the course of therapy. A good alternative to penicillin is metronidazole (250 mg tid) for not more than 7 days. Although it has more side effects than penicillin, metronidazole is particularly active against spirochetes and *Prevotella* and a good clinical response can be expected.

If treatment of ANUGP is initiated when the infection is limited to the gingiva, tissue destruction and deformity are minimal and no further corrective treatment is required. However, the disease frequently creates marked interdental defects and surgical procedures to correct them are necessary for long-term maintenance of gingival and periodontal health. Necessary surgical procedures range from routine gingivoplasty to improve papillary contour to osseous resection to reduce interproximal craters. If uncorrected these defects may dispose patients to chronic periodontitis or recurrence of ANUGP.

Another problem in the management of ANUGP is patient attitude and compliance. Affected patients often have long-standing poor oral hygiene, chronic gingivitis or periodontitis, an erratic history of dental care, and apparent low interest in oral or general health. These patients are likely to be heavy smokers and lead an overtly stressful lifestyle. Once their initial symptoms are relieved, they believe they are "cured" and do not return for follow-up evaluation and continued care. Recurrence of ANUGP is highly likely. Such patients likely will exhibit a similar pattern of behavior at subsequent exacerbations.

PERICORONITIS

A healthy, fully erupted tooth is surrounded by gingival tissue that typically extends not more than 2 to 3 mm coronally. For a variety of anatomical reasons—partial eruption, malposition, the immediate proximity of the anterior border of the ramus—the crowns of third molars and occasionally other teeth may be covered to a considerably greater extent with gingiva and sometimes mucosa. The potential space between the soft tissue and crown is in effect a gingival or pseudopocket that can be of considerable depth and volume. A diverse and extensive subgingival microflora colonizes these pockets and gingival inflammation is almost always present. Not unlike pockets elsewhere in the mouth, these sites may become acutely infected and produce symptoms; they then are defined as *pericoronitis*. Although these lesions resemble periodontal abscesses, they differ in several respects.

Clinical Features and Diagnosis   Pericoronitis overwhelmingly affects mandibular third molars and to a much lesser extent maxillary third molars primarily because of their frequent partial impaction and proximity to the anterior border of the mandible.[112] This predilection for third molars largely explains the usual age of occurrence. The majority of cases of pericoronitis occur in young adults. A recent study of 245 patients found that 81% were 20 to 29 years of age and 13% were 30 to 39 years old.[112]

Acute pericoronitis typically begins as localized pain and gingival tenderness. Pain may occasionally radiate to the face, ear, or angle of the mandible. Visual inspection and palpation quickly reveal the affected site: an enlarged, inflamed, and tender segment of soft tissue covering one or more of the coronal surfaces, including the occlusal surface, of the involved tooth (Plates 25 and 26). The affected tissue may be gingiva, mucosa, or both. On mandibular molars, little coverage of the facial and lingual surfaces and an inflamed pedicle-like mass of tissue (operculum) projecting from the retromolar area onto the occlusal surface may exist. This configuration usually is found when the tooth essentially is upright with the distal aspect embedded into the soft tissue of the anterior border of the ramus.

With mesioangular impaction the tissue usually covers much of the facial, lingual, distal, and occlusal surfaces.

Inspection of the lesion usually reveals accumulated plaque and other debris on the exposed portion of the affected tooth and its near neighbor because tissue tenderness restricts toothbrushing. Pus may be observed exuding beneath the margin of the pericoronal tissue or expressed by gentle palpation. Depending on the degree of edema and tenderness the affected tissue can be retracted and the pocket explored to a variable extent. This maneuver may cause copious bleeding. It may also result in release of considerable soft oral debris, particulate fragments, such as a popcorn hull, or pus. Even when the infection is suppurative, pericoronitis does not commonly create fistulous tracts. Drainage occurs through the opening of the pericoronal space, but if this path is blocked an acute abscess can form or the infection may spread into adjacent tissue spaces such as the masticator.

The severity of pericoronitis varies. Many sites remain in a primarily symptom-free state of chronic, low-grade inflammation indefinitely and, like other sites with chronic gingivitis, progress to periodontitis. Because the patient is often unaware of the infection the lesions are not treated. In other cases a chronically inflamed site abruptly becomes more intensely inflamed and produces symptoms, which may consist of only mild to moderate tenderness and swelling of pericoronal tissue. In mandibular third molars the more occlusal portion of the affected tissue may begin to be traumatized by the opposing tooth. As infection increases, so do the local signs of inflammation and tissue tenderness. Suppuration may be notable. The buccal mucosa immediately adjacent to the pericoronal tissue may be erythematous and edematous. Dull pain in the area is a common complaint. The patient also often reports pain on maximal opening or limited jaw movement. Further worsening of the infection exacerbates these signs and symptoms. An overt abscess can be present or appears imminent. In addition, submandibular lymph node enlargement and tenderness, facial swelling, and pain or difficulty in swallowing are common. In extreme cases, fever, general malaise, and extension of the infection into the masticator or other fascial spaces is present.[56,120]

Etiology   Pericoronitis undoubtedly is an infectious process. However, the specific organisms responsible for this infection have not been identified. Relatively few studies have addressed the issue of the bacterial flora associated with pericoronitis. These studies suggested that *S. viridans*,[60] a mixed oral flora,[54] and spirochetes and fusobacteria[112] were involved. More recent studies detected some bacteria associated with periodontitis, such as *Prevotella intermedia, Peptostreptococcus micros, F. nucleatum, A. actinomycetemcomitans,* and *Veillonella* and *Capnocytophaga* spp., in pockets of acute pericoronal lesions.[98,166] *Porphyromonas gingivalis* and *Eubacterium* spp., both strongly implicated in periodontitis, were not found. Although pericoronitis apparently is an infection related to a highly anaerobic bacterial flora, the key organisms may

differ from those in periodontitis. The contribution of the ubiquitous spirochetes and fusiforms to pericoronitis remains unknown. Some investigators believe these organisms are involved fundamentally in the pathogenesis.[112] Conversely, these organisms may simply be opportunistic residents of the anaerobic, nutrient-rich, and inflamed pericoronal space.

As in ANUGP, several secondary or contributory factors have been suggested as the cause of pericoronitis.[112,145] Trauma from an opposing tooth is commonly cited. Although such an injury could trigger an acute exacerbation in chronically inflamed pericoronal tissue, the trauma also could be subsequent to exacerbation and enlargement of the tissue. Other suggested factors are emotional stress, smoking, chronic fatigue, general debilitating illnesses, and recent upper respiratory tract infection. Supporting evidence for association of any of these factors with pericoronitis is anecdotal; little objective evaluation has been done.

Treatment   Treatment of pericoronitis focuses on infection control. Strategies depend on initial assessment of two issues. The first is the severity of the infection and extent to which it has disseminated beyond the primary site. An infection that affects regional lymph nodes, spreads into fascial spaces, or causes fever is serious and requires more intensive therapy than one that is localized. The second is the relative importance of the affected tooth and whether the pericoronal tissue can be returned to and maintained in a healthy state.

Well-localized mild to moderate pericoronitis affecting a tooth that is to be retained is managed conservatively. Treatment consists of debridement and drainage of the pericoronal pocket by gentle curettage and external pressure. During and after curettage the pocket should be irrigated with sterile saline solution using a syringe and large-gauge blunt needle. Caution is necessary during irrigation to avoid penetration of tissue with the needle or high pressure, which may force fluid into tissue or tissue spaces. Some clinicians advocate irrigation with an antimicrobial solution, such as 10% povidone-iodine or 1% gentian violet,[145] but whether this action provides additional benefit is not known. If a fluctuant abscess is present and does not drain well through the pocket, drainage should be accomplished by incision. The placement of a device to maintain patency of the incision usually is not necessary. The patient should be instructed to rinse the area vigorously with warm water or saline solution at frequent intervals until symptoms subside. Posttreatment monitoring is necessary to ensure resolution of the acute phase. When signs and symptoms have regressed the need for corrective surgery should be considered. Resection of some or all pericoronal tissue, depending on tooth position in the jaw and soft tissue relationships, reduces the chance of recurrent infection.

In most cases, debridement and drainage of well-localized pericoronitis leads to resolution of the initial signs and symptoms within a few days. However, many clinicians also routinely use systemic antimicrobial therapy in such cases and some use only topical antimicrobial therapy. Neither practice is prudent or cost effective. Antimicrobial use should be reserved for localized cases that do not respond to mechanical therapy and for severe disseminating cases. Effective agents are penicillin (500 mg q6h) or amoxicillin (500 mg q6h); clindamycin (300 mg q6h) is used in the event of hypersensitivity. Regardless of the agent, drug therapy should be continued for at least 5 days after remission of the infection.

If an opposing third molar is hypererupted or will require removal in the near future and is in contact with inflamed tissue over the lower third molar, it can be removed to help decrease pain and hasten recovery from the pericoronitis. If the affected tooth is nonfunctional or considered unsalvageable because of malposition or other reasons, extraction usually is appropriate. If pericoronitis is localized with no evidence of abscess, extraction may proceed or be delayed until the acute inflammation has subsided. If pus is present the best treatment is drainage and resolution of the acute phase before elective extraction. If immediate extraction is necessary, perioperative and systemic antimicrobial therapy should be used.

More severe pericoronitis with evidence of regional dissemination (lymphadenitis, fever, or cellulitis) should be treated as described previously. In addition, antimicrobial chemotherapy should be started immediately. Penicillin or amoxicillin are appropriate choices. Chemotherapy is especially important if cellulitis is present because of the proximity of most pericoronitis to the pharynx and the base of the tongue. Close monitoring of treatment outcome is necessary. Extraction should be postponed until the infection shows definite signs of localization or has completely resolved.

PERIODONTAL DISEASES AND HIV INFECTION

The concept that the incidence, severity, and course of chronic inflammatory periodontal diseases and their acute exacerbations can be altered by host status is well established. Thus particularly severe and destructive inflammatory periodontal diseases are associated with the profoundly compromised immune state resulting from HIV infection. Chapter 24 provides a detailed discussion of HIV infections and acquired human immunodeficiency syndrome (AIDS). Patients with HIV infection or AIDS are subject to a variety of opportunistic bacterial infections in the oral cavity; the majority are caused by a spectrum of increasingly aggressive periodontal diseases.[104] These diseases are not truly unique but appear to represent altered forms of gingivitis, periodontitis, and ANUGP in a particular immunodeficiency state. The terms *HIV-associated gingivitis* (HIV-G) and *HIV-associated periodontitis* (HIV-P) are used to distinguish these two diseases from their counterparts in otherwise healthy individuals. In addition, a severe ulcerative-necrotizing infection that begins in the gingiva and spreads extensively

(necrotizing stomatitis) occasionally is seen in patients with HIV infection.

Clinical Features and Diagnosis   Diagnosis of inflammatory periodontal diseases in individuals with HIV infection does not differ greatly from diagnosis of these diseases in a healthy person. The basic features and diagnostic criteria for gingivitis, periodontitis, and ANUGP are the same regardless of HIV status and diagnosis usually is uncomplicated. However, HIV immunosuppression can cause subtle or overt changes in the presentation of inflammatory periodontal diseases. Knowledge of these changes is especially important when examining patients whose HIV status is not known.

Gingivitis in a person with HIV infection may be indistinguishable clinically from that in a perfectly healthy individual. However, individuals with HIV infection frequently have a narrow, well-delineated zone of intense erythema at the gingival margin extending into the papilla, which may exist despite apparently good personal dental hygiene. An increased tendency for gingival bleeding may exist. Small erythematous areas scattered in the attached gingiva occur frequently; these areas have been described as punctate.[174] In other cases a diffuse redness affects much or all of the gingiva and may extend into the vestibular mucosa. Approximately 75% of individuals with HIV infection have a punctate or diffuse pattern of gingival erythema.[154] Another difference is that gingivitis in HIV infection appears less responsive to conventional therapy (plaque control and scaling) than other forms of gingivitis.[173]

Like gingivitis, HIV-P may show no unusual features. In other cases, HIV-P may occur as a severe, rapidly destructive form of periodontitis that can result in tooth loss within a few months. Unlike uncomplicated adult periodontitis a generalized distribution of disease in more likely in HIV-P. Patients with HIV infection frequently report large interproximal defects that developed quickly, may bleed spontaneously, and are associated with pain often described as "deep" or "gnawing."[174] These defects are intensely inflamed at the marginal and papillary gingiva and often extend well into attached gingiva and even into vestibular mucosa (Plate 27). Plaque and debris fill the defects to the extent that the patient has abandoned cleaning efforts. Calculus may not be notable. Tissue destruction in HIV-P usually affects both the gingiva and underlying attachment and bone, which minimizes pocket formation. Together with pain, this characteristic imparts an ANUGP-like aspect to HIV-P. ANUGP does occur in HIV infection and may be superimposed on periodontitis, but HIV-P is distinct in that ulceration and overt necrosis do not occur.

Although no data are available, ANUGP is common in patients with HIV or AIDS (Plate 28). Given the association of ANUGP with other systemic diseases or conditions that impair resistance to infection, its occurrence in HIV infection is not surprising. The clinical features at presentation are similar to the disease in uninfected individuals.

The primary differences are its more widespread extent, aggressiveness, and lower response to treatment.[42]

The most threatening periodontal infections associated with HIV-infection or AIDS may be necrotizing stomatitis. It is less common than ANUGP and apparently results from a progression of ANUGP or even HIV-P. However, establishment of the cause is difficult because patients often do not seek treatment until the lesion is fully developed. Findings at the initial examination may range from large areas of gingiva and mucosa undergoing necrosis to areas of exposed alveolar bone surrounded by severely inflamed tissue with an overtly necrotic margin. If necrotizing stomatitis is treated successfully in the early stage, bone involvement and loss are minimal; otherwise, bony sequestra are likely and sizable defects may remain after healing. A resemblance of necrotizing stomatitis in HIV infection to noma (cancrum oris) has been noted.[169,175]

Etiology Although the bacteria responsible for the various forms of inflammatory periodontal disease in HIV infection are not certain, the progressively more profound immunosuppression caused by the virus is the fundamental pathogenic phenomenon. Patients infected with HIV are increasingly depleted of T4 lymphocytes and their ability to mount a normal immune reaction is reduced or lost. The severity and aggressiveness of destructive inflammatory periodontal disease is related to the severity of the systemic manifestations of HIV infection. T4/T8 cell ratios in HIV-P are lower than in HIV-G.[44] The severity of HIV-P also is inversely correlated with the number of T4 cells in peripheral blood.[89]

The microbiota associated with periodontal disease in HIV infections has not been extensively investigated. One study found *P. gingivalis, P. intermedia, F. nucleatum,* and *A. actinomycetemcomitans* in 60% to 80% of sites sampled in both HIV-G and HIV-P.[105] This flora resembles that typically found in uncomplicated periodontitis but is quite different from that found in uncomplicated gingivitis. This finding suggests that HIV-G may be an immediate precursor of HIV-P, with the transition triggered by a further decrease in the number of T4 cells In addition to the previous organisms, other studies have reported *W. recta, E. corrodens, P. micros, Capnocytophaga* spp., and other gram-negative species.[89,127] Spirochetes, motile rods, and *Candida albicans* also were detected.

Currently gingivitis and periodontitis associated with HIV infection do not represent opportunistic infection caused by organisms not ordinarily found in the mouth. The hypothesis that the usual periodontal pathogenic bacteria simply overwhelm the increasingly deficient immune response of the host is reasonable.[105,107]

Treatment Treatment of HIV-G, HIV-P, and ANUGP uses the same antiinfective strategies used to treat these diseases in patients who are immunocompetent: debridement and chemotherapy. However, the response to the strategies may be notably less effective, primarily because of the immune impairment. In addition, the patient may not keep appointments or comply with prescribed medications or home care measures because of other more urgent systemic manifestations of HIV infection or mental depression and apathy. Relapses are common for the same reasons.

Debridement should be prompt and thorough. The use of ultrasonic instruments is not advised because of the generation of infectious aerosol. Gingival tenderness and heavy bleeding during scaling may limit the extent of debridement that can be accomplished in a single visit. If so, additional visits should be scheduled daily until debridement is complete. The patient should be instructed in techniques for gentle mechanical self-cleaning with a soft brush.

Several types of chemotherapy are helpful. Twice-daily use of 0.4% chlorhexidine oral rinse reduces plaque and gingival inflammation. This preparation may not be well tolerated if gingival or mucosal ulcerative lesions are present. For symptomatic lesions or severely inflamed sites in HIV-P or in ANUGP, office irrigation with 10% povidone-iodine (Betadine) has been used with good results.[42,174] Irrigation can be combined with mechanical debridement and should be continued at daily intervals until the acute phase wanes. Systemic chemotherapy may be necessary for control of ANUGP and almost certainly is necessary for necrotizing stomatitis. Clindamycin and metronidazole are rational choices based on their activity against gram-negative anaerobes. When an acute periodontal infection is diagnosed in a patient who is HIV positive or who has AIDS, the physician of record should be consulted if possible before systemic chemotherapy is initiated.

PULPAL INFECTIONS

Pulpal infections occur for many reasons and can be difficult to detect and control. Because most major odontogenic infections begin in the dental pulp, management of these conditions requires understanding of the pathophysiology of infections in this area.

Numerous factors cause pulpal inflammation and subsequent pulpal infection and necrosis. These insults to the pulpal tissues include physical, thermal, and chemical irritants, and most important, microbial organisms. Even basic restorative procedures often cause reversible to irreversible pulpal damage. Kakehashi et al.[17] demonstrated a direct relationship between pulpal inflammation and microorganisms. In addition, Sundqvist et al.[35] noted the significant role of anaerobes in the pathogenesis of endodontic infections. However, before an in-depth examination of pulpal microorganisms, their path of entry into pulpal tissues must be considered.

CLASSIFICATION OF PULPAL DISEASES

The classification of diseases of pulpal tissue is divided into several categories. Pulpal diagnosis is based primarily on objective clinical tests and subjective patient responses to these tests. Radiographs usually are of little, if any, aid in determining pulpal states. The diagnosis of pulpal disease relies almost entirely on the clinician's interpretation of patient responses to various "objective" tests. The word *objective* must be noted—although the test is objective, the response of the patient is entirely "subjective" and therefore open to interpretation by the clinician performing the tests.

Several studies have demonstrated the lack of correlation between the histological findings in pulpal tissue and the clinical signs and symptoms associated with pulpal diseases.[3,13,14] An understanding of the response of "normal" pulp to various clinical tests is necessary to comprehend the "abnormal" states of pulpal diseases.

NORMAL PULP

Healthy normal vital pulp generally responds to various stimuli (heat or cold) without an exaggerated response. Normal pulp responds to cold or heat stimulation with a mild painful response that lingers no longer than 10 seconds. In addition, percussion of the tooth causes no painful reaction. However, normal pulp may not respond to thermal tests. If the pulp chamber or root canal is calcified because of the aging process, trauma (restorative procedures, caries), masticatory forces, or other causes, thermal tests may not yield a response from the patient yet the pulp is vital and healthy.

Electric pulp testers usually elicit a response from a patient with vital pulp. The clinician must be aware the numbers on pulp testers are arbitrary and do not necessarily indicate the health or inflammatory status of a vital pulp.

REVERSIBLE PULPITIS

A defensive inflammatory response is common after mild to moderate mechanical, chemical, or bacterial insults to healthy pulp. This histological change in the pulpal tissue often is reflected in the clinical response of the patient to various stimuli. Most commonly, patients report the inability to tolerate cold or hot liquids in a region of reversible pulpitis. The painful response to these thermal changes usually lasts no longer than 10 to 15 seconds. Once the painful response has subsided, no additional pain or discomfort is noted. This short pain duration is significant clinically because a painful spontaneous response after removal of the stimulus and subsidence of the initial painful response indicate that the pulp is no longer considered in a reversible state.

Although the electric pulp test is useful for determining the "responsiveness" or vitality of the pulpal tissues, it is the least desirable clinical test for vitality testing because it provides no indication of the "clinical status" of the pulp. The astute clinician uses thermal stimulation to indicate the need for a more careful assessment. Positive responses to percussion tests may indicate periradicular inflammation; however, in the case of a diagnosis of reversible pulpitis, the periradicular inflammation has a

cause other than pulpal tissues (excessive occlusal forces, periodontal problems, high restorations).

IRREVERSIBLE PULPITIS

Irreversible pulpitis is a clinically based term that indicates the clinical status of a pulp. It usually occurs when reversible pulpitis can no longer be contained by the inflammatory or immunological response of pulpal tissues and begins to degenerate into an irreversible pathological condition. The patient commonly describes prolonged sensitivity to cold or hot foods and liquids. The pain lasts typically from 15 seconds to several minutes and often persists much longer. Patients report spontaneous pain with this condition and the pain may be so severe that it awakens them at night. Patients with irreversible pulpitis commonly use analgesics, although in most cases they do not completely alleviate the symptoms.

The tooth with an irreversible pulpitis may be sensitive to mastication (percussion). This sensitivity depends solely on whether the inflammation has proceeded into the periradicular area. If the inflammation is confined to the pulp chamber, no sensitivity to mastication exists. However, if the inflammatory products and immunological response to the irritation have advanced throughout the coronal and radicular pulpal tissue, the tooth causes symptoms and the patient cannot use the tooth normally.

Histologically the pulp may exhibit areas of increased vascular stasis, and sometimes, small areas of necrosis or abscess formation. These circumscribed areas of inflammation, vascular stasis, and local necrosis eventually proceed throughout the pulpal tissue.[41]

NECROTIC PULP

Pulpal necrosis has a variety of causes. The most common cause is continuation of an irreversible pulpal state. The disease process may occur rapidly (within several weeks) or over many months to years. Other causes such as dental trauma result in almost immediate pulpal necrosis depending on the nature of the trauma. In addition, operative procedures, attrition, and caries, if left untreated, may result in necrosis of the pulpal tissue. Pulpal necrosis proceeds in a more chronic rather than acute fashion.

The pulp environment is unique with respect to most other body tissues. Because pulp is contained in a "noncompliant" environment, inflammatory products cannot be removed in the same rapid manner as in other soft tissues of the body, resulting in many areas of localized destruction within the pulpal tissue. Ultimately this environment leads to pulpal destruction.

Symptoms vary and wide-ranging presentations of pulpal necrosis are possible. For example, a patient may relate a history of acute pain in a tooth that no longer causes discomfort. The tooth probably has become necrotic, but the inflammatory and immunological defense mechanism maintains a balance so that the patient is asymptomatic. When the inflammatory response is severe, periradicular pain is acute and although the pulp is necrotic, severe peri-radicular pain is present because of the ensuing immuno-logical response. Patients cannot differentiate periradicular pain from pulpal pain (because of the common source of innervation for both) and therefore often question why they experience pain from a "dead" tooth.

Mastication sensitivity is an inconsistent finding with pulpal necrosis. Acute inflammation of the periodontal lig-ament results in mastication sensitivity. This acute inflam-matory response does not occur in every case of pulpal necrosis and may resolve without clinical intervention. If the periradicular response is severe and causes loss of the cortical bone adjacent to a necrotic tooth, the inflamma-tion and resultant products are eliminated into the oral cavity through a sinus tract. This clearance often results in immediate abatement of acute symptoms and mastication sensitivity with no clinical intervention.

PORTALS OF ENTRY TO PULPAL TISSUES

DENTINAL TUBULES

Dentinal tubules exposed as a result of operative proce-dures are one of the most common methods for bacteria to gain access to pulpal tissues. Bacterial infection occurs as a result of operative procedures, fractures in the enamel from excessive occlusal forces, exposed dentin from cervi-cal abrasion, and factitial and other injuries. Anatomical defects from within the enamel such as dens invaginatus also provide a means for bacterial entry.

DIRECT PULPAL EXPOSURE

Direct pulpal exposure from operative procedures or trauma can allow entry of bacteria into the pulp. Whenever dentin is exposed to the oral environment—from simple Class I procedures to more complex crown preparations—the potential for bacterial invasion is great. Depending on the patient's age the dentinal tubules may not yet be scle-rotic and therefore direct entry to the pulp is highly proba-ble. However, because healthy pulp can prevent irreversible damage to itself, these transient exposures to microorgan-isms during restorative procedures usually are insignificant. For traumatic injuries the type of trauma is directly related to long-term pulpal prognosis. For example, although a Class II fracture is limited to only enamel and dentin, this type of trauma often occurs in younger patients with large, patent dentinal tubules that provide an excellent portal of entry for bacteria into the pulp.

Class III fractures that affect not only the enamel and dentin but also cause direct pulpal tissue exposure to the oral environment provide a rapid transport method for mi-croorganisms to pulpal tissues. Often avulsion and luxa-tion injuries, particularly extrusive and lateral luxations, allow bacteria to enter the pulp directly from the peri-radicular area, specifically the apical foramen. In younger patients the apex is immature and provides a large and di-rect access to pulpal tissues from the periradicular tissues.

The most common and significant contamination and subsequent penetration into pulpal tissues occur from dental caries. This process may proceed over several weeks to several years. During this insult and as the caries progress increasingly closer to the pulp chamber, the pulp's defense mechanism responds with the formation of reparative dentin directly under the dentinal tubules af-fected by caries. Sclerotic dentin also is formed and the pulp chamber becomes smaller because of the carious in-sult. If the carious process proceeds more rapidly than the pulp's ability to form reparative dentin, the pulp is re-versibly inflamed, irreversibly inflamed, or both.

ACCESSORY AND LATERAL CANALS

Accessory canals (canals that branch from the main canal, usually in the apical third of the root canal system) and lat-eral canals (canals usually located at a right angle to the main root canal system) provide direct channels of entry for bacteria to pulpal tissues. When bacteria enter the pulp from a lateral or accessory canal, periodontal disease usu-ally has a direct or an indirect effect on degradation of the pulpal tissue.

ANACHORESIS

Robinson and Boling[29] discovered that blood-borne mi-croorganisms have the ability to preferentially concen-trate or collect, specifically in areas of acute inflamma-tion. They determined that after injection of known microorganisms into the systemic vasculature of cats, the same bacteria were concentrated in pulpal tissues of teeth intentionally irritated or inflamed with croton oil. Thus systemic bacteria may enter previously inflamed pulpal tissues if present in the vasculature. However, Delivanis et al.[11] questioned the concept of anachoresis. In their study, instrumented but unfilled root canals in five cats were analyzed for the presence of systemically injected bacteria. Bacteremia was induced in these animals for a minimum of 2 hours; however, no microorganisms were discovered in the periradicular area of the instrumented but unfilled teeth. Even up to 48 hours after the induc-tion of the bacteremia, no test bacteria were cultured from the canals in these animals. The concept of ana-choresis inducing pulpal infections in humans is still questioned.

MICROBIAL VIRULENCE FACTORS

Various microbial virulence factors are important because of the pathogenetic role of bacteria in pulpal disease. Vir-ulence is a measure of the pathogenicity of a microorgan-ism given specific host conditions. At least six major fac-tors contribute to the virulence of a microorganism:

1. Motility is the ability of bacteria to evade macro-phages and therefore to establish new areas of infec-tion within the pulpal tissues.

2. Adherence is the ability of the microorganism to attach itself to certain types of host tissues. Laminin, fibronectin, and M protein play a major role in this process.
3. The ability of the microorganism to multiply and increase its population is considered a growth virulence factor. The increased growth rate often overwhelms host defense mechanisms and leads to infection of host tissues.
4. The capsule of bacteria is another virulence factor that allows the microorganism to overpower the host tissue. This capsule is an exterior coat or defense mechanism that prevents or inhibits phagocytosis.
5. Invasins also play a major role in the spread of bacteria through tissues. These bacterial enzymes facilitate the spread of the infective process. They include collagenase, hyaluronidase, chondroitin sulfatase, kinases, hemolysins, leukocidins, DNAase, gelatinase, and coagulase.
6. Bacterial toxins are perhaps the most significant of the virulence factors among the various microbes that invade the pulpal tissues. These toxins are proteins that stimulate tissue damage and promote pulpal tissue degradation. Two types of toxins cause soft tissue damage. Some microorganisms secrete exotoxins externally, which may result in fever, stimulation of T-helper cells, resorption of bone, and vasomotor shock.

Endotoxins reside within the gram-negative cell walls and are known as lipopolysaccharides. Schonfeld et al.[30] determined that the major components of the toxic and tumor-destroying material in microorganisms consisted of both lipid and polysaccharides, coining the term *lipopolysaccharides*. These endotoxins generally are released after destruction of the gram-negative bacteria. They can produce systemic changes such as vasomotor shock, bone resorption, and systemic responses to the release of epinephrine.[15,37] Rietschel and Brade[28] presented an excellent review on the mechanism of actions of endotoxins. They found lipopolysaccharides on the walls of gram-negative bacteria. The lipopolysaccharides consisted of lipid A, which constitutes a majority of the external half of the membrane. A small string of sugars connects the lipid to the O-specific chain (core oligosaccharide). The O-specific chain projects from the core as the outermost aspect of the endotoxin. This side chain also is the most variable part that initiated the specific immune response. When bacteria multiply or die, the lipopolysaccharides are released from the cell wall. They then bind to a specific binding protein that circulates systemically. This circulating complex in turn binds to a CD14 receptor on a circulating macrophage. The specific binding protein then stimulates the macrophage, activates complement, and causes mast cell degranulation.

ANTIBIOTIC THERAPY IN ENDODONTICS

Few indications for antibiotic therapy exist in endodontics. Unfortunately, many clinicians believe that a patient with moderate to severe pain should begin antibiotic therapy to reduce the "infection" that may (or may not) be the cause of the pain. Mere pain from a tooth is not an indication for antibiotic therapy. Although antibiotics may help alleviate pain, they should be used only when specific indications warrant their prescription. These indications include systemic involvement of infection; generally the patient is febrile (temperature $\geq 100°$ F) and has palpable lymph nodes with or without cellulitis.

Antibiotics should be prescribed prophylactically in some cases for patients with compromised host immunity. Antibiotic coverage also should be considered in all patients with compromised immune systems (e.g., patients with AIDS or specific blood dyscrasias). However, clinicians should use discretion in prescribing antibiotics because absolute rules regarding their administration are few and seldom indicated.

Frequently a patient has irreversible pulpitis and antibiotics are administered in an attempt to alleviate the problem. This poor clinical practice should be avoided because expedient emergency endodontic treatment resolves the patient's symptoms without the need for adjunctive antibiotic therapy. In addition, the patient's symptoms are derived from vital or nonvital pulp, not from a fulminating infection, thus contraindicating drug therapy.

Some clinicians routinely prescribe antibiotics before and/or after endodontic surgical procedures. However, Paterson et al.[26] and Pendrill and Reddy[27] suggested that routine use of antibiotics before surgical procedures may increase the patient's risk of postoperative infection. The incidence of infection after surgery is extremely low. Most postoperative infections are a direct result of poor reapproximation of the surgical flap and therefore lack of proper closure, and poor aseptic techniques.[10]

COMMON MICROORGANISMS IN PULPAL TISSUE

Bacteria in the dental pulp were identified as early as 1919 when Henrici and Hartzell[16] discovered that the majority of pulpal bacteria were streptococci and staphylococci. Winkler and Van Amerongen[45] corroborated these findings when they discovered that almost 80% of the bacteria from more than 4000 root canal tissue cultures were streptococci or staphylococci. They also discovered the presence of gram-negative rods, lactobacilli, and *Corynebacterium* spp. in the cultured teeth. Unfortunately, the early culture studies determined only the aerobic bacteria because sophisticated methods of bacterial culturing had not yet been refined.

Kantz and Henry[18] were among the first to use anaerobic culturing techniques from intact pulp chambers in nonvital teeth. They discovered that more than 25% of their samples contained obligate anaerobes, which included *Actinomycosis, Peptococcus, Veillonella, Fusobacterium, Bacteroides,* and *Campylobacter.* Bystrom and Sundqvist[9] discovered that almost 90% of the bacteria cultured in their study were anaerobic.

Sundqvist[34,36] was one of the first researchers to investigate traumatized teeth and the relationship of microorganisms in patient symptoms, periradicular inflammation, and bone resorption. Sundqvist is credited with the discovery of the significant role of *P. melaninogenica* in the development of symptoms and periradicular abscesses from necrotic teeth.

MICROORGANISMS IN THE PERIRADICULAR REGION OF INFECTED TEETH

Although some investigators claim that the periradicular area of abscessed or infected teeth is more often sterile than infiltrated with microorganisms,[20] the significant role of bacteria in the pathogenesis of periradicular tissue destruction has been well documented.[38] Baumgartner and Falkler[4] discovered that the majority of bacteria in the apical 5 mm of infected teeth were strict anaerobes. Bacteria also have been isolated in the periradicular tissues of cysts, granulomas, and abscesses. Wayman et al.[44] determined that the majority of the microorganisms in the periradicular tissues were strict anaerobes with more than 25% facultative anaerobes and less than 10% aerobes.

NEUROPHYSIOLOGY OF PULPAL PAIN

Dental caries are the primary cause of pulpal pain. Initially the tooth is sensitive to thermal changes, mechanical stimulation, and sweet substances but no spontaneous pulpal pain is present. As the carious lesion advances and the pulp is invaded by the bacteria and bacterial by-products, pulpal inflammation (pulpitis) develops, which causes acute intermittent and spontaneous pain. As the inflammatory process progresses a throbbing and poorly localized pain continues long after a stimulus such as thermal change is applied to the tooth. Therefore as the intensity of acute dental pain increases, its spatial distribution in the maxilla or mandible is not sufficient as a diagnostic tool for identifying the source of pain.[33]

Under certain conditions, stimulation of the pulpal tissues can evoke sensations other than pain.[37] Several studies questioned whether the painful or nonpainful sensations are carried by two distinct populations of afferent nerves. McGrath et al.[22] investigated the quality and magnitude of sensations evoked by pulpal stimulation from an electrical source. They concluded that the nonpainful sensations evoked in the pulp were mediated by a distinct population of afferents not involved in the coding of pain. However, Virtanen et al.[42] favored the theory of single-modality innervation. They concluded that perception and pain thresholds were modified by temporal summation and that activation of A-fiber populations was responsible for production of prepain and painful sensations.

The underlying mechanism for dentinal sensitivity and pulpal pain conduction has been investigated extensively.[1,7,12,23,25] Byers and Kish[8] demonstrated that dental nerves end freely below the odontoblast layer, form gap junctions on the odontoblast cell body, or penetrate along its dentinal process for 150 to 200 μm. This limited innervation of dentin and the fact that dentinal pain can be evoked only by mechanical stimulation, temperature, or changes in osmotic pressure led to the development of the hydrostatic pressure theory by Brannstrom et al.[6] They hypothesized that with the exception of direct electrical stimulation, all procedures known to produce dentinal pain may distort mechanically the structure of pain-sensitive nerves in the pulp and predentinal area. This effect is mediated by a hydrodynamic link: the movement of dentinal fluid within the dentinal tubules activates pain-sensitive mechanoreceptors to produce pain.

The mechanism for pulpal pain as a result of direct pulpal inflammation and a host of other mediators such as prostaglandins, serotonin, and bradykinin has been hypothesized.[25,31,39] Two populations of nociceptive fibers are present in the pulp, the C fibers and the A fibers. C fibers are more sensitive to the inflammatory mediators, increased intrapulpal pressure, and damaged microcirculation than A fibers. However, leukotriene B$_4$ can sensitize all nociceptors within the pulp and may act as a long-lasting hyperalgesic factor contributing to pulpal pain.[21] Regardless of the mechanisms involved in pulpal pain the clinician can gather tangible evidence for pulpal and periradicular diagnosis only from a patient's subjective response to a stimulus of pain.

CLASSIFICATION OF PERIRADICULAR DISEASES

ACUTE PERIRADICULAR PERIODONTITIS

The term *acute periradicular periodontitis* is used to describe a patient's response to a percussion test performed on an affected tooth. If the tooth is sensitive to percussion, acute periradicular periodontitis is diagnosed. This purely descriptive term provides no indication of pulpal vitality or other periradicular conditions that may be associated with a particular tooth.

ASYMPTOMATIC CHRONIC PERIRADICULAR PERIODONTITIS

Chronic periradicular periodontitis is a term used to describe a long-standing periradicular lesion that is apparent radiographically. The radiographic appearance varies from a slightly widened periodontal ligament space to a large, radiolucent periradicular lesion that has eroded significant amounts of cortical bone. Patients do not display symptoms and often are unaware that any pathosis is present. The condition may have been preceded by a symptomatic period but the patient often is unaware of any acute history of pain.

A periradicular histological diagnosis cannot be made on the basis of symptoms or radiographic appearance. Studies have demonstrated the difficulty and inability to determine a histological diagnosis based solely on radiographic appearances of periradicular lesions.[2,43] Most (approximately 80% to 90%) periradicular lesions are cysts or granulomas[5,19,24] (Plates 29 and 30). Furthermore, periradicular cysts are more common in males than in females. In addition, the incidence of occurrence in the maxilla was nearly 10 times more frequent than in the mandible.[5]

SYMPTOMATIC CHRONIC PERIRADICULAR PERIODONTITIS

Because chronic periradicular periodontitis also may produce symptoms, another category of periradicular states is needed under this same heading. Essentially all characteristics of chronic periradicular periodontitis are present radiographically; however, the patient displays symptoms and may have chronic low-grade pain in the region or mastication sensitivity. Regardless of the presence of mastication sensitivity the patient experiences pain from the tooth, usually as spontaneous, low-grade pain that often exacerbates into more severe discomfort requiring immediate clinical intervention. Histologically, chronic inflammatory cells such as lymphocytes, plasma cells, and macrophages are noted.

Depending on the chronicity of the lesion, associated resorption of the root may exist. Resorption usually is minor and of little consequence clinically. In some cases the resorption may be severe and produce significant root resorption that ultimately may result in the inability to perform adequate conventional endodontic therapy.

PHOENIX ABSCESS

A phoenix abscess classically occurs in a patient with chronic periradicular periodontitis who does not display symptoms. Host factors, increased numbers of microorganisms, increased virulence of the microorganisms in the root canal system, or a combination of these factors produces symptoms. Often swelling is present and purulence is obtained on opening the tooth. However, whether the purulent drainage is from the offending tooth depends on many variables and drainage does not occur in every case. The patient usually needs acute care; relief generally is obtained on initial entry into the tooth once drainage has been obtained. This "abscess" literally "rises from the ashes" and a patient who previously was asymptomatic becomes acutely aware of the ensuing endodontic problem.

The radiographic appearance of a phoenix lesion is similar to chronic periradicular periodontitis in that a "frank" periradicular lesion usually is present on the radiograph. The lesion is sufficiently large to be discernible from the radiograph and is not limited solely to a widened periodontal ligament space.

CHRONIC SUPPURATIVE PERIRADICULAR PERIODONTITIS

Chronic suppurative periradicular periodontitis is a chronic periradicular lesion that has established a pathway through the cortical bone and periosteum into the oral cavity or extraorally through the skin. In some cases this pathway may traverse coronally through the periodontal ligament space. When this occurs, clinical findings often confound the diagnostic ability of the clinician because a periodontal problem now appears to be associated with the asymptomatic tooth. However, in most cases a single deep probing indicates a vertical root fracture or, more likely in the case of a nonendodontically treated tooth, a "vertical" sinus tract. In all cases in which the cause of the periodontal pocket is a nonvital tooth, deep probing resolves to a normal depth almost immediately after biomechanical instrumentation of the root canal system. Although lesion may be evident radiographically for 3 to 6 months after removal of the necrotic tissue from the root canal, the sinus tract heals immediately in most instances. However, depending on the duration of the sinus tract, it may epithelialize forming a fistula. The longer the duration of the sinus tract, the greater is the likelihood of epithelialization.[40]

Most sinus tracts are preceded by a slight swelling on the attached gingiva or mucosa and may have a parulis (pimple) on the soft tissue. In some cases this lesion begins to drain without clinical intervention or additional treatment may be required to establish drainage.

Many practitioners mistakenly believe that a patient with a sinus tract has a greater likelihood of symptoms if treatment is delayed. However, the opposite is true. Patients generally do not display symptoms and may report only a "bad taste" or odor from their mouth. The chronic suppurative periradicular periodontitis constantly drains purulence or necrotic polymorphonuclear cells from the sinus tract. Although antibiotics may resolve temporarily the clinical presentation, because the cause is necrotic pulpal tissue, endodontic therapy must be initiated before resolution can occur. The use of antibiotics alone to treat suppurative periradicular periodontitis is contraindicated in most cases.

CONDENSING SCLEROSING OSTEITIS

Chronic inflammation in the pulpal tissue may result in a condition known as *condensing sclerosing osteitis*. Although some clinicians consider this condition a true periradicular disease, it is primarily a chronic inflammatory reactive state of the periradicular bone associated with a specific tooth. The bone adjacent to inflamed or necrotic pulp becomes reactive and begins to lay down additional bone. This increase in bone density results in increased radiopacity of the cancellous bone usually directly around one or more roots of a tooth with a chronically inflamed or necrotic pulp. Patients do not display symptoms and are unaware of any bony changes. This state is often noted in the periradicular area of teeth with large restorations or crowns. The condition cannot be resolved by endodontic therapy; once the bone has been deposited the radiographic appearance generally does not change with respect to the opacity of the periradicular area even after successful endodontic therapy.

TREATMENT OF PULPAL AND PERIRADICULAR DISEASES

Treatment of pulpal and periradicular diseases depends on the severity of the patient's symptoms and the pulpal and periradicular diagnosis of the affected tooth. In some cases, several treatment options are available; however, usually only one method will remedy the patient's distress in the most expedient manner. Two factors are vital in the treatment of endodontic problems. First, the type of treatment should result in the greatest relief of symptoms. This seemingly obvious statement correlates with the pulpal and periradicular diagnosis and the specific treatment options for each diagnosis. Second, the specific tooth type (anterior, premolar, molar) must be considered with a thorough understanding of the anatomy and morphology of the roots and the root canal system. The astute clinician recognizes specific limitations to treatment based solely on tooth type. For example, although pulpotomy often alleviates the patient's symptoms the more appropriate treatment in anterior vital teeth is complete pulpectomy.

REVERSIBLE PULPITIS

The symptoms of reversible pulpitis usually are present only briefly and resolve without clinical intervention. However, in some cases once a recently placed composite or amalgam is established as the cause, the clinician may consider removal of the restoration and placement of a temporary restoration such as intermediate restorative material (IRM) in an attempt to resolve the symptoms. Unless the patient's symptoms dictate otherwise, this procedure should not be considered until at least 2 to 3 weeks after the original insult to the pulp.

Because inflammation of pulpal tissue is reversible, the use of IRM generally causes an immediate reduction of symptoms and uneventful healing. However, whenever a restoration is replaced in a tooth, additional inflammatory changes are likely in the pulp. In most instances the additional irritation is minor and does not cause a reversible situation to become irreversible.

IRREVERSIBLE PULPITIS

Localized Symptoms Because a tooth with an irreversibly inflamed pulp often is vital throughout the entire pulp chamber and root canal system, the most expedient treatment is removal of the affected pulpal tissue. In most instances a pulpotomy procedure is performed. This technique does not remove or disturb the tissue within the root canals but treats only the pulp chamber contents. This method is used primarily in posterior teeth because of the difficulty in debridement of small and sometimes calcified canals. Because the symptoms are caused primarily by the pulp chamber tissue and not the tissue in the root canal system, pulpotomy is the method of choice in posterior teeth.

In general, anterior teeth possess a larger root canal system; therefore pulpectomy is the preferred treatment for irreversibly inflamed pulpal tissue. This procedure involves complete removal of the pulp chamber contents and soft tissue within the root canal system. In most anterior teeth, little additional time is required to perform a pulpectomy versus a pulpotomy. However, pulpotomy is an acceptable treatment option if no periradicular inflammation is present. If the patient has an irreversible pulpitis and acute periradicular periodontitis, the soft tissue should be removed completely from the canal system. Pulpotomy procedures are contraindicated in these cases.

During pulpectomy in anterior teeth, the clinician should attempt total removal of the soft tissue from within the root canal system in one step. Files should be turned clockwise into the pulpal tissue and the tissue literally twisted around the instrument with simultaneous removal of both tissue and instrument. Often the inadvertent laceration and gouging of the soft tissue prevents its complete removal, resulting in a high likelihood of continued patient symptoms or, more important, exacerbations of the current symptoms.

Mastication Sensitivity In patients with irreversible pulpitis and mastication sensitivity the pulpal inflammatory products have traversed the entire pulp chamber and entered the root canals. In some cases, inflammation may affect every root in a tooth with multiple roots or canals. Mastication sensitivity is a direct consequence of periradicular inflammation of the periodontal ligament. Therefore appropriate treatment requires removal of the tissue within the pulp chamber and the root canals to resolve symptoms.

However, instrumentation of all root canals often is impractical, particularly during an emergency appointment. Expedient treatment dictates that the largest canal of multirooted teeth be cleaned, leaving the other root canal systems undisturbed. In many situations the palatal root of maxillary posterior teeth or the distal root of mandibular molars is affected. This approach is ideal when the emergency patient or clinician has little time available for therapy.

Nonlocalized Symptoms Occasionally a patient initially is seen with long-standing chronic pain, often spontaneous in nature but adequately severe to require clinical intervention. The patient reports discomfort to hot and cold foods and liquids but not to mastication. In these cases the pain to thermal stimulation often diminishes or abates completely. The patient responds normally to objective clinical testing of thermal stimulation and exhibits no percussion sensitivity. Essentially all clinical test results are within normal limits yet the patient relates a history of moderate to severe pain associated with a particular area or a specific tooth. The patient may believe that he or she can identify the tooth causing the discomfort.

In some cases, patients may be adamant about their ability to identify the tooth causing the pain yet the clinician is unable to identify objectively a specific cause. Radiographs are not clinically valuable because the periradicular anatomy typically is within normal limits. Because patients have had varying degrees of pain for some time, they expect treatment immediately to relieve the impending symptoms. Such situations often present the most difficult clinical decisions.

Clinicians should not begin endodontic therapy on any tooth unless they are 80% to 90% confident of an appropriate diagnosis. Although patients may be totally convinced of a specific tooth as the cause of their pain, no treatment should be instituted unless the clinician can reproduce the symptoms, especially if no tangible radiographic evidence of pathosis is apparent. The histopathological process of pulpal inflammation usually results in pain localized to a specific tooth at which time the clinician can perform appropriate treatment. However, endodontic therapy often is initiated on a "suspected" tooth with the unfavorable outcome that the patient, clinician, or both were inaccurate in their ability to determine the cause. In these cases the patient should be given the option of over-the-counter analgesics and provided assurance that the pain will localize eventually. Several days to several weeks may elapse before the affected tooth can be identified.

NECROTIC PULP

Necrotic Pulp without Swelling   A diagnosis of necrotic pulp may be based on clinical tests, history of symptoms, and radiographic findings. Unlike the treatment of teeth with irreversible pulpitis, necrotic pulp, regardless of its location in the oral cavity, is treated similarly. Because the symptoms relate to the periradicular area of the tooth and not the pulpal tissue, complete removal of all necrotic debris is necessary for symptom relief. Therefore pulpotomy is contraindicated in necrotic pulp; the procedure leaves a significant amount of necrotic tissue and bacteria within the root canal system. The by-products of the microorganisms (endotoxins and exotoxins) within the root canal are released from the root through the apical foramen and into the periradicular area, resulting in mild to moderate or severe pain. Thus pulpectomy or complete debridement of both the pulp chamber and the root canals must be performed.

Localized Intraoral Swelling   Patients with necrotic pulp with localized intraoral swelling must be treated similar to patients without swelling: the necrotic pulpal tissue must be removed. Because of the localized swelling, some clinicians suggest prescription of antibiotics. However, this practice is contraindicated because no systemic infection is present and removal of the cause, the infected pulpal tissue, is the only treatment required.

The root canal systems must be chemomechanically debrided once complete swelling begins to resolve. Depending on the type of swelling (fluctuant versus diffuse), several days to a week may be required for complete resolution.

Four basic scenarios may exist in the treatment of localized intraoral swelling:

1. The soft tissue is fluctuant and drainage has been obtained through the tooth—In such cases the tooth should be opened and thoroughly cleaned. Incision and drainage of the fluctuant soft tissue area is completed with a No. 12 or No. 15 scalpel blade. A drain may be placed; however, a drain generally is not necessary because adequate drainage usually is obtained within the first 12 hours after incision of the lesion.
2. The soft tissue is fluctuant but no drainage is obtained through the tooth—The tooth should be opened and thoroughly cleaned. Because no drainage is obtained through the tooth, incision of the fluctuant area is mandatory. The placement of a drain is not required.
3. The soft tissue is nonfluctuant but drainage is obtained through the tooth—Biomechanical instrumentation of the tooth is required; however, no incision or surgical intervention is indicated. Because drainage has been obtained through the tooth, no additional treatment is required since the tissue is nonfluctuant. However, warm saline solution rinses may be suggested to aid in localizing the swelling.
4. The soft tissue is nonfluctuant with no drainage through the tooth—After biomechanical instrumentation of the tooth, warm saline solution rinses are indicated. Antibiotic treatment may be indicated if the swelling is more diffuse. In most cases, removal of the cause results in healing and resolution of the swelling.

Diffuse Extraoral Swelling   Often patients have not only diffuse extraoral swelling but also are febrile and may exhibit lymphadenopathy. These patients require immediate attention, and appropriate endodontic therapy adjunctive antibiotic therapy should be instituted. In most cases, endodontic therapy must be initiated with thorough cleaning and shaping of the canals at the emergency appointment.

In addition to endodontic treatment, if the patient is not allergic to penicillin a loading dose of 1 to 2 g of penicillin with subsequent 500 mg every 6 hours is indicated immediately on diagnosis of this condition. Depending on the duration of the condition aggressive treatment is mandatory to prevent exacerbation of the infection and avoid hospitalization and administration of intravenous antibiotics.

The patient should return for follow-up within 24 to 48 hours. Although the response to antibiotics may not be immediate, no change or augmentation of the initial antibiotic regimen is indicated before 48 to 72 hours have elapsed. A patient's initial presentation often does not change within the first 48 hours with respect to extraoral swelling or fever. However, if the swelling, fever, or both do not increase the antibiotics likely are performing appropriately and no treatment change is necessary. Clinicians often augment antibiotic therapy or change antibiotics if response to this therapy occurs within the first 24 to 48 hours; this practice is inappropriate and misuses antibiotic therapy.

REFERENCES

Periodontal Infections

1. Ainamo J, Lahtinen A, Uitto VJ: Rapid periodontal destruction in humans with poorly controlled diabetes: a report of two cases, *J Clin Periodontol* 17:22, 1990.
2. American Academy of Periodontology: Consensus report, discussion section I. In Nevins R, Becker W, Kornman K, editors: *Proceedings of the World Workshop in Clinical Periodontics,* Chicago, 1989, American Academy of Periodontology.
3. Armitage GC: *The biologic basis of periodontal maintenance therapy,* Berkeley, Calif, 1980, Praxis.
4. Armitage GC: Development of a classification system for periodontal diseases and conditions, *Ann Periodontol* 4:1, 1999.
5. Axelsson P, Lindhe J: Effect of controlled and hygiene procedures on caries and periodontal disease in adults, *J Clin Periodontol* 5:133, 1978.
6. Beck J, Garcia R, Heiss G, et al: Periodontal disease and cardiovascular disease, *J Periodontol* 67:1123, 1996.
7. Bergenholtz G: Periodontics and endodontics. In Lindhe J, editor: *Textbook of clinical periodontology,* ed 2, Copenhagen, 1989, Munksgaard.
8. Bergström J, Eliasson S: Noxious effect of cigarette smoking on periodontal health, *J Periodontal Res* 22:513, 1987.
9. Bergström J, Eliasson S, Dock J: A 10-year prospective study of tobacco smoking and periodontal health, *J Periodontol* 71:1338, 2000.
10. Brown LJ, Oliver RC, Loe H: Periodontal disease in the U.S. in 1981: prevalence, severity, extent and role in tooth mortality, *J Periodontol* 60:363, 1989.
11. Buchanan SA, Robertson PB: Calculus removal by scaling/root planing with and without surgical access, *J Periodontol* 58:159, 1987.
12. Capilouto ML, Douglass CW: Trends in the prevalence and severity of periodontal diseases in the US: a public health problem? *J Public Health Dent* 48:245, 1988.
13. Carranza F: Radiographic and other aids in the diagnosis of periodontal disease. In Carranza F, Newman MG, editors: *Carranza's clinical periodontology,* ed 8, Philadelphia, 1996, WB Saunders.
14. Carranza F: Gingival enlargement. In Newman MG, Carranza F, Takei H, editors: *Carranza's clinical periodontology,* ed 9, Philadelphia, 2002, WB Saunders.
15. Carranza F: The periodontal pocket. In Newman MG, Carranza F, Takei H, editors: *Carranza's clinical periodontology,* ed 9, Philadelphia, 2002, WB Saunders.
16. Chilton NW, Miller MF: Epidemiology. a position paper and review of literature. In Klaven B, Genco R, Löe H, et al, editors: *International Conference of Research in the Biology of Periodontal Disease,* Chicago, 1977, University of Illinois College of Dentistry.
17. Reference deleted in proofs.
18. Christersson LA, Rosling BG, Dunford RG, et al: Monitoring of subgingival *Bacteroides gingivalis* and *Actinobacillus actinomycetemcomitans* in the management of advanced periodontitis, *Adv Dent Res* 2:382, 1988.
19. Cianciola LJ, Genco RJ, Patters MP, et al: Defective polymorphonuclear leukocyte function in human periodontal disease, *Nature* 265:445, 1977.
20. Clark RA, Kimball HR: Defective chemotaxis in Chediak-Higashi syndrome, *J Clin Invest* 50:2645, 1971.
21. Cohen DW, Morris AL: Periodontal manifestations of cyclic neutropenia, *J Periodontol* 32:159, 1961.
22. Darveau RP, Tanner A, Page RC: The microbial challenge in periodontitis, *Periodontol* 2000 14:12, 1997.
23. Dennison DK, Van Dyke TE: The acute inflammatory response and the role of phagocytic cells in periodontal health and disease, *Periodontol* 2000 14:54, 1997.
24. Douglas CW, Fox CH: Cross-sectional studies in periodontal disease: current status and implications for dental practice, *Adv Dent Res* 7:25, 1993.
25. Elders PJ, Habets LL, Netelenbos JC, et al: The relation between periodontitis and systemic bone mass in women between 46 and 55 years of age, *J Clin Periodontol* 19:492, 1992.
26. Reference deleted in proofs.
27. Enwonwu CO: Epidemiological and biochemical studies of necrotizing ulcerative gingivitis and noma (cancrum oris) in Nigerian children, *Arch Oral Biol* 17:1357, 1972.
28. Epstein S, Scopp I: Antibiotics and the intraoral abscess, *J Periodontol* 48:236, 1977.
29. Frank RM: Bacterial penetration in the apical pocket wall of advanced human periodontitis, *J Periodontal Res* 15:563, 1980.
30. Garrett S, Adams DF, Bogle G, et al: The effect of locally delivered controlled-release doxycycline on scaling and root planing on periodontal maintenance patients over nine months. *J Periodontol* 71:22, 2000.
31. Gemmel E, Marshall RI, Seymour GJ: Cytokines and prostaglandins in immune homeostasis and tissue destruction in periodontal disease, *Periodontol* 2000 14:112, 1997.
32. Genco RJ, Slots J: Host responses in periodontal diseases, *J Dent Res* 63:441, 1984.
33. Genco RJ, Zambon JJ, Christersson LA: The origin of periodontal infections, *Adv Dent Res* 2:245, 1988.
34. Giddon DB, Zackon SJ, Goldhaber P: Acute necrotizing ulcerative gingivitis in college students, *J Am Dent Assoc* 68:381, 1964.
35. Gold SI: Periodontics. The past. Part I. Early sources, *J Clin Periodontol* 12:79, 1985.
36. Goldberg MH: The changing nature of acute dental infection, *J Am Dent Assoc* 80:1048, 1970.
37. Goldhaber P, Giddon DB: Present concepts concerning the etiology and treatment of acute necrotizing ulcerative gingivitis, *Int Dent J* 14:468, 1964.
38. Goodson JM: Clinical measurements of periodontitis, *J Clin Periodontol* 13:446, 1986.
39. Goodson JM, Offenbacher S, Farr DH, et al: Periodontal disease treatment by local drug delivery, *J Periodontol* 56:265, 1985.
40. Goodson JM, Tanner AC, Haffajee AD, et al: Patterns of progression and regression of advanced periodontal disease, *J Clin Periodontol* 9:472, 1982.
41. Gottlieb B: Die diffuse atrophie des alveolarknochens, *Z Stomatol* 31:195, 1923.
42. Grassi M, Williams CA, Walker JR, et al: Management of HIV-associated periodontal disease. In Robertson PB, Greenspan JS, editors: *Perspectives on oral manifestations of AIDS,* Proceedings of a symposium held Jan. 18-20, 1988 in San Diego, Littleton, Mass, PSG, 1988.
43. Greene JC: General principles of epidemiology and methods for measuring prevalence and severity of periodontal disease. In Genco RJ, Goldman H, Cohen DW, editors: *Contemporary periodontics,* St Louis, 1990, Mosby.

44. Greenspan D, Schiodt M, Greenspan JS, et al: *AIDS and the mouth: diagnosis and management of oral lesions,* Copenhagen, 1990, Munksgaard.

45. Greenstein G: The role of bleeding upon probing in the diagnosis of periodontal disease, *J Periodontol* 55:684, 1984.

46. Greenstein G: Nonsurgical periodontal therapy in 2000: a literature review, *J Am Dent Assoc* 131:1580, 2000.

47. Haffajee AD, Socransky SS: Attachment level changes in destructive periodontal diseases, *J Clin Periodontol* 13:461, 1986.

48. Haffajee A, Socransky S: Microbial etiological agents of destructive periodontal diseases, *Periodontol* 2000 5:78, 1994.

49. Haffajee AD, Socransky SS, Goodson JM: Clinical parameters as predictors of destructive periodontal disease activity, *J Clin Periodontol* 10:257, 1983.

50. Heijl L, Dahlen G, Sundin Y, et al: A 4-quadrant comparative study of periodontal treatment using tetracycline-containing drug delivery fibers and scaling, *J Clin Periodontol* 18:111, 1991.

51. Hugoson A, Thorstensson H, Falk H: Periodontal conditions in insulin-dependent diabetics, *J Clin Periodontol* 16:215, 1989.

52. Hujoel PP, Drangholt MT, Speikerman C, et al: Periodontal disease and risk of coronary heart disease, *JAMA* 284:1406, 2000.

53. Hujoel PP, Drangholt MT, Speikerman C, et al: Examining the link between coronary heart disease and the elimination of chronic dental infections, *J Am Dent Assoc* 132:883, 2001.

54. Ingham HR: Metronidazole compared with penicillin in the treatment of acute dental infections, *J Oral Surg* 14:364, 1977.

55. Ishikawa I, Nakashima K, Koseki T, et al: Induction of the immune response to periodontopathic bacteria and its role in the pathogenesis of periodontitis, *Periodontol* 2000 14:79, 1997.

56. Jacobs MH: Pericoronal and Vincent's infections: bacteriology and treatment. *J Am Dent Assoc* 30:392, 1943.

57. Jeffcoat MK, Geurs NC, Reddy MS: Periodontal infection and preterm birth: results of a prospective study, *J Am Dent Assoc* 132:875, 2001.

58. Jimenez LM, Baer PN: Necrotizing ulcerative gingivitis in children: a 9-year clinical study, *J Periodontol* 46:715, 1975.

59. Johnson BD, Engel D: Acute necrotizing ulcerative gingivitis: a review of diagnosis, etiology and treatment, *J Periodontol* 57:141, 1986.

60. Kay LW: Investigations in the nature of pericoronitis—II, *Br J Oral Surg* 62:1025, 1966.

61. Kelstrup J, Theilade E: Microbes and periodontal disease, *J Clin Periodontol* 1:15, 1974.

62. Killoy WJ: Treatment of periodontal abscesses. In Genco RJ, Goldman HM, Cohen DW, editors: *Contemporary periodontics,* St Louis, 1990, Mosby.

63. Knowles JW, Burgett FG, Nissle RR, et al: Results of periodontal treatment related to pocket depth and attachment level: eight years, *J Periodontol* 50:225, 1979.

64. Kornman KS: The role of supragingival plaque in the prevention and treatment of periodontal disease: a review of concepts, *J Periodontal Res* 21(suppl 16):5, 1986.

65. Kornman KS, Loesche WJ: The subgingival microflora during pregnancy, *J Periodontal Res* 15:111, 1980.

66. Kornman KS, Newman MG, Alvarado R, et al: Clinical and microbiological patterns of adults with periodontitis, *J Periodontol* 62:634, 1991.

67. Lang NP, Brecx MC: Chlorhexidine digluconate: an agent for chemical plaque control and prevention of gingival inflammation, *J Periodontal Res* 21(suppl 16):74, 1986.

68. Lang NP, Cumming BR, Loe H: Toothbrushing frequency as it relates to plaque development and gingival health, *J Periodontol* 44:396, 1973.

69. Lang NP, Kiel RA, Anderhalden K, et al: Clinical and microbial effects of subgingival restorations with overhanging or clinically perfect margins, *J Clin Periodontol* 10:563, 1983.

70. Linden G, Mullaly BH: Cigarette smoking and periodontal destruction in young adults, *J Periodontol* 65:718, 1994.

71. Lindhe J, Svanberg G: Influence of trauma from occlusion on progression of experimental periodontitis in the beagle dog, *J Clin Periodontol* 1:3, 1974.

72. Listgarten MA: Electron microscopic observation on the bacterial flora of acute necrotizing ulcerative gingivitis, *J Periodontol* 36:328, 1965.

73. Listgarten MA, Lewis DW: The distribution of acute necrotizing ulcerative gingivitis: an electron microscopic and statistical survey, *J Periodontol* 38:379, 1967.

74. Löe H: Human research model for the production and prevention of gingivitis, *J Dent Res* 50:256, 1971.

75. Löe H: Chlorhexidine in the prophylaxis of dental diseases, *J Periodontal Res* 8:5, 1973.

76. Löe H, Anerud A, Boysen H, et al: The natural history of periodontal disease in man: the rate of periodontal destruction before 40 years of age, *J Periodontol* 409:67, 1978.

77. Löe H, Anerud A, Boysen H, et al: Natural history of periodontal disease in man: rapid, moderate and no loss of attachment in Sri Lankan laborers 14-46 years of age, *J Clin Periodontol* 13:431, 1986.

78. Löe H, Brown LJ: Early onset periodontitis in the United States of America, *J Periodontol* 62:608, 1991.

79. Löe H, Morrison E: Epidemiology of periodontal disease. In Genco RJ, Goldman HM, and Cohen DW, editors: *Contemporary periodontics,* St Louis, 1990, Mosby.

80. Löe H, Schiott CR: The effect of chlorhexidine mouth rinses and topical application of chlorhexidine on the development of dental plaque and gingivitis in man, *J Periodont Res* 5:79, 1970.

81. Löe H, Silness J: Periodontal disease in pregnancy. I. Prevalence and severity, *Acta Odontol Scand* 21:533, 1963.

82. Löe H, Theilade E, Jensen SB: Experimental gingivitis in man, *J Periodontol* 36:177, 1965.

83. Loesche WJ: Periodontal disease and the treponemes. In Johnson RC, editor: *The biology of parasitic spirochetes,* New York, 1976, Academic Press.

84. Loesche WJ: The role of spirochetes in periodontal disease, *Adv Dent Res* 2:275, 1988.

85. Loesche WJ, Schmidt E, Smith BA, et al: Metronidazole therapy for periodontitis, *J Clin Periodontol* 22:224, 1987.

86. Loesche WJ, Syed SA: Bacteriology of human experimental gingivitis: effect of plaque and gingivitis score, *Infect Immun* 21:830, 1978.

87. Loesche WJ, Syed SA, Laughon BE, et al: The bacteriology of acute necrotizing ulcerative gingivitis, *J Periodontol* 53:223, 1982.

88. Lovdal A, Arno A, Schei O, et al: Combined effect of subgingival scaling and controlled oral hygiene on the incidence of gingivitis, *Acta Odontol Scand* 19:537, 1961.

89. Lucht E, Heimdahl A, Nord CE: Periodontal disease in HIV-infected patients in relation to lymphocyte subsets and specific micro-organisms, *J Clin Periodontol* 18:252, 1991.

90. Ludwig TG: An investigation of the oral flora of suppurative oral swellings, *Aust Dent J* 2:259, 1957.

91. MacCarthy D, Claffey N: Acute necrotizing ulcerative gingivitis is associated with attachment loss, *J Clin Periodontol* 18:776, 1991.

92. Marshall-Day CD: The epidemiology of periodontal disease, *J Periodontol* 22:13, 1951.

93. Mealey BL: Influence of periodontal infections on systemic health, *Periodontol 2000* 21:197, 1999.

94. Meitner SW, Zander HA, Iker HP, et al: Identification of inflamed gingival surfaces, *J Clin Periodontol* 6:93, 1979.

95. Merchant NE: Infections related to the jaws, *Practitioner* 209:679, 1972.

96. Miller AJ, Brunelle JA, Carlos JP, et al: *Oral health of United Stated adults: the national survey of oral health in U.S. employed adults and seniors:* 1985-1986 (NIH publication No. 87-2868), Bethesda, Md, National Institutes of Health, 1987.

97. Miller WD: *The micro-organisms of the mouth,* Philadelphia, 1890, SS White Dental Manufacturing.

98. Mombelli A, Buser D, Lang NP, et al: Suspected periodontopathogens in erupting third molar sites of periodontally healthy individuals, *J Clin Periodontol* 17:48, 1990.

99. Moore JR, Russell C: Bacteriological investigation of dental abscesses, *Dent Pract Dent Rec* 22:390, 1972.

100. Moore WEC: Microbiology of periodontal disease, *J Periodontal Res* 22:335, 1987.

101. Moore WEC, Holdeman LV, Cato EP: Bacteriology of moderate ("chronic") periodontitis in mature adult humans, *Infect Immun* 42:510, 1983.

102. Moore WEC, Holdeman LV, Cato EP, et al: Variation in periodontal floras, *Infect Immun* 46:720, 1984.

103. Moore WEC, Moore LH, Ranney RR, et al: The microflora of periodontal sites showing active destructive progression, *J Clin Periodontol* 18:729, 1991.

104. Murray PA: Periodontal diseases in patients infected by human immunodeficiency virus, *Periodontol 2000* 6:50, 1994.

105. Murray PA, Grassi M, Winkler JR: The microbiology of HIV-associated periodontal lesions, *J Clin Periodontol* 16:636, 1989.

106. Murray PA, Patters MR: Gingival crevice neutrophil function in periodontal lesions, *J Periodontal Res* 15:463, 1980.

107. Murray PA, Winkler JR, Sadowski L, et al: Microbiology of HIV-associated gingivitis and periodontitis. In Robertson PB, Greenspan JS, editors: *Perspectives on oral manifestations of AIDS, diagnosis and management of HIV-associated infections,* Littleton, Mass, 1988, PSG.

108. Nabers JM, Meador HL, Nabers CL, et al: Chronology, an important factor in the treatment of osseous defects, *Periodontics* 2:304, 1964.

109. Neely AL: Prevalence of juvenile periodontitis in a circumpubertal population, *J Clin Periodontol* 19:367, 1992.

110. Newman MG, Sanz M: Advanced diagnostic techniques. In Carranza F, Newman MG, editors: *Clinical periodontology,* ed 8, Philadelphia, 1996, WB Saunders.

111. Newman MG, Sims TN: The predominant cultivable flora of the periodontal abscess, *J Periodontol* 50:350, 1978.

112. Nitzan DW, Tal O, Sela MN, et al: Pericoronitis: a reappraisal of its clinical and microbiologic aspects, *J Oral Maxillofac Surg* 43:510, 1985.

113. Offenbacher S: Periodontal diseases: pathogenesis, *Ann Periodontol* 1:821, 1996.

114. Offenbacher S, Katz V, Fertik G, et al: Periodontal infection as possible risk factor for preterm low birth weight, *J Periodontol* 67:1103, 1996.

115. Overholser CD, Peterson DE, Williams LT, et al: Periodontal infection in patients with acute nonlymphocytic leukemia: prevalence of acute exacerbations, *Arch Intern Med* 142:551, 1982.

116. Page RC: Rapidly progressive periodontitis: a distinct clinical condition, *J Periodontol* 54:197, 1983.

117. Page RC, Bowen T, Altman L, et al: Prepubertal periodontitis. I. Definition of a clinical disease entity, *J Periodontol* 54:257, 1983.

118. Page RC, Schroeder HE: Pathogenesis of inflammatory periodontal disease: a summary of current work, *Lab Invest* 33:235, 1976.

119. Page RC, Schroeder H: *Periodontitis in man and other animals,* Basel, 1982, Karger.

120. Perkins AE: Acute infections around erupting mandibular third molar, *Br Dent J* 76:199, 1944.

121. Peterson DE, Minah GE, Overholser CD, et al: Microbiology of acute periodontal infection in myelosuppressed cancer patients, *J Clin Oncol* 5:1461, 1987.

122. Pihlstrom BL, McHugh RB, Oliphant TH, et al: Comparison of surgical and nonsurgical treatment of periodontal disease: a review of current studies and additional results after 6½ years, *J Clin Periodontol* 10:524, 1983.

123. Pindborg JJ, Bhat M, Devanath KR, et al: Occurrence of acute necrotizing gingivitis in South Indian children, *J Periodontol* 37:14, 1966.

124. Pindborg JJ, Holmstrupp P: Acute necrotizing ulcerative gingivitis related to HIV infection, *Afr Dent J* 1:5, 1987.

125. Polson AM, Meitner SW, Zander HA: Reversibility of bone loss due to trauma alone and trauma superimposed upon periodontitis, *J Periodontal Res* 11:290, 1976.

126. Ramfjord SP, Emslie RD, Green JC, et al: Epidemiological studies of periodontal disease, *Am J Public Health* 58:1713, 1968.

127. Rams TE, Andriolo M, Feik D, et al: Microbiological study of HIV-related periodontitis, *J Periodontol* 63:74, 1991.

128. Ranney RR: Diagnosis of periodontal disease, *Adv Dent Res* 5:21, 1991.

129. Ranney RR, Best AM, Breen TJ, et al: Bacterial flora of progressing periodontitis lesions, *J Periodontal Res* 22: 205, 1987.

130. Rehwinkel FH: Pyhorrha alveolaris, *Dent Cosmos* 29:572, 1877.

131. Reynolds RJ, Meikle MC: Mechanisms of connective tissue matrix destruction in periodontitis, *Periodontol 2000* 14:144, 1997.

132. Russell AL: International nutritional surveys: a summary of preliminary findings, *J Dent Res* 42:232, 1963.

133. Russell AL: The prevalence of periodontal disease in different populations during the circumpubertal period, *J Periodontol* 42:508, 1971.

134. Saglie R, Carranza FA Jr, Newman MG, et al: Bacterial invasion of gingiva in advanced periodontitis in humans, *J Periodontol* 53:217, 1982.

135. Saglie R, Marfany A, Camargo P: Intragingival occurrence of *Actinobacillus actinomycetemcomitans* and *Bacteroides gingivalis* in active destructive periodontal lesions, *J Periodontol* 59:259, 1988.

136. Salvi GE, Lawrence HP, Offenbacher S, et al: Influence of risk factors on the pathogenesis of periodontitis, *Periodontol 2000* 14:173, 1997.

137. Sanz M, Newman MG, Nisengard R: Periodontal microbiology. In Carranza F, editor: *Glickman's clinical periodontology,* ed 7, Philadelphia, 1990, WB Saunders.

138. Schei O, Waerhaug J, Lovdal A, et al: Alveolar bone loss as related to oral hygiene and age, *J Periodont* 30:7, 1959.

139. Schenkein HA, Gunsolley JC, Koertge TE, et al: Smoking and its effects on early-onset periodontitis, *J Am Dent Assoc* 126:1107, 1995.

140. Schiott CR, Briner WW, Kirkland JJ, et al: Two years' oral use of chlorhexidine in man. Part 3. Changes in sensitivity of the salivary flora, *J Periodontal Res* 11:153, 1976.

141. Schiott CR, Briner WW, Loe H: Two years' oral use of chlorhexidine in man. Part 2. The effect on the salivary bacterial flora, *J Periodontal Res* 11:145, 1976.

142. Schiott CR, Loe H, Briner WW: Two years' oral use of chlorhexidine in man. Part 4. Effect on various medical parameters, *J Periodontal Res* 11:158, 1976.

143. Schluger S, Yuodelis R, Page RC, et al: *Periodontal diseases. Basic phenomenon, clinical management, and occlusal and restorative relationships,* Philadelphia, 1990, Lea & Febiger.

144. Schwartz Z, Goultschin J, Dean DD, et al: Mechanisms of alveolar bone destruction in periodontitis, *Periodontol* 2000 14:158, 1997.

145. Seward GR, Harris M, McGowan DA, et al: *Killey and Kay's outline of oral surgery. Part I,* Bristol: 1987, Wright.

146. Slots J: Microflora in the healthy gingival sulcus in man, *Scand J Dent Res* 85:247, 1977.

147. Slots J: The predominant cultivable microflora of advanced periodontitis, *Scand J Dent Res* 85:114, 1977.

148. Slots J: Subgingival bacteria and periodontal disease, *J Clin Periodontol* 6:351, 1979.

149. Slots J, Genco RJ: Black-pigmented *Bacteroides* species, *Capnocytophaga* species, *Actinobacillus actinomycetemcomitans* in human periodontal disease: virulence factors in colonization, survival, and tissue destruction, *J Dent Res* 63:412, 1984.

150. Slots J, Listgarten MA: *Bacteroides gingivalis, Bacteroides intermedius* and *Actinobacillus actinomycetemcomitans* in human periodontal disease, *J Clin Periodontol* 15:85, 1988.

151. Slots J, Moenbo D, Langeback J, et al: Microbiota of gingivitis in man, *Scand J Dent Res* 86:174, 1978.

152. Slots J, Rams TE: Antibiotics in periodontal therapy: advantages and disadvantages, *J Clin Periodontol* 17:479, 1990.

153. Slots J, Rams TE: Microbiology of periodontal disease. In Slots J, Taubman MA, editors: *Contemporary oral microbiology and immunology,* St Louis, 1992, Mosby.

154. Slots J, Ting M: *Actinobacillus actinomycetemcomitans* and *Porphyromonas gingivalis* in human periodontal disease: occurrence and treatment, *Periodontol* 2000 20:82, 1999.

155. Socransky SS: Microbiology of periodontal disease: present status and future considerations, *J Periodontol* 48:497, 1977.

156. Socransky SS: Criteria for infectious agents in dental caries and periodontal disease, *J Clin Periodontol* 6:16, 1979.

157. Socransky SS, Haffajee AD, Goodson JM, et al: New concepts of destructive periodontal disease, *J Clin Periodontol* 11:21, 1984.

158. Stamm JW: Epidemiology of gingivitis, *J Clin Periodontol* 13:360, 1986.

159. Tanner ACR, Haffer C, Bratthall GT, et al: A study of the bacteria associated with advancing periodontitis in man, *J Clin Periodontol* 6:278, 1979.

160. Theilade E: The non-specific theory in microbial etiology of inflammatory periodontal diseases, *J Clin Periodontol* 13: 905, 1986.

161. Theilade E, Wright WH, Jensen SB, et al: Experimental gingivitis in man. II. A longitudinal clinical and bacteriological investigation, *J Periodontal Res* 1:1, 1966.

162. Tomar SL, Asma S: Smoking-attributable periodontitis in the United States: findings from NHANES III, *J Periodontol* 71:743, 2000.

163. Topoll HH, Lange DE, Muller RF: Multiple periodontal abscesses after systemic antibiotic therapy, *J Clin Periodontol* 17:268, 1990.

164. Van der Velden U: The onset age of periodontal destruction, *J Clin Periodontol* 18:380, 1991.

165. Van Palenstein Heldermann WH: Is antibiotic therapy justified in the treatment of human chronic inflammatory periodontal disease? *J Clin Periodontol* 13:932, 1986.

166. Wade WG, Gray AR, Absi EG, et al: Predominant cultivable flora in pericoronitis, *Oral Microbiol Immunol* 6:310, 1991.

167. Waerhaug J: *Epidemiology of periodontal disease—a review of the literature.* World Workshop in Periodontics, Ann Arbor, Mich, University of Michigan, 1966.

168. Watanabe K: Prepubertal periodontitis: a review of diagnostic criteria, pathogenesis and differential diagnosis, *J Periodontal Res* 25:31, 1990.

169. Williams CA, Winkler JR, Grassi M: HIV-associated periodontitis complicated by necrotizing stomatitis, *Oral Surg Oral Med Oral Pathol* 3:351, 1990.

170. Williams RC: Periodontal disease, *N Engl J Med* 322:373, 1990.

171. Williams CE, Davenport ES, Sterne JA, et al: Mechanisms of risk in preterm low-birth weight infants, *Periodontol* 2000 23:142, 2000.

172. Winkler JR, Grassi M, Murray PA: Perspectives on oral manifestations of AIDS. Clinical description and etiology of HIV-associated periodontal disease. In Robertson BB, Greenspan JS, editors: *Proceedings of a symposium held Jan. 18-20, 1988 in San Diego,* Littleton, Mass, 1988, PSG.

173. Winkler JR, Murray PA, Grassi M, et al: Diagnosis and management of HIV-associated periodontal lesions, *J Am Dent Assoc* Nov(suppl):25-S, 1989.

174. Winkler JR, Murray PA, Hammerle C: Gangrenous stomatitis in AIDS: a complication of HIV-associated periodontal disease? *Lancet* 2:108, 1989.

175. Wright WE: Periodontium destruction associated with oncology therapy: five case reports, *J Periodontol* 58:559, 1987.

176. Zambon JJ: Microbiology of periodontal disease. In Genco RJ, Goldman HM, Cohen DW, editors: *Contemporary periodontics,* St Louis, 1990, Mosby.

177. Zambon JJ, Christersson LA, Genco RJ: Diagnosis and treatment of localized juvenile periodontitis, *J Am Dent Assoc* 113:295, 1986.

178. Zambon JJ, Umemoto T, DeNardin E, et al: *Actinobacillus actinomycetemcomitans* in the pathogenesis of human periodontal disease, *Adv Dent Res* 2:269, 1988.

179. Zander HA, Polson AM: Present status of occlusion and occlusal therapy in periodontics, *J Periodontol* 48:540, 1977.

Pulpal Infections

1. Anderson DJ, Hannam AG, Mathews B: Sensory mechanisms in mammalian teeth and their supporting structures, *Physiol Rev* 50:171, 1970.

2. Baumann L, Rossman S: Clinical, roentgenologic, and histopathologic findings in teeth with apical radiolucent areas, *Oral Surg* 9:1330, 1956.

3. Baume LJ: Diagnosis of diseases of the pulp, *Oral Surg* 29:102, 1970.

4. Baumgartner JC, Falkler WA Jr: Bacteria in the apical 5 mm of infected root canals, *J Endod* 17:380, 1991.

5. Bhaskar SN: Oral surgery–oral pathology conference No. 17, Walter Reed Army Medical Center. Periapical lesions: types, incidence, and clinical features, *Oral Surg* 21:657, 1966.

6. Brannstrom M, Johnson G, Linden LA: Fluid flow and pain response in the dentine produced by hydrostatic pressure, *Odontol Revy* 20:15, 1969.

7. Brannstrom M, Johnson G, Nordenvall KJ: Transmission and control of dentinal pain: resin impregnation for the desensitization of dentin, *J Am Dent Assoc* 99:612, 1979.

8. Byers MR, Kish SJ: Delineation of somatic nerve endings in rat teeth by radioautography of axon-transported protein, *J Dent Res* 55:419, 1976.

9. Bystrom A, Sundqvist G: Bacteriologic evaluation of the effect of 0.5 percent sodium hypochlorite in endodontic therapy, *Oral Surg* 55:307, 1983.

10. Curran JB, Kennett S, Young AR: An assessment of the use of prophylactic antibiotics in third molar surgery, *Int J Oral Surg* 3:1, 1974.

11. Delivanis PD, Snowden RB, Doyle RJ: Localization of blood-borne bacteria in instrumented unfilled root canals, *Oral Surg* 52:430, 1981.

12. Dubner R: Neurophysiology of pain, *Dent Clin North Am* 22:11, 1978.

13. Garfunkel A, Sela J, Ulmansky M: Dental pulp pathosis: clinicopathologic correlations based on 109 cases, *Oral Surg* 35:110, 1973.

14. Hasler JE, Mitchell DF: Painless pulpitis, *J Am Dent Assoc* 81:671, 1970.

15. Hausmann E, Weinfeld N, Miller WA: Effects of lipopolysaccharides on bone resorption in tissue culture, *Calcif Tissue Res* 9:272, 1972.

16. Henrici A, Hartzell T: The bacteriology of vital pulps, *J Dent Res* 1:419, 1919.

17. Kakehashi S, Stanley HR, Fitzgerald RJ: The effects of surgical exposures of dental pulps in germ-free and conventional laboratory rats, *Oral Surg* 20:340, 1965.

18. Kantz WE, Henry CA: Isolation and classification of anaerobic bacteria from intact pulp chambers of non-vital teeth in man, *Arch Oral Biol* 19:91, 1974.

19. Lalonde ER, Luebke RG: The frequency and distribution of periapical cysts and granulomas: an evaluation of 800 specimens, *Oral Surg* 25:861, 1968.

20. Langeland K, Block RM, Grossman LI: A histopathologic and histobacteriologic study of 35 periapical endodontic surgical specimens, *J Endod* 3:8, 1977.

21. Madison S, Whitsel EA, Suarez-Roca H, et al: Sensitizing effects of leukotriene B4 on intradental primary afferents, *Pain* 49:99, 1992.

22. McGrath PA, Gracely RH, Dubner R, et al: Non-pain and pain sensations evoked by tooth pulp stimulation, *Pain* 15:377, 1983.

23. Narhi MV: The characteristics of intradental sensory units and their responses to stimulation. *J Dent Res* 64 Spec No:564, 1985.

24. Nobuhara WK, del Rio CE: Incidence of periradicular pathoses in endodontic treatment failures, *J Endod* 19:315, 1993.

25. Olgart LM: The role of local factors in dentin and pulp in intradental pain mechanisms, *J Dent Res* 64 Spec No:572, 1985.

26. Paterson JA, Cardo VA Jr, Stratigos GT: An examination of antibiotic prophylaxis in oral and maxillofacial surgery, *J Oral Surg* 28:753, 1970.

27. Pendrill K, Reddy J: The use of prophylactic penicillin in periodontal surgery, *J Periodontol* 51:44, 1980.

28. Rietschel ET, Brade H: Bacterial endotoxins, *Sci Am* 267:54, 1992.

29. Robinson H, Boling L: The anachoretic effect in pulpitis. I. Bacteriologic studies, *J Am Dent Assoc* 28:268, 1941.

30. Schonfeld S, Greening A, Glick D, et al: Endotoxic activity in periapical lesions, *Oral Surg* 53:82, 1982.

31. Seltzer S, Farber PA: Microbiologic factors in endodontology, *Oral Surg* 78:634, 1994.

32. Sessle BJ, Bradley RM, Dubner R, et al: Dental neuroscience, *New Dent* 10:32, 1979.

33. Sharav Y, Leviner E, Tzukert A, et al: The spatial distribution, intensity and unpleasantness of acute dental pain, *Pain* 20:363, 1984.

34. Sundqvist G: Ecology of the root canal flora, *J Endod* 18:427, 1992.

35. Sundqvist GK, Eckerbom MI, Larsson AP, et al: Capacity of anaerobic bacteria from necrotic dental pulps to induce purulent infections, *Infect Immun* 25:685, 1979.

36. Sundqvist G, Johansson E, Sjögren U: Prevalence of black-pigmented bacteroides species in root canal infections, *J Endod* 15:13, 1989.

37. Tani N, Osada T, Watanabe Y, et al: Comparative immunohistochemical identification and relative distribution of immunocompetent cells in sections of frozen or formalin-fixed tissue from human periapical inflammatory lesions, *Endod Dent Traumatol* 8:163, 1992.

38. Torabinejad M: Mediators of acute and chronic periradicular lesions, *Oral Surg* 78:511, 1994.

39. Trowbridge HO: Pathogenesis of pulpitis resulting from dental caries, *J Endod* 7:52, 1981.

40. Valderhaug J: A histologic study of experimentally produced intra-oral odontogenic fistulae in monkeys, *Int J Oral Surg* 2:54, 1973.

41. Van Hassel H: Physiology of the human dental pulp, *Oral Surg* 32:126, 1971.

42. Virtanen AS, Huopaniemi T, Narhi MV, et al: The effect of temporal parameters on subjective sensations evoked by electrical tooth stimulation, *Pain* 30:361, 1987.

43. Wais F: Significance of findings following biopsy and histological study of 100 periapical lesions, *Oral Surg* 11:650, 1958.

44. Wayman BE, Murata SM, Almeida RJ, et al: A bacteriological and histological evaluation of 58 periapical lesions, *J Endod* 18:152, 1992.

45. Winkler K, Van Amerongen J: Bacteriologic results from 4000 root canal cultures, *Oral Surg* 12:855, 1959.

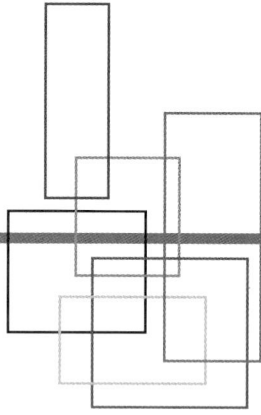

Odontogenic Infections and Deep Fascial Space Infections of Dental Origin

Morton H. Goldberg
Richard G. Topazian

Dentistry is largely the treatment of dental infection or the restoration and replacement of dentition lost to bacterial infection. The prevention and treatment of orofacial infection involve every aspect of dental care: caries, pulpal disease, gingivoperiodontal pathological conditions, trauma, and reconstructive and implant surgery. The surgeon routinely faces the realities of the potentially pathogenic flora of odontogenic infection when surgical procedures are performed in or around the oral cavity.

Dental infection has plagued humankind for as long as our species has existed. Little imagination is required to picture a primitive man suffering pain and swelling of the face because of fractured teeth, dental caries, or periodontal disease. Indeed, infection of dental origin is one of the most common diseases of humans and in underdeveloped countries a frequent cause of death. The remains of pre-Columbian Indians, unearthed in the American Midwest, and the remains of people who lived in early Egypt have revealed the bony crypts of dental abscesses, sinus tracts, and the ravages of osteomyelitis of the jaws.

Treatment of localized infection was probably the first primitive surgical procedure performed, and it most likely involved the opening of bulging abscesses with sharp stones or pointed sticks. Today the principle remains the same; fortunately, the technique has improved.

Not until the early twentieth century, however, was a causal relationship definitely established between dental infection and the severe life-threatening neck swelling that Ludwig described nearly 70 years earlier.[10] Although therapy has progressed, the scalpel, extraction forceps, and the endodontic reamer remain the keystones of therapy for odontogenic infections, along with the judicious use of antibiotics.

Despite great advances in dental care in Western society, including fluoridation of water, early interception of caries, and periodontal prophylaxis, infection remains a major problem of dental practice. Although penicillin was considered the long-awaited panacea for dental infection, the bacteriological spectrum of the oral flora and the understanding of its complexities have undergone rapid evolution since penicillin was introduced.

Before the antibiotic era, most serious odontogenic infections were known to be streptococcal; but the problem of bacterial resistance to antibiotics soon became obvious in the oral cavity, as elsewhere. The serious epidemic of penicillin-resistant staphylococcal infections of the 1950s and 1960s finally was resolved by the development of the semisynthetic antibiotics, which are not metabolized by the penicillinase enzyme of the staphylococci. The widespread use of these drugs has resulted in the current plague of human infection from enteric (gram-negative) and opportunistic organisms, including vancomycin-resistant enterococci and methicillin-resistant staphylococci. Mutation and selective genetic pressure have resulted in species that now exhibit resistance to multiple antibiotics, a situation complicated by deoxyribonucleic acid exchange among species.

Nature abhors a vacuum, even a biological one. The empty ecological niche created by the decline of certain pathogenic bacterial species soon is filled by other organisms. The human oral cavity is a biological system that supports life for many species of microorganisms. Bacterial infection of dental origin is a constantly changing but measurable reflection of the modern evolution of the oral flora.

During the past four decades, dangerous and life-threatening dental infections have been reported and are related to a variety of bacterial species, some opportunistic, others nosocomial, and a few anaerobic. These include *Pseudomonas, Proteus, Escherichia coli, Serratia, Acinetobacter (Mima), Klebsiella, Eikenella, Bacteroides (Prevotella), Coryne-bacterium,* and other less common organisms. For example, *Pseudomonas,* once thought to be a rare transient in the oral cavity, currently is found in the saliva of 5% to 10% of healthy subjects. Similar changes have been observed in the pharyngeal flora that are probably related to antibiotic-induced reduction of normal flora, acquiring of new flora during hospitalization, and use of immunosuppressive drugs. Aerobic gram-negative rods inhabit the pharynges of 5% of normal nonhospitalized persons but colonize the pharynges of more than 60% of institutionalized elderly and hospitalized patients with serious illnesses, those who have undergone surgical procedures, and critical care health workers.

Nevertheless, aerobic and anaerobic streptococci, *Bacteroides, Fusobacterium,* and *Eikenella,* and mixed aerobic-anaerobic flora are the organisms most commonly identified in odontogenic infections in otherwise healthy patients. Quantitative estimations of the number of microorganisms in saliva and plaque range as high as 10^{11}/mL. In the depths of a periodontal pocket, the number of anaerobes per gram of curetted material may reach 1.8×10^{11}/mL, approximately the same concentration of anaerobes in human feces. Considering the plethora of microorganisms that grow luxuriantly in this wet, warm, dark, and debris-strewn cavity, the effectiveness of the systemic and oral host defense mechanisms in preventing serious infection from commonplace minor trauma such as cheek biting or the shedding of deciduous teeth is remarkable.

PRINCIPLES FOR EXAMINATION

Patients with an infection may have signs and symptoms ranging from the trivial to the extremely serious. A rapid initial assessment of the patient's status should be made to determine the presence of an acute illness requiring urgent care or a less severe problem treatable in a more deliberate manner. Individuals who display signs of toxicity, central nervous system changes, or airway compromise should be considered for immediate hospitalization with aggressive medical and surgical intervention, including intubation and tracheostomy (see Chapter 23). Indications of possibly fatal infections are respiratory impairment; difficulty in swallowing; impaired vision, eye movement, or both; change in voice quality; lethargy; and decreased level of consciousness. Toxicity is suggested by paleness, tachypnea, tachycardia, fever, appearance of illness, shivering, lethargy, and diaphoresis. Significant central nervous system changes associated with infection are decreased level of consciousness, evidence of meningeal irritation (severe headache, stiff neck, vomiting), eyelid edema, and abnormal eye signs.

The basic principles of patient evaluation must be observed if an accurate diagnosis and appropriate treatment are to be achieved. Inaccurate diagnoses and inappropri-

ate therapy complicate or prevent proper care, and almost always result from failure to identify properly the major problem that caused the patient to seek care. Departure from an orderly approach often occurs. For example, an inadequate oropharyngeal examination in a patient with hypoxia may not discover pharyngeal space infection of odontogenic origin, a mistake that can be fatal.

Patient evaluation is based on a careful history, including a review of systems, physical examination, appropriate laboratory and imaging studies, and proper interpretation of the findings. In the patient with infection the likely pathogens and host factors must be considered early in the evaluation. Whether a patient has been hospitalized or is an outpatient, recognition of each initial problem is of great value in directing attention to all of the patient's needs. A problem list is derived from the database, consisting of a complete history, physical examination, and imaging and laboratory data. The database is used to identify the problems requiring attention. Treatment plans then are derived by isolating each problem and its parameters from the mass of data in the database.

Important findings in the database must be understood in the light of the pathophysiology of infection and in terms of the mechanisms responsible for signs and symptoms. Accordingly, the inflammatory response and signs of infections are discussed briefly.

PATHOPHYSIOLOGY OF INFECTION: THE INFLAMMATORY RESPONSE

The body's response to infectious agents is inflammation, which is essentially protective. Toxic substances are diluted, neutralized, localized, or dissipated. Ultimately, repair of the tissues ensues. In the patient whose immune system is competent to deal with infection the following events transpire:

1. Hyperemia caused by vasodilation of arterioles and capillaries, and increased permeability of venules with slowing of the venous blood flow
2. Passage of exudate rich in plasma proteins, antibodies, and nutrients, and the escape of leukocytes into the surrounding tissues
3. Release of a permeability factor, leukotaxin, which allows migration of polymorphonuclear leukocytes (and later monocytes) into the area
4. Precipitation of a network of fibrin from the exudate, tending to wall off the region
5. Phagocytosis of bacteria, other organisms, and dead cells
6. Disposal by macrophages of necrotic debris

SIGNS OF INFECTION

The cardinal signs of inflammation are present to some degree in nearly all patients with infection. Their absence may indicate that the acute phase of infection is subsiding, infection is spreading through deeper tissues, drug therapy is effective (analgesics, antibiotics), or the patient is a compromised host. *Rubor,* or redness, is seen when infection is close to the tissue surface in individuals with light complexions and is the result of vasodilation. *Tumor,* or swelling, results from the accumulation of fluid exudate or pus. *Calor,* or heat, is the result of inflow of relatively warm blood from the deeper tissues, increased quantity of blood flow caused by vasodilation, and increased rate of metabolism. *Dolor,* or pain, results from pressure on sensory nerve endings from distention of tissues caused by edema or spread of infection. The action of liberated or activated factors such as kinins, histamine, metabolites, or bradykinin-like substances on nerve endings also is responsible for pain, as is the loss of tonicity of injured tissues. *Functio laesa,* or loss of function, is reflected in difficulty in chewing, swallowing, and respiratory embarrassment. Loss of function of the inflamed part is caused by mechanical factors and reflex inhibition of muscle movements associated with pain.

Fever   The normal oral temperature ranges from 97.7° F to 99.5° F, with an average of 98.6° F. In children the oral temperature averages 0.3° F higher. The rectal temperature is approximately 1° F higher, and axillary or inguinal temperature is 1° to 3° F lower. Increased temperature ordinarily is one of the most consistent signs of infection, but it also may be a manifestation of neoplastic disease such as lymphoma, noninfectious inflammatory disorders such as rheumatoid arthritis, or excess catabolism as in thyrotoxicosis. Normal or subnormal temperatures in the presence of infection may be caused by metabolic abnormalities such as myxedema or uremia.

Body temperature results from a balance between heat production and heat loss and is maintained by the movement of heat from sites of metabolic heat production (deep organs, heart, viscera, and brain) in the body core to the skin through the circulation. Temperature is controlled by complex systems involving the hypothalamus and the vasomotor, sudomotor, and shivering systems. In clinical fever the hypothalamic thermoregulating centers are stimulated by endogenous pyrogen, which is activated by bacterial endotoxins and released from granulocytes, monocytes, and macrophages.

Young patients often have a high temperature even during trivial infection, whereas elderly patients may have little temperature change even during severe infections. Variables affecting temperature are concurrent antipyretic or corticosteroid therapy, site of temperature determination, recent oral intake of warm or cold beverages, and length of time in determining the temperature. The use of antipyretics often is responsible for misleading the clinician. Not all patients require antipyretics. Temperatures lower than 102° F probably do not harm the patient and may indeed be helpful because increases in temperature enhance phagocytic activity. Antipyretics do not alter the course of an infection, and their use deprives the clinician of one clear way of monitoring the patient's response to therapy. Therefore when the patient does not complain of temper-

ature elevation or has a temperature less than 102° F, many clinicians prefer not to prescribe antipyretics during the acute phase of the infectious disease.

Oral temperature may vary by as much as 3° F from one side of the mouth to the other when infection is localized to one side. The oral temperature also is altered by recent cold drinks and mouth breathing. The thermometer should be placed on the side of the mouth opposite the infection. The thermometer should be left in place for at least 3 minutes for rectal and 5 minutes for oral readings if not using a digital thermometer. Temperature assessment probes that use the auditory canal are of value, especially in children. Rectal thermometers, although inconvenient, are quite accurate. The patient's temperature should be interpreted with caution, especially if it is inconsistent with laboratory and clinical findings.

A history of repeated chills is common in bacteremias and pyogenic abscesses. Headache, which commonly accompanies infection, usually is associated with fever and results from stretching of sensitive structures surrounding dilated intracranial arteries.

Lymphadenopathy   Lymphadenopathy may be present as a result of odontogenic infections. In acute infection, lymph nodes are enlarged, soft, and tender. The surrounding skin is red and the associated tissues are edematous. In chronic infection the enlarged nodes generally are less firm (depending on the degree of inflammation), often are not tender, and edema of the surrounding skin is unusual. The location of enlarged nodes often indicates the site of infection.

Suppuration of nodes occurs when the infecting organism overwhelms the local defense mechanism in the node and produces excessive cellular reaction and collection of pus. This process may subside spontaneously, require incision and drainage, or lead to destruction of the node with spontaneous rupture and drainage. Suppuration may occur in a single node or in a coalescence of multiple nodes.

HISTORY AND REVIEW OF SYSTEMS

Any aspect of the history may provide clues to the nature and location of the problem and the possibility of host factors affecting the disease process. Thus information about the origin, extent, location, and potential severity of the problem is obtained by a careful history.

The clinician should obtain the following information: the history of the present illness as it relates to the onset; history of toothache or headache; nature, location, and duration of pain and chills; and previous treatment and its effects, including possible trauma to the soft and hard tissues of the region. Of special importance are a history of recurrent or frequent infections, previous hospitalizations with infection, or an infection without an appropriate response, all of which suggest a host disorder. The presence of draining fistulas or sinuses, difficulty in opening the mouth, difficulty in swallowing, increased salivation, changes in phonation, any difficulty in breathing, or foul breath odor should be noted.

PHYSICAL EXAMINATION

A comprehensive regional examination of the patient should include inspection, palpation, and percussion. The skin of the face, head, and neck should be examined carefully for swelling, injuries, and areas of tenderness, especially over the maxillary and frontal sinuses. Swellings, fluctuation, erythema, fixation of skin or mucosa to underlying bone, sinus or fistula formation, and subcutaneous crepitus occur often. Any swelling should be carefully assessed and described, and simple line drawings of the swelling should be made, showing size in centimeters, and extent and relationship to regional anatomical structures. Palpation is used to confirm size, note tenderness, assess local temperature, determine fluctuance and crepitus, and assess enlargement of underlying bone and salivary glands.

Assessment of regional nodes should include visible and palpable enlargement, tenderness, redness and warmth, and softness or firmness of the overlying skin. The group of nodes involved often helps determine the structure involved.

Intraorally, any trismus and its degree should be noted, with measurement of the interincisal opening. Special attention should be directed to the teeth. The clinician should check their number, the presence of caries and large restorations, localized swellings and fistulas, altered color, increased mobility, and sites of tooth extractions. Percussion with a metallic instrument or tongue blade is useful in determining hypersensitivity. When the cause of the disease is not obvious, heat and cold and electrical pulp testing of teeth provide helpful information for determining the cause of the patient's symptoms. The ducts of the parotid and submandibular glands should be visualized, and fluid (either pus or saliva) should be expressed from them if possible. Attention should be directed to the soft palate, tonsillar fossae, and oropharynx, noting displacement of tissues, presence of swelling, or drainage of pus.

Ophthalmological examination should include assessment of extraocular muscle function, proptosis, or swelling of the eyelids and dorsum of the root of the nose. The cranial nerve examination should be thorough, with special attention to nerves III, IV, and VI, particularly if ascending infection is suspected (see Chapter 15).

General examination of the thorax and extremities, with attention directed especially to any areas in which a problem was suspected during the review of systems, may yield additional useful information, especially in regard to the heart. Murmurs, for example, if not present in the patient's past history, may suggest septicemia or endocarditis, indicating the need for blood cultures.

Checking the temperature, pulse, respiratory rate, and blood pressure is vital in proper assessment of the patient, and serves as a useful baseline for noting progression or regression of the disease process. Rigors, tachypnea, and tachycardia should be noted. The pulse rate tends to increase 10 beats/min for each degree (° F) of increased temperature; therefore tachycardia commonly accompanies fever and infection, regardless of the cause or anatomical location.

The differential diagnosis of odontogenic infection is broad but should include pathological study of soft and hard tissues, including congenital, inflammatory, or developmental cysts, benign and malignant tumors, salivary gland infections and neoplasms, undiagnosed trauma, and metabolic disorders. Adequate imaging of teeth, bone, and soft tissue is essential for diagnosis and therapy. Basic laboratory studies, when indicated, include complete blood cell count, C-reactive protein, erythrocyte sedimentation rate, blood glucose levels, blood cultures, Gram staining, and culture and sensitivity of any exudate or pus from the infection site.

Inflammatory swelling of the face in adults represents odontogenic infection until proven otherwise. However, facial infections in children admitted to hospitals are odontogenic in only 11% in the upper face and 22% in the lower face. Gingivostomatitis, sinus infection, and skin infections, frequently of staphylococcal or *Haemophilus* origin, are more common and therefore require special consideration in any differential diagnosis in children.

PATHWAYS OF DENTAL INFECTION

The cause, diagnosis, and therapy for bacterial infection limited to the dental pulp or periodontal tissue are not described at length here (see Chapter 7).

The narrow pulpal foramen at the root apex, although of insufficient diameter to permit adequate drainage of infected pulp, does serve as a reservoir of bacteria and permits egress of bacteria into periodontal tissue and bone. This access explains the occasional problem when antibiotics alone are used to treat draining fistulas from abscessed teeth. Once the drainage ceases the bacteria harbored in the pulp chamber subsequently repopulate the periapical tissues from the untreated pulp, thus reinitiating the infection. Serious dental infection, spreading beyond the socket, is more commonly the result of pulpal infection than of periodontal infection. Once infection extends past the apex of the tooth, the pathophysiological course of a given infectious process can vary, depending on the number and virulence of the organism, host resistance, and anatomy of the involved area (Figure 8-1).

If the infection remains localized at the root apex, a chronic periapical infection may develop. Frequently

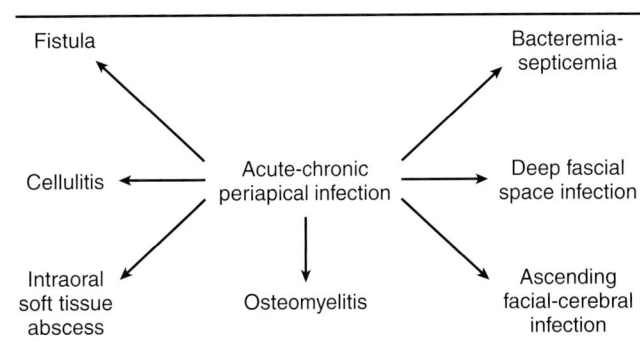

Figure 8-1 Pathways of dental infection.

sufficient destruction of bone develops to create a well-corticated radiolucency observable on dental radiographs. This process represents a focal bone infection, but "garden variety" radiolucencies associated with carious teeth should not be confused with true osteomyelitis.

Once infection extends beyond the root apex, it may proceed into deeper medullary spaces and evolve into widespread osteomyelitis. More commonly, these processes form fistulous tracts through alveolar bone and exit into the surrounding soft tissue. This phenomenon often is associated with sudden soft tissue swelling and a reduction in intrabony pressure, resulting in a lessening of pain. The fistula may penetrate the mucosa or skin, and thus serve as a natural drain for the abscess (Figure 8-2). The puckered, ulcerated, and chronically indurated appearance of such dentocutaneous fistulae frequently leads the unwary or inexperienced examiner to diagnoses ranging from chancre to cancer. Unnecessary, time-consuming and costly diagnostic procedures, including biopsy can be avoided if dental radiographs and careful examinations are performed. Dental infection should lead the list of possible diagnoses when facial swelling or a fistula is the initial sign.

Once beyond the confines of the dentoalveolar bone, infection may localize as an abscess or spread through soft tissue as cellulitis or both. In common clinical usage, these terms are often confused or used interchangeably. An *abscess* is a thick-walled cavity containing pus, whereas *cellulitis* is a diffuse, erythematous submucosal or subcutaneous infection. Staphylococci frequently are associated with abscess formation. These microorganisms produce coagulase, an enzyme that can cause fibrin deposition in citrated or oxalated blood. Streptococci are associated more often with cellulitis because they produce enzymes such as streptokinase (fibrinolysin), hyaluronidase, and streptodornase. These enzymes break down fibrin and connective tissue ground substance, and lyse cellular debris, thus facilitating rapid spread of the bacterial invaders. These organisms are not restricted to one or the other type of reaction. Oral infections frequently are composed of a mixed flora, or the bacteria behave in an untraditional fashion. Thick-walled abscesses, with little or no blood supply to their lumen, respond slowly or poorly to antibiotic therapy, whereas cellulitis usually responds well without surgical drainage.

Erysipelas is a specific form of cellulitis (lymphangitis) caused by β-hemolytic streptococci. A discrete entry injury usually occurs on the face, violating this barrier to bacteria. Marked interstitial edema of the subcutaneous tissues occurs, but relatively little evidence of necrosis is present. Characteristically the tissues have a sharply demarcated, brawny, edematous swelling that is intensely red as a result of vasodilation. The lesion often is associated with a profound toxemia.

TREATMENT OF ODONTOGENIC INFECTIONS

Treatment of odontogenic infections may involve medical, surgical, or dental therapy, or combinations thereof. Any infection of dental origin requires definitive treatment of the affected tooth if the source of the infection is to be eliminated. Once the tooth has been identified, endodontic elimination of the infected pulp, deep periodontal scaling, or extraction must be performed. The method of tooth treatment is a question of judgment, determined by factors such as the extent of the infection, patient's general health status, degree of trismus present, and biomechanical necessity of retaining the tooth. However, the last factor must not sway the surgeon's judgment to the detriment of the patient's well-being. The clinician must avoid "tunnel vision" when diagnosing dental disease because it can have serious consequences if a major infection is present. Extraction of the involved tooth is the most rapid method of establishing drainage while simultaneously removing the nidus of microorganisms within the pulp chamber and canals. Alternatively, endodontic therapy may be used to eliminate the source of infection.

For many decades the question of whether an abscessed tooth should be extracted in the presence of acute infection has been controversial. Concern over potential iatrogenic spread of infection by manipulation of the tooth has been challenged by those who believe that early extraction leads to early resolution of the infection by eliminating the source of infection and providing a portal for drainage. Although numerous clinical studies on this subject suggest that immediate extraction does not cause extension of the infection and may, indeed, result in fewer postoperative problems than late extraction, these studies are not conclusive. Reliable evidence indicates that extractions of lower molar teeth in the presence of infection increase the incidence of alveolar osteitis. Therefore antibiotic therapy should be used when a tooth is to be extracted during the acute stage of diffuse or deep infections, especially those involving the mandibular third molars.

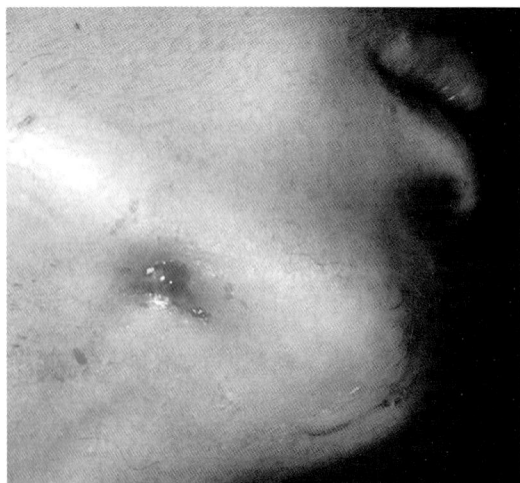

Figure 8-2 Chronic cutaneous submandibular fistula of dental origin (mandibular molar).

INCISION AND DRAINAGE

Incision and drainage rid the body of toxic purulent material and decompress the tissues, allowing better perfusion of blood containing antibiotics and defensive elements and increased oxygenation of the infected area.

The abscess should be drained surgically at the same time that dental therapy is performed. Incision and drainage are the oldest and usually the simplest surgical procedures. Rapid, sharp incision through the oral mucosa adjacent to the alveolar bone usually is sufficient to produce "laudable pus," an eighteenth and nineteenth century phrase that is both descriptive and exclamatory. The surgeon who could produce instant relief and probably cure by the evacuation of pus from an abscess was also praiseworthy and, therefore, was more renowned than less skillful colleagues who incised prematurely or in the wrong place.

A thorough knowledge of facial and neck anatomy is necessary to properly drain a deep abscess, but an abscess confined to the dentoalveolar region presents no anatomical mysteries to the surgeon. Only the thin, bulging mucosa separates the scalpel from the infection. Ideally, abscesses should be drained when fluctuant before spontaneous rupture and drainage. Incision and drainage are best performed at the earliest sign of this "ripening" of the abscess, although surgical drainage also may be effective early, before the development of classic fluctuance.

The following principles should be used when possible with incision and drainage:

1. Incise in healthy skin and mucosa when possible. An incision placed at the site of maximum fluctuance where the tissues are necrotic or beginning to perforate may result in a puckered, unesthetic scar.
2. Place the incision in an esthetically acceptable area, such as under the shadow of the jaw or in a natural skin fold or crease.
3. When possible, place the incision in a dependent position to encourage drainage by gravity.
4. Dissect bluntly, with a closed surgical clamp or finger, through deeper tissues and explore all portions of the abscess cavity thoroughly so that compartmentalized areas of pus are disrupted and excavated. Extend the dissection to the roots of teeth responsible for the infection.
5. Place a drain (sterile latex or catheter) and stabilize it with sutures.
6. Consider use of through-and-through drains in bilateral, submandibular space infections.
7. Do not leave drains in place for an overly extended period; remove them when drainage becomes minimal. The presence of the drain itself may produce some exudate and can be a portal for secondary bacterial invaders.
8. Clean wound margins daily under sterile conditions to remove clots and debris.

Another approach to drainage of well-localized abscesses is the use of a computed tomographic (CT)-guided catheter. It is introduced percutaneously and guided into the abscess cavity. This procedure is useful especially for deep neck abscesses. CT-guided catheterization allow precise location of the lesion without extensive dissection and subsequent scarring. In selected patients, it can be performed in a radiology suite. Specimens for Gram staining and culture are readily obtained, and the catheter may be left in place to serve as a drain.

The use of heat and poultices to "draw" an abscess to the surface have been discussed and debated extensively. The physiology of heat application to infection appears rational because the resulting dilation of small vessels intensifies host defenses through increased vascular flow and diffusion. However, the hope of converting an extraoral abscess into an intraoral one by the use of warm mouth rinses is not well based; no scientific evidence exists that any application of heat will produce the desired effect.

If no purulent flow is obtained from incision of a dentoalveolar abscess, the drainage procedure may have been ill-timed or a cellulitis may have been incised. *Fenestration* of the alveolar bone with a high-speed dental drill, although uncommon, occasionally may be used to relieve pain. Fenestration is best accomplished through the soft tissue drainage wound at the level of the root apex. Medical therapy for localized dentoalveolar abscesses consists mainly of supportive care: hydration, soft diet, analgesics, and good oral hygiene.

ANTIBIOTIC THERAPY

The use of antibiotics in the treatment of a well-localized and easily drained dentoalveolar abscess probably is unnecessary because surgical drainage and dental therapy resolve the infection in most patients. Abscesses and cellulitis in patients who are immunocompromised and in those with systemic signs and symptoms such as trismus or elevated temperature usually indicate the need for antibiotics. Poorly localized, extensive abscesses and those associated with diffuse cellulitis require antibiotic therapy.

In patients with diminished host defenses, such as those with poorly controlled diabetes, patients who are immunosuppressed or immunoincompetent, those receiving renal dialysis, or the seriously ill hospitalized patient, supplemental antibiotics are required for dentoalveolar infection because of the fear of sudden, overwhelming sepsis spreading from even a small focus. Fatal dental infection may be observed in patients who are immunosuppressed.

Ideally the choice of antibiotic for the therapy of odontogenic infection depends on the definitive laboratory results of culture and sensitivity testing. Inasmuch as most dentoalveolar infections occur in otherwise healthy outpatients seen in offices and clinics, cultures are not routinely performed and usually are not needed. A pragmatically rational approach to empirical antibiotic selection is acceptable, both ethically and legally, if the choice is based on scientific data and on contemporary experience with the microbiology of the flora of oral infection.

The constantly evolving flora of oral infection has been well documented. Numerous studies indicate that the majority of infections consist of mixed aerobic and anaerobic flora (65% to 70%), or are exclusively anaerobic (25% to 30%), whereas only 5% are exclusively aerobic. More than 90% contain some anaerobes. The most frequently and consistently isolated organisms are aerobic streptococci (α-, β-, and γ-), anaerobic streptococci *(Peptostreptococcus)*, Bacteroides *(Porphyromonas, Prevotella)*, Fusobacterium, *and* Eikenella. Less frequently, *Bacteroides fragilis,* the gram-negative anaerobic rod that normally inhabits the bowel and pelvis, is found. Skin organisms such as *Staphylococcus aureus* and *Staphylococcus epidermidis* currently are reported less frequently than in previous decades of the antibiotic era, but have a high incidence in nonodontogenic facial infections in children. Aerobic *Corynebacterium* and anaerobic *Propionibacterium,* both gram-positive rods, are encountered occasionally.

Penicillin has been the antibiotic of empirical choice for dental infections for nearly five decades with a proven record of efficacy. However, the microorganism and macroorganism population of any ecosystem can and does evolve in response to environmental selection or through mutatory influences, whether on the floor of a tropical rain forest or in the gingival sulcus of *Homo sapiens.* The population of some oral microspecies has demonstrated a profound and measurable change in its susceptibility to penicillin, and β-lactamase–producing organisms such as *Bacteroides* now are frequently noted to be insensitive to penicillin, with some published series reporting 40% resistance. Even streptococci, which historically have been exquisitely sensitive to penicillin, are occasionally reported as penicillin resistant. Several strains of clindamycin-resistant *Bacteroides* also have been observed.[8]

Facial surgeons should read and interpret these data with a very critical eye. If some 40% of *Bacteroides* are reported to be resistant, 60% must be sensitive, a ratio that still has therapeutic validity in a mixed aerobic-anaerobic infection.

The validity of in vitro sensitivity testing on a laboratory agar plate also should be viewed cautiously. Most laboratories test bacterial isolates for susceptibility to antimicrobial drugs with a disk diffusion test, although semiautomated methods are available. These methods determine the minimum inhibitory concentration of different antibiotics for each isolate or convert those data to designations of susceptibility testing. Laboratory antibiotic testing for anaerobes may be less accurate than for aerobes.

The humoral and cellular host defense mechanisms, if normal, are far more essential to the demise of invading organisms than is the antibiotic disk applied in the laboratory. In addition, obtaining material (pus) for culture usually implies that surgical drainage (or aspiration) has been performed, a procedure that ranks equal in importance to the presence of normal defenses in the successful therapeutic outcome of dentoalveolar infection.

Inasmuch as most of these infections are a mixed flora of aerobes and anaerobes, the bacterial synergism that enhances growth of these different types of organisms may be disrupted by the use of penicillin. Whether the aerobic streptococci produce essential nutrients for the anaerobes, provide enzymes, clear metabolites, or reduce the oxygen tension in the tissue, their destruction by penicillin secondarily diminishes the growth and reproduction of the anaerobes.

Therefore penicillin remains the empirical antibiotic of choice in treatment of most dentoalveolar infection in the noncompromised host. Stated succinctly and scientifically by Moenning, "it would seem presumptuous to state that penicillin is currently not effective against most odontogenic infections and premature to consider substituting another antibiotic as the drug of first choice for mild to moderate odontogenic infections, especially when cost and lack of toxicity are also considered."[11] That statement remains as valid in 2002 as it was in 1989. For more severe or recalcitrant infections seen in an outpatient environment, culture and antibiotic sensitivity studies may be necessary. Metronidazole is an effective supplement to penicillin and enhances killing of anaerobes. Oral clindamycin is an excellent choice for both aerobic and anaerobic killing, but its cost and potential side effects must be considered. If a β-lactam antibiotic (i.e., penicillin) has been used for 2 to 3 days without any resolution of an odontogenic infection, the use of another non–β-lactam or β-lactamase–stabile antibiotic (i.e., clindamycin) should be considered.

The paradox of antibiotic therapy often leads to clinical situations in which the solution to problem A creates problem B. Recent observations show that the use of antianaerobic antibiotics (clindamycin, metronidazole, amoxicillin-clavulanate) may create high-density colonization of the stools by vancomycin-resistant enterococci in patients already colonized by these organisms (i.e., patients in intensive care units), thus enhancing the infection's morbidity and mortality, and placing other patients and intensive care unit personnel at greater risk of colonization.[3]

Erythromycin is poorly absorbed and less effective in odontogenic infection than penicillin or clindamycin, but newer macrolides (azithromycin) are tolerated better than erythromycin, resulting in higher compliance rates. Amoxicillin-clavulanic acid (Augmentin), a potent inhibitor of β-lactamases, is efficacious, but its cost and usefulness in severe infections should inhibit its use in routine odontogenic infections. First- and second-generation cephalosporins also are quite useful in odontogenic infection. Tetracycline is not recommended for severe anaerobic infection therapy, but its analogues minocycline and doxycycline may be useful in low-grade dentoalveolar infection.

For the patient ill enough to require hospitalization for odontogenic infection and for the compromised host (including patients with insulin-dependent diabetes, those with chronic alcoholism, intravenous drug abusers, recently hospitalized patients, and those receiving prophylactic antibiotics in the previous 4 weeks), clindamycin alone or in combination with metronidazole or gentamicin, or a first- or second-generation cephalosporin can be used, as can parenteral ampicillin-sulbactam (Unasyn). Quinolones have limited activity against anaerobes; thus justifying their use for odontogenic infections is difficult.

Fourth-generation quinolones, although useful against anaerobes, have created serious hepatic toxicity in some patients. For the recalcitrant infection that does not respond rapidly to penicillin therapy and in the compromised host, aerobic and anaerobic culturing and sensitivity studies are necessary to determine whether antibiotics other than penicillin are indicated.

The use and abuse of antibiotic therapy and the indications for therapy are discussed at length in Chapters 5 and 6. Antibiotics are indicated in combination with surgery both therapeutically and prophylactically in the following situations:

1. Acute cellulitis of dental origin
2. Acute pericoronitis with elevated temperature and trismus
3. Deep fascial space infections
4. Open (compound) fractures of the mandible and maxilla, or other facial bones
5. Extensive, deep, or old (>6 hours) orofacial lacerations
6. Dental infection or oral surgery in the compromised host
7. Prophylaxis for dental surgery in the patient with valvular cardiac disease or a prosthetic valve; also for some class II and all class III and IV operative wounds (see Chapter 17).

Whether treatment is medical (antibiotics), surgical (incision and drainage, extraction or endodontics), or both, another important decision is whether hospitalization for the therapy is warranted or ambulatory (office) care is sufficient. Although the number of odontogenic infections treated in the United States has never been determined, conservative extrapolation shows 21,000 hospital admissions and at least 150 deaths occur annually from such infections.

The decision to hospitalize a patient depends on evaluation of risk factors, which include the anatomical location of the infection (i.e., buccal vs. lateral pharyngeal spaces), health status (insulin-dependent diabetes, immunosuppression), duration (acute vs. chronic) of the infection, temperature, the presence of trismus, level of hydration, need for anesthesia or intubation, and the response to orally administered antibiotics. The use of contemporary imaging (CT imaging) may reveal deep but obscure infection that certainly may influence the decision.

The following case reports illustrate management of dentoalveolar infections against the background of the modern changing bacterial spectrum and in the compromised host.

■ CASE REPORT

A healthy 24-year-old man underwent extraction of a partially impacted mandibular third molar because of a history of intermittent pain and swelling. Penicillin was prescribed postoperatively for 10 days. Seventeen days after surgery, pain and swelling recurred. Penicillin again was prescribed but had no effect. Surgical drainage of the dentoalveolar abscess was performed, and the culture report revealed the presence of *Acinetobacter calcoaceticus* var. *lwoffi (Mima polymorpha),* which is sensitive to ampicillin, gentamicin, and carbenicillin. The infection rapidly resolved with ampicillin therapy.

The causative organism in this patient may have been an oral transient that became an opportunistic invader of the pericoronal culture media, or it may have been a secondary virulent aggressor whose growth was stimulated by penicillin suppression of the normal flora. Culture contamination is always a consideration when an unusual organism is encountered, but the response of the infection to the culture-specific antibiotic suggests otherwise.

■ CASE REPORT

A 26-year-old man was admitted to the hospital for chemotherapy for acute lymphocytic leukemia of 3 months' duration. A previous attempt at chemotherapy had been discontinued because of the development of *Escherichia coli* sepsis and pneumonia.

On the first hospital day the patient reported mandibular pain and submandibular adenopathy was palpable. His temperature was 100° F and the white blood cell count was 1250/mm^3 with numerous blast forms present, but platelet counts were well above normal levels. Oral examination revealed pericoronal swelling and tenderness but no erythema or purulence.

Blood cultures were performed and antibiotic therapy was started (tobramycin, 60 mg tid, and ticarcillin, 3 g q4h). By the patient's third hospital day, his temperature was normal and the white blood cell count was 3800/mm^3.

Dental radiographs revealed three partially impacted third molars. All three were extracted with the patient under local anesthesia, the wounds were irrigated with bacitracin solution, and the margins were loosely sutured. No further signs of infection were observed and chemotherapy was instituted.

Comments Patients whose immune systems are compromised or suppressed are at great risk from odontogenic infection. The lack of erythema and purulence, or even a lack of temperature elevation, is typical of patients with neutropenia who do not demonstrate the classic signs of infection, often until serious generalized sepsis has focused attention on the original site. The patient with leukemia who is receiving chemotherapy has both quantitative and qualitative abnormalities of granulocytes.

The choice of antibiotics for this patient was based on his previous episode of gram-negative sepsis and on the hope of providing the widest possible spectrum of antibacterial activity. The optimal time to perform exodontia for patients with leukemia during remission is when the white blood cell count is above 2000/mm^3, and antibiotics, which are considered therapeutic rather than prophylactic, should be used. Some investigators further advocate that impacted teeth should be removed as a prophylactic measure in patients with leukemia.[12] However, it is difficult to justify

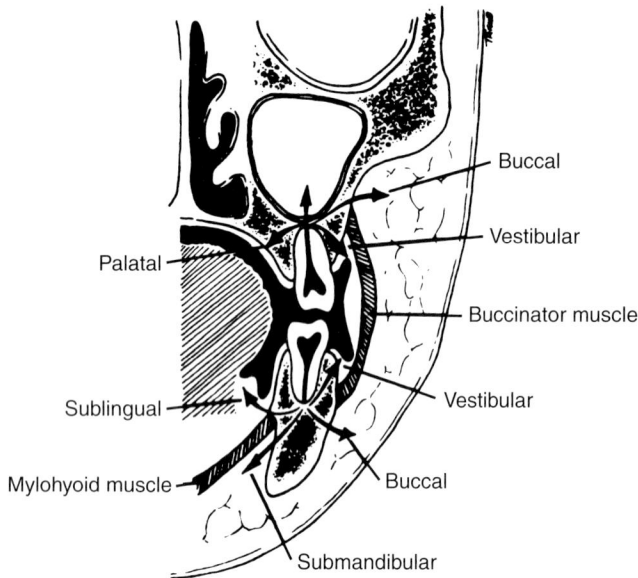

Figure 8-3 Diagram of potential routes of spread of pulpal infection from root apices. Muscle and fascial attachments determine direction of spread. Extension beyond muscle and fascial restrictions leads to fascial (deep) space infections.

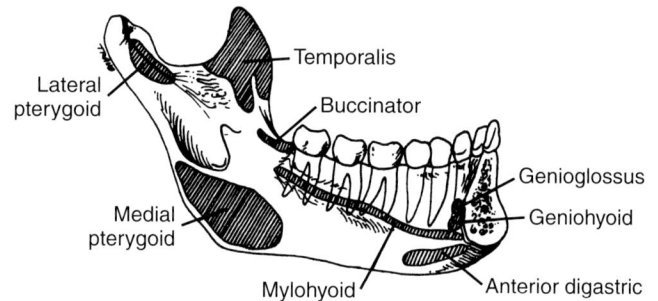

Figure 8-4 Lingual surface of the mandible showing muscle attachments. The relationship of the mylohyoid muscle attachment to the apices of the teeth is an important factor in determining whether a sublingual or a submandibular abscess will form.

TABLE **8-1**

Localization of Dental Abscesses

Teeth	Common Abscess Site	Less Common Site
Mandibular incisors	Labial/lingual	Lingual
Mandibular canines	Labial	Labial
Mandibular premolars	Buccal	Lingual
Mandibular molars	Buccal	Lingual
Maxillary incisors	Labial	Palatal
Maxillary canines	Labial	Palatal
Maxillary first premolars	Labial (buccal roots)	—
	Palatal (palatal roots)	—
Maxillary second premolars	Buccal	Palatal
Maxillary molars	Buccal (buccal roots)	—
	Palatal (palatal roots)	—

subjecting patients who are severely ill or immunocompromised (e.g., leukemia, human immunodeficiency virus infection) to prophylactic surgery when the potential complications of that surgery—the risk of sepsis and the possibility of toxic side effects from high-dose antibiotics—are basically the same as those for an infection in the unextracted third molar. This situation is in contrast to the much better risk/benefit ratio for the extraction of asymptomatic impacted third molars in healthy patients.

The universal extraction of impacted teeth in all compromised hosts has been suggested, but the cost and potential morbidity and mortality suggest otherwise. Careful observation, antibiotic therapy, and selective exodontia seem more prudent in the compromised host.

ANATOMICAL CONSIDERATIONS IN DENTOALVEOLAR INFECTIONS

Localization of a dentoalveolar abscess is related to the anatomical position of the dental root from which it originated, especially in relationship to muscle attachments and particularly the buccinator and mylohyoid muscles (Figures 8-3 and 8-4). Although a diffuse infection may cause some diagnostic consternation, the appearance of an acute dental abscess or fistula distant from its site of origin is rare. Familiarity with dental root anatomy is helpful in the occasional case in which an abscess develops in a less common position. Infection usually follows the path of least resistance, and the data presented in Table 8-1 represent clinical experience and anatomical realities. For example, any acute swelling or fistulous formation of the posterior hard palate should prompt an investigation of the palatal roots of the adjacent maxillary molar.

Infection of mandibular incisors and canines usually appears as a bulging erythematous mass deep in the labial sulcus. These infections are quite obvious to the surgeon and are accessible to drainage by a scalpel. Ideally, the incision should be carried down to bone, but deep sharp dissection at the lower canine region should be avoided because of the presence of the sensory (mental) nerve to the lip. If the infection spreads from bone deep to the origin of the mentalis muscle, the submental space becomes involved. A lingual site for infection of the mandibular anterior teeth is less common and is usually caused by periodontal sepsis rather than periapical sepsis. Simple gingival incision usually is adequate for drainage on the lingual surface, unless the sublingual space is involved.

The mandibular premolars generally demonstrate buccal infection. Incision into the buccal vestibule is indicated, but again discretion must be used because of the presence of the mental nerve and its foramen. If the infection extends inferior to the buccinator muscles laterally or infe-

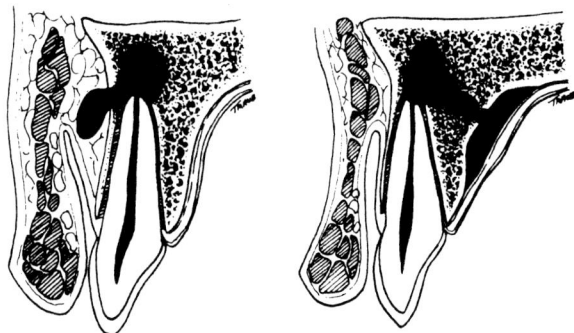

Figure 8-5 Schematic illustration of maxillary incisor periapical infection with labial *(left)* and palatal *(right)* surface dentoalveolar abscess formation.

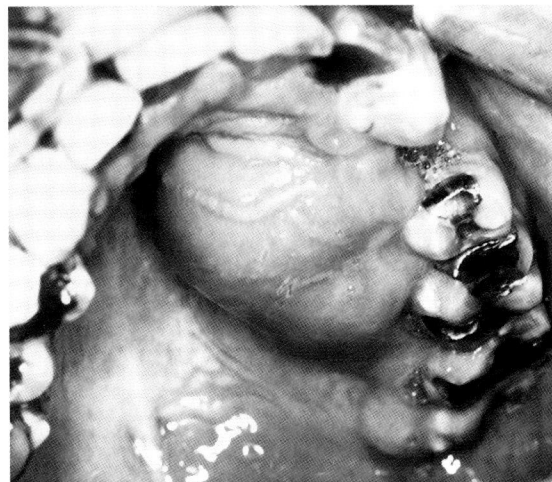

Figure 8-6 Palatal dentoalveolar abscess originating from premolar (root) infection.

rior to the mylohyoid muscle lingually, deep infections of the buccal space and submandibular space may occur.

Infection of mandibular third molars frequently is periodontal (pericoronitis) but can be related to the root apices if caries has invaded the pulp of an erupted or partially erupted tooth. The pathways of infection from mandibular third molars may involve the buccal vestibule, buccal fascial space, masticator space, and pharyngeal space. Drainage of these deep spaces is discussed in the section on fascial spaces (see Chapter 9).

The manifestation of infections of the upper teeth also depends on the anatomical location of their root apices (Figure 8-5). Maxillary incisor and canine roots lie closer to the thin labial plate of bone than to the thicker palatal bone, and infections therefore usually are observed as bulging submucosal (vestibular) abscesses or fistulas in the labial sulcus. The muscles of the upper lip, arising from the alveolar bone, are quite thin and have little influence on the spread of infection. Generalized cellulitis of the upper lip or midface may occur, but penetration of infection into the floor of the nose is quite rare. Drainage is accomplished easily by sharp incision into the labial sulcus. When palatal migration of infection does occur from an anterior tooth, it may vary in appearance from minimal swelling to massive bulging of the anterior palate (Figure 8-6). Incision of the palatal mucosa provides adequate drainage. The palatal vessels may be avoided by making the incision parallel to the vessel.

Maxillary premolar and molar infection may extend buccally or palatally because multiple roots usually are present (Figure 8-7). Infection from maxillary premolars usually extends into the connective tissue of the buccal vestibule and may spread superiorly, causing cellulitis to the level of the eyelids. This situation is best resolved by incision high in the buccal vestibule, which usually is the area of dependent fluctuance. The attachment of the buccinator muscle usually is well above the root apex of maxillary premolars, but penetration into the buccal space may occur.

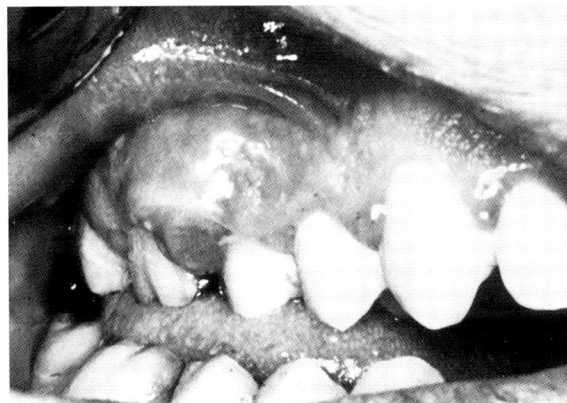

Figure 8-7 Dentoalveolar abscess originating from buccal roots of premolar or molar.

Maxillary molar infection may exit from the alveolar bone buccally, palatally, or posteriorly. The buccal vestibule is the most common site for appearance of abscesses but invasion of the buccal space occurs commonly. Molar infection of the palatal region is surprisingly uncommon, considering the length of most molar palatal roots; superior spread of pus into the maxillary sinus also is uncommon. Posterior spread of infection may involve the masticator and pharyngeal spaces, and superior extension into the infratemporal space also may occur.

In all odontogenic infections, examination usually reveals the presence of deep caries, periodontal inflammation, or impacted or fractured teeth as the cause. Bone fractures or gingival trauma should not be overlooked in the search for the causative factors of abscesses or cellulitis. Careful examination of the oral cavity, radiographs, and a high index of suspicion for all restored teeth help to localize the origin of the infection accurately. An easily overlooked cause of facial infection is the eruption of the maxillary third molar in an extreme buccal or posterior position, thereby causing erosion of the buccal mucosa, cellulitis, deep space infection, and severe trismus. Because of the difficulties of performing adequate examination of the posterior oral cavity in such circumstances and the inadequacies of radiographs, frequently only the suspicious, experienced, and persistent examiner is successful in discovering the cause of the infection.

FASCIAL SPACE INFECTION

When dental infection spreads deeply into soft tissue rather than exiting superficially through oral or cutaneous routes, fascial spaces may be affected (Box 8-1). Following the path of least resistance through connective tissue and along fascial planes, infection may spread quite distantly from its dental source, causing considerable morbidity and occasionally death. A thorough knowledge of the anatomy of the face and neck is necessary to predict the pathways of spread of these infections accurately and drain these deep spaces adequately. Excellent anatomical descriptions are provided in Chapter 9.[5,6,9,13,14]

Spread of infection through deep fascial spaces is determined by the presence and patterns of loose connective tissue. Fasciae develop in planes of connective tissue subjected to muscular movement and contraction. Surrounding or separating muscles, the fasciae and fascial planes offer an anatomically defined highway for infection to spread from superficial to deep parts of the face and neck. A description of deep fascial spaces essentially is an anatomical discussion of the various fasciae that surround or separate the anatomical boundaries of a given space. The concept of fascial "spaces" is based on the anatomist's knowledge that all "spaces" exist only potentially, until fasciae are separated by pus, blood, drains, or a surgeon's finger.

BOX 8-1

Fascial Spaces of Clinical Significance

Face
Buccal
Canine
Masticator
   Masseteric compartment
   Pterygoid compartment
   Zygomaticotemporal compartment
Suprahyoid
Sublingual
Submandibular
   Submaxillary
   Submental
Lateral pharyngeal
Peritonsillar
Infrahyoid
Anterovisceral (pretracheal)
Space of total neck
Retropharyngeal
Danger space
Space of carotid sheath

Infections of fascial spaces are discussed primarily in terms of their odontogenic origins. Teeth are the most common cause of these infections, and therapy is incomplete without definitive dental treatment. However, deep fascial space infections of the neck also may occur as a result of pharyngeal and tonsillar infections, trauma, reconstructive surgery, cancer surgery, and sialadenitis of major salivary glands.

Each fascial space infection described in this chapter is a clinical entity; the accompanying case reports illustrate the unique characteristics of each situation. In the treatment of infections of fascial spaces, including surgical treatment, the principles discussed earlier should always be considered. The following points also are germane:

1. Diffusion of antibiotics into close fascial spaces is limited because of poor vascularity. Penetration of antibiotics through thick-walled abscesses is minimal. "Average" doses may be inadequate.
2. Therapy of fascial space infections depends on adequate, open, and dependent drainage.
3. Large surgical incisions are necessary to obtain adequate exposure of deep compartments.
4. Fascial spaces are contiguous and infection spreads readily from one space to another. Multiple incisions may be necessary because frequently more than one space is involved in the infection.
5. Secondary spaces and the primary one must be drained.
6. The anatomy of the face or neck may be grossly distorted by the swelling of the infectious process.
7. Repeat surgical drainage may be necessary.
8. The fascial spaces most commonly involved in dentigerous infections are the submandibular, submental, and buccal spaces. Less common are the masticator space compartments, lateral pharyngeal, and temporal spaces. Least common are the retropharyngeal and canine spaces.

Although observation and palpation can elicit the presence of superficial dentoalveolar and fascial space infections (i.e., buccal, canine, submental spaces), the presence of deep infections must always be a suspicion. The presence of dysphagia, dyspnea, prolonged white blood cell and temperature elevation, and unresolved trismus suggests the need for repeat imaging (CT, magnetic resonance imaging) of deep spaces, inasmuch as the presence of or even surgical drainage of superficial infection may obscure a concomitant or secondary deep space involvement.

CANINE SPACE

The canine space is involved infrequently in odontogenic and is implicated even less frequently in nasal infection. Infections of the maxillary canine teeth usually appear as labial sulcus swelling and less commonly as palatal swelling. However, the levator muscle of the upper lip overlies the apex of the canine root. The origin of the muscle is high in the canine fossa of the maxillary wall, whereas its insertion is the angle of the mouth, intermingling with the fibers of the orbicular muscle of the mouth and the zygomatic muscle.

If the canine infection perforates the lateral cortex of maxillary bone superior to the origin of the muscle, the potential canine space is affected. Whether this represents a true fascial space or simply a muscular compartment is debatable, but abscess of this space requires surgical intervention. Canine space infections may cause marked cellulitis of the eyelids (Figure 8-8). Drainage is accomplished best through an intraoral approach, high in the maxillary labial vestibule by sharp and blunt dissection. This approach is an extension of that used for fenestration or apicoectomy of the canine root apex. Percutaneous drainage may be performed lateral to the nose, but this procedure does not afford dependent drainage and results in a visible scar.

■ CASE REPORT

A 52-year-old man underwent extraction of the maxillary left canine tooth 1 month before the onset of swelling lateral to the nares (Figure 8-9). Nasal infection had been the diagnosis, and his physician had prescribed penicillin for the swelling.

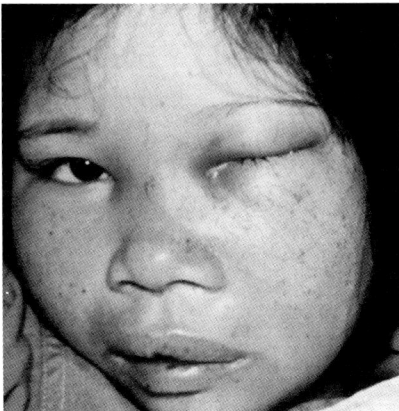

Figure 8-8 Canine space infection after extraction of maxillary canine. Note swelling lateral to the nose.

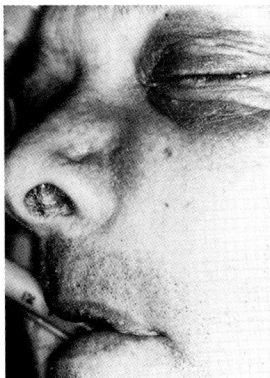

Figure 8-9 Abscess from canine space infection manifesting lateral to the nose.

When the swelling spread to the labial sulcus, the patient could no longer wear his denture and sought a dental consultation. Examination revealed a fluctuant mass lateral to the nares and firm swelling under the upper lip. Dental radiographs revealed a bone radiolucency in the area of the previously extracted canine root.

With the patient under general anesthesia, an incision into the labial sulcus produced drainage of pus. Blunt dissection superiorly with a small clamp produced greater egress of pus as the lateral nasal abscess (canine space) was entered. The mass collapsed, a drain was placed, and the purulent granulation tissue was curetted from the bony fossa over the canine root.

A culture report later revealed growth of *Citrobacter freundii,* a gram-negative enteric rod. Penicillin therapy was discontinued and further healing was uneventful.

■ CASE REPORT

A 29-year-old woman had been examined in numerous hospital clinics because of intermittent swelling and drainage from a fistula "below her eye" (Figure 8-10). Otolaryngologic, ophthalmologic, and dermatologic examinations had failed to reveal the cause of the lesion, as had radiographs of the sinuses, fungal cultures, chest radiography, and tuberculosis testing. Biopsy of the lesion was scheduled after dental consultation.

Dental examination revealed a carious pulpal exposure of the maxillary canine tooth, and a dental radiograph demonstrated an apical radiolucency at the root tip. Culture of the fistula revealed β-hemolytic streptococci. The tooth was extracted and the fistula promptly closed, terminating the chronic canine space infection.

CAVERNOUS SINUS THROMBOSIS

Although ascending infection (venous sinus thrombosis) is not a fascial space infection, it can be of odontogenic origin. Cavernous sinus infection, ascending from the maxillary teeth, upper lip, nose, or orbit through the valveless

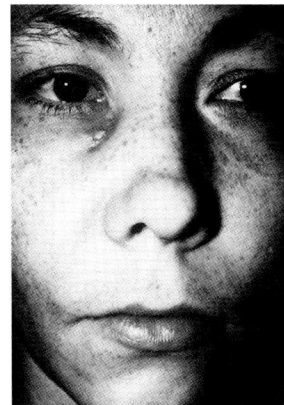

Figure 8-10 Chronic fistula high in canine space from periapical infection of maxillary canine tooth.

anterior and posterior fascial veins, carries an extremely high mortality rate. Any patient with initials signs of proptosis, fever, obtunded state of consciousness, ophthalmoplegia, or paresis of the oculomotor, trochlear, and abducens nerves, especially after maxillary infections and exodontia, should have an emergency neurosurgical consultation (see Chapter 16).

BUCCAL SPACE

Mandibular and maxillary premolar and molar teeth tend to drain in a lateral and buccal direction. The relation of the root apices to the origins of the buccinator muscle (the outer surfaces of the alveolar process of the maxilla and mandible) determines whether infection exits intraorally in the buccal vestibule or extends deeply into the buccal space. Molar infections exiting superiorly to the maxillary origin of the muscle or inferiorly to the mandibular origin of the muscle enter the buccal space.

The buccal space contains the buccal fat pad, Stensen's (parotid) duct, and the facial (external maxillary) artery. Infection of this space is diagnosed easily because of marked cheek swelling associated with a diseased molar or premolar tooth. When fluctuance occurs, it should be drained percutaneously. Attempts to direct fluctuance intraorally by warm rinses are futile, and intraoral drainage through mucosa, submucosa, and buccinator muscle may be difficult.

Cutaneous drainage should be performed inferior to the point of fluctuance with blunt dissection into the depth and extreme boundaries of the space. The purulent contents may expand the space to a surprising volume (Figures 8-11 and 8-12). The branches of the facial nerve should be avoided. The usual incision and drainage site is quite inferior to Stensen's duct. Aspiration of this space is performed easily.

Of special interest, and far from uncommon, is nonodontogenic buccal space infection or buccal cellulitis caused by *Haemophilus influenzae* (see Chapter 13). This infection, usually seen in infants or children younger than 3 years of age, is characterized by high fever for at least 24 hours before the appearance of clinical signs. The rapid onset of dark red swelling easily may be confused with odontogenic infection or erysipelas. Otitis media frequently also is present or has occurred recently. Now commonly resistant to ampicillin, *H. influenzae* infection may respond well to amoxicillin-clavulanate (Augmentin) or a cephalosporin such as cefaclor. This process can occur in older children (Figure 8-13).

Recurrent buccal space abscesses can occur as a complication of Crohn's disease. This segmental transmural intestinal disease, whose clinical course includes intermittent abdominal pain, fever, weight loss, and diarrhea, is

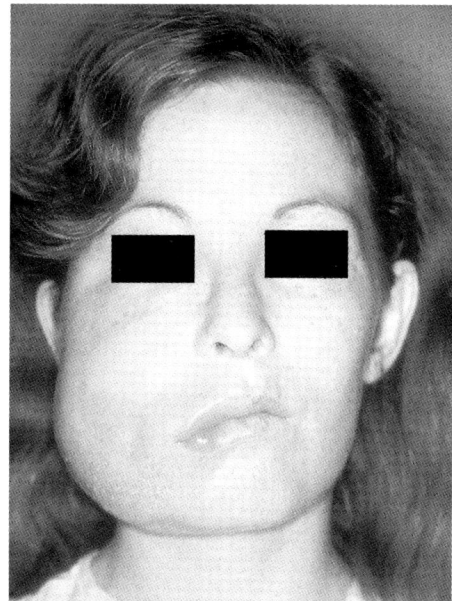

Figure 8-12 Buccal space infection. Note massive swelling, erythema, and early skin necrosis.

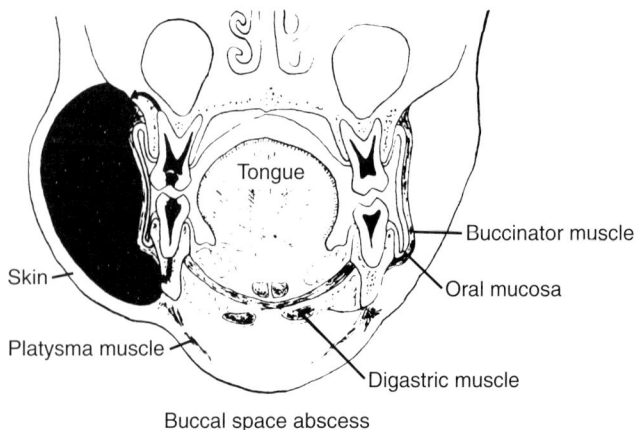

Figure 8-11 Buccal space abscess anatomy. (From Laskin DM: Anatomic considerations in diagnosis and treatment of odontogenic infections, *J Am Dent Assoc* 69:308, 1964.)

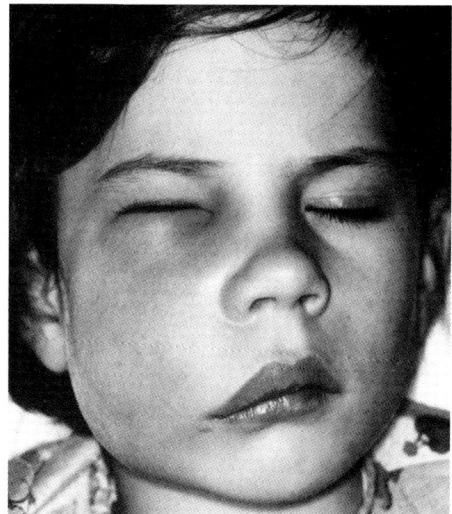

Figure 8-13 Buccal cellulitis caused by *Haemophilus influenzae* after recent otitis media.

characterized by inflammatory granulomas, which can occur throughout the entire length of the gastrointestinal tract, from the mouth to the anus. Granulomatous lesions and ulcerations of the buccal mucosa can progress to true buccal space abscesses. A high recurrence rate of the granulomas or new abscess formation is possible despite antibiotic, corticosteroid, or surgical therapy.

■ CASE REPORT

A 10-year-old boy had massive swelling of the cheek to the level of the eyelids. Before the onset of the swelling, he had a toothache in a molar tooth, but the commencement of the swelling was associated with diminution of pain. His temperature was 101° F, and the skin of his cheek was warm, tender, and erythematous. The affected tooth was treated by pulpal extirpation and penicillin therapy was started. Two days later, fluctuance was noted in the inferior portion of the cheek, and percutaneous incision and drainage were performed on an outpatient basis. Ten cubic centimeters of pus was obtained, and a culture later yielded streptococci. Penicillin therapy was continued for 10 days, and the infection resolved. Endodontic filling of the tooth was performed later.

MASTICATOR SPACES

The masticator spaces—*masseteric, pterygoid,* and *temporal*—are well differentiated but communicate with each other and with the buccal, submandibular, and parapharyngeal spaces. Infection may be confined to any one of these compartments or may spread rather readily to any or all of the others.

Of the muscles of mastication, only the outer surface of the masseter and the inner surface of the medial (internal) pterygoid are covered by true fascia. Sicher[14] states that the temporal "fascia" is really the suspensory bracing of the zygomatic arch, rather than a muscle sheath.

Although little space exists between the fibers of the masseter and temporalis muscles, considerable space is present between the temporalis muscle and the pterygoids. The fatty connective tissue in this space extends anteriorly to the border of the buccinator muscle at the pterygomandibular raphe.

The masticator space as a unit is bound by fascia. It contains the muscles of mastication and the internal maxillary artery and the mandibular nerve. If subdivided, the boundaries of the masseteric compartment are the masseter muscle laterally and the mandibular ascending ramus medially, whereas the pterygoid compartment is bounded medially by the pterygoid muscles and laterally by the mandible. Both compartments communicate freely with the superficial and deep temporal pouches superiorly, the buccal space anteriorly, and the lateral pharyngeal spaces posteriorly. Extension of infection into parotid and submandibular spaces also may occur.

Infection of the masticator space occurs most frequently from molar teeth, and infections of the third molars (wisdom teeth) are implicated most commonly as the cause. Pericoronitis of the gingival flap of third molars or caries-induced dental abscesses usually can be found in cases of masticator space infection. Infections of this space also have been reported as a result of contaminated mandibular block anesthetic injections, or infection may spread to this space from nearby contiguous spaces. Infection of the masticator space also may result from direct trauma to or through the muscles of mastication or surgery in the area (e.g., after temporocranial flaps are made for neurosurgery). Masticator space infection also has been reported as a complication of circumzygomatic wiring for midface trauma.

Infratemporal space infections also may occur as a result of temporomandibular joint surgery or arthroscopy. The postulated mechanism is contamination from the external auditory canal flora (streptococci, staphylococci, *Haemophilus, Proteus,* and *Pseudomonas* organisms).

Clinically the hallmark of masticator space infection is *trismus* (Figure 8-14), the sine qua non of masticator space infection. If trismus is not present, these spaces are uninvolved with the infectious process. An exception would be infection in a patient who is immunosuppressed, who may not exhibit the classic signs of inflammation or the unique signs of deep space infection.

Swelling may not be a prominent sign of masticator space infection, especially in the masseteric compartment. In this area the infectious process exists deep to large muscle masses that obscure or prevent much observable swelling. This process distinctly contrasts with infections of the buccal space, in which swelling is the cardinal sign of infection.

Surgical access to the various compartments of the masticator space is complicated by the containment of the

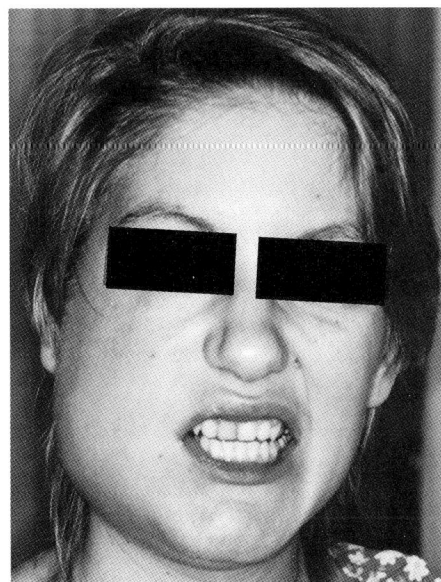

Figure 8-14 Severe trismus associated with masticator space infection. Observe the bulging of the masseter muscle overlying the deep space infection. Note the inability to open the mouth.

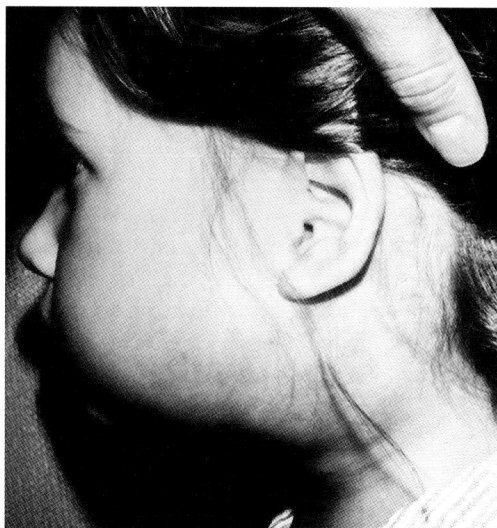

Figure 8-15 Masticator space infection in a 5-year-old child caused by infection from a deciduous mandibular molar.

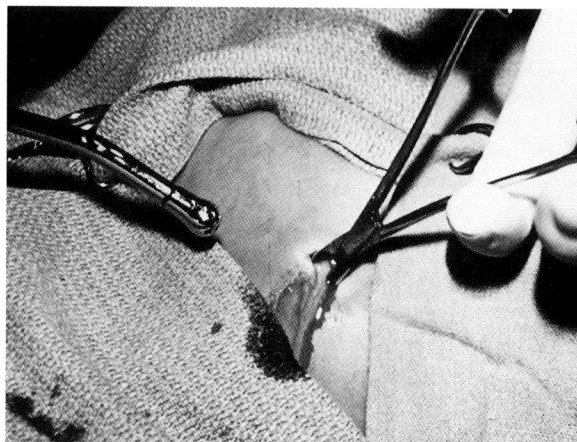

Figure 8-16 Incision and drainage of masticator space of child in Figure 8-15. Purulent flow occurred after blunt penetration of masseteric compartment.

infectious process by the muscle masses. Although drainage of the entire masticator space from the intraoral space is possible and occasionally practical, access from an extraoral incision is easier technically and more prudent. Sicher's[14] suggested approach to all compartments through an incision along the pterygomandibular raphe is technically possible in a cadaver, but is less feasible in an infected patient with trismus. In such patients the oral approach could compromise the airway postoperatively because of persistent bloody or purulent oozing, and intraoral drains may be difficult to maintain and can be aspirated if loosened inadvertently.

The masseteric and pterygoid compartments may be entered by superficial sharp and deep blunt dissection at the external angle of the mandible, avoiding the mandibular branch of the facial nerve. This approach allows dependent drainage of both spaces at the insertion of the muscle sling on the inferior border at the mandibular angle. Adequate local anesthesia can be accomplished at the mandibular angle (Figures 8-15 through 8-17).

The temporal spaces, although accessible through Sicher's intraoral incision, also may be drained percutaneously through an incision slightly superior to the zygomatic arch. The incision should be made parallel to the zygomatic arch and therefore parallel to the zygomatic branch of the facial nerve rather than perpendicular to it.

■ CASE REPORT

A 5-year-old girl underwent extraction of an "abscessed" mandibular deciduous molar associated with swelling of the buccal vestibule. Penicillin was prescribed but was never administered by the parent. Sixteen days later the child returned to the hospital with severe trismus, intense pain, brawny erythematous swelling involving the masseteric compartment of the masticator space, and a temperature

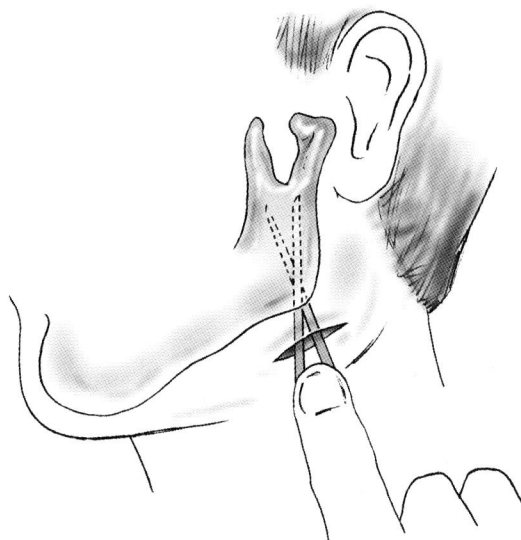

Figure 8-17 Schematic drawing of blunt dissection into masseteric (lateral) or pterygoid compartments through submandibular incision. (Courtesy William Bontempi.)

of 102.6° F (see Figure 8-15). Radiographs revealed "brushfire" osteomyelitis of the mandible. Her white blood cell count was 16,700/mm³, with 78% polymorphonuclear leukocytes.

Despite intravenous penicillin therapy the swelling and pain intensified and on the third hospital day the girl was taken to the operating room. After blind nasal intubation a curvilinear skin incision was made below the angle of the mandible, and blunt dissection was carried to bone at the mandibular angle. Blunt penetration of the masticator sling resulted in a profuse flow of foul-smelling pus (see Figures 8-15 and 8-16). Specimens for aerobic and anaerobic cultures were obtained and a drain was placed. A Gram stain

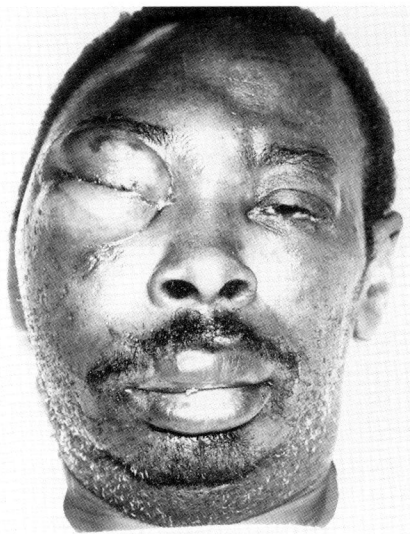

Figure 8-18 Infection of the temporal compartment of the masticator space. Note bulging of the temporalis muscle and cellulitis of the zygomaticoorbital region.

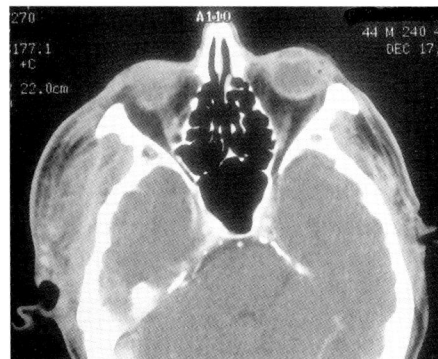

Figure 8-19 Diffuse infection of the temporal compartment of the masticator space. Note diffuse infection of the right side.

revealed gram-positive cocci, some in chain formation. Cultures later yielded anaerobic streptococci.

Medical evaluation for defective host defense mechanisms proved fruitless; penicillin therapy was continued orally and parenterally, sequestrectomy was performed later, and after many months the soft tissue and bone infection cleared completely.

Although unusual, this case illustrates masticator space infection and the problems of patient noncompliance. Intraoral incisions and drainage might have been technically difficult in a small child and would not have provided dependent drainage. Long-term intraoral purulent flow and the presence of drains might not have been well tolerated. The need for anaerobic and aerobic culturing of deep space infections also is illustrated by this case.

■ CASE REPORT

A 28-year-old male hospital employee underwent forceps extraction of a carious maxillary third molar. Four days later, he noted the onset of trismus, pain, and temporal area headache. By the sixth postextraction day, he had an oral opening of only 12 mm, and examination revealed tender firm swelling in the temporal area just superior to the zygomatic arch (Figure 8-18). His white blood cell count was 13,950/mm3, and his temperature was 101.8° F.

The patient was admitted to the hospital and underwent percutaneous incision and drainage of the temporal space the next day. A small amount of purulent material was obtained from the superficial temporal pouch, and culture later revealed mixed oral flora. Penicillin was administered and the infection resolved without further sequelae.

No antibiotic was used at the time of extraction, nor was any antibiotic therapy indicated for extraction of a noninfected maxillary molar. Drainage also could have been ac-

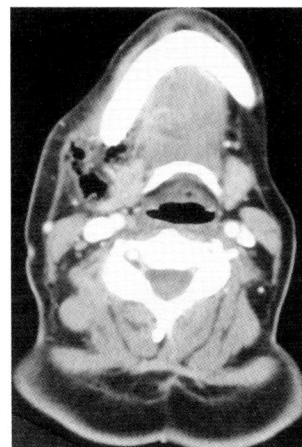

Figure 8-20 CT scan shows infection of the right masseteric and pterygoid compartments. Note gas formation from anaerobic pathogens.

complished intraorally at the insertion of the temporalis muscle at the mandibular coronoid process. Imaging (CT scan) of the masticator space confirms the diagnosis of infection, even if early or occult (Figures 8-19 and 8-20), and can delineate its extent.

SUBMANDIBULAR AND SUBLINGUAL SPACES

The submandibular (submaxillary) and sublingual spaces, although quite distinct anatomically, should be considered as a surgical unit because of their proximity and frequent dual involvement in odontogenic infection. Some confusion in nomenclature exists because some anatomists describe these spaces as compartments of the "submandibular space."

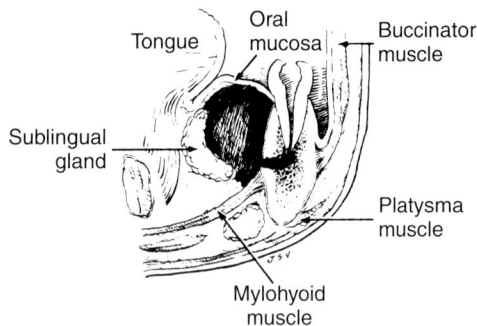

Figure 8-21 Sublingual space infection. Note the ease with which this space may be drained intraorally through the mucosa. (From Laskin DM: Anatomic considerations in diagnosis and treatment of odontogenic infections, *J Am Dent Assoc* 69:308, 1964.)

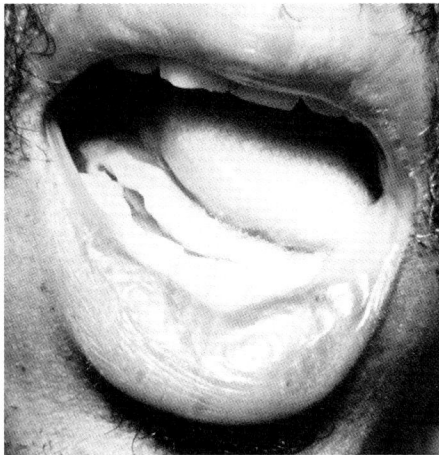

Figure 8-23 Schematic drawing of submandibular space infection originating from a mandibular molar tooth. Surgical drainage is accomplished through skin and platysma muscle. (From Archer WH: *Oral and maxillofacial surgery,* vol I, ed 5, Philadelphia, 1975, WB Saunders.)

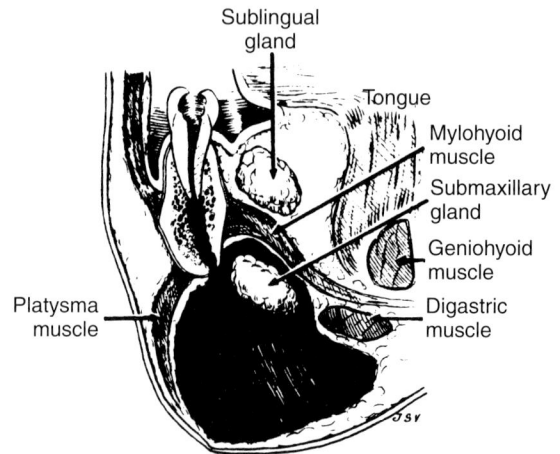

Figure 8-22 Clinical appearance of sublingual space infection with elevation of the tongue by indurated sublingual tissue.

The mylohyoid muscle, which forms the floor of the oral cavity, is the key to the diagnosis and surgical management of these space infections. Separating the sublingual space above from the submandibular space below is the mylohyoid muscle, which attaches to the lingual surface of the mandible in an obliquely downward line from posterior to anterior. Thus the root apices of the premolar and first molar teeth usually are superior to this attachment. As a result, lingual perforations of infections from these teeth penetrate into the more superior (sublingual) compartment (see Figure 8-4). Only loose connective tissue rather than true fascia actually separates one side of the floor of the mouth from the other, an anatomical situation that permits infection to spread bilaterally with ease (Figures 8-21 and 8-22).

Anteriorly the sublingual space communicates with the submental space. In this area the sublingual space may be invaded by infection from incisor teeth, especially from periodontal infection. Posteriorly the sublingual space communicates with the lateral pharyngeal spaces, in the neighborhood of the posterior edge of the mylohyoid muscle and the lesser wings of the hyoid bone.

Infection of the sublingual space appears clinically as brawny, erythematous, tender swelling of the floor of the mouth, beginning close to the mandible and spreading toward the midline or beyond. Some elevation of the tongue may be noted in late cases. Infection must be differentiated from the cellulitis that may accompany an impacted sialolith in Wharton's duct. Radiographs of the teeth and occlusal films of the oral floor should be used in diagnosis.

Surgical drainage of the sublingual space should be performed intraorally by an incision through the mucosa parallel to Wharton's duct bilaterally. If the submandibular space is to be drained, both spaces can be reached through a submandibular approach.

The submandibular space is separated from the overlying sublingual space by the fibers of the mylohyoid muscle. Odontogenic infections of this space commonly are caused by the second and third molar teeth (and, rarely, the first molar), inasmuch as their root apices lie inferior to the mylohyoid line of muscle attachment. The space is bounded laterally by the submandibular skin, superficial fascia, platysma muscle, superficial layer of deep cervical fascia, and the lower border of the mandible. The contents of the submandibular space include the submandibular salivary gland and its lymph nodes, the facial (external maxillary) artery, the proximal portion of Wharton's duct, and the lingual and hypoglossal nerves as they course deep to the submandibular gland on the inferior surface of the mylohyoid muscle (Figures 8-23 through 8-25).

Diagnosis of submandibular space infection is made by finding the typical swelling of the space, either brawny or soft, and correlating it with the presence of a diseased mandibular molar. Infection may be related to sepsis in an adjoining space such as the sublingual, the submental, or

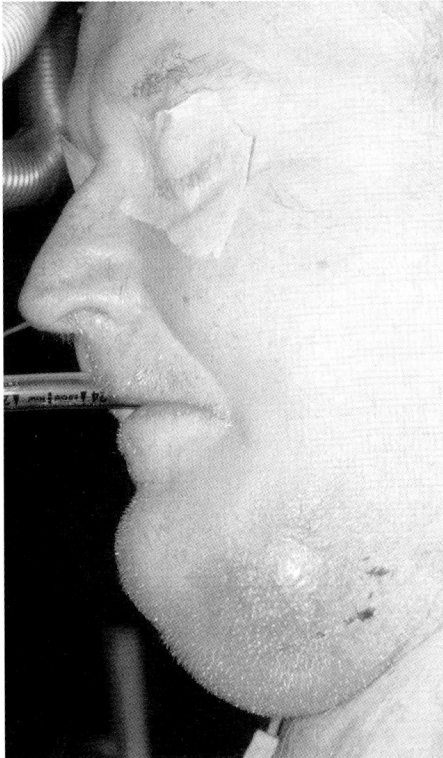

Figure 8-24 Clinical appearance of submandibular space infection. (Courtesy William Benzing.)

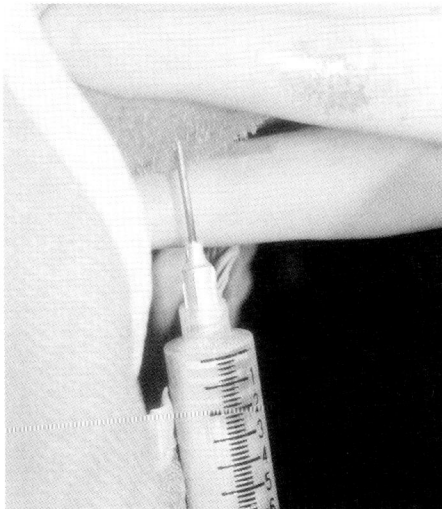

Figure 8-25 Aspiration of submandibular space infection (for anaerobic culture) before open incision and drainage. (Courtesy William Benzing.)

the masticator space. Conversely, infection may spread from the submandibular space into any contiguous space, including the pharyngeal spaces. The infectious process commonly spreads across the midline into the contralateral submandibular space. If spread is bilateral and involves all submandibular and sublingual spaces and the submental space, the result is the well-known Ludwig's angina.

Differential diagnosis should include acute sialadenitis, sublingual trauma or foreign body, and submandibular lymphadenitis. These may produce a secondary overlying cellulitis that further confuses the diagnosis.

Therapy of submandibular space odontogenic infection includes surgical drainage, antibiotics, and definitive care of the primary dental infection. Incision is performed through the skin below and parallel to the mandible. Blunt dissection is carried to the depths of the space and to its anterior and posterior margins. Deep abscess loculations should be entered with a small closed clamp, probing in all directions while attempting to avoid damage to the submandibular gland, the facial artery, and the lingual nerve. The contralateral space should not be entered unless it is involved in the infection; if necessary, however, a through-and-through drain can be placed into both sides, as in the treatment of Ludwig's angina.

■ CASE REPORT

A 47-year-old patient who had received a kidney transplant reported swelling under his tongue. The patient was receiving immunotherapy including cortisone therapy. Examination revealed erythematous, firm, tender swelling of the floor of the mouth. Two mandibular incisors were mobile; radiographs revealed diffuse bone loss consistent with periodontitis, and deep gingival pockets were present. His temperature was 100.4° F.

Penicillin and warm saline solution rinses were prescribed for this ambulatory patient. Two days later, with the patient under outpatient general anesthesia, the teeth were extracted and a mucosal incision parallel to Wharton's duct produced a small amount of purulent drainage from the sublingual space. Culture of specimens revealed streptococci, both aerobic and anaerobic; the infection resolved in 10 days.

SUBMENTAL SPACE

A potential fascial space exists in the chin and occasionally becomes infected, either directly from a mandibular incisor or indirectly from the submandibular space. The submental space is located below the chin and is bound above by the skin and the chin (mentalis) muscles, laterally by the anterior bellies of the digastric muscles, deeply by the mylohyoid muscle, and superiorly by the deep cervical fascia, the platysma muscle, the superficial fascia, and the skin. Submental infection may spread easily to either or both submandibular spaces.

If infection from the incisors exits labially through the mandibular bone, inferior to the muscle attachments, the submental space becomes involved. The chin appears grossly swollen and is quite firm and erythematous (Figure 8-26). Percutaneous surgical drainage is the most effective approach. A horizontal incision in the most inferior portion of the chin, in a natural skin crease, provides dependent drainage and the most cosmetically acceptable scar. The space may be drained

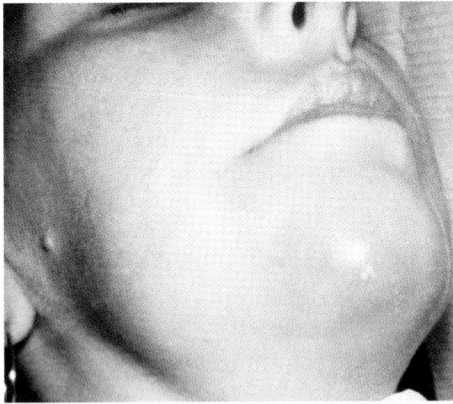

Figure 8-26 Prominent bulging of chin point with imminent fistulization *(white spot)* and peripheral cellulitis.

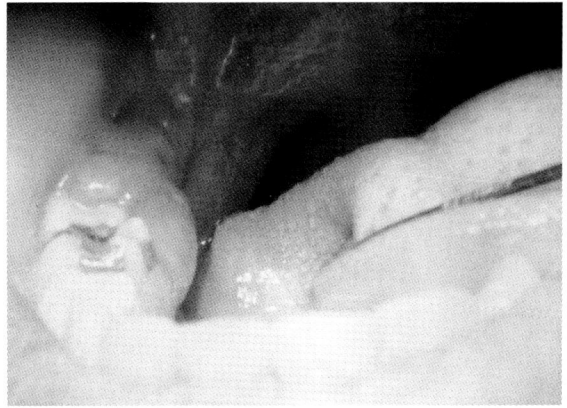

Figure 8-27 Swollen infected flap of pericoronitis of mandibular third molar. Also note swelling extending to lingual surface of the mandible.

orally through the mentalis muscle through the labial vestibule, but dependent drainage cannot be established from this approach.

■ CASE REPORT

A 63-year-old patient with insulin-dependent diabetes and a history of poorly controlled hyperglycemia was transferred from a rural hospital, where he had been treated with intravenously administered penicillin for 4 days because of massive swelling of the neck. The infection originally had been localized in the submental area after extraction of a mobile mandibular central incisor.

Examination revealed an obese, febrile man whose neck was swollen, intensely erythematous and tender, with palpable crepitus from the chin to the sternal notch. His white blood cell count was 27,400/mm^3, and the fasting blood glucose level was 280 mg/dL. CT scanning revealed gross swelling of the neck associated with profuse gas formation and tissue necrosis.

After fluid resuscitation and intubation the patient's neck was opened widely and necrotic fascia and muscle were removed. Brown necrotic tissue and fluid, with a fecal odor, extended from the submandibular and submental spaces to the superior mediastinum. After cultures were obtained, multiple drains were placed, small areas of necrotic skin were excised, and intravenous imipenem (Primaxin) therapy was started empirically when a Gram stain revealed a mixed flora of gram-positive cocci and gram-negative rods.

Culture later revealed aerobic and anaerobic streptococci and *Fusobacterium* and *Bacteroides* organisms. Healing progressed slowly but uneventfully after hyperglycemia was controlled, and the patient was discharged on the twenty-third hospital day.

In a grossly obese, hyperglycemic patient with insulin-dependent diabetes, periodontal infection is the norm and postextraction infection is commonplace. Whether standard penicillin therapy (or prophylaxis) would have avoided or aborted an infection is debatable. The early concomitant use of metronidazole (Flagyl) and clin-

damycin would have increased the chance of success in this mixed-flora infection.

In this patient a localized submental space infection spread to the submandibular spaces and into the neck, creating a life-threatening necrotizing fasciitis (see Chapter 13).

■ CASE REPORT

A 10-year-old child was brought to the emergency department 2 days after a fall from a bicycle. Examination revealed a markedly swollen chin, and imaging revealed a nondisplaced symphyseal fracture and a subcondylar fracture. The central incisors were slightly mobile. Despite rigid fixation and penicillin therapy, the submental area became fluctuant and required incision and drainage, from which streptococci and *Bacteroides* were cultured. After drainage the infection and fracture healed uneventfully.

Antibiotics do not penetrate well into fascial space infections, regardless of the primary source of infection; a scalpel blade often is the therapy of choice. Fractures and surgery may be the cause of space infections.

INFECTIONS ASSOCIATED WITH IMPACTED THIRD MOLAR TEETH

Lower third molars are a frequent cause of infection, even in otherwise healthy patients. In Western society, where contemporary dental care and the widespread use of fluoridated drinking water have resulted in the remarkable decrease of dental caries and prevention of early loss of first and second molar teeth, a high rate of impacted third molars has resulted. Impaction is often associated with pericoronal infection (Figure 8-27). Bacteriologically the profuse colonization under the moist, poorly oxygenated pericoronal flap consists of the usual mixed aerobic-anaerobic flora but may result in tissue destruction and pain to a level similar to that of acute necrotizing ulcerative gingivitis. The use of antibiotics is recommended for third molar pericoronitis if temperature is elevated or trismus or adenopathy is present. Initially, gentle mechanical irrigation and de-

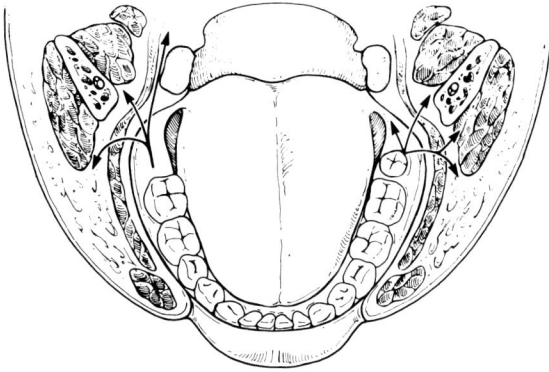

Figure 8-28 Spread of infection from third molar teeth. Infection may invade into masticator, submandibular, buccal, parapharyngeal, parotid, and other contiguous spaces. (From Rogerson KC, Topazian RG: Infections associated with impacted teeth. In Alling CC, Helfrick JF, Alling RD, editors: *Impacted teeth,* Philadelphia, 1993, WB Saunders.)

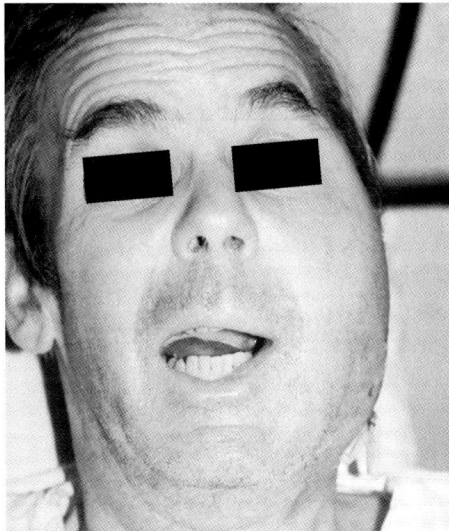

Figure 8-29 Pan-space infection from third molar, including buccal, parotid, masticator, submandibular, and sublingual spaces in patient with insulin-dependent diabetes.

bridement can be useful, as are incision and drainage, with extraction of the maxillary third molar (or cuspal reduction) if it is in occlusion with the edematous mandibular flap. Lower extraction usually is delayed until the trismus has resolved sufficiently to permit surgical access.

Pericoronitis occasionally spreads rapidly because of the anatomical location of the mandibular third molar at the crossroads of the masticator, submandibular, and buccal fascial spaces with adjacent anatomical access to contiguous parapharyngeal, parotid, submandibular, and other spaces (Figures 8-28 and 8-29). Unfortunately, the same potentially serious sequelae exist as postextraction complications, an important issue in the risk/benefit ratio and medicolegal areas of surgery.

The role of prophylactic antibiotics in third molar surgery is controversial. If pericoronitis is present at the time of surgery or has been present recently, antibiotic therapy is indicated. However, removal of the truly asymptomatic and completely impacted third molar fits the category of clean-contaminated rather than contaminated surgery, and data exist to support the efficacy of both the use and nonuse of prophylactic antibiotics. If the mandibular marrow space has been widely exposed, especially during a lengthy extraction, "prophylactic" postoperative antibiotics would seem prudent. However, for true prophylaxis, the antibiotic ideally should be administered preoperatively. The use of antibiotics after third molar extraction has not altered the infection rate. Advocates and dissenters continue the ongoing clinical debate.

Penicillin remains the antibiotic of choice, administered as 2 g of penicillin V orally 1 hour before the procedure and a second dose 2 hours after the initial dose, with no further doses given. Alternatively, 2 g of penicillin G may be given intravenously as a single dose. In patients who are allergic to penicillin, clindamycin, 300 mg orally or intravenously as a single dose, is suggested.

The overall third molar postoperative infection rate ranges from 4.2% to 6.3% with or without antibiotics, but most studies are subject to challenge because they fail to differentiate which patients have a history of pericoronitis and whether the extraction sites were profusely irrigated.

LUDWIG'S ANGINA

Ludwig's angina is a firm, acute, toxic cellulitis of the submandibular and sublingual spaces bilaterally and of the submental space. As early as 1796, extraction of abscessed teeth was considered contraindicated because "it might give rise to extensive inflammation and angina, in a dangerous degree." Three "*f*s" became evident even before the first written description of the disease: it was to be *feared,* it rarely became *fluctuant,* and it often was *fatal.* A sensation of choking and suffocation (angina) often was combined with the name of the author (Ludwig) who fully described it in 1836.[10]

The original description of the disease has not been improved since the observations of Wilhelm Friedrich von Ludwig were published while he was court physician to the King of Württemberg and president of that kingdom's medical association. His descriptive phrases ring true today, despite considerable improvements in therapy and mortality:

> . . . *amidst the symptoms which herald the approach—an erysepalous angina, temperature swings . . . discomfort upon swallowing, there develops on one or both sides of the neck a firm connective tissue with which in comes in contact . . . it extends uniformly about the periphery of the neck . . . to a marked degree. It advances in similar fashion to involve the tissues which cover the small muscles between the larynx and the floor of the mouth . . . the tongue rests upon a red, indurated mass which feels like a hard ring adjacent to the inner surface of the jaw bone. It becomes difficult and painful to open the mouth . . . speech is impaired and hoarse . . . this is because the tongue is pressed backward and upwards, there is pressure upon the*

larynx . . . as the disease progresses . . . externally certain areas become, at times, softer . . . at other times more prominent and apparently fluctuant. Fever increases with morning exacerbations . . . swallowing continues to be difficult and the patient opens the mouth only with effort; dyspnea appears usually in paroxysms . . . and on the tenth to twelfth day of the disease, death occurs, with the patient in a comatose state with evidence of respiratory paralysis . . . there are nuances in the typical picture of the disease . . . particularly the onset and severity of the local lesion. . . . Among the cases in which autopsy was permitted . . . there were found abscess cavities whose walls were made up of gangrenous partly decomposed masses of muscle . . . the periosteum of the inner surface of the jaw was loosened from the bone and was discolored.

Ludwig refrained from suggesting a "scientifically valid" hypothesis of the cause of the disease, but stated that "it differentiates itself from other neck inflammations with symptomatic or idiopathic swelling of the salivary glands." As therapy, he recommended local and general bloodletting, softening poultices, and external and internal use of mercurials, vesicants, cathartics, and diuretics. He described the case of Fräulein N.N., who suffered both the disease and the therapy, including leeches, bran poultices, tartar emetic, dry heat, a gargle of althea and honey, almond oil, ipecac, and finally, "a piece of silver nitrate the size of a six Krenzer coin over the middle of the swelling . . . which had created a splendid necrosis." Because of or despite the therapy (chemical incision and drainage), N.N. survived, and "three weeks after the onset, when the last traces of the induration could still be felt, the patient felt well and strong."

Almost 60 years passed before the causative relationship between dental disease and Ludwig's angina was established. Carious rotten teeth were ubiquitous in Ludwig's era, whereas his eponymous angina was comparatively uncommon; hence, he never recognized the association. Considering that the germ theory of disease had yet to be postulated, antibiotics were undiscovered, anesthesia did not exist, and contemporary surgeons were reluctant to incise without the certainty of finding "laudable pus," N.N. was indeed fortunate to have survived. Curiously, Ludwig did not survive a throat inflammation and he died in 1865 at the age of 75.

Today, Ludwig's angina is a disease primarily of dental origin. Dental infection has been reported as the causative factor in 90% of cases in some series, either as primary dental infection or as a postextraction phenomenon. As Williams and Guralnick[15] stated in 1943, "The dentist who is unfortunate enough to have performed extraction on a patient who subsequently develops Ludwig's angina is more likely to have been incidental to the train of events than to have been the responsible agent."

Other causative factors include submandibular gland sialadenitis, compound mandibular fracture, oral soft tissue lacerations, puncture wounds of the oral floor, and secondary infections of oral malignancies. Ludwig's angina infection has been reported in a newborn. The term *pseudo–Ludwig's angina* has been applied to these cases of nondental origin; they also are referred to as pseudo–Ludwig phenomena.

Fortunately, the incidence of Ludwig's angina remains low in this modern era of preventative dental care and antibiotic therapy. In the preantibiotic era a mortality rate of greater than 50% was reported, but this was reduced to approximately 5% with the use of penicillin. Most early cases probably are aborted by the use of antibiotics before rapid, deep spread of infection occurs. Representing less than 1% of all admissions to oral-maxillofacial services, Ludwig's angina is observed most frequently in the contemporary compromised host. If the disease is untreated the mortality rate is close to 100%.

Bilateral infection of the sublingual and submandibular spaces with brawny edema, an elevated tongue, airway obstruction, and a paucity of pus are the clinical hallmarks of Ludwig's angina. The submental space also is swollen, and sepsis may spread rapidly to involve the masticator and pharyngeal spaces (Figure 8-30).

A veritable host of organisms have been implicated as the causative agents of this disease. Because Ludwig's angina is commonly of dental origin, streptococci or mixed oral flora are the most commonly reported organisms from cultures of whatever exudate can be obtained after surgical drainage. Contemporary reports of Ludwig's angina have demonstrated the presence of staphylococci, gram-negative enteric organisms such as *E. coli* and *Pseudomonas,* and anaerobes, including *Bacteroides* and *Peptostreptococcus* spp. The isolation of these organisms may indicate the changing oral flora of the antibiotic era or may reflect more sophisticated modern culture techniques. *Prevotella melaninogenicus, Prevotella oralis,* and *Prevotella corrodens* also have been isolated from patients with Ludwig's angina or other odontogenic infections. Experimental data from studies of cutaneous infections similar to the ulcer of Meleney suggest that a synergistic or obligatory synergistic relationship may exist among anaerobes such as *Prevotella (P. melaninogenicus),* anaerobic streptococci, and fusospirochetes, all common organisms. Mixtures of oral

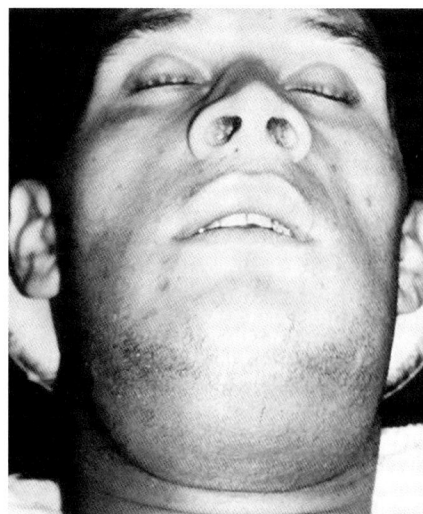

Figure 8-30 Ludwig's angina. Brawny diffuse swelling of bilateral submandibular, sublingual, and submental spaces.

organisms that did not include *Prevotella* could not create transmissible subcutaneous infections in experimental animals, whereas an infection was produced by the addition of that organism. Whatever the role of anaerobes, primary or synergistic, a search for them should not be omitted when culturing specimens from Ludwig's angina or other serious odontogenic infections. (See Geisler et al.[4] and Chow et al.[1])

Treatment of Ludwig's angina includes early diagnosis of the incipient cases, maintenance of a patient airway, intense and prolonged antibiotic therapy, extraction of the affected teeth, hydration, and early surgical drainage (with a life in the balance, a quick extraction is more rational than time-consuming tooth salvage). Empirical antibiotic therapy (intravenous) for Ludwig's angina should be intense; choices include penicillin plus metronidazole or clindamycin or imipenem used as single agents.

Establishment and maintenance of an adequate airway are the sine qua non of therapy. Death is more likely to occur early from airway obstruction than from sepsis. Tracheostomy has been almost routine during most of the twentieth century but may prove difficult to perform in the late stage of the disease because of massive neck edema and tissue distortion. Attempts at blind endotracheal intubation may be time consuming, unsuccessful, and fraught with danger, especially if attempted by an inexperienced anesthesiologist, because of the swollen elevated tongue and glottic edema. The danger of rupturing a bulging lateral pharyngeal or retropharyngeal abscess exists if the infection involves these fascial spaces. Cervical soft tissue plain films and CT scanning should be done before attempted tracheostomy, if time permits. Fiber-optic laryngoscopy is useful in the airway management of Ludwig's angina but requires an anesthesiologist skilled in its use, and the patient must be cooperative and premedicated. Tracheal intubation with the patient under deep inhalation anesthesia may be successful, usually obviating the need for tracheostomy. The use of sedative and narcotic agents, which may cause more rapid respiratory deterioration, is not recommended (see Chapter 23).

Although some authorities advocate high doses of antibiotics without surgery until fluctuance develops, in most surgeons' experience, fully developed Ludwig's angina requires prompt and deep surgical incision because fluctuance is uncommon and late. Ludwig's angina is a diffuse cellulitis of deep fascia. Seventy percent of cases still require surgical intervention and drainage. The submandibular and sublingual spaces and secondarily involved spaces must be explored bilaterally. The masticator spaces must be drained if trismus is present. The prudent and experienced surgeon recognizes the wisdom of the maxim "a chance to cut is a chance to cure" when confronted with Ludwig's angina.

A horizontal incision midway between the chin and the hyoid bone was the classic approach to the surgical drainage of Ludwig's angina, but this "cut-throat" incision has proved unnecessary and unaesthetic. Bilateral incision into the submandibular spaces with blunt dissection to the midline suffices if a through-and-through drain or bilateral drains meeting in the midline are placed. This maneuver, combined with drainage of the sublingual spaces, relieves the intense pressure of edematous tissue on the airway and provides specimens for Gram staining and culture (Figure 8-31).

The platysma muscle and suprahyoid fascias are incised by this approach, and the fascia of the submandibular gland also is entered. The mylohyoid muscle should be divided and the sublingual spaces entered. A closed clamp should be inserted through the median raphe of the mylohyoid muscle and advanced to the hyoid bone at the base of the tongue. Generally, little pus is obtained because the infection often represents cellulitis of the fascia spaces rather than true abscess formation. In some cases, especially late or fully developed ones, purulent flow is produced.

Needle aspiration of deep fascial space infections has been attempted, sometimes obviating open drainage procedures. However, Ludwig's angina, basically a rapid-spreading, deep cellulitis without localization of pus or formation of fluctuance, is not amenable to this technique, even if the needle is CT guided.

Sequelae after adequate drainage and antibiotic therapy are uncommon. However, inadequate drainage or premature closure of the surgical wounds may lead to reinfection. Late spread to other fascial spaces or generalized sepsis may occur and are ever-present dangers. Failure to extract the offending tooth could cause reinfection. Secondary revision of scarring may be necessary for cosmetic reasons or to repair stenosis of Wharton's duct.

The mortality rate for Ludwig's angina has decreased since the advent of prompt surgical intervention, airway maintenance techniques, and antibiotic therapy. However, three fatal cases are discussed in the following case reports to illustrate the potential or actual lethality of this disease.

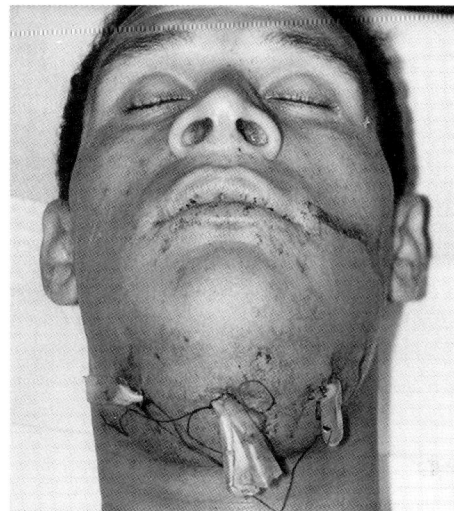

Figure 8-31 Surgical therapy for Ludwig's angina involves incisions and placement of drains bilaterally into submandibular spaces, meeting in the midline and draining the submental space.

■ CASE REPORT ■

A 9-year-old girl in severe respiratory distress was brought to the emergency department by ambulance. Four days earlier a diagnosis of "submaxillary mumps" had been made by the family physician because of unilateral swelling beneath the mandible. Despite progressive swelling, pain, and temperature elevation, only symptomatic therapy was used. A few hours before the patient's hospital admission, the swelling had spread bilaterally and respiratory distress had developed. Examination in the emergency department revealed a cyanotic, semicomatose child with a large firm swelling of the anterior neck. Her tongue was displaced superiorly and posteriorly by wooden-hard erythematous sublingual edema. Laryngoscopy in the emergency department was unsuccessful.

Tracheostomy was attempted but was difficult because of massive edema and displacement of the trachea. The child died within a few minutes while the tracheostomy was being performed, and resuscitation efforts proved fruitless. Postmortem examination confirmed the diagnosis of Ludwig's angina and a deeply carious mandibular molar as its cause.

Submaxillary mumps without parotid involvement is rare, if it exists at all, whereas untreated Ludwig's angina is lethal. Had the association of submandibular swelling with a diseased tooth been noted, the child's death could have been prevented. The rapidly lethal course of the infection, once it had crossed the submandibular midline, illustrates the clear danger of ignoring early signs of this disease. Ludwig's angina leaves little room for misdiagnosis or procrastination, especially in children. Although the overall incidence of Ludwig's angina is decreasing, as is the frequency of mortality, contemporary (1990s') series of cases reveal that as many as 24% of patients in hospitals with this diagnosis are admitted to the pediatric service. Tonsillitis is a more common cause of deep neck infections in children than is odontogenic infection, and airway compromise is less well tolerated than in adults.

■ CASE REPORT ■

A 25-year-old woman, in apparently good health, underwent extraction of a painful, partially impacted third molar teeth in a dental office. No antibiotics were prescribed because there were no obvious clinical signs of infection at the time of surgery.

Low-grade temperature elevation and facial swelling developed during the evening after surgery. By the following day a firm bilateral submandibular swelling, mild trismus, and temperature elevation to 100.8° F were noted. The patient experienced chills, and the swelling had increased and trismus had intensified later that day. Symptomatic therapy in the form of analgesics and oral rinses was used.

By the morning of the third postoperative day the patient was obtund and cyanotic. The family physician called to her home was unable to obtain a recordable blood pressure and observed that she was cold, cyanotic, and barely arousable. He noted the presence of purpura and that massive swelling extended from "the jaw to the clavicle."

She was transferred by ambulance to a hospital emergency department and admitted with the diagnosis of Ludwig's angina and septicemia. Laboratory studies at the time of admission revealed visible blood in the urine, red blood cell casts, hemoglobin level of 15.2 g/100 mL, and a white blood cell count of 8300/mm³. Platelets were absent from the peripheral blood smear, and the prothrombin time was markedly prolonged. Because of the presence of shock, acral cyanosis, purpura, thrombocytopenia, and obvious coagulopathy, the diagnosis was modified to disseminated intravascular coagulation secondary to Ludwig's angina of dental origin.

Further laboratory data in the intensive care unit revealed a blood urea nitrogen level of 75 mg/100 mL, platelet count of 39,000/mm³, partial thromboplastin time of 52 seconds, and a moderately decreased fibrinogen level associated with a severe depletion of other hemostatic factors. Gram stain of the buffy coat demonstrated large numbers of gram-positive cocci, whereas blood cultures later grew β-hemolytic *Streptococcus* colonies.

Tracheostomy was performed and oxygen administered; fluids, fresh plasma, and blood were infused; penicillin and oxacillin were administered; and heparin therapy was started. Despite all therapy, neck swelling increased, temperature increased to 105° F, urine output decreased, and the blood pressure could be maintained no higher than 90/60 mm Hg with the continuous infusion of vasopressors. A purulent exudate was noted in the oral cavity, and gram-positive cocci were seen on Gram stain.

By the morning of the fourth postoperative day (second hospital day), the shock syndrome and renal failure appeared irreversible and the patient was comatose. The purpura became generalized and bleeding persisted around the tracheostomy and intravenous catheter sites. Immunoelectrophoresis studies supported the diagnosis of consumption coagulopathy, as did serial coagulation tests.

Assisted respiration and use of plasma, serum albumin, and mannitol infusions were continued. Chest radiography revealed diffuse infiltrates bilaterally, and bloody sputum was obtained from tracheal suctioning. Unremitting deterioration continued, and late on the fourth postoperative day fatal cardiopulmonary arrest occurred.

Disseminated intravascular coagulation is a well-recognized but fortunately uncommon sequela of severe infection. It occurs as a result of gram-negative sepsis far more commonly than as a result of streptococcal infection, but severe complications are possible with dental infection. The possible preventive effect of antibiotic use at the time of surgery is purely speculative, inasmuch as the 50% to 70% fatality rate of patients with disseminated intravascular coagulation includes many who were receiving antibiotics at the time of the onset of the consumptive coagulopathy. Generalized sepsis can be the cause of death in Ludwig's angina.

■ CASE REPORT

A 60-year-old woman with a diagnosis of Ludwig's angina and septicemia was admitted to the intensive care unit by a clinician in the hematology section. The patient had a 13-year history of chronic lymphocytic leukemia, which had required chemotherapy only during the last year. She had complained to her dentist about painful swollen gingiva 3 days before admission, and penicillin had been prescribed for the periodontal infection. By the date of admission, her mouth and neck were markedly swollen, airway obstruction was present, and she was in septic shock.

Examination revealed an intubated, obtunded patient with temperature of 101° F. The tongue was elevated over erythematous indurated sublingual tissue, and the gingivae were edematous and red, especially adjacent to the mandibular incisors. The upper neck was bilaterally swollen and firm. The white blood cell count was 52,000/mm^3, consisting exclusively of immature lymphocytes and a few blast forms.

Blood and oral cultures grew *Pseudomonas aeruginosa.* Incision and drainage of the neck were performed and cultures also revealed *Pseudomonas.* High-dose, intravenous multiple-antibiotic therapy was instituted, but the patient died of generalized sepsis on the fifth hospital day.

Despite a secure airway, the patient died of Ludwig's angina. The compromised host is the contemporary patient most at risk from deep fascial space infection, usually from opportunistic organisms. Although the death certificate listed chronic lymphocytic leukemia, septicemia, and Ludwig's angina as causes of death, the initiating factor was gingivitis.

Alternative treatment for Ludwig's angina has been described. Glucocorticoids have been added to antibiotic therapy when the latter did not halt the inexorable progression of the infection. The rationale is to combat the inflammatory edema with resolution finally accomplished without surgery.[7] However, extreme caution is recommended when considering the administration of corticosteroids to a patient with an already established infection.

PHARYNGEAL SPACE INFECTION

The *lateral pharyngeal space* (pharyngomaxillary space) is a lateral neck space shaped like an inverted cone, with its base at the skull and its apex at the hyoid bone. Its medial wall is contiguous with the carotid sheath, and it lies deep to the pharyngeal constrictor muscle. It is divided, for surgical and anatomical purposes, into anterior and posterior compartments.

Infections of the lateral pharyngeal space may result from pharyngitis, tonsillitis, parotitis, otitis, mastoiditis, and dental infection, especially if the masticator spaces are primarily infected. Herpetic gingivostomatitis involving pericoronal tissue has also been reported as a cause of the lateral pharyngeal abscess. If the anterior compartment becomes infected, the patient exhibits pain, fever, chills, me-

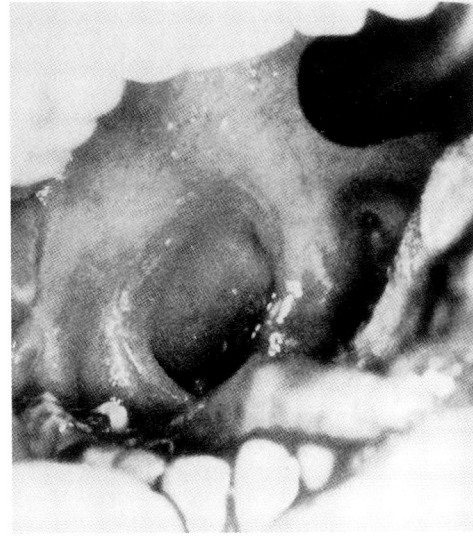

Figure 8-32 Lateral pharyngeal space abscess occurring late after third molar extraction. Note bulging of the lateral pharyngeal wall, soft palate, and tonsillar area with displacement of the uvula. (Courtesy William Marco III.)

dial bulging of the lateral pharyngeal wall with deviation of the palatal uvula from the midline, dysphagia, swelling below the angle of the mandible, and usually trismus (Figure 8-32). Infection of the posterior compartment is noted for absence of trismus and visible swelling, but respiratory obstruction, septic thrombosis of the internal jugular vein, and carotid artery hemorrhage may occur in patients at a late stage of infection. CT may prove useful in diagnosing lateral pharyngeal infections and may reveal confluence with other deep space infections and septic erosion of the wall of the great vessels. CT is more useful than standard radiographs in viewing the lateral neck spaces and has become the contemporary standard.

Therapy consists of antibiotics, surgical drainage, and tracheostomy if indicated. The surgical approach may be oral, by incision of the lateral pharyngeal wall (Figure 8-33), or external, by exposure of the carotid sheath near the lateral tip of the hyoid bone after retraction of the sternocleidomastoid muscle. Blunt dissection along the posterior border of the digastric muscle leads to the lateral pharyngeal space. In the combined intraoral and extraoral approach a mucosal incision is made lateral to the pterygomandibular raphe, and a large curved clamp is passed medial to the medial pterygoid muscle in a posterior-inferior direction. The tip of the clamp is delivered through the skin by a cutaneous incision between the angle of the mandible and the sternocleidomastoid muscle.

■ CASE REPORT

A 19-year-old man was seen with trismus and dysphagia. Historically, he had multiple episodes of pericoronitis controlled by antibiotics, but he had refused third molar extraction. Examination was difficult because of trismus and

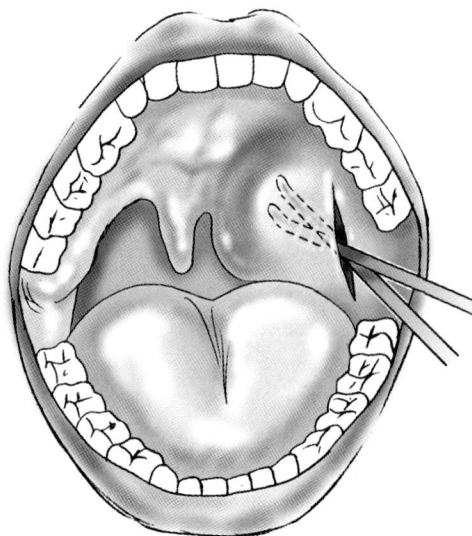

Figure 8-33 Incision and blunt drainage of lateral pharyngeal space. (Courtesy William Bontempi.)

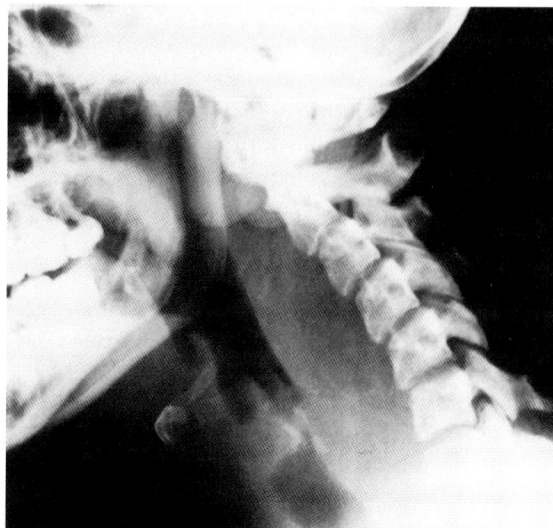

Figure 8-34 Retropharyngeal space abscess after extraction of mandibular third molar. Note massive soft tissue swelling with tracheal displacement. (Courtesy John F. DuPont, Jr.)

pain, but bulging of the lateral pharyngeal wall and soft palate with deviation of the uvula was observed, in addition to tenderness and slight swelling at the mandibular angle. CT imaging confirmed the diagnosis of lateral pharyngeal space and masticator space (pterygoid compartment) infection.

After cautious blind nasal intubation, a mucosal incision at the pterygomandibular raphe and an angle skin incision, with deep blunt dissections, released pus from the spaces and relieved the trismus. Mixed oral flora were treated with intravenous penicillin and metronidazole, but persistent pharyngeal swelling and inadequate drainage, confirmed by CT, necessitated second incision and drainage 5 days later, which resolved the infection. The affected tooth was removed.

Medically and legally, a patient must be fully informed of the risks of recurrent pericoronitis. In such situations, the procedure is not elective, but rather is better categorized as urgent.

Dysphagia, like dyspnea, is an alarm in the presence of odontogenic infection. Anesthesia consultation, prompt imaging, and rapid surgical decompression are necessary.

Failure to respond quickly to incision and drainage, demonstrated by defervescence of fever, lowered white blood cell count, and relief from dysphagia or dyspnea, requires reevaluation by examination and reimaging to determine adequacy of drainage or possible late involvement of other spaces. A second trip to the operating room during the initial hospitalization is medically and legally superior to a later readmission.

RETROPHARYNGEAL SPACE

The esophagus and trachea are enclosed by the middle layer of deep cervical fascia. A thick strand of connective tissue extends laterally from the esophagus to the carotid sheath, thus creating an anterior neck compartment known as the *pretracheal* (previsceral) space and a posterior or *retropharyngeal* (retrovisceral) space. The posterior space lies behind the esophagus and pharynx and extends inferiorly to the upper mediastinum and superiorly to the base of the skull.

Clinically, retropharyngeal space infections may result from nasal and pharyngeal infections in children, dental infection diffusing through contiguous spaces, esophageal trauma or foreign bodies, and tuberculosis. Infection also may reach this space through the lymphatics to involve the retropharyngeal lymph nodes. Dysphagia, dyspnea, nuchal rigidity, esophageal regurgitation, and fever characterize infections of the retropharyngeal space. If the pharynx can be visualized, a bulging of the posterior wall may be observed and is usually more prominent unilaterally because of the adherence of the median raphe of the prevertebral fascia. Lateral soft tissue radiographs of the neck are extremely useful and may reveal considerable widening of the retropharyngeal space, well beyond the 3- to 6-mm width in normal adults at the second vertebra (or >14 mm in children) (Figure 8-34). In adults the space width/vertebra ratio is 6 mm at C2 and 20 mm at C6. The presence of gas in the prevertebral soft tissues and the loss of the normal lordotic curvature of the cervical spine also may be observed on plain films and CT scan. CT scans reveal the presence of the infection in the retropharyngeal space and its inferior extent.

Although some reports indicate that 10% to 40% of retropharyngeal infections resolve with only medical management, these cases reflect early diagnosis and antibiotic therapy. Infection of the retropharyngeal space usually requires prompt surgical drainage and allows little time for delay, debate, or decision by committee. Because many anesthesiologists are reluctant to risk aspiration or airway obstruction by pus pouring from the ruptured space during passage of an endotracheal tube, tracheostomy is usually indicated. However, drainage has been performed transorally with the patient under local anesthesia in the extreme Trendelenburg position and with constant suctioning. In the transoral technique an incision is made through the midline of the posterior pharyngeal mucosa, and the abscess is opened by blunt dissection.

An external approach generally provides more dependent drainage. An incision is made along the anterior border of the sternocleidomastoid muscle and parallel to it, inferior to the hyoid bone. This muscle and the carotid sheath are retracted laterally, and blunt finger dissection is carried deeply, avoiding the hypoglossal nerve, to the level of the hypopharynx. Blunt finger dissection deep to the inferior constrictor muscles opens the retropharyngeal space abscess. Deep drains are placed and maintained until all clinical and laboratory signs of infection are no longer apparent. Needle aspiration with CT scan guidance has avoided open surgical drainage in a few cases. The overall mortality rate for retropharyngeal infections of all causes is approximately 10%.

■ CASE REPORT

A 60-year-old man was admitted to the hospital from the emergency department with a diagnosis of multiple space infections and parotitis. Facial swelling had been present for 4 days before admission. His medical history revealed the presence of hepatic cirrhosis and steroid therapy for peripheral neuropathy.

Admission examination demonstrated unilateral facial swelling extending from the temporal region to the angle of the mandible; moderate trismus, bulging of the soft palate, and purulent discharge from Stensen's duct orifice, which was macerated. The mandibular second molar was mobile, and bloody purulent exudate could be expressed from the adjacent gingiva. His temperature was 102° F and the white blood cell count was 14,850/mm³. Gram stain results suggested streptococci from the gingival purulence and staphylococci from the duct. Specimens for culture were sent to the laboratory, and high-dose intravenous cephalosporin therapy was started. Steroid therapy was reduced gradually and then discontinued during his hospitalization.

Despite treatment the patient's swelling and pain persisted, and by the second hospital day he reported dysphagia and dyspnea. Soft tissue radiographs revealed narrowing of the upper airway because of expansion of the posterior pharyngeal space.

On the evening of the second hospital day, tracheostomy was performed with the patient under local anesthesia, and general anesthesia then was administered. Drainage of the buccal, masticator, infratemporal, lateral pharyngeal, and retropharyngeal spaces was accomplished intraorally. Profuse purulent flow was obtained and drains

were placed. External drainage of the parotid gland was performed by a preauricular approach. Repeat drainage of the temporal spaces was performed on the fourth day; drainage was performed percutaneously because of persistent pain and bulging in the area. Two mandibular molars were extracted. Rapid resolution of the space infections and parotitis followed, but osteomyelitis of the mandible (mixed oral flora) subsequently developed.

Cortisone was a major contributing factor in the rapid and deep spread of this dental infection. The parotitis may have been a result of dehydration or caused by occlusal trauma to the bulging buccal mucosa and duct orifice. It also may have been the result of spread of infection from neighboring spaces. The infection was exacerbated by the antiinflammatory effects of the steroids. This case is a prime example of an overwhelming minor infection in a compromised host.

■ CASE REPORT

A 40-year-old man underwent extraction of an infected third molar and penicillin was prescribed and taken. However, on the third postextraction day the patient was seen at an emergency department with fever, shaking chills, trismus, and dysphagia. His physician ordered blood cultures and intravenous antibiotics. By the third day of his hospitalization and after two further changes of antibiotics, the patient remained febrile and blood culture revealed *Fusobacterium*. No imaging was performed.

Surgical drainage of the masticator and lateral pterygoid spaces on the fourth hospital day resulted in diminished swelling and defervescence. The patient was discharged the following day taking oral penicillin. Eight days later, he was sent from work back to the emergency department where he reported chills, headache, and nuchal rigidity. The antibiotic regimen was changed again, but he returned to the emergency department 2 days later semicomatose.

Blood cultures again grew *Fusobacterium* and streptococci, and MRI revealed a posterior pharyngeal space abscess and an epidural brain abscess near the brain stem. Surgical drainage of both sites and 10 days of intensive intravenous antibiotic therapy resolved all signs of infection, but the patient has severe neurological deficits, including deafness and hemiparesis. Legal action ensued against the physician, the surgeon, the emergency physician, and the hospital, with a final settlement of almost $2 million.

Fusobacterium, an oral organism, can be virulent, especially when causing generalized sepsis. Patients with positive blood culture results should not be discharged until cultures are sterile or after 10 days of appropriate intravenous antibiotic therapy. Even a lateral plain film might have revealed an incipient posterior pharyngeal space infection. Shaking chills, headache, and neck stiffness should have been strong indicators, especially with the patient's history of recent drainage of a lateral pharyngeal space.

MEDIASTINITIS

Extension of infection from deep neck spaces into the mediastinum is heralded by chest pain and severe dyspnea, unremitting fever, and radiographic demonstration of mediastinal widening. Rarely, mediastinitis also may be caused by odontogenic infection that spreads directly along the great vessels in the perivascular space of the carotid sheath. Intravenous drug abusers who inject into the major blood vessels of the neck are at risk for deep neck infections, including the carotid space, and may have septic thrombosis of the jugular veins.

Spread of odontogenic infection to the mediastinum also is noteworthy because it is preceded by infection of other fascial spaces that may have been drained quite adequately. Therefore mediastinitis may be a very late complication and should be suspected in patients with exacerbation of fever associated with substernal pain. Progressive septicemia, mediastinal abscesses, pleural effusion, empyema, compression of mediastinal veins with decreased venous return to the heart, and pericarditis may occur, with death as the final outcome.

Necrotizing mediastinitis of dental origin may be related to the synergistic effect of aerobic and anaerobic bacteria invading susceptible tissue far from their normal oral environment.[2,16] Passively commensal in the mouth, the bacteria may become synergistically aggressive and invasive elsewhere.

Treatment of suppurative mediastinitis consists of extensive, long-term antibiotic therapy and surgical drainage of the mediastinum. Specimens for culture should be obtained regularly during long-term therapy.

■ CASE REPORT

A 20-year-old student underwent extraction of bilateral painful impacted mandibular third molar teeth in an outpatient facility. His medical history was significant for numerous episodes of staphylococcal pneumonitis and skin infections during childhood. A chronic fungal infection of his nail beds resisted treatment. No antibiotics were used or prescribed at the time of surgery.

Eight days after extraction of the teeth, he was admitted to the hospital because of dyspnea, dysphagia, swelling of the left side of the neck and face, and temperature of 103.4° F. The diagnosis at the time of admission was lateral pharyngeal space abscess, left submandibular space abscess, and left buccal space infection. Dehydration was clinically apparent, and the white blood cell count was 19,700/mm³ with a marked shift to the left.

Intravenous fluids and clindamycin were administered. On the second hospital day, spontaneous drainage from the buccal space occurred, and Gram-stained smears of specimens revealed gram-positive cocci and gram-negative rods. Culture yielded *Bacteroides* species and peptostreptococci.

Despite extensive antibiotic therapy, his condition worsened, and lateral neck radiographs revealed widening of the retropharyngeal space. On the fourth hospital day, he underwent tracheostomy and exploration of the suprahy-

oid spaces, carotid sheath, lateral pharyngeal spaces, and posterior pharyngeal spaces through submandibular and sternocleidomastoid approaches. Three drains were placed, and mixed aerobic and anaerobic floras were cultured from the heavy purulent fluids suctioned from these spaces.

The patient's condition improved considerably after surgery, with relief of respiratory distress, lowered temperature, and lessened leukocytosis. Blood glucose, B- and T-lymphocyte counts, complement assay, and white blood cell chemotaxis studies were performed and yielded normal findings. Blood cultures yielded *Peptostreptococcus* on two occasions.

On the thirteenth hospital day the patient reported chest pain, his temperature spiked to 104° F, and radiographs revealed a widened mediastinum and pleural effusions (Figure 8-35). Thoracentesis produced a cloudy aspirate that yielded *Eikenella corrodens* when cultured. Ampicillin was added to the antibiotic regimen. Sputum cultures later yielded *P. aeruginosa;* tobramycin therapy was instituted, and clindamycin was discontinued.

On the seventeenth hospital day the mediastinum and a large empyema cavity were drained. Two ribs were resected and drains were inserted.

The patient slowly recovered, but on the twenty-seventh hospital day, swelling of the neck and exacerbation of the fever occurred. His neck was reexplored, a small amount of pus was obtained, and drains were inserted. Cultures revealed *E. corrodens* and peptostreptococci.

All signs of infection resolved, all drains were removed, and the patient was discharged on the fifty-third hospital day.

This patient's history was strongly suggestive of compromised host defenses. Although he underwent testing while he had an infection, no defects in the defense system

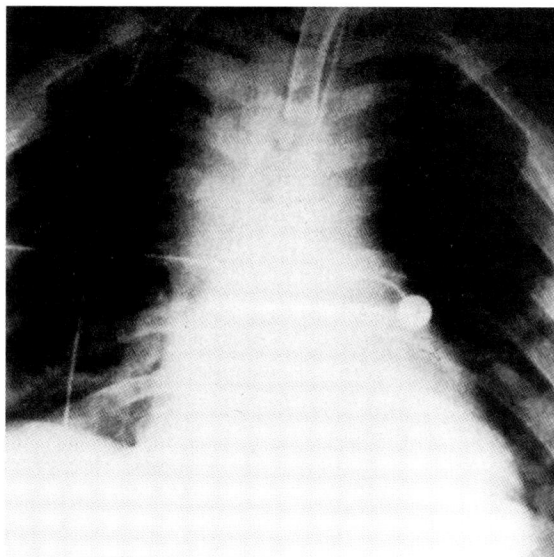

Figure 8-35 Mediastinitis caused by retropharyngeal space infection.

were found, based on contemporary knowledge. Such was the state of the art. His progressive and persistent infectious course may have been related in part to the well-documented failure of clindamycin to destroy *E. corrodens*.

SUMMARY

The incidence and severity of odontogenic infections have diminished since the advent of antibiotic therapy. However, significant morbidity and mortality of these infections continue. Dentists and physicians constantly must be alert to the potential seriousness of these infections, which should never be dismissed as simple dental abscesses. Odontogenic infection therapy—dental, medical, or surgical, outpatient or inpatient—is based on the severity and anatomical location of the infection, the patient's general health status, his or her response to therapy, and the assumed or laboratory-determined pathogenic microflora of the infection. Small superficial odontogenic infections different greatly from deep space infections despite their common origins.

Deep space infections must be recognized promptly and treated as an emergency. Underlying medical problems must be controlled, a patent airway established, contemporary diagnostic imaging done, and deep drainage performed. Repeat diagnostic and therapeutic measures may be necessary until the end point—absence of clinical, radiographic and laboratory signs of infection—has been reached.

REFERENCES

1. Chow AW, Roser SM, Brady FA: Orofacial odontogenic infections, *Ann Intern Med* 88:392, 1978.
2. Colmenero Ruiz C, Labajo AD, Yanez Vilas I, et al: Thoracic complications of deeply situated serious neck infections, *J Craniomaxillofac Surg* 21:76, 1993.
3. Donskey CJ, Chowdhry TK, Hecker MT, et al: Effect of antibiotic therapy on the density of vancomycin-resistant enterococci in the stool of colonized patients, *N Engl J Med* 343:1925, 2000.
4. Geisler PJ, Wheat P, Williams RA, et al: Isolation of anaerobes in Ludwig's angina, *J Oral Surg* 37:60, 1979.
5. Grodinsky M, Holyoke EA: Fasciae and fascial spaces of head, neck and adjacent regions, *Am J Anat* 63:367, 1938.
6. Hollinshead WH: *Anatomy for surgeons*, vol 1, ed 2, New York, 1968, Harper & Row.
7. Hutchinson IL, James DR: New treatment of Ludwig's angina, *Br J Oral Maxillofac Surg* 27:83, 1989.
8. Kuriyama T, Nakagawa K, Karasawa T, et al: Past administration of beta-lactam antibiotics and increase in the incidence of beta-lactamase–producing bacteria in patients with odontogenic infections, *Oral Surg Oral Med Oral Pathol Oral Radiol Endod* 89:186, 2000.
9. Laskin DM: Anatomic considerations in diagnosis and treatment of odontogenic infections, *J Am Dent Assoc* 69: 308, 1964.
10. Ludwig WF: Medicinishe correspondenz, *Blatt de Würtembergischen Arztlichen Vercins*, 6:26, 1836.
11. Moenning JE, Nelson CL, Kohler RB: The microbiology and chemotherapy of odontogenic infections, *J Oral Maxillofac Surg* 47:976, 1989.
12. Segelman AE, Doku H: Treatment of oral complications of leukemia, *J Oral Surg* 35:469, 1977.
13. Shapiro HH, Sleeper EL, Guralnick WC: Spread of infection of dental origin-anatomical and surgical considerations, *Oral Surg* 3:1407, 1950.
14. Sicher H: *Oral anatomy*, St Louis, 1965, Mosby.
15. Williams AC, Guralnick WC: The diagnosis and treatment of Ludwig's angina, *N Engl J Med* 228:443, 1943.
16. Zeitoun IM, Dhanarajani PJ: Cervical cellulitis and mediastinitis caused by odontogenic infections: report of two cases and review of the literature, *J Oral Maxillofac Surg* 53:203, 1995.

SUGGESTED READINGS

1. Abramowicz M, editor: Antimicrobial susceptibility tests, *Med Lett* 28:2, 1986.
2. Aderhold L, Knothe H, Frenkel G: The bacteriology of dentogenous pyogenic infections, *Oral Surg* 52:583, 1981.
3. Allen D, Loughnan TE, Ord RA: A re-evaluation of the role of tracheostomy in Ludwig's angina, *J Oral Maxillofac Surg* 43:463, 1985.
4. Appleton JLT: *Bacterial infection with special reference to dental practice*, Philadelphia, 1933, Lea & Febiger.
5. Assael LA, McCravy LL: Use of soft tissue radiographs for assessing impending airway obstruction in head and neck infections: report of cases, *J Oral Maxillofac Surg* 44:398, 1986.
6. Baker CJ: Cervical lymphadenitis. In Oski FA, editor: *Principles and practice of pediatrics*, Philadelphia, 1990, JB Lippincott.
7. Bartlett JG, Garbuch SI: Anaerobic infection of the head and neck, *Otolaryngol Clin North Am* 9:655, 1976.
8. Beck AL: Deep neck infection, *Ann Otol* 51:592, 1942.
9. Beck AL: The influence of the chemotherapeutic and antibiotic drugs on the incidence and course of deep neck infections, *Ann Otol Rhinol Laryngol* 61:515, 1952.
10. Biederman GR, Dodson TB: Epidemiologic review of facial infections in hospitalized pediatric patients, *J Oral Maxillofac Surg* 52:1042, 1994.
11. Bodner L, Bar-Ziv J: Cutaneous sinus tract of dental origin-imaging with a dental CT software programme, *Br J Oral Maxillofac Surg* 36:311, 1998.
12. Bounds GA: Subphrenic and mediastinal abscess formation: a complication of Ludwig's angina, *Br J Oral Maxillofac Surg* 23:313, 1985.
13. Briggs PC: Submandibular duct stenosis as a complication of Ludwig's angina, *Oral Surg* 47:14, 1979.
14. Britt JC, Josehson GD, Gross GW: Ludwig's angina in the pediatric population: report of a case and review of the literature, *Int J Pediatr Otorhinolaryngol* 52:79, 2000.
15. Bryan CS, King BG, Bryant RE: Retropharyngeal infection in adults, *Arch Intern Med* 134:127, 1974.
16. Burton DJ, Scheffer RB: *Serratia* infection in a patient with bilateral subcondylar impacted third molars and associated dentigerous cysts, *J Oral Surg* 38:135, 1980.
17. Caruso VG: Masticator space abscess complicating removal of suspension wires, *Ann Otol Rhinol Laryngol* 87:266, 1978.

18. Chandrasekar PA, Molinari JA: Endogenous anaerobes in orofacial infections, *Infect Surg* 5:217, 1986.

19. Chapman RM, Crosby WH: Elective dental extractions in leukemia, *N Engl J Med* 295:114, 1976.

20. Cogan MIC: Necrotizing mediastinitis secondary to descending cervical infection. *Oral Surg* 36:307, 1973.

21. Cole DR, Bankoff M, Carter BL: Percutaneous catheter drainage of deep neck infections guided by CT, *Radiology* 152:224, 1984.

22. Collier FA, Yglesias L: The relation of the spread of infection to fascial planes in the neck and thorax, *Surgery* 1:323, 1937.

23. Cottrell DA, Bankoff M, Norris LH: Computed tomography–guided percutaneous drainage of a head and neck infection, *J Oral Maxillofac Surg* 50:1119, 1992.

24. Dean LW: The proper procedure for external drainage of retropharyngeal abscess secondary to caries of the vertebrae, *Ann Otol* 28:566, 1919.

25. DeMarie S, Tham RT, VanderMey AG, et al: Clinical infections and nonsurgical treatment of parapharyngeal space infections complicating throat infections, *Rev Infect Dis* 11:975, 1989.

26. DeMello FJ, Meyer SL: *Eikenella corrodens*: a new pathogen, *Oral Surg* 47:401, 1979.

27. Dingman RO: The management of acute infection of the face and jaws, *Am J Orthod Oral Surg* 25:780, 1939.

28. Dodson TB, Perrott DH, Kaban LB: Pediatric maxillofacial infections: a retrospective study of 113 patients, *J Oral Maxillofac Surg* 47:327, 1989.

29. Dzyak WR, Zide MF: Diagnosis and treatment of lateral pharyngeal space infections, *J Oral Maxillofac Surg* 42:243, 1984.

30. Edson RS, Rosenblatt JE, Lee DT, et al: Recent experience with anti-microbial susceptibility of anaerobic bacteria: increasing resistance to penicillin, *Mayo Clin Proc* 57:737, 1980.

31. Fein S, Mohnac AM: Ludwig's angina infection: a report of a case and associated systemic complication, *J Oral Surg* 31:785, 1973.

32. Feingold SM: *Anaerobic bacteria in human disease,* New York, 1977, Academic Press.

33. Feingold M, Gellis SS: Cellulitis due to *Haemophilus influenzae* type B, *N Engl J Med* 272:788, 1965.

34. Fischmann GE, Graham BS: Ludwig's angina resulting from the infection of an oral malignancy, *J Oral Maxillofac Surg* 43:795, 1985.

35. Flynn TR: Management of maxillofacial infections (discussion), *J Oral Maxillofac Surg* 51:873, 1993.

36. Flynn TR, Topazian RG: Infections of the oral cavity. In Waite DE, Kwon HJ, editors: *Practical oral surgery,* ed 3, Philadelphia, 1987, Lea & Febiger.

37. Freilander AH: *Proteus vulgaris* osteomyelitis of the mandible: report of a case, *Oral Surg* 40:39, 1975.

38. Gianoli G-J, Espinola TE, Guarisco JL, et al: Retropharyngeal space infection: changing trends, *Otolaryngol Head Neck Surg* 105:92, 1991.

39. Goldberg MH: Gram-negative bacteremia after dental extraction, *J Oral Surg* 26:180, 1968.

40. Goldberg MH: The changing biological nature of acute dental infections, *J Am Dent Assoc* 80:1048, 1970.

41. Goldberg MH: Infections of the maxillofacial regions. In Hayward JR, editor: *Oral surgery,* Springfield, Ill, 1976, Charles C Thomas.

42. Goldberg MH: The third molar as a cause of deep space infections (discussion), *J Oral Surg* 50:35, 1992.

43. Goldberg MH, Nemarich A, Marco W: Complications of third molar surgery: a statistical analysis of 500 consecutive procedures, *J Am Dent Assoc* 111:272, 1985.

44. Goldberg MH, Wong TY: Discussion of a nationwide survey of deaths from oral and maxillofacial infections: the Taiwanese experience, *J Oral Maxillofac Surg* 57:1300, 1999.

45. Goodman AD: *Eikenella corrodens* isolated in oral infections of dental origin, *Oral Surg* 44:128, 1977.

46. Gross BD, Roark DT, Meador RC, et al: Ludwig's angina due to bacteroides, *J Oral Surg* 34:456, 1976.

47. Hall HD, Gunter JW, Jamison HC, et al: Effect of time of extraction on resolution of odontogenic cellulitis, *J Am Dent Assoc* 77:626, 1968.

48. Halsband RR, Maloney PL, Doku HC: Gram-negative osteomyelitis, *Oral Surg* 29:806, 1970.

49. Har-El G, Aroesty JH, Shaha A, et al: Changing trends in deep neck abscesses: a retrospective study of 110 patients, *Oral Surg* 77:446, 1994.

50. Haug RH, Hoffman MJ, Indresano AT: An epidemiologic and anatomic survey of odontogenic infections, *J Oral Maxillofac Surg* 49:976, 1991.

51. Hawkins DB, Austin JR: Abscesses in the neck of infants and young children: a review of 112 cases, *Ann Otol Laryngol* 100:361, 1991.

52. Herzon FS: Needle aspiration of non-peritonsillar head and neck abscesses, *Arch Otolaryngol Head Neck Surg* 114:1312, 1988.

53. Hohl TR, Whitacre RJ, Hooley JR, et al: *Diagnosis and treatment of odontogenic infections: a self-instructional guide,* Seattle, 1983, Stoma Press.

54. Holt RG, McManus K, Newman RK, et al: Computed tomography in the diagnosis of deep neck infections, *Arch Otolaryngol* 108:693, 1982.

55. Hought RT, Fitzgerald BE, Latta JE, et al: Ludwig's angina: report of two cases and review of the literature from 1945 to January, 1979, *J Oral Surg* 38:849, 1980.

56. Hunt DE, Meyer RA: Continued evaluation of microbiology of oral infections, *J Am Dent Assoc* 107:52, 1983.

57. Indresano AT, Haug RH, Hoffman MJ: The third molar as a cause of deep space infections, *J Oral Maxillofac Surg* 50:33, 1992.

58. Iwu CO: Ludwig's angina: report of seven cases and review of current concepts in management, *Br J Oral Maxillofac Surg* 28:189, 1990.

59. Johnason WG, Pierce AK, Sanford JP: Changing pharyngeal bacterial flora of hospitalized patients: emergence of gram-negative bacilli, *N Engl J Med* 281:1137, 1969.

60. Kannangara DW, Thadepalli H, McQuirter JL: Bacteriology and treatment of dental infections, *Oral Surg* 50:103, 1980.

61. Kirner A, Gürtler E, Ruzicka A, et al: Die bakteriologischen Befunde aus den submandibulären Abszessen, *Dtsch Stomatol* 19:434, 1969.

62. Krisham V, Johnson JV, Helfrick JF: Management of maxillofacial infections, *J Oral Maxillofac Surg* 51:868, 1993.

63. Krogh HW: Extraction of teeth in the presence of acute infections, *J Oral Surg* 9:136, 1951.

64. Labriola JD, Mascaro J, Alpert B: The microbiologic flora of orofacial abscesses, *J Oral Maxillofac Surg* 41:711, 1983.

65. Lazare M: Oral temperatures, *Oral Surg* 23:446, 1967.

66. Lepore ML: Upper airway obstruction induced by warfarin sodium, *Arch Otolaryngol* 102:505, 1976.

67. Levitt GW: Cervical fasciae and deep neck infections, *Otolaryngol Clin North Am* 9:703, 1976.

68. Levy SP: *The antibiotic paradox: how miracle drugs are destroying the miracle,* New York, 1992, Plenum Press.

69. Loughnan TE, Allen DE: Ludwig's angina: the anesthetic management of nine cases, *Anesthesia* 40:295, 1985.

70. Lynch EP, Stuteville OH: Evaluation of the sensitivity disk method of testing and susceptibility of bacterial infections of dental origin of antimicrobial agents, *Oral Surg* 9:674, 1956.

71. Mackowiak PA: Microbial synergism in human infection, *N Engl J Med* 298:83, 1978.

72. Mason DA: Steroid therapy and dental infection, *Br Dent J* 128:271, 1970.

73. McDonald JB, Socransky SS, Gibbons RJ: Aspects of the pathogenesis of mixed anaerobic infections of mucous membranes, *J Dent Res* 42:529, 1963.

74. Meyers BR, Lawson W, Hirschman SZ: Ludwig's angina: case report with review of bacteriology and current therapy, *Am J Med* 53:257, 1972.

75. Molins TJ, Wilson A, Ward-Booth RP: Recurrent buccal space abscesses: a complication of Crohn's disease, *Oral Surg Oral Med Oral Pathol* 72:19, 1991.

76. Monaldo LJ, Bellome J, Zegarelli DJ, et al: *Bacteroides* infection of the mandible with secondary spread to the neck, *J Oral Surg* 32:370, 1974.

77. Moncada R, Warpeha R, Pickeman J, et al: Mediastinitis from odontogenic and deep cervical infection, *Chest* 73:497, 1978.

78. Morey E, Higgins TJ, Moule AJ: Microbial flora of acute dental infection, *J Dent Res* 63:479, 1984 (abstract).

79. Mosher HP: The submaxillary fossa approach to deep pus in the neck, *Trans Am Acad Ophthalmol Otolaryngol* 34:19, 1929.

80. Nitzan DW: Pericoronitis: a reappraisal of its clinical and microbiological aspects, *J Oral Maxillofac Surg* 43:510, 1985.

81. Osborn TP: A prospective study of complications related to mandibular third molar surgery, *J Oral Maxillofac Surg* 43:767, 1985.

82. Peters ES, Fong B, Wormuth DW, et al: Risk factors affecting hospital length of stay in patients with odontogenic maxillofacial infections, *J Oral Maxillofac Surg* 54:1391, 1996.

83. Peterson LJ: Contemporary management of deep infection of the neck, *J Oral Maxillofac Surg* 51:226, 1993

84. Piecuch JF, Arzadon J, Lieblich SE: Prophylactic antibiotics for third molar surgery, *J Oral Maxillofac Surg* 53:53, 1995.

85. Pogrel MA: Complications of third molar surgery, *Oral Maxillofac Surg Clin North Am* 2:441, 1990.

86. Powell KR: Infectious diseases. In Behrman RE, Kliegman RM, Jenson HB, editors: *Nelson textbook of pediatrics,* ed 16, Philadelphia, 2002, WB Saunders.

87. Quale AA: *Bacteroides* infections in oral surgery, *J Oral Surg* 32:91, 1974.

88. Quayle PA, Russel C, Hearn B: Organisms isolated from severe odontogenic soft tissue infections: their sensitivities to cefotetan and seven other antibiotics and implication for therapy and prophylaxis, *Br J Oral Surg* 25:34, 1987.

89. Roe CF: Fever and infections: fever in surgical patients. In Hardy JD, editor: *Rhodes textbook of surgery: principle and practice,* vol I, ed 5, Philadelphia, 1977, JB Lippincott.

90. Rogerson KC, Topazian RG: Infections associated with impacted teeth. In Alling CC, Helfrick JF, Alling RD, editors: *Impacted teeth,* Philadelphia, 1993, WB Saunders.

91. Rosen EA, Shulman RH, Shaw AS: Ludwig's angina: a complication of bilateral mandibular fracture, *J Oral Surg* 30: 196, 1972.

92. Sabiston CB, Grigsby UR, Segerstrom N: Bacterial study of pyogenic infections of dental origin, *Oral Surg* 41:430, 1976.

93. Schmitt BD: Cervical adenopathy in children, *Postgrad Med* 60:251, 1976.

94. Schroeder DC, Sarha ED, Hendrickson DA, et al: Severe head and neck infection from gas-forming organisms, *J Am Dent Assoc* 114:65, 1987.

95. Schwartz HC, Bauer RA, Davis NJ: Ludwig's angina: use of a fiber-optic laryngoscope to avoid tracheostomy, *J Oral Surg* 32:608, 1974.

96. Sethi DS, Stanley DE: Deep neck abscesses: changing trends, *J Laryngol Otol* 108:138, 1994.

97. Socransky SS, Gibbons RJ: Required role of *Bacteroides melaninogenicus* in mixed anaerobic infections, *J Infect Dis* 115:247, 1965.

98. Solnitsky OC, Jeghers H: Lymphadenopathy and disorders of lymphatics. In MacBryde CM, Blacklow RS, editors: *Signs and symptoms: applied pathologic physiology and interpretation,* ed 6, Philadelphia, 1983, JB Lippincott.

99. Spilka CJ: Pathways of dental infections, *J Oral Surg* 24:111, 1966.

100. Steinhauser PR: Ludwig's angina: report of a case in a 12 day old boy, *J Oral Surg* 25:256, 1967.

101. Strauss HR, Hankins J: Ludwig's angina, empyema, pulmonary infiltration, and pericarditis secondary to extraction of a tooth, *J Oral Surg* 38:223, 1980.

102. Sugata T, Myoken Y, Fujita Y: Cervical cellulitis with mediastinitis from an odontogenic infection complicated by diabetes mellitus, *J Oral Maxillofac Surg* 55:864, 1997.

103. Tung-Yiu W, Jehn-Shyun H, Ching-Hung C, et al: Cervical necrotizing fasciitis of odontogenic origin: a report of 11 cases, *J Oral Maxillofac Surg* 58:1347, 2000.

104. Valenti WM, Tandell RG, Bentley DW: Factors predisposing to oropharyngeal colonization with gram-negative bacilli in the aged, *N Engl J Med* 298:1108, 1978.

105. Van Hassel HJ, Short JP: Buccal cellulitis in infants, *Oral Surg* 49:217, 1980.

106. Virolainen E, Haapaniemi J, Aitasolo K, et al: Deep neck infections, *Int J Oral Surg* 8:407, 1979.

107. Weinberger BW: *Introduction to the history of dentistry, with medical and dental chronology and bibliography data,* vol 1, St Louis, 1948, CV Mosby.

108. Weinstein L, Swartz MN: Host response to infection. In Sodeman WA, Sodeman WA Jr, editors: *Pathologic physiology: mechanisms of disease,* ed 6, Philadelphia, 1985, WB Saunders.

109. Wong TY: A nationwide survey of deaths from oral and maxillofacial infections: the Taiwanese experience, *J Oral Maxillofac Surg* 57:1297, 1999.

110. Zeitler DL: Prophylactic antibiotics for third molar surgery: a dissenting opinion, *J Oral Maxillofac Surg* 53:61, 1995.

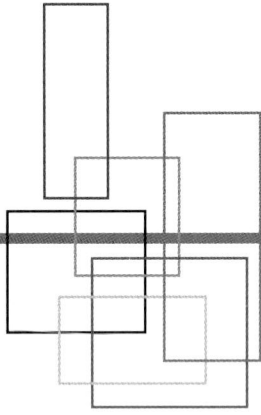

Anatomy of Oral and Maxillofacial Infections

Thomas R. Flynn

In 1939, Ashbel Williams[22] reported in the *New England Journal of Medicine* on a series of 31 cases of Ludwig's angina in which 54% of the patients died of their infections. In 1979, Hought et al.[11] reported several cases of Ludwig's angina and reviewed the literature on the topic up to that date. In their review the mortality rate of Ludwig's angina had decreased to 4%. Perhaps because of similar progress in the prevention and treatment of common dental diseases, the incidence of severe oral and facial infections also has decreased in similar proportions. Today's surgeons do not have the same repeated surgical experience with severe infections of the deep fascial spaces of the head and neck as their forebears. Thus modern facial surgeons must prepare for the unexpected need to manage deep fascial space infections by repeated study of the surgical anatomy of the head and neck.

HEAD AND NECK FASCIAE IN INFECTION

In the 1930s the classic anatomical studies of Grodinsky and Holyoke[5-7] established the modern understanding of the fascial layers and the potential anatomical spaces through which infections can spread in the head and neck. They injected dyed gelatin into cadaver specimens at selected portals of entry. Their hypothesis was that these infections spread primarily by hydrostatic pressure, with the flow of infected fluids guided by the resistance of certain tissues such as the fasciae, muscles, and bone. These concepts do explain the usual progress of abscess-forming infections in this region. Exceptions are actinomycotic and mycobacterial infections that may follow the bone in cases of osteomyelitis. Actinomycotic infections of the soft tissues tend to burrow directly toward the skin, whereas mycobacterial infections of the soft tissues generally follow lymphatic pathways.

The term *fascia* is used to describe broad sheets of dense connective tissue whose function is to separate structures that must pass over each other during movement, such as muscles and glands, and serve as pathways for the course of vascular and neural structures. The function of the fascia may be compared with the tissue paper in a shirt box. The tissue paper encloses the neatly folded shirt, allowing it to slide around inside the shirt box as it is jostled during transit. Because bacterial infections appear to spread by hydrostatic pressure, they follow the path of least resistance, which is the loose, areolar connective tissue that surrounds the muscles enclosed by the fascial layers. This type of tissue is destroyed easily by the hyaluronidases and collagenases elaborated by bacteria, thus opening the potential spaces surrounding the muscles. For example, an odontogenic infection beginning in a lower molar may erode through the thin lingual cortical plate of the mandible inferior to the attachment of the mylohyoid muscle. Once the invading organisms have eroded through the cortical bone and periosteum, they enter the submandibular space directly. The potential space of the submandibular triangle is filled primarily by areolar connective tissues surrounding the submandibular gland. As the infection enters the submandibular space the areolar connective tissue gradually undergoes necrosis; it is replaced first by cellulitic fluid and then by pus. Vascular dilation, transudation, and exudation draw fluid into the region, thus increasing the hydrostatic pressure. As this pressure is applied to the borders of the submandibular space, the advancing front of the infection may bypass the anterior belly of the digastric muscle to enter the submental space anteriorly, or the posterior belly of the digastric muscle to enter the lateral pharyngeal space posteriorly. This current theory explains the mechanisms by which suppurative infections of the head and neck can dissect from one anatomical space to another, thus allowing prediction of their course.

FASCIAE OF THE HEAD AND NECK

SUPERFICIAL FASCIA

The superficial fascia is a layer of dense connective tissue that courses deep to the subcutaneous tissue throughout the entire body. The subcutaneous space is defined as the tissues lying superficial to the superficial fascia. Subcutaneous space infections involve mainly the areolar and fatty connective tissues known to surgeons as subcutaneous tissue. Below the mouth the muscles of facial expression lie deep to the superficial fascia, whereas in the upper face the muscles of facial expression are positioned superficial to this layer.

DEEP CERVICAL FASCIA

Various authors have described the three main anatomical layers of the fasciae of the head and neck, generating multiple synonyms for the same structures.* Box 9-1 correlates some of these synonyms with the nomenclature used in this chapter. The nomenclature of Hollinshead[10] is used primarily with reference to commonly used synonyms as appropriate. Figures 9-1 and 9-2 show a visual overview of the deep cervical fasciae. The following outline provides a conceptual overview of their organization:

I. Superficial fascia
II. Deep cervical fascia
    A. Anterior layer
        1. Investing fascia (over the neck)
        2. Parotideomasseteric
        3. Temporal
    B. Middle layer
        1. Sternohyoid-omohyoid division
        2. Sternothyroid-thyrohyoid division
        3. Visceral division
            a. Buccopharyngeal
            b. Pretracheal
            c. Retropharyngeal
    C. Posterior layer
        1. Alar division
        2. Prevertebral division

Anterior Layer   The anterior layer of the deep cervical fascia is also called the *superficial* or *investing layer.* The anterior layer encircles the neck, splits to surround the sternocleidomastoid and trapezius muscles, and attaches posteriorly to the spinous processes of the cervical vertebrae. It forms the superficial border of the submandibular

*References 2, 4, 7, 10, 13, 15.

BOX **9-1**

Synonyms for Deep Fascial Spaces of the Head and Neck

Name	Synonym
Space of the body of the mandible	Mandibular space
Submandibular space	Submaxillary space Submylohyoid space
Masticator space	Masticatory space Masseteric space
Temporal spaces	Temporal pouches
Infratemporal space	Postzygomatic space
Buccal space	Buccinator space
Infraorbital space	Canine space
Lateral pharyngeal space	Parapharyngeal space Pharyngomaxillary space
Retropharyngeal space	Retroesophageal space
Pretracheal space	Perivisceral spaces Paravisceral space Paratracheal space
Carotid sheath	Visceral vascular space

Adapted from Granite EL: Anatomic considerations in infections of the face and neck: review of the literature, *J Oral Surg* 34:34, 1976.

space and splits to form the capsule of the submandibular gland. As the anterior layer approaches the inferior border of the mandible, it fuses with the periosteum of the horizontal ramus of the mandible. Over the ascending ramus of the mandible it splits to surround the muscles of mastication, thus forming the masticator space. Superficially the anterior layer is called the *parotideomasseteric fascia* in this region because it covers the superficial surface of the masseter muscle anteriorly and splits to surround the parotid gland posteriorly. On the medial side of the ascending ramus of the mandible, it covers the medial side of the medial pterygoid muscle and attaches to the base of the skull at the sphenoid bone and pterygoid plates. At the zygomatic arch the anterior layer of the deep cervical fascia fuses with the periosteum of the arch and then rises superiorly to cover the superficial surface of the temporalis muscle. It attaches to the cranium, terminating at the superficial temporal crest. Above the zygomatic arch the anterior layer is called the *temporal fascia.* For a distance of approximately 2 cm superior to the zygomatic arch, the temporal fascia divides into two layers, between which is the temporal fat pad, an extension of the buccal fat pad. Similarly the anterior layer splits at about 2 cm above the manubrium of the sternum to form the suprasternal space of Burns, which contains only areolar connective tissue.

Middle Layer   The middle layer of the deep cervical fascia can be divided into three divisions. The first two are the sternohyoid-omohyoid and the sternothyroid-thyrohyoid divisions. These two divisions surround the corresponding strap muscles of the neck between the hyoid bone and the clavicle. The primary surgical significance of these layers is

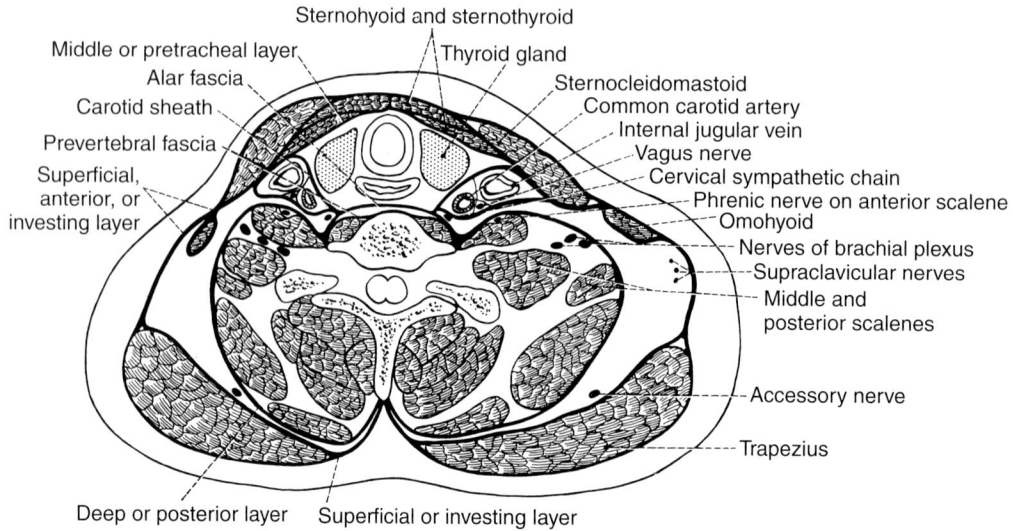

Figure 9-1 Transverse section of the neck at the level of the thyroid gland shows the three layers of the deep cervical fasciae and their enclosed structures. Note the relation of the carotid sheath to all three layers of the deep cervical fascia, and the compartmentalization within the carotid sheath for the carotid artery, internal jugular vein, and vagus nerve. (From Hollinshead WH: Anatomy for surgeons, vol 1, ed 2, *The head and neck,* Hagerstown, Md, 1968, Harper & Row.)

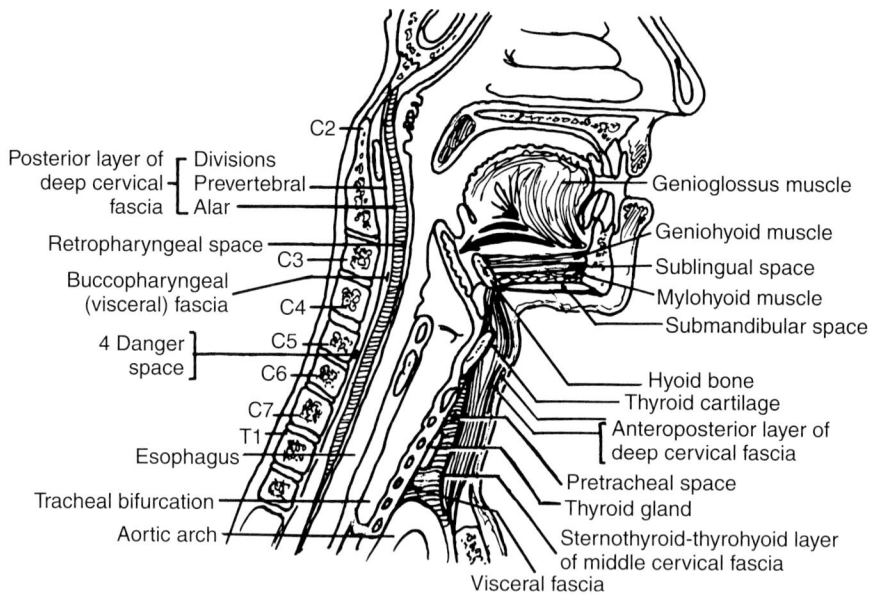

Figure 9-2 Sagittal section of the head and neck shows the relations of the three layers of the deep cervical fasciae and their enclosed structures. (From Flynn TR: Anatomy and surgery of deep fascial space infections. In Kelly JJ, editor: *Oral and maxillofacial surgery knowledge update 1994,* Rosemont, Ill, 1994, American Association of Oral and Maxillofacial Surgeons.)

that they must be divided in the midline in a surgical approach to the trachea or thyroid gland. They usually are not directly involved in head and neck infections because they do not lie on the major routes that an orofacial infection may follow to the mediastinum or chest wall.

The third division of the middle layer of the deep cervical fascia is clinically significant. Below the hyoid bone the visceral division surrounds the trachea, esophagus, and thyroid gland. Above the hyoid bone the visceral fascia wraps around the lateral and posterior sides of the pharynx, lying

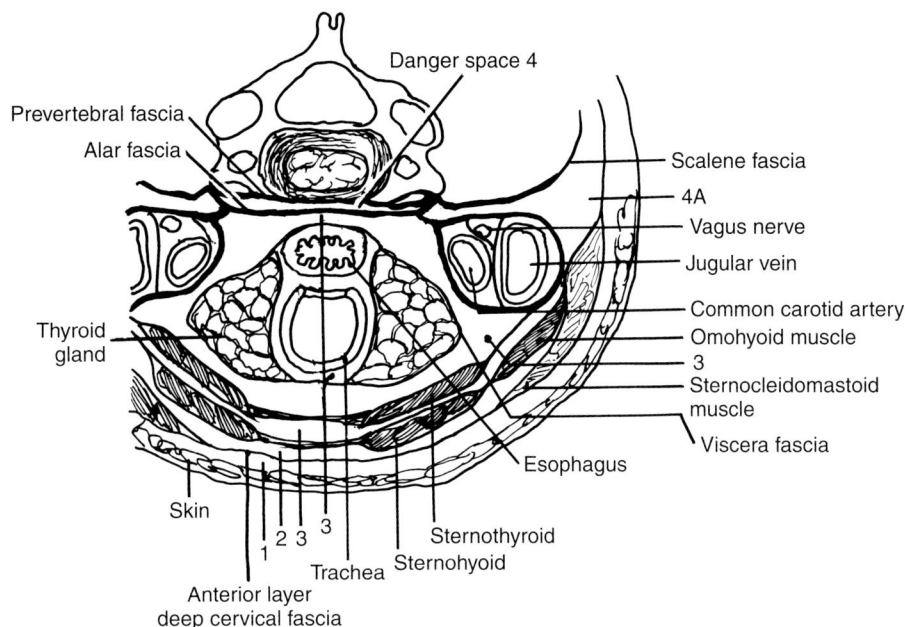

Figure 9-3 Transverse section of the neck at the level of the thyroid gland shows the numbered spaces of Grodinsky and Holyoke. (From Flynn TR: Anatomy and surgery of deep fascial space infections. In Kelly JJ, editor: *Oral and maxillofacial surgery knowledge update 1994,* Rosemont, Ill, 1994, American Association of Oral and Maxillofacial Surgeons.)

on the superficial (toward the skin) side of the pharyngeal constrictor muscles. In this region it is also called the *buccopharyngeal fascia.* The important deep neck spaces (i.e., the retropharyngeal, lateral pharyngeal, and pretracheal spaces) all lie on the superficial side of the visceral division of the middle layer of the deep cervical fascia (see Figure 9-1).

Posterior Layer The posterior layer of the deep cervical fascia has two divisions, the alar and the prevertebral. The alar fascia passes through the transverse processes of the vertebrae on either side, posterior to the retropharyngeal fascia.

In the vertical dimension the posterior layer extends from the base of the skull to the diaphragm. The alar fascia fuses with the retropharyngeal fascia at a variable level between the sixth cervical (C6) and the fourth thoracic (T4) vertebrae. This fusion forms the bottom of the retropharyngeal space. Infections of the retropharyngeal space may rupture the alar fascia, thus entering the danger space, which is continuous with the posterior mediastinum (see Figure 9-2).

The prevertebral fascia surrounds the vertebrae and the attached postural muscles of the neck and back. The prevertebral fascia lies just anterior to the periosteum of the vertebrae, and infections of the vertebrae, such as tuberculous osteomyelitis, may enter the prevertebral space. The prevertebral fascia usually is not invaded by infections arising in the maxillofacial regions.

Carotid Sheath Controversy exists as to which of the deep cervical fascia contribute to the carotid sheath. Some authors believe that the carotid sheath is formed from the alar division of the posterior layer of the deep cervical fascia,[10] whereas others attribute formation of this important structure to all three layers of the deep cervical fascia[7] (see Figure 9-1). Nonetheless, the carotid sheath begins at the origin of the carotid artery in the superior mediastinum and passes through the pretracheal space in an upward and posterior direction. Above the hyoid bone it lies at the junction of the lateral pharyngeal and retropharyngeal spaces. The carotid sheath terminates at the jugular foramen and carotid canal, where the internal jugular vein and carotid artery enter the base of the skull, respectively. The carotid sheath also contains the vagus nerve. The cervical sympathetic chain is attached to the posterior surface of the carotid sheath. The carotid, jugular, and vagus nerves each have compartments within the carotid sheath.

Numbered Spaces of Grodinsky and Holyoke In their landmark article of 1938 in which they described the deep fascial spaces of the head and neck, Grodinsky and Holyoke[7] used numbers to indicate the various deep neck spaces (Figure 9-3). Space 1 lies superficial to the superficial fascia and therefore is synonymous with the subcutaneous space. Space 2 is a group of spaces surrounding the cervical strap muscles, lying superficial to the sternothyroid-thyrohyoid division of the middle layer of the deep cervical fascia, or between the sternothyroid-thyrohyoid division and the sternohyoid-omohyoid division. Space 3 is the potential anatomical space lying superficial (toward the skin) to the visceral division of the middle layer of the deep cervical fascia. Space 3 contains the pretracheal, retropharyngeal, and lateral pharyngeal spaces. Space 3A is the carotid sheath. Space 4 is the potential space that lies between the alar and prevertebral divisions of the posterior layer of the deep cervical fascia; this is also known as the danger space. The term *danger space 4* is a misnomer resulting from the combination of two synonyms for the same anatomical space. Space 4A is in the posterior triangle of the neck, posterior to the carotid sheath. Space 5 is the prevertebral space, and Space 5A is enclosed by the prevertebral fascial, posterior to the transverse processes of the vertebrae, as it surrounds the scalene and the spinal postural muscles.

PATHWAYS OF SPREAD OF INFECTION FROM TEETH

PATHOPHYSIOLOGY OF ODONTOGENIC INFECTION

Once an infection has passed beyond the dental apex and apical periodontal ligament, a very localized apical osteomyelitis occurs. Bone destruction in osteomyelitis is similar to the process of necrosis of the inflamed dental pulp. Essentially, as the interstitial hydrostatic pressure increases as a result of the transudation of extracellular fluid, followed by the exudation of inflammatory cells, the flow of new blood into the region is compromised. In soft tissues the increased interstitial fluid pressure is relieved by swelling. When the soft tissues are contained within an unyielding mineralized structure, such as the medullary spaces of bone or the pulp canal, the increased pressure cannot be relieved. Therefore the pulpal or medullary soft tissues die as a result of ischemia. Tissue breakdown products recruit circulating macrophages and histiocytes by the process of chemotaxis. As mineralized tissue is encountered these circulating macrophages coalesce and differentiate into osteoclasts, which resorb mineralized bone.

The process of bone necrosis and resorption expands in a roughly spherical pattern until a bony cortex is reached. At this point the process of bone resorption is slowed by the densely mineralized tissue, thus changing the shape of the bony cavity that is produced. When the bony cortical layer finally is breached the infectious process then may enter the soft tissues.

The invading bacterial pathogens that trigger this autolytic inflammatory process persist throughout its extent. Not only can they spread the inflammatory process by continued antigen production, but they also can cause direct tissue destruction. Streptococci, commonly found in the early stages of infection, can invade tissues by their elaboration of hyaluronidases, which break down the extracellular glycoproteins of connective tissue. As the streptococci flourish in their exponential growth phase, they create an environment conducive to the subsequent growth of the anaerobic flora of odontogenic infections. They consume local oxygen supplies and metabolize nutrients to create a more acidic environment. They also may produce essential nutrients for the anaerobes present after about 3 days of clinical symptoms. The anaerobes, including *Prevotella* and *Porphyromonas* spp., produce collagenases, which destroy

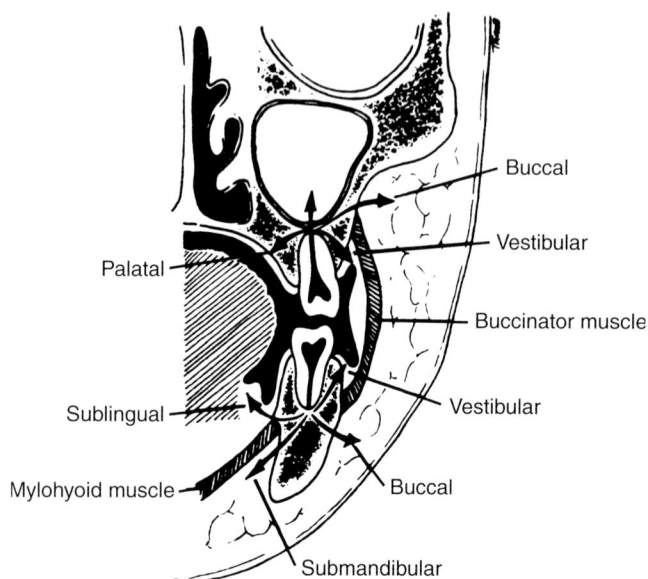

Figure 9-4 Potential pathways of the spread of infection from the teeth.

collagen, the most plentiful extracellular matrix protein of connective tissue.[14]

As the infection perforates the bony cortical plate the process of bacterial inoculation, followed by inflammation and necrosis, begins anew in the soft tissues. The most vulnerable tissue is areolar connective tissue that is not well vascularized. It is loose and easily dissected by relatively low hydrostatic pressures. Thus the spreading infection follows the path of least resistance, deflected by denser and better vascularized structures such as muscle, fascia, organs, and bone.[12] The deep fascial infections are deflected or contained by the structures that define the anatomical deep fascial spaces. For example, if a dental infection that recently breached the bony cortex is restrained by the dense periosteum surrounding the bone, a subperiosteal abscess may result. This process may result in an infection of the space of the body of the mandible or a subperiosteal palatal abscess. Conversely, if the periosteum also has been breached the local muscle attachments may direct the spread of the infection into the soft tissues. For example, if the buccinator attachment on the lateral surface of the maxilla is inferior to the cortical perforation arising from the mesiobuccal root of the maxillary first molar, then the infection would enter and spread throughout the buccal space. However, if the infection perforates the bone and periosteum inferior to that muscle attachment, the infection would pass between the oral surface of the buccinator muscle and the oral mucosa to enter the vestibular space (Figure 9-4).

STAGES OF INFECTION

The inflammatory tissue-destructive events also explain the stages of infection in the clinical course of odontogenic infections[19] (Table 9-1). Initially the inoculation stage is caused by the early spread, probably of streptococci, into the soft tissues. This stage can be recognized by a soft, doughy,

TABLE 9-1

Stages of Infection

Characteristic	Inoculation	Cellulitis	Abscess
Duration	0-3 days	3-7 days	>5 days
Pain	Mild-moderate	Severe and generalized	Moderate-severe and localized
Size	Small	Large	Small
Localization	Diffuse	Diffuse	Circumscribed
Palpation	Soft, doughy, mildly tender	Hard, exquisitely tender	Fluctuant, tender
Appearance	Normal color	Reddened	Peripherally reddened
Skin quality	Normal	Thickened	Centrally undermined and shiny
Surface temperature	Slightly heated	Hot	Moderately heated
Loss of function	Minimal or none	Severe	Moderately severe
Tissue fluid	Edema	Serosanguineous, flecks of pus	Pus
Levels of malaise	Mild	Severe	Moderate-severe
Severity	Mild	Severe	Moderate-severe
Percutaneous bacteria	Aerobic	Mixed	Anaerobic

From Flynn TR: The timing of incision and drainage. In Piecuch JF, editor: *Oral and maxillofacial surgery knowledge update 2001,* Rosemont, Ill, American Association of Oral and Maxillofacial Surgeons.

mildly tender soft tissue swelling with little redness. During the cellulitis stage the process of inflammation is paramount, resulting in a deeply reddened, hard, exquisitely painful swelling with loss of function, such as trismus or the inability to protrude the tongue. During the third stage, abscess formation, necrosis predominates. A central softening of the cellulitic region, which may become fluctuant, is present. The term *fluctuant* is misused to describe a soft edema. Rather, fluctuance is the bimanual or bidigital palpation of a fluid wave by one hand or finger as the lesion is compressed with the other hand or finger. The fluid wave is caused by the flow of pus within the abscess cavity. The final stage in odontogenic infections is resolution, which occurs after spontaneous or therapeutic drainage.

The stages of infection can be used as a conceptual framework to understand the progression of untreated severe odontogenic infections through the anatomical deep fascial spaces of the head and neck. For example, if a virulent odontogenic infection originating in a lower molar has flourished in the submandibular space, producing an abscess, it may have progressed through the inoculation stage to the cellulitis stage in the neighboring lateral pharyngeal space. The retropharyngeal space already may have been inoculated by bacteria carried along the advancing front of inflammatory edema. These concepts may explain why "unsuccessful" incision and drainage procedures that yield no pus still abort the spread of the infection and result in cure.

CLINICAL ANATOMY OF THE DEEP FASCIAL SPACES OF THE HEAD AND NECK

The deep fascial spaces are presented according to their association with maxillary or mandibular odontogenic sources. However, this division is arbitrary. Infections do not always follow the patterns described, yet they often spread from more superficial locations and affect deeper

anatomical spaces along a common pathway toward vital structures, such as the brain or the mediastinum.

DEEP SPACES ASSOCIATED WITH ODONTOGENIC INFECTIONS

The facial surfaces of the maxilla and mandible share a common anatomical organization in relation to the nearby muscles of facial expression. In the posterior parts of the alveolar processes the buccinator muscle attaches along the facial surface of the maxilla and mandible. Anteriorly the elevator muscles of the upper lip and the depressor muscles of the lower lip attach to the maxilla and mandible, respectively, but usually in a position beyond the apices of the anterior teeth. The buccinator attachment is often at the midroot level of the posterior teeth. Therefore infections that begin in the posterior teeth often rupture through the cortical plate and periosteum on the superficial (skin) side of the buccinator to enter the buccal space. Conversely, infections arising in the anterior teeth usually perforate the bone on the oral side of the nearby muscle of facial expression to enter the vestibular space. This difference may explain the tendency of anterior dental infections to affect the vestibular space whereas posterior dental infections tend to propagate into the buccal space (Tables 9-2 and 9-3).

Vestibular Space The vestibular space is the potential space between the oral vestibular mucosa and the nearby muscles of facial expression (Figure 9-5, *A*). The term *dentoalveolar abscess* describes an infection between the alveolar process and the alveolar mucosa on the facial wall of the alveolar process. Because no anatomical structure limits the spread of a dentoalveolar abscess or cellulitis into the oral vestibule and the attachment of the nearby muscle of facial expression is apical to the infection, dentoalveolar abscesses occupy a portion of the vestibular space.

T A B L E 9-2

Borders of the Deep Spaces of the Head and Neck

Space	BORDERS					
	Anterior	Posterior	Superior	Inferior	Superficial or Medial*	Deep or Lateral†
Buccal	Corner of mouth	Masseter muscle Pterygomandibular space	Maxilla Infraorbital space	Mandible	Subcutaneous tissue and skin	Buccinator muscle
Infraorbital	Nasal cartilages	Buccal space	Quadratus labii superioris muscle	Oral mucosa	Quadratus labii superioris muscle	Levator anguli oris muscle Maxilla
Submandibular	Anterior belly of digastric muscle	Posterior belly of digastric muscle Stylohyoid muscle Stylopharyngeus muscle	Inferior and medial surfaces of mandible	Digastric tendon	Platysma muscle Investing fascia	Mylohyoid, hyoglossus, superior constricting muscles
Submental	Inferior border of mandible	Hyoid bone	Mylohyoid bone	Investing fascia	Investing fascia	Anterior bellies of digastric muscles†
Sublingual	Lingual surface of mandible	Submandibular space	Oral mucosa	Mylohyoid muscle	Muscles of tongue*	Lingual surface of mandible†
Pterygomandibular	Buccal space	Parotid gland	Lateral pterygoid muscle	Inferior border of mandible	Medial pterygoid muscle*	Ascending ramus of mandible†
Submasseteric	Buccal space	Parotid gland	Zygomatic arch	Inferior border of mandible	Ascending ramus of mandible*	Masseter muscle†
Lateral pharyngeal	Superior and middle pharyngeal constrictor muscles	Carotid sheath and scalene fascia	Skull base	Hyoid bone	Pharyngeal constrictors Retropharyngeal space*	Medial pterygoid muscle†
Retropharyngeal	Superior and middle pharyngeal constrictor muscles	Alar fascia	Skull base	Fusion of alar and prevertebral fasciae at C6-T4		Carotid sheath and lateral pharyngeal space†
Pretracheal	Sternothyroid-thyrohyoid fascia	Retropharyngeal space	Thyroid cartilage	Superior mediastinum	Sternothyroid-thyrohyoid fascia	Visceral fascia over trachea and thyroid gland

*Lateral border.
†Medial border.

TABLE 9-3

Relations of Deep Spaces in Infections

Space	Likely Causes	Contents	Neighboring Spaces
Buccal	Upper premolars Upper molars Lower premolars	Parotid duct Anterior facial artery and vein Transverse facial artery and vein Buccal fat pad	Infraorbital Pterygomandibular Infratemporal
Infraorbital	Upper canine	Angular artery and vein Infraorbital nerve	Buccal
Submandibular	Lower molars	Submandibular gland Facial artery and vein Lymph nodes	Sublingual Submental Lateral pharyngeal Buccal
Submental	Lower anteriors Fracture of symphysis	Anterior jugular vein Lymph nodes	Submandibular (on either side)
Sublingual	Lower premolars Lower molars Direct trauma	Sublingual glands Wharton's ducts Lingual nerve Sublingual artery and vein	Submandibular Lateral pharyngeal Visceral (trachea and esophagus)
Pterygomandibular	Lower third molars Fracture of angle of mandible	Mandibular division of trigeminal nerve Inferior alveolar artery and vein	Buccal Lateral pharyngeal Submasseteric Deep temporal Parotid
Submasseteric	Lower third molars Fracture of angle of mandible	Masseteric artery and vein	Buccal Pterygomandibular Superficial temporal Parotid
Infratemporal and deep temporal	Upper molars	Pterygoid plexus Interior maxillary artery and vein Mandibular division of trigeminal nerve Skull base foramina	Buccal Superficial temporal Inferior petrosal sinus
Superficial temporal	Upper molars Lower molars	Temporal fat pad Temporal branch of facial nerve	Buccal Deep temporal
Lateral pharyngeal	Lower third molars Tonsils Infection in neighboring spaces	Carotid artery Internal jugular vein Vagus nerve Cervical sympathetic vein	Pterygomandibular Submandibular Sublingual Peritonsillar Retropharyngeal

Posteriorly the local muscle of facial expression is the buccinator; anteriorly the intrinsic muscles of either lip, such as the orbicularis oris, quadratus labii superioris, mentalis (depressor labii inferioris), or risorius (depressor anguli oris), limit the vestibular space. The vestibular space is filled with submucosal and areolar connective tissues is crossed by the long buccal and mental nerves. It communicates, between gaps in the muscles of facial expression, with the buccal and subcutaneous spaces. Vestibular swellings may elevate the overlying facial structures, distorting the externally visible features (Figure 9-5, *B*). Spontaneous drainage often occurs through the oral mucosa (Figure 9-5, *C*).

Subcutaneous Space In the head and neck the subcutaneous space occupies the potential space between the su-

perficial fascia, along with the muscles of facial expression, and the skin. Infection in almost any deep fascial space may point through the subcutaneous space to the skin.

Necrotizing fasciitis, a rapidly spreading infection, causes necrosis of the tissues in the subcutaneous space by thrombosis of vessels that supply the superficial muscles and skin. In the neck, necrotizing fasciitis may follow the platysma muscle inferiorly to its terminus on the anterior chest wall (Figure 9-6). Necrotizing fasciitis also may affect the deeper fascial spaces, resulting in a particularly aggressive spread through those spaces to deeper structures, as in descending necrotizing mediastinitis.[13,15,18]

Buccal Space The buccal space occupies the portion of the subcutaneous space between the facial skin and the buccinator muscle. Anteriorly the buccal space ends at the

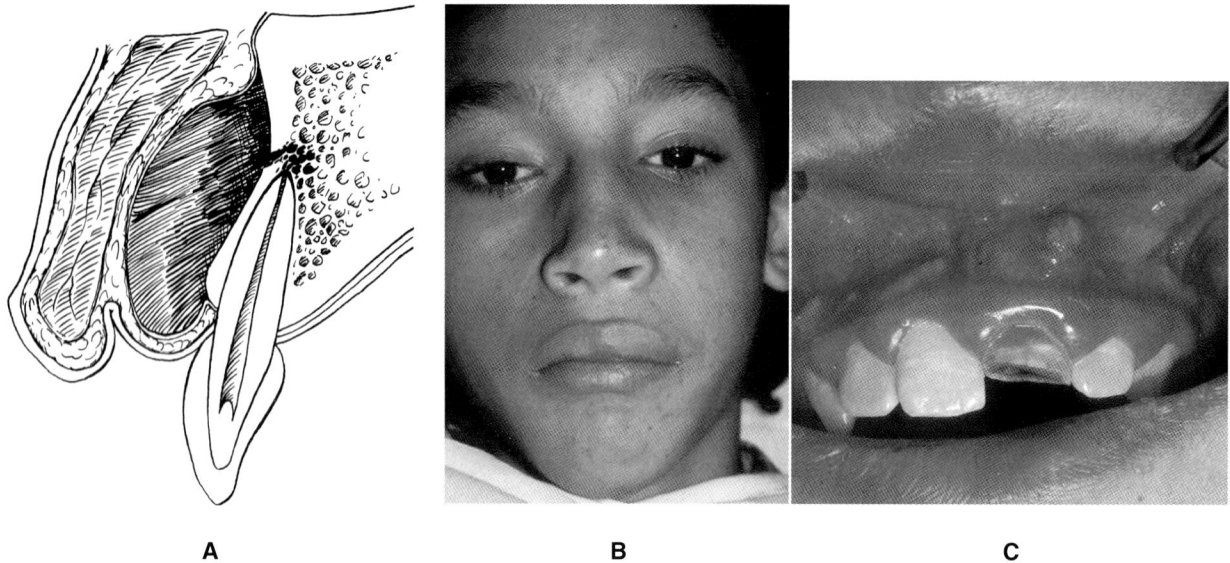

A

B

C

Figure 9-5 A, Diagram of a vestibular space abscess occupying the potential space between the oral mucosa and the muscles of the upper lip. (From Archer WH: *Oral and maxillofacial surgery,* vol 1, ed 5, Philadelphia, 1975, WB Saunders.) **B,** Frontal view of a patient with a vestibular space abscess arising from the upper left central incisor, causing elevation of the overlying upper lip and the left ala of the nose. **C,** Intraoral view of the same patient with discoloration and fracture of the upper left central incisor caused by a basketball injury. The swelling over the alveolar process extends into the labial vestibule with pointing of the infection into the oral mucosa.

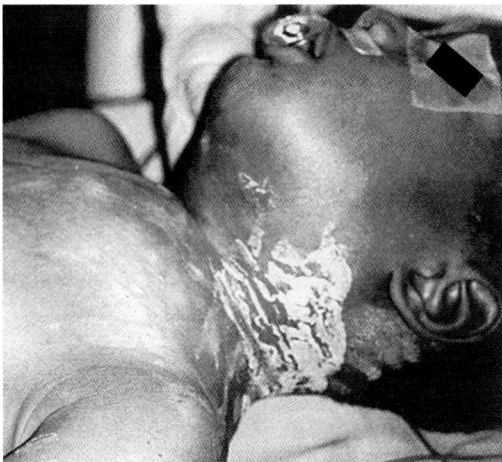

Figure 9-6 Lateral view of a patient with necrotizing fasciitis. The infection followed the platysma muscle onto the anterior chest wall. (From Flynn TR, Piecuch JF, Topazian RG: Infections of the oral cavity. In Feigin RD, Cherry JD, editors: *Textbook of pediatric dentistry,* vol 1, ed 4, Philadelphia, 1998, WB Saunders.)

modiolus, which is the aponeurotic junction of the buccinator and orbicularis oris muscles just posterior to either oral commissure (Figure 9-7, *A*).

At its posterior extent the buccinator muscle sweeps around the anterior border of the mandible to join the superior pharyngeal constrictor muscle at the pterygomandibular raphe. This formation leads to important anatomical pathways for the spread of infection into other

spaces. The superficial (skin) side of the buccinator becomes its posterior surface as it sweeps around the anterior border of the mandibular ramus. Superficially this creates the communication of the buccal space with the submasseteric space. On the medial side of the mandible the buccal space communicates with the pterygomandibular space inferiorly and the infratemporal space superior to the lateral pterygoid muscle. An infection may continue its spread along the posterior surface of the buccinator–superior pharyngeal constrictor junction (the pterygomandibular raphe) and enter the lateral pharyngeal space. Extensions of the buccal fat pad allow buccal space infections to enter the superficial temporal space (Figure 9-7, *B*); extension along the buccal fat pad, transverse facial vein, and pterygoid plexus allows infections to enter the infratemporal space (Figure 9-8). Buccal space infections that erode into the transverse facial vein or pterygoid plexus may follow the posterior route to the cavernous sinus, as described in the section on cavernous sinus thrombosis.

Because the buccal space is a portion of the subcutaneous space, buccal infections can spread through the subcutaneous space into the periorbital space (see Figure 9-7, *B*) and past the inferior border of the mandible to the subcutaneous tissues lying superficial to the submandibular space. This spread may confuse or obscure the diagnosis of a submandibular space abscess. A swelling in the subcutaneous space has no inferior limiting structure in the neck, where a submandibular space infection is limited inferiorly by the attachment of the anterior (investing) layer of the deep cervical fascia and the mylohyoid muscle to the

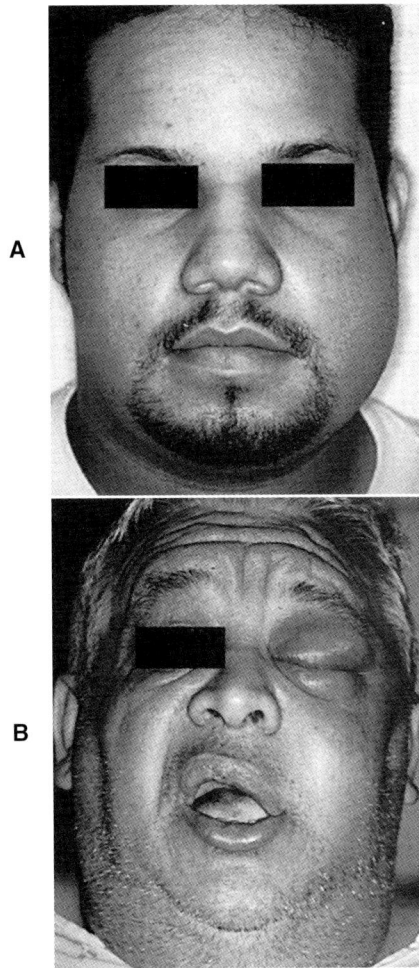

A

B

Figure 9-7 A, Buccal space abscess with swelling extends from the midcheek to the inferior border of the mandible, and from the oral commissure to the anterior edge of the masseter muscle. (From Flynn TR: The swollen face, *Emerg Med Clin North Am* 15:481, 2000.) **B,** Buccal space abscess extending into the periorbital and superficial temporal spaces and the subcutaneous space in the upper left neck. The swelling is restricted over the zygomatic arch, caused by the dense attachment of the superficial fascia to the zygomatic arch. (From Flynn TR: Surgical management of orofacial infections, *Atlas of the Oral and Maxillofacial Surgery Clinics of North America* 8:77, 2000.)

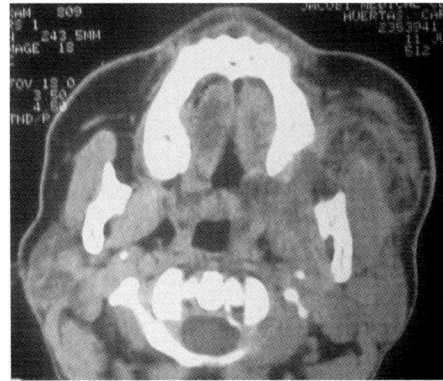

Figure 9-8 Axial CT scan of buccal space abscess spreading into the infratemporal space. The radiolucent region posterior to the maxilla extends around the maxillary tuberosity into the soft palate. (From Flynn TR: The swollen face, *Emerg Med Clin North Am* 15:481, 2000).

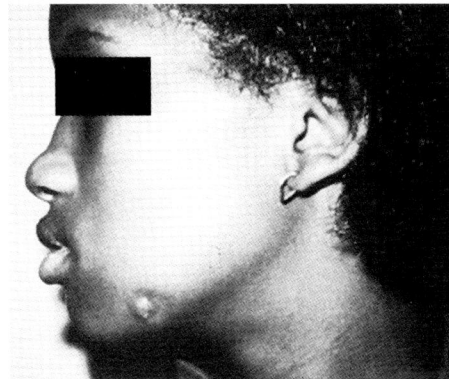

Figure 9-9 This cutaneous sinus tract at the inferior portion of the buccal space can leave an unsightly scar. (From Flynn TR, Topazian RG: Infections of the oral cavity. In Waite D, editor: *Textbook of practical oral and maxillofacial surgery,* Philadelphia, 1987, Lea & Febiger.)

hyoid bone. Undrained buccal space infections tend to point subcutaneously near the inferior border of the mandible inferior border below and just posterior to the oral commissure (Figure 9-9).

DEEP SPACES ASSOCIATED WITH MANDIBULAR ODONTOGENIC INFECTIONS

Space of the Body of the Mandible Mandibular dental infections that perforate the bony cortical plate, but not the overlying periosteum, commonly originate in the mandibular premolar and molar teeth. These infections often are quite painful because the richly innervated periosteum is dissected from the bone by the increasing abscess volume.

The borders of the space of the body of the mandible are the periosteal envelope and the cortical surface of that bone. This potential anatomical space has no contents because of the intimate adaptation of the periosteum to the mandible during health. However, the mental nerve may cross this space if it is distended by an abscess near the mental foramen. The mandible itself appears enlarged in a patient with an infection of the space of the body of the mandible (Figure 9-10).

Sublingual Space The sublingual space is defined superiorly by the mucosa of the mouth floor and inferiorly by the mylohyoid muscle. Anteriorly and laterally the lingual surface of the mandible comprises its bony border. Medially the intrinsic muscles of the tongue and the genioglossus muscles divide the right and left sublingual spaces. The posterior border of the sublingual space is the superior, posterior, and medial portion of the submandibular space. The styloglossus muscle passes between the superior and middle pharyngeal constrictor muscles in this region to

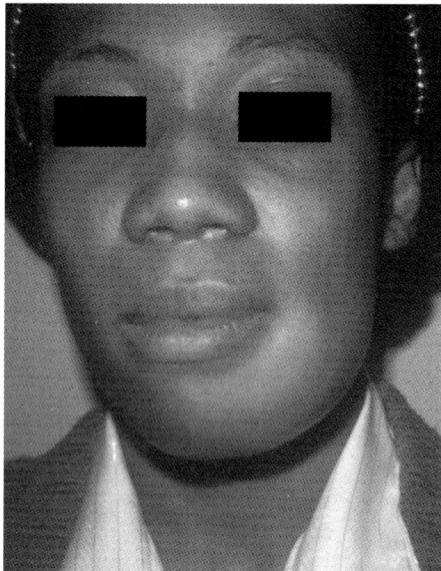

Figure 9-10 An abscess of the space of the body of the mandible. The mandible itself appears enlarged by the subperiosteal infection. (From Flynn TR: The swollen face, *Emerg Med Clin North Am* 15:481, 2000.)

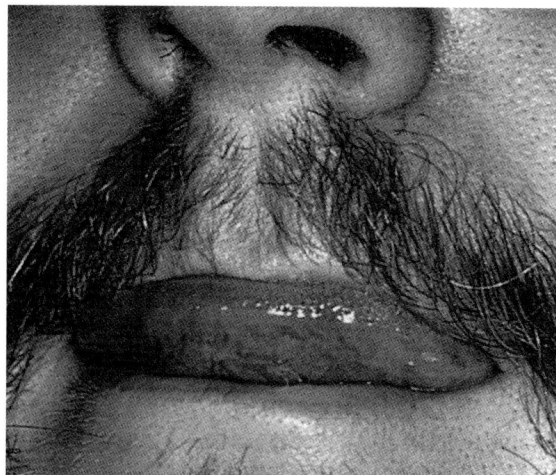

Figure 9-11 This patient's ability to protrude his tongue to the vermilion border of the upper lip indicates no significant sublingual space infection. (From Flynn TR: The swollen face, *Emerg Med Clin North Am* 15:481, 2000.)

enter the tongue. The separation between these two pharyngeal constrictors formed by the styloglossus muscle is termed the *buccopharyngeal gap*. Infections may pass through this gap to enter the lateral pharyngeal space directly from the sublingual space. The sublingual space also is continuous with the submandibular space at the posterior edge of the mylohyoid muscle, where the submandibular gland curves around the free edge of that muscle to enter the sublingual space. The contents of the sublingual space are the sublingual gland, submandibular duct, hilum of the submandibular gland, lingual nerve, and sublingual artery and vein.

Elevation of the tongue is the clinical hallmark of a sublingual space infection. Significant involvement of the sublingual space can be ruled out if the patient can protrude the tongue to or beyond the vermilion border of the upper lip (Figure 9-11).

Sublingual space infections can pass readily from the sublingual space into the submandibular space around the posterior border of the mylohyoid muscle (Figure 9-12). When dyed gelatin was injected into the sublingual space, Grodinsky and Holyoke[7] found that the material flowed into dissection planes between the intrinsic muscle of the tongue extending back to the epiglottis. These dissection planes may account for the epiglottis occasionally associated with severe sublingual space infections (Figure 9-13). For example, the patient in Figure 9-14 had a greatly enlarged epiglottis at intubation. The abscess ruptured during intubation and pus followed the endotracheal tube into the trachea in the moments before the tube's cuff was inflated. Because the anesthesiologist informed the surgeon of this fact immediately, tracheobronchial suction and lavage was helpful in preventing aspiration pneumonitis.

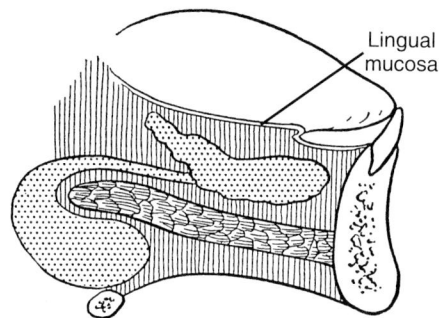

Figure 9-12 Parasagittal diagram of submandibular and sublingual spaces showing the free communication of these spaces around the posterior border of the mylohyoid muscle. The hilum and duct of the submandibular gland occupy a portion of both spaces. (From Hollinshead WH: Anatomy for surgeons, vol 1, ed 2, *The head and neck,* Hagerstown, Md, 1968, Harper & Row.)

Submandibular Space In their classic anatomical studies from the 1930's, Grodinsky and Holyoke[5-7] used the term *submandibular space* to describe all of the perimandibular spaces, which this text defines separately as the submandibular, submental, and sublingual spaces. Grodinsky and Holyoke used the term *submaxillary space* to identify what is now termed the *submandibular space*. These landmark authors believed the perimandibular spaces were truly one anatomical fascial space because of the ready flow of injected gelatin into all three spaces. Clinical experience indicates that these spaces often become infected separately. When the right and left submandibular and sublingual spaces, along with the submental space, are infected in the cellulitis stage, the term *Ludwig's angina* may be ap-

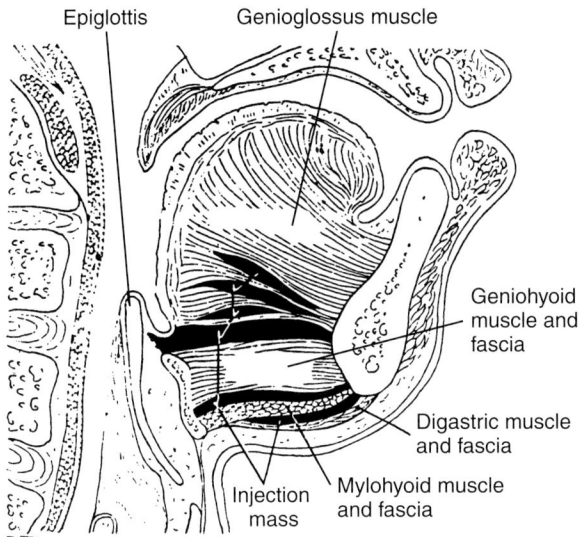

Figure 9-13 Sagittal diagram of dissection planes between the mylohyoid muscle and intrinsic muscles of the tongue, which terminate at the epiglottis. (From Grodinsky M: Ludwig's angina: an anatomical and clinical study with review of the literature, *Surgery* 5:678, 1939.)

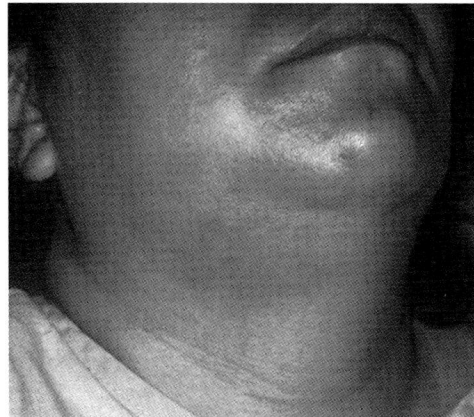

Figure 9-15 Oblique view of a patient with a submandibular space abscess. The redness and swelling are limited by the inferior border of the mandible, the anterior and posterior bellies of the digastric muscle, and the hyoid bone. (From Flynn TR: Surgical management of orofacial infections, *Atlas of the Oral and Maxillofacial Surgery Clinics of North America* 8:77, 2000.)

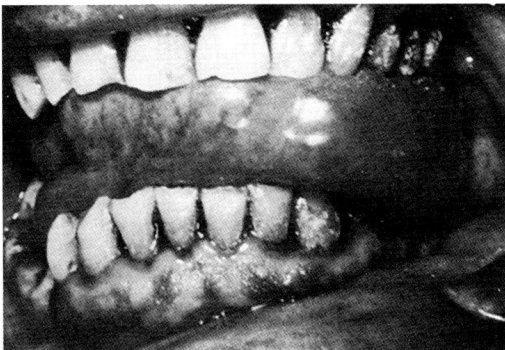

Figure 9-14 Oral view of a patient with severe elevation of the tongue caused by a sublingual space infection. On intubation the anesthesiologist noted epiglottitis. (From Flynn TR, Topazian RG: Infections of the oral cavity. In Waite D, editor. *Textbook of practical oral and maxillofacial surgery,* Philadelphia, 1987, Lea & Febiger.)

plied. No unique bacterial pathogen is associated with Ludwig's angina. The severity of this condition is related to anatomical factors because it hinders access to the airway and may directly compress it. In addition, a fulminant infection involving these spaces can spread rapidly to involve the lateral pharyngeal spaces and the retropharyngeal space, thus encircling the airway and threatening the mediastinum. In 1939, Ashbel Williams[22] reported a 54% mortality rate in Ludwig's angina. Four years later, a series of 20 cases Ludwig's angina was published in which only two (10%) patients died. The increased survival of the patients with this dreaded infection was the result of early establishment of a secure airway by tracheotomy and early

aggressive surgery.[23] In a recent prospective case series of hospitalized patients with odontogenic infections, the submandibular space was the second most frequently involved space (22/37 [59%] of cases).[3]

The anterior and posterior borders of the submandibular space are defined by the anterior and posterior bellies of the digastric muscle (Figure 9-15). The posterior border of this space also includes the stylohyoid muscle and the middle and superior pharyngeal constrictors at the superior, medial, and posterior corner of this space. An infection of the submandibular space can pass easily around the posterior belly of the digastric or the stylohyoid muscle, or along the lateral surface of the pharyngeal constrictor muscles, to the lateral pharyngeal space. Anteriorly, infection may pass around the anterior belly of the digastric to the submental space. The superior border of the submandibular space is the inferior border and lingual surface of the mandible, inferior to the attachment of the mylohyoid muscle at the mylohyoid line. The mylohyoid line slopes inferiorly as it passes anteriorly. Therefore infection beginning in the mandibular molars is likely to perforate the thin lingual plate of the mandible to enter the submandibular space directly. Infection of the premolar teeth may perforate the lingual cortical plate above the mylohyoid line and enter the sublingual space. The medial border of the submandibular space is the mylohyoid muscle, which extends from the mylohyoid line to the hyoid bone. Submandibular infections can pass readily around the posterior border of the mylohyoid muscle, following the submandibular gland and duct, to the sublingual space (see Figure 9-12).

The submandibular gland largely fills the submandibular space. The five branches of the facial artery in the

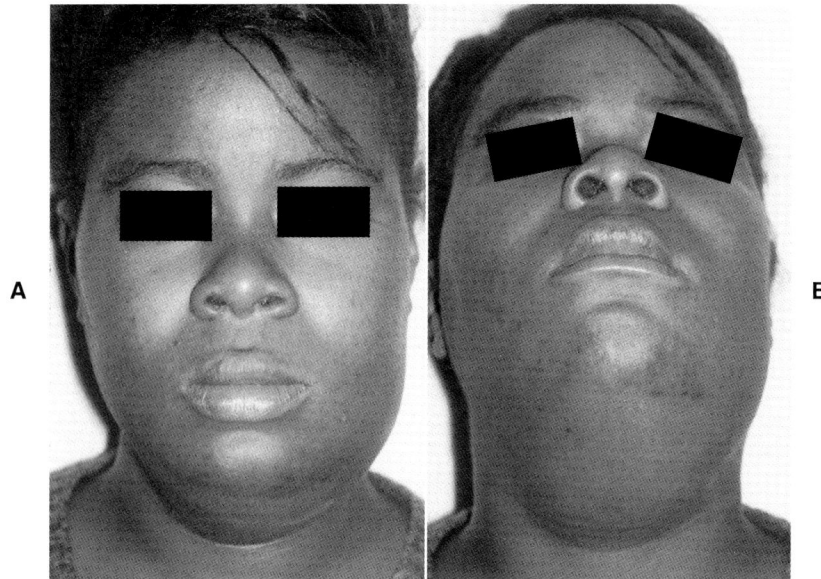

Figure 9-16 A, Frontal view of patient with a left submandibular space abscess spreading into submental space. **B,** Submentovertex view of the same patient illustrating fullness of the submental space and limitation of the swelling by attachment of the anterior layer of the deep cervical fascia to the hyoid bone. (From Flynn TR: Surgical management of orofacial infections, *Atlas of the Oral and Maxillofacial Surgery Clinics of North America* 8:77, 2000.)

submandibular space are the ascending palatine, tonsillar, sublingual, muscular (multiple), glandular (multiple), and submental.[10] The main trunk of the facial artery and vein enter the submandibular space deep to the submandibular gland, and the digastric and stylohyoid muscles inferiorly, and leave the submandibular space between the submandibular gland and the inferior border of the mandible in the antegonial notch. Perivascular lymph nodes accompany the facial artery and vein. They drain the anterior mandible, submental region, floor of the mouth, tonsillar pillars, and tongue.

Submental Space The submental space is a midline structure bordered laterally by the anterior bellies of the digastric muscle. The superficial border is the anterior layer of the deep cervical fascia between the hyoid bone and the inferior border of the mandible. The submental space is filled with areolar connective tissue, submental lymph nodes, and the anterior jugular veins in the lower portion of the space.

Infections of the submental space may begin in the anterior mandibular teeth but occur more commonly by the spread of infection from the submandibular space on either side. Infected skin wounds or anterior mandibular fractures also may cause infections of the submental space. Figure 9-16 shows a patient with a submental space cellulitis caused by spread of infection from the left submandibular space.

Masticator Space Like the perimandibular spaces, the masticator space is one anatomical compartment enclosed by the splitting of the anterior layer of the deep cervical fas-

cia around the muscles of mastication, following those muscles to their attachments to the cranium and skull base (Figure 9-17, *A*). Infections generally affect discrete portions of the masticator space, defined as the *submasseteric, pterygomandibular, superficial temporal,* and *deep temporal spaces.* Figure 9-17, *B* illustrates a patient with infection of the entire masticator space. The patient had a 60-day history of right facial swelling caused by infected upper molar teeth.

Submasseteric Space The submasseteric space lies between the anterior layer of the deep cervical fascia, locally referred to as the *parotideomasseteric fascia,* and the lateral surface of the ascending ramus of the mandible. The inferior border is the pterygomasseteric sling. The superior border of this space is the dense attachment of the parotideomasseteric fascia to the lateral surface of the zygomatic arch, the inferior border of the zygomatic arch, and the bottom of the superficial temporal space medial to the arch. The submasseteric space communicates with the pterygomandibular space through the sigmoid notch, through which passes the submasseteric artery. No separating structure exists between the submasseteric space and the superficial temporal space as they communicate deep to the zygomatic arch and superficial to the temporalis muscle.

The only major structures in the submasseteric space are the masseter muscle and the submasseteric artery and vein. A small amount of easily dissected areolar connective tissue is present between the masseter muscle and the periosteum of the ascending ramus of the mandible. Infections in this space typically cause inflammation and edema of the

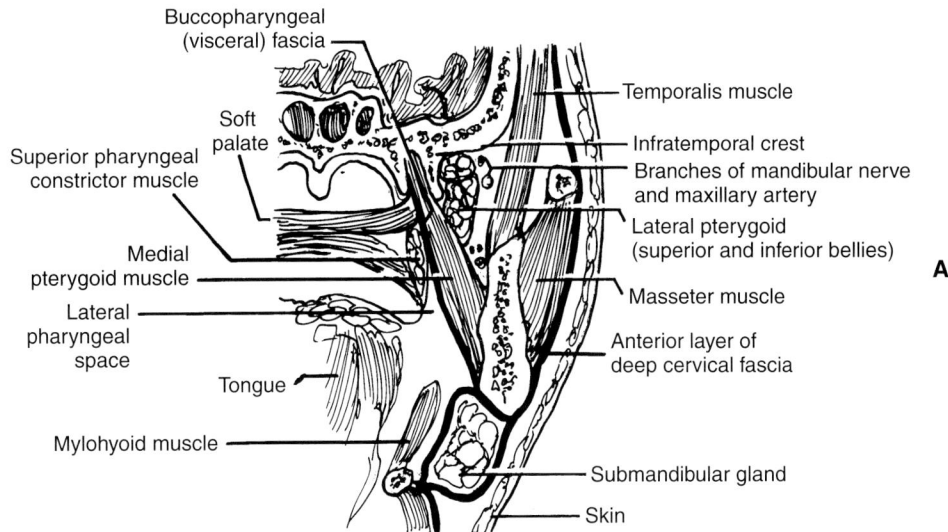

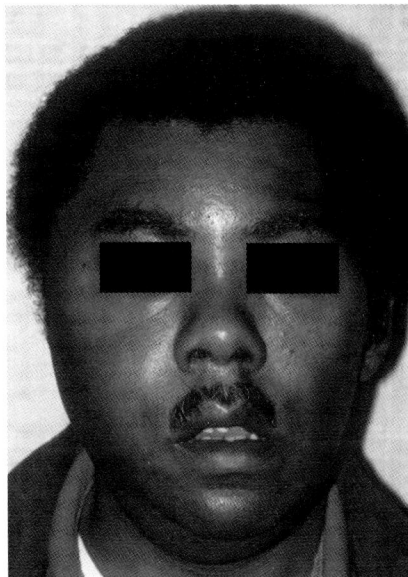

Figure 9-17 A, Coronal section of the left neck illustrating the borders, contents, and relations of the masticator space. (From Flynn TR: Anatomy and surgery of deep fascial space infections. In Kelly JJ, editor: *Oral and maxillofacial surgery knowledge update 1994,* Rosemont, IL, 1994, American Association of Oral and Maxillofacial Surgeons.) **B,** Frontal view of patient with a 60-day history of right facial swelling. The entire masticator space is distended. The temporal region is bulging and the right ear is obscured by the submasseteric swelling. (From Flynn TR: The swollen face, *Emerg Med Clin North Am* 15:481, 2000.)

overlying masseter muscle (Figure 9-18). The inflammatory process results in significant trismus, the hallmark of this condition. Submasseteric swellings can be differentiated from parotid swellings because submasseteric swellings obscure the ear lobe, whereas parotid swellings elevate it. The marked submasseteric swelling may obscure the ear lobe in frontal view (Figure 9-19; see Figure 9-17, *B*).

Pterygomandibular Space   In a recent prospective study of severe odontogenic infections the pterygomandibular space was the most frequently affected anatomical compartment; abscess or cellulitis was present in the pterygo-

mandibular space in 23 (62%) of 37 cases.[3] Infection of the pterygomandibular space correlated highly with pericoronitis of the mandibular third molar. Trismus, caused by edema and inflammation of the medial pterygoid muscle, hinders the view of the swollen anterior tonsillar pillar and the deviation of the uvula to the opposite side that are characteristic of infection in this space. Figure 9-20 illustrates these findings in a pterygomandibular space infection caused by a carious, partially erupted mandibular third molar. The photographic visualization was aided by a mandibular fracture in the region, which was distracted for access while the patient was under general anesthesia.

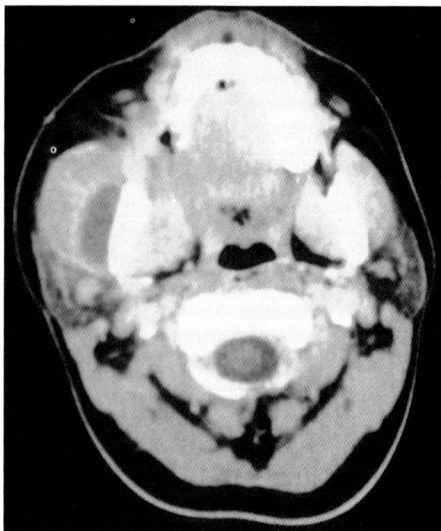

Figure 9-18 Axial CT scan of submasseteric space abscess demonstrating radiolucent collection of fluid between the ascending ramus of the mandible and the edematous masseter muscle.

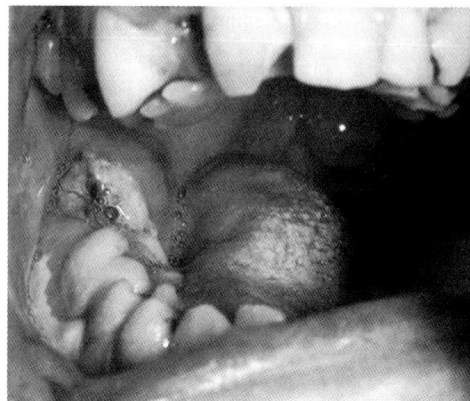

Figure 9-20 Oral view of a right pterygomandibular space abscess caused by a fracture of the mandibular angle involving the carious lower third molar. Swelling of the anterior tonsillar pillar and deviation of the edematous uvula to the opposite side are present. (From Flynn TR, Topazian RG: Infections of the oral cavity. In Waite D, editor: *Textbook of practical oral and maxillofacial surgery,* Philadelphia, 1987, Lea & Febiger.)

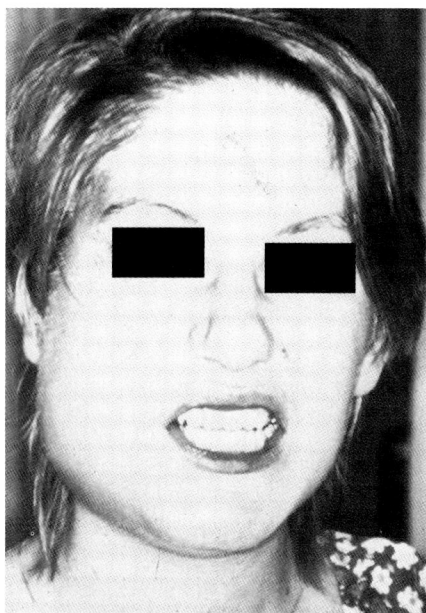

Figure 9-19 Marked trismus is present and the swelling partially obscures the lobe of the ear in this patient with a right submasseteric space abscess.

The borders of the pterygomandibular space are the ascending ramus of the mandible laterally, the medial pterygoid muscle medially, the pterygomasseteric sling inferiorly, and the lateral pterygoid muscle superiorly. The parotid gland and its capsule form the posterior border, and the anterior border is formed by the buccinator and superior pharyngeal constrictor muscles as they meet at the pterygomandibular raphe. Infections may spread into the infratemporal portion of the deep temporal space by passing superiorly around the lateral pterygoid muscle,

which runs from the mandibular condylar neck and articular disk to the medial pterygoid plate. More commonly, however, pterygomandibular space infections spread to the lateral pharyngeal space by passing around the anterior border of the medial pterygoid muscle, following the posterolateral surface of the buccinator and superior pharyngeal constrictor muscles. Figure 9-21 is a computed tomographic (CT) scan of a pterygomandibular space infection with an edematous, distended pterygoid muscle and early involvement of the lateral pharyngeal space in a young adult with a mandibular third molar pericoronitis.

The contents of the pterygomandibular space include the inferior alveolar neurovascular bundle and the vascular and motor supply of the medial pterygoid and masseter muscles, whose arteries are branches of the internal maxillary. The sensory portion of the mandibular division of the trigeminal nerve is also found in the pterygomandibular space, including the lingual, inferior alveolar, mylohyoid, and auriculotemporal nerves. Needle track infections occur most often in the pterygomandibular space because of attempts to anesthetize the inferior alveolar nerve before dental procedures. Figure 9-22 is a CT scan of a well-encapsulated pterygomandibular space abscess near the mandibular condyle in a middle-aged woman who had received several inferior alveolar nerve blocks for restorative dentistry approximately 6 weeks earlier.

Superficial Temporal Space The superficial temporal space lies between the temporal fascia, which is the continuation of parotideomasseteric fascia, and the temporalis muscle. The temporal fascia rises from the zygomatic arch to terminate at the superficial temporal crest of the tem-

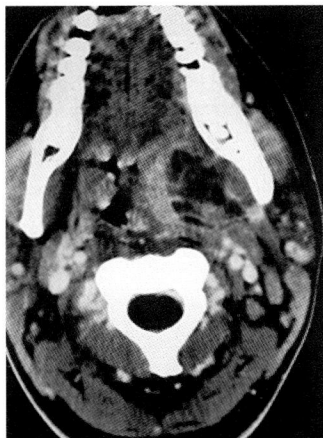

Figure 9-21 Axial CT scan of pterygomandibular space abscess in a female adolescent with pericoronitis of the left lower third molar showing radiolucent collection between the ascending ramus of the mandible and distended medial pterygoid muscle. The lateral pharyngeal space and airway are distorted by the mass effect of the pterygomandibular space infection. (From Flynn TR: The swollen face, *Emerg Med Clin North Am* 15:481, 2000.)

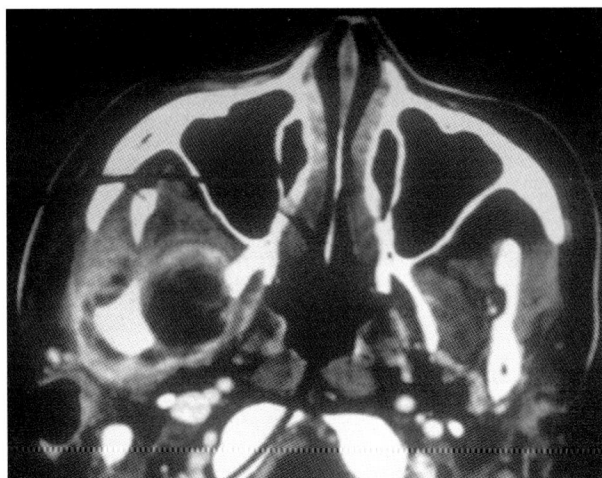

Figure 9-22 Contrast-enhanced axial CT scan of pterygomandibular space abscess. The collection is high in the pterygomandibular space at the level of the pterygoid plates and surrounding the condylar neck of the mandible. The well-vascularized capsule shows ring enhancement of this abscess, which produced acute symptoms 6 weeks after inferior alveolar nerve blocks for restorative dentistry.

poral bone. The anterior border of the superficial temporal space is the posterior surface of the lateral orbital rim, and its posterior border is the fusion of the temporal fascia with the pericranium at the posterior edge of the temporalis muscle. The inferior border of the superficial temporal space is the zygomatic arch and the areolar connective tissues medial to the arch, where this space communicates with the submasseteric space. For approximately 2 cm su-

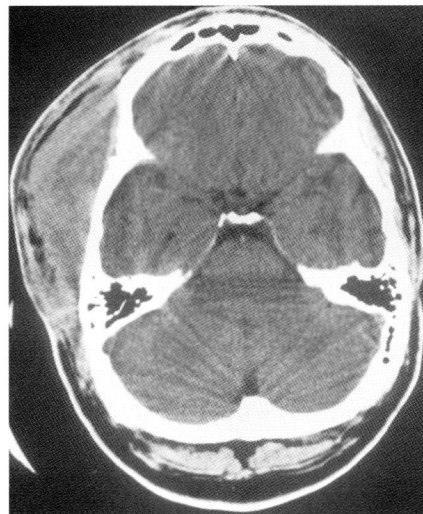

Figure 9-23 Axial CT scan of a large deep temporal space abscess in the patient in Figure 9-17, *B* shows distention of the temporalis muscle.

perior to the zygomatic arch a small compartment is formed by the splitting of the temporal fascia into two layers that pass lateral and medial to the zygomatic arch. This compartment contains a leaflet of the buccal fat pad and three small veins that drain the temporal region. Buccal space infections may follow the buccal fat pad into this space (see Figure 9-7, *B*).

Deep Temporal Space The lateral border of the deep temporal space is the temporalis muscle, and its medial border is the squamous temporal bone and the skull base, formed mainly by the sphenoid bone (Figure 9-23). The infratemporal space is the portion of the deep temporal space that lies inferior to the infratemporal crest of the sphenoid bone. The inferior border of the deep temporal space is the superior surface of the lateral pterygoid muscle. The superior, posterior border is formed by the attachment of the temporalis muscle to the cranium at the temporal crest. The anterior border of the temporal space is composed of the posterior wall of the maxillary sinus, the pterygomaxillary fissure, and the posterior surface of the orbit, including the inferior orbital fissure. The important contents of the deep temporal space are found in the infratemporal portion. These include the terminal division of the internal maxillary artery and the mandibular division of the trigeminal nerve.

Thrombophlebitis may ascend into the cavernous sinus through the infratemporal space, which is the posterior pathway of cavernous sinus thrombosis. The pterygoid plexus lies within the infratemporal space and receives venous tributaries from the transverse facial vein, which passes through the buccal space. Buccal space infections that erode into the transverse facial vein may cause ascending thrombophlebitis of the pterygoid venous plexus. Emissary veins from the pterygoid plexus pass through the foramina of Vesalius, ovale, and lacerum to enter the

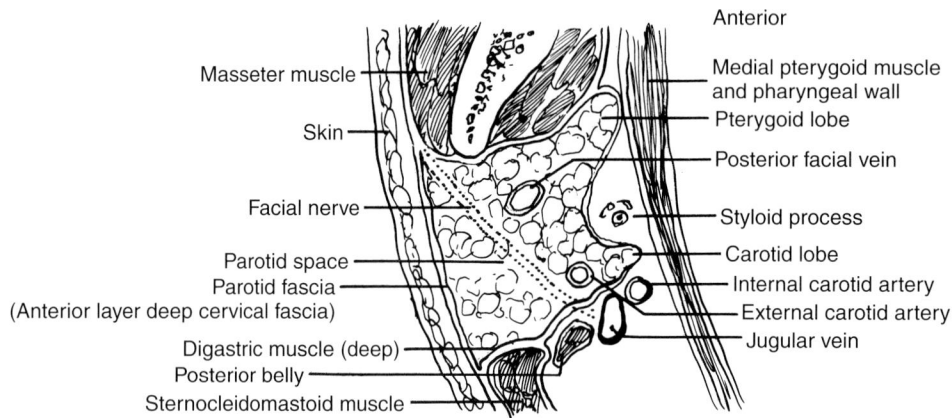

Figure 9-24 Transverse section just above the angle of the mandible illustrating the borders, contents, and relations of the parotid space. (From Flynn TR: Anatomy and surgery of deep fascial space infections. In Kelly JJ, editor: *Oral and maxillofacial surgery knowledge update 1994,* Rosemont, IL, 1994, American Association of Oral and Maxillofacial Surgeons.)

cavernous sinus within the cranial cavity. A buccal space infection may pass around the posterior surface of the maxilla to enter the infratemporal portion of the deep temporal space (see Figure 9-8).

Parotid Space   The parotid space is formed by the splitting of the anterior (investing) layer of the deep cervical fascia to form the capsule of the parotid gland. In this region the fascia is called the *parotideomasseteric fascia.* The parotid space contains the parotid gland, facial nerve, posterior facial lymphatics, the external carotid artery and its terminal branches, and the posterior facial (retromandibular) vein.[9] The parotid capsule is thick on the lateral surface of the gland, but it is less well defined medially where the parotid gland abuts the styloid process and carotid sheath in the lateral pharyngeal space. The temporomandibular joint capsule and external auditory meatus are the superior relations of the parotid space, whereas the mastoid process, sternocleidomastoid muscle, and the posterior belly of the digastric muscle are its posterior and inferior relations. Within the parotid space the facial nerve courses superficially and anteriorly as it divides into its five main branches. Just above the angle of the mandible the posterior facial vein is deep to the facial nerve, and the external carotid artery lies more deeply within the substance of the gland (Figure 9-24). Just below the condylar neck of the mandible the external carotid terminates in the internal maxillary artery, which courses deeply between the mandible and the sphenomandibular ligament to enter the pterygomandibular space, and the superficial temporal artery, which rises to cross the zygomatic process of the temporal bone.

Lateral Pharyngeal Space   The lateral pharyngeal space is shaped like an inverted pyramid with its base at the base of the skull and its apex at the hyoid bone. The pharyngeal constrictor muscles form its medial border; the overlying visceral division of the middle layer of the deep cervical fascia is termed the *buccopharyngeal fascia* in this location (Figure 9-25). The lateral border is the medial pterygoid muscle superiorly and the anterior layer of the deep cervical fascia inferiorly. The anterior border is the palatal musculature superiorly, the buccinator and superior pharyngeal constrictor muscles in the middle, and the stylohyoid muscle and the posterior belly of the digastric muscle inferiorly. Free communications exist along this anterior border with the sublingual and submandibular spaces. The posterior border is the carotid sheath posterolaterally and the retropharyngeal space posteromedially. A short layer of fascia runs from the anterior layer of the deep cervical fascia overlying the medial pterygoid muscle, across the styloid process and the styloid muscles to the buccopharyngeal fascia. This fascial condensation is called the *aponeurosis of Zuckerkandl and Testut,* which divides the lateral pharyngeal space into anterior (prestyloid) and posterior (poststyloid) compartments.[1] The anterior compartment has little content except areolar connective tissue. The posterior compartment of the lateral pharyngeal space contains cranial nerves IX (glossopharyngeal), X (vagus), XI (spinal accessory), and XII (hypoglossal), the carotid sheath and its contents, and the cervical sympathetic chain, attached to the posterior surface of the carotid sheath. These structures give rise to the ominous clinical signs of cranial nerve and carotid sheath involvement that can occur in severe infections of the lateral pharyngeal space.

The relations of the lateral pharyngeal space explain the most frequent causes of lateral pharyngeal space infections. Peritonsillar infections that penetrate the pharyngeal constrictor muscles enter the lateral pharyngeal space. Sublingual space infections can enter the lateral pharyngeal space in the posterior part of the floor of the mouth through the buccopharyngeal gap. Submandibular space infections can pass around the posterior belly of the digastric muscle or the stylohyoid muscle to enter the lateral pharyngeal space. Retropharyngeal space infections, pos-

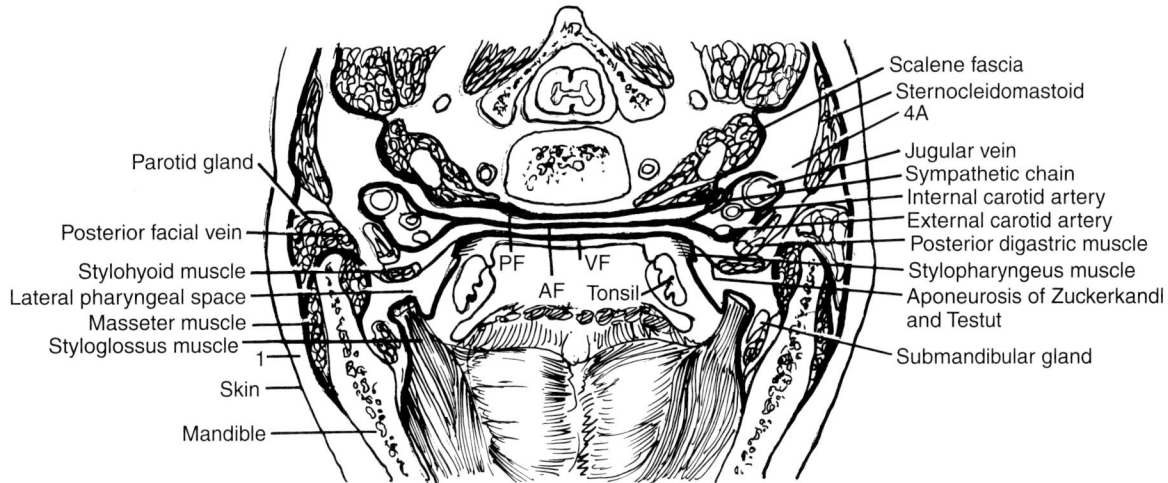

Figure 9-25 Transverse section through the ascending ramus of the mandible illustrating the borders, contents, and relations of the lateral pharyngeal and retropharyngeal spaces. *PF,* Prevertebral fascia; *VF,* visceral fascia, *AF,* alar fascia. (From Flynn TR: Anatomy and surgery of deep fascial space infections. In Kelly JJ, editor: *Oral and maxillofacial surgery knowledge update 1994,* Rosemont, IL, 1994, American Association of Oral and Maxillofacial Surgeons.)

sibly caused by necrotic breakdown of retropharyngeal lymph nodes, can spread easily into the lateral pharyngeal space because no membranous or muscular barrier exists between these two spaces. Infections may encircle the airway by spreading from one lateral pharyngeal space to the other through the retropharyngeal space. A postoperative CT scan can reveal this type of airway encirclement after drainage of an odontogenic abscess of the pterygomandibular space (Figure 9-26). Figure 9-27 shows the clinical and radiographic features of patients with lateral pharyngeal space infections. In the frontal view the only visible swelling may be between the posterior belly of the digastric and the anterior border of the sternocleidomastoid muscles, just superior to the hyoid bone. On palpation a tender fullness of this region also suggests the correct diagnosis. Intraorally only mild to moderate trismus may be noted unless the masticator space also is involved. The palatoglossal arch is blunted on the affected side with deviation of the uvula to the unaffected side. The anterior tonsillar pillar is edematous and tender, along with the lateral pharyngeal wall, if it is visible. The patient's head may tilt toward the shoulder of the unaffected side to position the upper airway over the deviated trachea and larynx (Figure 9-27, *C*). Contrast-enhanced CT is a valuable aid in confirmation of the diagnosis of deep cervical space infections, and in determination of the extent and the stage of the infection. When correlated with clinical signs a correct diagnosis of abscess or cellulitis of the lateral and retropharyngeal spaces can be made with a sensitivity of 95% and a specificity of 80%.[16]

Retropharyngeal Space The retropharyngeal space extends vertically from the base of the skull to the fusion of the retropharyngeal fascia, a local name for the visceral division of the middle layer of the deep cervical fascia with

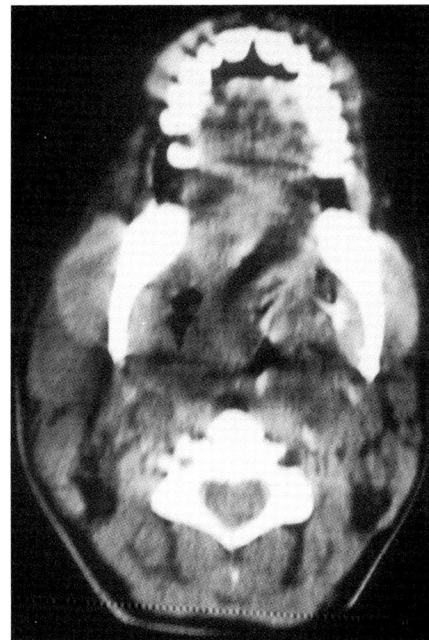

Figure 9-26 Postoperative axial CT scan of a previously drained left pterygomandibular space abscess. Infection extends into the right and left lateral pharyngeal spaces and the retropharyngeal space with constriction and deviation of the airway. (From Flynn TR: Surgical management of orofacial infections, *Atlas of the Oral and Maxillofacial Surgery Clinics of North America* 8:77, 2000.)

the alar fascia.[8] These two fascial layers unite at a variable level between the sixth cervical and fourth thoracic vertebrae. Therefore these two fascial layers compose the anterior, posterior, and inferior borders of the retropharyngeal space. The lateral borders of the retropharyngeal spaces on either side are the lateral pharyngeal space and the carotid

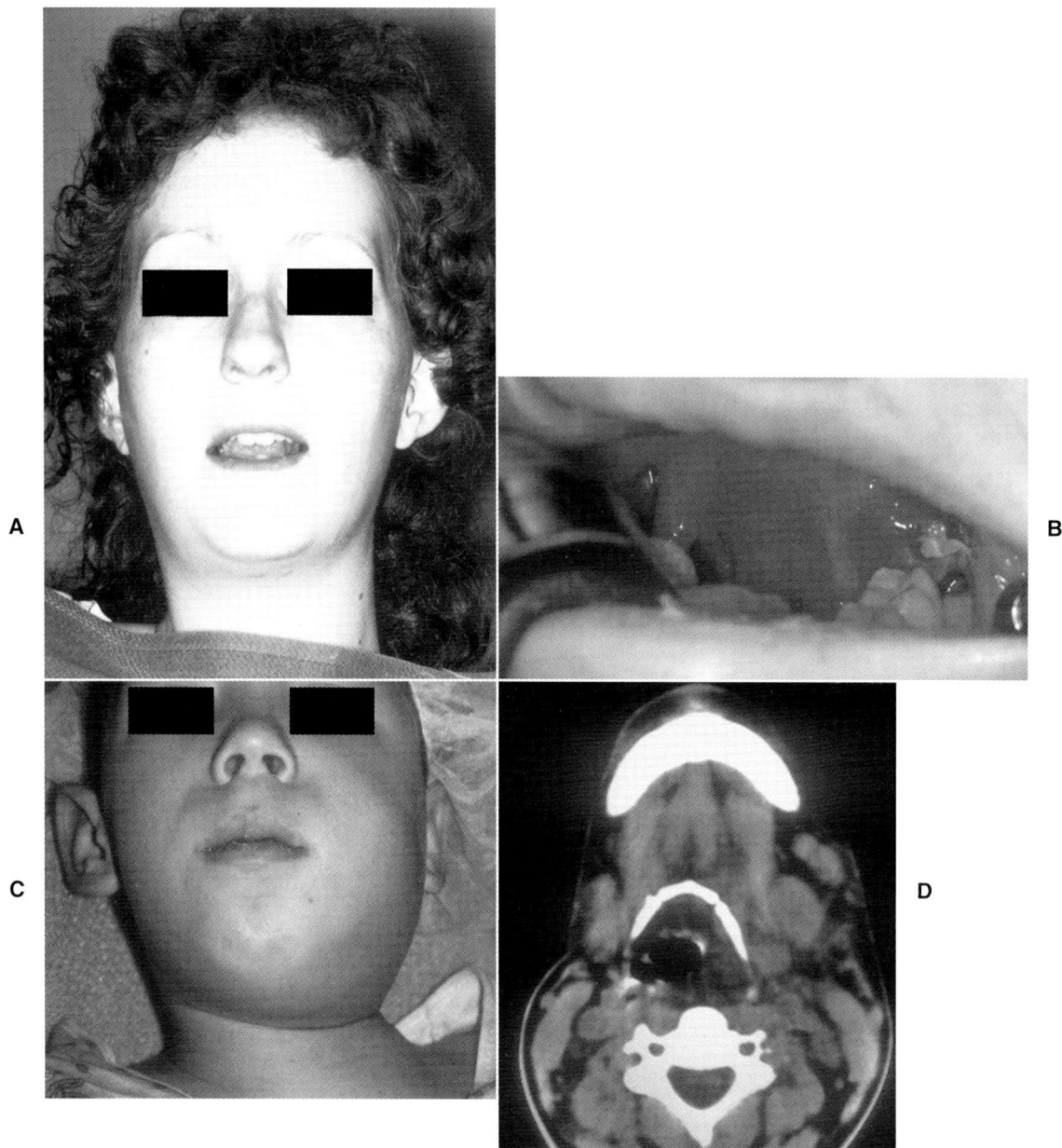

Figure 9-27 A, Frontal view of right lateral pharyngeal space abscess after third molar removal showing mild trismus and external swelling just anterior to the sternocleidomastoid muscle and above the hyoid bone. **B,** Oral view of the same patient showing swelling of the anterior tonsillar pillar and blunting of the left palatouvular fold. **C,** A boy with a left lateral pharyngeal space abscess has swelling just anterior to the sternocleidomastoid muscle with deviation of the head toward the right shoulder in an attempt to place the upper airway directly over the deviated trachea. **D,** Axial CT scan at the level of the hyoid bone demonstrating cellulitis of the left lateral pharyngeal space deviating the airway to the opposite side and spreading into the retropharyngeal space.

sheath. A midline septum exists between the right and left retropharyngeal spaces that is crossed easily. Thus surgeons and anatomists conceptualize the retropharyngeal space as a unitary structure (see Figures 9-1 to 9-3).

The retropharyngeal space contains areolar connective tissue and lymph nodes that drain the adenoidal tissues of the posterior pharyngeal wall. The adenoids and tonsils encircle the oropharynx in a structure referred to as *Waldeyer's ring.* The lateral and retropharyngeal spaces contain a rich supply of lymph nodes that drain Waldeyer's ring. When

these nodes are overwhelmed or necrotic, a fascial space infection may develop.

Infections of the retropharyngeal space are ominous because of their ability to impinge on the airway directly and potential involvement of the danger space. The alar fascia divides the retropharyngeal space from the danger space, and once an aggressive necrotizing infection has fully distended the retropharyngeal space, pressure necrosis and enzymatic destruction of the alar fascia may allow the infection to perforate into the danger space.

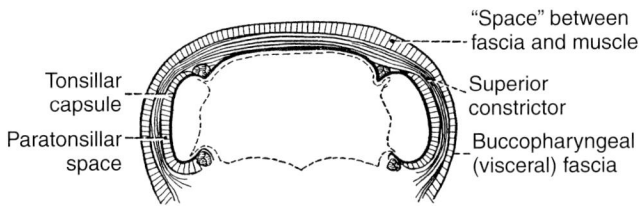

Figure 9-28 Transverse section of the peritonsillar space illustrating its borders, contents, and relations. (From Hollinshead WH: *Anatomy for surgeons,* vol 1, ed 2, *The head and neck,* Hagerstown, Md, 1968, Harper & Row.)

Pretracheal Space The pretracheal space is the anterior portion of space 3 described by Grodinsky and Holyoke[7] (see Figure 9-3). Its superior border is the fusion of the visceral division and the sternothyroid-thyrohyoid division of the middle layer of the deep cervical fascia at the thyroid cartilage and hyoid bone. Inferiorly the pretracheal space is continuous with the superior and anterior mediastinum at the level of the aortic arch, where the pericardium and the posterior surface of the sternum are joined by dense connective tissue. The pretracheal space lies between the deep surface of the sternothyroid-thyrohyoid fascia and the superficial surface of the visceral fascia, which surrounds the trachea, esophagus, and thyroid gland. Laterally the pretracheal space is continuous with the retropharyngeal space between the thyroid cartilage superiorly and the inferior thyroid artery inferiorly. Because of the fairly dense fusion of the fascial layers at the superior extent of this space, infections that begin above in the jaws and oral cavity usually do not descend into the pretracheal space.

Visceral Space The visceral space is enclosed by the visceral division of the middle layer of the deep cervical fascia. The visceral space contains the pharynx, larynx, trachea, esophagus, and thyroid glands (see Figure 9-3). Anteriorly the visceral space begins at the thyroid cartilage and follows the trachea and esophagus into the mediastinum. Posteriorly the visceral space begins at the base of the skull. Above the hyoid bone it is the space enclosed by the buccopharyngeal fascia, which includes the nasopharynx and oropharynx. Below the hyoid bone the visceral fascia encloses the larynx, trachea, thyroid gland, and esophagus like a tubular sheath that descends into the mediastinum. Within the visceral space, each organ is surrounded by a thin layer of areolar connective tissue. Infections of these organs drain into the lumen of the pharynx, esophagus, or trachea or pierce the visceral fascia anteriorly to enter the pretracheal space.

The visceral space encloses the peritonsillar space, which is analogous to the vestibular space intraorally (Figure 9-28). The peritonsillar space lies between the oropharyngeal mucosa and the superior pharyngeal constrictor muscle. It contains and surrounds the palatine tonsil. Peritonsillar infections may drain through the mucosa into the oropharynx or may perforate the superior constrictor and visceral (buccopharyngeal) fascia to enter the lateral pharyngeal space. Rather than spreading laterally to encircle the oropharynx, peritonsillar infections ascend vertically toward the hard palate or eustachian tube, or descend inferiorly toward the piriform recess.

Danger Space The deep fascial space known as the danger space is aptly named because of its communication with the mediastinum (see Figures 9-1 and 9-2). The danger space extends from the base of the skull superiorly to the diaphragm inferiorly. Its lateral extent is at the fusion of the alar and prevertebral fasciae at the transverse processes of the cervical and thoracic vertebrae. The only content of the danger space in the cervical region is areolar connective tissue. However, in the chest the danger space is continuous with the posterior mediastinum, which contains the vena cava, aorta, thoracic duct, trachea, and esophagus. Therefore, infections that pass through the danger space into the mediastinum can erode into or compress major vessels, lower airway, and upper digestive tract.

In 1921 Pearse[18] described the anatomical routes of head and neck infections in a series of 110 cases of mediastinitis. In 8% of the cases, pretracheal space infections descended directly into the anterior mediastinum. Infections followed the carotid sheath to the mediastinum in 21% of cases. However, in 71% of cases infections passed from the retropharyngeal space to the mediastinum through the danger space.

Carotid Sheath The carotid sheath encloses the common and internal carotid arteries, internal jugular vein, and vagus nerve (see Figure 9-1). It extends from the jugular foramen and carotid canal in the occipital bone to the mediastinum, where it divides to surround the major vessels that contribute to its contents. The cervical sympathetic chain attaches to the posterior surface of the carotid sheath. Infections that have eroded into the carotid sheath may cause disruption of any of the structures associated with it, including expanding hematoma in the neck, bleeding episodes ("herald bleeds"), variations in heart rate or speech function, or septic emboli. Involvement of the cervical sympathetic chain may cause Horner's syndrome on the affected side, which is characterized by miosis (pupillary constriction), ptosis (drooping of the lid caused by inactivation of Müller's muscle), and anhidrosis (decreased sweating of the affected side of the head, neck, and upper extremity).

Mediastinum The mediastinum can be visualized as the facade of a Greek temple, with the superior mediastinum sitting atop the three columns formed by the anterior, middle, and posterior mediastinum (Figure 9-29). All of the cervical structures that pass into the mediastinum traverse the superior mediastinum that begins at the first rib and the manubrium of the sternum. The inferior border is an imaginary line drawn from the bottom of the fourth thoracic vertebra (T4) to the angle of Louis (the manubriosternal junction). The structures in the superior mediastinum, in order from anterior to posterior, are the origins of the sternohyoid and sternothyroid muscles; the thymic remnant; the major vessels, including the carotid, brachiocephalic, subclavians, aortic arch (inferiorly), thoracic duct; the trachea; the vagus,

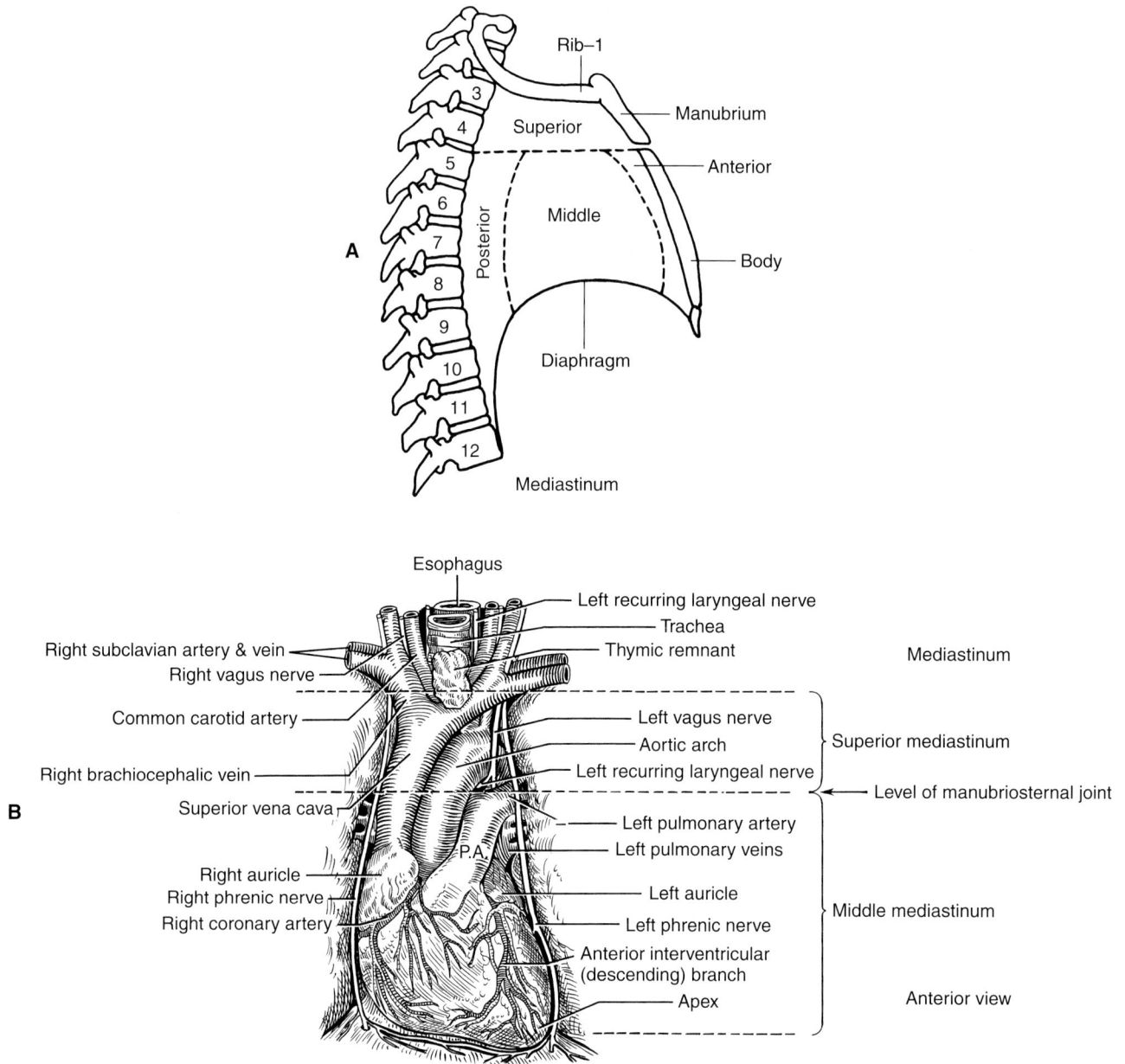

Figure 9-29 A, Sagittal section of the mediastinum illustrating its subdivisions. **B,** Cut-away view of the middle mediastinum, containing the heart and phrenic nerves, and the posterior mediastinum, containing the great vessels, thymus, trachea, esophagus, and various nerves. (From Pansky B, House EL: *Review of gross anatomy,* ed 2, New York, 1969, MacMillan.)

recurrent, cardiac and phrenic nerves; the esophagus; and the longus colli muscle. Cervical dissection into the mediastinum follows a plane posterior to the esophagus in the danger space, thus avoiding the vital structures anterior to the esophagus.

The anterior mediastinum is a potential space filled with areolar connective tissue, a few small lymph nodes, and vessels that lie between the pericardium and the posterior surface of the sternum. Superior to the anterior mediastinum lies the superior mediastinum and the pretracheal space is above. The inferior margin of the anterior mediastinum is the diaphragm. It is bounded laterally by the visceral pleura on either side. The middle mediastinum

contains the heart, pericardium, and the phrenic nerves, which course inferiorly on either side of the heart to the diaphragm.

The posterior mediastinum contains all of the noncardiac major structures of the mediastinum, including the thoracic aorta, superior and inferior venae cavae, azygos vein, thoracic duct, vagus nerves, trachea, esophagus, and the splanchnic nerves in the inferior portion. The posterior mediastinum is bounded anteriorly by the pericardium, posteriorly by the alar fascia, and laterally by the visceral pleura on either side. The inferior border is the diaphragm; superiorly it is bounded by the superior mediastinum, with the danger space above.

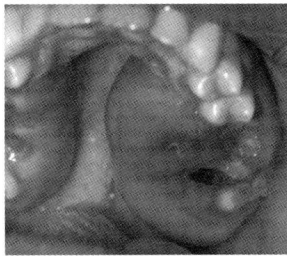

Figure 9-30 Intraoral view of a left palatal abscess arising from carious upper molar teeth.

INFECTIONS ASSOCIATED WITH MAXILLARY ODONTOGENIC INFECTIONS

Although the division of the deep fascial spaces of the head and neck into those associated with maxillary infections versus those associated with mandibular infections is arbitrary, maxillary infections generally rise toward the brain and mandibular infections descend toward the chest. Maxillary infections may ascend through the valveless venous drainage of the face by the anterior or posterior route or through the sinuses to the orbit or brain. Exceptions to these patterns occur.

Palatal Space Infections that begin in the lateral incisor or the palatal roots of upper posterior teeth tend to cause infections of the palatal space because their roots are located closer to the palatal cortical plate (Figure 9-30). The palatal space essentially is the subperiosteal space of the palate, and infections in this region can be exquisitely painful because of the rich innervation of the periosteum.

No structures exist between the bone and periosteum in this region, but surgeons must consider that the greater palatine neurovascular bundle runs in a groove at the junction of the horizontal and vertical portions of the hard palate, running anteriorly from the second molar region to the first premolar region. The submucosal portion of the hard palate also contains minor salivary glands, fat, and minor aggregates of lymphoid tissue. Anteriorly the nasopalatine nerve exits from the incisive foramen. Its branches radiate from this foramen to provide sensation to the soft tissue of the hard palate anterior to and including the canine teeth.

Because the palatal periosteum is bound tightly to the underlying bone, abscesses in this region are localized discretely. Spontaneous drainage, although uncommon, usually occurs through the gingival sulcus of the infected tooth.

Infraorbital Space The quadratus labii superioris muscle defines the infraorbital space. The four heads of the muscle arise from the region of the infraorbital rim (Figure 9-31). The levator labii superioris attaches to the midportion of the infraorbital rim, and the levator anguli oris (caninus) muscle attaches inferior to the former muscle on the anterior maxillary wall. The other two heads of the quadratus labii superioris, the zygomaticus major and minor, originate laterally along the zygomatic arch and insert into the lateral part of the upper lip.

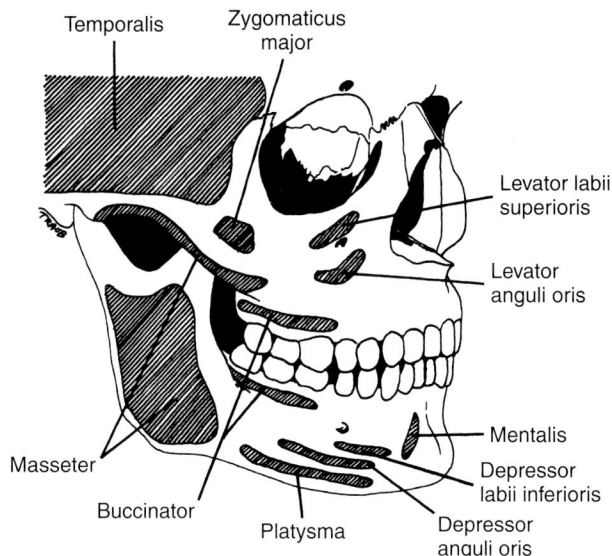

Figure 9-31 Origins of the facial muscles on the bony skeleton showing the relations of the attachments of the levator labii superioris and the levator anguli oris muscles, between which is found the infraorbital space. Infraorbital space infections may point into the lower eyelid on either side of the attachment of the levator labii superioris muscle.

Infections that begin in the maxillary anterior teeth and premolars can affect the infraorbital space. Because of the length of its root, dental infections of the maxillary canine may perforate the facial cortical plate of the maxilla at a point superior to the attachment of the levator anguli oris muscle. The infection may spread directly into the infraorbital space because it forms the space between the levator anguli oris muscle and the levator labii superioris. The nasal cartilages and subcutaneous tissue lie medially and the buccal space is found laterally.

Spontaneous intraoral drainage of the infraorbital space may be delayed because an abscess in this region must pass through or around the levator anguli oris muscle to reach the vestibular space and the oral mucosa. Alternatively, infraorbital space infections burrow toward the skin on either side of the quadratus labii superioris muscle. Thus the abscess may point through the medial or lateral aspect of the lower eyelid (Figure 9-32).

Cavernous sinus thrombosis is a rare but dreaded complication of infraorbital space abscess caused by ascending thrombophlebitis of the angular vein, which passes through the infraorbital space. The facial veins generally are valveless and thus allow bidirectional flow. The only venous valves in the head and neck are found at the superior jugular bulb, where the internal jugular passes through the jugular foramen, and the inferior jugular bulb, just above the terminus of this vein at the subclavian and brachiocephalic veins. Thus a septic thrombophlebitis of the angular vein may ascend to the cavernous sinus through the inferior ophthalmic vein, which passes through the orbit. The infraorbital space also contains the infraorbital nerve and its lateral nasal, inferior palpebral, superior labial, and anterior superior alveolar branches.

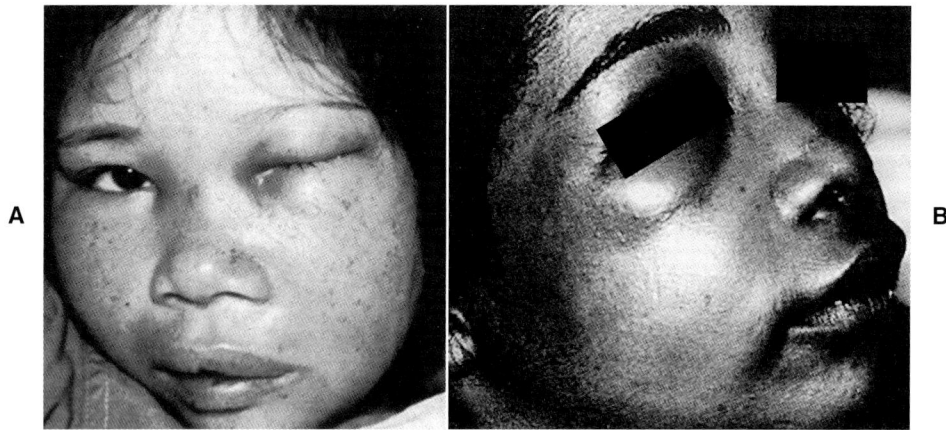

Figure 9-32 A, An infraorbital space abscess about to point in the lower eyelid, medial to the attachment of the levator labii superioris muscle. **B,** An acute infraorbital space abscess about to point in the lower eyelid, lateral to the attachment of the levator labii superioris muscle on the infraorbital rim. (From Flynn TR: The swollen face, *Emerg Med Clin North Am* 15:481, 2000.)

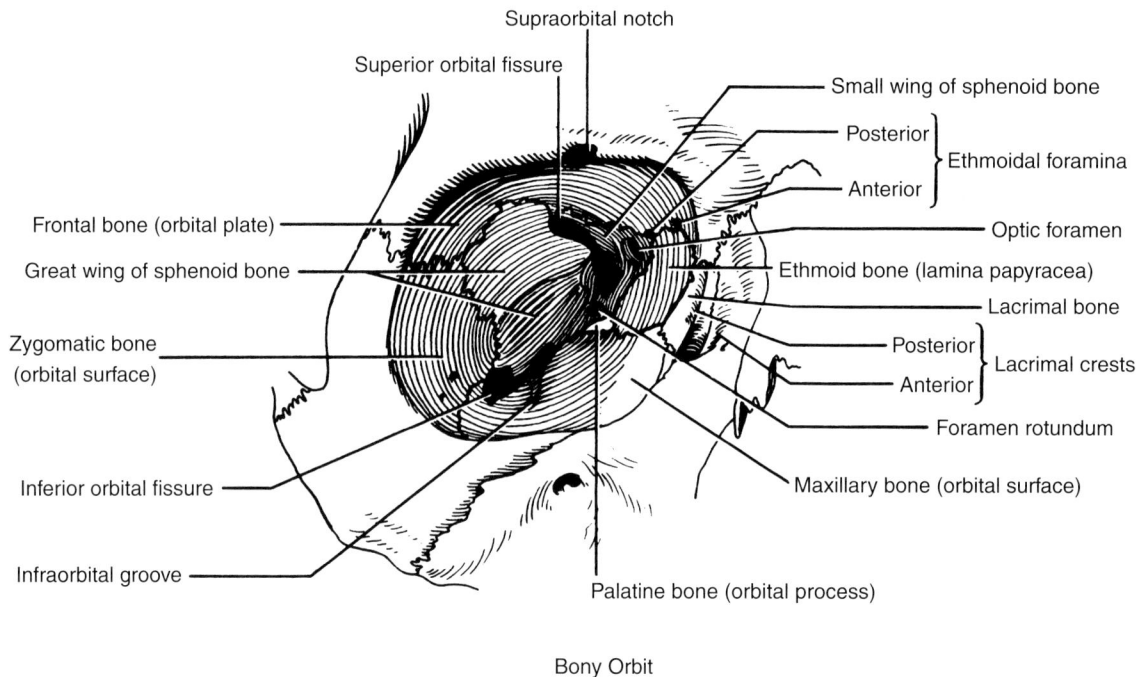

Bony Orbit

Figure 9-33 Frontal diagram of bony orbit illustrating the superior and inferior orbital fissures and the optic foramen. (From Pansky B, House EL: *Review of gross anatomy,* ed 2, New York, 1969, MacMillan.)

Periorbital Space   The periorbital, or preseptal, space lies between the orbicularis oculi muscle and the orbital septum, which is a leaflet arising from the periosteum of the orbital rim, extending and attaching to the tarsal plates. The periorbital space is divided into upper and lower compartments by the medial and lateral canthal ligaments as they attach to the orbital rim. Fat and areolar connective tissue fill the periorbital space very loosely, which accounts for the propensity of the eyelids to accommodate edema fluid (see Figure 9-7, *B*) or extravasated blood, as in periorbital ecchymosis. The zygomatic branch of the facial nerve provides motor innervation to the orbicularis oculi muscle, entering at a point just inferior to the lateral canthus of the eye. Periorbital space infections may enter the orbital space by penetration of the orbital septum and may drain through the thin overlying skin.

Orbital Space   The orbital space is bounded by the bony walls of the orbit peripherally and posteriorly (Figure 9-33). The anterior border of the orbital space is the orbital septum, which divides it from the periorbital space. This space is cone shaped with its base at the orbital septum and its apex posteromedially at the optic foramen. The lateral wall of the orbit is perforated by the orbital fissures. The superior orbital fissure runs inferiorly from lateral to medial and the inferior orbital fissure runs inferiorly from medial to lateral. Important structures pass through the superior orbital fissure: the ophthalmic division of the trigeminal nerve (cranial nerve V), the trochlear nerve (IV), the oculomotor nerve (III), the ophthalmic vein, and the abducens nerve (VI). Damage to the structures passing through the superior orbital fissure results in superior orbital fissure syndrome, characterized by paresthesia of the upper eyelid and forehead, and paralysis of the extraocular and pupillary muscles.[20] Because the optic nerve is not involved in superior orbital fissure syndrome, the direct and consensual ocular reflexes are lost in the affected eye, but the consensual reflex is retained in the unaffected eye.

Damage to the structures passing through the superior orbital fissure and those passing through the optic foramen results in orbital apex syndrome. Because the optic foramen contains the optic nerve and artery, vision is lost in the affected eye. Therefore the direct and consensual reflexes are lost in the affected eye and the consensual reflex also is lost in the unaffected eye.

Thin layers of bone separate the orbital space from the maxillary sinus inferiorly and the ethmoid sinus medially.[17] The medial orbital wall is termed the *lamina papyracea* (Latin for "paper-thin layer"). Infection may spread into the orbital space by resorption of these bony layers or through tiny emissary veins that perforate the bone. For example, a subperiosteal orbital abscess may originate in a carious primary molar and pass into the orbit through the maxillary and ethmoid sinuses (Figure 9-34). Additional emissary veins pass from the orbital space to the infratemporal space through the inferior orbital fissure. Infections can pass between these two spaces through the inferior orbital fissure.

Cavernous Sinus Thrombosis   The cavernous sinuses are bilateral venous drainage channels for the contents of the middle cranial fossa, particularly the pituitary gland (Figure 9-35). Therefore part of the function of the cavernous sinus is absorption of endocrine secretions of that gland. Anteriorly the cavernous sinus is bordered by the superior orbital fissure and it receives a tributary from the ophthalmic vein. The orbit is drained by the superior and inferior ophthalmic veins. They may pass through the superior orbital fissure separately or join in the posterior orbit to form the ophthalmic vein. Orbital infections may follow these veins into the cavernous sinus. Posteriorly the cavernous sinus is bounded by the trigeminal ganglion. The ophthalmic (V1) and maxillary (V2) divisions of the trigeminal nerve pass through the cavernous sinus on their way to the superior orbital fissure and the foramen rotundum, respectively. The sphenoid bone, surrounding the sphenoid sinus, lies between the two cavernous sinuses.

The dura mater is at the superior and lateral borders of the cavernous sinus. The ophthalmic vein (or the superior and inferior ophthalmic veins separately), the central retinal vein, and the middle meningeal vein drain into the cav-

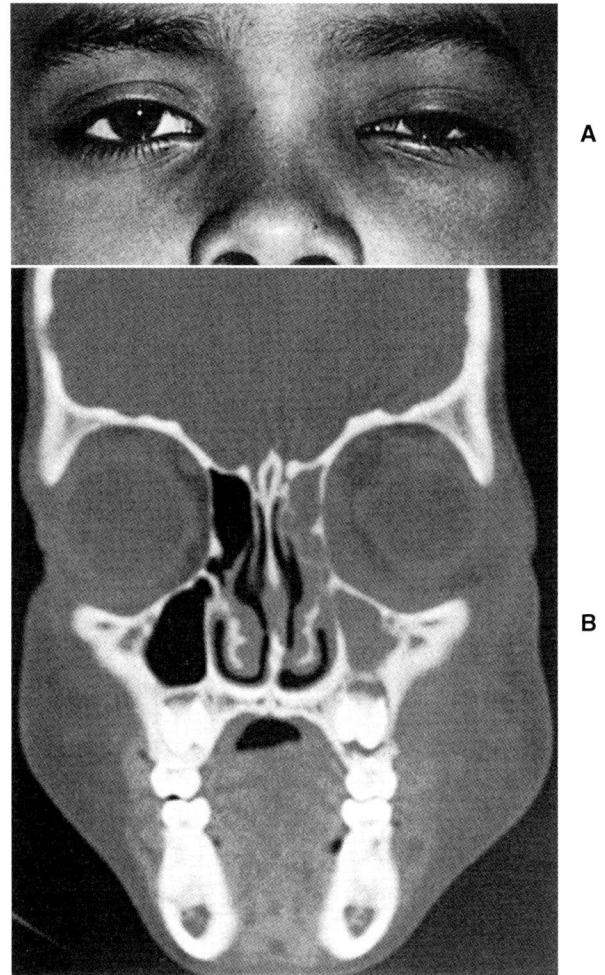

Figure 9-34 A, Frontal view of a boy with a left subperiosteal orbital abscess on its medial wall showing periorbital redness, partial ptosis, and lateral displacement of the globe. (From Flynn TR, Piecuch JF, Topazian RG: Infections of the oral cavity. In Feigin RD, Cherry JD, editors: *Textbook of pediatric infectious diseases,* ed 4, Philadelphia, 1998, WB Saunders.) **B,** Coronal CT scan of the same patient showing opacification of the left maxillary and ethmoid sinuses and thickening of the soft tissues on the medial orbital wall. The origin of this infection may have been a carious upper primary molar. (From Flynn TR, Piecuch JF, Topazian RG: Infections of the oral cavity. In Feigin RD, Cherry JD, editors: *Textbook of pediatric infectious diseases,* ed 4, Philadelphia, 1998, WB Saunders.)

ernous sinus. In turn the cavernous sinus is drained by superior and inferior petrosal sinuses, which empty into the internal jugular vein. Additional drainage pathways are by three emissary veins passing through the base of the skull at the foramina of Vesalius, ovale, and lacerum. These veins drain into the pterygoid plexus and then into the posterior facial (retromandibular) vein and the external jugular vein. Because the valveless veins of the face and anterior skull base allow blood flow in either direction, an ascending septic thrombophlebitis may follow the anterior route to the cavernous sinus through the ophthalmic veins or the posterior route through the pterygoid plexus and emissary veins passing through the base of the skull.

Venous Drainage of Head

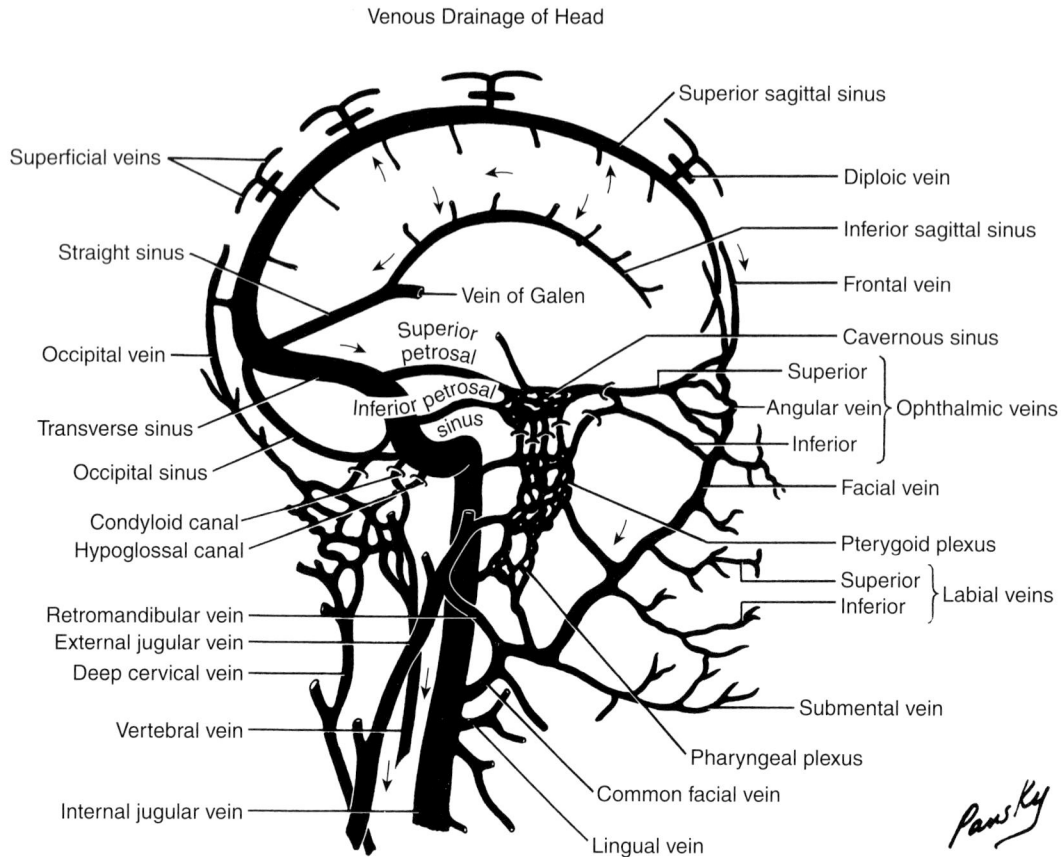

Figure 9-35 Venous drainage of the head including the dural sinuses. (From Pansky B, House EL: *Review of gross anatomy,* ed 2, New York, 1969, MacMillan.)

The cavernous sinus may not be a venous sinus at all, but rather a complex of interconnected veins maximizing the drainage of the pituitary gland. Therefore the internal carotid artery and abducens nerve may pass among these veins rather than through a large venous sinus. This concept is based on anatomical research by Swanson.[21]

The relations of the structures in the cavernous sinus to its walls vary considerably. The carotid artery and abducens nerve are usually described as lying within the cavernous sinus, whereas the third, fourth, and fifth cranial nerves are described as lining its lateral wall (Figure 9-36). The hypothesis that the cavernous sinus actually is a venous plexus may explain this variability. The constant factor among the relations of these structures is that the carotid artery is most medial, followed by the abducens nerve (cranial nerve VI), and then the oculomotor (III), trochlear (IV), trigeminal (V1 and V2) nerves in or near the lateral wall of the cavernous sinus. The third, fourth, and fifth nerves are oriented vertically in numerical order along the lateral side of the cavernous sinus. The maxillary division of the trigeminal nerve (V2) is found only in the posterior portion of the cavernous sinus because it courses inferiorly toward the foramen rotundum soon after leaving the trigeminal ganglion. If the cavernous sinus actually is a venous plexus, then the constant relations among the internal carotid artery and cranial nerves III through VI may vary only by their mediolateral position relative to the mass of interconnected veins.

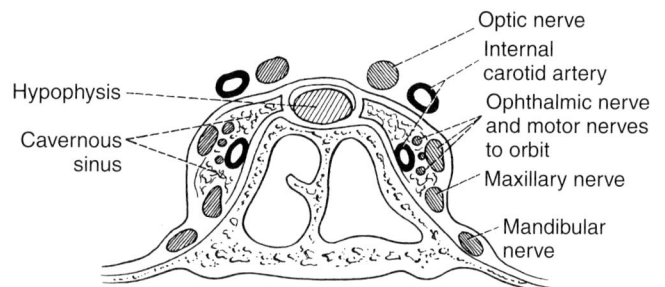

Figure 9-36 Coronal section of the cavernous and sphenoid sinuses showing the borders, contents, and relations of the cavernous sinus. (From Hollinshead WH: Anatomy for surgeons, vol 1, ed 2, *The head and neck,* Hagerstown, Md, 1968, Harper & Row.)

The cranial nerve most likely to be affected in cavernous sinus thrombosis is the abducens (VI), probably because its exposure to the cavernous sinus is greatest. The other cranial nerves occupy the lateral side of the cavernous sinus. On the other hand, the earliest clinical sign of cavernous sinus thrombosis most likely is congestion of the retinal veins of the eye on the unaffected side. This effect is the result of the rich interconnections of the right and left cavernous sinuses by the veins draining the pituitary gland anteriorly and posteriorly, which collectively are termed

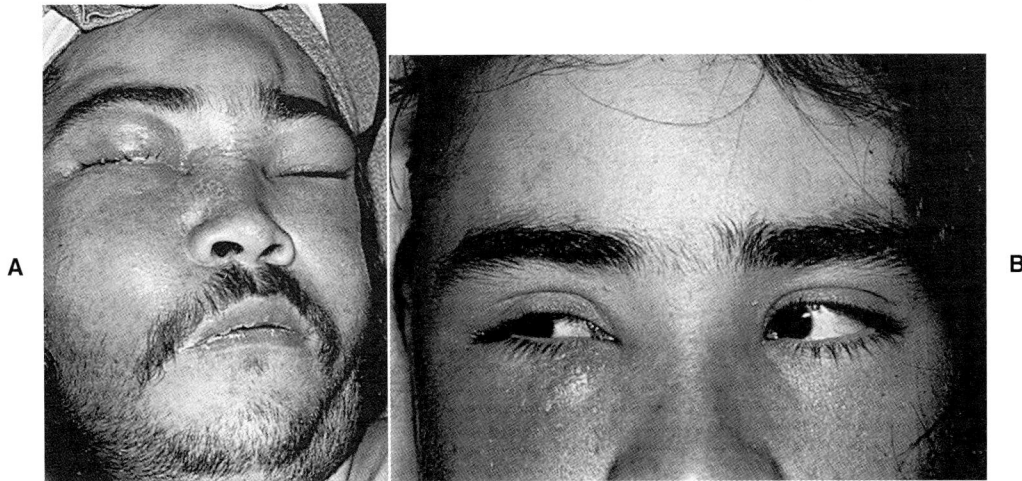

Figure 9-37 A, Frontal view of patient with right cavernous sinus thrombosis showing venous congestion in the fundus of the left eye. (From Flynn TR, Topazian RG: Infections of the oral cavity. In Waite D, editor: *Textbook of practical oral and maxillofacial surgery,* Philadelphia, 1987, Lea & Febiger.) **B,** The same patient 2 weeks later. Right abducens nerve function is intact. (From Flynn TR: The swollen face, *Emerg Med Clin North Am* 15:481, 2000.)

the *intercavernous sinus.* The right and left cavernous sinuses also are connected by the sinus of the dorsum sellae within the bony sella turcica and the basal plexus, which connects the right and left inferior petrosal sinuses. The patient shown in Figure 9-37 demonstrates this process. The infection involved the right cavernous sinus and the left retinal veins were congested. Early aggressive treatment was instituted. Two weeks later the right abducens nerve was intact. Contrast-enhanced CT also may facilitate early diagnosis of cavernous sinus thrombosis by demonstrating a filling void in the affected cavernous sinus.

REFERENCES

1. Dzyak WR, Zide MF: Diagnosis and treatment of lateral pharyngeal space infections, *J Oral Maxillofac Surg* 42:243, 1984.
2. Flynn TR: Anatomy and surgery of deep fascial space infections. In Kelly JJ, editor: *Oral and maxillofacial surgery knowledge update 1994,* Rosemont, Ill, 1994, American Association of Oral and Maxillofacial Surgeons.
3. Flynn TR, Wiltz M, Adamo AK, et al: Predicting length of hospital stay and penicillin failure in severe odontogenic infections, *Int J Oral Maxillofac Surg* 28(suppl 1):48, 1999 (abstract).
4. Granite EL: Anatomic considerations in infections of the face and neck: review of the literature, *J Oral Surg* 34:34, 1976.
5. Grodinsky M: Retropharyngeal and lateral pharyngeal abscesses, *Ann Surg* 110:177, 1939.
6. Grodinsky M: Ludwig's angina: an anatomical and clinical study with review of the literature, *Surgery* 5:678, 1939.
7. Grodinsky M, Holyoke EA: The fasciae and fascial spaces of the head, neck, and adjacent regions, *Am J Anat* 63:367, 1938.
8. Haug RH, Picard U, Indresano AT: Diagnosis and treatment of the retropharyngeal abscess in adults, *Br J Oral Maxillofac Surg* 28:34, 1990.
9. Healey JE, Hodge J: *Surgical anatomy,* ed 2, Toronto, 1990, BC Decker.
10. Hollinshead WH: Anatomy for surgeons, vol 1, ed 2, *The head and neck,* Hagerstown, Md, 1968, Harper & Row.
11. Hought RT, Fitzgerald BE, Latta JE, et al: Ludwig's angina: report of two cases and review of the literature from 1945 to January 1979, *J Oral Surg* 38:849, 1980.
12. Laskin DM: Anatomic considerations in diagnosis and treatment of odontogenic infections, *J Am Dent Assoc* 69:308, 1964.
13. Levitt GW: The surgical treatment of deep neck infections, *Laryngoscope* 81:403, 1970.
14. Lewis MAO, MacFarlane TW, McGowan DA: A microbiological and clinical review of the acute dentoalveolar abscess, *Br J Oral Maxillofac Surg* 28:359, 1990.
15. Lindner HH: The anatomy of the fasciae of the face and neck with particular reference to the spread and treatment of intraoral infections (Ludwig's) that have progressed into adjacent fascial spaces, *Ann Surg* 204:6, 1986.
16. Miller WD, Furst IM, Sandor GK, et al: A prospective, blinded comparison of clinical examination and computed tomography in deep neck infections, *Laryngoscope* 109:1873, 1999.
17. O'Ryan F, Diloreto D, Barber HD, et al: Orbital infections: clinical and radiographic diagnosis and surgical treatment, *J Oral Maxillofac Surg* 46:991, 1988.
18. Pearse HE: Mediastinitis following cervical suppuration, *Ann Surg* 108:588, 1938.
19. Peterson LJ: Principles of management and prevention of odontogenic infections. In Peterson LJ, Ellis E, Hupp JR, et al, editors: *Contemporary oral and maxillofacial surgery,* ed 2, St Louis, 1993, Mosby.
20. Pogrel MA: The superior orbital fissure syndrome: report of case, *J Oral Surg* 38:215, 1980.
21. Swanson MW: Neuroanatomy of the cavernous sinus and clinical correlations, *Optom Vis Sci* 67:891, 1990.
22. Williams AC: Ludwig's angina, *Surg Gynecol Obstet* 70:140, 1940.
23. Williams AC, Guralnick WC: The diagnosis and treatment of Ludwig's angina: a report of twenty cases, *N Engl J Med* 228:443, 1943.

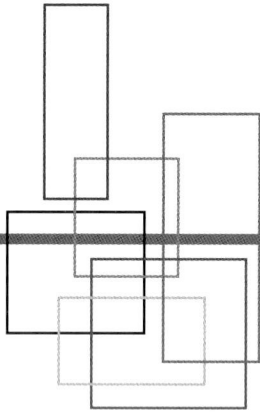

Osteomyelitis of the Jaws

Richard G. Topazian

Osteomyelitis of the jaws is a challenging disease for clinicians and patients despite many advances in diagnosis and treatment. In the past, osteomyelitis was encountered frequently and dreaded because of its prolonged course, uncertainty of outcome, and occasional disfigurement resulting from loss of teeth and bone, and the accompanying facial scarring. Today jaw osteomyelitis is much less common; improved nutrition and dental care, the availability of antibiotic therapy, and earlier diagnosis and intervention based on new imaging modalities have been major factors in lessening the morbidity of this disease.

The development of organisms resistant to commonly used antibiotics, existence of more individuals who are medically compromised, lack of experience with managing the disease by many practitioners, and its unique manifestations when the jaws are affected have made the effective management of osteomyelitis increasingly difficult. An apparent increase in the incidence of osteomyelitis caused by resistant organisms has been noted, adding to the treatment challenge.

By strict definition, *osteomyelitis* is an inflammation of the medullary portion of bone. However, the process rarely is confined to the endosteum. Osteomyelitis usually also affects the cortical bone and periosteum. Therefore osteomyelitis may be considered an inflammatory condition of bone that usually begins as an infection of the medullary cavity, rapidly involves the haversian systems, and quickly extends to the periosteum of the area. The infection becomes established in the calcified portion of bone when pus in the medullary cavity and beneath the periosteum compromises or obstructs the blood supply. Following ischemia the infected bone becomes necrotic.

In the past, osteomyelitis of the jaws, like that of the long bones, was believed to be caused primarily by *Staphylococcus aureus, Staphylococcus epidermidis,* or hemolytic streptococci. In recent years, several anaerobic bacteria have been identified, thus altering understanding of the microbiology of the disease as it affects the jaws.

CLASSIFICATION

Osteomyelitis of the jaws may be classified as suppurative or nonsuppurative, and as originally proposed by Lew and Waldvogel,[35] related to a contiguous focus of infection or hematogenous in origin. A more comprehensive classification proposed by Cieny et al.[10] and Mader and Calhoun[37] divides the disease into 4 stages combining 4 anatomical disease types and 3 physiological host categories to define 12 discrete clinical stages of osteomyelitis. Such a classification system, although important in dealing with numerous sites and allowing intrainstitutional studies, is unnecessarily complex for jaw infections that are classified readily as suppurative and nonsuppurative and as acute, subacute, and chronic (Box 10-1).

A variety of special and less common forms of the disease, such as syphilitic, tuberculous, brucellar, fungal, viral, chemical, *Escherichia coli,* and *Salmonella* osteomyelitis, are described in other sections of this book, and in textbooks of infectious disease and pathology. The basic principles of diagnosis and treatment in this chapter apply generally to

---

BOX **10-1**

Classification of Osteomyelitis of the Jaws

Suppurative Osteomyelitis	Nonsuppurative Osteomyelitis
Acute suppurative osteomyelitis	Diffuse sclerosing osteomyelitis
Chronic suppurative osteomyelitis	Focal sclerosing osteomyelitis (condensing osteitis)
Primary—no acute phase preceding	Proliferative periostitits (periostitis ossificans, Garré's sclerosing osteomyelitis)
Secondary—follows acute phase	
Infantile osteomyelitis	Osteoradionecrosis

these types of osteomyelitis and to osteomyelitis of the jaws caused by more common organisms. Osteomyelitis of the jaws differs in several important aspects from osteomyelitis of long bones. Therefore extrapolation from long bone disease with respect to etiology, microbiology, pathogenesis, and treatment to disease of the jaw should be done with caution.

PREDISPOSING FACTORS

Given the frequency and severity of odontogenic infections and the intimate relationship of the root ends of teeth to the medullary cavity, the relative infrequency of osteomyelitis of the jaws is remarkable. Its low incidence is largely a result of host resistance. In addition to the virulence of microorganisms, conditions affecting host resistance and alteration of jaw vascularity are important in the onset and severity of osteomyelitis.

Systemic disease with concomitant alterations in host defenses may influence profoundly the course of osteomyelitis. An underlying alteration of host defenses probably occurs in the majority of patients with osteomyelitis of the jaws regardless of whether such deficiencies can be detected, given the current state of knowledge of host defenses. Osteomyelitis has been associated with diabetes, autoimmune disease, agranulocytosis, leukemia, severe anemia, malnutrition, syphilis, cancer chemotherapy, steroid drug use, sickle cell disease, and acquired immunodeficiency syndrome.[38] Tobacco and alcohol use frequently are associated with the condition.[29] The clinician should consider host compromise and treat any compromising condition, when feasible, concomitantly with the infection. Conditions that alter the vascularity of bone predispose patients to the onset of osteomyelitis and include radiation, osteoporosis, osteopetrosis, Paget's disease of bone, fibrous dysplasia, bone malignancy, and bone necrosis caused by mercury, bismuth, and arsenic.

ETIOLOGY AND PATHOGENESIS

Osteomyelitis is initiated by a contiguous focus of infection or hematogenous spread. In long bone disease, primary hematogenous osteomyelitis occurs mainly in infants and children because of the anatomy of the metaphyseal region. A single pathogenic species almost always is recovered from the bone.[37] *Staphylococcus* spp. are the most common organisms isolated in adults and are prominent in children and infants. In contrast, hematogenous osteomyelitis of the jaws is infrequent; the disease is caused primarily by contiguous spread of odontogenic infections originating from pulpal or periodontal tissues. Trauma, especially compound fractures, is the second leading cause of jaw osteomyelitis. Infections derived from periostitis after gingival ulceration, lymph nodes infected by furuncles or lacerations, or hematogenous origin account for an additional small number of jaw infections.

Osteomyelitis of the maxilla is much less frequent than that of the mandible because the maxillary blood supply is more extensive. Thin cortical plates and a relative paucity of medullary tissues in the maxilla preclude confinement of infections within bone and permit the dissipation of edema and pus into the soft tissues and paranasal sinuses. In the mandible the regions affected, in decreasing frequency, are the body, symphysis, angle, ramus, and condyle.[7]

The mandible resembles long bones: it has a medullary cavity, dense cortical plates, and a well-defined periosteum. Bone marrow is composed of sinusoids rich in reticuloendothelial cells, erythrocytes, granulocytes, platelets and osteoblastic precursors, and cancellous bone, fat, and blood vessels. The marrow space is lined by the endosteum, a membrane of cells containing large numbers of osteoblasts. Bone spicules radiate centrally from cortical bone to produce a scaffold of interconnecting trabeculae.[12] The distinctive architecture of cortical bone includes longitudinally oriented haversian systems (osteons), each with a central canal and blood vessel that provide nutrients by means of canaliculi to osteocytes contained within lacunae. Central canals communicate among adjunct haversian systems and with the periosteum and marrow space by Volkmann's canals to provide a complex interconnecting vascular and neural network that nourishes bone and allows for repair, regeneration, and functional demands. The cortical bone is enveloped by the periosteum, which consists of an outer fibrous layer and an inner layer of osteogenic cells.

Compromise of the blood supply is a critical factor in the establishment of osteomyelitis. Except for the coronoid process, which is supplied primarily from temporalis muscle, the mandible receives its major blood supply from the inferior alveolar artery. A secondary source is the periosteal supply, which generally runs parallel to the cortical surface of the bone, giving off nutrient vessels that penetrate the cortical bone and anastomose with branches of the inferior alveolar artery. The richness of the vascular supply is demonstrated readily (Figure 10-1). Mandibular venous drainage proceeds upward to the pharyngeal plexus through the inferior dental veins and downward to the external jugular veins.

Most periapical and periodontal infections are localized by the production of a protective pyogenic membrane or soft tissue abscess wall. If sufficiently virulent, microorganisms may destroy this barrier. Reduced host resistance during surgery or repeated movement of unreduced fractures may contribute to development of suppurative osteomyelitis. Mechanical trauma burnishes bone, causing ischemia, and introduces organisms deeply into underlying tissues.

The process leading to osteomyelitis is initiated by acute inflammation: hyperemia, increased capillary permeability, and infiltration of granulocytes. Tissue necrosis occurs as proteolytic enzymes are released and as destruction of bacteria and vascular thrombosis ensue. When pus, composed of necrotic tissue and dead bacteria within white blood cells, accumulates, intramedullary pressure increases resulting in

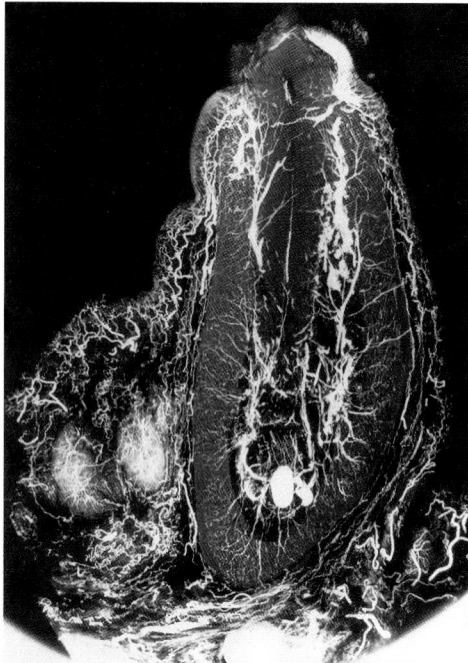

Figure 10-1 Microangiogram of rhesus monkey mandible demonstrates rich, complex interconnecting network of vessels. (Courtesy Dr. William H. Bell.)

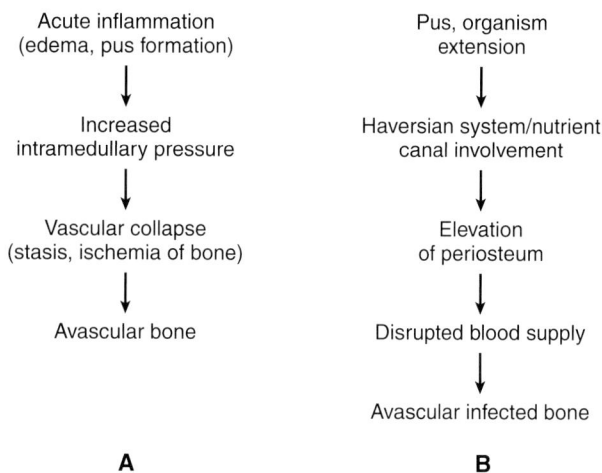

Figure 10-3 Lateral oblique radiograph shows appearance of chronic osteomyelitis of the mandible demonstrating sequestrum, bed of granulation tissue and involucrum, the sheath of new bone at the periphery. Teeth had loosened and had been removed earlier.

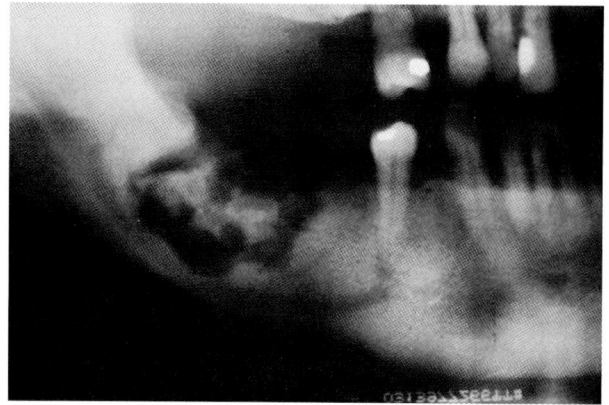

Figure 10-2 Pathogenesis of osteomyelitis. **A,** Inflammation leading to avascular bone. **B,** Extension of pus and microorganisms.

vascular collapse, venous stasis, and ischemia. Pus travels through the haversian and nutrient canals and accumulates beneath the periosteum, elevating it from the cortex and thereby further reducing the vascular supply (Figure 10-2). Compression of the neurovascular bundle accelerates thrombosis and ischemia and results in osteomyelitis-mediated inferior alveolar nerve dysfunction. Extensive periosteal elevation occurs more frequently in children, presumably because the periosteum is bound less firmly to bone than in adults. If pus continues to accumulate, the periosteum is penetrated and mucosal and cutaneous abscesses and fistulas may develop.

As the effectiveness of host defenses and therapy increases the osteomyelitic process may become chronic. Inflammation regresses, granulation tissue forms, and new blood vessels lyse bone, thus separating fragments of necrotic bone *(sequestra)* from viable bone. Small sections of bone may be lysed completely, whereas larger ones may be isolated by a bed of granulation tissue encased in a sheath of new bone *(involucrum)* (Figure 10-3). Sequestra may be revascularized, remain quiescent, resorb, or be infected chronically and require surgical removal before the infection subsides completely. Occasionally the involucrum is penetrated by channels *(cloacae)* through which pus escapes to an epithelial surface. Bone surrounding a sequestrum sometimes appears radiographically as less densely mineralized than the sequestrum itself because increased vascularity of adjacent vital bone creates a relative demineralization.

MICROBIOLOGY OF OSTEOMYELITIS

The establishment of an infection in bone is related to the virulence of the organisms, integrity and effectiveness of host defenses, and anatomical and structural factors. Until recently estimates of the involvement of *S. aureus* and *S. epidermidis* in osteomyelitis of the jaws ranged between 80% and 90%; *Staphylococcus* continues to be listed frequently in connection with osteomyelitis of the jaws. Mixed bacterial cultures, hemolytic streptococci, pneumococci, typhoid and acid-fast bacilli, *Escherichia coli,* and *Actinomyces* organisms accounted for the remaining infections.

A decrease in the frequency of *S. aureus* osteomyelitis in recent reports is attributable to the use of more sophisticated culture methods that result in more accurate identification of responsible organisms. Consequently, organisms not previously associated with osteomyelitis are now known to be responsible for many bone infections. For example, the previous estimate of anaerobic involvement for all instances of osteomyelitis was less than 1%. The number of sterile cultures from many series of patients with osteomyelitis was significant. Failure to isolate organisms may have resulted from an inability to culture anaerobes. Conversely, anaerobes now are associated frequently with aerobic organisms in osteomyelitis, and anaerobic osteomyelitis also may occur alone. Findings helpful in recognition of pure anaerobic or mixed aerobic-anaerobic infections in osteomyelitis of the jaws are presence of a foul-smelling exudate, sloughing of necrotic tissue, gas in soft tissues, black discharge from the wound, Gram stain revealing multiple organisms of different morphological characteristics, failure to grow organisms from clinical specimens, particularly when gram-negative organisms are seen on the smear, and presence of sequestra.[54]

The appropriate collection and transportation of cultures described earlier are essential for accurate diagnosis and initiation of proper therapy. At the same time the difficulties in obtaining pus and representative specimens in cases of osteomyelitis of the jaws must be acknowledged. Repeated cultures are important especially in osteomyelitis because antibiotic therapy often is prolonged and occasionally results in development of resistant strains. Repeated sampling of bone specimens and culture of all sequestra sometimes is required; specimens should be transported and cultured anaerobically and aerobically. Organisms do not grow well in bone and proper handling of specimens is important. Hand-carrying the specimen to the laboratory and requesting that bone specimens be ground or minced may increase the culture yield.

Although penicillin is effective for most undiagnosed anaerobic infections, it is ineffective against *Prevotella* and *Porphyromonas* spp., the organisms responsible for some cases of anaerobic osteomyelitis. Exacerbations of chronic osteomyelitis treated for long periods may be explained by the development of a preponderance of anaerobes.

Osteomyelitis of the jaws now is recognized as a disease caused primarily by streptococci (α-hemolytic) and oral anaerobes, particularly *Peptostreptococcus, Fusobacterium,* and *Prevotella (Bacteroides),* the organisms responsible for odontogenic infections.[16,52] Antibiotic therapy therefore should be directed toward streptococci and anaerobes and not staphylococci.

Only occasional cases of osteomyelitis of the jaws are caused by *S. aureus.* When found in cultures of jaw osteomyelitis, *S. aureus* originates from the skin through wounds and fistulas. A few organisms apparently are derived from perimandibular space infections that also may involve *Eikenella corrodens* in a relatively high percentage of patients.[53] Occasionally, anaerobic or microaerophilic cocci and gram-negative organisms such *as Klebsiella, Pseudomonas,* and *Proteus* spp., are found. In addition, *Mycobacterium tuberculosis, Treponema pallidum,* and *Actinomyces* spp. produce specific forms of osteomyelitis. Various organisms are responsible for the few remaining variants of the disease. Culture reports should be interpreted carefully because of possible skin and oral contaminants in the specimen. When osteomyelitis follows extraoral trauma with involvement of soft tissues, staphylococcal infection is likely. The rational selection of appropriate antibiotics, based on valid culture data, is critical for cure and reduced morbidity.

CLINICAL FINDINGS

Four types of osteomyelitis of the jaws are observed clinically: (1) acute suppurative; (2) secondary chronic, a form that begins as acute osteomyelitis and becomes chronic; (3) primary chronic, a form that has manifested no acute phase previously, having always been a low-grade infection; and (4) nonsuppurative. A subacute stage also exists in which acute symptoms such as elevated temperature and white blood cell count are nearly normal but in which production of pus and extension into adjacent bone continues. The clinical findings differ among these various disease conditions.

Early acute suppurative osteomyelitis (acute intramedullary osteomyelitis) of the mandible usually is characterized by four findings: (1) deep, intense pain, (2) high intermittent fever, (3) paresthesia or anesthesia of the lower lip (inferior alveolar nerve), and (4) a clearly identifiable cause, usually deep caries in an involved tooth. Conventional radiographs do not show changes early in the disease process, but strongly positive radionuclide scan results (discussed in the following text) together with these clinical findings strongly support the diagnosis of acute suppurative intramedullary osteomyelitis. In the initial phase of the acute form of the disease, teeth are not loose, swelling is minimal, and fistulas are not present.

Immediate antibiotic therapy at this stage may prevent progression to involvement of the periosteum. Hospitalization should be considered with aggressive intravenous antibiotic therapy (see the "Treatment" section) to avoid involvement of the periosteum (subperiosteal osteomyelitis). Identification and correction of immunocompromising conditions such as diabetes mellitus should be attempted. Results of laboratory studies generally are negative except for slight leukocytosis and conventional radiographs essentially appear normal. Because material for culture rarely is available at this early stage, empirical selection of antibiotics is necessary.

If the disease is not controlled within 10 to 14 days after onset, subacute suppurative osteomyelitis is established. Pus extends through the haversian canals to accumulate under the periosteum and then may penetrate and extend into the soft tissues. Deep pain, malaise, fever, and anorexia are present. The teeth begin to loosen and become sensitive to percussion. Pus exudes around the gingival sulcus and through mucosal and, possibly, cutaneous fistulas; a fetid oral odor often is present. Firm cellulitis of the cheek, expansion of the bone from increased periosteal activity, abscess formation with localized warmth, erythema, tenderness to palpation, and mental nerve paresthesia also may be noted. Trismus is not always present, but regional lymphadenopathy is a constant finding. The patient's temperature may reach 101° to 102° F and the patient often is dehydrated. Unlike acute osteomyelitis of the long bones, in which systemic reactions are often marked, in osteomyelitis of the jaws laboratory studies show only moderate evidence of acute infection. Leukocytosis consisting of a white blood cell count in the range of 8,000 to 15,000 cells/mm³ with a shift to the left occurs. The count rarely reaches 20,000 cells/mm³. The erythrocyte sediment rate may be slightly elevated, but unlike in long bone disease, it rarely is a valid indicator of the extent or the course of the disease in the jaws.

Inadequately treated acute osteomyelitis progresses to a subacute or chronic form. In chronic secondary osteomyelitis, the type observed in incompletely treated acute osteomyelitis, the clinical findings usually are limited to fistulas, induration of soft tissues, and a thickened or "wooden" character to the affected area with pain and tenderness on palpation. Primary chronic osteomyelitis, the form not preceded by an episode of acute symptoms, is insidious in onset with slight pain, slow increase in jaw size, and gradual development of sequestra, often without fistulas.

IMAGING

Imaging of suspected osteomyelitis of the mandible is accomplished by conventional radiography, supplemented as needed by computed tomography (CT), magnetic resonance imaging (MRI), and radionuclide bone scanning (see Chapter 4). Proper imaging aids in determining the extent and degree of disease, the location of sequestra, and in planning the approach and extent of surgery. Imaging also helps to determine when treatment may be stopped and assists in distinguishing osteomyelitis from bone tumors.

An estimated 30% to 60% of the mineralized portion of bone must be destroyed before significant radiographic changes can be distinguished. This degree of bone alteration requires a minimum of 4 and up to 14 days after onset of acute osteomyelitis. The full extent of bone dissolution cannot be determined radiographically until 3 weeks after initiation of the osteomyelitic process. Therefore in the early stages of disease the history and clinical findings may constitute the sole basis for diagnosis. Radiographic changes later may confirm and establish the rate of progression and a possible need to alter treatment. Radiographic changes clearly lag behind the actual clinical situation in both early and late stages of the disease process.

Once osteomyelitis has become well established, radiographic changes usually demonstrate one of the following groups of characteristics described by Worth[69] (Figures 10-4, 10-5, and 10-6).

1. Scattered areas of bone destruction vary in size and number, are separated by variable distances and by bone with normal or nearly normal appearance. Bone has a "moth-eaten" appearance because of enlargement of medullary spaces and widening of Volkmann's canals resulting from destruction by lysis and replacement with granulation tissue.

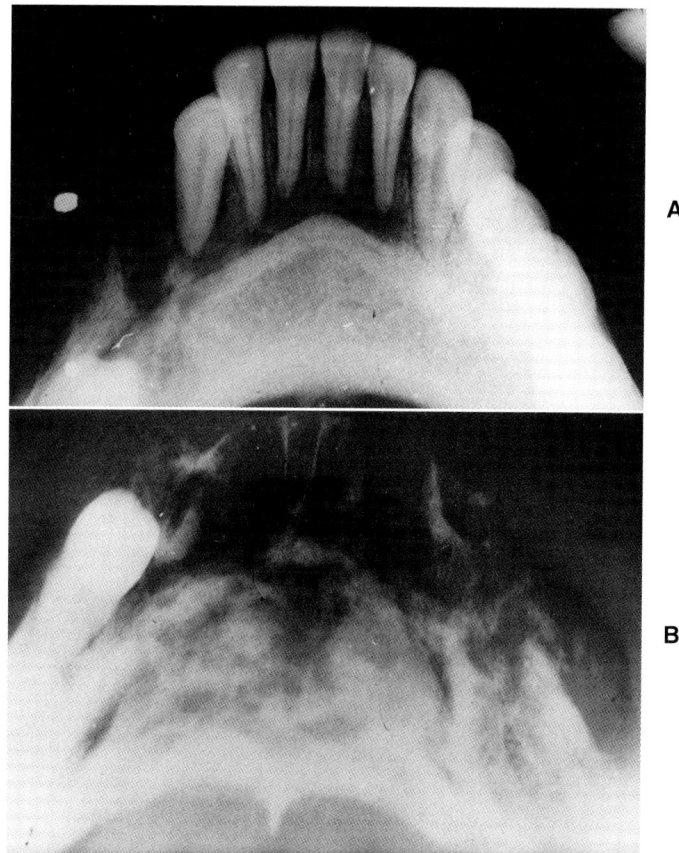

Figure 10-4 A, Occlusal radiograph of the anterior mandible with subacute, suppurative osteomyelitis shows a large sequestrum containing several anterior teeth. **B,** Subacute, chronic suppurative osteomyelitis of the anterior mandible demonstrates "moth-eaten" appearance resulting from bone destruction and replacement with granulation. Numerous sequestra are present.

2. Bone destruction of varying extent, in which there are "islands," that is, sequestra, with evidence of a trabecular pattern and marrow spaces. A sheath of new bone (involucrum) often is found, separated from the sequestra by a zone of radiolucency.

3. Stippled or granular densification of bone caused by subperiosteal deposition of new bone obscuring the intrinsic bone structure or deposition of new bone on surfaces of existing trabeculae at the expense of marrow spaces. The central sequestra usually present in osteomyelitis help to distinguish it from fibrous dysplasia.

Fibrous dysplasia, osteoid osteoma, Paget's disease of bone, and malignant bone-producing tumors (such as osteosarcoma) may be confused with osteomyelitis, particularly when marked periosteal bone production is seen as can occur in preadolescent patients. The laminated or "onion-skin" appearance of bone in osteomyelitis is seen only rarely with tumors. Destructive jaw lesions such as lymphosarcoma, Ewing's tumor, and intraosseous squamous cell carcinoma also may mimic infection. Secondary infection may occur in bone tumors and potentially confuse the true di-

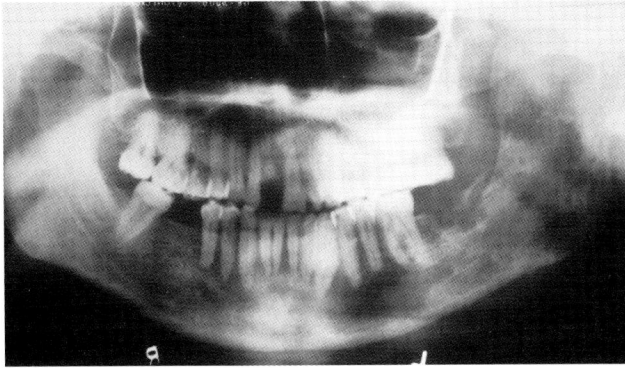

Figure 10-5 Subacute suppurative osteomyelitis involving the body, angle, and ramus of the mandible.

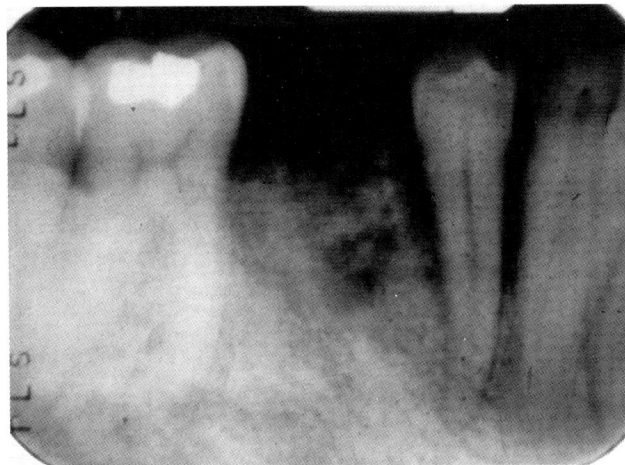

Figure 10-6 Chronic osteomyelitis with sequestrum seen in periapical film. (Courtesy Stephen Rozen and Ellen Eisenberg.)

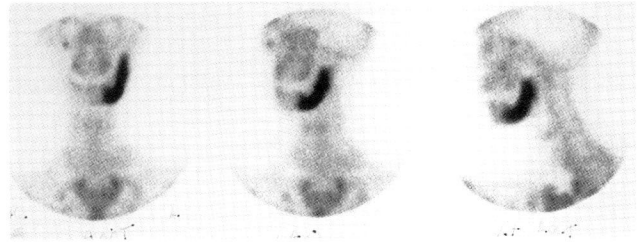

Figure 10-7 Scintigram of jaws of a patient with suspected early osteomyelitis of the mandible. From left to right are the posteroanterior, left lateral oblique, and lateral projections showing a dark or "hot" area in the left angle and ramus indicative of increased bone activity. Bone scanning shows activity in osteomyelitis well before it is reflected in conventional radiographs, thus allowing vigorous early treatment. A similar picture may be seen in other forms of bone disease including neoplastic disease; therefore the diagnosis of osteomyelitis must be based on clinical and laboratory findings and imaging. (Courtesy John M. Alexander and Louis G. Mercuri.)

agnosis. The possibility of neoplasm as the primary disease always must be considered. The radiographic similarities and differences among osteomyelitis, malignant disease, and fibrous dysplasia are well described.[70]

Careful history, physical examination, and radiographs adequate for visualization of the complete process with delineation of surface contours are necessary to distinguish osteomyelitis from neoplasms. Biopsy should be considered when history, physical findings, and radiographs are equivocal and resolution does not occur as expected. For example, biopsy should be done in a child with no dental disease and marked but atypical proliferative periostitis (Garré's sclerosing osteomyelitis; periostitis ossificans) to distinguish the periostitis from sarcoma and to prevent delay of appropriate treatment. Repeated biopsy may be necessary until a definitive diagnosis is obtained.

TYPES OF IMAGING

Radionuclide Imaging Bone scanning, radionuclide imaging, or skeletal scintigraphy is useful in determining the presence of reactive bone; thus it is particularly help-

ful in the diagnosis of bone disease. Although not specific for inflammation, radionuclide imaging often is important in the diagnosis and management of osteomyelitis of the jaws. The application of scanning to osteomyelitis and other maxillofacial disease has been reviewed.[56,66] Approximately half of bone mineral must be altered before changes are observed on conventional radiographs; the change process requires 10 to 14 days or longer after infectious onset. In a study of 18 patients, conventional radiographs were definitively diagnostic of osteomyelitis in all patients only after 4 weeks.[59]

Radiopharmaceuticals that are absorbed by bone provide particularly useful information based on the presence of reactive bone formation rather than demineralization. Changes are seen as early as 3 days after the onset of symptoms of osteomyelitis. In most applications, bone is scanned using ^{99m}Tc-labeled methylene diphosphonate administered intravenously. The radioisotope is distributed to the entire skeleton and concentrated in areas of increased blood flow and osteoblastic activity. A rectilinear scanner or a scintillation camera, both of which contain sodium iodide, a crystal nuclide that emits light, then is used to obtain images of the isotope-containing areas. The resulting image shows the distribution of radionuclide in areas of increased bone activity (Figure 10-7).

The complete ^{99m}Tc bone scan has three phases. The first phase (flow study) consists of serial 3- to 4-second images during the 1 to 2 minutes after injection of the drug. The second phase (blood pool study) consists of a single image obtained 5 to 10 minutes after injection. The third phase (delayed study) includes multiple views obtained 2 to 4 hours after injection.[19]

Positive ^{99m}Tc scan results can be useful in confirming the diagnosis of acute osteomyelitis, although bone scan findings may be negative very early in the disease. Addition of a ^{67}Ga study to the ^{99m}Tc scans aids in distinguishing osteomyelitis from malignancy and trauma. If neoplastic disease is not suspected as the cause of symptoms by reason of age or clinical and laboratory studies, a positive ^{99m}Tc scan result alone is sufficient to diagnose osteomyelitis. When the patient's age and clinical findings make the diagnosis equivocal, as when a neoplasm is suspected, the ^{99m}Tc scan may be followed by a ^{67}Ga scan. Positive findings on both tests usually confirm the infectious nature of the disease. When the ^{99m}Tc scan result is positive and the ^{67}Ga scan result is negative, osteomyelitis probably is not the primary disease. ^{67}Ga uptake that exceeds ^{99m}Tc uptake indicates active inflammatory disease. In chronic osteomyelitis, reduced ^{67}Ga accumulation in the follow-up scan is a useful indicator for termination of therapy in osteomyelitis. ^{111}In white blood cell scintigraphy also is useful in determining when the lesion is inactive and therapy may cease. A decision tree for selection of imaging studies for the diagnosis of osteomyelitis is helpful[1] (Figure 10-8).

Scintigraphy can confirm a diagnosis of very early osteomyelitis (before the occurrence of conventional radiographic bone changes) in which signs, symptoms, and physical findings are nearly conclusive. Early interceptive antibiotic and supportive therapy can be instituted. Thus established typical fulminant disease with its associated morbidity can be prevented. Bone scanning also may be useful in monitoring chronic osteomyelitis when a decision must be made regarding the need for and the extent of additional surgery or the duration of antibiotic therapy. Negative scintigraphic findings indicate that bone activity has ceased and support the discontinuation of therapy. Cessation of bone activity usually occurs several weeks after the inflammatory process subsides. Similarly, in patients with early symptoms suggestive of relapse, positive scan findings allow early diagnosis and immediate resumption of therapy before symptoms worsen and bone involvement is more extensive.

Computed Tomography   Because of its sensitivity, high-resolution CT detects early bone changes before they can be seen on conventional films. Changes visible on CT scans include increased attenuation in the medullary cavity, destruction of cortical bone, new bone formation, and the appearance of sequestra.[1] CT scanning has special value over plain radiography in revealing the extent of the lesion, extent of cortical erosion, and identification of sequestra.

Magnetic Resonance Imaging   When ^{99m}Tc bone scan and ^{67}Ga or ^{111}In white blood cell scan findings are negative or equivocal and osteomyelitis still is highly suspected, MRI or CT may provide useful information in selected cases, aiding the decision to intervene surgically.[59]

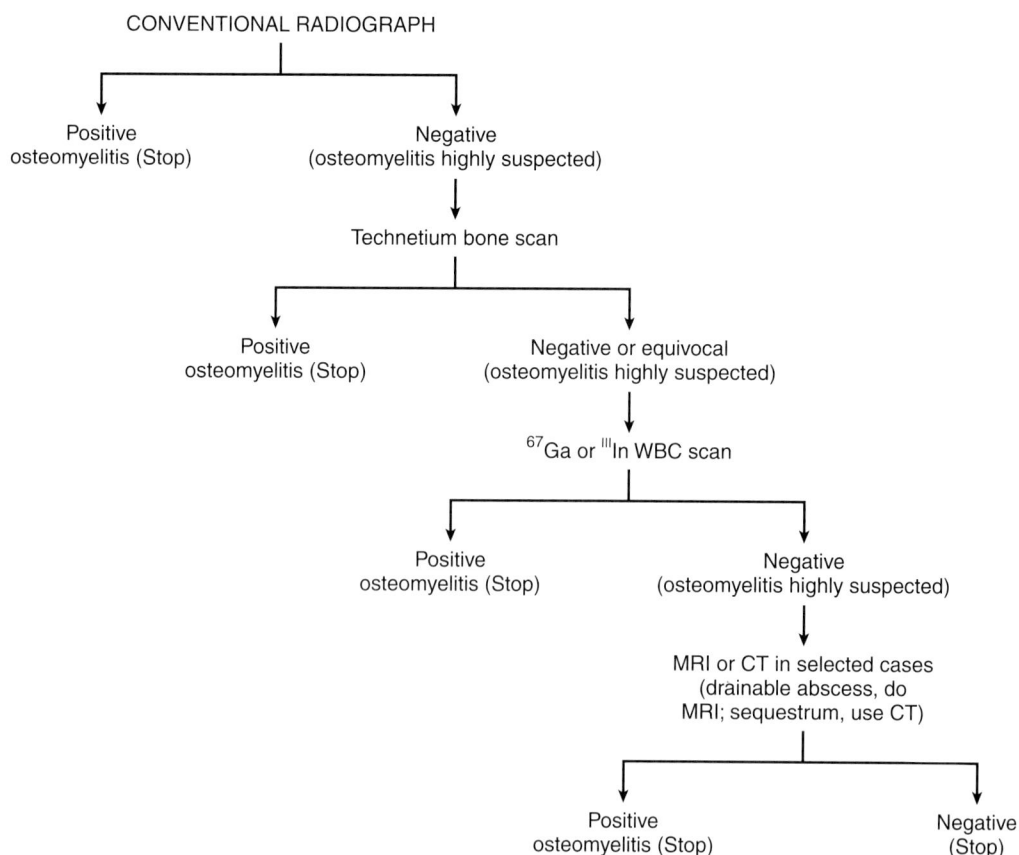

Figure 10-8 Decision tree for use of imaging studies in the diagnosis of osteomyelitis. *WBC,* White blood cells; *MRI,* magnetic resonance imaging; *CT,* computed tomography. (From Aliabadi P, Nikpoor J: Imaging osteomyelitis, *Arthritis Rheum* 37:617, 1994.)

TREATMENT

Osteomyelitis of the jaws usually requires medical and surgical treatment, although occasionally antibiotic therapy alone is successful. The principles of treatment are (1) evaluation and correction, to the extent possible, of compromised host defenses, (2) Gram staining and culture and sensitivity testing, (3) imaging of the region to determine the extent of the lesion and to rule out the presence of tumors, (4) empirical administration of Gram stain–guided antibiotics, (5) removal of loose teeth and sequestra, (6) prescription of culture-guided antibiotic therapy; and (7) sequestrectomy, debridement, decortication, resection, or reconstruction as indicated (Box 10-2). Intermaxillary fixation should be considered when the continuity of the mandible is questionable and the possibility of pathological fracture exists. The role of adjunctive hyperbaric oxygen (HBO) treatment for nonradiation osteomyelitis has not been well defined but may be considered, especially in refractory infections and in patients who are seriously medically compromised with no HBO contraindications.

TREATMENT

Acute Suppurative Osteomyelitis Early acute suppurative osteomyelitis usually is diagnosed by the findings of deep intense pain, paresthesia of the inferior alveolar nerve, fever, a clearly identified cause, and positive bone scan findings.[47] The initial management of affected patients often is aided by hospitalization to administer high-dose intravenous antibiotic therapy, identify and correct host compromise factors, and treat the cause. Underlying alteration of host defenses is present in some patients with osteomyelitis of the jaws. Careful inquiry and investigation may reveal diabetes, autoimmune disease, alcohol-starvation syndrome, intravenous drug abuse, severe anemia, leukemia, agranulocytosis, acquired immunodeficiency syndrome, syphilis, sickle cell disease, or steroid or cancer chemotherapy drug use. Factors that may delay recovery should be identified and corrected. Corrective measures involve treatment of anemia with iron or transfusion, man-

agement of malnutrition with dietary supplementation and vitamins, control of diabetes, and discouraging smoking and alcohol intake.[7] Once the infection is controlled, treatment may be continued on an outpatient basis using home intravenous therapy with percutaneous indwelling catheters and antibiotic pumps.

Whenever possible, specimens should be obtained for Gram staining, aerobic and anaerobic cultures, and antibiotic sensitivity testing. Appropriate mucosal and skin preparation is vital in specimen collection. Sterile, large-gauge needles should be used to aspirate areas of suspected pus deposits. Material removed by debridement such as sequestra should be transported and cultured under anaerobic conditions. Gram stain should be used to determine initial therapy until laboratory results are available. Biopsy of bone, granulation tissue, and fistulas also may be indicated. The consistency, color, and odor of pus may provide important clues to diagnosis and initial treatment. For example, thick creamy pus from a localized abscess indicates a staphylococcal infection. A foul-smelling, dark exudate accompanying slough of necrotic tissues, gas in soft tissues, and multiple organisms of variable morphological characteristics strongly suggest anaerobic osteomyelitis. At the same time, obtaining culture material from the contaminated oral environment that accurately reflects the actual causative organisms is difficult. Conventional radiographs and possibly bone scans should be obtained to determine the extent of the disease, the existence of causative factors such as periapical abscesses and fractures, and the presence and location of sequestra.

Extremely loose teeth and readily accessible sequestra should be removed early in the disease course. Pus should be evacuated and drains placed whenever fluctuance exists. After acute stages of the disease have subsided with intravenous or parenteral antibiotics and supportive measures, other treatment options include sequestrectomy and saucerization, debridement, direct placement of antibiotics into the wound by means of indwelling catheters or antibiotic-impregnated beads, HBO, decortication, resection of infected bone, and immediate or late bone graft reconstruction.

ANTIBIOTIC THERAPY

The severity or duration of disease, status of host defenses, presence of systemic involvement, and ability to obtain material for a laboratory diagnosis all affect the use of antibiotic treatment of osteomyelitis of the jaws. Antibiotics of value in the treatment of osteomyelitis are penicillin, extended-spectrum penicillins, semisynthetic penicillins, clindamycin, cephalosporins, and metronidazole. Principles of antibiotic selection and use are discussed in Chapters 5 and 6. Monitoring the clinical course of the disease, repeated antibiotic sensitivity testing when possible, and surgical measures such as drainage and sequestrectomy must be performed to achieve a cure. Dependence on antibiotics alone may prolong the disease course. An antibiotic usually should not

---

BOX 10-2

Principles of Treatment of Osteomyelitis

1. Evaluation and correction of host defense deficiencies
2. Gram staining, culture and sensitivity
3. Imaging to rule out bone tumors
4. Administration of stain-guided empirical antibiotics
5. Removal of loose teeth and sequestra
6. Administration of culture-guided antibiotics; repeated cultures
7. Possible placement of irrigating drains/ polymethylmethacrylate-antibiotic beads
8. Sequestrectomy, debridement, decortication, resection, reconstruction

be used until culture material is obtained and Gram stain examination and culture and sensitivity tests have been performed. However, time is critical in patients with acute osteomyelitis or those with clear systemic involvement; empirical antibiotic choices often must be made without aid of laboratory results.

Many organisms responsible for osteomyelitis of the jaws are now penicillin resistant, including *Prevotella, Porphyromonas,* and *Fusobacterium.* Therefore a drug effective against these resistant organisms, such as metronidazole, should be added to penicillin thus covering aerobic streptococci as well as penicillin-resistant anaerobes. Penicillin alone may be effective in some cases. Examples of such combinations are penicillin plus metronidazole, amoxicillin plus metronidazole, amoxicillin/clavulanate potassium (Augmentin), and ampicillin/sulbactam sodium (Unasyn-IV). Other drugs effective against jaw osteomyelitis are clindamycin alone, clindamycin plus metronidazole, and cephalosporins (Box 10-3).

Once valid culture and sensitivity information has been obtained, antibiotic therapy may be modified accordingly, particularly if the infection appears refractory to the treatment instituted. If a favorable clinical response has occurred, no change is indicated because in vivo effectiveness is the ultimate guide to treatment.

BOX 10-3

Antibiotic Regimen for Osteomyelitis of the Jaws

Regimen I: For Hospitalized/Medically Compromised Patient or When Intravenous Therapy Is Indicated
Aqueous penicillin, 2 million U IV q4h, *plus* metronidazole, 500 mg, q6h
When improved for 48 to 72 hours, switch to:
Penicillin V, 500 mg PO q4h, *plus* metronidazole, 500 mg PO q6h, *for an additional 4 to 6 weeks*
OR
Ampicillin/sulbactam (Unasyn), 1.5 to 3.0 g IV q6h
When improved for 48 to 72 hours, switch to:
Amoxicillin/clavulanate (Augmentin), 875/125 mg PO bid, *for an additional 4 to 6 weeks*

Regimen II: For Outpatient Treatment
Penicillin V, 2 g, *plus* metronidazole, 0.5 g q8h PO, for 2 to 4 weeks after last sequestrum removed and patient without symptoms
OR
Clindamycin, 600 to 900 mg q6h IV, then:
Clindamycin, 300 to 450 mg q6h PO
OR
Cefoxitin (Mefoxin), 1.0 g q8h IV or 2 g q4h IM or IV, until no symptoms, then switch to:
Cephalexin (Keflex), 500 mg q6h PO, for 2 to 4 weeks
For penicillin-allergic patients:
Clindamycin (as above)
Cefoxitin as above, if allergy not of anaphylactoid type

In patients who are allergic to penicillin, clindamycin is recommended because of its effectiveness against penicillinase-producing staphylococci, streptococci, and anaerobic bacteria, including *Prevotella (Bacteroides).* When used intravenously for the acute phase, a dose of 600 to 900 mg every 8 hours should be given. Once the acute phase has passed, therapy is continued with an oral dose of 300 to 450 mg four times daily. Clindamycin is not recommended as the first-choice antibiotic because it is bacteriostatic and occasionally causes diarrhea and pseudomembranous colitis.

A cephalosporin such as cefoxitin is the third-choice drug for patients who have had only mild allergic reactions to penicillins. The oral cephalosporins generally are safe. Cephalosporins also are useful in patients who may have had side effects of clindamycin therapy or those with gram-negative infections from intestinal flora. As a result of cephalinosporinase production by many *Prevotella* and *Fusobacterium* spp., some second-generation cephalosporins, particularly cefoxitin, resistant to this enzyme, are effective against many anaerobic gram-negative bacilli.[6] Cefoxitin (Mefoxin), 1.0 g intramuscularly or intravenously every 8 hours, is effective against most gram-positive cocci, including penicillinase-producing staphylococci and many strains of gram-negative aerobic bacilli such as *Escherichia coli, Klebsiella,* and *Proteus.* Once acute symptoms have subsided an oral cephalosporin, such as cephalexin (Keflex), 500 mg every 6 hours, is used. Cephalosporins are not recommended as the first choice in the management of osteomyelitis because they are only moderately effective against oral anaerobes and their broad-spectrum coverage increases antibiotic complications. Patients with a history of immunoglobulin E–mediated allergic reactions to a penicillin (e.g., anaphylaxis, angioneurotic edema, immediate urticaria) should not receive a cephalosporin because of possible cross-sensitivity.[18]

Erythromycin and the other macrolides, clarithromycin (Biaxin) and azithromycin (Zithromax), are not recommended for the treatment of osteomyelitis because they are no longer reliably effective against the oral streptococci and anaerobes. The recommended antibiotic regimen for osteomyelitis of the jaws is summarized in Box 10-3.

Chronic Suppurative Osteomyelitis   Chronic osteomyelitis requires surgical procedures such as sequestrectomy and removal of foreign bodies such as wires, bone plates, and screws, and repeated culturing and improvement of host defenses. Any excised bone or soft tissue should be cultured. When an uncontaminated specimen is difficult to obtain for culture, injection of sterile saline solution (without a bacteriostatic agent) into the involved area, followed by aspiration may be helpful. Treatment of suppurative osteomyelitis should begin with intravenous therapy and continue even after discharge using home intravenous therapy, usually with Unasyn, because it is stable for 24 hours after mixing with the intravenous fluid. Intravenous therapy generally is continued for 2 weeks or until the patient has shown improvement for 48 to 72 hours. Oral therapy should be continued for 4 to 6 weeks after the patient has no symptoms or from the date of the last debridement. Clindamycin therapy is recommended if Unasyn is ineffective and a specimen cannot be obtained. Radionuclide imaging may be used to determine when to discontinue antibiotic therapy.

LOCAL ANTIBIOTIC THERAPY

Closed Wound Irrigation-Suction   Determination of the extent of chronic infection of residual bone after debridement is not always possible. Placement of tubes against the bone may be desirable to allow drainage of pus and serum and to provide a route for irrigation, thus reducing the number of remaining organisms. Irrigation without surgical debridement to the point of bleeding bone is unlikely to be effective, prolongs the process, and delays definitive treatment (Figure 10-9).

The following technique of closed wound irrigation is suggested. After intraoral debridement, saucerization or decortication, small pediatric nasogastric feeding tubes, French catheters, or polyethylene irrigation tubes 3 to 4 mm in diameter and 6 to 10 inches in length are perforated along a distance of 3 to 4 cm from the tip.[63] The tubes are placed into the bone bed through separate skin incisions along the lateral bony surface and are affixed to the bone with catgut sutures through holes drilled in the bone. These drains are held to the skin with sutures or tape. Alternatively, two tubes may exit from one stab incision or a single tube may be used for instillation and suction (Figure 10-10). Continuous irrigation obviously cannot be achieved if a single drain is placed.

After tube placement a watertight closure of the wound is achieved, the tubes are flushed with saline solution, and the irrigating solution is introduced through one tube while the other tube is connected to low-pressure suction.

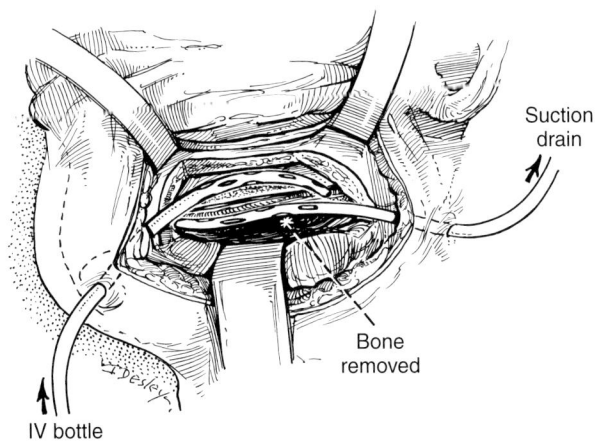

Various irrigating solutions may be used and often contain antibiotics, wetting agents, and proteolytic enzymes. One to 2 L of solution is instilled through the afferent tube and the solution is evacuated by suction through the efferent drain every 24 hours. Cultures are performed from specimens taken from the efferent tube at the end of each cycle and irrigation is continued for 1 week and until three successive cultures are sterile.

Antibiotics in high concentrations also may be placed in direct contact with the bone manually or with an implantable pump.[4,51] Various antibiotics have been used

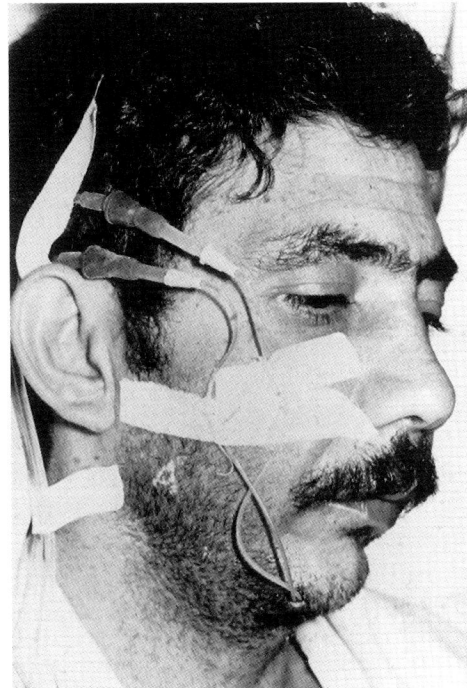

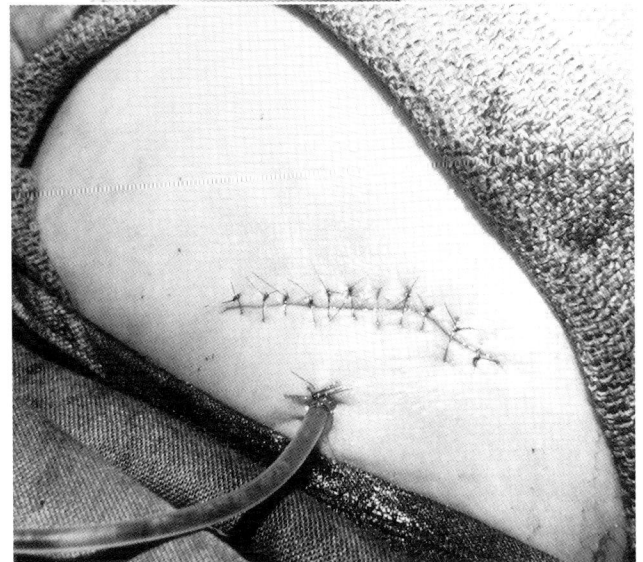

Figure 10-9 Diagram of placement of tubes for closed wound irrigation. One tube is used to infuse the irrigating solution, and the other tube serves as the efferent limb. (From Turlington EG: *Transactions of the IV International Conference on Oral Surgery,* Copenhaven, Denmark, 1973, Munksgaard.)

Figure 10-10 A, Patient with closed irrigation tubes, both of which exit from a single puncture wound. **B,** Use of single tube after decortication. (Courtesy Arie Shteyer and the Department of Oral and Maxillofacial Surgery, Hadassah Medical Center, Jerusalem, Israel.)

for this purpose including clindamycin. Alternatively, Neosporin G.U. irrigant (bacitracin zinc–neomycin sulfate–polymyxin B sulfate solution for irrigation) or a solution of 1% neomycin with 0.1% polymyxin B in equal volumes may be instilled on a 12-hour cycle. The drug is left in place for 3 hours; then low-pressure intermittent suction is used for 9 hours, followed by culture of specimens. This process is repeated until successive sterile cultures are obtained.[28] The wound must not be overfilled. The volume should be decreased gradually to allow for filling of the wound by healthy granulation tissue and to avoid neomycin toxicity. Other solutions including normal saline solution also have been used for irrigation. Systemic antibiotics should be continued throughout irrigation and for at least 2 months after cessation of clinical evidence of disease.

Because of the labor-intensive, time-consuming aspects of continuous antibiotic infusion, irrigation, and suction drainage techniques, other approaches have been suggested, including the use of antibiotic-impregnated acrylic beads placed in the wound bed or HBO therapy.

Antibiotic-Impregnated Beads   Antibiotic-impregnated acrylic beads have been used in the treatment of osteomyelitis to deliver high concentrations of antibiotics into the wound bed and in immediate proximity to the infected bone[2,9,21] (Figure 10-11). The antibiotic is leached from the beads, producing high local concentrations but low systemic concentrations thus reducing the risk of toxicity. Tobramycin or gentamicin is contained in acrylic resin (polymethylmethacrylate) bone cement beads. Impregnated chains of beads are useful especially in chronically infected bone associated with fractures and in chronic sclerosing osteomyelitis refractory to systemic antibiotics. In the latter situation, after decortication the chain of beads is applied against the bleeding surface, a drain is inserted, and the wound is closed. The beads and drain are left in place 10 to 14 days and then removed through a small incision. Systemic antibiotics are administered si-

multaneously. When fracture is associated with chronic osteomyelitis, foreign bodies are removed, the bone ends are debrided, a rigid reconstruction plate is placed, and a string of antibiotic-impregnated beads is placed against the bone. The beads subsequently are removed before final reconstruction.[9] Clindamycin is effective against most streptococci and oral anaerobes and can be combined with and released from methylmethacrylate.

Hyperbaric Oxygen Therapy   HBO therapy has been used to promote healing in refractory chronic osteomyelitis and osteoradionecrosis. Its use is discussed in the following text.

SURGICAL MANAGEMENT

Surgical intervention as an adjunct to medical treatment usually is necessary. In the acute stage, surgery should be limited to removal of severely loose teeth and bone fragments and incision and drainage of fluctuant areas and may proceed, if necessary, to sequestrectomy, with or without saucerization, decortication, or resection, and then reconstruction.

Unless abscesses are extensive or pus is located deeply, initial drainage and debridement may be accomplished with the patient under local anesthesia and sedation. Deeply located or extensive abscesses may require treatment with the patient under general anesthesia. Heat should be avoided in such cases because it may encourage extension of infection through bone.

Treatment of systemic diseases and supportive therapy consisting of a high-protein, high-vitamin diet with adequate hydration achieved either orally or by infusion should be instituted. Once chronic infection is established a decision is required concerning further surgical intervention, including removal of persistently loose teeth and sequestra. If drainage persists despite appropriate antibiotic treatment, as demonstrated by repeated cultures and sensitivity testing, debridement, local antibiotic therapy, sequestrectomy, saucerization, decortication, or resection and subsequent reconstruction must be considered.

SEQUESTRECTOMY

Sequestra usually are cortical but may be cancellous or cortical-cancellous and generally are not seen until at least 2 weeks after the onset of infection. Once fully formed, sequestra persist for several months before they are resorbed, removed, or spontaneously expelled through the mucosa or skin. Resorption occurs by lytic activity of osteoclasts in granulation tissue ingrowing sequestra. If partial healing occurs before the sequestrum is fully resorbed, exacerbations follow because of pus accumulation. In the chronic state the involucrum, or shell of bone produced by the periosteum, may be perforated by tracts (cloacae) through which pus escapes to epithelial surfaces. Sequestra are avascular and therefore poorly penetrated by antibiotics. Pathological fractures may occur in the region of the infection because of bone loss from sequestration or diminution in bone

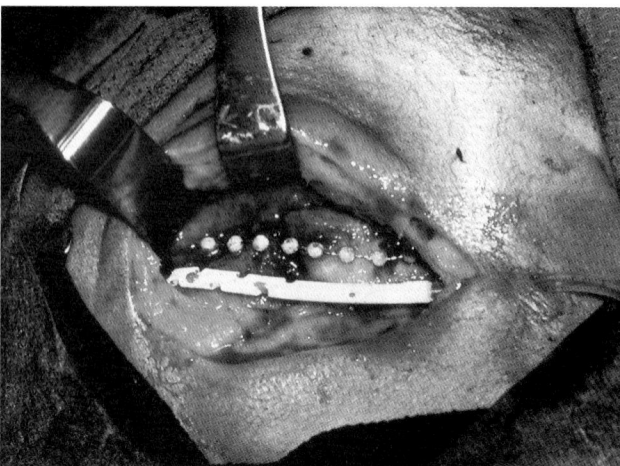

Figure 10-11 Gentamicin-impregnated polymethylmethacrylate beads with drain in place in close contact with infected bone. (Courtesy Brian Alpert.)

strength. Rarely do sterile abscesses (Brodie's abscess), common to long bones, occur in the jaws.

Some authors urge conservative treatment of developing sequestra in conjunction with supportive and antibiotic therapy. Once the sequestrum has formed completely, it can be removed with a minimum of surgical trauma. This method prevents the spread of infection and minimizes tooth and bone loss. However, the patient is subjected to a chronic infection with a protracted course of antibiotics, attendant complications, draining fistulas, and hygienic problems. Consequently a more aggressive approach is advised.

SEQUESTRECTOMY AND SAUCERIZATION

Saucerization is the "unroofing" of the bone to expose the medullary cavity for thorough debridement. The margins of necrotic bone overlying the focus of osteomyelitis are excised allowing visualization of sequestra and excision of affected bone. Saucerization is useful in chronic osteomyelitis because it permits removal of formed and forming sequestra. Saucerization should be performed intraorally whenever possible. This approach provides direct access to the bone and avoids facial scarring. The defect is packed open to allow subsequent exfoliation of unrecognized sequestra. The procedure can be performed as soon as acute infection has resolved with the aim of decompressing the bone to allow ready extrusion of pus, debris, and avascular fragments. The patient is more comfortable and ultimate bone loss is minimized. Local or general anesthesia may be used and the following steps employed (Figure 10-12):

1. A buccal mucoperiosteal flap is reflected to expose infected bone. Extensive tissue reflection should be avoided to preserve blood supply.
2. Loose teeth and bony segments and particles are removed.
3. The lateral cortex of the mandible is reduced using burs or rongeurs until bleeding bone is encountered at all margins, approximately to the level of the unattached mucosa, thus producing a saucerlike defect.

4. All granulation tissue and loose bone fragments are removed from the bone bed using curettes and the area is thoroughly irrigated; the region is usually hyperemic, but bleeding is readily controlled by packing.
5. The buccal flap is trimmed and a medicated ¼- or ½-inch pack (such as iodoform gauze lightly covered with triple-antibiotic ointment) is inserted for hemostasis and to maintain the flap in a retracted position until initial healing occurs. The pack is placed firmly but without pressure. The pack is retained by several nonresorbable interrupted sutures, extending over the pack from the lingual to the buccal flap, for 3 to 6 days and may be replaced several times until the surface of the bed of granulation tissue is epithelialized and the margins have healed.

Unlike treatment of weight-bearing long bone osteomyelitis in which bone strength is critical and primary closure is required over bone grafts, healing by secondary intention usually leaves a mandible of adequate strength.

Reduction of the lingual cortex rarely is necessary except to remove obviously necrotic bone and sharp crestal margins. The mylohyoid muscle attachments provide a rich blood supply and usually maintain vascularity of the bone lingually. When saucerization is performed extraorally, the defect also may be packed open. However, the soft tissue usually is closed primarily and closed irrigation-suction is used. Saucerization rarely is needed in the maxilla with its thin cortex because sequestra usually form rapidly and creation of a wide defect may cause oroantral fistulas.

DECORTICATION

Decortication of the mandible refers to the removal of chronically infected cortex of bone. The lateral and inferior border cortex is removed 1 to 2 cm beyond the affected area thus providing access to the medullary cavity (Figure 10-13). First advocated for jaw osteomyelitis in 1917 and further described by Mowlem,[48] decortication

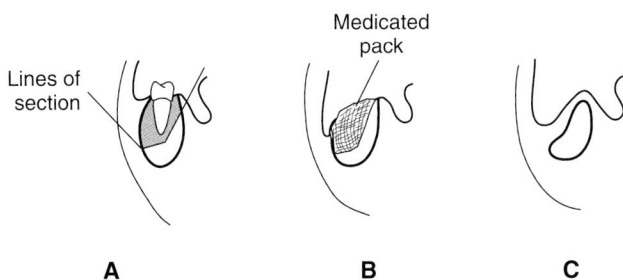

Figure 10-12 Diagram of saucerization. **A,** Outline of bone removed; after reflection of the mucoperiosteum, loose teeth are removed and the superior aspect of the buccal cortical plate is excised along the extent of the involved area. The bone is trimmed until bleeding is noted from all margins. Sequestra are removed. **B,** A medicated pack is placed within the saucer, slightly overfilling the defect; the mucosa is trimmed and several sutures are tied over the pack to maintain its position. **C,** After healing the bone remodels and is covered by normal mucosa.

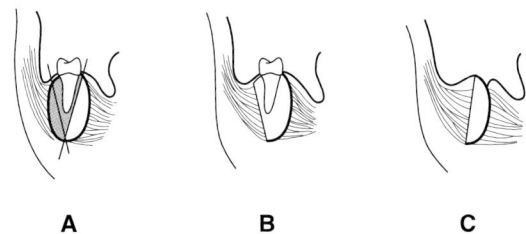

Figure 10-13 Decortication of the mandible. **A,** The lateral cortical plate and a portion of the inferior cortical plate are removed a distance of 1 to 2 cm beyond the involved area. Usually bone that supports teeth is involved, which necessitates tooth removal. **B,** Vascular muscle flap is shown approximating the bony surface when teeth are retained, and **C,** when they are removed.

in the antibiotic era has been well described.[25] Once the disease is in its subacute or chronic stages, use of decortication promotes resolution based on the premise that the affected cortical bone is avascular and harbors microorganisms. Usually granulation tissue and pus exist within the medullary cavity that antibiotics cannot penetrate. Waiting for formation of sequestra risks extension, abscess formation, cellulitis, and the hazards associated with prolonged antibiotic therapy and convalescent periods.

Decortication may be used as initial treatment of primary and secondary chronic osteomyelitis or, more commonly, when initial conservative regimens have failed. Although decortication originally was performed extraorally, today it is achieved through an intraoral approach that prevents facial scarring.

The steps in decortication are (1) creation of a buccal flap by a crestal incision extending along the necks of the teeth, (2) reflection of the mucoperiosteum to the inferior border; (3) removal of teeth in the involved area, and (4) removal of the lateral cortical plate and inferior border with chisels (see Figure 10-13). The lateral cortex may be scored with burs and removed in sections with an osteotome. Bone must be cut back to uninvolved areas as demonstrated by bleeding points along the bone margins.

The bone bed is debrided thoroughly, the flap is closed primarily, and dead space is eliminated by reapproximation of the flap and use of a pressure bandage for 24 to 48 hours to maintain close contact between the vascular soft tissue flap and the bone bed. Irrigation tubes may be placed through separate cutaneous stab incisions, and closed irrigation-suction may be used or antibiotic-impregnated acrylic beads placed for 10 to 14 days. Specimens should be obtained for aerobic and anaerobic culture and sensitivity testing, and antibiotic therapy should be continued.

In secondary chronic osteomyelitis (the sequel of acute osteomyelitis), removal of the lateral cortical plate exposes the medullary cavity occupied by granulation tissue, pus, and sequestra. In primary chronic osteomyelitis the cavity usually is not found; rather dense sclerotic bone is present with occasional small areas of granulation tissue.

If the affected area is extensive and the lingual plate of bone is affected, the possibility of mandible fracture during debridement should be anticipated. The surgeon should be prepared to stabilize and reconstruct the jaw.

RESECTION AND RECONSTRUCTION

Resection of osteomyelitic area with immediate or delayed reconstruction may be necessary to resolve low-grade, persistent chronic osteomyelitis. This technique has been used successfully in cases of pathological fracture, persistent infection after decortication, and marked disease of both cortical plates.

Using an extraoral approach, bone is debrided until bleeding surfaces are encountered distally and proximally. For immediate reconstruction, single or multiple blocks of

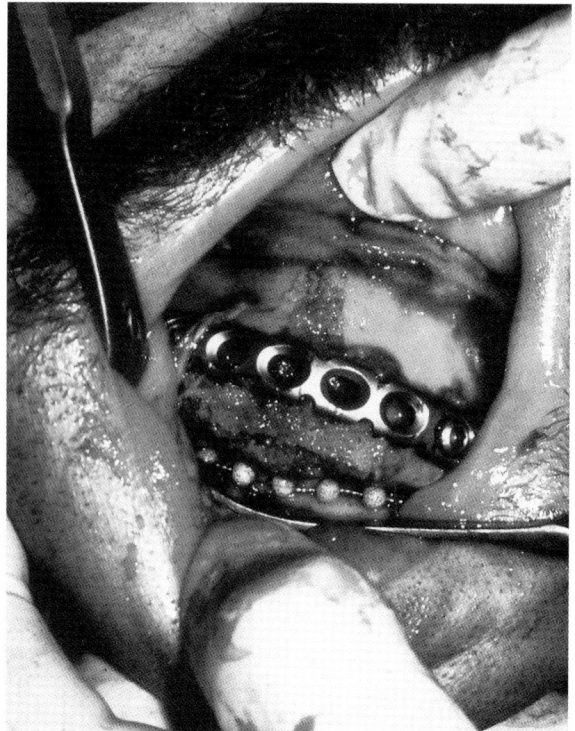

Figure 10-14 Reconstruction plate with autologous particulate marrow graft placed after debridement of fracture sustained 4 weeks earlier. A chain of antibiotic-impregnated acrylic beads was also placed and removed after 4 days. (Courtesy Brian Alpert.)

autologous corticocancellous bone grafts are secured to a reconstruction plate, particulate cancellous bone graft material is packed around the plate (Figure 10-14), split ribs forming a crib are packed with cancellous bone and wired into place, or metallic or other alloplastic trays are secured proximally and distally and packed with cancellous bone[34,44] (Figure 10-15).

TYPES OF OSTEOMYELITIS

OSTEOMYELITIS ASSOCIATED WITH FRACTURES

Failure to use effective methods of reduction, fixation, and immobilization may lead to osteomyelitis as debris and microorganisms gain access to the fracture site. Overzealous use of intraosseous wiring, bone plates, or screws that devascularize bone segments predisposes patients to osteomyelitis (Figures 10-16 and 10-17). Once osteomyelitis caused by fractures becomes established, intermaxillary fixation should be instituted as soon as possible. Fixation enhances patient comfort and minimizes ingress of microorganisms and debris caused by movement of bone fragments.[36,45] Loose teeth and foreign materials in the line of fracture should be removed and initial debridement performed as soon as possible. Internal fixation with reconstruction plates accompanied by high-dose antibiotic therapy produces the rigid immobilization necessary to

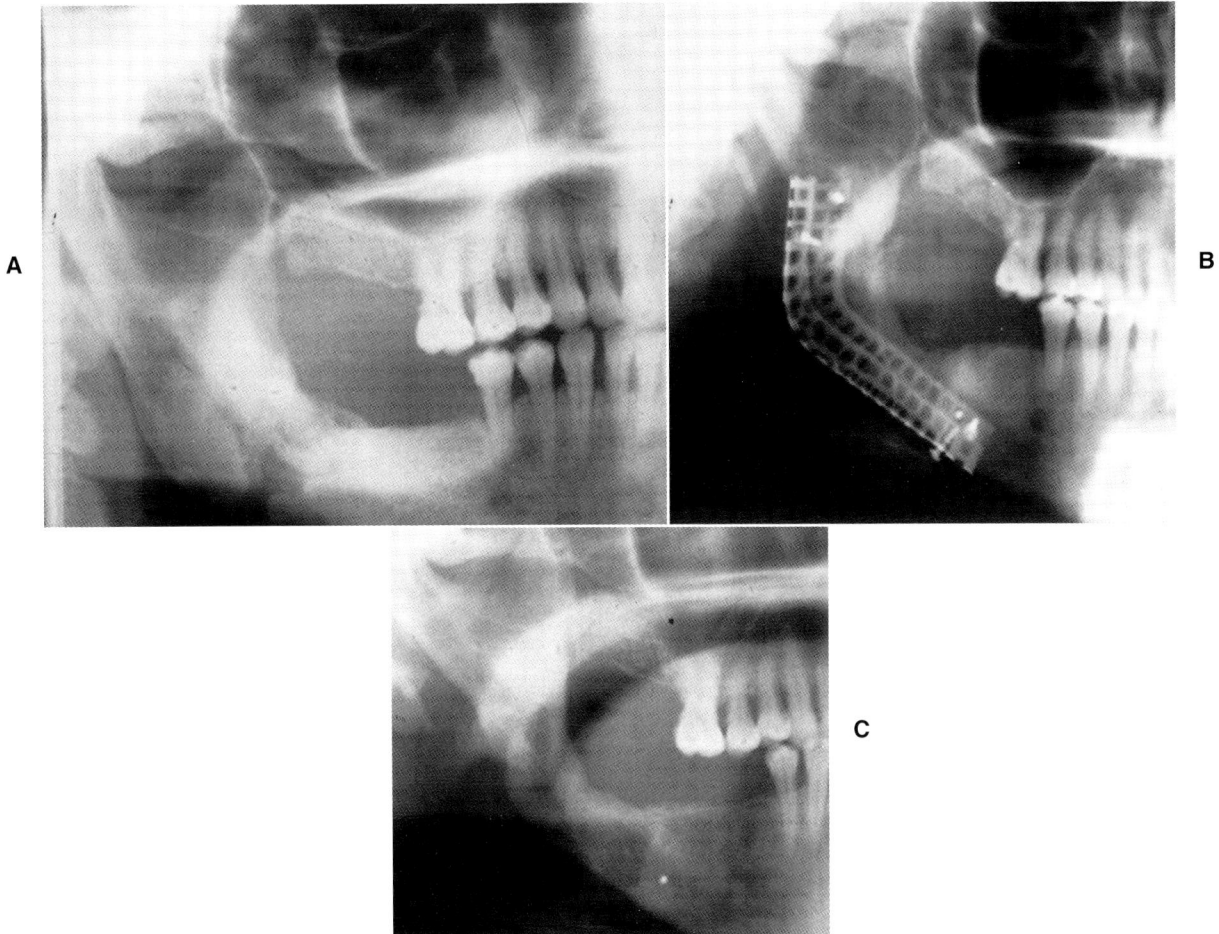

Figure 10-15 Persistent chronic osteomyelitis in a patient after extension of infection from an extraction site. **A,** Radiograph showing presence of osteomyelitis 26 months after various modes of treatment, one of which was completely successful. Both cortical plates were involved. **B,** Radiograph taken 9 months after segmental resection of chronic osteomyelitis and replacement with an autologous cancellous bone graft in a titanium mesh tray. **C,** Radiograph taken 4 years later after the tray was removed because of a small persistent mucosal fistula.

eliminate the infection and encourage bony healing[30] (see Chapter 17).

INFANTILE OSTEOMYELITIS

Osteomyelitis of the jaws in infants is an uncommon disease but merits special mention because of the risks of involvement of the eye, extension to the dural sinuses, and the potential for facial deformities and loss of teeth resulting from delayed or inappropriate treatment. Infantile osteomyelitis occurs most often a few weeks after birth and usually affects the maxilla. Before the advent of antibiotics the mortality rate approached 30%. Infantile osteomyelitis is believed to occur by the hematogenous route or from perinatal trauma of the oral mucosa from the obstetrician's finger or the mucus suction bulb used to clear the airway immediately after birth. Infection involving the maxillary sinus and contaminated human or artificial nipples also have been implicated as sources of infant infection.

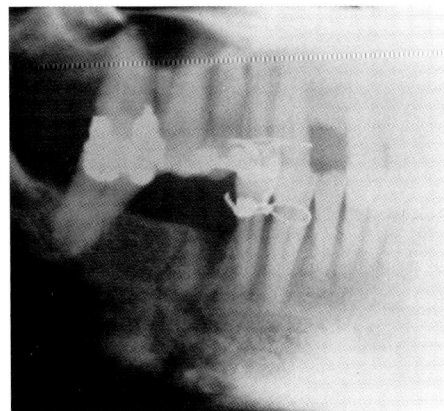

Figure 10-16 Radiograph of osteomyelitis resulting from inadequate immobilization of a fracture of the mandible. Ivy loops with intermaxillary elastics did not provide adequate immobilization.

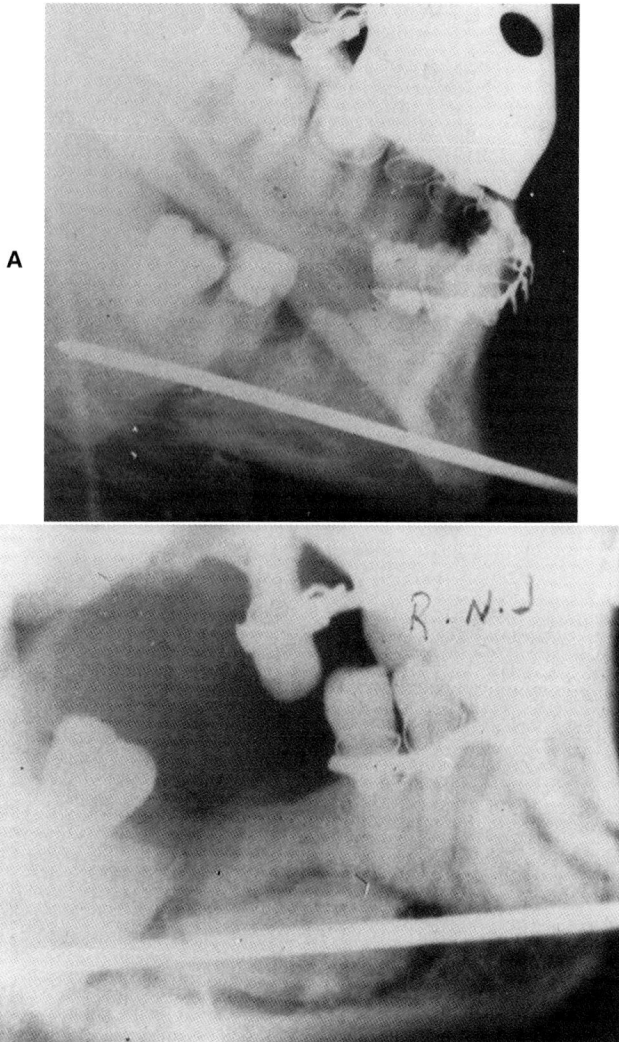

Figure 10-17 A, Use of an intramedullary Kirschner wire in the treatment of a mandibular fracture. Inadequate reduction and fixation resulted in osteomyelitis. **B,** Large sequestrum formed in association with the application of a Kirschner wire. (Courtesy Arie Shteyer and the Department of Oral and Maxillofacial Surgery, Hadassah Medical Center, Jerusalem, Israel.)

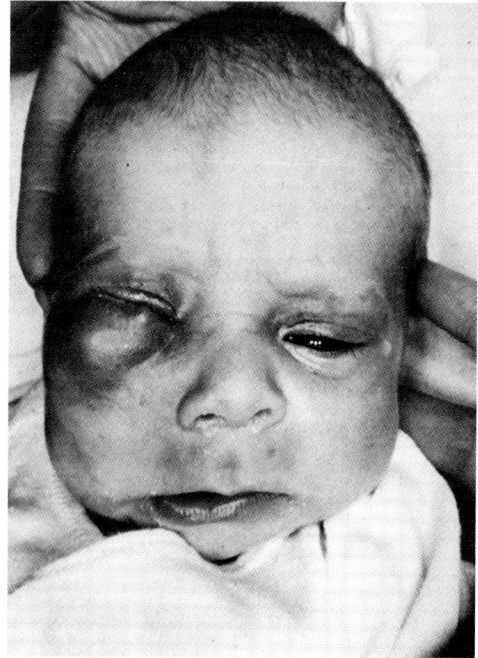

Figure 10-18 A 3-week-old infant with osteomyelitis of the newborn of unknown origin. Treatment with antibiotics alone was successful. (Courtesy M. Michael Cohen, Sr.)

Clinically the patient has facial cellulitis centered about the orbit (Figure 10-18). Irritability and malaise precede frank cellulitis and are followed by hyperpyrexia, anorexia, and dehydration. Convulsions and vomiting may occur. Pus is often present in the nostril on the affected side.

Inner and outer canthal swelling, palpebral edema, closure of the eye, conjunctivitis, and proptosis may result. A purulent discharge may be associated with the nose or with an inner canthal sinus. A concomitant subperiosteal abscess caused by acute ethmoiditis may be present. CT imaging is indicated to determine the extent of orbital involvement, presence, location and extent of orbital abscess, and possible dural sinus involvement.[61]

Intraorally the maxilla on the affected side is swollen both buccally and palatally, especially in the molar region. Fluctuance often is present and fistulas may exist in the alveolar mucosa. During the early acute phase, little radiographic change is noted. Leukocytosis is present with a shift to the left. *S. aureus* usually is the offending organism, although many other organisms, particularly streptococci, can occasionally be found.

Treatment should be prompt and aggressive to prevent permanent optic damage, neurological complications, and loss of tooth buds and bone. Treatment consists of intravenous antibiotics and drainage of all abscesses. Intravenous penicillin and a penicillinase-resistant penicillin, ampicillin/sulbactam (Unasyn), or clindamycin should be given, and drainage of all fluctuant areas should be established. Specimens should be obtained repeatedly for sensitivity testing with appropriate adjustment of the antibiotic regimen. Supportive treatment consists of antipyretics, fluids, and proper diet. Antibiotics should be continued orally for 2 to 4 weeks after all signs of infection have subsided. A conservative approach to sequestrectomy is advisable because of the danger of damage to tooth buds. Occasionally tooth buds are extruded and sequestra form. When teeth in the area eventually erupt they may be discolored. Scarring beneath the eyelid also has been noted, causing an ectropion. Corrective lid surgery sometimes is required for correction.

CHRONIC RECURRENT MULTIFOCAL OSTEOMYELITIS OF CHILDREN

An inflammatory disease of bone, chronic recurrent multifocal osteomyelitis of children resembles infectious osteomyelitis and affects children averaging 14 years of age

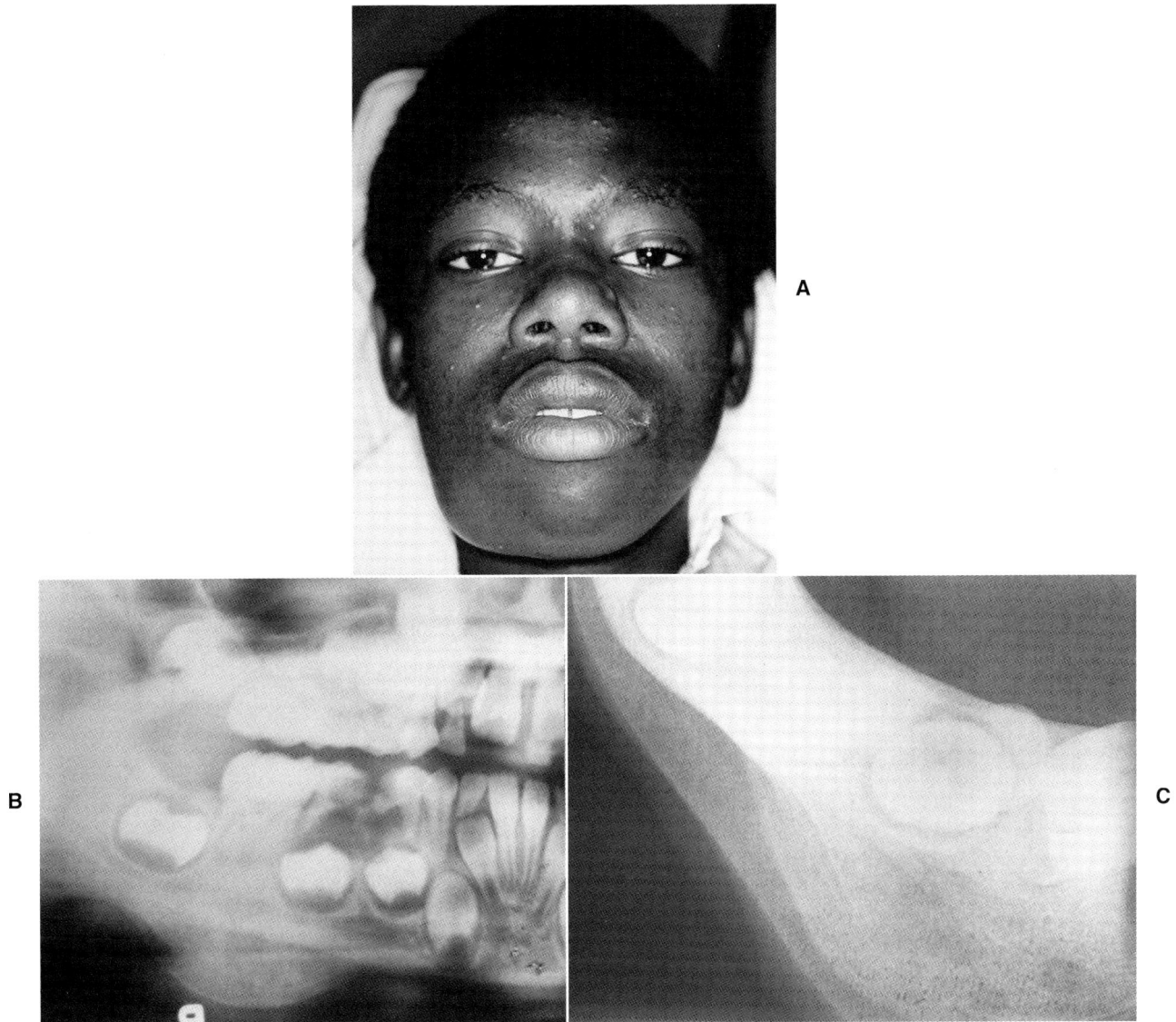

Figure 10-19 A, Facial deformity caused by proliferative periostitis (Garré's sclerosing osteomyelitis) in an 8-year-old child. Apical infection associated with the primary molars was the apparent cause. **B,** Panographic film shows marked periosteal reaction. **C,** Occlusal film shows the "onion skin" appearance of the newly formed bone. (Courtesy Larry J. Peterson.)

but has no obvious infectious origin.[61] Sites include the tibia, clavicle, fibula, spine, femur, and mandible. Mandibular lesions are bilateral, irregular, mottled, and multilocular and are located in the mandibular rami. Treatment is controversial.[3] Antibiotics and debridement have little effect on the prolonged course of the disease and spontaneous remission is frequent.[50]

PROLIFERATIVE PERIOSTITIS (GARRÉ'S SCLEROSING OSTEOMYELITIS)

Proliferative periostitis, also known as chronic nonsuppurative sclerosing osteomyelitis, proliferative periostitis of Garré, Garré's sclerosing osteomyelitis, and periostitis ossificans, was first described in 1893 by Carl Garré as an irritation-induced focal thickening of the periosteum and cortical bone of the tibia. The disease occurs primarily in children and young adults and occasionally in older individuals.

Proliferative periostitis is characterized clinically by a localized, hard, nontender, unilateral bony swelling of the lateral and inferior aspects of the mandible. The skin overlying the lesion is normal. Lymphadenopathy, fever, and leukocytosis usually do not occur. Proliferative periostitis commonly is associated with a carious lower first molar tooth, with a history of past toothache (Figure 10-19). On occasion no dental cause is detectable.

Radiographically a focal area of well-calcified bone proliferation may be seen that is smooth and often has a laminated or "onion skin" appearance. Radiolucency may be associated with the apices of the involved tooth.

Proliferative periostitis is considered a response to a low-grade infection or irritation that influences the potentially active periosteum of young individuals to lay down new bone. *S. aureus* and *S. epidermidis* organisms have been found in specimens of bone biopsy of lesions.

Ewing's sarcoma, osteosarcoma, and cortical hyperostosis (Caffey's disease) are similar in radiographic appearance and must be differentiated from proliferative periostitis.[13] When no dental disease exists or when lesions persists after treatment of the dental pathological condition, biopsy should be considered to establish the diagnosis. Histologically the lesion consists of new bone formation with a fibrous marrow containing chronic inflammatory cells.

Treatment is directed toward removal of identifiable sources of inflammation. When the affected tooth is not restorable, extraction is indicated. Endodontic therapy has been used successfully with resolution of the mass.[14] Antibiotic administration is not useful. Posttreatment follow-up is essential. If the lesion continues to increase in size after apparently successful treatment of the infection, early biopsy is indicated. Remodeling of the mandible generally occurs after successful treatment of the dental condition, but the deformity may remain static and surgical recontouring may be required.

CHRONIC SCLEROSING OSTEOMYELITIS

The nature and cause of sclerosing lesions of the jaws have been a matter of disagreement over the years. Two distinct types of lesions exist; one is diffuse and affects only the mandible (chronic diffuse sclerosing osteomyelitis), and the other is characterized by opaque masses, limited to the alveolar process that may be present in both jaws (florid osseous dysplasia). A third entity, chronic tendoperiostitis, has been described. Many studies have attempted to clarify the nature and classification of these entities but disagreement persists.[22,58,64] The clinician must know when (and when not) to intervene and how to advise patients.

Chronic Diffuse Sclerosing Osteomyelitis True or primary chronic diffuse sclerosing osteomyelitis is an inflammatory, nonsuppurative, painful disease with a protracted course. It occurs only in the mandible and affects both the basal bone and the alveolar process, that is, it involves the entire height of the mandible simultaneously, and is usually unilateral. In addition to the body of the mandible, it may affect the angle, ramus, and even the condyle (Figure 10-20). The bone often is mildly expanded and tender. Episodes of recurrent swelling and pain occur. The disease is seen mainly in adults in their third decade, although its occurrence in patients in their 60s has been reported.[22] Approximately two thirds of patients are women with no apparent racial predilection. Radiographically a diffuse intramedullary sclerosis with poorly defined margins is noted with occasional focal areas of radiolucency and radiopacity. Radionuclide bone scans show increased uptake corresponding to the area of sclerosis. Fever and leukocytosis usually do not occur,

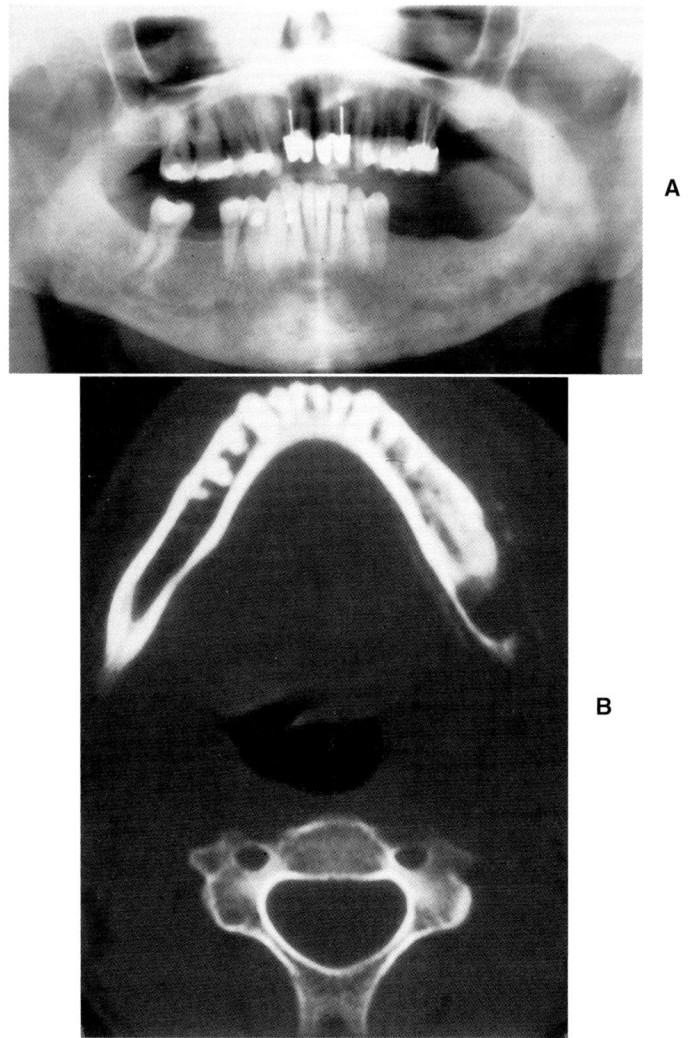

Figure 10-20 A, Panoramic radiograph of patient with chronic diffuse sclerosing osteomyelitis shows involvement of the inferior portion and ramus of the mandible on the patient's left side. B, CT scan demonstrates subperiosteal bone enlargement, sclerosis, and lytic area posteriorly. The soft tissue swelling commonly associated with this form of the disease is also seen. (Courtesy Robert E. Marx.)

although the erythrocyte sedimentation rate may be increased.

The cause of diffuse sclerosing osteomyelitis is controversial. Some believe that the condition is infectious, whereas others believe that some cases are noninfectious and result from overuse of the jaw, malocclusion, and abnormal jaw positing habits causing chronic tendoperiostitis.[22] A study by Marx et al.[41] showed a bacterial cause when great care is taken in obtaining tissue samples and transporting specimens within minutes for aerobic and anaerobic culture. In such circumstances, *E. corrodens, Actinomyces, Arachnia,* and *Bacteroides* spp. were recovered in all patients. Thus true diffuse sclerosing osteomyelitis may be indeed infectious.

Treatment is essentially the same as for chronic suppurative osteomyelitis: high doses of antibiotics for pro-

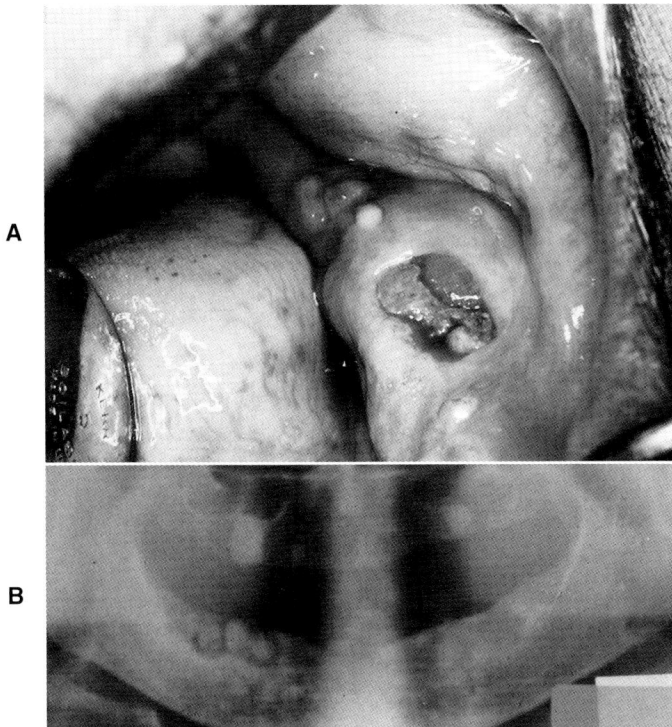

Figure 10-21 A, Clinical appearance of florid osseous dysplasia exposed in the oral cavity in a 40-year-old woman. **B,** Radiograph showing lesions in all quadrants. Lesions should not be removed unless secondarily infected. Masses in the lower right quadrant were exposed into the oral cavity and with chronic infection. They were removed surgically without complication. (Courtesy Larry J. Peterson.)

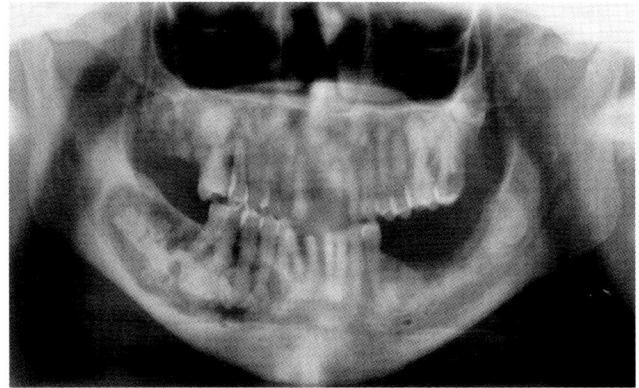

Figure 10-22 Chronically infected florid osseous dysplasia demonstrates masses limited to the alveolar processes in both jaws. (Courtesy Robert A. Ord.)

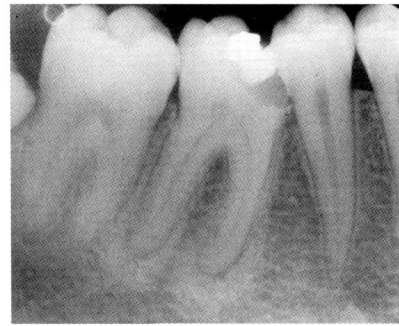

Figure 10-23 Condensing osteitis (chronic focal sclerosing osteomyelitis). (Courtesy David J. Krutchkoff.)

longed periods as in treatment of actinomycotic osteomyelitis, removal of the source of infection, repeated culture and sensitivity testing, wound irrigation, antibiotic-impregnated acrylic beads, and debridement. Decortication, resection, and reconstruction may be needed in extensive and long-standing cases. HBO therapy should be considered in refractory cases.[35]

Florid Osseous Dysplasia Florid osseous dysplasia has been confused with diffuse sclerosing osteomyelitis. Multiple, exuberant (florid), lobulated densely opaque masses are restricted to the alveolar process in either or both jaws (Figures 10-21 and 10-22). It occurs most often in black women. The lesions should be treated only when symptoms are present. Infection results from bacterial invasion by periapical infection, advanced periodontal disease, extraction of teeth, attempts at surgical excision, or ulceration of mucosa when the lesions become superficial as when residual ridge resorption proceeds. Fistulas and sequestra may form (see Figure 10-22). Secondarily infected florid osseous dysplasia is a suppurative, mildly painful condition of the mandible without expansion.[8] The masses, sequestra, and associated granulation tissue are excised and the wound debrided and irrigated, followed by primary or secondary closure.[58]

CONDENSING OSTEITIS (FOCAL SCLEROSING OSTEOMYELITIS)

Condensing osteitis is a localized area of bone sclerosis associated with the apex of a carious tooth and periapical periodontitis (Figure 10-23). Treatment consists of endodontic therapy or extraction; the lesion then regresses or remains as a bone scar.

ACTINOMYCOTIC OSTEOMYELITIS OF THE JAWS

Actinomycosis is a chronic, slowly progressive infection with both granulomatous and suppurative features; it usually affects soft tissue and, only occasionally, bone. It forms external sinuses that discharge distinctive sulfur granules and spreads unimpeded by anatomical barriers when endogenous oral commensals invade the tissues of the oral-cervicofacial, thoracic, pelvic, and abdominal (ileocecal) regions. Tissues may be invaded by direct extension or by hematogenous spread. About two thirds of cases are cervicofacial.[67]

Cervicofacial disease may affect the mandible and overlying soft tissues, parotid gland, tongue, and maxillary sinuses. Nearly every structure and space of the head and neck may be the initial site of involvement.[32] Secondary spread to other areas of the head and neck readily occurs.

In 1891 J. Israel isolated a gram-positive organism belonging to the genus *Actinomyces.* Historically, such organisms were considered fungi and were associated with a disease in humans analogous to lumpy jaw disease of cattle. At least three species have been related to disease: *A. israelii,* responsible for the disease in humans; *A. bovis,* causing the disease in cattle but only rarely in humans; and *A. baudetii,* causing actinomycosis in cats and dogs. *A. naeslundii, A. odontolyticus, A. meyeri,* and *Propionibacterium propionicum* are established but less common causes of the disease. Other organisms including *E. corrodens, Fusobacterium, Bacteroides, Staphylococcus, Streptococcus,* and Enterobacteriaceae often are found in association with actinomycotic infections and may be potential copathogens that aid in the inhibition of host defenses or reduce oxygen tension.[57] They are found in tonsillar crypts, salivary and dental calculus, and on mucosa of the oropharyngeal and gastrointestinal regions.

Actinomyces are not highly virulent pathogens but are endogenous oral saprophytes present in periodontal pockets, carious teeth, and tonsillar crypts that take advantage of infection, trauma, or surgical injury to penetrate normal intact mucosal barriers and invade adjacent tissues.[5] When actinomycosis occurs, it is certain to be endogenous in origin; pathogenicity is attributed to changes in the local or systemic substrate that permit the establishment of disease. The early hypothesis that organisms gain access to the oral cavity when humans chew contaminated straw has not been substantiated. Although the disease has been connected with steroid use and chemotherapy, lung and renal transplantation, renal failure, metastatic carcinoma, and human immunodeficiency viral infection, *Actinomyces* are rarely opportunistic in compromised hosts.[57,67]

Actinomycetes are not fungi, but rather gram-positive, microaerophilic, non–spore-forming, non–acid-fast bacteria. Their morphological characteristics vary, with filamentous cocci of bacillary forms. Early confusion concerning correct classification resulted because they are slow growing in culture and sometimes appear as "sulfur granules," that is, clumps of filamentous masses. Like *Nocardia* and mycobacteria, actinomycetes share characteristics of both bacteria and fungi. However, they are not sensitive to antifungal drugs and, unlike fungi, are sensitive to antibiotics. Cell wall, electron microscope, and other studies confirm their bacterial nature.

Infections with *A. israelii* occur in areas of tissue damage or inflammation in concert with other oral organisms. The organism gains access to the soft tissues directly or by extension from bone through periapical or periodontal lesions, fractures, or extraction sites. In some patients, no injury can be identified. When established the infection spreads without regard for fascial planes and typically appears on cutaneous rather than mucosal surfaces.

Firm, soft tissue masses are present on the skin; they have purplish, dark red, oily areas with occasional small zones of fluctuance. Spontaneous drainage of serous fluid containing granular material may occur (Figure 10-24). When expressed onto a piece of gauze, these granular, yellowish substances, the sulfur granules, may be seen clearly and represent colonies of bacteria. Microscopically, granules show closely packed branching filaments 1 μm in diameter. Regional lymph nodes occasionally are enlarged, but trismus is not common unless secondary infection has occurred. The patient usually has no fever and does not feel ill.

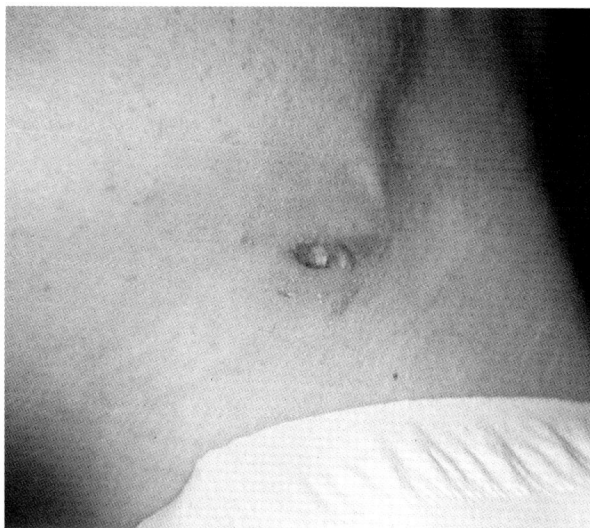

Figure 10-24 Spontaneous drainage from a mass in the submandibular region. Sulfur granules were seen on gauze in this instance of cervicofacial actinomycosis.

Radiolucencies of varying size and delay in healing of extraction sites are common (Figure 10-25). Periostitis, diffuse mandibular lucencies, or marked bone sclerosis also may be apparent on radiographs. Occasionally sequestra form. Laboratory findings in the absence of secondary infection usually are normal, although the erythrocyte sedimentation rate and white blood cell count may be elevated slightly.

Whenever any firm mass that is considered infectious does not respond to conventional antibiotic therapy, actinomycosis, a mycotic or mycobacterial infection, or a neoplasm should be considered in the diagnosis. Cervicofacial actinomycosis should be distinguished from parotitis, parotid tumors, cervical tuberculosis, and suppurative osteomyelitis.

Diagnosis is based on culture or biopsy of the lesion. Initially aspiration of a specimen for a Gram-stain smear and antimicrobial sensitivity testing for aerobic and anaerobic organisms are imperative. In actinomycosis the smear reveals gram-positive organisms of various morphological types, particularly diphtheroid and filamentous forms. Specific immunofluorescent staining to distinguish among the various species of actinomycosis is available.[26,31] It also may be used with formalin-fixed and paraffin-embedded biopsy specimens, even retrospectively in case of prolonged infection.[24] Biopsy of the wall of an abscess or fistula is useful in making the diagnosis when material is not available for smear and culture or when laboratory data are equivocal.

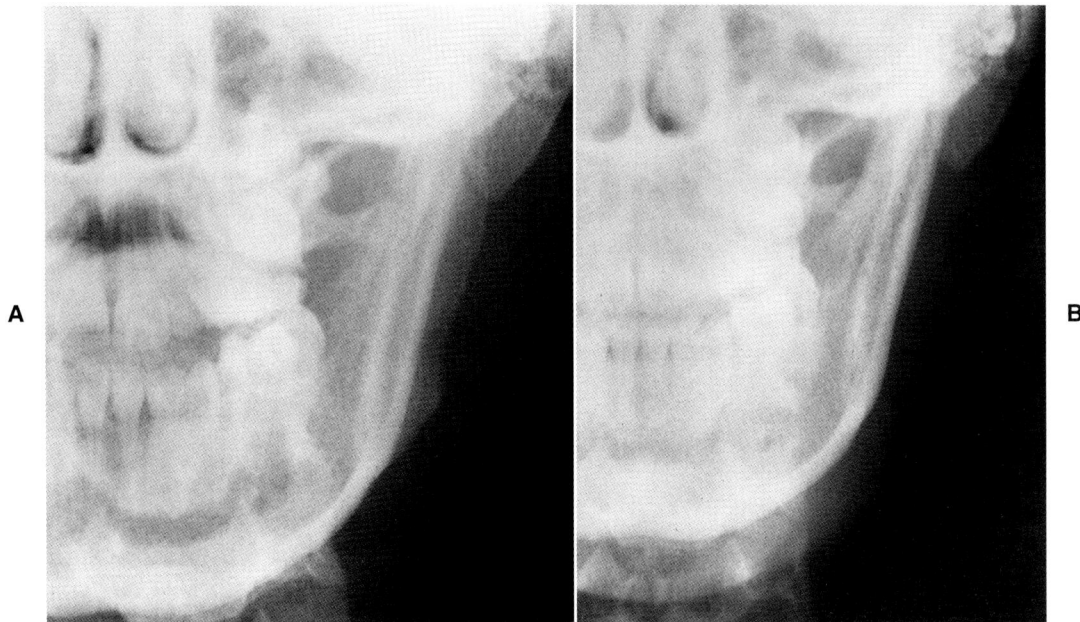

Figure 10-25 A, Radiograph of mandible shows marked periosteal reaction in a 14-year-old girl with actinomycotic osteomyelitis. **B,** Response 13 months after penicillin therapy shows complete remodeling of bone.

Treatment Many therapeutic agents and techniques have been used in the treatment of actinomycosis, including iodides, radiation, incision and drainage, excision of soft tissue and bone, and use of various antibiotics. *Actinomyces* infections produce dense bone and scarring of soft tissue and have been described by the term *lumpy jaw* (Figure 10-26). Scar tissue produces a harbor for organisms and reduces the blood supply to the affected region, reducing penetration of antibiotics. Consequently after aspiration for culture and sensitivity, all abscesses, regardless of size, should be disrupted surgically with a hemostat and all loculations penetrated and rendered contiguous.

Antibiotic Therapy In actinomycosis the dosage and duration of therapy that are effective for most infections may result in only temporary resolution followed by recurrence. Therefore antibiotics must be administered in high doses and for prolonged periods. Intravenous antibiotics should be administered for 4 to 6 weeks, followed by oral therapy for 6 to 12 months. Initially hospitalization may be indicated to begin intravenous antibiotic therapy and surgical procedures. Then intravenous therapy at home can be instituted. Numerous drugs are effective including the penicillins and macrolides, doxycycline and ceftriaxone, and clindamycin. The suggested regimen is penicillin G, 10 to 20 million units per day intravenously for 4 to 6 weeks, followed by penicillin V, 1 g four times a day for 6 to 12 months; or ampicillin, 50 mg/kg per day intravenously for 4 to 6 weeks, then amoxicillin 500 mg three times a day for 6 to 12 months.

For patients who are allergic to penicillin, doxycycline, 100 mg twice daily for 6 months, is effective. When bone is not affected and the infection is confined to soft tissues, treatment for 2 to 4 months usually is sufficient. With

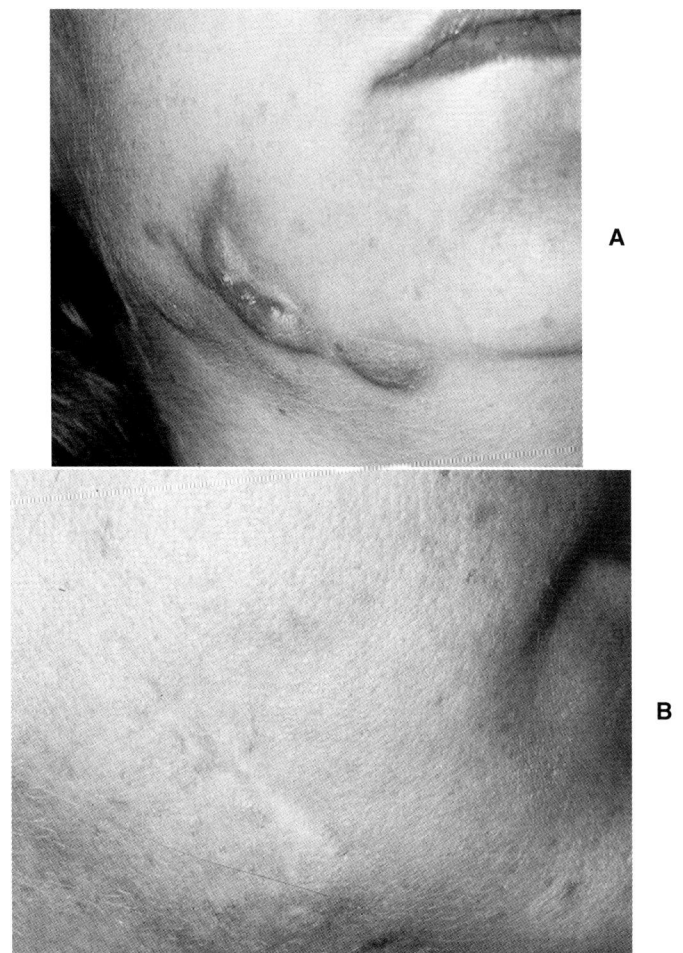

Figure 10-26 A, Soft tissue scars associated with actinomycosis. Scarring may be extensive and deforming. **B,** Appearance of face 6 months after antibiotic therapy. The patient elected not to have the scars revised.

home intravenous therapy a drug such as ceftriaxone (Ro-cephin), 1 g, may be given once a day.[18]

Imaging should be used throughout treatment to monitor healing of bone and the possible need for additional surgical procedures such as sequestrectomy and saucerization. Residual facial scars may be revised for cosmetic purposes. The following case report illustrates many features of this disease.

■ CASE REPORT

A 36-year-old woman had a 3-month history of drainage from a very firm tissue mass on the left side of the face (Figure 10-27, *A*). She first noticed a small swelling of her cheek approximately 0.5 cm in diameter opposite the lower left second premolar tooth. She was seen in a dental clinic and told that the lower left second premolar was abscessed. The root canal was opened, drainage was established, and the patient was told to return for definitive treatment. She returned 2 months later with a larger, more painful soft tissue swelling in the same area. The lower left second premolar tooth was extracted. No antibiotics were prescribed. Four days later she returned with increased swelling that was painful and indurated. Penicillin was given for 8 days and the swelling decreased slightly. No lymphadenopathy was present. Dental radiographs showed a periapical radiolucency. The patient then was referred to the oral-maxillofacial surgery clinic where 1 mL of fluid was aspirated from the mass and sent for culture and sensitivity testing. Immunofluorescence testing and a Gram-stain smear showed *A. israelii*. She was admitted to the hospital and given 3 million U of penicillin G intravenously every 4 hours for 14 days resulting in diminished swelling. Because the lesion was small, surgery was not performed. She was discharged and received 500 mg of penicillin V with 500 mg of probenecid orally every 4 hours for 4 months. Radiographs taken 1 year after commencement of antibiotic treatment showed persistent radiolucency in bone despite the absence of symptoms (Figure 10-27, *B*).

After having no symptoms for 6 years the patient underwent extraction of the lower left second molar tooth and hemisection of the distal root of the first molar for advanced periodontal disease. She continued to have no symptoms for 3 years thereafter; she then was evaluated for a small elevated swelling at the site of the scar from the earlier sinus tract. The adjacent mucobuccal fold was swollen. She was given 1 g of penicillin V with 500 mg probenecid orally three times a day. Three days later the extraoral fistula drained spontaneously. Specimens were taken for culture, Gram straining, and fluorescent antibody tests for *A. israelii* and *A. naeslundii*. Bone scan indicated infection of the posterior body of the left mandible. Intermittent drainage occurred over the next 14 days, and the fistula and skin became bound down to the mandible in the apical region of the hemisected tooth. The patient was admitted to the hospital and received intravenous penicillin and oral probenecid and underwent incision and drainage, debridement, and extraction of the lower left first molar mesial root. Actinomycosis never was demonstrated despite numerous cultures and Gram stains, but the clinical findings and course strongly suggested it. She received ampicillin and probenecid intravenously for 2 weeks. Antibiotic therapy was continued orally on discharge for 4 additional months. Eighteen months later the patient was still free of symptoms. This case illustrates the indolent nature of actinomycosis of the jaw and demonstrates that it may recur months or years after an apparent cure.

NOCARDIAL OSTEOMYELITIS

Nocardiosis is a chronic disease that resembles actinomycosis. Although it occurs primarily in the lungs, from which it may spread hematogenously to the nervous system and soft tissues, it occasionally involves the cervicofacial region in-

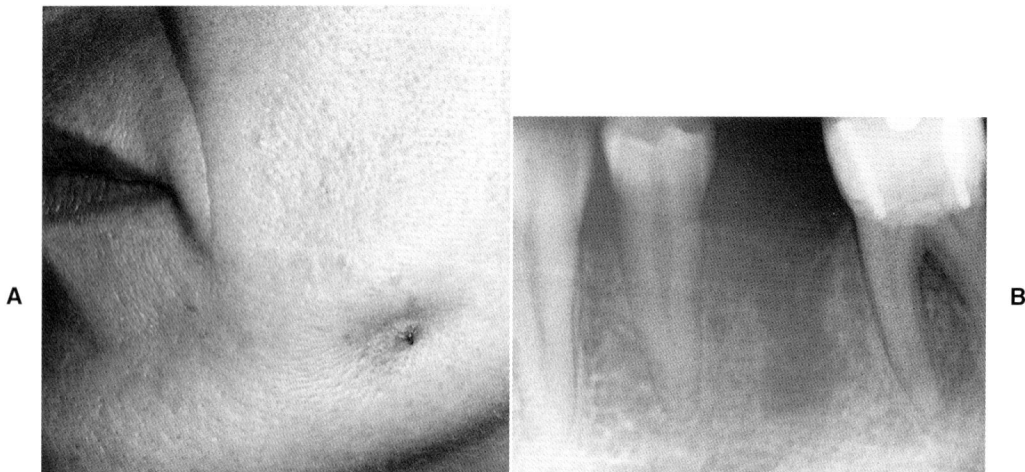

Figure 10-27 A, Indurated swelling of and fistula associated with actinomycosis that drained spontaneously but persisted after extraction of an abscessed lower left second premolar tooth. **B,** Persistence of radiolucency in bone seen 1 year after all clinical symptoms of the disease were absent.

cluding bone.[60] Nocardiosis is caused by organisms of the genus *Nocardia,* order Actinomycetales, earlier considered an aerobic form of actinomycosis, which it resembles in many respects. However, nocardiosis differs sufficiently, especially in its antibiotic sensitivity, that it must be distinguished from actinomycosis. Human disease usually is caused by *Nocardia asteroides,* an aerobic, delicate, gram-positive, beaded, branching filamentous, variably acid-fast organism[33] (Figure 10-28). Human nocardiosis also is caused by *N. farcinica, N. brasiliensis, N. nova, N. transvalensis,* and *N. otitidiscaviarum.* It is a soil saprophyte and usually gains access to the body through inhalation or by direct inoculation of skin or soft tissues.[62] It occasionally is associated with inhalation of contaminated dust or is spread by the hands of health care workers or contaminated fomites.[27] It is not a normal oral inhabitant. Although nocardiosis occurs as an opportunistic infection in compromised hosts, it may be seen also in apparently healthy individuals. In the jaws it may occur with or without dental injury and forms suppurative lesions with acute necrosis and abscess formation. Treatment consists of drainage of pus and administration of sulfonamides such as sulfisoxazole (2 g PO q6h) or trimethoprim-sulfamethox-azole (TMP/SMX DS, 1 tablet po bid) for up to 6 months.[18] The cervicofacial form often is manifested by pustules with secondary involvement of regional lymph nodes.

The records of a patient with findings consistent with mandibular osteomyelitis after removal of an impacted third molar tooth were reviewed by the author. Penicillin administered for several weeks was ineffective. Smear and culture of bone and granulation tissue showed *N. asteroides,* which was successfully treated with saucerization and a prolonged course of trimethoprim-sulfamethoxazole.

MALIGNANCY MASQUERADING AS OSTEOMYELITIS

Signs and symptoms of chronic osteomyelitis and malignancy with secondary infection share many similarities, leading at times to delay in definitive diagnosis and appropriate treatment.[65] Lesions believed to be osteomyelitis that do not respond to treatment as expected within a short time should be viewed with concern, and imaging studies and biopsies should be performed to establish the diagnosis. The following case report illustrates many features of osteomyelitis in the presence of malignancy.

■ CASE REPORT

A 58-year-old man underwent extraction of the lower right third molar tooth, which was painful, partially erupted, slightly mobile, and associated with 2 weeks of trismus and swelling. Penicillin was prescribed and the patient was compliant with its use in the postextraction period. Pain, trismus, and swelling persisted. Three weeks after surgery a radiograph was taken and interpreted as "compatible with osteomyelitis." Irrigation and curettage of the unhealed site produced neither pus nor sequestra. Culture findings were reported as "normal flora." The patient was admitted to his local hospital and received intravenous antibiotics, followed by oral antibiotics after discharge. CT scan confirmed the diagnosis of "diffuse osteomyelitis."

Anesthesia of his lip developed and 4 weeks later another CT scan showed "progression and possible pathological fracture." The patient was transferred to another hospital where review of the CT scans by both the radiology and oral and maxillofacial surgery services resulted in a unanimous diagnosis of severe, diffuse osteomyelitis. In an attempt to obtain an adequate specimen for culture and sensitivity a percutaneous submandibular approach was performed, which revealed a thin, perforated, necrotic-appearing buccal cortex and a nondisplaced fracture. When the body of the mandible was entered a thick mass of yellow, curdlike material was found.

Culture later was reported as sterile but pathological examination of the excised material revealed keratin and invasive epidermoid carcinoma. Further imaging demonstrated that the tumor had extended into the infratemporal fossa. Despite extensive surgery and a long course of radiation therapy the patient died of malignant disease that had masqueraded as osteomyelitis.[20]

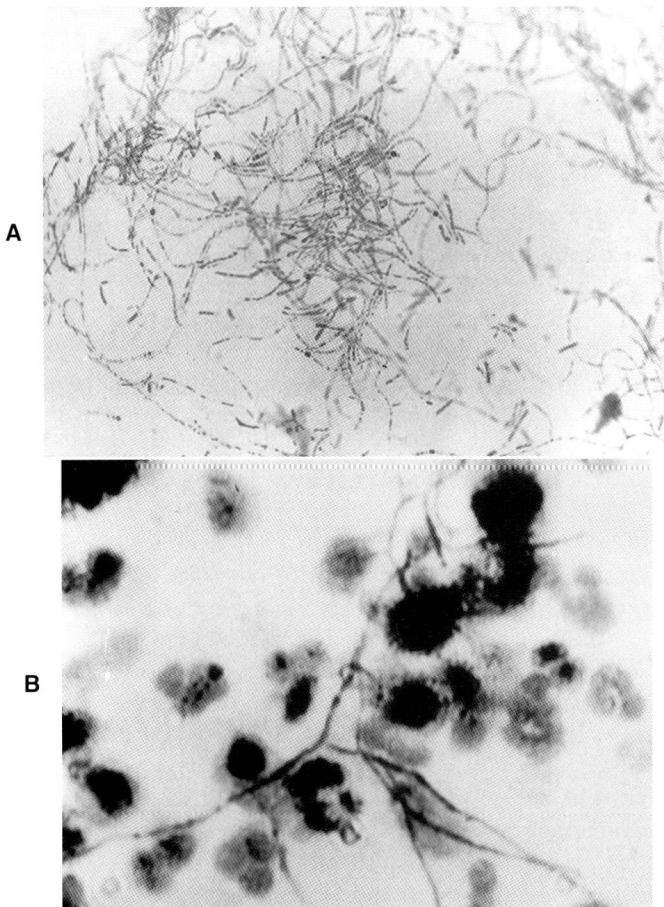

Figure 10-28 A, Gram stain of *Nocardia asteroides* in pure culture shows the delicate, beaded, weakly gram-positive filaments (×1200). (Courtesy L.R. Brettman.) **B,** Gram stain of *N. asteroides* demonstrates filamentous growth with true branching in a clinical specimen.

OSTEORADIONECROSIS

Cancer of the maxillofacial region usually is treated by radiation, surgery, or combined therapy. Radiation often has serious effects on soft and hard tissues adjacent to neoplasms: mucositis, atrophic mucosa, xerostomia, and radiation caries are common. Because of its mineral composition, bone absorbs more energy than soft tissue and is more susceptible to secondary radiation. An additional major complication is osteoradionecrosis, a disease of irradiated bone that may lead to marked pain, bone loss, and functional and cosmetic disability. For many years, osteoradionecrosis was considered an infection initiated by injury to irradiated bone. In more recent times, work by Marx[38] has shown that it is a chronic, nonhealing wound caused by hypoxia, hypocellularity, and hypovascularity of irradiated tissue.

The effects of radiation on bone depend on the quality and quantity of radiation, the size of the portals used, the location and extent of the lesion, and the condition of the teeth and periodontium. Before the 1960s, orthovoltage was used routinely for cancer therapy. Although effective against neoplasms it was highly deleterious to bone and resulted in an incidence of radiation necrosis of the jaws ranging from 17% to 37%. Radiation from implant sources also seriously damages adjacent bone. In recent years, orthovoltage has been supplanted by megavoltage and other techniques believed to be bone sparing. Dose fractionation, meticulous collimation, shielding of normal tissues, and maintenance of preirradiation and postirradiation dental health have been effective in further reducing the occurrence of osteoradionecrosis to the 2% to 5% range.

The mandible is affected more commonly than the maxilla because most oral tumors are perimandibular. The absence of dense cortical plates and the presence of a more extensive vascular network in the maxilla also lessen its likelihood of radiation necrosis effects compared with the mandible.

Radiation to the jaws in excess of 50 Gy kills bone cells and results in a progressive obliterative arteritis (endarteritis, periarteritis, hyalinization, and fibrosis and thrombosis of vessels). The periosteal vessels and larger vessels such as the inferior alveolar artery are affected markedly, resulting in aseptic necrosis of the portion of bone directly in the beam of radiation, with compromised vascularity of adjacent bone and soft tissue. Effective response to infection is diminished greatly. As long as the overlying soft tissues do not break down, irradiated bone may function normally. Formerly osteoradionecrosis was believed to be associated with the triad of radiation, trauma, and infection as microorganisms were introduced into bone with subsequent development of osteoradionecrosis. Marx et al.[39-44] have shown that microorganisms are merely contaminants and trauma is only one of several factors involved in the disease. When trauma is the precipitating factor, tooth extraction usually is the cause; fewer instances are caused by mucosal ulcers (denture sores) and lacerations, scaling of teeth, compound fractures, periodontal disease, and injudicious root canal

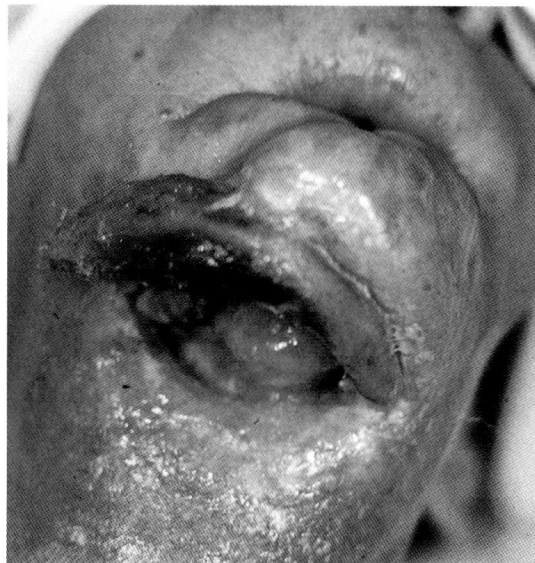

Figure 10-29 Orocutaneous fistula with pathological fracture of the mandible in a patient with osteoradionecrosis. This condition followed orthovoltage radiation.

instrumentation. Approximately one third of osteoradionecrosis cases occur spontaneously.

Osteoradionecrosis is a radiation-induced, nonhealing, hypoxic wound rather than true osteomyelitis of irradiated bone. The net effect of radiation is that tissues become less vascular (hypovascular), less cellular (hypocellular), and more hypoxic with time. The viable, radiation-damaged cells are not replaced by cells of the same type, resulting in less cellular, more extracellular elements such as collagen. The fibrotic and poorly vascularized tissue has reduced or absent healing ability. Breakdown occurs because the tissues cannot maintain normal cellular turnover and collagen synthesis. Such tissue is susceptible to spontaneous breakdown, breakdown from minor injury, or breakdown from other trauma especially tooth extraction.[40]

Cultures of affected bone show only surface organisms, predominantly streptococci, *Candida* spp., and gramnegative organisms. No organisms are found deep in bone. Staphylococci are found rarely unless in communication with the skin. When skin is affected the organisms most commonly found, as expected, are *S. aureus* and *S. epidermidis*.

Pain and evidence of exposed bone are the chief clinical features of osteoradionecrosis of the jaws. Initially the patient may have trismus, fetid breath, and an elevated temperature, although acute infection usually is not present. Exposed bone with a gray to yellow color is seen in association with intraoral and extraoral fistulae. Pathological fractures may be present (Figure 10-29). The exposed bone often has a rough surface texture that abrades adjacent soft tissue and causes further discomfort (Figure 10-30). The tissues surrounding the exposed bone may be indurated or ulcerated from infection or recurrent tumor. If induration persists after infection has been controlled by irrigation and antibiotics, or if ulceration is present, a biopsy should be performed.

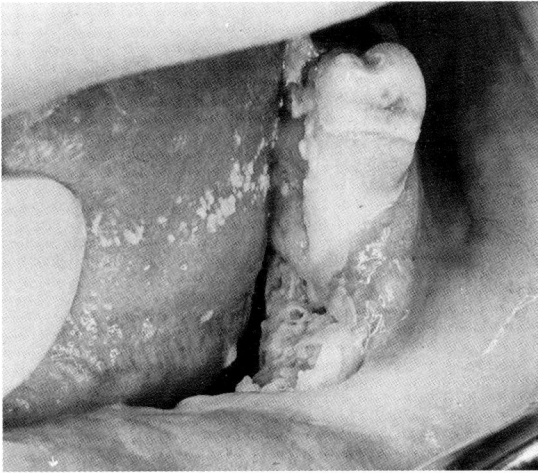

Figure 10-30 Osteoradionecrosis of the mandible with exposed bone intraorally caused marked pain and abrasion of the tongue. (Courtesy Arie Shteyer and the Department of Oral and Maxillofacial Surgery, Hadassah Medical Center, Jerusalem, Israel.)

Little radiographic change occurs early in the disease. The characteristic changes seen in osteomyelitis of nonirradiated bone (i.e., formation of sequestra or involucra) occur late or not at all in irradiated bone because of the severely compromised blood supply.

Treatment Initial treatment is directed at controlling frank infection, if present. Ambulatory care is appropriate except in patients who have symptoms of toxicity and are dehydrated; in such patients, hospitalization is recommended to allow supervised administration of parenteral antibiotics and fluids. Penicillin plus metronidazole, or clindamycin alone is recommended. Gentle irrigation of the soft tissue margins is useful in removing debris and reducing inflammation. If discrete abscesses or cutaneous fistulae are present, aerobic and anaerobic cultures should be obtained for sensitivity testing. Supportive treatment with fluids and a liquid or semiliquid diet, high in protein and vitamins, is desirable.

Some practitioners believe that conservative treatment of the bone is indicated initially. Consequently, irrigation of exposed bone is performed. A pulsating irrigation device is useful, but high pressures should be avoided because debris might be forced deeply into tissues. Exposed bone then is mechanically debrided and smoothed with large round or barrel-shaped burs and covered with a pack saturated with zinc peroxide and neomycin. Irrigation and packing are repeated weekly until sequestration occurs or the bone is penetrated by granulation tissue. If mucosal and muscle attachments are present lingually a series of holes may be drilled into the lingual cortical plate to the depth at which bleeding bone is encountered to encourage revascularization. This approach has been beneficial in selected cases.[23]

Ultrasound Therapy Another conservative approach is the use of ultrasound combined with local debridement. Ultrasound treatment is noninvasive and reportedly pro-

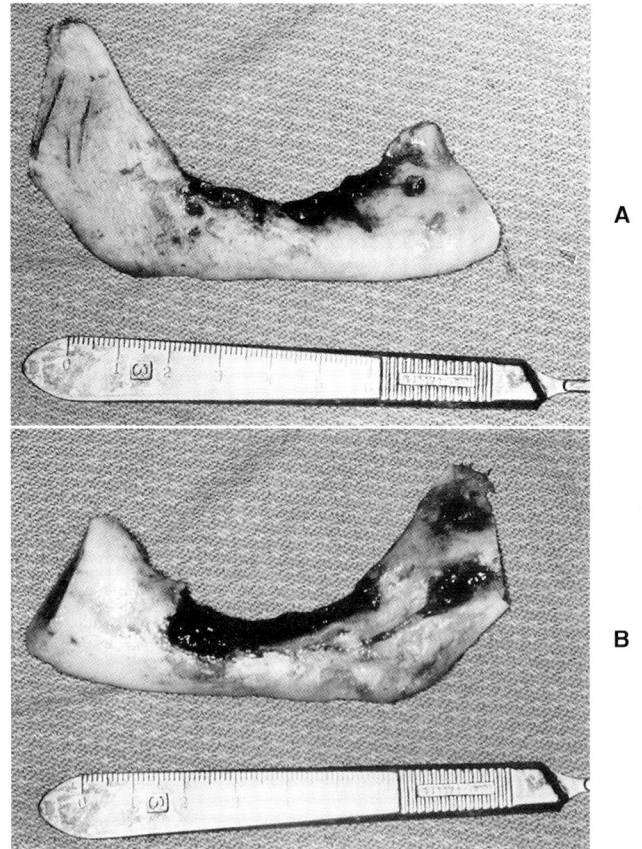

Figure 10-31 A, Lateral view of resected mandible after right partial mandibulectomy in a 60-year-old man in whom osteoradionecrosis developed in the body region after extraction of several mandibular teeth 2 days before beginning radiation treatment. He received 4500 rads for squamous cell carcinoma of the base of the tongue. Conservative management (including injection of bupivacaine) for 18 months resulted in no relief of marked pain; a decision then was made to perform a transoral partial mandibulectomy. **B,** Lingual view of mandible after right partial mandibulectomy. The process affects much of the lingual cortical plate in the midbody region.

motes neovascularity and neocellularity of ischemic tissues and has been used successfully in treating osteoradionecrosis of the jaws.[55]

Although pain associated with osteoradionecrosis may be controlled with narcotic analgesics, nerve blocks with bupivacaine (Marcaine) or alcohol, nerve avulsion, or rhizotomy, definitive treatment should be directed toward either revascularization of the bone or excision of the affected bone, with or without reconstruction, depending on the condition of the patient. Adjunctive treatment with HBO or other modalities may be necessary and feasible in selected patients.

Bone resection Patients who are not candidates for extensive treatment because of their medical condition may achieve pain relief by resection of the segment of involved bone. Intraoral resection usually is possible to reduce the likelihood of an orocutaneous fistula in radiation-compromised skin.[49] The soft tissue wound usually heals by secondary intention (Figure 10-31).

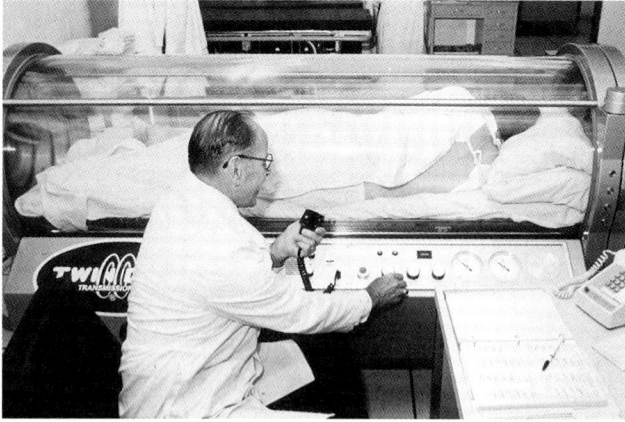

Figure 10-32 Monoplace hyperbaric chamber. The patient is constantly monitored. (Courtesy Eric B. Kindwall.)

HYPERBARIC OXYGEN IN TREATMENT OF OSTEOMYELITIS

HBO therapy consists of breathing 100% oxygen through a face mask or hood in a monoplace (Figure 10-32) or large chamber at 2.4 absolute atmospheres pressure for 90-minute sessions or "dives" for as many as 5 days a week totaling 30 or more sessions often followed by another 10 or more sessions. HBO treatment causes an increase in arterial and venous oxygen tension; the additional oxygen is carried in physical solution in the plasma. Oxygen under increased tension enhances healing by a direct bacteriostatic effect on microorganisms that renders them susceptible to lower antibiotic concentrations and by enhancing phagocytic killing. In addition, neoangiogenesis, fibroblastic proliferation, and collagen synthesis occur. Proliferation of granulation tissue increases and advances under increased oxygen tension from the nondiseased periphery into necrotic bone. As resorption and replacement of devitalized bone with healthy tissue progresses, formation of sequestra that may undergo resorption is enhanced.

Osteomyelitis and osteoradionecrosis of the jaws in some patients is refractory to usual medical and surgical treatment; these patients may be candidates for HBO treatment in conjunction with antibiotic and surgical care (Figure 10-33). Patients with refractory chronic suppurative osteomyelitis and those with chronic diffuse sclerosing osteomyelitis with marked pain often benefit from adjunctive HBO therapy.[42] The greatest value of HBO is in the treatment of osteoradionecrosis of the mandible. Marx[38,39] described a protocol for its effective use in several situations especially for the prevention, treatment, and reconstruction of the mandible where resection was indicated. HBO treatment may account for marked decreases in pain and trismus, closure of fistulas, and complete clinical and radiographic healing.

Marx–University of Miami Protocol HBO therapy without adjunctive surgery occasionally is successful for the definitive care of patients with osteoradionecrosis (Fig-

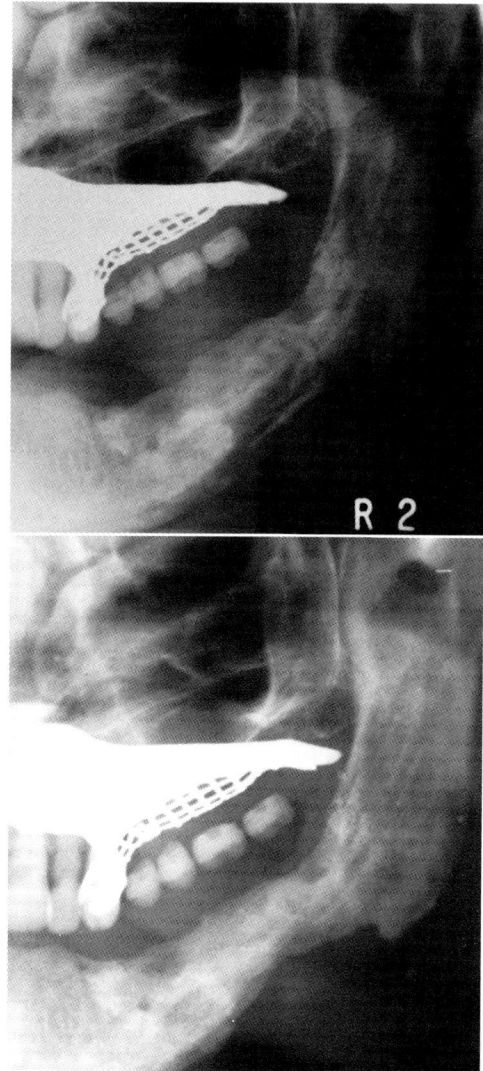

Figure 10-33 A, Radiograph of mandible in a 54-year-old man treated with 85 Gy of cobalt therapy for squamous cell carcinoma of the right floor of the mouth. Approximately 18 months later, osteoradionecrosis developed. Despite intensive conservative therapy, trismus, pain, and exposed bone persisted. Note sequestrum and pathological fracture. **B,** Follow-up radiograph 10 months later, after 120 hours of hyperbaric oxygen at 2 absolute atmospheres (ATA) over a 60-day period. The sequestrum had resorbed and the fracture had healed. (Courtesy Elgene G. Mainous.)

ure 10-33). Combined with surgical measures, it often helps provide a cure. Marx[39] described an HBO protocol for the treatment of osteoradionecrosis under various scenarios with an algorithm for use with dental extractions, dental implants, and for bone graft reconstruction (Figure 10-34). All patients entering this protocol receive 30 sessions of HBO (stage I). Those with a pathological fracture, an orocutaneous fistula, or osteolysis to the inferior border of the mandible as viewed by panoramic radiographs or a CT scan are placed in stage III category and have a continuity resection of the mandible. The mandible is stabilized with a reconstruction plate or external skeletal pins, and a myocutaneous or free vascular flap is used in cases

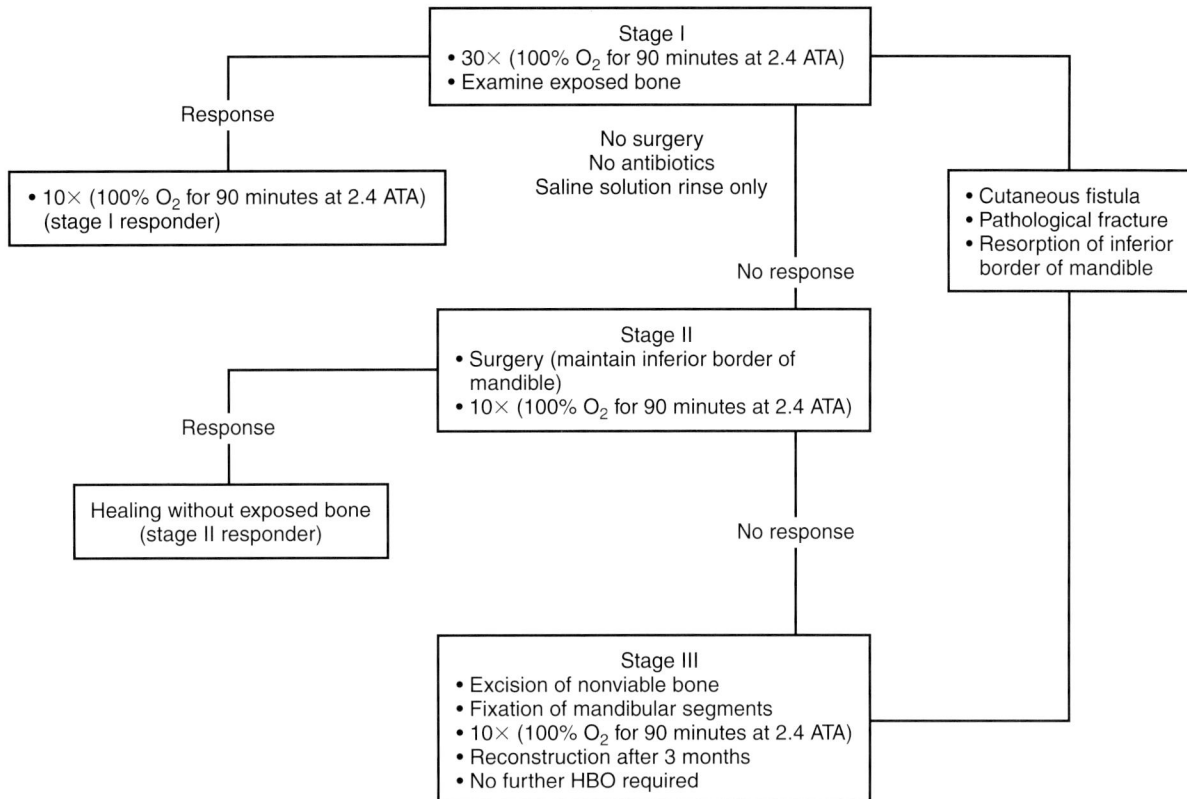

Figure 10-34 Marx–University of Miami Protocol for treatment of osteoradionecrosis of the mandible. *ATA,* Absolute atmosphere pressure. (From Marx RE: Hyperbaric oxygen: its role after radiation therapy. In Booth PW, Schendel SA, Hausamen J-E, editors: *Maxillofacial surgery,* New York, 1999, Churchill Livingstone.)

with soft tissue deficiency. Surgery is followed by 10 postoperative HBO sessions. Bony reconstruction may be accomplished after 3 or more months without the need for further HBO treatment.

Stage I   If individuals with osteoradionecrosis have none of the criteria to place them in stage III, they also undergo the initial 30 HBO sessions. If softening of the exposed bone results (an attempt at spontaneous sequestration and formation of healthy granulation), the wound is debrided and 10 more HBO sessions are provided. If no changes occur in the exposed bone after the initial 30 sessions, patients are reclassified as stage II.

Stage II   Stage II HBO treatment involves a noncontinuity resection of exposed bone to bleeding margins by alveolar bone resection or decortication followed by 10 HBO sessions. If the tissue heals completely with no exposed bone the patient is considered a stage II responder. If wound dehiscence results in exposure of nonviable bone the individual is considered a stage II nonresponder, and together with stage I nonresponders enters stage III treatment.

Stage III   Patients whose condition does not respond to either stage I or II treatment undergo a continuity re-

section and 10 postoperative sessions of HBO and reconstruction after 3 months.

HBO facilities currently are limited, treatment is expensive, and complications and contraindications to use of HBO exist. Reported problems include oxygen toxicity, seizures, high-pressure nervous syndrome, decompression sickness, pneumothorax, arterial gas embolism, tooth and sinus pain, visual changes, and gastric distress.[17] Optic neuritis and immunosuppressive disorders are two absolute contraindications. Relative contraindications are chronic obstructive pulmonary disease and claustrophobia. Most of these conditions are uncommon and can be anticipated and controlled. The need for preextraction HBO treatment continues to be a matter that is debated with regard to the real need and effect on the outcome.[11,46]

PREVENTION OF OSTEORADIONECROSIS

PREIRRADIATION DENTAL CARE

Preventive dental measures are effective in reducing the risk of osteoradionecrosis.[15,68] The radiotherapist should seek dental consultation sufficiently early before initiation of radiation therapy to allow achievement of optimal oral health. Failure to do so may result in bone necrosis months or years after completion of radiation therapy. Although recommendations for dental care differ, the following measures are based on both research and clinical experience:

1. All nonrestorable teeth in the direct beam of radiation and teeth with significant periodontal disease should be extracted 10 to 14 days before radiation therapy begins. In patients with poor oral health and poor motivation to maintain oral hygiene, extraction of all teeth is recommended. Judicious alveoloplasty should be performed to permit a linear closure of the mucoperiosteum. All sharp bone margins should be removed because irradiated bone does not remodel spontaneously.

2. All remaining teeth should be restored and periodontal therapy completed within this 2-week interval. Complete instructions and an opportunity to practice oral hygiene should be provided. Custom trays should be provided to permit application of 0.4% stannous fluoride gel, 1% sodium fluoride gel, or 1% acidulated fluorophosphate gel. After flossing, fluoride treatment should be performed for 15 minutes twice a day for 2 weeks followed by once daily thereafter (Figure 10-35).

POSTIRRADIATION DENTAL CARE

1. Dentures should not be used in the irradiated arch for 1 year after radiotherapy. Subsequently, patients must recognize the need for denture adjustment at the first sign of irritation. If natural teeth are present the oral hygiene and fluoride therapy recommended previously should be followed.

2. A saliva substitute may be used to lubricate the mouth to replace diminished flow from irradiated mucous and salivary glands. When residual salivary gland function is present, pilocarpine may be useful to stimulate salivary flow.

3. If postirradiation pulpitis develops and the involved tooth is restorable, endodontic therapy should be undertaken. Caution must be exercised not to introduce organisms beyond the apex by instrumentation. Treatment should be performed in conjunction with administration of a prophylactic antibiotic.

4. Necessary extractions should be limited to one or two teeth per appointment. Removal of teeth should be performed as atraumatically as possible, with trimming of sharp bone margins only. No attempt should be made to raise flaps or obtain linear closure. A nonlidocaine, low epinephrine concentration or nonepinephrine local anesthetic should be used and antibiotics should be administered. A suggested regimen is 2 g penicillin V plus 500 mg metronidazole orally 1 hour before surgery and 500 mg of both drugs given four times a day for 1 week after extraction. Alternately, 600 mg of clindamycin 1 hour before surgery and 300 mg three times a day for a week is recommended.

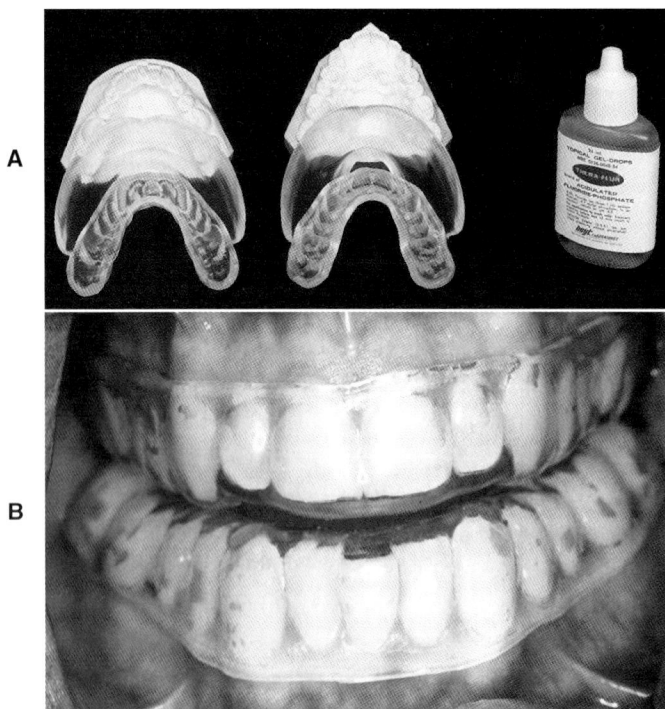

Figure 10-35 A, Photograph shows dental casts, stock plastic trays, and custom-made trays with a bottle of acidulated fluorophosphate solution. **B,** After the teeth have been flossed, the solution is placed in the tray and applied to the teeth as shown for 15 minutes. Treatment is performed twice a day for 2 weeks and then once daily thereafter for an indefinite period.

SUMMARY

Osteomyelitis of the jaws is a disease with significant morbidity unless it is recognized promptly and treated vigorously. In recent years understanding of its microbiology has changed, along with that of other oral infections. Unless communication with the skin occurs, osteomyelitis of the jaws is essentially a disease of streptococci and oral anaerobes, particularly *Peptostreptococcus, Fusobacterium,* and *Prevotella.* Antibiotics should be chosen to control those organisms specifically and not the broad array of other organisms rarely seen in oral infections. When possible, repeated aerobic and anaerobic cultures should be obtained to identify involved organisms since the microbiology of the infection may change over time.

Early recognition of osteomyelitis followed by appropriate antibiotic treatment can prevent extensive loss of bone and teeth. Nevertheless, surgery usually is necessary to drain abscesses and encourage sequestration and removal of nonvital bone. Excision of nonvital bone may result in discontinuity defects of the mandible requiring bone grafting. When properly used in chronic osteomyelitis and osteoradionecrosis, bone grafting usually leads to complete restoration of function. HBO therapy offers new hope for resistant osteomyelitis and has resulted in resolution of infections not amenable to conventional techniques. Despite all advances, however, proper management of osteomyelitis continues to depend on careful clinical and imaging examination, proper assessment of findings, an understanding of the nature of the disease, and a repeated review of the effectiveness of therapy in the individual patient.

REFERENCES

1. Aliabadi P, Nikpoor J: Imaging osteomyelitis, *Arthritis Rheum* 37:617, 1994.
2. Alpert B, Colosi T, van Fraunhofer JA, et al: The in vivo behavior of gentamicin-PMMA beads in the maxillofacial region, *J Oral Maxillofac Surg* 47:46, 1989.
3. Bjorksten B, Gustavson KH, Eriksson B, et al: Chronic recurrent multifocal osteomyelitis and pustulosis palmoplantaris, *J Pediatr* 93:227, 1978.
4. Boda A: Antibiotic irrigation-perfusion treatment of chronic osteomyelitis, *Arch Orthop Trauma Surg* 95:31, 1979.
5. Bowden GHW: Pathogenesis of *Actinomyces israelii* infections. In Ortiz-Ortiz L, Bojalil FF, Yakoleff V, et al, editors: *Biological, biochemical and biomedical aspects of actinomycetes,* Orlando, Fla, 1984, Academic Press.
6. Brook I: Oropharyngeal anaerobes. In Johnson JT, Yu VL, editors: *Infectious diseases and antimicrobial therapy of the ears, nose and throat,* Philadelphia, 1997, WB Saunders.
7. Calhoun KH, Shapiro RD, Stiernberg CM, et al: Osteomyelitis of the mandible, *Arch Otolarygol Head Neck Surg* 114:1157, 1988.
8. Carlson ER: Chronic nonsuppurative osteomyelitis; current concepts, *Oral and Maxillofacial Surgery Knowledge Update,* 1:61, 1994.
9. Chisholm BB, Lew D, Sadasivan IK: The use of tobramycin-impregnated polymethylmethacrylate beads in the treatment of osteomyelitis of the mandible, *J Oral Maxillofac Surg* 51:444, 1993.
10. Cieny G, Mader JT, Pennick H: A clinical staging system of adult osteomyelitis, *Contemp Orthop* 10:17, 1985.
11. Clayman L: Management of dental extractions in irradiated jaws: a protocol without hyperbaric oxygen therapy, *J Oral Maxillofac Surg* 55:275, 1997.
12. Copehhaver WM, Kelly DE, Wood RL: *Bailey's textbook of histology,* ed 17, Baltimore, 1978, Williams & Wilkins.
13. Ellis DJ, Winslow JR, Indovina AA: Garré's osteomyelitis of the mandible: report of a case, *Oral Surg* 44:183, 1977.
14. Ferreira BA: Garré's osteomyelitis: a case report, *Int Endod J* 25:165, 1992.
15. Findlay PM: Prosthetic rehabilitation and implantology after cancer ablation. In Booth PW, Schendel SA, Hausman JE, editors: *Maxillofacial surgery,* London, 1999, Churchill Livingstone.
16. Flynn TR: Anatomy and surgery of deep space infections of the head and neck. In *Knowledge update,* Rosemont, Ill, 1993, American Association of Oral and Maxillofacial Surgeons.
17. Foster JH: Hyperbaric oxygen therapy: contraindications and complications, *J Oral Maxillofac Surg* 50:1081, 1992.
18. Gilbert DN, Moellering RC Jr, Sande MA: *The Sanford guide to antimicrobial therapy,* ed 30, Hyde Park, Vt, 2000, Antimicrobial Therapy Inc.
19. Gold R: Diagnosis of osteomyelitis, *Pediatr Rev* 12:292, 1991.
20. Goldberg MH: Personal communication, October 2000.
21. Grime PD, Bowerman JE, Weller PJ: Gentamicin-impregnated polymethylmethacrylate (PMMA) beads in the treatment of chronic osteomyelitis of the mandible, *Br J Oral Maxillofac Surg* 28:367, 1990.
22. Groot RH, van Merkesteyn JPR, Bras J: Diffuse sclerosing osteomyelitis and florid osseous dysplasia, *Oral Surg* 81:333, 1996.
23. Hahn GW, Corgill DA: Conservative treatment of radionecrosis of the mandible, *Oral Surg* 24:707, 1967.
24. Happonen RP, Viander M: Comparison of fluorescent antibody technique and conventional staining methods of diagnosis of cervicofacial actinomycosis, *J Oral Pathol* 11:417, 1982.
25. Hjorting-Hansen E: Decortication in treatment of radionecrosis of the mandible, *Oral Surg* 29:641, 1970.
26. Holmberg K: Diagnostic methods for human actinomycosis, *Microbiol Sci* 4:72, 1987.
27. Houang ET, Lovett IS, Thompson FD, et al: *Nocardia asteroides* infection: a transmissible disease, *J Hosp Infect* 1:31, 1980.
28. Khosla VM: Chronic osteomyelitis of the mandible, *J Oral Surg* 29:649, 1971.
29. Koorbusch GF, Fotos P, Goll KT: Retrospective assessment of osteomyelitis: etiology, demographics, risk factors and management in 35 cases, *Oral Surg* 74:149, 1992.
30. Koury M, Ellis E III: Rigid internal fixation for the treatment of infected mandibular fractures, *J Oral Maxillofac Surg* 50:434, 1992.
31. Lambert FW Jr, Brown JM, Georg LK: Identification of *Actinomyces israelii* and *Actinomyces naeslundii* by fluorescent antibiody and agar gel diffusion techniques, *J Bacteriol* 94:1287, 1967.
32. Lerner PI: The lumpy jaw. Cervicofacial actinomycosis, *Infect Dis Clin North Am* 2:203, 1988.
33. Lerner PI: Nocardiosis, *Clin Infect Dis* 22:891, 1996.
34. Lew DP, Hinkle RM: Bony reconstruction of the jaws. In Peterson LJ, Indresano AT, Marciani RD, et al, editors: *Principles of oral and maxillofacial surgery,* Philadelphia, 1992, JB Lippincott.
35. Lew DP, Waldvogel FA: Osteomyelitis, *N Engl J Med* 336:999, 1997.
36. Lieblich SE, Topazian RG: Infection in the patient with maxillofacial trauma. In Fonseca RJ, Walker RV, Betts NJ, et al, editors: *Oral and maxillofacial trauma,* ed 2, Philadelphia, 1997, WB Saunders.
37. Mader JT, Calhoun J: Osteomyelitis. In Mandell GL, Bennett JE, Dolin R, editors: *Mandell, Douglas and Bennett's principles and practice of infectious diseases,* ed 5, Philadelphia, 2000, Churchill Livingstone.
38. Marx RE: Chronic osteomyelitis of the jaws, *Oral Maxillofac Surg Clin North Am* 3:367, 1991.
39. Marx RE: Hyperbaric oxygen: its role after radiation therapy. In Booth PW, Schendel SA, Hausamen JE, editors: *Maxillofacial surgery,* New York, 1999, Churchill Livingstone.
40. Marx RE: Osteoradionecrosis: a new concept of its pathophysiology, *J Oral Maxillofac Surg* 41:283, 1983.
41. Marx RE, Carlson ER, Smith BR, et al: Isolation of *Actinomyces* species and *Eiikenella corrodens* from patients with chronic diffuse sclerosing osteomyelitis, *J Oral Maxillofac Surg* 52:26, 1994.
42. Marx RE, Johnson RP: Hyperbaric oxygen in oral and maxillofacial surgery. In Davis JC, Hunt TD, editors: *Problem wounds,* New York, 1986, Elsevier Science.
43. Marx RE, Johnson RP, Kline SN: Prevention of osteoradionecrosis: a randomized prospective clinical trial of hyperbaric oxygen versus penicillin, *J Am Dent Assoc* 111:49, 1985.
44. Marx RE, Stevens MR: Reconstruction of avulsive maxillofacial injuries. In Fonseca RJ, Walker RV, Betts NJ, editors: *Oral and maxillofacial trauma,* ed 2, Philadelphia, 1997, WB Saunders.

45. Mathog RH, Toma V, Clayman L, et al: Nonunion of the mandible: an analysis of contributing factors, *J Oral Maxillofac Surg* 58:746, 2000.

46. Maxymiw WG, Liu FF: Postradiation dental extractions without hyperbaric oxygen, *Oral Surg* 72:270, 1991.

47. Mercuri LG: Acute osteomyelitis of the jaws, *Oral Maxillofac Surg Clin North Am* 3:355, 1991.

48. Mowlem R: Osteomyelitis of the jaws, *Proc R Soc Med* 38:452, 1945.

49. Obwegeser HL, Sailer HF: Experiences with intra-oral partial resection and simultaneous reconstruction in cases of mandibular osteomyelitis, *J Maxillofac Surg* 6:34, 1978.

50. Otsuka K, Hamakawa H, Kayahara H, et al: Chronic recurrent multifocal osteomyelitis involving the mandible in a 4-year-old girl: a case report and a review of the literature, *J Oral Maxillofac Surg* 57:1013, 1999.

51. Perry CR, Davenport K, Vossen MK: Local delivery of antibiotics via an implantable pump in the treatment of osteomyelitis, *Clin Orthop* 226:222, 1988.

52. Peterson LJ: Microbiology of head and neck infections, *Oral Maxillofac Clin North Am* 3:247, 1991.

53. Peterson LR, Thomson RB Jr: Use of the clinical microbiology laboratory for the diagnosis and management of infectious diseases related to the oral cavity, *Infect Dis Clin North Am* 13:775, 1999.

54. Raff MJ, Melo JC: Anaerobic osteomyelitis, *Medicine* 57:83, 1978

55. Reher P, Harris M: Ultrasound for the treatment of osteoradionecrosis, *J Oral Maxillofac Surg* 55:1195, 1997.

56. Rohlin M: Diagnostic value of bone scintigraphy in osteomyelitis of the mandible, *Oral Surg* 75:650, 1993.

57. Russo TA: Agents of actinomycosis. In Mandell GL, Bennett JE, Dolin R, editors: *Mandell, Douglas and Bennett's principles and practice of infectious diseases,* ed 5, Philadelphia, 2000, Churchill Livingstone.

58. Schneider LC, Mesa ML: Differences between florid osseous dysplasia and chronic diffuse sclerosing osteomyelitis, *Oral Surg* 70:308, 1990.

59. Schuknecht BF, Carls FR, Valavanis A, et al: Mandibular osteomyelitis: evaluation and staging in 18 patients, using magnetic resonance imaging, computed tomography and conventional radiography, *J Craniomaxillofacial Surg* 25:24, 1977.

60. Schwartz JG, Tio FO: Nocardial osteomyelitis: a case report and review of the literature, *Diagn Microbiol Infect Dis* 8:37, 1987.

61. Skouteris CA, Velegrakis G, Christodoulou P, et al: Infantile osteomyelitis of the maxilla with concomitant subperiosteal orbital abscess: a case report, *J Oral Maxillofac Surg* 53:67, 1995.

62. Sorrell TC, Iredell JR, Mitchell DH: Nocardia species. In Mandell GL, Bennett JE, Dolin R, *Mandell, Douglas and Bennett's principles and practice of infectious diseases,* ed 5, Philadelphia, 2000, Churchill Livingstone.

63. Turlington EG: *Chronic sclerosing nonsuppurative osteomyelitis.* Transactions of the IV International Conference on Oral Surgery, Munksgaard, Copenhagen, 1973.

64. Van Merkesteyn JPR, Groot RH, Bras J, et al: Diffuse sclerosing osteomyelitis of the mandible: a new concept of its etiology, *Oral Surg* 70:414, 1990.

65. Vezeau PJ, Koorbusch GF, Finkelstein M: Invasive squamous cell carcinoma of the mandible presenting as a chronic osteomyelitis: report of a case, *J Oral Maxillofac Surg* 48:1118, 1990.

66. Weber PC, Seabold JE, Graham SM, et al: Evaluation of temporal and facial osteomyelitis by simultaneous In-WBC/Tc-99m-MDP bone SPECT scintigraphy and computed tomography scan, *Otolargygol Head Neck Surg* 113:36, 1995.

67. Weese WC, Smith JM: A study of 57 cases of actinomycosis over a 36-year period, *Arch Intern Med* 135:1562, 1975.

68. Worrall SF: Avoiding and managing complications in minor oral surgery. In Booth PW, Schendel SA, Hausman JE, editors: *Maxillofacial surgery,* London, 1999, Churchill Livingstone.

69. Worth HM: *Principles and practice of radiology,* Chicago, 1969, Year Book Medical.

70. Worth HM, Stoneman DW: Osteomyelitis, malignancy disease, and fibrous dysplasia. Some radiologic similarities and differences, *Dent Radiogr Photogr* 50:1, 1977.

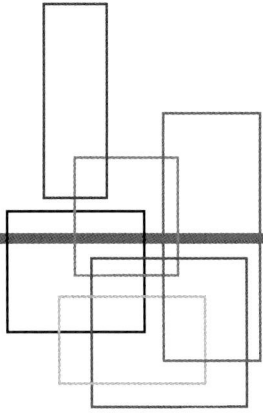

Fungal, Viral, and Protozoal Infections of the Maxillofacial Region

Stewart A. Bergman

FUNGAL INFECTIONS

Fungal infections are a major source of morbidity and mortality. Patients increasingly are at risk of infection, invasion, and dissemination. Significant risk factors include long-term, broad-spectrum antibiotic therapy; immunosuppression, whether iatrogenic (i.e., patients who have undergone organ transplantation or with cancer undergoing immunosuppressive chemotherapy) or acquired (i.e., patients with acquired immunodeficiency syndrome [AIDS]); and critical injuries.

Medically important fungi are divided into two basic categories: pathogenic and opportunistic. Pathogenic fungi cause infection even in hosts with normal immune function, whereas opportunistic fungi, because of low virulence, produce invasive infections primarily in immunocompromised hosts. Pathogenic fungal infections occur in endemic areas. These virulent fungi include *Histoplasma capsulatum* (histoplasmosis), *Blastomyces dermatitidis* (North American blastomycosis), *Paracoccidioides brasiliensis* (South American blastomycosis, paracoccidioidomycosis), and *Coccidioides immitis* (coccidioidomycosis). These organisms are infectious but not contagious. Only the airborne spores are infectious. The opportunistic fungi include *Candida albicans* (candidiasis), *Aspergillus fumigatus* and *Aspergillus flavus* (aspergillosis), *Mucor* and *Rhizopus* organisms (mucormycosis), *Sporothrix schenckii* (sporotrichosis), *Cryptococcus neoformans* (cryptococcosis), and *Pneumocystis carinii* (pneumocystosis).

PATHOGENIC FUNGAL INFECTIONS

HISTOPLASMOSIS

Histoplasmosis has a worldwide distribution but is more prevalent in certain parts of North and Latin America.[93] Endemic areas in the United States include the eastern and central regions, especially the Mississippi and Ohio River valleys.

Although most cases of histoplasmosis occur in the endemic areas, cases have been identified outside those areas.[25] Once primarily a disease of rural communities, histoplasmosis has emerged as a problem in many urban areas[26] (Box 11-1).

Pathogenesis Spores (microconidia) or mycelial fragments are inhaled by patients. Usually they cause a localized or patchy pneumonitis. However, if the patient inhales a large inoculum, severe, often fatal pneumonitis can result.[96] In addition, hematogenous dissemination from the lungs to other tissues frequently occurs before specific immunity has developed, usually during the first 2 weeks after infection.[72] Dissemination is believed to occur through intracellular transport by macrophages and neutrophils that have phagocytosed the organism.

Cellular immunity develops 10 to 14 days after exposure. Immunity develops first in the lungs and mediastinal lymph nodes and then throughout the reticuloendothelial system.[28] CD4[+] T lymphocytes are activated by antigen-presenting cells that have phagocytosed and processed fungal antigens. These activated T lymphocytes interact with the antigen-presenting cells and cause upregulation of myeloperoxidase enzymes, allowing them to assume fungicidal properties. These defense mechanisms are potent enough to control the infection in individuals who are immunocompetent. This factor explains the subclinical or self-limited course characteristic of acute histoplasmosis. More than 40 million Americans have had histoplasmosis; most cases have been subclinical. Fewer than 5% of exposed individuals develop symptomatic disease after low-level exposure.[93] However, after heavy exposure most patients develop symptomatic infection. In the absence of intact cellular immunity, progressive illness occurs characterized by hematogenous dissemination and involvement of extrapulmonary tissues.

Reactivation of old foci of infection in histoplasmosis may occur as a consequence of immunosuppression,

243

BOX 11-1

Histoplasmosis

Endemic area
United States: Mississippi and Ohio River valleys
Africa, Southeast Asia, Caribbean, Central and South
America

Pathogenesis
Inhalation of microconidia, mycelial fragments; not
transmitted person to person

Clinical Characteristics
Primary disease
Low-level exposure: asymptomatic
High-level exposure: flulike URI
Fever, chills, headache, myalgia, chest pain, cough,
arthralgias
Mediastinal granuloma and fibrosis
Airway obstruction, eosphageal constriction
Chronic disease
Cavitary pulmonary disease: low-grade fever, produc-
tive cough, dyspnea, weight loss
Disseminated disease
Patients who are immunosuppressed, infants
Fever, malaise, weight loss, cough, diarrhea, he-
patosplenomegaly, cervical lymphadenopathy, ane-
mia, leukopenia
Focal and diffuse CNS disease
Oral and skin lesions: granulomatous nodules and ul-
cers on lips, tongue, buccal mucosa, and palate

Diagnosis
Isolation of organism from body fluids or tissues, serology, PCR

Treatment
Treatment usually not necessary
Severe disease
Itraconazole (200 mg/day × 4-6 wk PO)
Disseminated disease, CNS disease
Amphotericin B (0.4 to 0.6 mg/kg/day)

URI, Upper respiratory tract infection; *CNS,* central nervous system; *PCR,* polymerase chain reaction.

primarily as a result of reduced cellular immunity. Typically such cases are recognized outside endemic areas in
patients who previously lived in endemic regions. Reinfection also occurs in histoplasmosis. Evidence for reinfection includes the occurrence of acute histoplasmosis
in individuals with radiographic, skin test, or laboratory
evidence of past infection. Reinfection histoplasmosis
may be less severe than first episodes as a result of protective immunity induced by the primary episode.[93]

Clinical Characteristics   The most common manifestations of histoplasmosis in the normal host after heavy exposure include flulike pulmonary illnesses, pericarditis,
and arthritis or arthralgia with erythema nodosum. Acute
pulmonary histoplasmosis is characterized by fever, chills,
headache, myalgia, anorexia, cough, and chest pain. Chest

radiographs usually reveal enlarged hilar or mediastinal
lymph nodes associated with patchy infiltrates. Most patients recover within a few weeks but some report fatigue
for several months. In more severe cases, patients often develop respiratory insufficiency caused by diffuse pulmonary involvement, characterized by reticulonodular or
miliary pulmonary infiltrates suggestive of tuberculosis.
Some patients have progressive extrapulmonary dissemination. Obstructive syndromes caused by enlarged mediastinal lymph nodes encroaching on either the airway or
pulmonary arteries may occur in patients with acute pulmonary histoplasmosis. Symptoms include chest pain,
cough, hemoptysis, and dyspnea. In addition, compression
with erosion of the esophagus may occur resulting in
esophagobronchial or tracheoesophageal fistulas. Symptoms include chest pain and dysphagia. Pericarditis has
been reported in approximately 10% of symptomatic cases
and is caused by an immunological reaction initiated by
the histoplasma organisms. In rare cases, pericarditis may
be a complication of disseminated histoplasmosis. Patients
commonly have chest pain, pericardial friction rub, pulsus
paradoxus, and fever. Hemodynamic compromise may occur as a result of pericardial effusion. Rheumatological
manifestations also occur in approximately 10% of patients
with symptoms, the majority of whom are women. The
arthritis is polyarticular and symmetrical and affects joints
of the upper and lower extremities with equal frequency.
Nearly half of such patients develop erythema nodosum.
Joint radiographs usually reveal normal findings.[93]

Disseminated histoplasmosis as a result of hematogenous spread is rare. Progressive illness occurs most frequently in patients who are immunocompromised, and elderly or very young patients. Severity varies with degree of
immune deficiency and extent of exposure. An acute,
rapidly fatal course with widespread involvement characterizes the infection in infants and patients who are severely immunocompromised. A chronic course with a
more focal organ distribution is characteristic of children
and adults who are immunocompetent. Clinical findings
are nonspecific and usually include fever, weight loss, hepatosplenomegaly, and lymphadenopathy. Less frequently
skin and mucosal lesions occur. The oral lesions occur on
the lips, buccal mucosa, palate, and tongue. The lesions are
granulomatous and can persist as nodular lesions and ulcerate. Skin lesions manifest as subcutaneous nodules,
papules, and ulcers. Abscesses and cellulitis may develop.
Eczematous dermatitis, erythema nodosum, and erythema
multiforme also have been reported. Chronic meningitis
occurs in approximately 10% of cases. Less commonly
granulomas develop in the brain or spinal cord. Addison's
disease is an uncommon finding.[93]

Diagnosis   Because the clinical manifestations of
histoplasmosis are similar to many other diseases, definitive diagnosis depends on detection of the organisms
by microscopy, culture, and isolation. Diseases most frequently confused with histoplasmosis include tuberculosis, carcinoma, leukemia, sarcoidosis, and Hodgkin's
disease. Other laboratory tests useful in diagnosis are

antigen detection and serological tests for antibodies. These tests are reasonably specific and serve as the basis for diagnosis in patients with compatible clinical manifestations. Culture results are positive in 85% of patients with disseminated infections. Similar success rates are achieved in patients with AIDS and severe immunosuppression. The highest yield is achieved from bone marrow samples. Blood culture results are positive in 50% to 70% of patients. In patients with diffuse interstitial or miliary pulmonary infiltrates, *Histoplasma capsulatum* may be isolated from the sputum, alveolar lavage specimens, or lung tissue. Urine culture findings are positive in approximately 40% of cases. Biopsy results of lesions of the mouth, skin, and enlarged lymph nodes are positive in 25% of cases. *H. capsulatum* organisms typically require several weeks to grow in culture. Multiple specimens often are needed, especially in patients with mild disease. Recent nucleic acid probes using polymerase chain reactions (PCRs) have been developed, which have shortened the time necessary to identify a fungus as *H. capsulatum* to only a few hours.[93]

Culture results infrequently are positive in patients with acute pulmonary histoplasmosis, mediastinal granuloma, pericarditis, and rheumatic disease. In these cases, antigen detection may be useful. Cross-reactions have occurred in patients with penicilliosis, paracoccidioidomycosis, and blastomycosis since these organisms share similar antigens. Cross-reactions do not occur with *Aspergillus, Candida,* and *Cryptococcus* organisms. However, diagnosis often can be made based on the clinical presentation and epidemiological features.

Treatment The majority of cases of acute pulmonary histoplasmosis do not require treatment. Bed rest and antipyretics usually suffice. However, for patients with high inocula, those with fever for more than 1 week, or patients with respiratory compromise, anorexia, and malaise, the administration of itraconazole (200 mg PO qd for 4 to 6 weeks) is appropriate and sufficient for most patients. Alternatively, ketoconazole (400 mg PO qd) can be used. Fluconazole is less active than the other drugs and should not be used. If the patient cannot tolerate azole drugs, amphotericin B (0.4 to 0.5 mg/kg IV qd) is preferred until symptoms subside. The azole drugs are highly lipophilic agents that inhibit the cytochrome P-450 enzyme systems. Consequently, numerous drug interactions are possible. Caution is needed for patients who are taking concomitant drugs to ensure the avoidance of any adverse drug interactions.[14]

Disseminated histoplasmosis is a life-threatening disease. Prompt amphotericin B therapy is essential. The mortality rate without treatment is high. Mortality with antifungal therapy can be reduced significantly. Patients should receive 25 mg as the initial dose, followed by increasing dosages to 0.7 to 1.0 mg/kg per day. Symptoms improve in most patients within 1 week. When the patient becomes afebrile and is in clinically stable condition, the amphotericin B dosage can be reduced to 0.4 to 0.5 mg/kg per day. After resolution of symptoms, itraconazole (400 mg/day) is administered for up to 6 months in place of am-

photericin B. In patients with mild forms of disseminated histoplasmosis or who have intact immune systems, itraconazole (400 mg qd) is efficacious. The success rate approaches 90%. Patients who develop meningitis or central nervous system (CNS) involvement must be treated with amphotericin B because the azoles itraconazole and ketoconazole do not cross the blood brain barrier.[14]

COCCIDIOIDOMYCOSIS

Pathogenesis The primary pathogen of coccidioidomycosis is *C. immitis,* which lives in soil. The infectious particle is the arthroconidium (arthrospore). When the arthroconidia become airborne (e.g., in dust storms) they can be inhaled into the lungs. In the lungs the arthroconidia transform into spherical cells (spherules) that undergo multiple cell divisions, dividing the spherule into multiple compartments, each containing a viable daughter cell or endospore. In tissue the spherules may become as large as 75 μm in diameter. The spherule ruptures when it matures, releasing the endospores that spread to adjacent tissues and repropagate. *C. immitis* is endemic to the southwestern United States, principally the states of California, Arizona, and Texas, and Mexico and Central and South America (Box 11-2).

Clinical Characteristics Sixty percent of individuals infected by *C. immitis* have no symptoms or develop symptoms indistinguishable from other upper respiratory tract infections. The only indication that they have had coccidioidomycosis is a positive coccidioidal skin test result. The remaining 40% develop symptoms characteristic of a lower respiratory tract infection approximately 3 weeks after exposure. Symptoms include fever, sweating, anorexia, weakness, arthralgias, cough, sputum production, and chest pain. As with histoplasmosis, erythema nodosum or erythema multiforme may develop. Chest radiographic findings include infiltrates, pleural effusion, and hilar adenopathy.[86] In patients with normal immune competence the symptoms resolve without any specific therapy, although the illness may last several weeks. In approximately 5% of these cases, patients have residual nodules or thin wall cavities in the lungs. In rare cases the acute pulmonary infection does not resolve and progressive pneumonia or chronic lung infection results. Infection occurs most commonly in patients with diabetes and patients who are immunocompromised.

Disseminated Disease Disseminated extrapulmonary disease develops in approximately 1 in 200 people infected with *C. immitis.* Common extrapulmonary sites are the meninges, bone, joints, skin, and soft tissue organs. Widespread miliary dissemination is rare and when it occurs usually results in death. Hematogenous spread is a common occurrence, probably as a result of intracellular residence in migrating macrophages. However, widespread disease is unlikely, indicating the potency of the host's immune response. As with histoplasmosis the T lymphocytes play a critical role in the development of cell-mediated immunity that is

Coccidioidomycosis

Endemic Area
Southwestern United States: California, Arizona, and Texas
Mexico, Central and South America

Pathogenicity
Inhalation of arthroconidia (spores)

Clinical Characteristics
Primary disease
Majority asymptomatic or mild URI
Remainder lower respiratory tract infection: fever, sweating, anorexia, weakness, arthralgias, cough, sputum production, and chest pain
Chronic disease
Pulmonary nodules and cavities, progressive pneumonia, pleuritic pain, cough, hemoptysis
Disseminated disease
Immunosuppressed patients, predilection for skin, joints, and bone
Skin: maculopapular, keratotic, verrucous ulcers (nasolabial fold), subcutaneous abscesses, cervical lymphadenopathy
Joints: synovitis, effusions (knees, hands, feet)
Bone: lytic lesions long bones, vertebra
CNS: meningitis

Diagnosis
Isolation of organism in body fluids and tissues, serology, PCR

Treatment
Treatment usually not necessary
Severe disease
Itraconazole (200 mg/day × 4 to 6 wk PO) or ketoconazole (400 mg/day × 4 to 6 wk PO)
Disseminated disease, CNS disease
Amphotericin B (0.4 to 0.6 mg/kg/day)

URI, Upper respiratory tract infection; *CNS,* central nervous system; *PCR,* polymerase chain reaction.

responsible for resolution of the infection. Disseminated infections occur most commonly in men, pregnant women, individuals who are immunocompromised, and nonwhite people, especially those of Filipino ancestry.

In disseminated diseases the bones most frequently involved are the skull, hands, feet, and spine. In addition, the tibia frequently is involved. Joint lesions usually are unifocal with prominent synovitis and effusions. The ankles and knees are the most common joints affected. The most frequent site of dissemination is the skin. Lesions vary from maculopapular to wartlike, verrucous keratotic ulcers. Subcutaneous fluctuant cold abscesses or nodules often develop. These lesions usually occur in the nasolabial fold. Supraclavicular and cervical lymphadenopathy frequently is present. Meningitis is the most serious manifestation of disseminated disease. The basilar meninges are the most common sites of meningeal disease. The initial symptoms

are headache, vomiting, and altered mental status rather than signs of meningeal irritation. Early diagnosis of meningitis is essential, because without treatment 90% of patients are likely to die within 12 months.[86]

Diagnosis   Failure to consider coccidioidomycosis is the major reason for failure of diagnosis. Culture and serological testing remain the primary methods of diagnosis. Culture requires 3 to 4 days for growth of colonies. However, *C. immitis* cannot be definitively identified in the mycelial form. Conversion to the arthrospore and inoculation of animals, special cultures, or the detection of extracellular coccidioidal antigens are required to identify the fungus. Specific deoxyribonucleic acid (DNA) probes can shorten significantly the time necessary for identification by PCR. Alternatively, identification of a mature spherule of *C. immitis* with endospores in a tissue specimen is pathognomonic.

The mycelial-phase antigen, coccidioidin, can be used to reliably detect antibody. Immunoglobulin M (IgM) antibody can be detected for a short period in 75% of individuals with primary infection.[68] IgG antibodies appear later and are present for several months after resolution of the infection. High titers of IgG antibodies occur in patients with disseminated disease and can be used as a marker of treatment effectiveness. Most affected individuals have positive skin test results after infection. Skin testing rarely is useful clinically because a positive test results merely indicates prior infection. Anergy commonly develops in progressive disease; consequently, a false-negative test result can occur.

Treatment   Most patients recover without treatment. However, patients with severe primary infection or high antibody titers should receive treatment. The oral azoles are effective and allow outpatient treatment. Treatment for a few weeks is likely to resolve signs and symptoms of acute infection. Ketoconazole (200 to 400 mg qd for 4 to 6 weeks) can be prescribed. Prolonged therapy is always indicated in patients with disseminated disease. Amphotericin B in doses similar to those used for disseminated histoplasmosis should be administered until the disease becomes inactive, or for a total of 2 to 3 months. Because of its more rapid onset, amphotericin B is the drug of choice in patients with severe pulmonary compromise or those whose condition is deteriorating rapidly. Lipid-complex amphotericin B, which provides high serum levels and fewer adverse effects, may be an acceptable alternative. In patients with chronic or less severe disseminated disease, the oral azoles itraconazole (200 mg bid) or fluconazole (400 mg qd) are proven effective alternatives to amphotericin B.[9,36,46] Therapy should continue for at least 6 months after the disease becomes inactive to prevent relapse.

Surgical intervention depends on the nature of the specific lesions. Pulmonary resection should be considered in patients with severe hemoptysis or cavities that rupture or enlarge during chemotherapy. Surgery also is indicated to drain empyemas, close persistent bronchopleural fistulas, and expand lungs restricted by residual disease. Surgery is indicated in patients with extensive musculoskeletal involvement. Local debridement and drainage of infected sites may be critical to control the infection. Surgery also may be necessary to stabilize pathological fractures or prevent vertebral compression.

NORTH AMERICAN BLASTOMYCOSIS

Pathogenesis North American blastomycosis, also known as Gilchrist's disease, is caused by the organism *B. dermatitidis*. The disease is endemic to specific areas of the United States, primarily the Mississippi and Ohio River basins, and specific areas of Africa and India. Males are affected predominantly, especially between the ages of 25 and 50 years. Infection occurs primarily through inhalation of the fungal conidium into the lung parenchyma. Infection usually is confined to the lungs, but disseminated disease may occur. The most frequent sites of involvement include the skin, bone, genitourinary tract, and CNS. Between 40% and 80% of patients with pulmonary disease develop skin lesions.[92] Cell-mediated immunity plays a critical role in the host's defense against disease. In contrast to other systemic fungal infections the risk of disseminated disease is not increased in patients with AIDS or others who are immune suppressed[67] (Box 11-3).

Clinical Characteristics More than half of patients with blastomycosis have no symptoms. When symptoms are present, they resemble those of chronic atypical pneumonia. Pulmonary radiographs frequently show normal findings. However, in patients with more severe disease, radiographic findings resemble those of bronchiogenic carcinoma and granulomatous processes (e.g., tuberculosis, sarcoidosis, histoplasmosis, silicosis). Often cavitary lesions, hilar adenopathy, fibronodular infiltrates, and rarely, pulmonary fibrosis are seen. Skin and mucous membrane lesions are common in disseminated disease. The skin of the face and unclothed areas are the more common sites. Characteristic lesions have a verrucous border and white to yellow cribriform atrophic centers. Pustules and a yellow crust often are present at the border of the lesion. Less commonly lesions are ulcerative. They begin as small, ulcerative pustules with a granulomatous base.[15]

Diagnosis Definitive diagnosis of blastomycosis depends on growth in culture of the organism derived from clinical specimens. *B. dermatitidis* can be identified by its characteristic thick-walled, broad-based budding yeast cells in tissue samples. Serological studies usually are not used because of poor sensitivities and possible false-positive results related to cross-reactivity with other fungi. Enzyme-linked immunosorbent assay with the A-antigen of *B. dermatitidis* provides increased sensitivity but is not available in most laboratories.

Treatment Treatment of blastomycosis depends on the severity of disease and patient immune status. No treatment is necessary in mild cases. Antifungal therapy is required in more severe cases or in those in which signs and

---

BOX 11-3

North American Blastomycosis

Endemic Area
United States: Mississippi and Ohio River valleys
Parts of Africa and India

Pathogenesis
Inhalation of arthroconidia (spores)

Clinical Characteristics
Primary disease
Most patients asymptomatic
Symptoms similar to atypical pneumonia: fever, nonproductive cough, chest pain, myalgias, arthralgias
Chronic disease
Productive cough, hemoptysis, pleuritic pain, low-grade fever; pulmonary nodules and cavities possible
Disseminated disease
Skin lesions most common: papulopustular verrucous lesions, crusted, gray to violaceous on exposed skin; subcutaneous nodules, ulcers; mucosal lesions: nose, mouth, larynx; bone, and joint often with draining sinuses; prostatitis, epididymitis; CNS; liver, spleen (immunocompromised host)

Diagnosis
Isolation of organism from clinical specimens: pus, secretions, and so on; serology helpful but not diagnostic; PCR

Treatment
Mild cases
No treatment necessary
Severe cases
Itraconazole (200-400 mg/day × 2 mo)
Disseminated disease, life-threatening disease
Amphotericin B (0.4-0.6 mg/kg/day IV)

CNS, Central nervous system; *PCR*, polymerase chain reaction.

---

symptoms persist or progress. Amphotericin B is the drug of choice in life-threatening disease, in cases with CNS involvement, and in patients who are immunosuppressed. The oral azole drugs, ketoconazole, fluconazole, and itraconazole, are efficacious in treatment of mild to moderate disease. Itraconazole (200 to 400 mg/day) was successful and well tolerated in 95% of patients treated for a minimum of 2 months.[21] Surgery has little role in the treatment of blastomycosis. Drainage of abscesses and empyema fluid and debridement of devitalized bone are important when fluid accumulation is present.

SOUTH AMERICAN BLASTOMYCOSIS (PARACOCCIDIOIDOMYCOSIS)

Pathogenesis Paracoccidioidomycosis is an uncommon systemic mycosis caused by *P. brasiliensis*. The disease is restricted to Latin America and found throughout South America. Endemic areas are tropical and subtropical forests where temperatures are mild and humidity high. The largest number of cases are reported in Brazil, Colombia,

South American Blastomycosis (Paracoccidioidomycosis)

Endemic Area
Throughout Latin America, especially Brazil, Colombia, Argentina, and Venezuela

Pathogenesis
Inhalation of arthroconidia (spores)

Clinical Characteristics
Primary disease
Most cases asymptomatic, rare in children and teenagers; organism possibly dormant for years; lung primary site of involvement: URI, fever, productive cough, chest pain, myalgias, arthralgias
Disseminated disease
Mucosal painful ulceration of upper respiratory and gastrointestinal tract common, especially mouth (lips, gingiva, tongue, and nose), tooth loss, dysphagia, change in voice; verrucous skin lesions on face and upper limbs; bone, liver, spleen, and urogenital tract frequently affected

Diagnosis
Identification of organism in biopsy of infected tissue, serology useful adjunct, PCR

Treatment
Fluconazole or ketoconazole (200-400 mg/day × 6-18 mo, amphotericin B (0.4-0.6 mg/kg/day) for severe or disseminated disease

URI, Upper respiratory tract infection.

Argentina, and Venezuela. In endemic areas, more than 70% of the population have positive skin test results to paracoccidioidin, suggesting a high incidence of asymptomatic or undiagnosed cases. The disease is rare in children and teenagers, and is most common in men older than 30 years of age. Agricultural workers are at greatest risk. Inhalation of the infectious arthroconidia appears to be the method of infection (Box 11-4).

Clinical Characteristics   Like other mycotic diseases, the majority of cases of paracoccidioidomycosis are asymptomatic. Unlike other mycoses, *P. brasiliensis* may remain dormant for long periods. Years later, when the patient becomes immunosuppressed or debilitated, the fungus multiplies and causes clinical disease. Cell-mediated immunity, as with other mycoses, plays a critical role in host defense.

Paracoccidioidomycosis is often a severe, progressive polymorphic disease that causes more severe disease in young people and a more chronic condition in adults. The lungs are the site of primary infection. In the juvenile form, respiratory complaints are minimal, whereas in the adult respiratory symptoms predominate. In the adult form of the disease, painful mucosal ulceration in the upper respiratory and digestive tracts, especially in the mouth (lips,

gingiva, and tongue) and nose, occurs frequently. Tooth loss is common. Patients usually report difficulty in swallowing and changes in voice. Verrucous skin lesions occur predominantly on the face and limbs. Cervical and axillary lymph nodes often are enlarged. Respiratory symptoms include shortness of breath, productive persistent cough, and chest pain. Pulmonary cavitation occurs in approximately one third of patients. Other sites of dissemination include bones, urogenital tract, brain, liver, spleen, and adrenal glands.[80]

Diagnosis   The primary method of diagnosis of paracoccidioidomycosis is biopsy of infected tissue. The presence of round, double-contoured, single-budding organisms, usually within multinucleated giant cells surrounded by a granulomatous cellular infiltrate, is characteristic. Adjunctive serological tests are useful to confirm clinical impressions and helpful in monitoring treatment effectiveness. The agar gel immunodiffusion test demonstrates circulating antibodies in nearly 95% of cases and has high specificity. Complement fixation is unreliable because of a high incidence of false-negative results and cross-reactivity with *H. capsulatum.* DNA probes with PCR can detect even small amounts of *P. brasiliensis* DNA and may replace these tests.

Treatment   Several antimicrobial agents are effective in the treatment of paracoccidioidomycosis. Sulfadiazine or sulfisoxazole therapy can arrest disease progress, but relapse often occurs unless continuous therapy is maintained for 3 to 5 years. All oral azole drugs are effective. Fluconazole (200 to 400 mg/day) resulted in a response rate of more than 90%. Ketoconazole (200 to 400 mg/day) also provided effective therapy. Because of its lower toxicity, itraconazole ultimately may prove to be the drug of choice. Oral azole therapy must be maintained for at least 6 months or as long as 18 months to prevent relapse.[80] Amphotericin B should be used only in cases of severe life-threatening disease.

OPPORTUNISTIC FUNGAL INFECTIONS

CANDIDIASIS *(Candida albicans)*

Invasive opportunistic fungal infections rarely were diagnosed before the 1960s. For example, the isolation of *Candida* species from human tissue or body fluids was viewed as a contaminant and of little clinical importance. The invasive potential of *C. albicans* was not appreciated until 1968. Krause et al.[48] recovered *C. albicans* in urine and blood after ingestion of the organism into a normally functioning intestine. Autopsy reports showed that *C. albicans* can invade solid organs. In the 1980s, *Candida* infections were shown to significantly increase the morbidity and mortality of critically injured patients and patients who are immunosuppressed.[39] In the last decade, *Candida* has become the fourth most likely nosocomial pathogen to be isolated in the blood of hospitalized patients[27,56] (Box 11-5).

BOX 11-5

Candidiasis

Pathogenesis
Commensal organisms: colonization of skin and mucosa of gastrointestinal and genitourinary tracts
Endogenous invasion caused by breach of host defenses
Natural: multiorgan failures, shock, HIV
Iatrogenic: multiple intravascular catheters, broad-spectrum antibiotic therapy, immunosuppression for transplant patients or cases caused by chemotherapy for malignancy

Clinical Characteristics
Mucocutaneous
Oral mucosal lesions:
Pseudomembranous—creamy white, curdlike patches affecting lips, tongue, gingiva, and oral mucosa
Acute atrophic—nonspecific atrophy of mucosa of tongue
Chronic atrophic—chronic inflammation and epithelial thinning
Angular cheilitis—symmetrical inflammatory lesions of corners of mouth
Candida leukoplakia—firm, white, hyperkeratotic plaques surrounded by erythematous mucosa
Similar lesions possible anywhere in gastrointestinal tract—esophagus, small and large intestines
Deep organs
Common manifestation of disseminated disease
Involvement of almost any organ possible
Microabscesses: brain, bone and joints, liver, spleen, and urinary tract
Diagnosis
Clinical presentation and location
Biopsy and identification of organism and isolation in culture, PCR

Treatment
Mucocutaneous
Tropical antifungal agents—nystatin, clotrimazole, and miconazole
Systemic
Oral azole drugs—ketoconazole and fluconazole
Disseminated disease
Amphotericin B

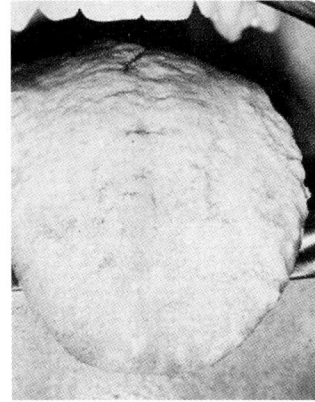

Figure 11-1 Pseudomembranous candidiasis of the tongue. (From Weinert M, Grimes RM, Lynch DP: Oral manifestations of HIV infection, *Ann Intern Med* 125:485, 1996.)

activation, is critical to the effectiveness of phagocytosis. Neutrophils and monocytes lacking myeloperoxidase fail to kill *C. albicans* efficiently.[51] Humoral factors, although incapable of killing *Candida* directly, are significant because of the facilitation of phagocytosis by the phagocytes' Fc immunoglobulin and complement receptors. *Candida* activates both the classic and alternate complement pathways. Other humoral factors inhibit candidal growth.[54] As expected, the CD4$^+$ T lymphocyte plays a critical role in activating cell-mediated host immunity to candidal infection.[39] Host defense mechanisms are so effective that *Candida* infections occurs only when these mechanisms are breached. Two types of factors are responsible for immune compromise: naturally occurring and iatrogenic. Natural factors include shock and multiple organ failure, especially the kidneys, liver, and lungs in patients with critical injuries. Another major factor is the presence of human immunodeficiency virus (HIV) infection. Iatrogenic factors are the most important because they predispose patients to candidal infection, especially disseminated candidiasis. The most common iatrogenic factors include more intense therapeutic efforts involving intravascular catheters, administration of broad-spectrum antibiotics, and immunosuppression for neoplastic disease and allograft preservation.

Clinical Characteristics

Mucocutaneous Candidiasis Mucous membrane infections include oral candidiasis (thrush), *Candida* esophagitis, gastrointestinal candidiasis, and *Candida* vaginitis. Thrush or oral candidiasis is a common disease. Classic lesions are characterized by creamy white, curdlike patches on the tongue, gingiva, lips, and oral mucosa. The uvula, soft palate, and tonsillar pillars also may be affected. Scraping of the mucosal surface easily removes the patch but leaves a raw, bleeding, and painful surface. The patch is a pseudomembrane consisting of *Candida*, desquamated epithelial cells, leukocytes, bacteria, keratin, necrotic tissue, and food debris (Figure 11-1). Other

Pathogenesis *C. albicans* is a commensal organism that colonizes the skin and mucosal tissues of the gastrointestinal and genitourinary tracts. Although person-to-person transmission of disease technically is possible, the majority of *Candida* infections are of endogenous origin. An intact integument is an effective barrier to *Candida* invasion. Maceration of the integument or the placement of indwelling catheters provides sites for opportunistic invasion even in healthy hosts. As with the more virulent fungi, phagocytosis is critical to host defenses against infection. The generation of reactive oxygen radicals, hydrogen peroxide and superoxide through myeloperoxidase

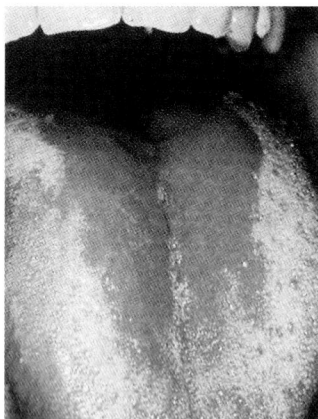

Figure 11-2 Atrophic candidiasis of the tongue. (From Weinert M, Grimes RM, Lynch DP: Oral manifestations of HIV infection, *Ann Intern Med* 125:485, 1996.)

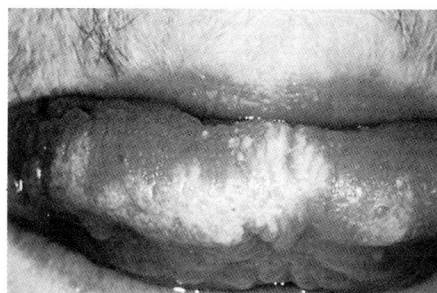

Figure 11-4 Hyperkeratotic candidiasis of the tongue. (From Weinert M, Grimes RM, Lynch DP: Oral manifestations of HIV infection, *Ann Intern Med* 125:485, 1996.)

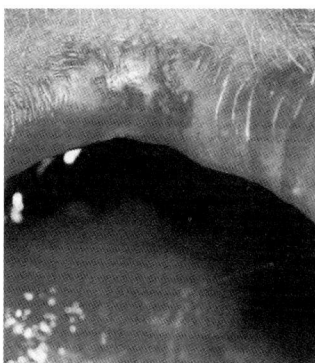

Figure 11-3 Angular cheilitis candidiasis. (From Weinert M, Grimes RM, Lynch DP: Oral manifestations of HIV infection, *Ann Intern Med* 125:485, 1996.)

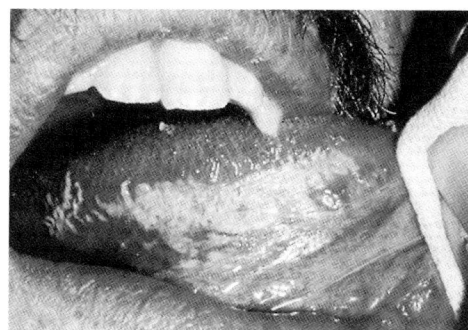

Figure 11-5 Hairy leukoplakia of the tongue. (From Weinert M, Grimes RM, Lynch DP: Oral manifestations of HIV infection, *Ann Intern Med* 125:485, 1996.)

forms of oral candidiasis include (1) acute atrophic candidiasis characterized by nonspecific atrophy of the tongue believed to be a sequela of pseudomembranous candidiasis; (2) chronic atrophic candidiasis characterized by chronic inflammation and epithelial thinning, usually under a denture (Figure 11-2); (3) angular cheilitis, an inflammatory symmetrical reaction at the corners of the mouth (Figure 11-3); and (4) *Candida* leukoplakia, firm white plaques surrounded by an erythematous area affecting the lips, cheeks, and tongue (Figure 11-4). A marked increase has occurred in the incidence of oral candidiasis in patients with AIDS, users of inhaled corticosteroids, patients who are immunosuppressed organ transplant recipients, and patients with cancer. The development of candidiasis in a patient who is HIV positive highly suggests progression to AIDS (Figure 11-5).

Candidal esophagitis is common in patients with AIDS and patients who are immunosuppressed. Candidal esophagitis often occurs in patients with thrush but can occur independently. Painful swallowing, a sensation of esophageal obstruction, and substernal chest pain are the most common symptoms. Esophagoscopy reveals lesions

similar to those in the oral cavity. Patients who are severely immunocompromised have concomitant herpes simplex or cytomegalovirus (CMV) infection. Esophageal perforation or esophageal obstruction rarely occurs.

Gastrointestinal candidiasis usually occurs in patients with neoplastic disease. The stomach is the most common site of involvement. The most frequent lesions consist of single or multiple ulcerations containing *Candida* deep in the ulcer beds. Infections of the small and large intestine also occur. As in the stomach, ulcers are the most common lesions. Endoscopic examination may reveal pseudomembranes, superficial erosions, and rarely, perforation.

Candida vaginitis is a common infection and most frequently occurs in women with diabetes mellitus, those receiving antibiotic therapy, or those who are pregnant. Most women develop *Candida* vaginitis sometime during their lifetime and usually have no predisposing factors. Symptoms include a thick, curdlike vaginal discharge containing desquamated epithelial cells, and masses of hyphae and pseudohyphae. Often little discharge occurs. Edema and pruritus of the vulva usually is present. The vagina and labia usually are erythematous, and extension onto the skin of the perineum can occur. In rare cases, extension of infection results in endometritis and urethritis. Recurrent vulvovaginal candidiasis has been associated with defects in cell-mediated and local mucosal immunity.

Cutaneous candidiasis can affect almost any area of the skin and adnexa.[11] Warm, moist areas are the most common sites. Candidal infection is one of the most frequent causes of paronychia. Lesions consist of well-localized areas of inflammation that extend well under the nail. Transverse ridges often develop and the nails become brown and thickened. *Candida* is a common cause of balanitis. Vesicular or exudative lesions that develop into white patches occur on the penis. Severe itching and burning often accompanies these lesions. The scrotum, thighs, gluteal folds, and buttocks may be affected by spreading infection. *Candida* folliculitis is a rare condition but may become extensive. *Candida* also occurs between fingers and toes. Painful lesions have a red base and may extend onto the sides of the digits.

Chronic mucocutaneous candidiasis is a syndrome of chronic candidal infection of mucosal and cutaneous structures. Most patients have defects in cell-mediated immunity. This condition may develop in any patient with T-lymphocyte defects. Chronic candidal infection rarely develops in patients with no apparent immune deficiency. Classic lesions are verrucous and associated with extensive epithelial hyperplasia. Most patients first develop oral thrush followed by nail and skin involvement. About half of patients develop significant endocrinopathies, most commonly hypoparathyroidism and Addison's disease. Less commonly hypothyroidism and diabetes mellitus develop.

Deep Organ Candidiasis   Almost any organ can be the site of candidal infection. Deep organ infection usually is a manifestation of disseminated disease.[12] For example, *Candida* may infect both the brain parenchymal tissue, where it forms multiple abscesses, and the meninges. Other organs frequently involved include the heart, urinary tract, bone and joints, liver, spleen, and eye. The lungs, gastrointestinal tract, skin, and endocrine glands are infected less commonly. Multiple organ involvement usually occurs. Diffuse microabscesses of organs usually are present. These lesions may be complicated by acute suppurative and granulomatous reactions. Despite intensive therapy the morbidity and mortality associated with disseminated disease remain high.[52]

Diagnosis   The diagnosis of candidal infection often is difficult. *Candida* is a normal part of the commensal flora. Hence, a positive culture result may not be sufficient cause to treat the patient. Furthermore, disseminated disease may occur in the absence of positive blood culture results because of the efficient clearing of organisms by the host. Conversely, an isolated episode of fungemia does not ensure that disseminated disease is present. Because *Candida* infection often is an opportunistic infection, the host's normal defenses are impaired; therefore clinical presentation may be blunted or atypical. Fever is the most common

finding, followed by leukocytosis. Diagnosis usually is based on the location and appearance of the lesions. Biopsy and identification of the organism in tissue section is the most reliable diagnostic tool. Isolation of the organism in culture can be a useful adjunct.

Because of the difficulty in diagnosis great need exists for reliable serological tests. Various methods have been developed to detect *Candida*-related antibodies, antigens, and cell wall components in the blood. Mannan, a cell wall polysaccharide, is released into the serum of patients with invasive candidiasis and can be identified reliably by immunological assays.[79] However, because of the lack of adequate sensitivity, this assay is not used widely. Cytoplasmic protein antigens and cytoplasmic proteins are found in many patients infected with invasive candidiasis. However, these assays also are limited by low sensitivity and a high false-positive response rate. Assays for *Candida* antigens and antibodies are of little use clinically. PCR assays, which can detect very small amounts of *Candida* DNA, have been used but yield a significant number of false-negative results.[77]

Treatment   Topical nystatin, clotrimazole, and miconazole have been efficacious in the treatment of mucocutaneous candidiasis. Itraconazole and fluconazole also are effective. Oral administration of ketoconazole and fluconazole is efficacious in the treatment of mucocutaneous infections, especially chronic cutaneous candidiasis syndrome, thrush, and esophagitis. The oral azole drug fluconazole is effective in some types of deep organ candidiasis such as renal and hepatosplenic disease. Amphotericin B remains the cornerstone for the treatment of refractory, disseminated, and deep organ disease.[14]

ASPERGILLOSIS *(Aspergillus fumigatus)*

Aspergillosis is an opportunistic infection that usually affects the lungs, sinuses, and the tracheobronchial tree and occurs most commonly in patients with severe immunocompromise. Affected patients include those with inherited abnormalities of granulocyte and T-lymphocyte function, patients undergoing cytotoxic chemotherapy for malignancies, patients with AIDS, and transplant recipients who are iatrogenically immunosuppressed. The risk of invasive aspergillosis in the normal healthy and immunocompetent host is negligible. *Aspergillus* infections can occur in immunocompetent hosts and include superficial infections such as onychomycosis and external otitis, and infection of damaged tissue as in keratitis or after surgery. Host defenses against infection are similar to those of other fungal infections and include the skin and mucous membrane barriers. Second-line defense is mediated by phagocytosis by neutrophils and monocytes facilitated by complement fixation. Oxidative killing of phagocytosed fungus is essential for recovery from invasive aspergillosis (Box 11-6).

Pathogenesis   In hosts who are immunosuppressed, vascular invasion is prominent and accompanied by

BOX 11-6

Aspergillosis

Pathogenesis
Opportunistic infection that occurs primarily in immunocompromised host
Infection characterized by vascular invasion, necrotizing
inflammation, and infarction
Frequent initiation of IgE and IgG allergic reactions and
eosinophilia

Clinical Characteristics
Allergic disease
Lung primarily site of involvement: bronchiolitis and
chronic eosinophilic pneumonia often associated with
asthma, cystic fibrosis
Allergic sinusitis
Aspergilloma
Fungal balls in maxillary and ethmoid sinuses and in lung
cavities produced by other disease processes (i.e.,
tuberculosis)
Lung parenchymal invasion: productive cough, hemopty-
sis, wheezing, hypoxia
Superficial disease
Patients immunocompetent
External otitis: pain, itching, blocked external auditory
canal
Cutaneous and nail bed infection rare

Invasive disease
Patients immunocompromised
Lung and airways primary sites of involvement
Lung: focal and diffuse disease, pleuritic pain, cough, he-
moptysis, dyspnea, hypoxia
Airways: tracheobronchitis, sinusitis, otomastoiditis
Oral lesions: yellow-black necrotic ulcers

Diagnosis
Identification of organism in aspirates, bronchoalveolar
lavage fluid, tissue biopsy, confirmed with culture

Treatment

Allergic and Pulmonary Disease
Steroids and oral itraconazole
Aspergilloma
Surgical drainage or resection
Superficial disease
Topical antifungal agent—clotrimazole, or flucytosine and
amphotericin B
Invasive disease
Amphotericin B alone and in combination with rifampin
or flucytosine

necrotizing inflammation. Infarction follows with necrosis, edema, and hemorrhage. Hyphae are abundant in these
tissues. Necrotizing granulomas become a prominent feature after development of T-lymphocyte–mediated acquired immunity. *A. fumigatus* also can cause an allergic
form of aspergillosis. Hypersensitivity reactions are prominent. Eosinophilia and precipitating IgG and IgE antibodies against *Aspergillus* are present.

Clinical Characteristics

Allergic Disease   Exudative bronchiolitis and chronic
eosinophilic pneumonia are common pathological features. Patients with allergic bronchopulmonary aspergillosis usually have underlying asthma or cystic fibrosis and are hypersensitive to the *Aspergillus* organism.
Central bronchiectasis eventually develops. Allergic aspergillus sinusitis has many features of sinus aspergilloma.
It differs in that the sinus is filled with eosinophil-rich
mucin that often contains Charcot-Leyden crystals (de-
generated eosinophils).[76] Steroids alone or in combination
with oral itraconazole are useful in treatment of allergic
bronchopulmonary aspergillosis but have little value in allergic aspergillus sinusitis.

Aspergilloma   Fungal balls sometimes develop in the
maxillary and ethmoid sinuses after endodontic therapy
of a maxillary tooth. No mucosal invasion is apparent and
surgical drainage usually is curative. Aspergillomas also

may develop in pulmonary cavities, cysts, or ectatic
bronchi resulting from other disease processes such as tuberculosis, sarcoidosis, or *Pneumocystis carinii* in patients
with AIDS. Some patients have no symptoms but most develop persistent productive cough, hemoptysis, wheezing,
weight loss, and clubbing of the fingers. *Aspergillus* organisms are detected in sputum cultures, and IgG antibodies
are present in the serum. Invasion into the lung parenchyma occurs and is most likely in patients who are immunosuppressed. Approximately 10% of aspergillomas resolve spontaneously.[32] Surgical resection and amphotericin
B and oral itraconazole therapy are useful in selected cases.

Superficial Aspergillosis   *Aspergillus* infection can cause
chronic otitis externa. Lesions may consist of a white mat
of fungal mycelia with black conidiophores throughout,
but the appearance often is similar to common external
otitis. Itching, pain, and blockage of the external auditory
canal are the most frequent symptoms. Treatment consists
of thorough cleansing of the external auditory canal and
application of a topical antifungal agent (e.g., clotrimazole,
flucytosine, amphotericin B). Cutaneous infection or onychomycosis rarely is caused by *Aspergillus*. *Aspergillus* has
been a frequent cause of posttraumatic ocular keratitis.
Topical antifungal agents usually are successful treatment.

Invasive Aspergillosis   Most patients who develop invasive aspergillosis have pulmonary disease. The disease

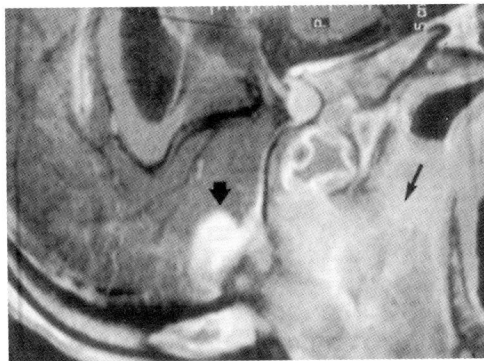

Figure 11-6 Magnetic resonance imaging scan of sinocerebral aspergillosis. Thin arrow shows lesion in nasal cavity and ethmoid sinus and broad arrow shows cerebral lesion. (From Lewis MB, Henderson B: Invasive intracranial aspergillosis secondary to intranasal corticosteroids, *J Neurol Neurosurg Psychiatry* 67:416, 1999.)

manifests differently depending on the severity of immunosuppression. Patients who are severely immunocompromised (i.e., bone marrow transplant recipients) have few symptoms initially but the disease progresses rapidly. Patients who are less immunocompromised (i.e., patients with AIDS) often initially have respiratory symptoms and the progression of the disease is slow. The earliest symptoms are dry cough and low-grade fever. Often pleuritic chest pain is present and sometimes is associated with hemoptysis. A pleural friction rub may exist. In patients with neutropenia the earliest manifestation may be pneumothorax. Dyspnea primarily occurs in patients with diffuse disease. Hypoxemia usually occurs in patients with diffuse disease and patients with extensive consolidation.

Other sites of invasive aspergillosis include the airways. For example, *Aspergillus* tracheobronchitis is common in patients with AIDS and transplant recipients. Invasive *Aspergillus* sinusitis occurs primarily in patients who are severely immunocompromised. A chronic form of the disease may occur in patients with diabetes, alcoholism, or AIDS. Localized oral lesions appear as yellow-black necrotic ulcerations on the soft palate, tongue, and pharynx. Bleeding, pain, and dysphagia are common. Cerebral aspergillosis occurs in approximately 10% to 20% of patients with invasive aspergillosis[16]; it is more common in patients with severe immunocompromise. Symptoms usually are nonspecific. Alteration of mental status and seizures are most common. Focal neurological signs and headache may develop in patients whose immune systems are less compromised (Figure 11-6). Deep organ involvement usually is a manifestation of disseminated disease. The heart, bone, kidney, gastrointestinal tract, and skin also may be affected.

Diagnosis   Several concurrent diagnostic studies should be performed rapidly if invasive aspergillosis is suspected. These tests include detailed radiological evaluation of lungs, sinuses, and brain. Other useful studies depending

on presentation include echocardiography, bronchoscopy, and nasal endoscopy. Bronchoalveolar lavage fluid and endotracheal aspirates should be processed for microscopy and culture. Definitive proof of invasive aspergillosis requires culture of the *Aspergillus* organism from a sterile site (i.e., abscess or brain aspirate). Identification of the organism in a biopsy specimen coupled with positive culture findings also is diagnostic. Serological tests are useful adjuncts and may permit early diagnosis. The presence of circulating galactomannan antigen is useful. Recent immunosorbent assays have provided high sensitivity and few false-positive results.[18]

Treatment   Invasive aspergillosis is nearly 100% fatal if untreated. The earlier the diagnosis and initiation of therapy the more likely is the success of treatment.[18] Amphotericin B, alone and in combination with rifampin or flucytosine, has been used with highly variable results; failure rates vary from 13% to 100%.[14] Lower failure rates occurred in patients whose disease was diagnosed and treated earlier and patients who recovered from a severe immunocompromised state. Other studies have suggested that efficacy of itraconazole is similar to that of amphotericin B.[19]

MUCORMYCOSIS (Mucoralis *Rhizopus*)

Pathogenesis   Mucormycosis is a rare opportunistic fungal infection most frequently caused by *Mucor* and *Rhizopus* spp. Depending on the immunological status of the host, the disease may manifest in six different ways depending on the affected site: rhinocerebral, pulmonary, cutaneous, gastrointestinal, central nervous system, or miscellaneous. For example, patients with diabetes mellitus usually have the rhinocerebral and pulmonary forms of disease.[50] Patients who are malnourished usually have the gastrointestinal form of disease. The primary mechanism of infection is through inhalation of spores. In the cutaneous form, spores enter through damaged skin. Once entry is gained and the fungus begins to grow, hyphae invade tissue, especially blood vessels, causing thrombosis and tissue necrosis. Disseminated disease most frequently occurs as an extension from a primary site in patients who are severely immunocompromised (Box 11-7).

Clinical Characteristics

Rhinocerebral Mucormycosis   Patients with rhinocerebral mucormycosis almost always report facial pain or headache. Often their mental state is impaired (Figure 11-7). Fever and orbital cellulitis frequently occur. Orbital invasion results in loss of extraocular muscle function followed by proptosis. Conjunctival swelling also is prominent. Loss of vision may result, suggesting retinal artery thrombosis. Cranial nerve involvement manifests by pupillary dilation and ptosis and is a poor prognostic sign. Meningoencephalitis, brain abscess, and cavernous sinus thrombosis may occur. Involvement of the nasal cavity results in rhinorrhea, bloody discharge, and necrosis of nasal

Mucormycosis

Pathogenesis
Opportunistic infection primarily in patients who are
immunocompromised
Infection characterized by vascular invasion, necrotizing
inflammation, and infarction
Inhalation of spores or entry through damaged
skin/mucosa

Clinical Characteristics
Rhinocerebral disease
Fever, pain, headache, impaired mental state
Necrosis of nasal septum or turbinates, rhinorrhea,
hemorrhage, palatal necrosis
Orbital cellulitis, proptosis, blindness
Cavernous sinus thrombosis, meningoencephalitis
Pulmonary disease
Fever, dyspnea, cough, hemoptysis, pulmonary infarct,
infiltration, consolidation
Cutaneous disease
Superficial painful erythematous patches with central
necrosis, pustules, and papules
Gastrointestinal disease
Abdominal pain and distention, nausea, vomiting, and
fever
CNS disease
Extension from primary disease of nasal cavity and
paranasal sinuses
Decreasing levels of consciousness, focal neurological
signs, hemiplegia, hemiparesis, and cranial nerve
involvement

Diagnosis
Identification of organism in biopsy

Treatment
Amphotericin B, surgical resection, and debridement

CNS, Central nervous system.

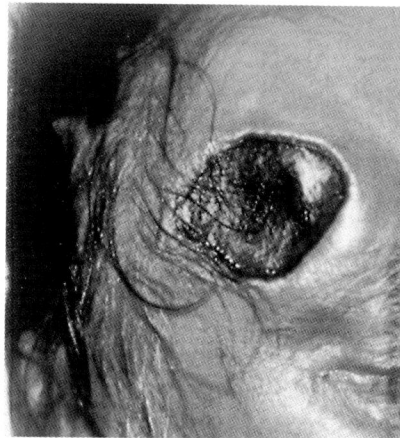

Figure 11-7 Mucormycosis lesion of the forehead. (From Carpenter CF, Subramian AK: Cutaneous zygomycosis [mucormycosis], *N Engl J Med* 341:1891, 1999.)

Gastrointestinal Mucormycosis   Gastrointestinal disease arises from organisms that enter the gastrointestinal tract in contaminated food. All portions of the gastrointestinal tract are susceptible to infection. The disease is acute and rapidly fatal. Initial manifestations include abdominal pain and distention, nausea, vomiting, and fever.

Central Nervous System Mucormycosis   CNS involvement usually is the result of extension from primary disease of the nasal cavity and paranasal sinuses. CNS involvement is characterized by decreasing levels of consciousness, focal neurological signs, hemiplegia, hemiparesis, and cranial nerve involvement. Isolated brain involvement has been reported in intravenous drug abusers with AIDS and patients with leukemia.[2]

Diagnosis   The hallmark of diagnosis is demonstration of the organism in a biopsy specimen. Serological assays for *Mucor* antigens have been developed. However, these assays remain investigational.

Treatment   Relatively high doses of amphotericin B are required because the fungus is relatively resistant to the drug. None of the oral azole drugs are efficacious. The lipid formulations of amphotericin B can maintain high blood levels with lower toxicity and may be more efficacious. Radical surgical resection and debridement with antibiotic therapy provide the best chance for survival. In addition, vigorous treatment directed against the cause of the underlying immunosuppression is essential.[2] Overall survival is poor, less than 50% in a recent review.[50]

PNEUMOCYSTOSIS (*Pneumocystis carinii*)

Pathogensis   *P. carinii* is a fungus of low virulence commonly found in the lungs of humans and other mammals. It is ubiquitous in the environment and infects the host primarily by inhalation of the organism in its trophic

septum and turbinates. Necrotic lesions of the hard and soft palate may be present and appear as sharply demarcated black eschars on the mucosa.

Pulmonary Mucormycosis   Most patients have significant neutropenia as a result of chemotherapy for hematological malignancies. Many patients also are taking broad-spectrum antibiotics. Patients initially may have few symptoms. Fever, dyspnea, and possibly cough usually are present, followed by hemoptysis and pulmonary infarcts. Fatal pulmonary hemorrhage sometimes occurs as a result of erosion of a major blood vessel. Pulmonary infiltration, consolidation, and cavitation occur in a high percentage of patients.

Cutaneous Mucormycosis   Primary cutaneous lesions appear as superficial painful erythematous patches with central necrosis, pustules, and papules. Secondary cutaneous lesions frequently occur as a manifestation of disseminated disease.

Pneumocystosis

Pathogenesis
Opportunistic infection in patients who are immuno-compromised
Organism ubiquitous in environment, aerosolized spores inhaled

Clinical Characteristics
Pneumonia: shortness of breath, nonproductive cough, fever, hypoxia

Diagnosis
Identification of organism in respiratory secretions, serology, PCR

Treatment
Trimethoprim-sulfamethoxazole, dapsone, clindamycin, primaquine

PCR, Polymerase chain reaction.

form. Unlike other fungi, *P. carinii* does not synthesize ergosterol, which is the primary target of most antifungal antibiotics. Instead it synthesizes distinct C27 to 32 alkylated sterols.[45] *P. carinii* causes pneumonia and is the most common opportunistic infection in patients with HIV infection, occurring in nearly 85% of patients who do not receive prophylactic treatment.[73] Infection occurs primarily in patients whose CD4+ lymphocyte counts decrease below 200/mm³. *P. carinii* infection also is prevalent in patients with severe immune suppression of congenital or iatrogenic origin. CD4+ lymphocyte activation of macrophages is critical for host defense against infection. The organism attaches to type I alveolar cells and begins to proliferate shortly after host defenses are compromised. The organism soon fills the alveolar lumen. This process initiates an inflammatory host response characterized by release of inflammatory cytokines and formation of a foamy, eosinophil cell–rich exudate. Eventually hyalin membrane formation and interstitial fibrosis occur. Patients become hypoxic and alkalotic, and lung compliance, total lung capacity, and vital capacity decrease (Box 11-8).

Clinical Characteristics The major initial symptoms of *P. carinii* pneumonia in compromised hosts are shortness of breath, fever, and nonproductive cough. Sputum production, chest pain, and rarely, hemoptysis may occur. In many patients the onset of symptoms is insidious and others may have no symptoms. Tachypnea and tachycardia characterize the acutely ill patient. Children often are cyanotic with alar flaring and intercostal retraction. Chest radiographs classically demonstrate bilateral diffuse infiltrates extending from the prehilar region. In some patients, unilateral infiltrates, nodules, cavities, pneumatoceles, lymphadenopathy, and effusion may be seen. Hypoxia is the most common finding.

Extrapulmonary pneumocystosis occurs mainly in patients with advanced HIV infection. The primary affected sites are lymph nodes, spleen, liver, bone marrow, gastrointestinal tract, eyes, thyroid, adrenal glands, and kidneys.

Diagnosis *P. carinii* pneumonia should be considered in any patient who is immunocompromised and who develops respiratory symptoms, fever, or has abnormal chest radiographic results. Diagnosis is made by identification of the organism in respiratory secretions or tissue sections. Immunofluorescence is the most widely used technique. Serological tests include demonstration of *P. carinii* antigens in the serum by immunoblotting techniques. A PCR assay efficiently identifies *P. carinii* DNA in respiratory specimens and provides high sensitivity and specificity.[89,91]

Treatment Optimal management of pneumocystosis depends on early diagnosis and institution of appropriate therapy. Severely ill patients require mechanical ventilation for respiratory support, administration of effective antifungal therapy, and intensive critical care. These supportive factors alone reduced the mortality rate from 80% to 90% to 50%.[30] Trimethoprim-sulfamethoxazole (TMP-SMX) is the antimicrobial drug of choice for all forms of pneumocystosis. This agent inhibits folic acid synthesis. TMP-SMX is relatively inexpensive, available in both oral and parenteral forms, and well tolerated. The usual intravenous dose is 15 to 20 mg/kg per day. Alternative drugs include dapsone, which has been proved safe and effective. Dapsone (100 mg/day PO) has been used alone and in combination with TMP-SMX for treatment of moderate infections. Other effective drugs include clindamycin and primaquine.

Because of the high morbidity and mortality of *Pneumocystis* infection in patients with AIDS, chemoprophylaxis is recommended in all patients with CD4+ counts below 200/mm³, those who develop oral candidiasis, have unexplained fever (>100° F for more than 2 weeks), or who recovered from a previous episode of pneumocystosis. TMP-SMX is the drug of choice (160 mg of trimethoprim and 800 mg of sulfamethoxazole per day) Chemoprophylaxis is continued for life. With the recent introduction of highly active antiviral treatment (HAART), many patients with AIDS have regained immunocompetence, with CD4+ counts increasing well above 200/mm³. This has resulted in a significant decrease in the incidence of several opportunistic infections (i.e., CMV, mycobacteriosis, cryptococcosis). In contrast, the incidence of pneumocystosis has increased, suggesting that prophylaxis remains necessary.[55]

CRYPTOCOCCOSIS *(Cryptococcus neoformans)*

Pathogenesis Cyptococcosis is a rare disease caused primarily by *C. neoformans* infection. *C. neoformans* is ubiquitous in the environment and not confined to any endemic area. The organism frequently is isolated in pigeon droppings, decaying wood, and soil. Infection is spread primarily by inhalation of aerosolized spores. Person-to-person transmission has not been demonstrated. The organism has low virulence and produces disease primarily in individuals who are severely immunocompromised, including patients with AIDS, hematological malignancies, congenital defects primarily of T-lymphocyte function, and transplant patients who are immunosuppressed iatrogenically, especially those taking steroids. Approximately 6% to 10% of patients with AIDS develop cyptococcosis.[61] *C. neoformans* grows in the tissues of the host in large distinctive capsules. The major constituent of this capsule is a polysaccharide containing unbranched α1-3–linked mannose units substituted with xylose and β-glucuronyl groups. This polysaccharide may have immunosuppressive properties and inhibits phagocytosis.[65] Often no inflammatory reaction exists around these capsules in the tissues of the host.[23] Although neutrophils are important, T-lymphocyte cell–mediated immunity appears to play a critical role in host defense against infection. AIDS-associated cryptococcosis usually occurs when the CD4$^+$ lymphocyte count decreases below 200/mm^3. *C. neoformans* produces no known exotoxins. Little necrosis or organ dysfunction is present until late in the course of infection (Box 11-9).

Clinical Characteristics   *C. neoformans* has a predilection for the CNS and primarily affects the meninges, basal ganglia, and cortical gray matter. Meningitis is the most common initial manifestation of infection, affecting 72% to 90% of patients.[61] Onset of CNS cryptococcosis may be acute or insidious. Acute symptoms occur primarily in patients who are severely immunocompromised, especially patients with AIDS, those receiving corticosteroids, and those with lymphoreticular malignancies. Symptoms include cranial nerve involvement resulting in decreased visual acuity, diplopia, and facial palsy. Seizures may occur. Patients often have minimal or no nuchal rigidity. Papilledema occurs in more than one third of patients. Some patients initially have hyperreflexia, ankle clonus, or extensor plantar responses. Focal signs may occur in patients with large cerebral granulomas. When the onset is more insidious, symptoms are nonspecific and include headache, nausea, dizziness, irritability, somnolence, clumsiness, confusion, or obtundation.

Pulmonary cryptococcosis may cause no symptoms or may cause production of blood-streaked sputum. Pulmonary involvement has been documented in 30% to 45% of patients with AIDS.[61] Patients with AIDS often have fever, cough, dyspnea, and a dull ache in the chest. Chest radiographs show diffuse interstitial infiltrates. These patients also may have severe, rapidly progressive pneumonia that frequently is fatal.[20]

In addition to the respiratory system, cryptococcosis may involve other sites outside the CNS. Cutaneous lesions occurs in 5% to 10 % patients. Lesions frequently occur on the scalp and face.[64] Lesions usually are painless, nonspecific, and often ignored but frequently are the first signs of infection. Lesions consist of small erythematous papules, pustules, erythematous indurated plaques, soft subcutaneous masses, draining sinus tracts, or large ulcers

---

BOX 11-9

Cryptococcosis

Pathogenesis
Opportunistic infection in patients who are immunocompromised
Organism ubiquitous in environment, aerosolized spores inhaled

Clinical Characteristics
Pulmonary
May be asymptomatic; in patients with AIDS: fever, cough, dyspnea, and chest pain likely
CNS
Predilection for meninges and basal ganglia; onset of symptoms acute or insidious; nuchal rigidity rare, cranial nerve involvement characterized by decreased visual acuity, diplopia, facial palsies, and hyperreflexia; nonspecific symptoms—headache, nausea, dizziness, irritability, somnolence, clumsiness, confusion, or obtundation
Cutaneous/mucosal lesions
Small erythematous papules, pustules, erythematous indurated plaques, soft subcutaneous masses, draining sinus tracts, or large ulcers with rolled edges surrounding a base of granulation tissue

Diagnosis
CT and MRI scans of brain, CSF, or secretions to identify organism using India ink stain, confirmed by culture, serology to identify cryptococcal polysaccharide capsular antigen

Treatment
CNS or disseminated disease
Amphotericin B with flucytosine for a period of 4 to 6 weeks followed by fluconazole prophylaxis thereafter for prevention of relapse
Pulmonary and cutaneous disease
Fluconazole

AIDS, Acquired immunodeficiency syndrome; *CNS,* central nervous system; *CT,* computed tomography; *MRI,* magnetic resonance imaging; *CSF,* cerebrospinal fluid.

---

with rolled edges surrounding a base of granulation tissue. Oral mucosal lesions also may occur. Regional lymph nodes usually are not affected. Some patients develop thrombocytopenic purpura. Cellulitis and vasculitis also may occur. In the disseminated form of the disease, almost any organ can be affected, including heart, bone and joints, kidney, gastrointestinal tract, liver, spleen, and endocrine glands.

Diagnosis   Any patients with neurological abnormalities who is HIV positive should have computed tomographic and magnetic resonance imaging scans of the brain to rule out a space-occupying lesion, infection, or neoplasm. In addition, any patient with extraneural cryptococcosis (i.e., skin or pulmonary infection) should be evaluated for CNS involvement. A lumbar puncture should be performed and evaluated for opening pressure, glucose, protein levels, and lymphocytes. The opening pressure usually is elevated, glucose levels are decreased, and protein concentration is increased. In addition, the cerebrospinal fluid (CSF) should be examined in an India ink preparation for the presence of cryptococcal capsules. The presence of the organism must be verified by culture. These tests can be supplemented by serological assays. Detection of the cryptococcal polysaccharide capsular antigen in CSF or other body fluids is a sensitive and specific assay. The antigen is present in CSF or serum in more than 90% of patients with cryptococcal meningitis.[61] However, the sensitivity of the assay decreases with extraneural disease.

Treatment   In patients with AIDS, cryptococcosis invariably is fatal in the absence of effective treatment. A combination of amphotericin B and flucytosine administered for a period of 4 to 6 weeks is the treatment of choice for cryptococcal meningitis. Because of the high incidence of adverse side effects with this regimen, alternative therapies have been sought. Fluconazole was used in one study and was less effective than amphotericin B and flucytosine.[49] A more recent multicenter study randomized treatment to either amphotericin B alone (0.7 to mg/kg per day) or combined with flucytosine (100 mg/kg per day) for 14 days. No significant difference existed between the two groups at 2 weeks. However, more patients had sterile CSF cultures at 2 weeks when both drugs were used than when amphotericin B alone was used. Lipid formulations of amphotericin B may be less toxic and have shown activity in patients with AIDS with cryptococcal meningitis.[84] Relapse is common in patients with severe immunosuppression; thus prolongation of therapy beyond 6 weeks is indicated. Fluconazole (200 mg/day) successfully prevented recurrence after initial therapy.[61] In patients who are HIV negative, fluconazole (200 to 800 mg/day) is as effective in treatment of cryptococcal meningitis and cryptococcosis outside the CNS as amphotericin B with and without flucytosine.[24]

Treatment of patients with pulmonary cryptococcosis without an immunocompromising underlying disease remains controversial. One investigator has reported that such patients do not require specific antifungal therapy.[26] However, this recommendation was based on analysis of only a few patients. With the development of relatively nontoxic oral azole drugs, other investigators recommend treatment. Further prospective studies are needed.[1]

SPOROTRICHOSIS (*Sporothrix schenckii*)

Sporotrichosis is a fungal infection that occurs worldwide. However, a predilection exists in tropical and subtropical regions of the Americas. In the United States the Mississippi and Missouri River valleys are the endemic areas. *S. schenkii* most often is isolated from soil and plant products such as straw and wood. Infection usually occurs by inoculation of the organism at the site of injured skin, although inhalation of spores also occurs. Exposure usually

occurs as result of injury from sharp vegetation such as rosebushes, barberry, sphagnum moss, and contaminated wood. Exposure also may occur as result of contact with animals such as horses, dogs, cats and rats. Most patients are farmers, gardeners, or veterinarians whose occupations expose them to this organism[81] (Box 11-10).

Clinical Characteristics

Cutaneous Sporotrichosis   Cutaneous lesions occur at the site of inoculation. The initial lesions are papulonodular, erythematous, and vary in size from a few millimeters to 2 to 4 cm. The lesions are smooth or verrucous. Ulceration frequently occurs. The borders are raised and erythematous. Lesions usually are painless even after ulceration. Secondary lesions may develop along the linear path of lymphatic drainage and appear similar to the primary lesions. Lymph node involvement is unusual but lymphadenopathy may occur. A fixed or plaquelike form of disease may occur in patients who live in endemic areas

---

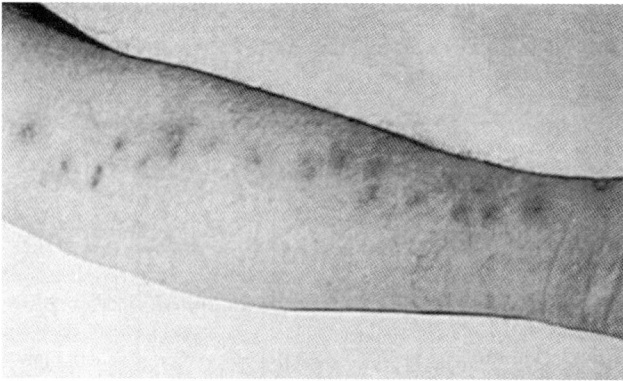

Figure 11-8 Multiple firm, violaceous, necrotic nodules and papules of disseminated sporotrichosis. (From Mandell GL, Bennett JE, Dolin R: *Mandell, Douglas, and Bennett's principles and practice of infectious diseases,* ed 5, vol 2, Philadelphia, 2000, Churchill Livingstone.)

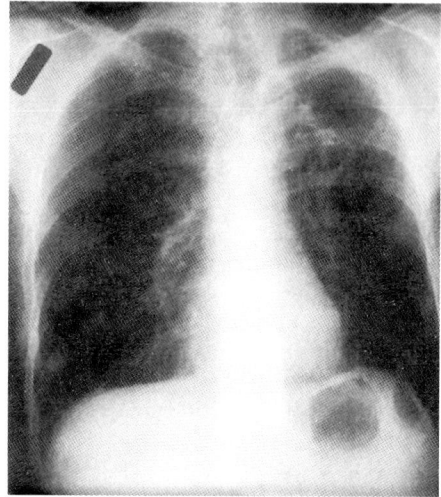

Figure 11-9 Posteroanterior chest radiograph demonstrating larger upper left lobe cavity caused by sporotrichosis. (From Byrd RP, Hourany J, Cooper C, et al: False-positive antineutrophil cytoplasmic antibodies in a patient with cavitary pulmonary sporotrichosis, *Am J Med* 104:101, 1998.)

with previously activated immunological states; this form of the disease differs in that local spread does not occur. The lesions wax and wane over months to years. Mucosal sporotrichosis most commonly affects the nose, mouth, or pharynx. Lesions appear erythematous and frequently ulcerate and become suppurative. Spread to regional lymph nodes frequently occurs. Oral lesions also may occur in the disseminated form of the disease.

Extracutaneous Sporotrichosis The most frequent sites of extracutaneous sporotrichosis are the joints of the hands, elbow, ankle, and knee. Skin lesions may or may not be present. The involved joint is swollen and painful with motion. An effusion usually is present and osteomyelitis and sinus tracts may occur. Systemic symptoms are minimal.

Pulmonary sporotrichosis is characterized by productive cough, low-grade fever, and weight loss. Chest radiographs usually reveal cavitary lesions associated with parenchymal infiltrates. Pleural effusion and hilar lymphadenopathy also may be present. Progressive pulmonary dysfunction occurs if the disease is untreated. Other organs may be affected but the incidence is rare.

Disseminated Sporotrichosis Severe immunosuppression such as HIV infection predisposes patients to disseminated disease. Disseminated disease occurs primarily in patients with CD4$^+$ T-lymphocyte counts less than 200/mm^3. Often these patients have widespread ulcerative cutaneous lesions frequently associated with polyarthritis (Figure 11-8). Visceral involvement is widespread and includes meningitis, parenchymal brain lesions, lung abscess, liver, spleen, and ocular manifestations (Figure 11-9). Fungemia may spread to the esophagus, colon, bone marrow, and lymph nodes. Sinusitis with invasion of bone has been reported.[63]

Diagnosis Diagnosis depends on culture of the organism from an infected site. Often multiple cultures are necessary. In patients with disseminated disease, positive blood culture results are diagnostic. Detection of the yeast form of the organism in tissue biopsy is helpful. However, such detection often is difficult and multiple sections of the specimen are required.[78] No standard serological testing method is available.

Treatment Potassium iodide is the treatment of choice for cutaneous lesions. Therapy begins with 5 to 10 drops of saturated solution taken orally three times a day. The dosage is gradually increased to 40 to 50 drops three times a day. The maximal tolerated dose should be continued until all lesions have resolved, which usually takes at least 6 to 12 weeks.[81] Oral itraconazole (100 to 200 mg/day) has been effective but therapy must be maintained for 3 to 6 months to prevent relapse. Amphotericin B with and without flucytosine is the treatment of choice for the extracutaneous and disseminated forms of the disease. This treatment should be followed by lifelong itraconazole therapy to prevent relapse. Joint involvement often requires surgical debridement in addition to chemotherapy.

VIRAL INFECTIONS

HERPESVIRUS INFECTIONS

All members of this virus family are large DNA-containing enveloped viruses. Eight human viruses are recognized and include herpes simplex virus (HSV) types 1 and 2, varicella-zoster virus, Epstein-Barr virus, CMV, human herpesviruses 6 through 8, and simian herpes B virus. These viruses induce disease in three ways: by direct destruction of infected cells, initiation of an immunopathological response, and facilitation of neoplastic transformation (Table 11-1).

TABLE 11-1

Systemic DNA Viral Infections

Causative Agent	Pathogenesis	Clinical Characteristics	Diagnosis	Treatment
Herpessimplex virus serotypes 1 and 2	Transmission occurs by close contact with person shedding viruses. Virus infects target cells: mucosa, epidermis, and neurons of dorsal ganglia.	Both HSV-1 and HSV-2 cause primary genital and orofacial lesions. Lesions consist of small vesicles that rupture to form shallow ulcers surrounded by an erythematous halo. Lesions occur on anterior tonsillar pillars and pharyngeal wall, hard and soft palates, buccal mucosa, tongue, gingiva, and adjacent skin.	Disease is diagnosed by isolation and identification of virus by animal or tissue culture from biopsy of mucosal, skin, or genital lesion; serological procedures identifying viral antibodies; PCR to identify viral DNA in body fluids.	Acyclovir or other nucleoside analogues that block viral DNA synthesis, valacyclovir and famciclovir or the pyrophosphate foscarnet for resistant strains, are used.
Epstein-Barr virus	Transmission occurs by direct contact with secretions (usually saliva) of individual shedding virus. Virus infects target cells by binding CR2 complement receptors of B lymphocytes and epithelial cells followed by cellular endocytosis.	After a 2- to 7-week incubation period, onset of chills, fever, sore throat, headache, fatigue, malaise, exudative tonsillopharyngitis, and lymphadenopathy occurs. Hepatosplenomegaly and jaundice may be present.	Disease is diagnosed by clinical presentation, heterophil monospot agglutination test, immunofluorescence, and complement fixation tests for antibodies to viral capsid antigens.	Supportive therapy, antibiotics (penicillin or erythromycin) are used only if concurrent streptococcal infection is present.
Varicella-zoster virus (chickenpox)	Transmission occurs by direct contact with viral-contaminated secretions including respiratory droplets. Target cells are mucosal cells of upper respiratory tract and conjunctiva and dorsal ganglia.	Low-grade fever and malaise are followed by maculopapular rash that appears first on face and trunk, then spreads to extremities. Oropharyngeal and vaginal mucosal lesions may occur. Maculopapules develop into vesicles that become purulent and rupture.	Disease is diagnosed by clinical presentation, isolation of virus in tissue culture from lesion biopsy. Disease is diagnosed by identification of VZ antibodies in serum.	Supportive therapy is directed at preventing complications.
Varicella-zoster Herpes zoster (shingles)	Recurrent infection is caused by reactivation of latent virus in dorsal ganglia.	Vesicular lesions of skin and mucosa follow the distribution of one of the divisions of the trigeminal nerve or spinal nerves, usually cervical and thoracic.	Disease is diagnosed by clinical presentation, isolation of virus in tissue culture, or PCR.	Supportive therapy is directed at preventing complications. Acyclovir or famciclovir may be used for ophthalmic division involvement.

HSV, Herpes simplex virus; *PCR,* polymerase chain reaction; *DNA,* deoxyribonucleic acid; *VZ,* varicella-zoster.

Continued

TABLE 11-1

Systemic DNA Viral Infections—cont'd

Causative Agent	Pathogenesis	Clinical Characteristics	Diagnosis	Treatment
Cytomegalovirus	Transmission occurs by direct contact with viral-contaminated secretions including respiratory droplets.	Primary infection may be asymptomatic or result in an infectious mononucleosis syndrome similar to Epstein-Barr infection characterized by sore throat, pharyngotonsillitis, fever, lymphadenopathy, and mild hepatitis. Secondary infection is common in severely immunocompromised patients and includes retinitis, polyradiculopathy, and gastrointestinal involvement.	Disease is diagnosed by isolation and culture of virus from body fluids, identification of viral antigens with various monoclonal antibodies, identification of viral DNA with PCR.	Supportive therapy is provided for primary disease; for secondary disease: ganciclovir, foscarnet, and cidofovir.
Human papilloma viruses	Transmission occurs by close personal contact with individual shedding virus. Target cells are basal cells of epithelium including skin, mucosa, and conjunctiva. Infection is associated with malignant transformation.	Oral lesions include painful ulcers or erosions. Cutaneous and oral warts, papillomas can occur. Common warts consist of exophytic, hyperkeratotic papules. Plantar warts are raised bundles of soft keratotic fibers 2 mm to 1 cm in diameter, often painful, and most commonly occur in adolescents. Flat warts are multiple, slightly elevated papules with irregular contour and smooth surface and are most common in children. Anogenital warts are flesh or gray colored, hyperkeratotic exophytic papules and usually are attached to the skin by a broad peduncle.	Disease is diagnosed by clinical presentation, histopathological study of lesions, identification of virus DNA in lesions.	Treatment consists of surgical excision, laser removal, cryotherapy, application of salicylic and lactic acid paint or podophyllotoxin, application of imiquimod cream.

HSV, Herpes simplex virus; *PCR,* polymerase chain reaction; *DNA,* deoxyribonucleic acid; *VZ,* varicella-zoster.

HERPES SIMPLEX VIRUS

Herpes simplex viruses have a worldwide distribution. No known animal vectors exist, although experimental animals can be infected easily. Humans appear to be the only natural reservoirs of the viruses, and infections with these viruses are common. Almost all adults have antibodies to HSV-1 by the fifth decade of life, and 20% to 25% have antibodies to HSV-2. Much higher rates occur in certain populations that correlate well with their level of sexual activity.[82]

Pathogenesis HSVs are relatively fragile and are inactivated rapidly by drying, placement in an acid solution (pH <6.8), lipid solvents, cationic detergents, proteolytic enzymes, and exposure to ultraviolet radiation. Consequently, transmission of HSV infection occurs most frequently through close contact with a person who is shedding virus at a peripheral site, mucosal surface, or in genital and oral secretions. Aerosol and fomitic spread are unusual methods of transmission. Infection occurs by inoculation of the virus on susceptible mucosal surfaces and through small cracks in the skin. Once the virus enters the cells of the epidermis and dermis, replication is initiated and new virions are produced. The virions then are transported to the cell surface where they can infect adjacent cells resulting in contiguous spread. The process of viral replication initiates apoptosis in the host cell resulting in death of the cell. Initially, HSV infection is subclinical and no lesions are produced. Eventually, sensory or autonomic nerve endings are infected. The virus nucleocapsid then is transported up the axon to the cell body in the peripheral ganglia. For HSV-1 the trigeminal ganglia most commonly are infected after oral inoculation, and in genital infection the sacral nerve ganglia most commonly are involved. Viral replication occurs in the neuron and spreads to infect contiguous neurons. New virions also can be transported centrifugally down the axons where they can infect mucosal cells distant from the site of initial inoculation. Such transport accounts for the large surface area involved and the high frequency of new lesions distant from the site of initial inoculation characteristic of primary genital or orallabial HSV infection.

All herpesviruses can achieve a state of latency. This state can occur only in specific cell types depending on the virus. Latency is a state in which the viral genomes are maintained by the host cell in a repressed state, unable to synthesize viral DNA, and compatible with the survival and normal function of the host cell. Only a small number of viral genes are transcribed.[74] HSVs achieve the latent state in ganglion neurons but not epithelial cells. Reactivation of viral replication may occur at any time depending on host factors. Reactivation has been associated with host tissue release of prostaglandins. Hence, any type of tissue injury (i.e., mechanical or ultraviolet radiation) may result in HSV reactivation.[74] Both humoral and cell-mediated immunity are involved in host containment of HSV infection. T-lymphocytes, both CD4+ and CD8+, play critical roles in this process. Patients with impaired cell-mediated immunity are at risk for reactivation of viral infection and development of disseminated life-threatening disease.

Clinical Characteristics

Primary Disease (No Viral Antibodies in Acute-Phase Serum)[80] Both HSV serotypes can cause genital and orofacial infections that are clinically indistinguishable. Approximately 30% to 40% of genital infections are caused by HSV-1.[82] Recurrent clinical and subclinical genital infection with HSV-1 is much less frequent than with HSV-2; hence transmission of HSV-1 genital infection is much less likely. HSV-2 can cause orofacial disease, but because HSV-2 is transmitted almost exclusively through sexual contact, orofacial lesions rarely occur in the absence of genital involvement. Primary infection frequently is accompanied by systemic signs and symptoms and involves mucosa and extramucosal sites. Orofacial infection is characterized by gingivostomatitis and pharyngitis and occurs most commonly in children (see Figure 11-8). Signs and symptoms include fever, malaise, myalgias, inability to eat, irritability, and cervical lymphadenopathy. Symptoms may last 3 to 14 days.[3] Lesions are located on the hard and soft palate, gingiva, tongue, lip, and adjacent facial skin. Lesions start as small vesicles that rupture to form superficial ulcers surrounded by erythematous halos (Figure 11-10). Exudative, ulcerative lesions involving the posterior pharynx or tonsillar pillars, or both, occur initially followed by lesions on the tongue, buccal mucosa, and gingiva. The gingiva appears swollen and hypertrophic, and the gingival margin is bright red (Figure 11-11). Kaposi's varicelliform eruption is a severe dermal lesion characterized by a crop of vesicular eruptions that appear over several days. Significant loss of fluid and epithelium may occur when these vesicles rupture.

Primary genital infection is characterized by itching, dysuria, vaginal and urethral discharge, and tender inguinal lymphadenopathy. Widely spaced bilateral lesions of the external genitalia characteristically occur. Lesions consist of vesicles, pustules, or painful erythematous ulcers. Women commonly develop lesions of the cervix and urethra, but the vulva and vagina also may be affected. In men,

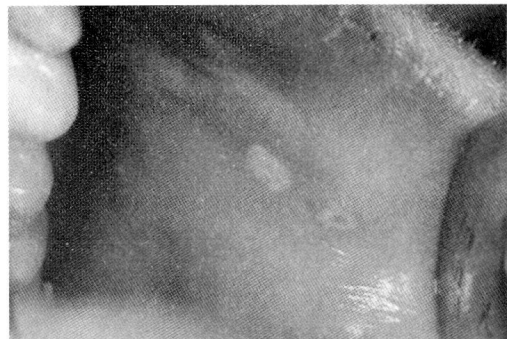

Figure 11-10 Oral primary herpes simplex ulcers. (From Coventry J, Griffiths G, Scully C, et al: Periodontal disease, *BMJ* 321:36, 2000.)

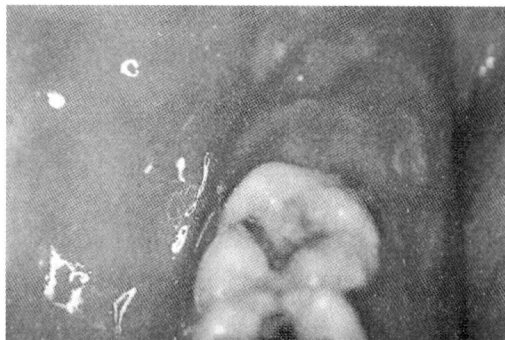

Figure 11-11 Primary herpetic gingivostomatitis. (From Coventry J, Griffiths G, Scully C, et al: Periodontal disease, *BMJ* 321:36, 2000.)

vesicles and ulcers occur anywhere on the penis, usually in clusters. Urethritis has been reported. Occasionally genital tract disease may occur characterized by endometritis and salpingitis in women and prostatitis in men. Proctitis also has been observed. Symptoms usually are severe, characterized by anorectal discharge, tenesmus, constipation, autonomic nervous system dysfunction, sacral paresthesias, impotence in men, and urinary retention.[3]

HSV encephalitis is the most common viral infection of the CNS in the United States. More than 95% of cases are caused by HSV-1. Clinical characteristics include acute fever, altered mental status, and focal neurological signs and symptoms usually involving the temporal lobes. If untreated, the prognosis is poor. Significant morbidity and mortality occurs even with antiviral therapy. In addition, 5% to 10% of patients experience relapse.[3]

Skin herpetic infection may occur at any site depending on the site of viral inoculation. Herpetic whitlow is HSV infection of the finger. It occurs most commonly in health care workers, often as a result of failure to use barrier isolation techniques when the hand is in contact with infected secretions. Because HSV can be shed asymptomatically in the saliva of patients with no active lesions, gloves should always be worn. Signs and symptoms include abrupt onset of edema, erythema, and localized tenderness of the infected finger. Vesicular lesions and pustules often develop and can be accompanied by fever and lymphadenopathy. HSV also may infect the eye and is the most frequent infectious cause of corneal blindness in the United States. Infection is characterized by acute onset of keratoconjunctivitis, pain, blurred vision, chemosis, and characteristic dendritic lesions of the cornea. The application of topical steroids may result in spread to the deeper structures of the eye. Recurrence of HSV is common. HSV chorioretinitis may occur in the disseminated form of the disease and is seen most commonly in patients with AIDS and in neonates.

Neonatal HSV infection is a devastating disease associated with high morbidity and mortality. More than 70% of infants develop disseminated or CNS disease unless antiviral therapy is initiated early. Other sites of infection include the skin, oral cavity, and eye. Lesions usually appear in the second to third weeks after birth. In 85% of cases of neonatal HSV, infection is acquired during the peripartum period from an infected mother.[3] Unfortunately, because many cases of primary genital HSV infection are asymptomatic many women are unaware they are transmitting the disease to their babies.

Reactivation Disease   Clinical manifestations of reactivated disease usually are much milder than those of primary disease. Prodromal symptoms occur 12 to 36 hours before the appearance of vesicles that quickly rupture and form shallow ulcers. Prodromal symptoms are described as tingling, itching, or burning at the site where the subsequent lesions appear. Intraoral lesions usually occur on keratinized tissues (i.e., gingiva and hard palate), whereas extraoral lesions occur primarily on or around the vermilion border of the lip.

Diagnosis   HSV-1 and HSV-2 can be isolated by virus culture from active mucosal, skin, eye, and genital lesions. Fluorescent antibodies then can be used to differentiate HSV-1 from HSV-2. Viral culture is not appropriate in all cases because recovery depends on the age of the cultured lesion, particularly in recurrent disease in which virus shedding may be brief. In addition, HSV rarely is recovered from the CSF of patients with encephalitis. Alternatively, fluorescent antibodies may be used to stain viral antigens in scrapings from active lesions and tissue samples. These assays are less sensitive and specific than culture. PCR, which can detect HSV DNA, is emerging as an acceptable procedure in the diagnosis of HSV encephalitis by CSF sampling.

Treatment   Acyclovir is the treatment of choice for most severe cases of HSV infection. Acyclovir is a synthetic acyclic guanosine analogue that inhibits viral DNA polymerase. Acyclovir is active only in virally infected cells because only viral-encoded thymidine kinase converts acyclovir to acyclovir monophosphate. Cellular enzymes then phosphorylate the monophosphate to the triphosphate, which is the active form of the drug. The recommended dosage is 200 mg five times a day. Acyclovir therapy shortens the duration of primary disease and reduces viral shedding. Acyclovir also is useful in the treatment of eye disease and patients who develop Kaposi's varicelliform eruptions and encephalitis. Acyclovir must be given during the prodromal state to be effective against recurrent disease. Acyclovir (400 mg q12h) has been effective as a prophylactic agent and in partial prevention of asymptomatic shedding of virus. This regimen is most useful in immunocompromised patients who are prone to develop severe mucocutaneous and disseminated disease. The regimen also has been effective in preventing genital herpes infection in pregnant women who can transmit the disease to the fetus. Newer drugs are available that provide better gastrointestinal absorption and long half-lives. Valacyclovir and famciclovir are effective drugs. Foscarnet, a pyrophosphate analogue that inhibits viral DNA polymerase, is not dependent on viral thymidine kinase for activation of the drug; hence, it is used for treatment of viruses that have developed resistance to acyclovir.[3]

EPSTEIN-BARR VIRUS (INFECTIOUS MONONUCLEOSIS)

Epstein-Barr virus (EBV) is a ubiquitous herpesvirus with worldwide distribution. More than 95% of adults in the world are seropositive for EBV antibodies. Once infected, the individual is a lifelong carrier. EBV is the causative agent in heterophile-positive infectious mononucleosis. In industrialized countries and higher socioeconomic groups, infectious mononucleosis occurs most frequently in late adolescence and early adulthood. However, in tropical and underdeveloped areas of the world, antibodies to EBV are commonly detected during childhood. Infection during childhood usually causes asymptomatic or mild disease.[75] In addition, EBV has been associated as a possible causative factor for Burkitt's lymphoma, nasopharyngeal carcinoma, some T-cell lymphomas, and Hodgkin's disease.

Pathogenesis EBV primarily infects B lymphocytes and nasopharyngeal epithelial cells by attachment to EBV receptors expressed by these cells. The EBV receptor is the CR2 complement receptor (CD21) that binds to the "d" region of the third complement component (C3d). After attachment the viral DNA enters the host cell nucleus where viral DNA synthesis is initiated. In host B lymphocytes, EBV may enter a state of latency in which only a few latent viral proteins are expressed. These latent proteins are believed to be responsible for the transformation or immortalization of the host cell.[87] Usually the B lymphocytes undergo DNA synthesis and begin to proliferate within 48 to 72 hours of EBV infection. Unlike the herpes simplex viruses, EBV does not activate the apoptosis program of the host cell, rather it suppresses it.[7,38] However, activation of the host cell (i.e., antigen stimulation of B lymphocytes) also results in activation of the virus genome. Viral replication and assembly occur and eventually result in lysis of the host cell.[7] Released viruses then infect other B lymphocytes. Hence B lymphocytes act as a reservoir of virus.

Like other herpesviruses, EBV transmission appears to be caused by direct contact with secretions, usually saliva, of individuals who are shedding virus. Individuals who have recovered from infectious mononucleosis continue to shed virus for up to 18 months.

Clinical Characteristics After exposure to the virus an incubation period of 2 to 7 weeks follows before the onset of symptoms. Prodromal symptoms include malaise, anorexia, and chills, which frequently occur before the onset of the classic signs and symptoms of infectious mononucleosis. These include fever, sore throat, headache, malaise, and fatigue accompanied by tonsillopharyngitis and lymphadenopathy. Periorbital edema often occurs. Fever may be as high as 102° to 104° F and last for 1 to

2 weeks. Nontender cervical adenopathy is common but generalized adenopathy may occur. Pharyngitis is diffuse, often with a thick tonsillar exudate. Palatal and gingival petechiae and ecchymosis may be present and often are accompanied by acute stomatitis, gingivitis, and gingival hyperplasia. Approximately 5% of patients develop a maculopapular, petechial, or urticarial rash on the trunk and extremities. Hepatosplenomegaly develops in about one fourth to one half of cases and usually occurs within the first 3 weeks of illness. Jaundice may be present.[75] Most patients with infectious mononucleosis recover uneventfully; however, complications may occur. These include autoimmune hemolytic anemia, mild thrombocytopenia, granulocytopenia, splenic rupture, hepatitis, and neurological disorders. Encephalitis, Guillain-Barré syndrome, Bell's palsy, and transverse myelitis have been reported.[75] Fortunately, most patients with neurological disorders recover spontaneously. Renal, pulmonary, and cardiac involvement is rare.

A close association exists among EBV infection and Burkitt's lymphoma and nasopharyngeal carcinoma. Virtually all African patients with Burkitt's lymphoma and most patients with nasopharyngeal carcinoma have high antibody titers to EBV. DNA hybridization studies have demonstrated the presence of the EBV genome in biopsy specimens. The virus also can be recovered from tissue cultures. In addition, in Burkitt's lymphoma EBV ribonucleic acids and EBV nuclear antigen 1 characteristic of EBV latency are expressed.[66] In contrast, a histologically identical Burkitt's lymphoma in the American population is not associated with EBV antigens or proteins.[97] This finding suggests that EBV may contribute to the pathogenesis of these malignancies but is not the only factor. Evidence indicates that EBV may be involved in the pathogenesis of Hodgkin's lymphoma. EBV DNA has been frequently isolated from Reed-Sternberg cells characteristic of this malignancy.[57]

Diagnosis CMV mononucleosis is the disease most commonly confused with EBV mononucleosis. Patients with CMV mononucleosis usually are older than those with EBV mononucleosis. Fever and malaise are more prominent in CMV and pharyngitis and lymphadenopathy less common than in EBV infectious mononucleosis. EBV infectious mononucleosis should be distinguished from other causes of pharyngitis. Group A β-hemolytic streptococci frequently are isolated from the throats of patients with infectious mononucleosis. Therefore isolation of this organism does not rule out EBV infectious mononucleosis. Other diseases that can cause signs and symptoms similar to infectious mononucleosis include malignancies, infection with adenoviruses, *Toxoplasma gondii*, rubella virus, HIV, hepatitis A and B, and diphtheria. Most of these diagnoses can be ruled out by appropriate laboratory tests. An increase in peripheral mononuclear cells including atypical lymphocytes usually exists in infectious mononucleosis. White blood cells counts may be as high as 20,000/mm³. Thrombocytopenia may occur. Often liver enzyme concentrations are mildly elevated.

Serological studies are diagnostic. The classic monospot heterophil agglutination test still is useful in adult disease and provides high specificity and sensitivity. Heterophile antibodies are IgM antibodies induced by EBV against antigens unrelated to the virus, found on sheep, horse, and cattle red blood cells. Children often do not develop a heterophile antibody response to EBV. Consequently viral-specific serological tests should be used in children, especially those younger than 4 years of age. Tests should include IgM and IgG antibody titers to viral capsid antigens. Antibodies to viral nuclear antigen and EBV early antigens also may be used.

Treatment   Supportive therapy usually is sufficient. Most patients are treated with bed rest, adequate fluids, and soft diet. Acetaminophen or ibuprofen usually is prescribed to reduce fever and symptoms associated with pharyngitis. Patients with concurrent streptococcal infection should receive either penicillin or erythromycin for a period of approximately 10 days to prevent streptococcal sequelae. Patients with splenomegaly are advised not to participate in contact sports until the spleen has returned to normal size to prevent rupture. Recovery from infectious mononucleosis often is gradual; some individuals report malaise or fatigue that persists for several months. For this reason, EBV was believed to be a causative agent in chronic fatigue syndrome. However, studies have not supported such an association.[42] Corticosteroid therapy has been advocated because it reduces the duration of fever and generally shortens the period of signs and symptoms. However, because of the many adverse effects, corticosteroid treatment is advocated only in the following situations: (1) impending airway obstruction, (2) severe thrombocytopenia, and (3) hemolytic anemia.

VARICELLA-ZOSTER VIRUS (CHICKENPOX AND SHINGLES)

Varicella-zoster virus (VZV) is a member of the herpesvirus family. It is a double-stranded enveloped DNA virus. The DNA consists of 125-kb pairs that codes for approximately 75 proteins. Five viral glycoproteins are present in the viral envelope, three of which are essential for viral infectivity. Monoclonal antibodies directed against these glycoproteins prevent infection.

Pathogenesis   Humans are the only known reservoirs for VZV. Infection occurs when the virus contacts the mucosa of the upper respiratory tract or conjunctiva. VZV is highly contagious, and infection can occur by direct contact with infected secretions including respiratory droplets. VSV binds to the heparin glycoproteins of the cell membrane. The viral glycoproteins then fuse with the cell membrane, allowing the virus to enter the cell. Similarly, newly synthesized VZV spreads to adjacent cells by direct contact. The virus also disseminates throughout the bloodstream in mononuclear cells.[5] Dissemination results in infection of other organs including the CNS. The virus thus infects and becomes latent in the dorsal root and cranial nerve ganglia.

Primary infection with VZV generally occurs in children younger than 13 years of age, producing varicella or chickenpox. The virus is endemic in the population at large but becomes epidemic during seasonal periods, usually late winter or early spring. After exposure the average incubation period is 14 days (range 10 to 20). Patients are infectious for a period of 48 hours before the onset of vesicles and for 4 to 5 days thereafter until all vesicles are crusted. The vesicles involve the corium and dermis. As viral replication occurs, the host cells undergo apoptosis. Multinucleated giant cells appear. Necrosis and hemorrhage occur in the dermis, resulting in formation of vesicles and an eventual influx of polymorphonuclear neutrophils. The vesicles then either rupture and form crusts or the vesicular fluid is resorbed.

Clinical Characteristics

Chickenpox   Initial signs and symptoms of chickenpox are maculopapular rash, low-grade fever, anorexia, and malaise. The maculopapules develop into vesicles, usually containing a clear fluid, and often are pruritic. Most lesions are small, round or oval, and approximately 5 mm in diameter but can become as large as 12 to 13 mm. Lesions have an erythematous base. Many vesicles become purulent and rupture, resulting in a crusted appearance. The lesions primarily occur on the trunk and face and then spread centripetally to other areas of the body. Lesions also may occur on the mucosa of the oropharynx and vagina but they are less common than skin lesions. The crusted lesions generally fall off within 2 weeks of onset. Prodromal symptoms may appear 1 to 2 days before the onset of the rash. In children who are immunocompetent, chickenpox is a benign illness lasting 3 to 5 days.

The most common extracutaneous involvement is the CNS. Acute cerebellar ataxia or encephalitis can manifest. Acute cerebellar ataxia is characterized by ataxia, vomiting, altered speech, fever, vertigo, and tremor. Most children recover from this complication, with resolution within 2 to 4 weeks. Encephalitis is a much more serious complication. Depressed levels of consciousness, progressive headaches, vomiting, altered thought patterns, fever, and frequent seizures often occur. Five percent to 20% of these patients die of the disease, and neurological sequelae may occur in as many as 15% of the survivors. Other CNS complications include meningitis, transverse myelitis, and Reye's syndrome.[44]

Varicella pneumonitis is a very serious sequela that occurs most frequently in adults and patients who are immunocompromised.[17] Varicella pneumonitis is characterized by cough, tachypnea, dyspnea, and fever. Chest radiographs reveal nodular or interstitial pneumonitis.

In children who are immunocompromised, the skin lesions are more numerous and often have a hemorrhagic base. Visceral organ involvement occurs in 30% to 50% cases and can be fatal in as many as 15% of cases. The lung, liver, and CNS are the most commonly affected sites. Superinfection with gram-positive bacteria, most commonly with type A streptococci, may occur. Streptococcal toxic shock is a rare but lethal complication.

Herpes Zoster After primary infection with VZV, latent infection of cranial nerve and dorsal root ganglia occurs. Reactivation of the virus, often decades later, may occur causing shingles, which often is followed by postherpetic neuralgia, especially in elderly patients who are immunocompetent (>50 years). Alternatively, the reactivated virus can cause zoster sine herpete, a condition characterized by dermatomal pain without an accompanying rash. More than 300,000 case of herpes zoster occur annually in the United States.[32] Zoster is characterized by severe sharp, lancinating, radicular pain and a rash that is indistinguishable from that of chickenpox. The pain often is associated with itching, dysesthesias, and allodynia. Any dermatome may be involved, but the thorax and face are the most common sites. The ophthalmic division of the trigeminal nerve distribution is the most common site of facial lesions. It frequently is associated with ophthalmic keratitis, which can result in blindness. Zoster of the maxillary and mandibular divisions of the trigeminal nerve may be associated with osteonecrosis and spontaneous exfoliation of teeth. Seventh cranial nerve involvement is characterized by a rash on the external ear and peripheral facial weakness (Ramsay Hunt syndrome). Zoster may involve the third cranial nerve resulting in ophthalmoplegia. Optic neuritis also may occur. Lower cranial nerve involvement is less common. Cervical zoster sometimes is associated with arm weakness. Less frequently diaphragmatic paralysis occurs. Similarly, lumbosacral zoster may be associated with leg weakness and bowel or bladder dysfunction. Complications of CNS involvement include myelitis characterized by paraparesis and sphincter impairment resulting from involvement of the spinal cord. Myelitis usually occurs within 2 weeks of the onset of rash; unfortunately, this condition may become chronic. Large- and small-vessel vasculopathies also may be caused by VZV. Large-vessel encephalitis (granulomatous arteritis) can result in hemorrhagic strokes. The disease is uncommon and occurs primarily in patients older than 60 years who are immunocompetent; encephalitis usually occurs 7 weeks after the development of zoster. Small-vessel encephalitis primarily occurs in patients who are immunocompromised (patients with AIDS). Small-vessel encephalitis is characterized by hemiplegia, aphasia, and visual field deficits and usually is fatal.

Postherpetic neuralgia is a frequent complication of herpes zoster. This condition is characterized by pain that persists more than 6 weeks after the development of the rash. Postherpetic neuralgia is more common in women. It does not occur in patients younger than 50 years of age and occurs in more than 40% of patients older than 60 years of age.[31]

Diagnosis The diagnosis of chickenpox and shingles usually is made based on history and physical examina-

tion. The presence of the characteristic skin rash and vesicles in all stages of development accompanied by fever, pruritus, and pain generally provides the basis for the diagnosis of chickenpox. The localization and distribution of the vesicular rash serves as the basis for the diagnosis of shingles. An infection sometimes confused with zoster is impetigo, which is caused by group A streptococci. Small vesicles may occur at the site of bacterial inoculation in injured skin. Often the vesicles progress to cellulitis and bacteremia. Demonstration of gram-positive cocci in scrapings from the lesions is diagnostic. Disseminated vesicular lesions also may be caused by herpes simplex viruses. However, these lesions often occur in combination with an underlying skin disorder (i.e., ectopic dermatitis or eczema). Diagnosis is made by isolation of the virus in tissue culture. Coxsackieviruses also may cause widespread distal vesicular lesions. However, the vesicles are morbilliform and hemorrhagic and occur more commonly in the oropharynx, palms of the hands, and soles of the feet. Isolation of the causative virus in tissue culture is the definitive method of diagnosis. Identification of VZV antibodies in acute or convalescent serum also is useful. For CNS infection, demonstration of VZV DNA in the CSF by PCR assay is most helpful.

Treatment Treatment of the normal host with chickenpox or shingles is directed toward reduction of the risk of complications. Prevention of secondary bacterial infection in patients with chickenpox is a primary goal. Frequent bathing, use of astringent soaks, and closely cropped fingernails are useful to prevent scratching of the pruritic lesions. Pruritus also can be decreased by application of a topical dressing or antipruritic drugs. Aluminum acetate or soaks with Burrow's solution are useful. Acetaminophen rather than aspirin should be used to reduce fever and prevent Reye's syndrome. Oral acyclovir therapy has been approved in the treatment of chickenpox and shingles. Acyclovir therapy helps to shorten lesion formation approximately 1 day, reduces the number of lesions, and reduces associated symptoms.[31] For children, the dosage is 20 mg/kg qid for 5 days (maximum dose 800 mg qid). For adolescents and adults, 800 mg five times per day is recommended. Alternatively, famciclovir (500 mg tid) also may be prescribed. Patients with ophthalmic division zoster should receive antiviral drugs for at least 7 days.

No universally accepted treatment for postherpetic neuralgia exists. Several types of neuroactive drugs have been used, including tricyclic antidepressants and the anticonvulsants carbamazepine and phenytoin. Some patients experience less pain with these drugs. A short course of steroids has been advocated to reduce inflammation. Ketamine therapy is effective but associated with intolerable side effects. The use of acyclovir alone or in combination with steroids reduces neuritis duration and improves quality of life.[94]

Prevention A vaccine containing a live attenuated Oka strain of VZV is available. Seroconversion occurs in 94% to

100% of children 12 months or older with one dose. Sero-conversion in adults is approximately 70% with two doses.[17] Subclinical infection occurs that is then protective. Whether administration of the vaccine to elderly patients at risk for herpes zoster will prevent an outbreak is unknown. For patients who are immunocompromised, administration of varicella-zoster immune globulin has been useful as a preventive and to ameliorate symptoms of chickenpox. Varicella-zoster immune globulin also is useful in pregnant woman who are seronegative and at high risk because the vaccine may result in fetal damage.

CYTOMEGALOVIRUS

Pathogenesis   CMV is a common viral pathogen that infects a large percentage of the population. In many U.S. cities, 60% to 70% of the population has been infected before adulthood.[98] CMV is a herpesvirus that consists of an enveloped double-stranded DNA genome. CMV is the largest virus to infect humans; its genome codes for approximately 230 proteins. Many viral glycoproteins are present in the envelope that are involved in viral entry into host cells; however, the host cell receptor or receptors necessary for viral attachment have not been identified. Host cell endocytosis is the primary mechanism of viral entry. CMV also produces several proteins that are directly involved in downregulation of the host immune response. One of the most important is a protein that prevents binding of processed viral protein antigens to human leukocyte antigen I proteins for antigenic display on the host cell membrane. Human leukocyte antigen I antigen complexes serve as the target recognition signal for CD8$^+$ cytotoxic lymphocytes. Similar to other herpesviruses, CMV can be latent in host cells for a lifetime. Reactivation can occur whenever favorable conditions exist. Primary infection with CMV results in highly variable disease, ranging from no disease in normal hosts who are immunocompetent, to a commonly fatal disease in neonates, to an infectious mononucleosis syndrome in young adults. In individuals who are immunocompromised, CMV produces severe disease that may affect the lung, liver, kidney, CNS, and gastrointestinal tract. CMV is the most common opportunistic viral pathogen detected and causes significant morbidity and mortality.[70]

Clinical Characteristics

Primary Disease   Infectious mononucleosis syndrome is one of the most common manifestations of primary disease in immunocompetent young adults. It is estimated that 79% of infectious mononucleosis is caused by EBV and the remaining 21% is caused by CMV.[47] In general, patients with CMV mononucleosis are older than patients with EBV disease. Systemic signs and symptoms of fever and malaise are major manifestations, whereas pharyngitis, tonsillitis, splenomegaly, and lymphadenopathy are less common in CMV than EBV mononucleosis.[75] Patients with CMV mononucleosis have negative heterophil test results and often have slightly elevated liver enzyme concentrations.

Complications in normal hosts include (1) interstitial pneumonia characterized by interstitial infiltrates on chest radiographs; (2) hepatitis, which usually is mild and rarely symptomatic; (3) Guillain-Barré syndrome, characterized by polyneuritis resulting in sensory and motor weakness that usually resolves within 3 months; (4) meningoencephalitis, characterized by severe headache, photophobia, lethargy, and pyramidal tract findings; (5) myocarditis; and (6) thrombocytopenia and hemolytic anemia, most commonly seen in children with congenital CMV.

Reactivation (Reinfection) Disease   Reactivation (reinfection) CMV primarily occurs in the setting of immunodeficiency. Most CMV disease is caused by reactivation of latent virus and is the result of defective cell-mediated immunity because many patients have adequate antibody titers. However, reinfection with new CMV viral subtypes has been reported in patients with AIDS.[37] Coinfection with CMV has been noted in more than 90% of homosexual men with HIV and is the most common viral opportunistic infection in this patient group.[13] Most patients with AIDS who develop CMV disease have CD4$^+$ lymphocyte counts less than 100/mm^3. CMV retinitis is the most common form of CMV disease in this patient group and occurs only rarely in transplant patients who are immunosuppressed.[43] CMV pneumonitis is the most common CMV disease in transplant recipients. CMV retinitis causes a complete-thickness infection of the retinal cells. Progressive irreversible retinal destruction occurs, resulting in severe visual impairment and eventual blindness.

The gastrointestinal tract frequently is affected by CMV disease in patients with AIDS and much less frequently in transplant patients. Gastrointestinal CMV infection is the most common cause of elective abdominal surgery in patients with AIDS.[33] Signs and symptoms include odynophagia with or without dysphagia; nausea and vomiting; abdominal pain; colitis, often with bloody diarrhea; painful oral erosions or ulcers; enlarged painful salivary glands; and ulcers of the esophagus, stomach, and small and large intestines.

CNS CMV disease also occurs frequently in patients with AIDS. CMV of the spinal cord is characterized by polyradiculopathy. Signs and symptoms include ascending weakness in the lower extremities and loss of deep tendon reflexes followed by loss of bowel and bladder control. The syndrome often begins with the onset of lower back pain with radicular or perianal radiation. CMV encephalitis has been reported in approximately 16% of patients with AIDS who died of their disease. CMV encephalitis also occurs in organ transplant patients.[4] The disease is characterized by fever, headache, confusion, seizures, coma, aphasia or dysphasia, and cranial nerve palsies. Fortunately, the recent introduction of HAART HIV antiviral therapy has significantly reduced the incidence of CMV end-organ disease in patients with AIDS.[6]

The incidence of opportunistic CMV disease in transplant patients is directly related to the degree of iatrogenic immunosuppression. The more severe the immune suppression, such as required after bone marrow transplantation, the more severe the opportunistic disease that occurs. Seronegative transplant patients also are at risk of developing primary disease, most commonly acquired from the transplanted organ and blood transfusions.

Diagnosis   Diagnosis of CMV infection depends on the growth of the virus from urine, CSF, or other body fluids or the demonstration of virion components such as viral antigens or DNA. Also useful is the identification of large nuclear inclusion–bearing cells, cytomegalic cells, in the sediment of body fluids such as the urine. Alternatively, a monoclonal antibody to the CMV matrix protein pp65 can be used to identify CMV antigen in the spinal fluid of patients in whom a CNS disease is suspected, or in the serum or leukocytes of patients with other suspected end-organ involvement. PCR assay provides a sensitive (79% to 100%) test for the detection of viral DNA.[4] Most commonly primers to the genes encoding immediate early proteins or DNA polymerase have been used. This technique reliably detects even small amounts of viral DNA in the CSF and other body fluids.

Treatment   Antiviral drugs that inhibit viral DNA polymerase have been effective in treating CMV end-organ disease. Ganciclovir, foscarnet, and cidofovir have been used successfully. Prophylactic ganciclovir treatment prevented gastrointestinal CMV in patients who had positive culture results after bone marrow transplantation.[34] Foscarnet has been effective in the treatment of CNS CMV.[40] In 80% to 90% of patients with CMV retinitis, intravenous ganciclovir or foscarnet administered twice daily for 14 to 21 days successfully arrested retinal-cell necrosis and reduced viral recovery from host urine and blood. Unfortunately, reactivation of CMV retinitis occurs in a high percentage of patients when drug therapy is discontinued. Cidofovir also is effective but may produce serious irreversible nephrotoxic effects.[43]

PAPILLOMAVIRUSES

Human papillomaviruses (HPVs) are ubiquitous and widespread throughout the world population. HPVs produce a wide spectrum of benign to malignant epithelial tumors of the skin and mucous membranes and have been associated closely with development of cervical cancers. Skin lesions vary from simple warts, which often occur on the hands and soles of the feet, to the rare epidermodysplasia verruciformis. The HPVs are small, nonencapsulated, circular, double-stranded DNA viruses of approximately 7800 bp. More than 100 different types have been identified. Each HPV type has a specific tissue tropism and different oncogenic properties. HPVs characteristically infect cells of the epithelium. The skin is the most common site of infection, but the mucosa of the genitalia, mouth, esophagus, larynx, trachea, and conjunctiva also may be affected.

Pathogenesis   HPVs characteristically infect the basal cells of the epithelium. Infection of the host cell may be permissive or persistent. Permissive infections follow the classic viral cycle: adsorption, penetration, transcription, translation, DNA replication, and maturation. A persistent infection occurs when HPV development is arrested at certain stages of its replication cycle. The persistent state appears to be involved in host cell transformation and development of malignancy. After viral penetration of the basal cell the virus may remain dormant depending on the differentiation program of the keratinocyte. Viral replication is initiated when the basal cell begins its differentiation into a squamous cell.[60] As the basal cells differentiate and progress to the surface of the epithelium, HPV DNA replicates and virions are assembled and released when the dead keratinocytes are shed. In a wart or condyloma, viral replication is associated with excessive proliferation of all layers of the epidermis except the basal layer, resulting in acanthosis, parakeratosis, and hyperkeratosis. Deepening of the rete ridges also occurs. Basal cell proliferation is characteristic of premalignant and malignant transformation.

Hyperplasia and hyperkeratosis are the hallmarks of skin infection with dermatotrophic HPVs. The characteristics of the lesion depend on the type of HPV causing the infection. Types 1, 2, and 4 are associated with common warts and plantar warts. Types 3, 10, 28, and 41 are associated with flat warts. Types 5, 8, 9, 12, 14, 15, 17, 19 through 25, 36, 46, and 47 are associated with epidermodysplasia verruciformis, which is characterized by disseminated cutaneous warts that undergo frequent malignant transformation. More than 25 mucosotropic HPVs exist. Laryngeal papillomatosis is caused by types 6 and 11. Papillomata of the mouth are caused by types 7, 16, and 32 in addition to types 6 and 11. Focal epithelial hyperplasia of the mouth is associated with types 13 and 32. Malignant tumors at these sites have been linked to types 16 and 18. Genital HPV infections produce venereal warts or condyloma acuminatum. Most infections are caused by types 6 and 11. Malignant transformation of these lesions is rare. Carcinomas of the anogenital region have been associated with lesions caused by types 16 and 18.

Close personal contact appears to be important for transmission of the virus in most cutaneous warts. Minor trauma at the site of inoculation also may be important because of the high incidence of these lesions in fish and meat handlers. Anogenital warts appear to be sexually transmitted.

Clinical Characteristics
Cutaneous Warts   Cutaneous warts include common, plantar, and flat warts. Common warts appear as well-demarcated, exophytic, hyperkeratotic papules with a rough surface. Common warts occur on the dorsum of the hand, between fingers, around nails, on the palms and soles, and rarely on mucous membranes. Morphological variants include mosaic warts—cobblestone patches several square centimeters in diameter rising slightly above an indurated base. Filiform warts usually occur on the head, and hyperproliferative, vegetating warts are seen primarily on the hands of fish and meat handlers. Plantar warts look like

raised bundles of soft keratotic fibers 2 mm to 1 cm in diameter. Lesions often are painful and most commonly occur in adolescents and young adults. Finally, flat warts appear as multiple, slightly elevated papules with an irregular contour and smooth surface. Flat warts are most common in children. Spontaneous resolution frequently occurs.

Epidermodysplasia Verruciformis   These warts appear as several morphological variants. The warts may resemble flat warts but more commonly resemble the lesion of pityriasis versicolor that covers the torso and upper extremities. The lesions occur most commonly in children. Many lesions, especially in sun-exposed areas, undergo malignant transformation to invasive squamous cell carcinomas. Patients usually have defects in cell-mediated immunity.

Anogenital Warts (Condylomata Acuminata)   Anogenital warts are flesh or gray colored hyperkeratotic exophytic papules usually attached to the skin by a broad peduncle. Lesions vary in size from less than 1 mm to several square centimeters when they merge into plaques. In men the penile shaft is involved most commonly. The urethral meatus also may be affected. Lesions may occur in the perianal area and in the mouth depending on the sexual practices of the patient. Lesions are most common in homosexual men and least common in heterosexual men. Lesions rarely occur on the scrotum, perineum, groin, and pubic areas. In women, most lesions occur on the posterior vulva introitus, the labia majora and minora, and the clitoris. Less commonly lesions may occur on the perineum, vagina, cervix, and urethra.

Approximately 75% of patients with anogenital warts display no symptoms. Itching and burning, pain, and tenderness are most common in symptomatic lesions. Spontaneous remission may occur. Malignant transformation to invasive or verrucous carcinoma rarely occurs.

The oral cavity also may be a site of HPV infection. Focal epithelial hyperplasia (Heck's disease) is caused predominantly by HPV type 13. Lesions appear on the lips and buccal mucosa as soft, multiple, 1- to 5-mm nodules of the same color as the adjacent mucosa. These lesions regress spontaneously. Laryngeal papillomas also may occur. They appear as soft, friable nodules that rarely exceed 1 cm in diameter.

Diagnosis   Diagnosis of warts usually is made on the basis of clinical examination. Histopathological examination may be useful. Lesions are characterized by acanthosis, parakeratosis, and hyperkeratosis. Virus inclusions sometimes can be seen in cells. PCR can be used to identify viral DNA in cells from the lesion.

Treatment   Safe and highly effective treatments of HPV diseases are not available. Most treatments are designed to decrease or eliminate undesirable clinical manifestations. Most approaches involve physical or chemical destruction of the lesions. These methods include excision, laser ablation and cryotherapy, and application of salicylic and lac-

tic acid paint or podophyllin resin. Podophyllotoxin, the active ingredient in podophyllin resin, now is available in the United States as the drug podofilox. With its standardized composition and potency, podofilox appears to be more efficacious with fewer adverse effects than podophyllin resin. However, determination of the efficacy of these treatments is difficult because many warts regress spontaneously. Recently imiquimod, an imidazoquinolineamine available as a 5% cream, has been used in the treatment of condyloma acuminatum. Imiquimod is an immune response modulator that increases production of both alpha and gamma interferons. In addition, imiquimod upregulates cell-mediated immunity.[90] Significant efficacy of imiquimod with acceptable adverse side effects has been shown in a well-controlled study.[62]

RIBONUCLEIC ACID VIRUSES

COXSACKIEVIRUSES GROUP A (HERPANGINA, HAND-FOOT-AND-MOUTH DISEASE)

The coxsackieviruses are members of the group of enteroviruses, all of which are picornaviruses. These viruses are small, nonenveloped, and contain a single linear strand of ribonucleic acid (RNA) of approximately 7.5 kb. The RNA is infectious and may function as a template for synthesis of RNA progeny or a messenger RNA that codes for a single polyprotein. The polyprotein then undergoes specific cleavages yielding structural polypeptides, an RNA replicase, viral proteases, and additional peptides needed for viral replication. These viruses commonly infect humans throughout the world and produce a broad range of diseases, including enanthems and exanthems, hemorrhagic conjunctivitis, myocarditis, pericarditis, CNS syndromes (most commonly aseptic meningitis), and febrile illnesses with or without respiratory symptoms (Table 11-2). Included in this group are polioviruses, group A and B coxsackieviruses, and echoviruses. Certain serotypes have been associated with particular syndromes. Coxsackievirus A16 usually is associated with hand-foot-and-mouth disease, and coxsackieviruses A2 through A6 are associated with herpangina. However, considerable overlap of diseases caused by these viruses exists. For example, a recent outbreak of hand-foot-and-mouth disease and herpangina in Taiwan was caused predominantly by enterovirus type 71 (61.9%), coxsackievirus type A16, (27.5%) and the remaining 10.6% of cases by other enteroviruses.[41]

Pathogenicity   Enteroviruses infect humans primarily as result of ingestion. The viruses then infect and replicate in cells of the pharynx and gut, which are believed to be mucosal cells. Eventually the lymphoid cells of the submucosal lymphatic tissues (e.g., Peyer's patches and tonsils) are infected. The virus then is passed to the regional lymph nodes, and a viremia may occur with spread to liver, spleen, bone marrow, and deep lymph nodes. Target organ

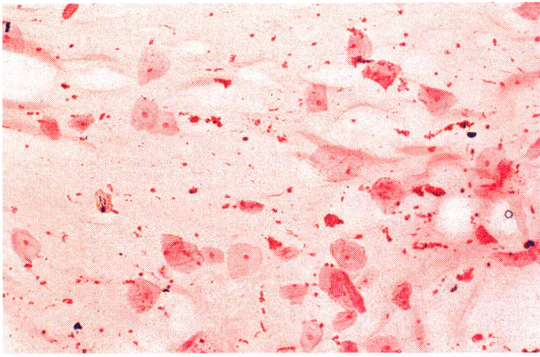

Plate 1 Squamous epithelial cells indicating superficial contamination. (Gram stain; ×100.)

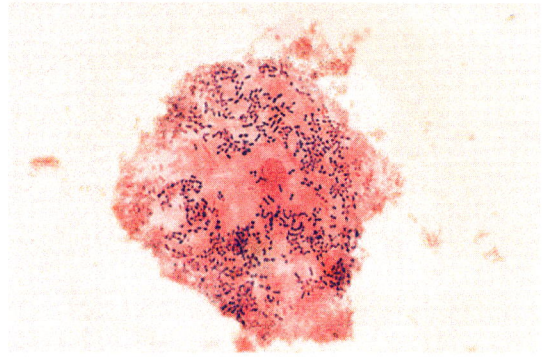

Plate 2 Squamous epithelial cell showing indigenous gram-positive and gram-negative organisms contained in specimens of superficial material. (Gram stain; ×1000.)

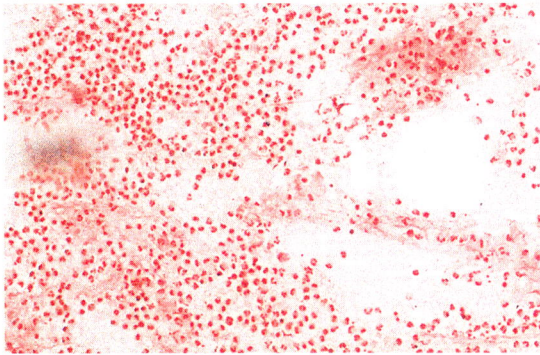

Plate 3 Inflammatory exudate containing neutrophils. (Gram stain; ×100.)

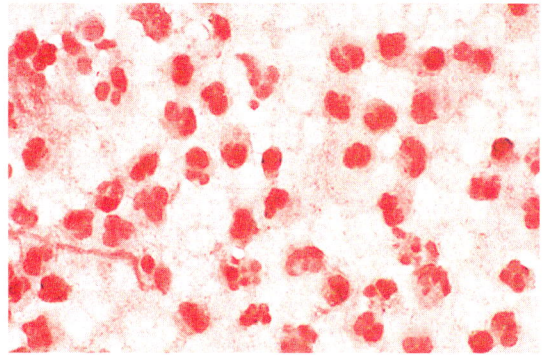

Plate 4 Neutrophils in inflammatory exudate. (Gram stain; ×1000.)

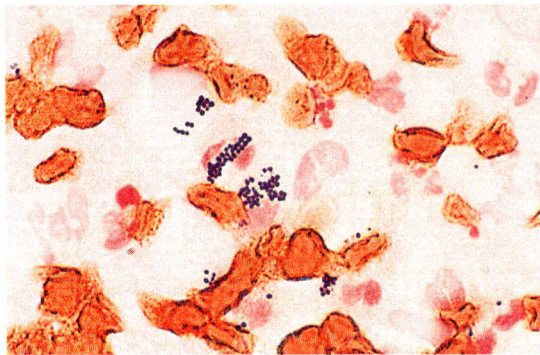

Plate 5 Direct smear of cyst fluid containing staphylococci. (Gram stain; ×1000.)

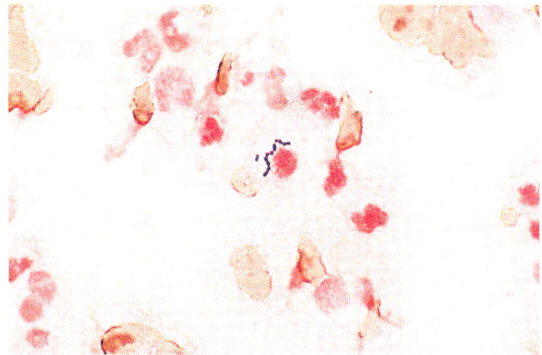

Plate 6 Direct smear demonstrating chains of streptococci. (Gram stain; ×1000.)

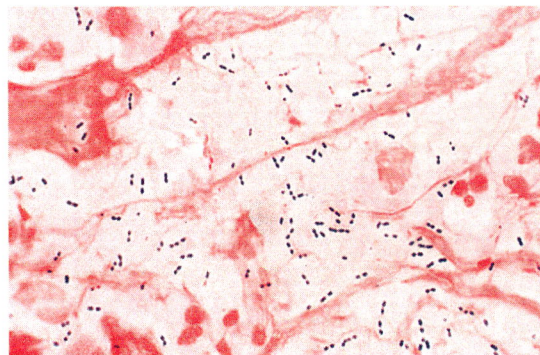

Plate 7 Direct sputum smear containing lancet-shaped gram-positive cocci suggestive of *S. pneumoniae*. (Gram stain; ×1000.)

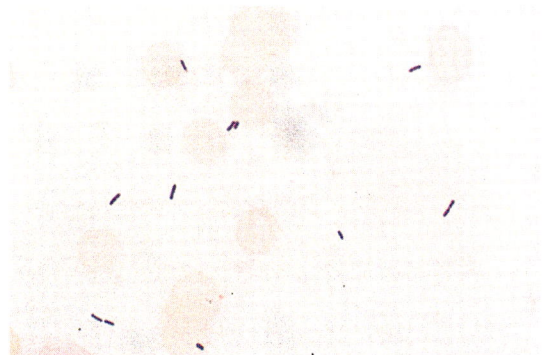

Plate 8 Direct smear of neck tissue containing plump gram-positive rods suggestive of *Clostridium*. Note the absence of spores in clinical material. (Gram stain; ×1000.)

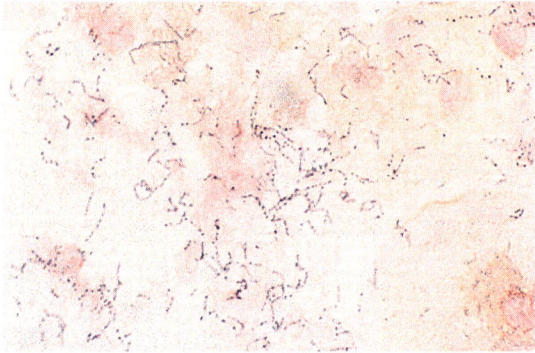

Plate 9 Direct smear of abscess fluid containing fine, sometimes branching gram-positive rods suggestive of *Actinomyces*. (Gram stain; ×1000.)

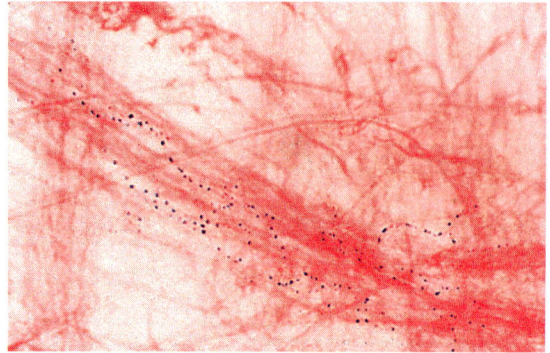

Plate 10 Direct smear containing fine, beaded, filamentous gram-positive rods suggestive of *Nocardia*. Note that the incomplete staining of the organism may result in its misinterpretation as streptococci. (Gram stain; ×1000.)

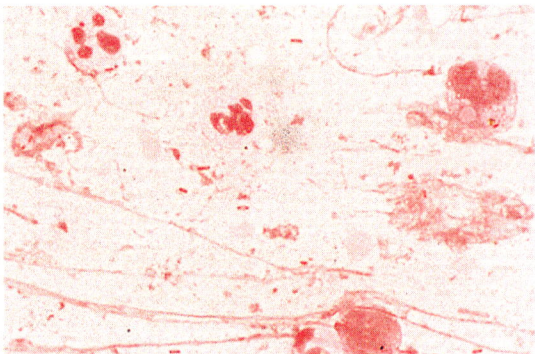

Plate 11 Direct smear containing plump gram-negative rods that demonstrate bipolar staining suggestive of Enterobacteriaceae. (Gram stain; ×1000.)

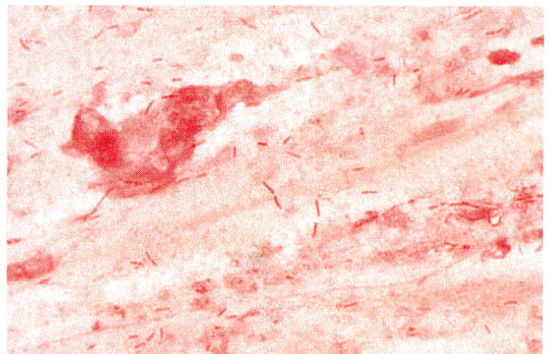

Plate 12 Direct smear containing slender, uniform-staining gram-negative rods suggestive of *Pseudomonas*. Note that organisms may be grouped end to end in pairs. (Gram stain; ×1000.)

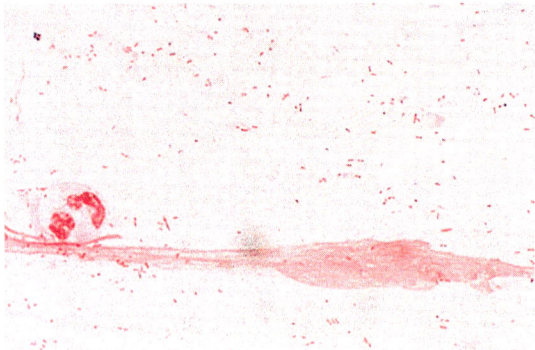

Plate 13 Direct smear containing small pleomorphic gram-negative rods suggestive of *Haemophilus* or *Bacteroides* infection. (Gram stain; ×1000.)

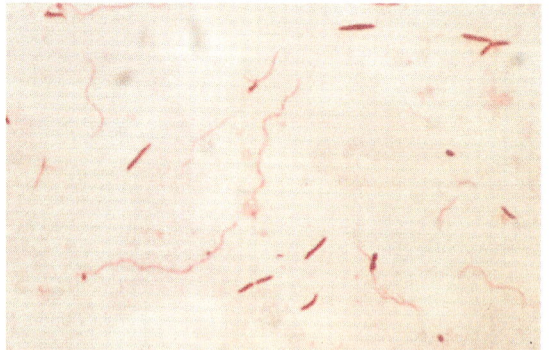

Plate 14 Direct smear of exudate from patient with Vincent's angina. Note the presence of spiral *T. vincentii* and long rods suggestive of *Fusobacterium*. (Gram stain counterstained with carbolfuchsin; ×1000.)

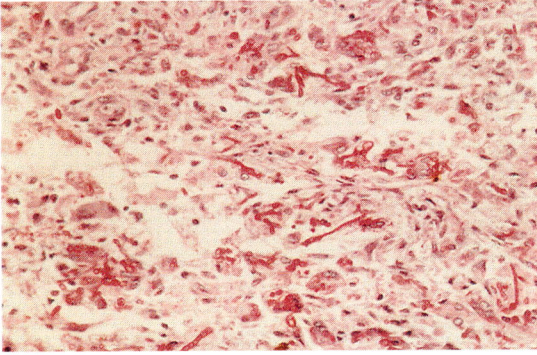

Plate 15 Tissue stained with periodic acid–Schiff (PAS) demonstrating red-staining fungal hyphae. (PAS; ×160.)

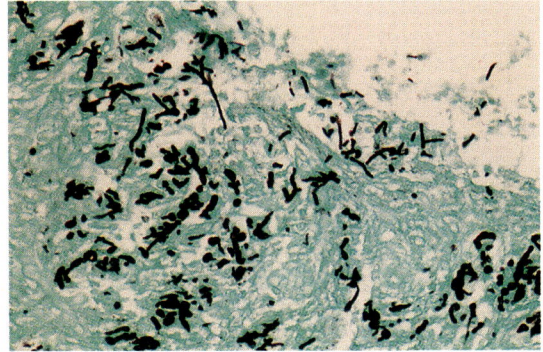

Plate 16 Tissue stained with Gomori's methenamine silver (GMS) demonstrating darkly stained (black) fungal hyphae. (GMS; ×160.)

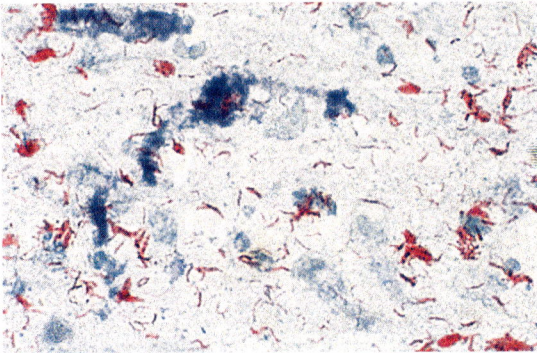

Plate 17 Direct smear of neck mass demonstrating numerous acid-fast bacilli. (Ziehl-Neelsen; ×1000).

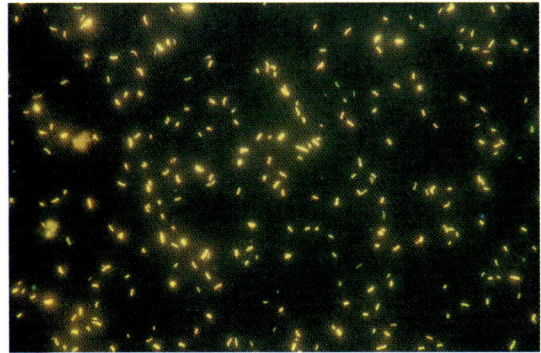

Plate 18 Direct smear of sputum demonstrating numerous acid-fast bacilli. The dark background facilitates the detection of fluorescing organisms. (Rhodamine-auramine; ×400.)

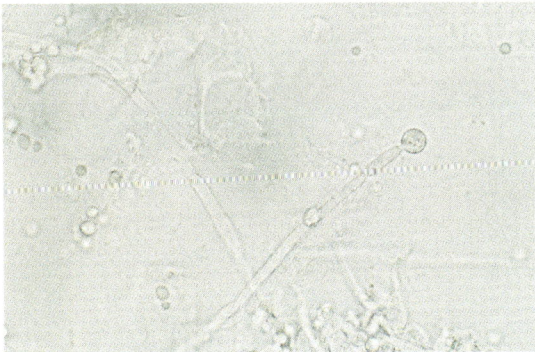

Plate 19 Direct smear of tongue scrapings from a patient with thrush. Note the presence of budding yeast and pseudohyphae suggestive of *Candida*. (Potassium hydroxide wet preparation; ×100.)

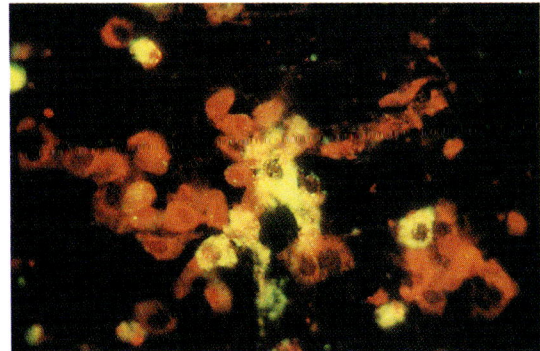

Plate 20 Direct smear of a nasopharyngeal aspirate from an infant stained with a monoclonal antibody specific for RSV. Note the presence of green fluorescence in RSV-infected cells. Other cells appear red because of the Evans blue counterstain. This method also allows for the determination of specimen adequacy. (Immunofluorescent stain; ×400.)

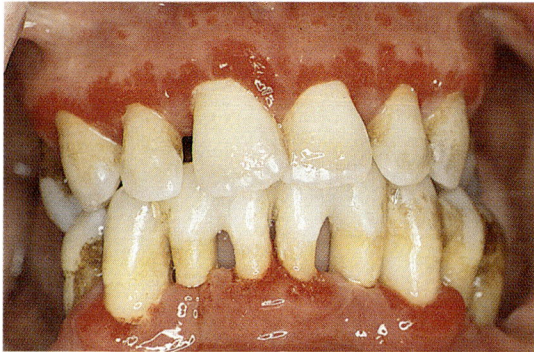

Plate 21 Severe aggressive periodontitis in a 29-year-old man with leukocyte adhesion deficiency syndrome.

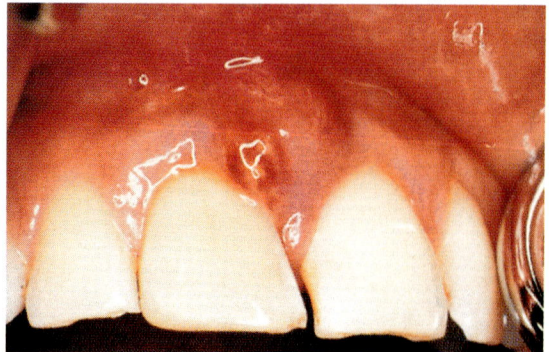

Plate 22 Acute periodontal abscess of right central incisor with advanced periodontitis.

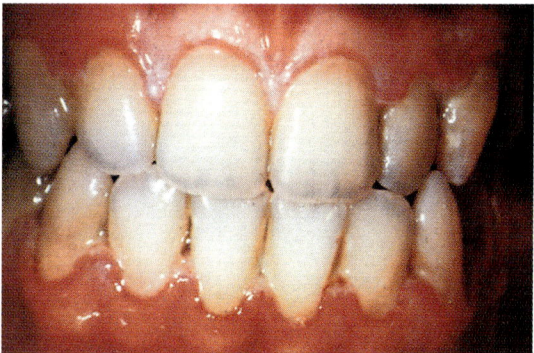

Plate 23 Early acute necrotizing ulcerative gingivitis involving only papillae.

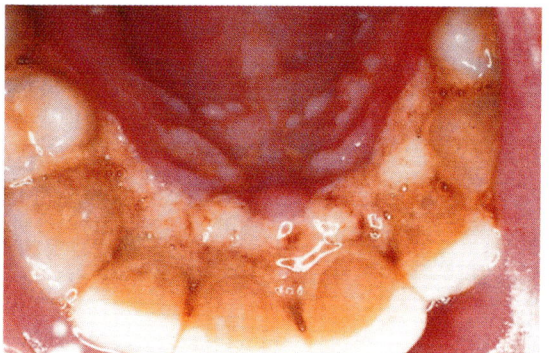

Plate 24 Acute necrotizing ulcerative gingivitis with extensive involvement of papillary and marginal gingiva.

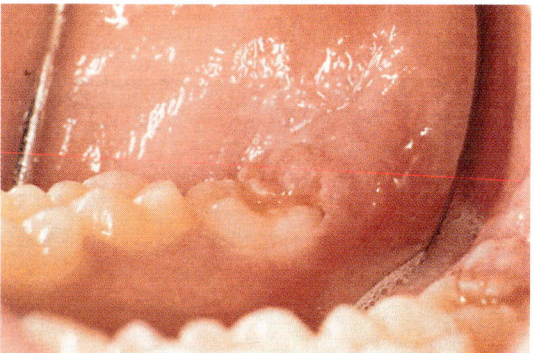

Plate 25 Acute pericoronitis with purulent exudation in mandibular third molar; extensive inflammation of pericoronal and adjacent mucosa is present.

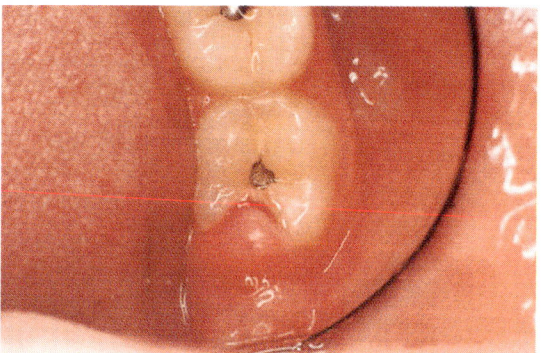

Plate 26 Acute pericoronitis of mandibular third molar; inflammation is confined to tissue on the occlusal surface.

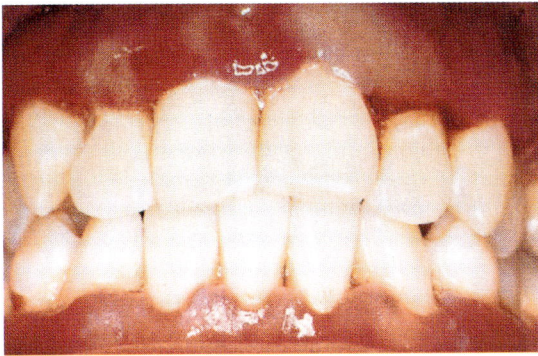

Plate 27 Severe aggressive periodontitis associated with AIDS.

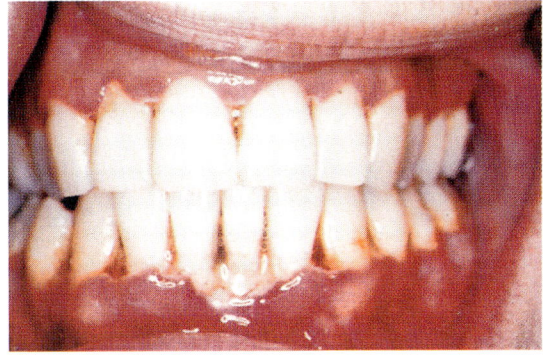

Plate 28 Acute necrotizing ulcerative gingivitis-periodontitis in a patient who is HIV positive.

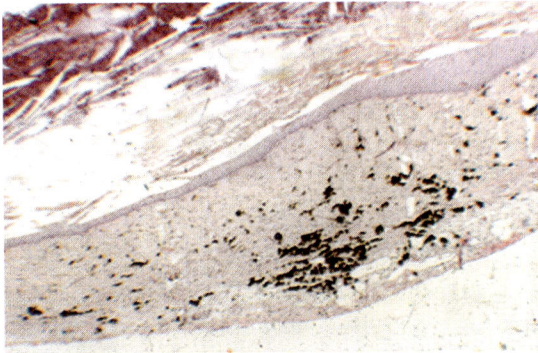

Plate 29 Histological section of a cyst with epithelium lining the border.

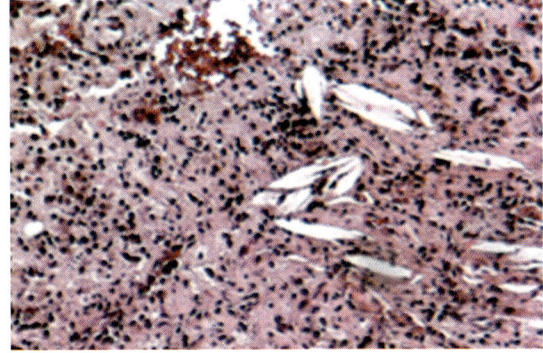

Plate 30 Histological section of a granuloma with infiltrate of lymphocytes and plasma cells and cholesterol slits in the tissue.

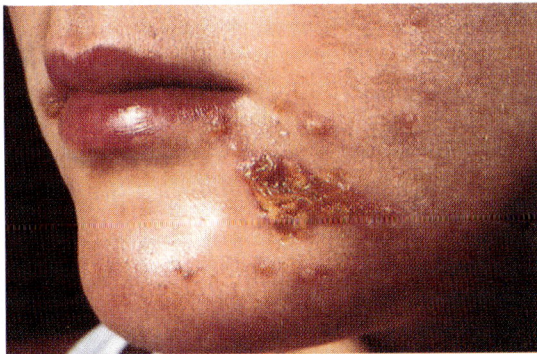

Plate 31 Streptococcal impetigo; typical presentation of perioral oozing and thickly crusted lesions with erythematous borders. Short-lived vesicles preceded the lesions shown here but ruptured.

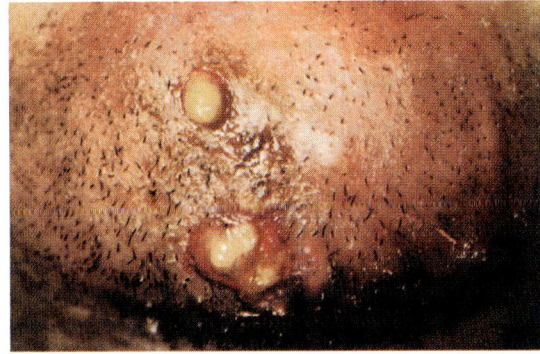

Plate 32 Staphyloccal carbuncle; a group of furuncles involving hair follicles of the chin have coalesced and spontaneously ruptured, leaving a raised, erythematous, tender lesion draining purulence.

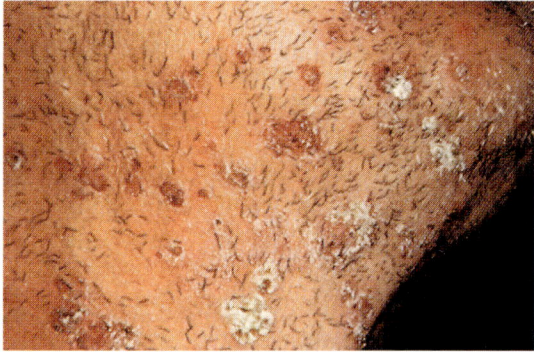

Plate 33 Folliculitis in bearded area of the face. (From Hall J, editor: *Sauer's manual of skin diseases,* ed 8, Lippincott, 2000.)

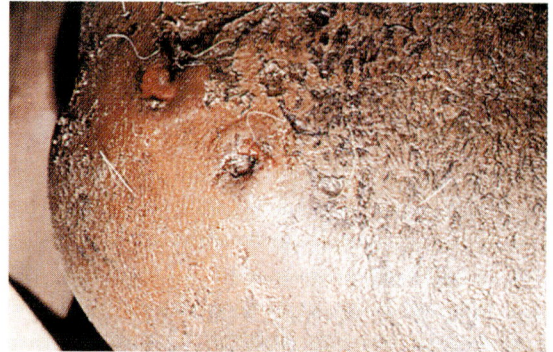

Plate 34 Cutaneous anthrax is characterized by marked erythema, edema, and vesicle eruption. (From Armstrong D, Cohen J: *Infectious diseases,* vol 2, London, 1999, Mosby.)

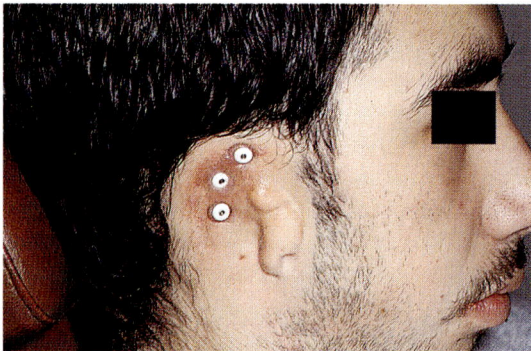

Plate 35 Local tissue infection after external implants for an ear prosthesis. Cultures grew methicillin-resistant *Staphylococcus epidermis,* demonstrating the need for sensitivity testing. The overhanging plastic healing caps further impeded adequate hygiene around the fixtures.

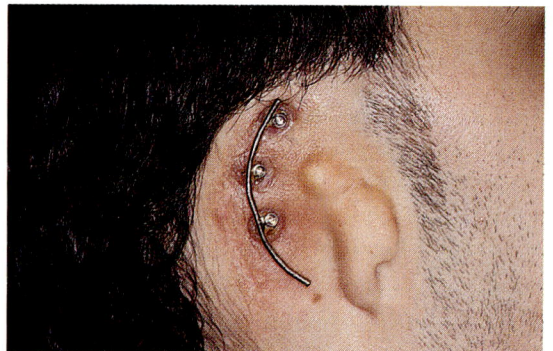

Plate 36 Same patient as in Plate 35. The infection resolved with appropriate antibiotics, local cleansing, and placement of the final bar prosthesis, which facilitated hygiene.

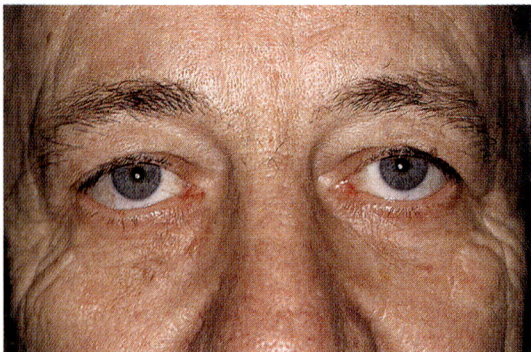

Plate 37 A patient with a previous mid-forehead lift is prepared for forehead dermabrasion and bilateral upper lid blepharoplasty and dermatochalasis and scar camouflage. This photo shows the patient before surgery.

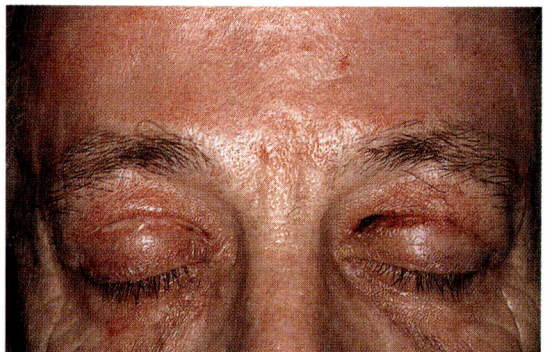

Plate 38 Patient in Plate 37 shown 5 days after surgery. The patient had rubbed his incisions and created a wound separation with superficial infection, which was treated with gentle wound care and antibiotic ointment.

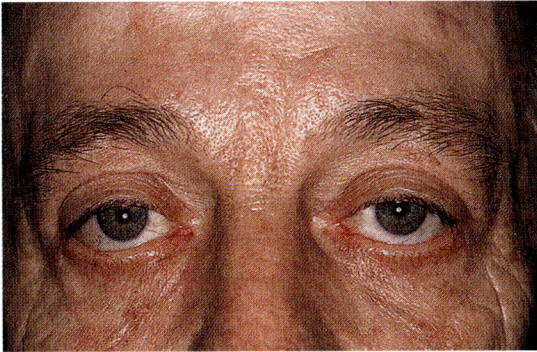

Plate 39 Patient in Plates 37 and 28 shown 9 months after surgery.

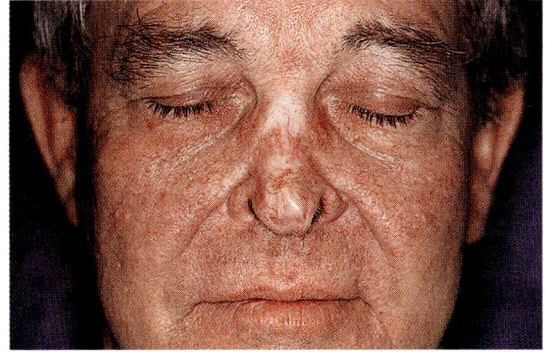

Plate 40 This patient had undergone carbon dioxide laser treatment of rhinophyma elsewhere approximately 5 years earlier. The skin–soft tissue envelope over the nose is densely scarred. This patient would be a poor candidate for alloplastic nasal augmentation because of scarring, hypovascularity, and decreased resistance to infection.

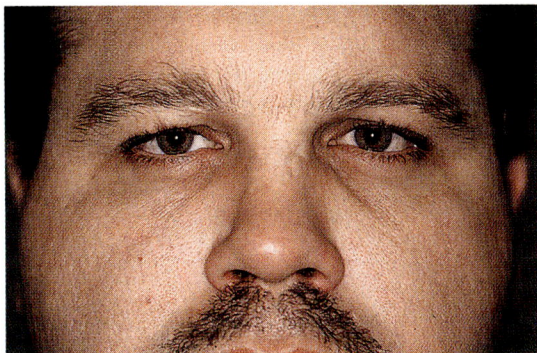

Plate 41 This patient had previously fractured and lacerated his nose and was prepared for nasal reconstructive surgery. This photo shows the patient before surgery with a visible nasal left lateral scar. (Plates 41 through 47 refer to the same patient.)

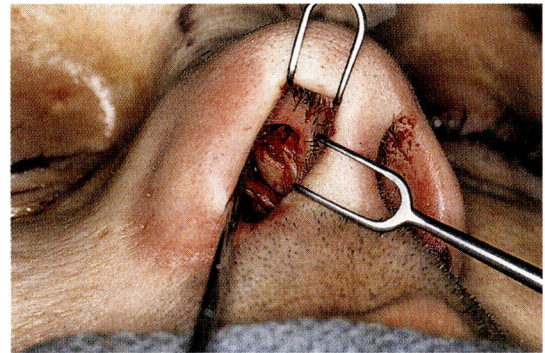

Plate 42 Endonasal nasal harvest of deflected septal cartilage.

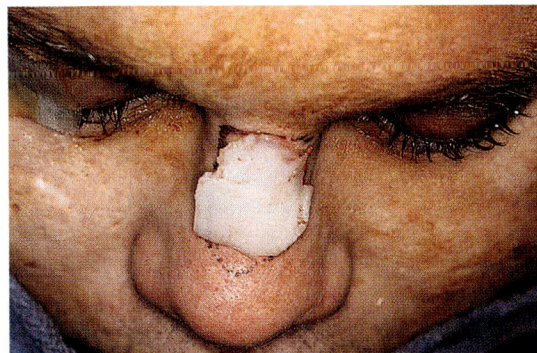

Plate 43 Planned position of cartilage for dorsal augmentation. The graft subsequently was divided longitudinally and the halves were glued together with a thin layer of n-butyl histocryl as a two-layer stack graft to elevate the dorsum. The patient was treated with a cephalosporin antibiotic before and for 5 days after surgery.

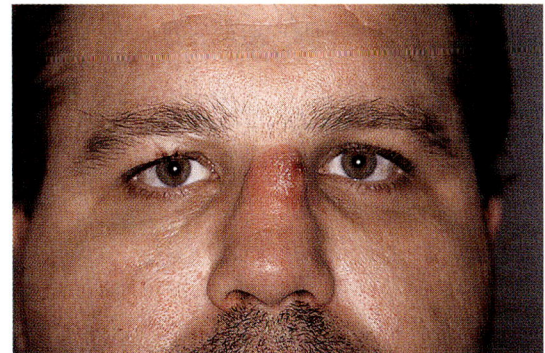

Plate 44 At 17 days after surgery the infected area was drained manually, the material was cultured, and the patient started amoxicillin-clavulanate therapy for presumed staphylococcal infection.

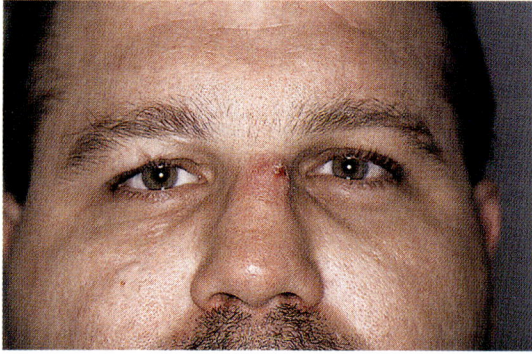

Plate 45 Frontal view at 21 days after surgery. The cultures from the dorsum and nasal septum grew *Enterobacter,* which was resistant to amoxicillin-clavulanate and cephalosporin antibiotic therapy. Based on sensitivities and incomplete response to empirical antibiotic therapy, the patient's antibiotic regimen was changed to ofloxacin and the infection resolved completely.

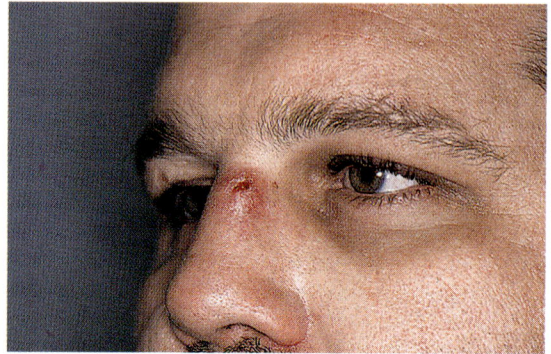

Plate 46 Oblique view at 21 days after surgery.

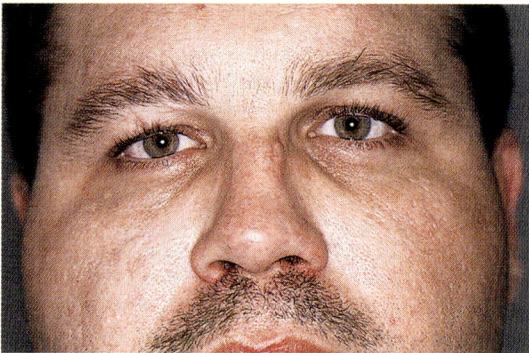

Plate 47 After surgery the original scar has widened and will likely require revision. Dorsal augmentation has been maintained despite infection.

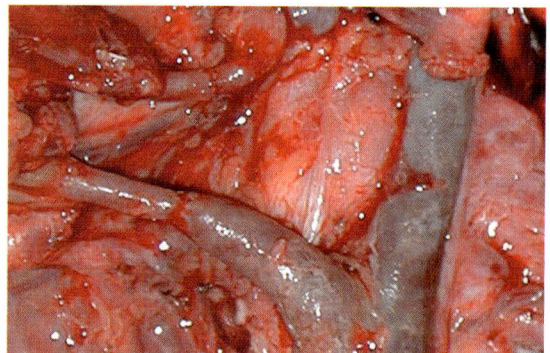

Plate 48 A free radial forearm flap microvascular anastomosis demonstrates the skeletonization of the flap vascular pedicle and recipient vessels required to complete the microvascular anastomosis. Such isolation of the vascular pedicle decreases resistance to the insults of wound infection and salivary fistulas.

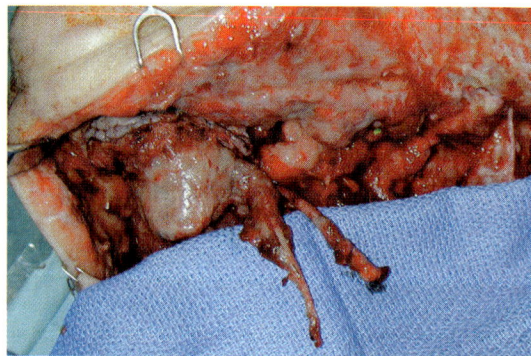

Plate 49 Salivary contamination of a wound after composite resection, neck dissection, and free radial forearm flap reconstruction. The cephalic vein is thrombotic (distended; clot is visible at site of transection) without compromise of the radial artery (collapsed) and the compromise of the flap. The adjacent tissues demonstrate fibrosis and a white-gray film resulting from exposure to saliva.

TABLE 11-2

Systemic RNA Viral Infections

Causative Agent	Pathogenesis	Clinical Characteristics	Diagnosis	Treatment
Coxsackie-viruses	Transmission is most commonly by ingestion of viral-contaminated food, inhalation of respiratory droplets, and direct contact with secretions. Target cells are mucosal cells of respiratory and gastrointestinal tract.	Febrile illness is characterized by sore throat, coryza, cough, and dysphagia. Herpangina is characterized by vesicular eruptions on fauces and soft palate. Hand-foot-and-mouth disease is characterized by papules and vesicular eruptions involving lips, tongue, hard palate, and buccal mucosa; lesions also present on feet and hands and rarely proximal extremities and buttocks.	Infection is diagnosed by clinical presentation, isolation of virus in tissue culture. Serological tests are useful for complement-fixing antibodies.	Care is supportive.
Mumps virus Paramyxovirus	Transmission is by direct contact, virally contaminated respiratory droplets, and fomites. Target cells are mucosal cells of upper respiratory tract.	Prodromal symptoms (headache, myalgias, arthralgias, anorexia, malaise, and low-grade fever) precede onset of major salivary gland swelling (usually parotid).	Infection is diagnosed by clinical presentation, elevated serum amylase; isolation of virus in tissue culture. Serological tests are useful for complement-fixing antibodies and antibody titers directed against viral nucleocapsid and surface hemagglutinin.	Care is symptomatic and supportive. Mumps immunoglobulin is useful in adult men to prevent orchitis.
Measles (rubeola) virus	Transmission is by inhalation of airborne virus contained in respiratory droplets. Target cells are respiratory mucosal cells.	10- to 14-day incubation is followed by onset of malaise, fever, anorexia, conjunctivitis, cough, and coryza. Koplik's spots appear in second molar region, buccal mucosa before onset of cutaneous erythematous maculopapular rash that begins on face and spreads to trunk and extremities including palms and soles.	Infection is diagnosed by clinical presentation. Serological tests for complement-fixing and viral antibodies are useful.	Care is supportive.
German measles (rubella) virus Togavirus	Transmission is by inhalation of airborne virus contained in respiratory droplets. Target cells are respiratory mucosal cells.	14- to 21-day incubation is followed by onset of fever, malaise, cough, and coryza. Variable cutaneous rash consisting of maculopapular to pinpoint papules begins on face and rapidly spreads to trunk and extremities, accompanied by markedly tender retroauricular, posterior cervical, and posterior occipital lymphadenopathy. Oral lesions consist of rose-colored macules that occur on soft palate and pharyngeal wall.	Clinical presentation is similar to many other conditions. Definitive diagnosis depends on isolation of virus in body secretions; serological tests often are helpful. PCR for viral RNA also is useful.	Treatment usually is not necessary. Exanthem resolves in 3 days.
Human immunodeficiency virus RNA retrovirus	Transmission is by sexual intercourse and contact with viral-contaminated body fluids or secretions. Target cells are dendritic cells through viral binding to CCR5 chemokine receptors and CD4+ T lymphocyte by binding CD4+ T-cell receptors.	Mononucleosis-like upper respiratory tract infection develops initially in 50% of patients, followed by variable incubation of 3 to 18 months and onset of night sweats, unexplained fever, chronic diarrhea, rapid weight loss, and regional lymphadenopathy. Opportunistic infections develop, usually fungal; candidiasis, Pneumocystis carinii, and mycobacteria often occur. Reactivation of herpes simplex and varicella-zoster may occur, producing oral and cutaneous aggressive lesions; CMV reactivation also is common.	Western blot detects antibodies to various viral proteins; PCR identifies viral RNA or provirus DNA in body fluids.	HAART consists of a combination of one or more nucleoside reverse-transcriptase inhibitors (zidovudine, didanosine, stavudine, zalcitabine, and lamivudine) and a protease inhibitor (indinavir, nelfinavir, ritonavir, and saquinavir).

PCR, Polymerase chain reaction; *RNA,* ribonucleic acid; *CMV,* cytomegalovirus; *DNA,* deoxyribonucleic acid; *HAART,* highly active antiretroviral therapy.

involvement may follow, including skin, heart, CNS, and lung. Small-particle aerosols of these viruses also may cause infection through the respiratory system. Direct transmission by fingers or fomites also has been implicated, especially in acute hemorrhagic conjunctivitis.

Clinical Characteristics   Many enteroviruses cause febrile illnesses characterized by sore throat, cough, or coryza. The majority of summertime upper respiratory tract infections are caused by enteroviruses. Coxsackieviruses A21 and A24 have been isolated frequently in adults with fever and coldlike symptoms. Tracheobronchitis and pneumonia are complications of these illnesses.

Herpangina   Herpangina, an illness characterized by vesicular eruptions (enanthem) of the fauces and soft palate, fever, sore throat, and pain on swallowing, frequently occurs in children 3 to 10 years of age, and less commonly in adolescents and adults, primarily during the summer months. Group A coxsackieviruses (serotypes 1 through 10, 16, and 22) are recovered most frequently. Less commonly type B coxsackieviruses and several echoviruses are involved. The illness has a sudden onset of fever (100° F to 104° F). Vomiting, myalgia, and headache are common at onset but usually do not persist. Sore throat and pain on swallowing, resulting in dysphagia, usually precedes the onset of the enanthem. Often erythema and a tonsillar exudate occur. The enanthem begins as punctate macules, which evolve into erythematous papules 2 to 4 mm in diameter. These papules eventually form vesicles that ulcerate. The ulcers, usually 6 to 12 in number, are quite painful and located primarily on the soft palate and uvula. Less commonly the buccal mucosa, tongue, posterior pharyngeal wall, and tonsils are affected. Fever usually subsides within 2 to 4 days but ulcers may persist for up to 1 week. A variant of herpangina, acute nodular pharyngitis, sometimes occurs. Lesions consist of tiny nodules containing packed lymphocytes that occur in the same distribution as the vesicular lesions. These lesions eventually resolve without ulceration.

Diagnosis   Herpangina often is confused with bacterial tonsillitis or other viral causes of pharyngitis. However, these infections do not produce the characteristic vesicles and ulcers. The vesicular enanthems caused by herpes simplex viruses and hand-foot-and-mouth disease characteristically occur in the anterior of the oral cavity, especially the lips, tongue, and buccal mucosa. Furthermore, herpes simplex virus commonly causes gingivostomatitis not seen in herpangina, and patients with hand-foot-and-mouth disease often have lesions on the hands and feet. Aphthous stomatitis also produces oral ulcers. These ulcers are larger and primarily affect the lips, tongue, and buccal mucosa; multiple recurrences are common.

Treatment   Treatment is symptomatic and supportive. Prompt recovery usually occurs.

Hand-Foot-and-Mouth Disease   Hand-foot-and-mouth disease generally is caused by coxsackievirus A16, but other serogroups have been isolated, including A5, A7, A9, A10, B2, and B5. Recently enterovirus 71 was isolated as a cause of hand-foot-and-mouth disease. Children younger than 10 years of age are affected most frequently.[42]

Clinical Characteristics   Many children initially complain of sore throat and mouth, and often refuse to eat. Most children develop fever between 100° and 102° F that lasts 1 to 2 days. Oral vesicles occur in essentially all cases and usually involve the lips, tongue, hard palate and buccal mucosa. Several lesions may coalesce to form bullae that frequently ulcerate. Cutaneous lesions occur in approximately 75% of patients. Most commonly they occur on the hands and feet, on the extensor surfaces, or palms and soles. Lesions rarely occur on the proximal extremities and buttocks. The lesions consist of mixed papules and clear vesicles with a surrounding area of erythema. These lesions occasionally ulcerate.

Diagnosis   Diagnosis usually is based on the clinical presentation. Vesicular lesions of chickenpox superficially may resemble those of hand-foot-and-mouth disease. However, oral lesions rarely are present in chickenpox and almost always are present in hand-foot-and-mouth disease. Furthermore, the lesions of chickenpox usually begin on the face and trunk and then spread to the extremities, whereas those of hand-foot-and-mouth disease start on the distal extremities and then spread toward the trunk. In addition, the lesions of chickenpox rarely involve the palms and soles. The enanthem of herpangina may be confused with that of hand-foot-and-mouth disease. However, the lesions of herpangina occur primarily in the posterior oral cavity and pharynx versus those of hand-foot-and-mouth disease, which occur in the anterior oral cavity. Definitive diagnosis depends on isolation of the virus in suckling mice. Serological tests of complement-fixing antibodies also may be useful but are not specific.

Treatment   Treatment is supportive because the majority of cases resolve in a few days without complications. In 1998 a large outbreak of more than 129,000 cases of herpangina and hand-foot-and-mouth disease occurred in Taiwan.[41] The majority of these cases were caused by enterovirus type 71 and most of the remaining cases by coxsackievirus A16. Severe disease occurred in 405 cases, most of which were in children younger than 15 years of age. Of these, 19% resulted in death. The majority of fatalities occurred in patients younger than 5 years of age and all were infected with the enterovirus type 71.[10,22] These patients often developed one of several CNS syndromes that included aseptic meningitis, encephalomyelitis, and flaccid paralysis. Pulmonary edema and hemorrhage were the most frequent complications resulting in death. Consequently, clinicians must be vigilant in follow-up of these patients because serious complications may occur, requiring aggressive antiviral therapy.

PARAMYXOVIRUSES

The paramyxoviruses are enveloped single-stranded RNA viruses. Viruses in this group include mumps, Newcastle disease, human parainfluenza, measles rubeola, and human respiratory syncytial virus.

MUMPS VIRUS

Mumps is a highly contagious disease that occurs worldwide. In the United States, epidemics occurred every 3 to 5 years before the introduction of the mumps vaccine. Approximately 85% of the cases occurred in children younger than 15 years old. Adults rarely were infected, and the disease was uncommon in infants younger than 1 year old as a result of passive maternal transfer of antibodies. The peak incidence was between the months of January and May, although the disease occurred throughout the year. After the introduction of the mumps vaccine in 1967, the number of reported cases in 1995 was 906 compared with 185,691 cases reported in 1968; this represents a decrease of 99%. Humans are the only known natural host. Persistent infection may occur, but a latent carrier state is not known to exist in humans.

Pathogenesis   The virus is transmitted by direct contact, through respiratory droplets or fomites, and enters primarily through the nose and mouth. The virus appears to infect and proliferate in the epithelial cells of the upper respiratory tract. After the incubation period, viremia ensues and the virus is disseminated throughout the body. Localization occurs primarily in glandular and neural tissues.

Clinical Characteristics   Persons with "classical mumps" have bilateral parotitis; however, in about one-fourth of cases, unilateral parotitis occurs. The incubation period from exposure to the onset of parotitis is approximately 16 to 18 days. Approximately one third of patients experience prodromal symptoms during this period consisting of headache, myalgias, arthralgias, anorexia, and malaise. These symptoms often are accompanied by low-grade fever. The onset of salivary gland involvement is accompanied by earache, glandular pain, trismus, and dysphagia. Pain often is exacerbated by stimulation of salivary flow. Often one parotid gland is involved followed a few days later by the other. Although the parotid glands most commonly are affected, other major salivary glands may be infected. However, submandibular or sublingual gland disease without concurrent parotid gland involvement is rare. Glandular swelling usually peaks within 2 to 3 days. Pain is most severe during this period. After the swellings peaks, pain, fever, and glandular tenderness rapidly resolve.

The CNS is the most common extrasalivary gland site of disease. Clinical meningitis occurs in 1% to 10% of patients with parotid disease. Conversely, mumps meningitis may occur in the absence of parotitis. Symptoms of meningitis may occur before, during, or as much as 1 to 2 weeks after the onset of parotitis. Typical symptoms of meningitis include headache, vomiting, fever, and nuchal rigidity. Resolution of symptoms generally occurs within 3 to 10 days after onset of illness. Complete recovery with no sequelae is the usual outcome. Encephalitis is a rare complication associated with mumps. Encephalitis has a bimodal distribution, occurring at the time of parotitis or 7 to 10 days after the onset of parotitis. Symptoms are those of nonfocal encephalitis and include marked decrease in level of consciousness, convulsions, paresis, aphasia and involuntary movements. High fever (104° F to 106° F) often is present. Neurological symptoms and fever gradually resolve within 1 to 2 weeks. Often sequelae of psychomotor retardation and convulsive disorders, cranial nerve palsies, paralysis, and hydrocephalus remain.

Epididymoorchitis is the most common extrasalivary gland manifestation in adults. It occurs in 20% to 30% of adult men. Testicular involvement usually is unilateral. Two thirds of the cases occur in the first week, and one-fourth occur within 2 weeks of the onset of parotitis. The involved testicle is warm, swollen two to three times normal size, and exquisitely tender. The scrotum often is erythematous. Fever is common and lasts 3 to 5 days. When the fever resides the testicular pain and swelling begin to resolve. However, long-term tenderness may persist for several weeks. Sterility rarely occurs even with bilateral involvement.

Oophoritis develops in about 5% of adult women. Symptoms include fever, nausea, vomiting, and lower abdominal pain. Impaired fertility and early menopause rarely have been reported. Fetal death often occurs in the presence of mumps in the first trimester. Congenital defects do not occur.[58]

Diagnosis   Diagnosis of mumps usually is made on the basis of clinical presentation. Mild leukopenia with relative lymphocytosis is common. The serum amylase level is elevated in the presence of parotitis and may remain elevated for 2 to 3 weeks. If mumps pancreatitis is suspected, isozyme analysis or pancreatic lipase determination should be done. In the presence of CNS involvement, CSF should be sampled. Often 10 to 2000 white blood cells are present per cubic millimeter, with lymphocytes the predominant cell type, although some patients may have polymorphs as the predominant cell type. Protein levels usually are normal to mildly elevated, and glucose levels are less than 40 mg/100 mL. The virus usually can be isolated from the saliva 2 to 3 days before and 4 to 5 days after the onset of parotitis and in the CSF when CNS disease is present.

Definitive diagnosis depends on serological studies or isolation of the virus. Complement-fixing antibodies to paramyxovirus "S" antigen, or soluble antibodies directed against the viral nucleoprotein core, appear within the first week of infection. Titers peak within 2 weeks and persist for 8 to 9 months. Antibodies directed against the surface hemagglutinin appear several weeks after those to the S antigen but persist for up-to 5 years. If results of serum studies are negative, a nonparamyxovirus responsible for the parotitis should be suspected. Coxsackieviruses, echoviruses, lymphocytic choriomeningitis viruses, parainfluenza virus, and HIV may cause parotitis.[58]

Treatment   Treatment is symptomatic and supportive. Acetaminophen usually is prescribed to reduce fever and provide some analgesia. Cold or warm packs over the parotid may relieve some discomfort. Patients with persistent vomiting caused by CNS involvement may require intravenous fluid replacement. Patients with orchitis often require narcotic analgesics. Application of ice packs may be beneficial. The efficacy of steroid therapy is unproved. Administration of mumps immune globulin to men with mumps has reduced the incidence of orchitis.

MEASLES VIRUS (RUBEOLA)

Before the introduction of the measles vaccine in 1963, approximately 400,000 cases of measles were reported each year in the United States. However, because virtually every child acquired measles, the number of cases actually approached 3.5 million, the average number of children born in the United States each year. Since the advent of the measles vaccine the reported incidence of measles has decreased more than 99%.

Pathogenesis   Measles is an airborne virus spread by direct contact with droplets from respiratory secretions of infected individuals. Measles is one of the most communicable infectious diseases. Patients are most infectious during the late prodromal phase of the illness, when cough and coryza are at their peak. However, viral transmission may occur for several days before and after the onset of rash. The virus infects by invasion of the respiratory epithelium where viral replication occurs, resulting in viremia. The virus then spreads within leukocytes, especially monocytes, to reticuloendothelial cells. Infection of these cells results in viral replication, necrosis of the host cells, secondary viremia, and further infection of the cells of the respiratory tract. This spread accounts for the onset of coryza and cough characteristic of measles.

Clinical Characteristics   After a 10- to 14-day incubation period after exposure, a prodromal phase lasting several days begins. This phase coincides with the onset of secondary viremia. Signs and symptoms include malaise, fever, anorexia, conjunctivitis, cough, and coryza. Toward the end of the prodromal phase, Koplik's spots appear followed by a rash. Koplik's spots are pathognomonic of measles and appear as blue-gray specks on an erythematous base located on the oral buccal mucosa, usually adjacent to the second molar region. In severe cases the entire oral mucosa is involved. This enanthem lasts for several days and begins to slough when the cutaneous rash appears. The measles rash usually begins on the face and then spreads to the entire body including the palms and soles. The rash is erythematous and maculopapular. After approximately 5 days the rash begins to clear, starting with the skin that was involved first.[59]

The most common complications of measles involve the respiratory tract or CNS. Bacterial superinfection in any part of the respiratory tract may occur. Pneumonia directly caused by the virus or bacterial superinfection is not uncommon, especially in adults, and frequently is the cause of death in infants who acquire the disease. Encephalitis may occur even in immunologically normal hosts. The resurgence of fever during the convalescent stage and the development of headache, seizures, and changes in state of consciousness are characteristic. Patients who recover often have neurological sequelae.

Measles during pregnancy, in contrast to German measles (rubella), does not cause congenital anomalies of the fetus. However, spontaneous abortion and premature delivery may occur.

Diagnosis   Diagnosis usually is made by the clinical presentation of the disease. Definitive diagnosis depends on the isolation of the virus or identification of viral antigens in the tissues of the host. This identification is useful particularly in patients who are immunocompromised whose antibody response may be minimal. Serological tests may be used to identify high titers of viral antibodies IgM and IgG. Neutralization, complement fixation, and enzyme-linked immunosorbent assays are used most commonly.

Treatment   Treatment generally is supportive. Antipyretics and fluids are administered as needed. Bacterial superinfection should be treated with appropriate antibiotics. Prophylactic use of antibiotics is of no value and should not be prescribed.

TOGAVIRUSES

The togaviridae are single-stranded RNA, lipoprotein-enveloped viruses. Togaviruses consist of four genera. The two main genera are the alphaviruses and the rubiviruses. These viruses enter their target cells by receptor-mediated endocytosis.

RUBELLA VIRUS (GERMAN MEASLES)

Pathogenesis   Rubella is an acute exanthematous infection of children and adults. The disease is transmitted through droplets of respiratory secretions of infected persons containing shed virus. Patients are most contagious when the rash is erupting, but the virus can be shed for a period beginning up to 10 days before the onset of rash to 15 days afterward. The incubation period after exposure is 14 to 21 days. However, 25% to 50% of rubella infections are subclinical.

Clinical Characteristics   Initial symptoms are those of an upper respiratory tract infection and often mild. The exanthem of rubella is variable. The rash usually begins as maculopapules but may become pinpoint papules resembling scarlet fever. Associated flushing is common. The eruption begins on the face and rapidly spreads to the trunk and extremities. Mild pruritus may be associated with the exanthem. The rash typically resolves within 3 days. A distinctive feature is the presence of markedly tender retroauricular, posterior cervical, and posterior occipital lymphadenopathy. Intraorally, just before eruption of the skin lesions, rose-colored macules may develop on the soft palate and posterior oropharynx. Primarily in adults, and especially women, transient polyarthralgia or polyarthritis frequently occurs.[59] Encephalitis is a rare complication of rubella infection and is more likely in adults. Thrombocytopenia is a more likely complication in children.

The most serious consequence of rubella infection occurs in pregnant women, especially in the first 16 weeks of pregnancy. Serious complications include miscarriage, abortion, stillbirth, and congenital rubella syndrome of the newborn.[29] A rubella pandemic occurred in the United States in 1964. Twelve million cases were reported, with 11,000 fetal deaths and 20,000 cases of congenital rubella syndrome in infants.[67] The most common anomalies associated with congenital rubella syndrome include auditory (neural deafness), ophthalmic (cataracts, microphthalmia, glaucoma, chorioretinitis), cardiac (patent ductus arteriosus, peripheral pulmonary artery stenosis, atrial or ventricular septal defects), and neurological (microcephaly, meningoencephalitis, and mental retardation) complications. In addition, radiolucent bone defects, hepatosplenomegaly, thrombocytopenia, and purpuric skin lesions have been observed.[59] After the widespread use of rubella vaccine the number of reported rubella cases decreased to less than 200 per year with only 4 confirmed cases of congenital rubella syndrome in 1995 and 2 in 1996. The majority of these cases occurred in young adults older than 20 years of age, indicating that continued surveillance is necessary.

Diagnosis   Rubella usually is a mild disease with non-specific symptoms. Hence, clinical diagnosis is difficult. Rubella often is confused with other diseases, including scarlet fever, mild rubeola measles, infectious mononucleosis, toxoplasmosis, roseola, and several enteroviral infections. Routine laboratory studies are of little value. Definitive diagnosis depends on isolation of the virus in throat swabs, urine, or other body secretions. Serological rubella antibody titers of IgM or IgG are helpful. Testing methods include enzyme-linked immunosorbent assay, passive latex agglutination test, and radial hemolysis test. Congenital rubella syndrome has been diagnosed by placental biopsy, demonstration of rubella antigen with monoclonal antibodies, and identification of viral RNA by PCR or in situ hybridization.

Treatment   Usually no treatment is necessary. Patients with high fever or arthralgia are treated symptomatically.

Prevention   All children without contraindications should receive the measles-mumps-rubella vaccine at age 12 to 15 months and again at age 4 to 6 years. All women of childbearing age should be vaccinated unless they have a documented history of vaccination or have titer evidence that they definitely had the disease.

RNA RETROVIRUSES (HUMAN IMMUNODEFICIENCY VIRUS)

The retroviruses consist of a diverse family of two enveloped single-stranded RNA viruses. Unlike other RNA viruses in which the genome acts as a messenger RNA serving as a template for the production of viral proteins and RNA duplication, the retroviruses contain a unique protein enzyme, an RNA-dependent DNA polymerase, or a reverse transcriptase. The virion RNA is duplicated into double-stranded DNA, which integrates with the host DNA genome. Consequently, the retroviruses have the survival advantage of the genetic diversity of an RNA virus (high frequency of mutation and recombination) and the advantage of latency provided by the DNA provirus integration into the host DNA. The infectious retroviruses have been classified into seven genera. The human retroviruses include the lentiviruses, HIV serotypes 1 and 2 (HIV-1 and -2); and the oncogenic viruses, human T-cell leukemia/lymphoma viruses I and II (HTLV-I and HTLV-II).

HUMAN IMMUNODEFICIENCY VIRUS

Pathogenicity   The most common mode of HIV infection is by sexual transmission. Alternatively, transmission may occur by exposure to infected fluids such as blood or blood products, from mother to fetus, and by accidental occupational exposure. Transmitted virus typically infects host cells by binding via the glycoprotein 120 envelop protein to one of two cellular receptors, the CD4 T-cell receptor of T lymphocytes or the CCR5 chemokine receptor, typically of monocytes and dendritic cells. After intravaginal or rectal inoculation, viral binding to primarily the CCR5 chemokine receptor of dendritic cells occurs; these cells are present in the lamina propria (other chemokine receptors also can be used). Rapid viral replication occurs in these cells. The dendritic cells then migrate to regional lymph nodes where released virions can infect CD4[+] T lymphocytes. Individuals who lack CCR5 receptors are resistant to infection by sexual transmission.[53] A plasma viremia soon follows with widespread dissemination primarily to lymphoid organs and the CNS (in which cells also express the chemokine receptors). A robust immunological response occurs in the host, and about half of infected individuals develop a mononucleosis-like acute syndrome. Plasma viral RNA levels rapidly decrease to reach a steady state, sometimes called a viral set-point. The level of plasma viral RNA achieved at this stage correlates well and is predictive of the subsequent disease. The course of the disease and the signs and symptoms that manifest depend on the balance between host production of primarily CD4[+] T lymphocytes (a critical cell required in the host's immune response to control viral replication) and viral destruction of these target cells.

Clinical Characteristics After HIV infection the incubation period before the onset of symptoms after the acute phase varies, ranging from 3 to 18 months. The initial signs are nonspecific and include night sweats, unexplained fever, chronic diarrhea, rapid weight loss, and regional lymphadenopathy. Patients often develop opportunistic infections and malignancy. The most common opportunistic infections are fungal; C. albicans and P. carinii are the organisms most frequently involved. Other frequently encountered infections are caused by atypical mycobacteria and herpes simplex viruses. The most common malignancy observed is Kaposi's sarcoma, but numerous cases of malignant lymphoma, oral warts, and squamous cell carcinoma also have been reported.

Lesions of the skin and oral cavity often occur in individuals with HIV infection.[71,85] Oral candidiasis frequently is observed in patients with HIV infection. Candidiasis is common in patients whose CD4+ T-lymphocyte counts are between 200 and 500/mm^3 and almost always is present when CD4+ counts decrease below 200/mm^3.[95] Oral candidiasis is rare in patients who are not infected with HIV. Usually such patients are receiving steroid immunosuppressive therapy or have taken broad-spectrum antibiotics. Oral candidiasis may appear in several clinical forms. The most common is pseudomembranous candidiasis (thrush), characterized by creamy, yellow-white, easily removed plaques. Removal of the plaques leaves a painful, bleeding surface. Thrush occurs most commonly on the palate, buccal and labial mucosa, and dorsal aspect of the tongue. Hyperplastic candidiasis usually is seen on the buccal mucosa. Hyperplastic candidiasis is characterized as a diffuse, white adherent plaque similar to oral leukoplakia. Lesions often are painful or burning but may be asymptomatic. Erythematous or atrophic candidiasis may occur on the palate, buccal and labial mucosa, and tongue. Lesions consist of diffuse or discrete red, nonremovable plaques. Oral hairy leukoplakia is another form of candidiasis that characteristically occurs on the lateral aspect of the tongue but may also occur on the buccal mucosa. The lesion is poorly demarcated, usually painless, white, and nonremovable and often has a corrugated surface. "Hairy" fingerlike projections frequently grow out of the center of the lesion as a result of reactivation of latent EBV infection. In the absence of iatrogenic immunosuppression the presence of oral hairy leukoplakia can be considered diagnostic of HIV infection. Finally, candidiasis may manifest as a macerated white or yellow-white, sometimes erythematous lesion located at the corners of the mouth (angular cheilitis). Angular cheilitis often is accompanied by intraoral lesions.

Oral ulcers occur in as many as half of individuals with HIV infection sometime during the course of the disease.[95] These ulcers may be the manifestation of reactivation of herpes simplex viruses, idiopathic ulcers (recurrent aphthous ulcers), or ulcers induced by drug therapy. Herpes simplex lesions in patients with HIV generally follow an aggressive and protracted course. Lesions are erosive, often painful, and may persist for several weeks. Often they extend into the esophagus. Lesions are seen occasionally in patients whose CD4+ T-lymphocyte counts are greater than 500/ mm^3, but are much more common in patients with more advanced disease. Other herpes viruses that can produce oral ulcers and cutaneous lesions include herpes varicella-zoster and CMV. Lesions caused by reactivation of these viruses primarily occur in advanced disease when CD4+ cell counts are less than 200/mm^3.

Recurrent aphthous ulcers frequently occur in patients with AIDS. Aphthous ulcers are described as minor or major according to size, depth of ulceration, and duration. Minor ulcers are less than 1 cm in diameter, shallow, and typically self-limiting. These ulcers rarely produce painful swallowing and dysphagia. Major aphthous ulcers are more than 1 cm in diameter, extend deep into the underlying tissue, are prolonged in duration, and heal with scarring. Major aphthous ulcers are painful and interfere with speech and swallowing.

Rapidly progressive and painful periodontitis is observed frequently in patients with HIV infection.[35] Periodontitis commonly occurs in patients with CD4+ T-lymphocyte counts less than 200/mm^3. Patients often have deep pain and spontaneous gingival bleeding. If untreated, severe, rapidly progressive, deep-space, life-threatening infection may develop. Initially the disease is characterized by severe linear erythema of gingival margin adjacent to the teeth. The erythema is followed by necrotizing gingivitis that may rapidly progress to involve the underlying alveolar bone and adjacent soft tissues.

Kaposi's sarcoma is a neoplastic proliferation of endothelial cells. Kaposi's sarcoma was a rare malignancy that occurred primarily in elderly men in the Mediterranean area and parts of Africa. However, it is the most common malignancy observed in patients with AIDS. The majority of patients with Kaposi's sarcoma have oral and perioral lesions. Intraoral lesions appear as blue or purple macules, papules, and nodules. Oral lesions frequently are asymptomatic but can progress to painful ulcers, often associated with bleeding, superinfection, and development of large bulky tumors. Oral lesions occur primarily on the hard palate or gingiva.

Diagnosis The diagnosis of HIV infection depends on the demonstration of antibodies to the HIV virion or its components, or the detection of HIV or one of its components. Antibodies to HIV generally appear in the serum within 4 to 6 weeks after infection. The Western blot test detects antibodies to several different HIV antigens (proteins derived from the gag, pol, and env components of the HIV genome) that are well characterized by their molecular weights. The antigens are separated on the basis of their molecular weights. The formation of discrete bands on the Western blot indicates that specific antibodies to these antigens are present in the test serum and is conclusive evidence of HIV infection. If Western blot results are indeterminate, PCR assay for viral RNA or provirus DNA can be used as a diagnostic test.

Treatment HAART was introduced in 1997. This therapy has revolutionized the treatment of HIV infection because it can reduce viral titers to virtually undetectable levels. This development has resulted in significant prolonged elevations of CD4$^+$ T lymphocytes and restoration of host immunity. HAART typically consists of a combination of one or more nucleoside reverse-transcriptase inhibitors (zidovudine, didanosine, stavudine, zalcitabine, and lamivudine) and a protease inhibitor (indinavir, nelfinavir, ritonavir, and saquinavir). HAART has reduced morbidity significantly and has prolonged the quality and length of life of many patients with HIV infection. HAART has not cured the disease because it does not remove latent or nascent virus from host cells, but it does prevent their multiplication and infectivity.

PROTOZOAL INFECTIONS

LEISHMANIASIS

Leishmaniasis consists of several clinically distinct diseases caused by *Leishmania* spp. *Leishmania* are protozoa that in their natural life cycle alternate between vertebrate and invertebrate hosts. The vertebrate hosts include humans, rodents, sheep, cattle, dogs, and cats, whereas the invertebrate hosts are sandflies of the genus *Lutzomyia* in the Americas and *Phlebotomus* elsewhere. In humans and other mammals, *Leishmania* organisms live in macrophages and cells of the reticuloendothelial system as intracellular amastigotes, and in gut of the sandfly as extracellular promastigotes. As expected with an intracellular pathogen, cell-mediated immune mechanisms are responsible for controlling leishmanial infections.

Leishmaniasis is divided into three syndromes: visceral (kala-azar), cutaneous, and mucosal. A single *Leishmania* species can produce different clinical syndromes, and each of the syndromes can be caused by more than one species. *Leishmania donovani* is involved primarily in causing visceral leishmaniasis that occurs in Asia, Africa, the Mediterranean area, and Central and South America. Cutaneous leishmaniasis is caused primarily by *L. tropica* and *L. major* in the Mediterranean area and southern Asia, and *L. braziliensis* and *L. mexicana* in South and Central America. Finally, mucosal leishmaniasis is caused by *L. braziliensis* in South and Central America. Oral lesions occur in both visceral and mucosal leishmaniasis.

Pathogenesis   Sandflies ingest amastigotes when they feed on infected mammals. The amastigotes convert to promastigotes in the sandfly gut, replicate, and differentiate into metacyclic promastigotes. The next time the sandfly feeds, the promastigote is transferred to the mammal in the saliva of the sandfly. The promastigote of several species can activate complement by the alternate pathway, thereby enabling attachment to the type 1 complement receptor of the macrophage. Other species require the presence of antibodies to activate complement by the classic pathway. In the absence of complement the promastigote may attach directly to the type III complement receptor. Once attached, the promastigote is phagocytosed by the macrophage. The phagosome fuses with lysosomes. The promastigotes that are resistant to the lysosomal enzymes convert within them to amastigotes. Parasitic replication follows. Amastigotes eventually are released and free to infect other mononuclear phagocytes.

Clinical Characteristics   The clinical manifestations of the disease depend on the species of *Leishmania* involved and on the immune response of the infected host.

Localized Cutaneous Leishmaniasis   Lesions most commonly occur in the skin of unclothed parts of the body, including the face, neck, and arms. The average incubation period after the sandfly bite is 1 to 3 months. Initially a red papule appears and enlarges to a plaque or nodule. The lesion commonly develops into an ulcer that is well circumscribed with a blue-red border. The margin of the ulcer is hypertrophic but not undermined, and the base is granulomatous and crusted. Often painless, rubbery subcutaneous nodules or cords develop around the ulcer as a result of the lymphatic spread of the *Leishmania.* Draining lymph nodes become enlarged. Satellite papules and subcutaneous induration may develop around the primary lesion. In rare cases a generalized papular rash develops, representing a hypersensitivity reaction of the host to the organism. Itching and pain are usually absent and mild if present. Secondary infection of the ulcer may occur. After 6 to 12 months the ulcer usually regresses spontaneously, leaving a hypopigmented or hyperpigmented atrophic scar.

Diffuse Cutaneous Leishmaniasis   Diffuse cutaneous leishmaniasis is a variant of localized cutaneous leishmaniasis in an anergic host. Lesions are disseminated and resemble lepromatous leprosy. *L. mexicana* appears to be the primary pathogen. The disease usually initially manifests as a solitary primary lesion. However, lesions soon disseminate and affect large areas of the skin. The lesions are nonulcerative nodules and usually scattered over the limbs, buttocks, and face (Figure 11-12). Unlike leprosy, nerve involvement does not occur in diffuse cutaneous leishmaniasis. Response to treatment is poor and chronic disease often develops. However, visceral invasion does not occur.

Mucocutaneous Leishmaniasis   The majority of patients who develop mucosal lesions had cutaneous lesions within the previous 2 to 10 years. Most patients had multiple, large or persistent cutaneous lesions that were treated inadequately. The disease commonly occurs in the Americas, and *L. braziliensis* usually is the causative organism. Mucous membrane involvement develops as a result of hematogenous or lymphatic spread of the pathogen. The disease has a predilection for the mucosa of the nasal septum. Initial symptoms usually are nasal stuffiness, discharge, pain, and epistaxis. Often the nasal septum is destroyed resulting in nasal collapse. Perforation can occur through the skin or soft palate. Bone usually remains intact. Other sites of involvement include the upper lip, gingiva, and buccal or pharyngeal mucosa. Occasionally the laryngeal mucosa is affected with extension into the trachea and bronchi. These lesions can be so extensive that dysphagia and fatal

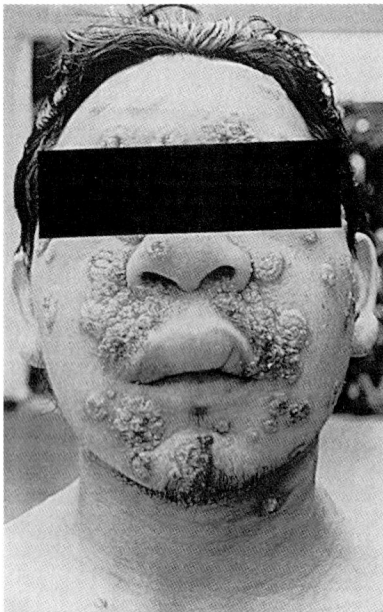

Figure 11-12 Cutaneous leishmaniasis demonstrating extensive disfiguring, verrucous facial lesions associated with bilateral ptosis and ectropion. (From Mandell GL, Bennett JE, Dolin R: *Mandell, Douglas, and Bennett's principles and practice of infectious diseases,* ed 5, vol 2, Philadelphia, 2000, Churchill Livingstone.)

pulmonary aspiration pneumonia occur. Rare dissemination to the mucosa of the eye and genitalia has been reported.[8]

Visceral Leishmaniasis   Visceral leishmaniasis or kala-azar (black fever) is a systemic disease caused by dissemination of pathogen throughout the reticuloendothelial system of the host. Characteristic signs and symptoms include fever, splenomegaly, lymphadenopathy, emaciation, pancytopenia, and hyperglobulinemia. During the active period of the disease, patchy, blackened skin, often with loss of hair, appears as a result of melanoblastic hyperpigmentation. Impaired cell-mediated immunity occurs, increasing the risk of opportunistic infections. Wound healing often is impaired.

Diagnosis   The differential diagnosis for leishmaniasis is extensive because several diseases manifest with similar lesions. However, in endemic areas diagnosis usually is based on its clinical presentation: (1) a small number of lesions (one to three) located in exposed areas of the skin, (2) presence of lesions for several months, (3) resistance of lesions to treatments, and (4) absence of pain or itching. Definitive diagnosis is made by identification of the amastigotes in tissue biopsy; specimens are best taken from the indurated border of the lesion. Fine-needle aspiration of a lesion after injection of saline solution also is useful. The biopsy specimen is cultured on Nicolle's modification of Novy-McNeal medium, blood agar, or rabbit blood agar. Growth of the promastigotes usually occurs within 2 to 14 days. In vivo culture can be done by injecting an aspirate into the footpad of a hamster. Identification of antibodies

to *Leishmania* in the serum using an enzyme-linked immunosorbent assay and positive leishmanin skin test results also are useful. Species-specific monoclonal antibodies and PCR are useful in identification of the species of *Leishmania* involved.[8]

Treatment   The drug of choice for the treatment of leishmaniasis is stibogluconate (Pentostam), a pentavalent antimony compound. The drug can be given intramuscularly or intravenously. The usual dosage is 20 mg/kg per day. Localized cutaneous leishmaniasis is treated for at least 2 weeks, whereas mucocutaneous leishmaniasis and visceral disease are treated for at least 1 month. Side effects include myalgias, arthralgias, abdominal pain, anorexia, nausea, and vomiting. Elevated concentrations of liver enzymes, lipase, and amylase often are present, and anemia, leukopenia, and thrombocytopenia occasionally occur. Electrocardiographic changes have been reported. In addition, drug resistance and treatment failures are more common.[83] Both pentamidine and amphotericin B have been successfully in the treatment of the cutaneous and visceral forms of leishmaniasis. Pentamidine is a highly toxic but effective drug. It is directly toxic to pancreatic β cells and can result in development of diabetes mellitus. Liposomal amphotericin B has been effective.[88] It is the only drug approved for the treatment of visceral leishmaniasis in the United States.

REFERENCES

1. Aberg J, Mundy LM, Powderly WG: Pulmonary cryptococcosis in patients without HIV infection, *Chest* 115:734, 1998.
2. Alleyne CJ, Vishteh AG, Spetzler RF, et al: Long-term survival of a patient with invasive cranial base rhinocerebral mucormycosis treated with combined endovascular, surgical and medical therapies: case report, *Neurosurgery* 45:1461, 1999.
3. Annunziato P, Gershon A: Herpes simplex virus infections, *Pediatr Rev* 17:415, 1996.
4. Arribas J, Storch GA, Clifford DB, et al: Cytomegalovirus encephalitis, *Ann Intern Med* 125:77, 1996.
5. Arvin A, Moffat JF, Redman R: Varicella-zoster virus: aspects of pathogenesis and host response to natural infection and varicella vaccine, *Adv Virus Res* 46:263, 1996.
6. Autran B, Carcelain G, Li TS, et al: Positive effects of combined antiretroviral therapy on CD4-cell homeostasis and function in advanced HIV disease, *Science* 277:112, 1997.
7. Baumforth K, Young LS, Flavel KJ, et al: The Epstein-Barr virus and its association with human cancers, *Mol Pathol* 52:307, 1999.
8. Berman J: Human leishmaniasis: clinical, diagnostic, and chemotherapeutic developments in the last 10 years, *Clin Infect Dis* 24:684, 1997.
9. Catanzaro A, Fierer J, Friedman PJ: Fluconazole in the treatment of persistent coccidioidomycosis, *Chest* 97:666, 1990.
10. Chang L, Lin TY, Huang YC, et al: Comparison of enterovirus 71 and coxsackievirus A16 clinical illnesses during the Taiwan enterovirus epidemic, *Pediatr Infect Dis J* 18:1992, 1999.
11. Chapman S, Daniel CR: Cutaneous manifestations of fungal infection, *Infect Dis Clin North Am* 8:879, 1994.

12. Chimelli L, Mahler-Araujo MB: Fungal infections, *Brain Pathol* 7:613, 1997.

13. Collier AC, Meyers JD, Corey L, et al: Cytomegalovirus infection in homosexual men. Relationship to sexual practices, antibody to human immunodeficiency virus, and cell-mediated immunity, *Am J Med* 82:593, 1987.

14. Como JA, Dismukes WE: Drug therapy: oral azole drugs as systemic antifungal therapy, *N Engl J Med* 330:263, 1994.

15. Cummins R, Romero RC, Mancini AJ: Disseminated North American blastomycosis in an adolescent male: a delay in diagnosis, *Pediatrics* 102:977, 1998.

16. Darras-Joly C, Veber B, Bedos JP, et al: Nosocomial cerebral aspergillosis: a report of 3 cases, *Scand J Infect Dis* 28:317, 1996.

17. De Vaul K, Garner CE: Varicella-zoster pneumonia in the adult patient, *J Emerg Nurs* 23:102, 1997.

18. Denning D: Early diagnosis of invasive aspergillosis, *Lancet* 355:423, 2000.

19. Denning D, Tucker RM, Hanson LH, et al: Treatment of invasive aspergillosis with itraconazole, *Am J Med* 86:791, 1989.

20. Derkering T, Duma RJ, Shadomy S: The evolution of pulmonary cryptococcosis: clinical implications from a study of 41 patients with and without compromising host factors, *Ann Intern Med* 94:611, 1981.

21. Dismukes W, Bradsher RW, Cloud GC, et al: Itraconazole therapy for blastomycosis and histoplasmosis, *Am J Med* 93:486, 1992.

22. Dolin R: Enterovirus 71: emerging infections and emerging questions, *N Engl J Med* 341:984, 1999.

23. Dong Z, Murphy JW: Intravascular cryptococcal culture filtrate (CneF) and its major component, glucuronoxylomannan, are potent inhibitors of leukocyte accumulation, *Infect Immun* 63:770, 1995.

24. Dromer F, Mathoulin S, Dupont B, et al: Comparison of the efficacy of amphotericin B and fluconazole in the treatment of cryptococcosis in human immunodeficiency virus–negative patients. Retrospective analysis of 83 cases, *Clin Infect Dis* 22(suppl 2):154, 1996.

25. Emmons C: Association of bats with histoplasmosis, *Public Health Rep* 73:590, 1958.

26. Emmons C: Isolation of *Histoplasma capsulatum* from soil in Washington, DC, *Public Health Rep* 76:591, 1961.

27. Eubanks P, Virgilio C, Klein S, et al: Candida sepsis in surgical patients, *Am J Surg* 166:617, 1993.

28. Fojtasek MF, Sherman MR, Garringer T, et al: Local immunity in lung-associated lymph nodes in a murine model of pulmonary histoplasmosis, *Infect Immun* 61:4607, 1993.

29. Freij B, South MA, Sever JL: Maternal rubella and the congenital rubella syndrome (CRS), *Clin Perinatol* 15:247, 1988.

30. Gatell J, Marrades R, El-Ebiary M, et al: Severe pulmonary infections in AIDS patients, *Semin Respir Infect* 11:119, 1996.

31. Gilden D, Kleinschmidt-DeMasters BK, LaGuardia JJ, et al: Medical progress: neurologic complications of the reactivation of varicella-zoster virus, *N Engl J Med* 342:635, 2000.

32. Giron J, Sans N, Poey C, et al: CT-guided percutaneous treatment of inoperable pulmonary aspergillomas: a study of 42 cases, *J Radiol* 79:139, 1998.

33. Goodgame R: Gastrointestinal cytomegalovirus disease, *Ann Intern Med* 119:924, 1993.

34. Goodrich J, Mori M, Gleaves CA, et al: Early treatment with ganciclovir to prevent cytomegalovirus disease after allogeneic bone marrow transplantation, *N Engl J Med* 325:1601, 1991.

35. Gravelink S, Lerner EA: Clinical reviews. Leishmaniasis, *J Am Acad Dermatol* 34: 257, 1996.

36. Graybill J, Stevens DA, Dismukes WE, et al: Itraconazole treatment of coccidioidomycosis, *Am J Med* 89:282, 1990.

37. Grundy J: Virologic and pathogenetic aspects of cytomegalovirus infection, *Rev Infect Dis* 12:S711, 1990.

38. Henderson S, Row M, Gregory C, et al: Induction of bcl-2 expression by Epstein-Barr virus latent membrane protein 1 protects infected B-cells from programmed cell death, *Cell* 65:1107, 1991.

39. Henderson V, Hirvela ER: Emerging and reemerging microbial threats: nosocomial fungal infections, *Arch Surg* 131:330, 1996.

40. Hengge U, Brockmeyer NH, Malessa R, et al: Foscarnet penetrates the blood-brain barrier: rationale for therapy of cytomegalovirus encephalitis, *Antimicrob Agents Chemother* 37: 1010, 1993.

41. Ho M, Chen E-R, Hsu K-H, et al: An epidemic of enterovirus 71 infection in Taiwan, *N Engl J Med* 341:929, 1999.

42. Horowitz C, Henle W, Henle G, et al: Long-term serological follow-up of patients for Epstein-Barr virus after recovery from infectious mononucleosis, *J Infect Dis* 151:1150, 1985.

43. Jacobson M: Drug therapy: treatment of cytomegalovirus retinitis in patients with the acquired immunodeficiency syndrome, *N Engl J Med* 337:105, 1997.

44. Johnson R, Milbourn PE: Central nervous system manifestation of chickenpox, *Can Med Assoc J* 102:831, 1997.

45. Kaneshiro ES, Wyder MA: C27 to 32 sterols found in *Pneumocystis,* an opportunistic pathogen of immunocompromised mammals, *Lipids* 35:317, 2000.

46. Klein N, Burke CA: New antifungal drugs for pulmonary mycoses, *Chest* 110:225, 1996.

47. Klemola E, Von Essen R, Henle G, et al: Infectious-mononucleosis-like disease with negative heterophil agglutination test: clinical features in relation to Epstein-Barr virus and cytomegalovirus and antibodies, *J Infect Dis* 121:608, 1970.

48. Krause W, Mateis H, Wulf K: Fungemia and funguria after oral administration of *Candida albicans, Lancet* 1:598, 1969.

49. Larsen R, Leal MA, Chan LS: Fluconazole compared with amphotericin B plus flucytosine for cryptococcal meningitis in AIDS: a randomized trial, *Ann Intern Med* 113:183, 1990.

50. Lee F, Mossad SB, Adal KA: Pulmonary mucormycosis: the last 30 years, *Arch Intern Med* 159:1301, 1999.

51. Lehrer R: The fungicidal mechanisms of human monocytes: evidence for myeloperoxidase-linked and myeloperoxidase-independent candidacidal mechanisms, *J Clin Invest* 55:338, 1975.

52. Lewis R, Klepser ME: The changing face of nosocomial candidemia: epidemiology, resistance, and drug therapy, *Am J Health Syst Pharm* 56:525, 1999.

53. Liu R, Paxton WA, Choe S, et al: Homozygous defect in HIV-1 co-receptor accounts for resistance of some multiply-exposed individuals to HIV infection, *Cell* 86:367, 1996.

54. Louria DB, Smith JK, Brayton RG, et al: Anti-Candida factors in serum and their inhibitors. I. Clinical and laboratory investigations, *J Infect Dis* 125:102, 1972.

55. Manfredi R, Chiodo F: Features of AIDS and AIDS defining diseases during the highly active antiviral therapy (HAART) era, compared with the pre-HAART period: a case-control study, *Sex Transm Infect* 76:145, 2000.

56. Mantuschak G, Lechner AJ: The yeast to hyphal transition following hematogenous candidiasis induces shock and organ injury independent of circulating tumor necrosis factor-alpha, *Crit Care Med* 25:111, 1997.

57. McCunney R: Hodgkin's disease, work, and the environment: a review, *J Occup Environ Med* 41:36, 1999.

58. McQuone S: Acute viral and bacterial infections of the salivary glands, *Otolaryngol Clin North Am* 32:793, 1999.

59. Measles, mumps, and rubella—vaccine use and strategies for elimination of measles, rubella, and congenital rubella syndrome and control of mumps: recommendations of the Advisory Committee on Immunization Practices, *MMWR Morb Mortal Wkly Rep* 47:1, 1998.

60. Meyers C, Mayer TJ, Ozbun MA: Synthesis of infectious human papillomavirus type 18 in differentiating epithelium transfected with viral DNA, *J Virol* 71 7381, 1997.

61. Minamoto G, Rosenberg AS: Fungal infections in patients with acquired immunodeficiency syndrome, *Med Clin North Am* 81:381, 1997.

62. Moore RA, Edwards JE, Hopwood J, et al: Imiquimod for the treatment of genital warts: a quantitative systematic review, *BMC Infect Dis* 1:3, 2001.

63. Morgan M, Reves R: Invasive sinusitis due to *Sporothrix schenckii* in a patient with AIDS, *Clin Infect Dis* 23:1319, 1996.

64. Murakawa G, Kerschmann R, Berger T: Cutaneous cryptococcus infection and AIDS: report of 12 cases and review of literature, *Arch Dermatol* 132:545, 1996.

65. Murphy J: Immunologic downregulation of host defenses in fungal infections, *Mycosis* 42(suppl 2):37, 1999.

66. Niedobitek G, Agathanggelou A, Row M, et al: Heterogeneous expression of Epstein-Barr proteins in endemic Burkitt's lymphoma, *Blood* 86:659, 1995.

67. Orenstein W, Bart KJ, Hinman AR: The opportunity and obligation to eliminate rubella from the United States, *JAMA* 251:1988, 1984.

68. Pappagianis D, Zimmer BL: Serology of coccidioidomycosis, *Clin Microbiol Rev* 3:247, 1990.

69. Pappas P, Potter JC, Powdrey WG, et al: Blastomycosis in patients with acquired immunodeficiency syndrome, *Ann Intern Med* 46:847, 1992.

70. Patel R, Snydman DR, Rubin RH, et al: Cytomegalovirus prophylaxis in solid organ transplant recipients, *Transplantation* 61:1279, 1996.

71. Patton L, McKaig R, Strauss R, et al: Changing prevalence of oral manifestations of human immunodeficiency virus in the era of protease inhibitor therapy, *Oral Surg Oral Med Oral Pathol* 89:299, 2000.

72. Paya C, Roberts GD, Cockerill FR 3rd: Transient fungemia in acute pulmonary histoplasmosis: detection by new blood-culturing techniques, *J Infect Dis* 156:313, 1987.

73. Payen M, De Wit S, Sommereijns B, et al: A controlled trial of dapsone versus pyrimethamine-sulfadoxine for primary prophylaxis of *Pneumocystis carinii* pneumonia and toxoplasmosis in patients with AIDS, *Biomed Pharmacother* 51:439, 1997.

74. Pereira F: Herpes simplex: evolving concepts, *J Am Acad Dermatol* 35:503, 1996.

75. Peter J, Ray CG: Infectious mononucleosis, *Pediatr Rev* 19:276, 1998.

76. Ponikau J, Sherris DA, Kern EB, et al: The diagnosis and incidence of allergic fungal sinusitis, *Mayo Clin Proc* 74:877, 1999.

77. Rand K, Houck H, Wolff M: Detection of candidemia by polymerase chain reaction, *Mol Cell Probes* 8:215, 1994.

78. Randhawa H, Budimulja U, Bazaz-Malik G: Recent developments in the diagnosis and treatment of subcutaneous mycoses, *J Med Vet Mycol* 32(suppl 1):299, 1994.

79. Repentigny L: Serodiagnosis of candidiasis, aspergillosis, and cryptococcosis, *Clin Infect Dis* 14:S11, 1992.

80. Sant'Anna G, Mauri M, Arrarte JL, et al: Laryngeal manifestation of paracoccidioidomycosis (South American blastomycosis), *Arch Otolaryngol Head Neck Surg* 125:1375, 1999.

81. Saxena M, Rest EB: An ulcerating nodule on the arm, *Arch Dermatol* 134:1279, 1998.

82. Schomogyi M, Wald A, Corey L: Emerging infectious diseases: herpes simplex virus-2 infection, *Infect Dis Clin North Am* 12:47, 1998.

83. Seaman J, Boer C, Wilkinson R, et al: Liposomal amphotericin B (Ambisome) in the treatment of complicated kala-azar under field conditions, *Clin Infect Dis* 21:188, 1995.

84. Sharkey P, Graybill JR, Johnson ES, et al: Amphotericin B lipid complex compared with amphotericin B in the treatment of cryptococcal meningitis in patients with AIDS, *Clin Infect Dis* 22:315, 1996.

85. Spira R, Mignard M, Doutre M-S, et al: Prevalence of cutaneous disorders in a population of HIV-infected patients: southwestern France, *Arch Dermatol* 134:1208, 1998.

86. Stevens D: Current concepts: coccidioidomycosis, *N Engl J Med* 332:1077, 1995.

87. Straus S, Cohen JI, Tosato G, et al: Epstein-Barr infections: biology, pathogenesis, and management, *Ann Intern Med* 118:45, 1992.

88. Sundar S, Murray HW: Cure of antimony-unresponsive Indian visceral Leishmaniasis with liposomal amphotericin B lipid complex, *J Infect Dis* 173:762, 1996.

89. Torres T, Goldman M, Wheat LJ, et al: Diagnosis of *Pneumocystis carinii* pneumonia in human immunodeficiency virus infected patients with PCR: a blinded comparison to standard methods, *Clin Infect Dis* 30:141, 2000.

90. Tyring S: Imiquimod: an immune response modifier, *J Am Acad Dermatol* 43:S18, 2000.

91. Weig M, Klinger H, Bogner B, et al: Usefulness of PCR for diagnosis of *Pneumocystis carinii* pneumonia in different patient groups, *J Clin Microbiol* 35:1445, 1997.

92. Weil M, Mercurio MG, Brodell RT, et al: Cutaneous lesions provide a clue to mysterious pulmonary process, *Arch Dermatol* 132:821, 1996.

93. Wheat J: Histoplasmosis. Experience during outbreaks in Indianapolis and review of the literature, *Medicine* 76:239, 1997.

94. Whitley R, Weiss H, Gnann JW Jr, et al: Acyclovir with and without prednisone for the treatment of herpes zoster: a randomized placebo-controlled trial. The National Institute of Allergy and Infectious Diseases. Collaborative Antiviral Study Group, *Ann Intern Med* 125:376, 1996.

95. Winkler J, Robertson PB: Periodontal disease associated with HIV infection, *Oral Surg Oral Med Oral Pathol* 73:145, 1992.

96. Wynne J, Olsen GN: Acute histoplasmosis presenting as the adult respiratory distress syndrome, *Chest* 66:158, 1974.

97. Young L, Dawson CW, Clark D, et al: Epstein-Barr virus gene expression in nasopharyngeal carcinoma, *J Gen Virol* 69:1051, 1988.

98. Zang L, Hanpf P, Rutherforrd C, et al: Detection of cytomegalovirus DNA, RNA, and antibody in normal donor blood, *J Infect Dis* 171:1002, 1995.

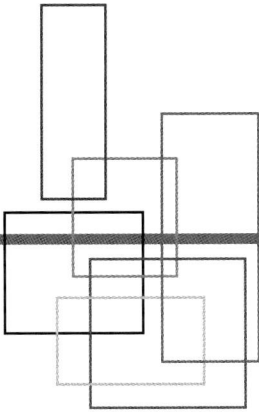

Salivary Gland Infections

Michael Miloro
Morton G. Goldberg

The majority of nonneoplastic diseases of the major salivary glands involve acute or chronic infections of the parotid, submandibular, and, rarely, sublingual glands. Infections of these glands may be bacterial, viral, or mycobacterial in origin. Although any of the major and minor salivary glands may be affected, the parotid and submandibular glands are involved most frequently as acute bacterial parotitis (ABP) and acute bacterial submandibular sialadenitis (ABSS). The cause of sialadenitis may be related to a variety of factors, including decreased salivary flow (dehydration, malnutrition, obstruction, and medications), trauma to the duct or ductal orifice (occupational, habitual, or dental), or obstruction to salivary flow (ductal trauma, mucous plug, sialolithiasis, or collagen-vascular disease). These factors form the basis for the classification of infectious disorders of the salivary glands (Box 12-1). A high index of suspicion is necessary to differentiate an infectious salivary gland process from other causes of salivary gland enlargement, including benign and malignant tumors. Infections of the submandibular gland usually are obstructive in origin, whereas those of the parotid gland result from nonobstructive causes. Sialodochitis, inflammation of the ductal system, also may follow episodes of acute sialolithiasis. Acute and chronic sialadenitis are influenced by several factors, including patient age, past medical and surgical history, immune status, total body fluid balance, medications, and allergies. Other causative factors of salivary gland infection include congenital or acquired ductal abnormalities; the presence of foreign bodies affecting the glands, ducts, or both; concomitant dental therapy; systemic granulomatous disease; human immunodeficiency virus (HIV); facial trauma; and recent hospitalization.

GENERAL CONSIDERATIONS

Routine patient evaluation includes a comprehensive medical history and physical examination. The medical history may provide relevant information regarding the assessment of the patient with salivary gland enlargement, because a variety of medical illnesses predispose patients to acute salivary gland infection (Box 12-2). Many cases of ABP occur in hospitalized patients who are debilitated with inadequate fluid intake and alteration of fluid balance with resultant dehydration. Patients who report postprandial submandibular edema and pain most likely have acute obstructive submandibular sialolithiasis. A previous history of salivary stone formation may aid in the diagnosis. Children with acute salivary gland edema and tenderness may have contracted epidemic mumps. Patients with acute

---

BOX 12-1

Classification of Salivary Gland Infections

Bacterial infections
Acute suppurative submandibular sialadenitis
Acute bacterial parotitis
Chronic recurrent submandibular sialadenitis
Chronic recurrent parotitis
Chronic recurrent juvenile parotitis
Acute allergic sialadenitis (radiological parotitis)
Actinomycosis
Cat-scratch disease
Viral infections
Epidemic parotitis (mumps)
Benign lymphoepithelial lesion (HIV disease)
Cytomegalovirus
Fungal infections
Mycobacterial infections
Tuberculosis
Atypical mycobacteria
Parasitic infections
Immunologically mediated infections
Collagen sialadenitis (systemic lupus erythematosus)
Sjögren's syndrome
Necrotizing sialometaplasia
Sarcoidosis

BOX **12-2**

Risk Factors Associated with Salivary Gland Infections

Dehydration
Recent surgery and anesthesia
Chronic medical illnesses
Advanced age
Premature infants
Radiation therapy
Immunocompromised status
Long-term institutionalization
Renal failure
Hepatic failure
Congestive heart failure
Diabetes mellitus
Hypothyroidism
Malnutrition
Sialolithiasis
Oral infection
Oral neoplasm
HIV disease
Sjögren's syndrome
Depression
Psychiatric disorders
Anorexia nervosa/bulimia
Hyperuricemia
Hyperlipoproteinemia
Cystic fibrosis (mucoviscidosis)
Lead intoxication
Cushing's disease
Medications
Others

BOX **12-3**

Medications Associated with Salivary Gland Infections

Antihistamines
Diuretics
Tricyclic antidepressants
Phenothiazines
Antihypertensives (β-blocking agents)
Barbiturates
Antisialagogues
Anticholinergics (atropine)
Chemotherapeutic agents

medications include diuretics, anticholinergics (e.g., atropine), antihistamines, tricyclic antidepressants, phenothiazines, β-blocking agents, antisialagogues, and some chemotherapeutic agents (Box 12-3). Any constitutional signs and symptoms should be determined, including fever, malaise, diaphoresis, chills, and nausea.

After a thorough history has been obtained, the physical examination should begin with inspection to ascertain any asymmetries in the appearance and size of the glands bilaterally before palpation and possible introduction of iatrogenic edema. Any cardinal signs and symptoms of inflammation should be identified, including edema, erythema, tenderness, and warmth. Evidence of facial trauma should be documented, including the presence of lacerations, ecchymosis, or abrasions (e.g., cat scratch or puncture). The examination should begin with an extraoral examination followed by an intraoral assessment. Palpation of the major salivary glands should be gentle with bimanual examination of the glands, ducts, and ductal orifices. The clinician must observe carefully for spontaneous and evoked salivary flow ("milking" of the gland bimanually), expulsion of mucous plugs or small stones or "sludge," and presence of purulence at the ductal orifice. Any potential odontogenic source of infection (secondary deep space involvement) for submandibular or posterior facial swelling must be ruled out by periapical radiographs and pulpal vitality testing.

The decision to perform instrumentation of the ductal orifice and probe the duct should not be made indiscriminately. The act of mechanical probing may be diagnostic, and therapeutic if a calculus is present, a mucous plug is dislodged, or a ductal stricture is dilated. Conversely, this procedure may introduce bacteria that normally colonize around the ductal orifice into the ductal system and allow retrograde contamination of the gland. Ductal probing generally is not indicated for epidemic mumps in children, and probably is contraindicated in the setting of ABP. Tumors and inflammation of the sublingual gland are rare; the most common lesion of this gland is a ranula. Finally, the head and neck examination should conclude with palpation of the facial and cervical regions for any signs of associated lymphadenopathy.

gland edema should be questioned about contact with animals, specifically cats. Musicians who play wind instruments who report bilateral parotid swelling after a concert may have acute air insufflation of the parotid gland and fascia in the classic "trumpet blower's syndrome." Patients who have undergone recent dental work, or more specifically, orthodontic bracket application, or with evidence of a cheek-biting habit and salivary gland enlargement may have been infected by traumatic introduction of bacteria into the ductal system with resultant retrograde sialadenitis. Although uncommon, any odontogenic source should be eliminated by dental and radiographic examination and tooth vitality testing. Evidence of facial trauma with facial lacerations may disrupt Stensen's duct and cause parotid region edema as a result of sialocele formation, or the presence of a foreign body (e.g., dirt, glass, toothbrush bristles) may cause a physical obstruction to salivary flow. A patient history significant for collagen-vascular disease or autoimmune disease may indicate the possibility of salivary gland obstruction as the cause of sialadenitis (e.g., a relationship between sarcoidosis and ranula formation in the sublingual glands). Finally, a proper medical history may reveal a variety of medications that can lead to decreased salivary flow with stasis and retrograde sialadenitis. Such

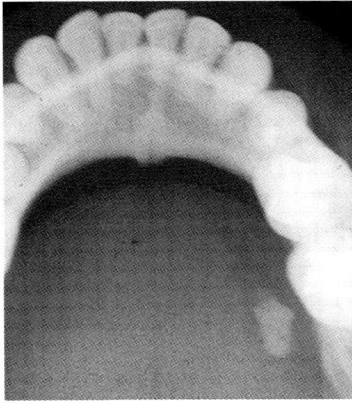

Figure 12-1 Salivary calculus in Wharton's duct on mandibular occlusal radiograph.

Salivary gland radiography is guided by the history and physical examination findings and is useful in the diagnostic assessment of salivary gland enlargement. Plain film radiography may be useful for detection of salivary gland calculi in the glands and the ductal system (Figure 12-1). The usefulness of this study is limited because only 80% to 85% of stones are radiopaque and therefore visible on plain films. A mandibular occlusal film can be used to detect calculi in the submandibular and sublingual glands and ducts. A "puffed cheek" view, in which the patient forcibly blows the cheek laterally to distend the soft tissues over the lateral ramus and zygoma, may detect parotid gland and Stensen's duct calculi. Periapical and panoramic radiographs occasionally show calculi of the major salivary gland systems.

Computed tomography (CT) allows better distinction between salivary gland tissue and adjacent soft tissue than sialography, and although radiation exposure is increased, it is a less invasive procedure. CT scanning can distinguish between intraglandular and extraglandular lesions. For example, the clinical appearance of a masticator space infection may mimic acute parotitis; however, a CT scan with soft tissue window attenuation differentiates the two entities. CT scanning may show posteriorly located submandibular hilar stones that were not visible on plain films. The use of three-dimensional CT scanning has been applied to the salivary glands, with the ability to visualize ductal irregularities and architectural alteration of the gland parenchyma in three dimensions with computer enhancement.[25]

Ultrasonography is a simple, noninvasive imaging technique that may be useful in the evaluation of mass lesions of the parotid and submandibular glands. Ultrasonography can distinguish solid from cystic (fluid-filled) masses. Parotid and submandibular gland cysts, stones, dilated ducts, and abscesses can be demonstrated. However, ultrasound images lack detailed image resolution.

Magnetic resonance imaging (MRI) provides excellent soft tissue image resolution without radiation or use of contrast media. The use of MRI in salivary gland infectious processes has been limited, but more recently MR sialography has gained popularity because of its excellent resolution of salivary gland ductal anatomy. Several studies have documented the use of fast T2-weighted MR images to delineate the ductal architecture and identify calculi.[51]

Over the past decade, sialoendoscopy has become a minimally invasive technique used in the diagnosis and treatment of obstructive salivary gland disorders.[33,37] This technique can be used in cases of difficult calculus access and removal (posterior Wharton's duct or submandibular gland hilum), to survey the ductal system after calculus removal, after positive findings from a sialogram or an ultrasound study, or as a screening examination in cases of recurrent gland edema without a diagnosis. This study shows promise in retrieval of salivary gland calculi and diagnosis of ductal inflammation and scarring without major complications.

Sialography had been considered the "gold standard" in diagnostic salivary gland radiology, although in recent years it has largely been replaced by CT scanning and MRI. Sialography is performed mostly in cases of obstructive or chronic sialadenitis. It is useful for detection of the 15% to 20% incidence of radiolucent calculi and mucous plugs, and provides excellent detail of the salivary gland parenchyma and ductal components. Sialography may demonstrate ductal strictures, foreign bodies, stones, and parenchymal abscess collections, and estimate the severity of ductal and parenchymal damage caused by obstructive, inflammatory, traumatic, and neoplastic diseases. Sialography is performed with water-soluble (or oil-based) contrast media that contain between 28% and 38% iodine concentration. Because of the high iodine content of the contrast media, sialography is contraindicated in the setting of acute sialadenitis because contrast may extravasate outside the capsule of inflamed or damaged glands and ducts and cause severe pain and possibly soft tissue damage, with possible foreign body reaction and glandular necrosis. Other contraindications to sialography include iodine sensitivity and use before a planned thyroid scan study. In addition to its diagnostic role in detection of calculi and, possibly, mucous plugs, sialography may be therapeutic by dislodging small calculi or mucous plugs, thereby relieving the physical obstruction to salivary flow. Most contrast media are considered bacteriostatic (some contain a combination of contrast and antibiotics), but their bacteriostatic activity within the glands has not been proved. Sialography may induce a transient systemic bacteremia. Sialography may be useful for determination of the degree of ductal and glandular destruction as a result of chronic and recurrent infectious or inflammatory processes. Sialadenitis, inflammation of the acinoparenchyma of the gland, results in saccular dilation caused by acinar atrophy that is visible as "pruning" of the normal full arborization of the ductal system (Figure 12-2). The contrast does not penetrate into the peripheral ductules of the gland. Sialodochitis, inflammatory damage to the ductal system, classically displays a "sausage link"

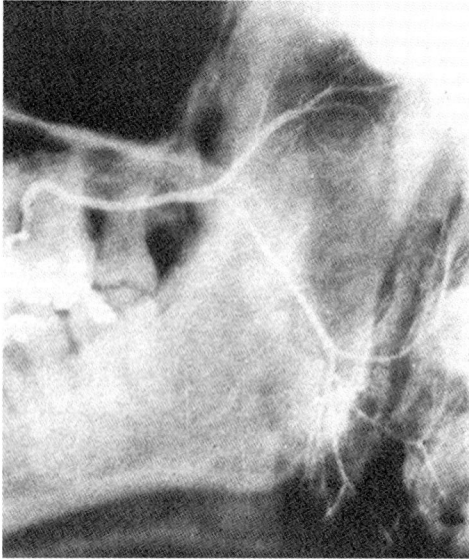

Figure 12-2 Sialogram of acute sialadenitis shows "pruning" of the ductal system.

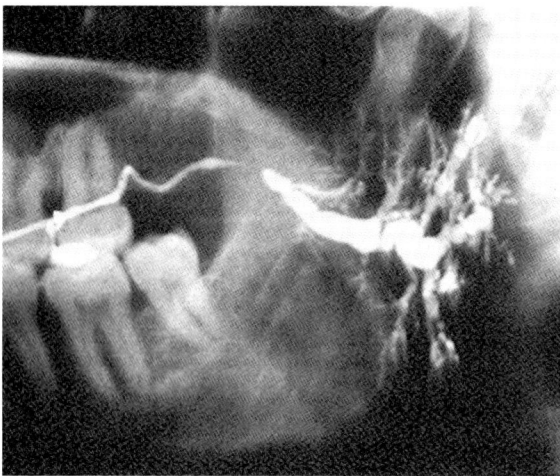

Figure 12-3 Sialogram of chronic sialadenitis shows the "sausage link" appearance of enlarged ducts.

appearance on sialograms (Figure 12-3). The saccular enlargement of the ductal system results from chronic inflammation, repetitive attempts to pump saliva out against a fixed obstruction, or both processes, with the resultant loss of ductal architecture and elasticity. Abscess cavities within the gland parenchyma may be seen as displacement and compression of the normal glandular architecture peripherally around a radiolucent area. Finally, the retention of contrast media in the glandular system after the study (postevacuation phase) may indicate a decrease in the amount of residual gland function. Recently sialography has been combined with both CT scanning and MRI to improve image resolution and detail of the study.[51]

Radioisotope scanning, or salivary scintigraphy, may be useful in the evaluation of salivary gland parenchyma. This study relies on the salivary glandular tissue's selective concentration of radioactive elements, such as radioactive iodine; this selectivity is similar to that of thyroid tissue. In general, intraglandular lesions, such as benign mixed tumors, Warthin's tumor, and malignant salivary gland tumors, may be detected on intravenous injection of a radioactive isotope (^{99m}Tc pertechnetate). Salivary scintigraphy may show increased uptake of ^{99m}Tc in an acutely inflamed gland or decreased uptake in a gland with poor function as a result of chronic inflammation and scarring. The advantage of salivary scintigraphy is that all glands may be imaged simultaneously; however, the main problem with scintigraphy is poor detail resolution.

Laboratory data may aid in the diagnosis of salivary gland infection. Peripheral leukocytosis may be expected in acute bacterial sialadenitis, and leukopenia and relative lymphocytosis may be present in cases of viral sialadenitis. Sialochemistry, the evaluation of the electrolyte composition of saliva, measures sodium and potassium ion concentration changes with alterations in salivary flow rates. In general, noninflammatory disorders of the salivary glands (sialadenosis) result in elevations in potassium levels (normal potassium levels: parotid, 25 mEq/L; submandibular, 20 mEq/L), whereas inflammatory sialadenitis results in a decrease in potassium and an increase in sodium concentrations (normal sodium concentrations: parotid, 7 mEq/L; submandibular 5 mEq/L). Recurrent parotitis also may exhibit elevations in protein concentration (>400 mg/dL), and collagen sialadenitis (e.g., systemic lupus erythematosus) results in elevations of chloride concentrations greater than two to three times normal. Salivary flow also may be decreased in sialadenitis.

Bacteriology is of paramount importance in the diagnostic assessment of salivary gland infection. Routine acquisition of purulent material (i.e., aspiration or spontaneous or evoked drainage) is evaluated rapidly by Gram stain and aerobic, anaerobic, and fungal culture and antibiotic sensitivity testing. Acid-fast staining techniques may be used for suspected mycobacterial infections. The differential diagnosis of salivary gland enlargement includes many disorders that may cause clinical confusion (Box 12-4). In general the presence of tumors and systemic diseases may be ruled out by the absence of any cardinal signs of inflammation. Sialadenosis, or noninflammatory salivary gland enlargement, may result from a variety of systemic conditions. The presence of a benign tumor usually manifests as a slow-growing, firm, painless mass, whereas a malignant tumor may enlarge more rapidly and include neurological deficits (e.g., facial nerve weakness), pain, or fixation to the underlying tissues. The presence of postprandial gland edema and pain generally suggests obstructive sialadenitis. A proposed algorithm for assessment of salivary gland enlargement is outlined in Figure 12-4.

BOX 12-4

Differential Diagnosis of Salivary Gland Enlargement

Salivary gland infection (see Box 12-1)
  Sialadenosis
  Hormonal
  Neurohumoral
  Dysenzymatic
  Malnutrition
  Mucoviscidosis (cystic fibrosis)
  Drug-Induced
Sialolithiasis
Sialocele
Ductal stricture
Mucocele
Ranula
Megastenon
Sialorrhea
Xerostomia
Trauma
Odontogenic infection (secondary space involvement)
Benign salivary gland tumors
  Pleomorphic adenoma (benign mixed tumor)
  Monomorphic adenoma

Warthin's tumor (papillary cystadenoma lymphomatosum)
Oxyphilic adenoma (oncocytoma)
Malignant salivary gland tumors
  Mucoepidermoid carcinoma
  Adenoid cystic carcinoma
  Malignant pleomorphic adenoma
  Acinic cell carcinoma
  Polymorphous low-grade adenocarcinoma
Lipoma
Fibroma
Mesenchymal tumors (hemangioma, neurofibroma, lipoma)
Lymph node hyperplasia
Reactive lymphadenitis
Infectious mononucleosis
Lymphoepithelial cyst
Dermoid cyst
Epidermoid cyst
Lymphoma

BACTERIAL SALIVARY GLAND INFECTIONS

ACUTE BACTERIAL PAROTITIS

The history of ABP parallels the history of modern medicine. The first reported case of ABP was in 1829 from the Hotel Dieu in Paris.[19] ABP was distinguished from viral mumps by Brodie in 1834.[4] This entity has been referred to as suppurative parotitis, pyogenic parotitis, and surgical mumps, because historically it has been attributed to postsurgical hypovolemia and dehydration. Before the modern surgical and antibiotic era of medicine, ABP was a common complication of abdominal surgery or intraabdominal trauma, with a mortality rate approaching 50%. Before the mid–twentieth century understanding of the physiology of fluid and electrolyte balance, postoperative dehydration was commonplace. The postoperative volume depletion caused by inadequate volume replacement to compensate for sensible and insensible surgical losses in addition to maintenance requirements resulted in salivary stasis and retrograde infection of the parotid gland through Stensen's duct. In July 1881, President Garfield suffered a gunshot wound to the abdomen in an assassination attempt. He underwent abdominal exploratory laparotomy surgery and developed peritonitis and dehydration. He died 10 weeks later as a result of sepsis, presumably as a result of suppurative parotitis.

Dehydration with resultant xerostomia has been associated with ABP in a report of seven cases caused by prolonged sun exposure in the Middle East in 1919.[8] By the late 1930s and during World War II, intravenous fluid resuscitation during and after surgery had become routine

practice, and the incidence of postsurgical ABP decreased dramatically. By 1955, with the routine use of perioperative prophylactic and therapeutic antibiotics, ABP was referred to by Robinson as ". . . a vanishing disease."[44] But by 1958, Petersdorf et al.[39] reported seven cases of penicillin-resistant staphylococcal parotitis, and by the early 1960s, large series of cases of ABP were reported.[27,49]

In the past several decades a dramatic change has occurred in the bacterial flora of the oral cavity. This change has been caused largely by the increased incidence of nosocomial and opportunistic infections in patients who are immunocompromised and those who are seriously ill in intensive care units whose mouths become colonized by microorganisms that were found rarely in the oral environment several decades ago. In addition, with the advent of antibiotics directed at some resident oral flora (e.g., streptococci), the voids became occupied by other bacterial species (e.g., gram-negative enteric organisms, *Escherichia coli, Proteus, Klebsiella, Haemophilus influenzae,* diphtheroids, *Neisseria gonorrhoeae*), and iatrogenically induced, genetically altered organisms (i.e., penicillin-resistant staphylococci). Finally, with the improvement in culture techniques and laboratory analyses, the identification of anaerobic organisms (e.g., *Peptostreptococcus, Fusobacterium, Prevotella,* and *Porphyromonas*) in Stensen's ductal discharge fluid and percutaneous needle aspiration material has increased.

ABP rarely occurs in children during the neonatal period beginning 2 weeks after birth. Similar to adult ABP, the cause is dehydration in the majority of cases. The classic clinical presentation of parotid edema and erythema, with purulence expressible at Stensen's duct, also may be

```
                          Salivary Gland Enlargement
                    ┌──────────────┴──────────────────────────┐
               Diffuse edema                              Discrete mass
          ┌────────┴────────┐                          ┌──────┴──────┐
      Unilateral         Bilateral                 Unilateral      Bilateral
     ┌────┴────┐        ┌────┴────┐                     │             │
   Acute    Chronic   Acute    Chronic              CT, MRI       Warthin's
     │                  │         │               ┌────┴────┐       tumor
   Pain               ABP      Sjögren's        Tumor       Rule
   Fever                       syndrome           │       out tumor
   Constitutional              SLE             Staging
   symptoms                    Sarcoid            │
   Purulence                   Other           Surgery

                               Medical
                               treatment

   Culture and
   sensitivity
   Hydration
   No antisialogogues
   Empiric antibiotics
   Incision and
   drainage
   Sialolithectomy

   No resolution ──────┐

              Reculture
              CT, MRI
              Repeat incision
              and drainage
              Sialoendoscopy
              Sialography
              (chronic)
          ┌──────┴──────┐
     Obstructive    Nonobstructive
          │
   Sialolithectomy/sialodochoplasty
   Sialoadenectomy (chronic)
```

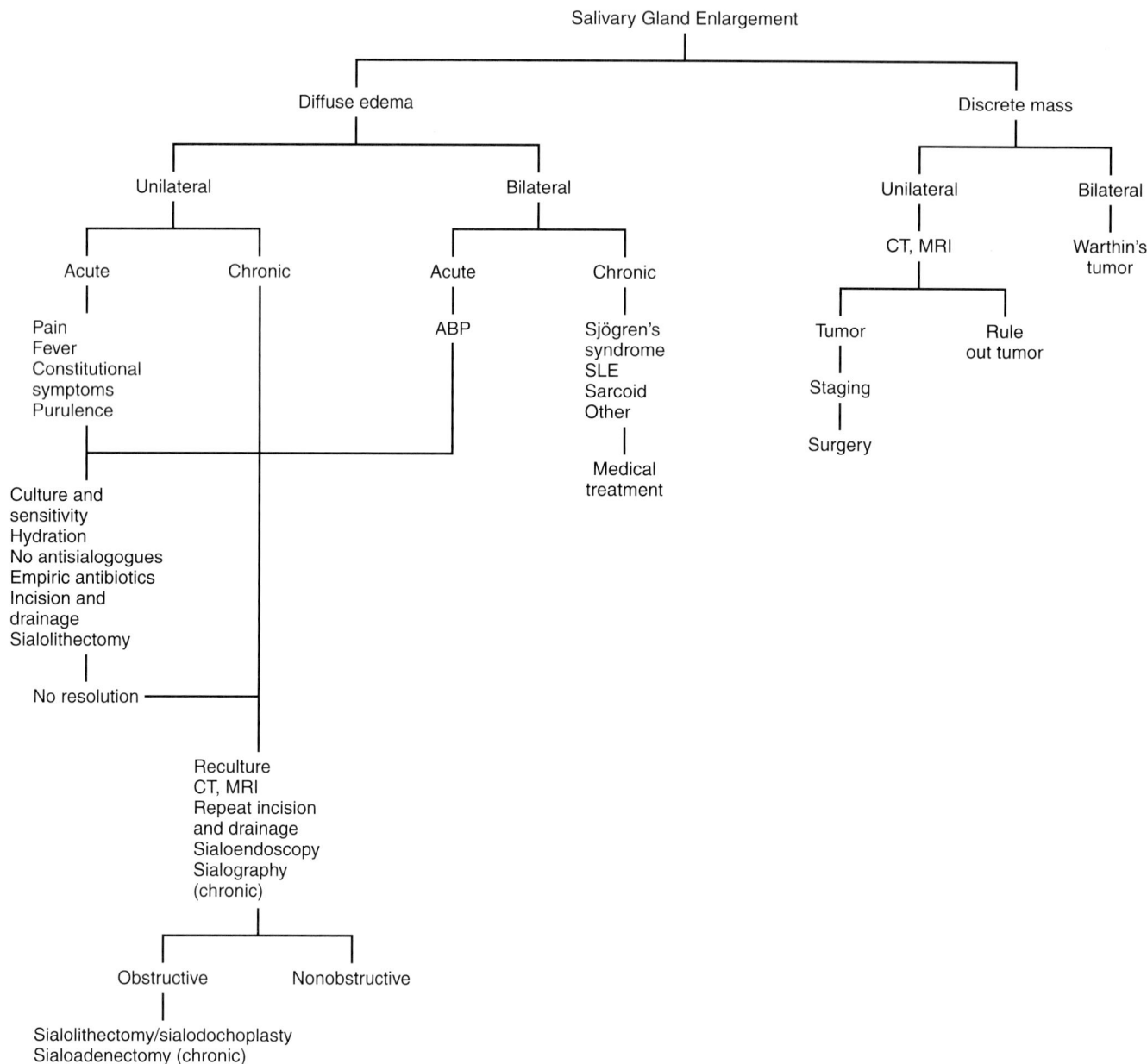

Figure 12-4 Algorithm for assessment and management of salivary gland enlargement. *SLE,* Systemic lupus erythematosus.

observed. Although *Staphylococcus aureus* is most commonly associated with neonatal ABP, *E. coli, Pseudomonas aeruginosa, Streptococcus pneumoniae,* and other organisms have been isolated. Systemic antibiotics and rehydration usually control the disease process, but some neonates may require surgical drainage.

In recent years ABP has manifest in one of two forms: nosocomial and community-acquired variants. Most previous clinical and reported evidence, however anecdotal, suggests that the most common organism cultured from hospital-acquired cases of parotitis is *S. aureus* (>50%). In many cases, parotitis in patients who are debilitated and immunocompromised has been caused by gram-negative enteric organisms, such as *Pseudomonas, Klebsiella, E. coli,*

Proteus, Eikenella corrodens, and *H. influenzae.*[21] Aerobic and anaerobic organisms may be cultured from patients with ABP.[5,6,34,40,42]

Several factors predispose the parotid gland to infectious processes. Retrograde infection of the parotid gland is postulated as the major cause of ABP. Dehydration, as a result of acute illness, surgery, trauma, or sepsis, may result in diminished salivary flow, thereby eliminating the normal "flushing action" of saliva as it traverses through Stensen's duct. Another hypothesis is that parotid saliva has less intrinsic bacteriostatic activity than saliva produced by the other major salivary glands. In healthy patients the content of parotid saliva includes high concentrations of fibronectin, which promote the adherence of

Streptococcus spp. and *S. aureus* around the ductal orifice of Stensen's duct.[23] Conversely, low levels of fibronectin promote the adherence of *Pseudomonas* and *E. coli*. This fact explains the clinical situation in which colonization as a result of dehydration leads to gram-positive parotitis versus the development of gram-negative parotid gland infections in patients who are debilitated or immunocompromised.[1,47,48] Adherence of gram-negative rods to oropharyngeal cells is increased in critically-ill patients.[21] Subsequent retrograde invasion of Stensen's duct and the parotid gland occurs with diminished salivary flow. The resultant ABP reflects the resident oral flora of the compromised host exposed to the opportunistic organisms of the hospital and intensive care unit.

Community-acquired ABP is much more common than hospital-acquired ABP. All of the organisms associated with nosocomial ABP can cause community-acquired ABP, but most frequently it is associated with gram-positive cocci, *Staphylococcus* and *Streptococcus*. Although obstructive phenomena such as sialoliths are uncommon in Stensen's duct compared with Wharton's duct, parotid duct obstruction may result from mucous plugs that form as a result of reduced salivary flow caused by dehydration or poor fluid balance. Salivary stasis may be the result of medications with antisialagogic side effects, such as diuretics, antihistamines, tricyclic antidepressants, antihypertensives (β-blocking agents), anticholinergics, tranquilizers, and phenothiazines. These drugs may lead to increased salivary viscosity that causes stasis of flow and, possibly, mucous plug formation. Hematogenous spread of infection to the parotid gland is unlikely. Trauma to Stensen's duct may be responsible for 5% to 10% of cases of ABP. Ductal trauma, with subsequent periductal edema, may cause partial obstruction of salivary flow. Trauma may be the result of dental trauma, orthodontic appliances, cheek biting, toothbrush trauma, air insufflation during dental therapy, and "trumpet blower's syndrome." This entity should be differentiated from ABP, because it is merely a pneumoparotid with tissue emphysema and crepitus on physical examination and lacks the constitutional symptoms of acute infection.[31] However, ABP may occur as a result of pneumoparotid if salivary stasis and bacterial infection are present. Finally, poor oral hygiene and immunocompromised states (e.g., diabetes mellitus, malnutrition, acute or chronic diarrhea) with resultant dehydration may be causative factors in ABP.

The diagnosis of ABP includes an assessment of history, physical examination, laboratory data, and radiographic studies. A history of recent surgery or previous episodes of ABP may be significant. In postoperative patients the onset usually occurs after the third postsurgical day following fluid redistribution. The presence of an immunocompromised state or use of medications with antisialagogic effects should be ascertained. The onset of ABP is sudden and rapid with painful swelling and erythema of the preauricular region, classically at mealtime. The physical findings of ABP usually are classic (Figure 12-5). The parotid gland is enlarged, possibly displacing the earlobe laterally,

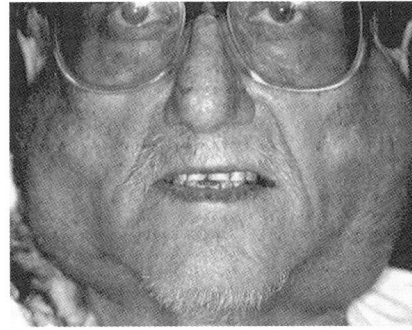

Figure 12-5 Clinical example of acute bacterial parotitis.

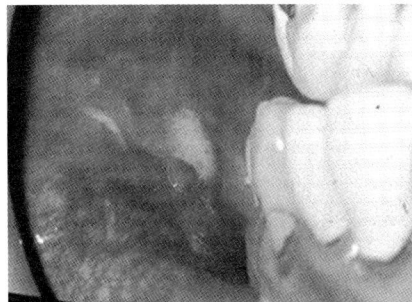

Figure 12-6 Purulence at Stensen's duct in acute bacterial parotitis.

and tender to palpation. Both parotid glands usually are affected (indicative of a systemic disorder), but if the infection is unilateral, the right gland seems to be affected more than the left side. A predilection for males exists for ABP, and the mean age of presentation is 60 years.

The act of "milking" of the parotid gland with bimanual pressure to Stensen's duct intraorally and extraorally, in the posterior to anterior direction, may express purulent material if the duct is patent (Figure 12-6). Probing of Stensen's duct (with lacrimal probes) and catheter irrigating generally is contraindicated in ABP. Although ductal strictures may be dilated and small mucous plugs relieved, the risk of introducing purulent material into the proximal duct and parotid gland should be considered. Constitutional symptoms, including fever, chills, and sweats, may occur if an established infection is present. Dehydration may be confirmed by the presence of xerostomia and poor skin turgor. Laboratory evaluation may reveal leukocytosis with a predominance of immature polymorphonuclear leukocytes and bandemia with true ABP. Further confirmation of dehydration is made by elevated hematocrit, increased blood urea nitrogen level, elevated urine specific gravity, decreased urinary flow rates, and possibly contraction alkalosis on electrolyte examination. Radiographic evaluation rarely demonstrates calculi in Stensen's ducts, and sialography is contraindicated in ABP. Ultrasonography may be useful for detection of stones when sialography is contraindicated. CT scanning may help visualization of abscess formation (Figure 12-7) or tumors, and can

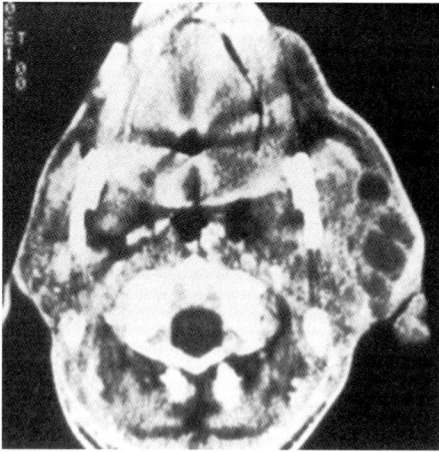

Figure 12-7 CT scan of left parotid abscess.

distinguish other secondary space infections (masticator, lateral pharyngeal, pterygomandibular spaces) from glandular ABP. MRI may be more useful for delineating soft tissue pathological conditions (tumors) and visualizing tissue planes. Bacteriological studies are essential in the diagnosis of ABP. A Gram stain of purulent discharge may identify potential pathogens quickly and easily; however, culture and sensitivity studies should be performed as soon as possible. The culture studies confirm the Gram stain findings and identify specific organisms, whereas the sensitivity determines the most appropriate choice of antimicrobial agent. If the empirical antibiotic that is chosen pending culture and sensitivity results does not control the infection, antimicrobial therapy is guided by the culture and sensitivity findings. The best collection method of material for bacteriologic examination is percutaneous needle aspiration or transductal aspiration using a small catheter introduced into Stensen's duct. Percutaneous aspiration prevents cross-contamination of the sample with normal resident oral flora. Unfortunately, in many circumstances obtaining sufficient material for examination percutaneously is difficult, and containing the sample for anaerobic analysis is problematic. If surgical drainage is required, direct needle aspiration through the exposed parotid fascia may be performed.[14,16]

The treatment of ABP consists of specific and nonspecific therapies. The historical description of nonspecific therapy included discontinuation of antisialagogic medications, increased fluid intake, heat packs, mouth rinses, sialogogues (such as lemon drops or glycerin swabs), analgesics as needed for pain, and Lugol's solution, which is an iodine compound that was efficacious only because it was administered with a large volume of water and addressed the dehydrated state of the patient. Radiation therapy, once considered a mainstay of therapy, no longer is warranted. The beneficial effects of radiation in cases of ABP in the early to mid-twentieth century actually were related to the simultaneous introduction and understanding of fluid and electrolyte balance. Rehydration remains a cornerstone of therapy for ABP, but caution must be exercised in

patients who are elderly and debilitated who may not be able to appropriately redistribute the fluid load and may be at risk for acute cardiac overload and failure with resultant pulmonary edema. Fluid overload should be avoided by careful monitoring of urine output and specific gravity, electrolytes, and possibly central venous pressure. Discontinuation of medications with antisialagogic side effects (or alteration of drug dosages) should be undertaken only after consultation with the prescribing physician and the determination of appropriate alternative medications. These measures (rehydration and drug alteration) should act together to increase salivary flow while decreasing salivary viscosity, resulting in the reestablishment of a "flushing action" of salivary flow. In addition, improvement in oral hygiene with the use of chlorhexidine rinses may decrease the oral bacterial load and the potential for continued retrograde colonization of the gland. Specific therapy of ABP involves removal of ductal obstructions such as mucous plugs (gentle ductal probing and irrigation) or sialoliths (open ductal surgery). These invasive procedures should be attempted only after the institution of empirical antimicrobial therapy.

Prompt species-specific antimicrobial therapy is the keystone of ABP treatment. Empirical therapy may be based on Gram stain results; alternatively, another antibiotic may be chosen based on knowledge of the contemporary flora of ABP discussed previously, including penicillinase-producing *Staphylococcus* and hemolytic *Streptococcus,* which normally colonize around the ductal orifice and may account for up to 40% to 50% of cases of ABP. In the past, community-acquired ABP and cases of suspected *Staphylococcus* involvement in nosocomial ABP, a semisynthetic antistaphylococcal penicillin (methicillin, oxacillin, or dicloxacillin) or a first-generation cephalosporin (cephalexin) was considered a reasonable choice for empirical therapy. If methicillin-resistant *Staphylococcus* organism was identified, vancomycin was the drug of choice. Current antimicrobial trends indicate that β-lactamase–inhibiting drugs such as amoxicillin with clavulanic acid (Augmentin) for outpatient oral administration in the less severe cases of ABP and ampicillin with sulbactam (Unasyn) for inpatient parenteral use in the more severe cases of ABP may be reasonable first-line choices for empirical therapy. Clindamycin also may be used in patients with severe penicillin allergy, but erythromycin should be avoided because of the high bacterial resistance. As alternatives, other newer macrolides antibiotics such as azithromycin (Zithromax) and clarithromycin (Biaxin) may be used in the outpatient setting of community-acquired ABP, because they have an appropriate bacterial spectrum for ABP and a dosage frequency that improves patient compliance. Combination antibiotic therapy may be necessary in consultation with the hospital infectious disease service in cases of hospital-acquired ABP, in community-acquired ABP in the immunocompromised host, or if generalized sepsis develops or nonroutine organisms are identified (e.g., *Pseudomonas*). Antibiotic therapy should be continued until at least 1 week after resolution of the signs and symptoms of ABP.

If the ABP is recalcitrant to therapy or recurs, repeated culture of the abscess and obtaining a CT scan to rule out possible parenchymal abscess formation should be considered (Figure 12-8).

Despite rehydration and antibiotic therapy, progressive infection may lead to local extension into adjacent fascial spaces, generalized hematogenous sepsis, airway obstruction (with involvement of the lateral pharyngeal-retropharyngeal spaces), generalized deterioration to a comatose state, and possibly death. Therefore if nonspecific and specific therapy fails to produce clinical improvement within 72 to 96 hours, if pain and edema increase, if temperature and white blood cell count increase, or if complications occur, surgical intervention may be necessary and lifesaving. Surgical drainage of ABP is performed much less frequently than in the past when antibiotic therapy was unavailable. However, as resistant strains of bacteria continue to develop because of the overuse of antibiotics, incision and drainage may become more necessary, and surgeons should be familiar with these techniques.[30] The parotid gland is surrounded by a dense fibrous soft tissue capsule that makes fluctuance on physical examination uncommon and spontaneous drainage an unlikely phenomenon. Surgical exposure is necessary to ensure drainage of all potential loculations that may have developed under the dense parotid fascia. The presence of loculations may be confirmed with CT scanning before surgery if time allows. If the parotitis is severe enough to warrant surgical intervention, needle aspiration (similar to the procedure for acute tonsillar abscesses) is unlikely to provide adequate surgical drainage and may place the terminal branches of the facial nerve at undue risk for injury.

Incision and drainage of the parotid gland usually is performed with the patient under general anesthesia, but monitored anesthesia care with local anesthesia may be used if the patient's condition precludes use of general anesthesia. Drainage usually is accomplished through a retromandibular incision (a modified superficial parotidectomy incision) through skin and subcutaneous tissue, which exposes the underlying parotid fascia. Multiple penetrations are made through the parotid fascia with blunt dissection (with a closed Kelly clamp) to prevent injury to major vascular hazards and branches of the facial nerve. Attention should be directed to any accessory parotid gland tissue that may contain abscess cavities and lie at or above the level of the zygomatic arch. This salivary gland tissue may require extension of the incision more cranially to gain access for adequate drainage. Although grossly purulent flow may not be obtained, serous drainage through the perforations in the parotid fascia may be sufficient to obtain "decompression" of the gland, which may result in immediate improvement in edema, pain, fever, and white blood cell count. The wound usually is packed open with saline gauze sponges that are changed twice or three times daily. Occasionally, rubber drains may be placed deep into the abscess cavities and advanced as necessary until the drains become nonproductive and granulation tissue appears and the wound closes spontaneously. This method

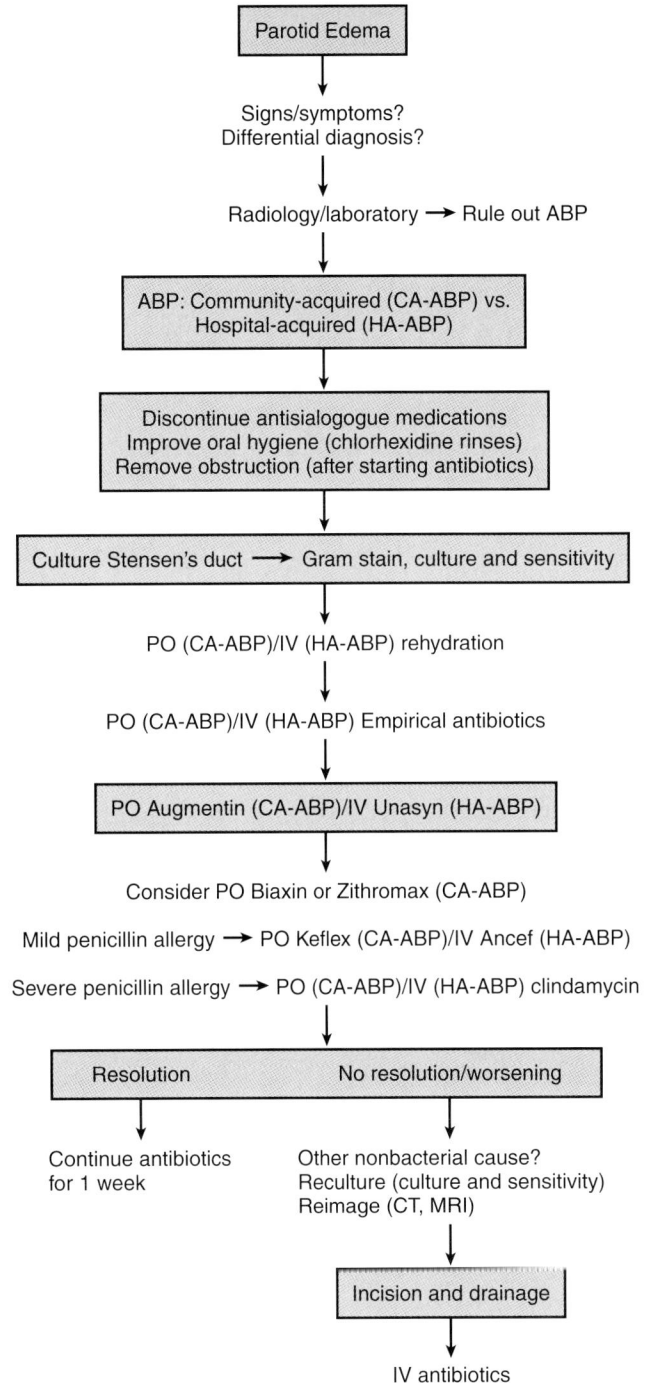

Figure 12-8 Algorithm for management of acute bacterial parotitis.

usually results in minimal scarring or cosmetic deformity, and the formation of sialoceles or persistent salivary fistulae are uncommon complications of surgery.

ACUTE BACTERIAL SUBMANDIBULAR SIALADENITIS

ABSS most commonly is associated with physical obstruction of Wharton's duct.[2,52] Sialolithiasis usually occurs in the submandibular gland and ductal system (85% of cases)

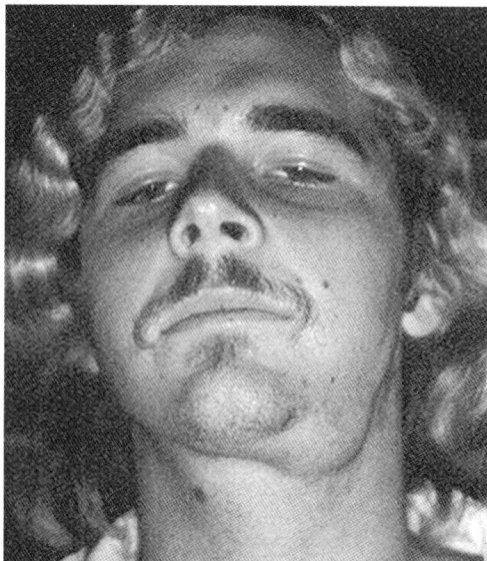

Figure 12-9 Acute bacterial submandibular sialadenitis of the left submandibular gland.

for several reasons. The submandibular gland lies inferior to the ductal system, so that in the erect *Homo sapiens,* flow must occur against the forces of gravity. The length of Wharton's duct contributes to increased transit time of saliva in the ductal system, which may result in the formation of microcalculi, and resultant coalescence causing mechanical obstruction to flow and eventual ABSS.[11] Two acute bends are present in Wharton's duct: one occurs as the gland courses posterior to the mylohyoid muscle, and the second occurs just proximal to the exit of the duct superiorly into the anterior floor of mouth. A sphincteric mechanism at the orifice of Wharton's duct acts as a physical narrowing at this portion of the duct. The alkaline submandibular gland saliva contains a higher concentration of calcium salts (carbonates, phosphates, and oxalates) than the other major salivary glands. All these factors may contribute to salivary stasis, crystallization of precipitated calcium salts with calculus formation, obstruction to salivary flow, and infection. This disease process occurs twice as often in males, with a peak age of occurrence between 30 and 50 years. Interestingly, the left submandibular gland more commonly is affected than the right, and bilateral involvement in the absence of another systemic disorder is rare. Multiple occurrences of sialolith formation in the same gland is common: two calculi are present in 20% of involved cases, and more than two calculi occur in approximately 5% of cases. Sialolithiasis may occur uncommonly in the parotid gland, sublingual glands, and minor salivary glands. Chronic stone formation may lead to ductal ulceration and strictures that may cause obstruction as a result of ductal stenosis.

The classic feature of ABSS is pain and swelling in the submandibular region that occurs at mealtime (Figure 12-9); that is, flow is stimulated against a fixed obstruc-

tion. Patients may report a history of previous similar episodes. Associated cervical lymphadenopathy may be present. ABSS is a community-acquired disease that less frequently is associated with dehydration and hospitalization than ABP. Purulence may be expressible from the orifice of Wharton's duct, but in many cases flow is completely obstructed. Any purulent material may be sent for Gram stain and culture and sensitivity studies, but any material collected intraorally is contaminated with resident oral flora. Therefore the majority of cultures from Wharton's duct demonstrate a mixed bacterial flora containing gram-positive cocci. As a result, empirical antimicrobial therapy consists of choices similar to those for ABP depending on the severity of the presentation. Choices include an extended-spectrum penicillin, a first-generation cephalosporin, clindamycin, or one of the newer macrolide antibiotics. The diagnosis of ABSS as a result of sialolithiasis may be confirmed with a mandibular occlusal radiograph (see Figure 12-1); however, only 80% to 85% of calculi are radiopaque and therefore visible on plain films. CT scans may be helpful in localization of a posterior stone in the proximal duct or at the hilum of the gland.

Treatment of ABSS consists of antibiotic therapy, maintenance of fluid intake, avoidance of antisialagogues, and removal of a sialolith, if present. Anterior calculi in the distal third of the duct may be removed in the office with the patient under local anesthesia. The procedure involves dilation of the ductal orifice with lacrimal probes, massage of the gland, and "milking" of the duct from proximal to distal in an attempt to expel the stone. A suture ligature should be placed proximal to the suspected location of the stone to prevent displacing the stone further proximally toward the gland hilum. If this method is unsuccessful, a sialolithotomy, or opening into the ductal system through the oral mucosa, is performed. Again an attempt is made to gently deliver the stone through the surgically created opening. A sialodochoplasty, or ductal revision surgery, is performed. This procedure involves suturing the edges of the duct to the oral mucosa in the area of the sialolithotomy. This approach provides several advantageous changes to the ductal anatomy in an attempt to prevent reoccurrence of the sialolithiasis. The sialodochoplasty effectively shortens the overall length of Wharton's duct and eliminates the narrow punctum and acute curvature at the orifice of the duct, so that flow can occur unimpeded through the new nonsphincteric opening. After a sialodochoplasty procedure a stent may be inserted in the new opening with a plastic catheter to ensure fistulization of the tract into the oral cavity. Patients are encouraged to use salivary stimulants such as lemon drops, glycerin swabs, and citrus fruits to encourage salivary flow postoperatively. In cases of posterior stones located in the middle or proximal third of Wharton's duct (and in cases of recurrent ABSS), access through an intraoral approach may be technically difficult, and in general, the submandibular gland and stone are removed through an extraoral approach with the patient under general anesthesia in the operating room. Although submandibular sialoadenectomy has several risks (extraoral scar, hypoglossal, marginal mandibular branch of facial and lingual nerve paresthesia, and facial and deep lingual artery vascular hazards), it is far less morbid than a parotidectomy.

CHRONIC RECURRENT BACTERIAL PAROTITIS

Chronic recurrent bacterial parotitis (CRBP) is defined as repeat episodes of ABP that are separated by intervening periods of remission. This disorder usually is caused by an episode of ABP, but it may be idiopathic or result from Sjögren's syndrome, congenital ductal malformations, strictures, trauma (e.g., from orthodontic appliances), foreign bodies within Stensen's duct (including toothbrush bristles, popcorn kernels, grass, straw, and fish bones), or as an aftereffect of viral parotitis (mumps).[15,35] Classically, two forms of CRBP have been described: an adult form and a juvenile form. The adult form has been associated more closely with infection from *S. aureus,* whereas *Streptococcus viridans* is the major pathogenic bacteria in the juvenile form, which usually occurs in children between the ages of 3 and 6 years. The juvenile form has a slight male predilection, is associated with unilateral parotid enlargement, and may resolve spontaneously at puberty with functional recovery of the parotid gland.[13,22,24,26,28] CT scanning or MRI is useful to distinguish chronic infection from parotid tumors in children. Although gram-positive cocci have been implicated most frequently in this disease process, other species, including opportunistic organisms in the immunocompromised host, have been identified in CRBP. Infection of the parotid gland may be subclinical at various times during the disease course, and therefore the gland may show evidence of latent infection during periods of clinical remission. CRBP may result in parenchymal destruction and loss of glandular function.

CRBP is characterized by unilateral or bilateral edema of the parotid gland that may last for days to months, with periods of exacerbation and remission. Constitutional symptoms may occur, and the white blood cell count and erythrocyte sedimentation rate may be elevated during times of exacerbation. Sialographic findings may include evidence of sialectasis with dilation of the ductal system and pooling of contrast media in the gland and ductal system, perhaps with cystic cavity formation (Figure 12-10).[38] Salivary gland scintigraphy with ^{99m}Tc pertechnetate may be used to assess the functional integrity of the gland and to monitor spontaneous functional recovery.

Treatment of CRBP should include species-specific systemic antibiotic therapy, guided by culture and sensitivity results when available. Any identified foreign bodies should be removed from the ductal system. Systemic antibiotics may be needed on an intermittent basis in the juvenile form of the disease until the patient reaches puberty.

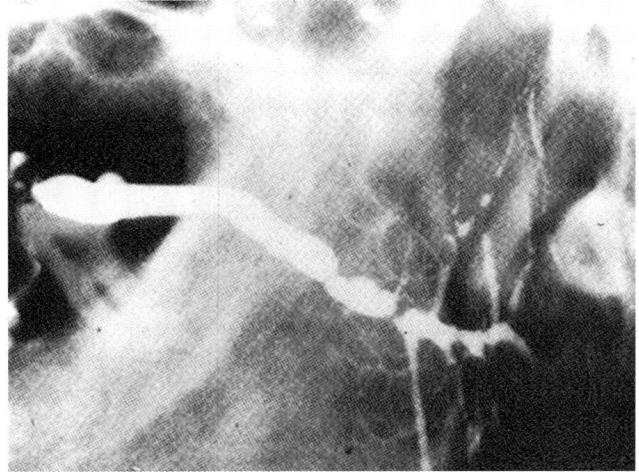

Figure 12-10 Sialogram of chronic sialadenitis shows pooling of contrast with cystic cavity formation.

Similar to treatment of ABP, analgesics may be necessary, and avoidance of dehydration and the discontinuance of antisialagogic medications is recommended. Intraductal instillation of antibiotics may be useful during periods of remission; such treatment is begun between 1 and 2 weeks after resolution of an acute episode.[41] The procedure involves cannulation of Stensen's duct with a No. 50 polyethylene tube. Local anesthesia with 2% lidocaine may be used to anesthetize the periductal tissues. The irrigant solution may contain tetracycline or erythromycin. Generally, in adults approximately 3 to 4 mL of 15 mg/mL solution is used; in children 1.5 to 2.5 mL of 10 mg/mL solution is instilled into the ductal system. The solution is allowed to remain in ductal system for between 5 and 10 minutes. This procedure may be repeated on a daily basis for 3 to 5 days. Historically, treatment was aimed at parotid gland destruction and atrophy using parotid duct ligation, glossopharyngeal nerve sacrifice, or low-dose radiation therapy to the gland. Current practice advocates parotidectomy with facial nerve preservation in cases recalcitrant to other forms of nonsurgical therapy.[17]

CHRONIC RECURRENT SUBMANDIBULAR SIALADENITIS

Chronic recurrent submandibular sialadenitis is associated with recurrent sialolithiasis and usually follows acute episodes of ABSS. Chronic recurrent submandibular sialadenitis occurs more commonly than CRBP. Sialography may be helpful in confirming the diagnosis by demonstrating evidence of sialadenitis and sialectasis, with decreased gland emptying rates indicative of poor gland function. Treatment of chronic recurrent submandibular sialadenitis consists of empirical antibiotic therapy, sialogogues, fluid replacement, and sialolithectomy if indicated. Ultimately, for recurrent episodes or if the submandibular gland is nonfunctional, sialoadenectomy is indicated.

Interestingly, long-standing chronic submandibular sialadenitis may produce a firm, tumorlike mass in the submandibular triangle, known as the Kuttner tumor.[50]

ACTINOMYCOSIS

On rare occasion, *Actinomyces* (*A. israelii*, *A. naeslundii*, *A. propionicus*, *A. viscosus*, *A. odontolyticus*, *A. meyeri*, and *A. eriksonii*) may invade the salivary glands and cause infection. Involvement of the salivary glands, the parotid gland most frequently, may occur in up to 10% of cases of cervicofacial actinomycosis. This organism is a member of the resident oral flora and may lead to acute or chronic infection that may be difficult to distinguish from other forms of sialadenitis. Bacterial invasion of the salivary gland parenchyma may be odontogenic in origin or arise from inflammation of the tonsils. Diagnosis is based on Gram stain and biopsy culture, and sensitivity testing. *Actinomyces* are gram-positive, microaerophilic, non–acid-fast bacteria that grow slowly in culture and may demonstrate the classic "sulfur granules," which are aggregates of the filamentous forms of the organisms. Culture material obtained from fistulous tracts may be contaminated and demonstrate a mixed bacterial flora. Sialography may show localized acinar destructive sialadenitis within the gland parenchyma. Treatment is the same as for cervicofacial actinomycosis, including incision and drainage if indicated, and long-term (6 to 24 months), high-dose penicillin therapy (other antibiotics have been used, including erythromycin and tetracycline). The avoidance of dehydration also is important in preventing the progression to chronic, irreversible sialadenitis.

CAT-SCRATCH DISEASE

Cat-scratch disease is caused by the pleomorphic, gram-negative bacillus, *Afipia felis*, and usually does not affect the salivary glands directly, but begins in the preauricular and cervical lymph node chains as a chronic lymphadenitis and subsequently involves the salivary glands, mostly the parotid gland, by contiguous spread.[10] A history of cat scratch or bite rarely is elicited, but the incubation period is generally 2 to 8 weeks after inoculation. Constitutional symptoms may be present, including fever, malaise, and headache. Diagnosis is made by the identification of lymphadenopathy, a positive Hanger-Rose intradermal skin test result for cat-scratch disease, the presence of a portal of entry (inoculation site), elimination of another cause, and characteristic stain findings (Warthin-Starry silver-staining bacteria on histopathological staining of an involved lymph node). The disease process in the cervicofacial region generally is self-limited and resolves spontaneously within 4 to 6 weeks. Antibiotics, including ciprofloxacin, gentamicin, and trimethoprim-sulfamethoxazole, have been used but generally are not indicated. Incision and drainage is performed rarely but may be necessary to release accumulated necrotic debris.[18]

ACUTE ALLERGIC SIALADENITIS/ RADIOLOGICAL PAROTITIS

On rare occasion, immunological disorders may lead to involvement of the major salivary glands. This may occur after therapeutic radiation to distant organs, with an allergic response to circulating metabolites. Although food allergies are rare, allergies to heavy metals and medications may occur more commonly (these include iodine, chloromycetin, terramycin, and thiouracil). The history generally is that of acute salivary gland enlargement, most commonly the parotid gland, and dyspnea after a contrast study such as an intravenous pyelogram (IVP). The course of this disease is self-limited.

VIRAL SALIVARY GLAND INFECTIONS

VIRAL SIALADENITIS/EPIDEMIC PAROTITIS/MUMPS

Viral mumps is an acute, nonsuppurative communicable infectious disease, primarily of the parotid gland tissue, that often occurs in epidemics during the spring and winter months. Although the disease usually is considered a childhood disease occurring between 6 and 8 years of age, with an equal sex predilection, it can occur in any age group, including adults who may have avoided childhood illness. The disease usually is caused by a paramyxovirus, a ribonucleic acid virus related to the influenza and parainfluenza virus groups. A variety of other nonparamyxoviruses may cause mumps, including coxsackie A and B viruses, Ebstein-Barr virus, influenza and parainfluenza (types 1 and 3) viruses, enteric cytopathic human orphan (ECHO) virus, lymphocytic choriomeningitis virus, and HIV (see following text).[3,7,36,46] The virus is transmitted by infected saliva and urine. The viral incubation period between exposure and the development of signs and symptoms is 15 to 18 days. The disease includes a prodromal period that lasts 24 to 48 hours and includes fever, chills, headache, and preauricular tenderness. The disease is characterized by rapid, painful, nonerythematous unilateral or bilateral swelling of the parotid glands that may be severe enough to displace the earlobe. Purulent discharge from Stensen's duct is rare. Because influenza and other viruses may infect the parotid gland, viral serum titers for mumps virus should help to confirm the suspected diagnosis. Laboratory evaluation generally is nonspecific but may show leukopenia with a relative lymphocytosis. Serum amylase levels also may be elevated, irrespective of an associated pancreatitis. Attempts to eradicate the disease have resulted in the routine administration of measles-mumps-rubella (MMR) vaccine in children at 12 months of age. The disease usually resolves spontaneously within 5 to 10 days; therefore symptomatic treatment of pain (analgesics) and fever (antipyretics) and the avoidance of dehydration is essential. Persistent or recurrent swelling may suggest the development of chronic bacterial sialadenitis of childhood.

Several untoward complications of viral mumps may result from generalized viremia. Mumps pancreatitis may manifest with abdominal pain and tenderness and elevated serum amylase levels. Diabetes mellitus is an uncommon complication of mumps pancreatitis. Orchitis, with testicular enlargement and tenderness, occurs in approximately 20% of adult men affected with mumps parotitis. Half of these individuals develop testicular atrophy, which, if bilateral, may lead to sterility. Priapism is an uncommon complication of mumps orchitis. Meningoencephalitis is an uncommon sequela of viral mumps, which may manifest as neck stiffness, lethargy, and headache. This disease generally is mild and self-limited but may lead to severe encephalitis. Other less common complications of viral mumps include mumps thyroiditis, mumps myocarditis, mumps nephritis, and mumps hepatitis.

HIV-ASSOCIATED SALIVARY GLAND INFECTION

The oral manifestations of HIV occur in approximately 5% to 10% of patients. These clinical findings have been well described and include xerostomia, associated parotid intraglandular, and possibly cervical, lymphadenopathy, and pulmonary insufficiency. Immunofluorescence shows that this siccalike syndrome is characterized by a diffuse lymphocytic infiltrate throughout the involved parotid gland acinar tissue, but without anti-Ro and anti-La autoantibodies, which are present in Sjögren's syndrome.[9,20] The development of benign lymphoepithelial lesions (BLL) in parotid glands affected by the HIV virus may occur. The BLL-diffuse lymphocytic infiltration later may progress to acinar atrophy, ductal proliferation, and production of epimyoepithelial islands. The CD8 lymphocytic infiltration of the parotid parenchyma also may lead to lymphoepithelial cyst formation.[32] In fact, in up to 5% of BLL lesions, malignant lymphomas may develop, most commonly non-Hodgkin's lymphoma, and up to 1% of BLL may progress to carcinoma. Therefore BLL must be included in the differential diagnosis of parotid enlargement.[43]

The possibility of HIV disease transmission from saliva remains controversial. After infection with HIV, low concentrations of HIV-1 viruses and IgA HIV-1 antibodies may be isolated from whole mouth saliva and from major salivary gland secretions. However, despite the presence of the virus the oral cavity may not be a route for spread of the disease,[12,29] perhaps because of the antiviral properties of saliva and inhibition of infectivity, although a specific factor has not been isolated. The xerostomia observed in patients with HIV may be caused by the virus itself or may be influenced by antiretroviral medications. The diagnosis may be aided with CT scanning, sialography, gallium-citrate scanning, and MRI, but ^{99m}Tc pertechnetate scanning is not useful.[45]

CYTOMEGALOVIRUS

Salivary gland inclusion disease may be caused by cytomegalovirus, a subgroup of herpesvirus that produces latent disease. Most infections produce no symptoms except in the immunocompromised host (especially the terminal stages of HIV disease). Transmission may occur from blood or organ transplantation, and the salivary glands frequently are involved in this disease process. A mononucleosis-like syndrome occurs including the triad of fever, pharyngitis, and lymphadenopathy, but results of the heterophile antibody test for infectious mononucleosis (Monospot test) are negative. No specific treatment is indicated, and cytomegalovirus is resistant to antiviral agents such as acyclovir.

MYCOBACTERIAL SALIVARY GLAND INFECTIONS

TUBERCULOSIS

Primary involvement of the salivary glands with *Mycobacterium tuberculosis* is uncommon. Tuberculosis may manifest in two different forms: an infiltrative, disseminated form or a circumscribed, nodular form. The disseminated form is spread hematogenously, whereas the circumscribed form spreads through lymphatics. The parotid gland and the preauricular lymph nodes usually are affected unilaterally, either in an acute or a chronic form. Secondary involvement of the salivary glands with *M. tuberculosis*, associated with active pulmonary tuberculosis, most commonly affects the submandibular gland and cervical lymph node chain, resulting in a draining lesion known as the scrofula (tuberculous cervical lymphadenitis). Diagnosis is made with chest radiography, positive findings from a purified protein derivative intradermal skin test, and the identification of acid-fast bacilli in sputum. Sialography may reveal "pooling" of contrast media in the affected parotid gland parenchyma. Treatment is similar to that for pulmonary tuberculosis with long-term, multidrug therapy.

ATYPICAL MYCOBACTERIAL INFECTIONS

Atypical mycobacteria also may affect the salivary glands, including both the submandibular and parotid glands. These infections are more common in the pediatric age groups and immunocompromised patients *(Mycobacterium avium-intracellulare)*. Skin testing may aid in the diagnosis. Surgical excision rarely is indicated as a treatment adjunct.

PARASITIC SALIVARY GLAND INFECTIONS

FILARIASIS

Helminthic infestations with filariasis worms have been reported in salivary glands. Filariasis is endemic in Africa and Central America. Definitive diagnosis is made by biopsy of the affected salivary gland nodule. Laboratory evaluation reveals eosinophilia. Treatment includes use of the antiparasitic drug, ivermectin (Stromectol), and excision of the salivary gland nodule.

IMMUNOLOGICAL SALIVARY GLAND DISORDERS

COLLAGEN SIALADENITIS (SYSTEMIC LUPUS ERYTHEMATOSUS)

The entire spectrum of collagen-vascular diseases may affect the salivary glands, including scleroderma, dermatomyositis, and polymyositis, but systemic lupus erythematosus is most common. This disease must be distinguished from Sjögren's syndrome. Collagen sialadenitis occurs most frequently in women in the fourth and fifth decades of life. The disorder may affect any of the major salivary glands and usually manifests as a slowly enlarging gland. The diagnosis is made by identification of the underlying systemic disorder, and sialochemistry studies may reveal sodium and chloride ion levels that are elevated two to three times normal values. Treatment involves addressing the causative systemic disease process.

SARCOIDOSIS

Sarcoidosis is a chronic, granulomatous disease characterized by noncaseating granulomas that may affect the salivary glands in up to 6% of cases. Heerfordt's syndrome, or uveoparotid fever, occurs in 10% of cases and consists of a triad of parotid enlargement, uveitis, and seventh cranial nerve palsy. The cause is unknown, and the disease is most common in the third and fourth decades of life and more common in black patients than white patients. The initial symptoms consist of prodromal constitutional symptoms of fever, malaise, weakness, nausea, and night sweats that may last from weeks to months. Typical chest radiographic features include symmetrical bilateral perihilar lymphadenopathy. Parotid enlargement usually is painless, firm, and bilateral, and the submandibular glands may be affected. The diagnosis can be confirmed with histopathological evidence of lack of caseation and acid-fast bacilli to distinguish the disease from tuberculosis. Laboratory evaluation may reveal hypercalcemia, elevation of serum alkaline phosphatase levels, and serum angiotensin-converting enzyme concentration. The Kveim test involves intradermal injection of human sarcoid tissue antigen, but results are positive in only 75% of cases. Therapy consists of early administration of corticosteroids, particularly if uveitis (which can lead to glaucoma) and facial paralysis are present.

REFERENCES

1. Aly RL, Levit S: Adherence of *Staphylococcus aureus* to squamous epithelium: role of fibronectin and teichoic acid, *Rev Infect Dis* S3(suppl):41, 1987.
2. Blair GS, Wood GD: Obstructive sialadenitis, *Int J Oral Surg* 9:63, 1980.
3. Brill SJ, Gilfillian RF: Acute parotitis associated with influenza type A: a report of 12 cases, *N Engl J Med* 296:1391, 1977.
4. Brodie BC: Inflammation of the parotid gland and salivary fistulae, *Lancet* 1:450, 1834.
5. Brook I, Finegold SM: Acute bacterial parotitis caused by anaerobic bacteria: report of two cases, *Pediatrics* 62:1019, 1978.
6. Brook I, Frazier EH, Thompson DH: Aerobic and anaerobic microbiology of acute suppurative parotitis, *Laryngoscope* 101:170, 1991.
7. Buckley JM, Poche P, McIntosh K: Parotitis and parainfluenza 3 virus, *Am J Dis Child* 124:789, 1972.
8. Cope VZ: Acute necrotic parotitis, *Br J Surg* 7:130, 1919.
9. DeVries EF, Kiapodi SB, Johnson JT: Salivary gland lymphoproliferative disease in acquired immune deficiency disease, *Arch Otolaryngol Head Neck Surg* 99:59, 1988.
10. English CK, Wear DJ, Margileth AM, et al: Cat-scratch disease, *JAMA* 259:1347, 1988.
11. Epivatianos A, Harrison JD, Dimitrov T: Ultrastructural and histochemical observations on microcalculi in chronic submandibular sialadenitis, *J Oral Pathol* 16:514, 1987.
12. Fox PC: Salivary gland involvement in HIV-1 infection, *Oral Surg* 73:168, 1992.
13. Galili D, Marmary Y: Spontaneous regeneration of the parotid salivary gland following juvenile recurrent parotitis, *Oral Surg* 60:605, 1985.
14. Goldberg MH, Harrigan WF: Acute suppurative parotitis, *Oral Surg* 20:281, 1965.
15. Gomez-Rodrigo J, Mendelsen J, Black M, et al: *Streptococcus pneumoniae* acute suppurative parotitis in a patient with Sjögren's syndrome, *J Otolaryngol* 19:195, 1990.
16. Guralnick WC, Donoff RB, Galdabini J: Parotid swelling in a dehydrated patient, *J Oral Surg* 26:669, 1968.
17. Hemenway WG, Smith RO, Harrison DG: Subtotal and total parotidectomy for chronic bacterial parotitis, *Rocky Mt Med J* 50:21, 1970.
18. Holley H: Successful treatment of cat-scratch disease with ciprofloxacin, *JAMA* 265:1563, 1991.
19. Hotel Dieu: parotitis terminating in gangrene, *Lancet* 2:540, 1829.
20. Itescu S, Brancato LJ, Winchester R: A sicca syndrome in HIV infection: association with HLA-DR5 and CD8 lymphocytosis, *Lancet* 2:466, 1989.
21. Johnson WG, Pierce AK, Sanford JP: Changing pharyngeal bacterial flora of hospitalized patients: emergence of gram-negative bacilli, *N Engl J Med* 281:1137, 1969.
22. Kaban LB, Mulliken JB, Murray JE: Sialadenitis in childhood, *Am J Surg* 135:570, 1978.
23. Katz J, Fisher D, Levine S: Bacterial colonization of the parotid duct in xerostomia, *Int J Oral Maxillofac Surg* 19:7, 1990.
24. Katzen M, DuPlessis DJ: Recurrent parotitis in children, *S Afr Med J* 38:122, 1964.
25. Kawamata A, Ariji Y, Langlais RP: Three-dimensional computed tomography imaging in dentistry, *Dent Clin North Am* 44:395, 2000.
26. Konno M, Ito E: A study on the pathogenesis of recurrent parotitis in childhood, *Ann Otol Rhinol Laryngol* 88(suppl):1, 1979.
27. Krippachne WW, Hunt TK, Dunphy J: Acute suppurative parotitis: a study of 161 cases, *Ann Surg* 156:251, 1962.
28. Leake DL, Krakowiak FJ, Leake RJ: Suppurative parotitis in children, *Oral Surg* 31:174, 1971.
29. Levy JA, Greenspan D: HIV in saliva, *Lancet* 2:1248, 1988.

30. Levy SB: *The antibiotic paradox: how miracle drugs are destroying the miracle,* New York, 1992, Plenum Press.
31. Mandel L: Wind parotitis, *N Engl J Med* 289:1094, 1973.
32. Mandel L, Kim D, Vy C: Parotid gland swelling in HIV diffuse infiltration CD8 lymphocytosis syndrome, *Oral Surg* 85:565, 1998.
33. Marchal F, Becker M, Dulguerov P, et al: Interventional sialendoscopy, *Laryngoscope* 110(2 Pt 1):318, 2000.
34. Masters RG, Carmier R, Saginot R: Nosocomial gram-negative parotitis, *Can J Surg* 29:41, 1986.
35. Matsuo T: Acute suppurative parotitis caused by a fish bone: a case report, *Int J Oral Maxillofac Surg* 26:54, 1997.
36. McAnnally T: Parotitis: clinical presentations and management, *Postgrad Med* 71:87, 1982.
37. Nahlieli O, Baruchin AM: Endoscopic technique for the diagnosis and treatment of obstructive salivary gland disease, *J Oral Maxillofac Surg* 57:1394, 1999.
38. Patey DH: Inflammation of the salivary glands with particular reference to chronic and recurrent parotitis, *Ann R Coll Surg Engl* 36:26, 1965.
39. Petersdorf RG, Forsyth BR, Bernanke D: Staphylococcal parotitis, *N Engl J Med* 259:1250, 1958.
40. Pruett TL, Simmons RL: Nosocomial gram-negative bacillary parotitis, *JAMA* 251:252, 1984.
41. Quinn JH, Graham R: Recurrent suppurative parotitis treated by intraductal antibiotics, *J Oral Surg* 31:36, 1973.
42. Raad II, Sabbagh NF, Caranasos GJ: Acute bacterial sialadenitis: a study of 29 cases and review, *Rev Infect Dis* 12:591, 1990.
43. Rubin MM, Ford HC, Sadoff RS: Bilateral parotid enlargement in a patient with AIDS, *J Oral Maxillofac Surg* 49:529, 1991.
44. Robinson JR: Surgical parotitis, a vanishing disease, *Surgery* 38:703, 1955.
45. Scully C, Davies R, Porter S, et al: HIV-salivary gland disease: salivary scintiscanning with technetium pertechnetate, *Oral Surg Oral Medicine Oral Pathol* 76:120, 1993.
46. Scully C, Samaranayake LP: *Clinical virology in dentistry and oral medicine,* Cambridge, 1992, Cambridge University Press.
47. Simpson WA, Courtney HS, Beachley EH: Fibronectin: a modulator of the oropharyngeal bacterial flora. In Schlesinger D, editor: *Microbiology,* Washington, DC, 1982, American Society for Microbiology.
48. Simpson WA, Harty DL, Beachley EH: Inhibition of the adhesion of *Escherichia coli* to epithelial cells by fibronectin. In Mergenhagen SF, Rosan B, editors: *Molecular basis of oral microbiologic adhesions,* Washington, DC, 1085, American Society for Microbiology.
49. Spratt JS: The etiology and therapy of acute pyonic parotitis, *Surg Gynecol Obstet* 112:391, 1961.
50. Yoshihara T, Kanda T, Yaku Y, et al: Chronic sialadenitis of the submandibular gland (so-called Kuttner tumor), *Auris-Nasus Larynx* 10:117, 1983.
51. Yousem DM, Kraut MA, Chalian AA: Major salivary gland imaging, *Radiology* 216:19, 2000.
52. Zachariades N: Bilateral recurrent submandibular obstructive sialadenitis, *J Oral Med* 40:86, 1985.

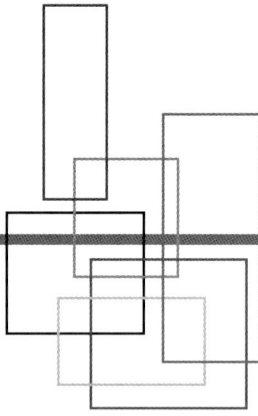

Infections of Soft Tissues of the Maxillofacial and Neck Regions

James R. Hupp

Epidermal tissues of the maxillofacial region present a formidable barrier to potentially infecting organisms. Moreover, if the barrier is breached and these underlying soft tissues become infected, the infection usually is contained quickly and spontaneously resolves. However, in certain circumstances an infection of the maxillofacial soft tissues becomes established. Such infections can cause significant morbidity and, if left unchecked, occasional mortality. The facial soft tissues are remarkably resistant to infection, but several disease entities can result from failures of soft tissues of the head and neck to limit the growth of infectious organisms.

ANATOMY OF FACIAL SKIN, FASCIA, AND MUSCLE

Skin represents the largest organ of the body and consists of two distinct layers that contain various appendages. The skin's components and architecture are important in the establishment and spread of infections. The outer, ectodermal layer, the epidermis, rests on a basement membrane and contains germinal cells, varying in degree of maturity and keratin formation, and dead desquamating cells that form an armor over the entire epidermal layer. The inner, mesodermal layer of skin, the dermis, lies just below the basement membrane of the epidermis. The dermis is divided into papillary and reticular regions, both consisting primarily of collagen fibers; the papillary dermis has a looser arrangement of fibers. The dermis contains most of the skin appendages, although many appendages extend into the superficial fascia on which the dermis lies (Figure 13-1).

The epidermis is devoid of blood vessels, nerves, and lymphatics; therefore it is relatively removed from cellular and humoral host defenses, particularly in the more superficial region. The arterial supply to the skin arises from a flat plexus of vessels located in the superficial fascia near its junction with the dermis. Smooth muscle cells in the precapillary arterioles control blood perfusion of the skin, thereby helping to regulate skin temperature. Venules and lymphatics accompany the arteries. Lymphatics in the dermis contain no valves, whereas those in the superficial fascia contain a few valves.[4,23]

Skin of the maxillofacial region contains hair follicles, and sweat and sebaceous glands. These appendages lie primarily in the dermal layer of skin, although epidermal cells line hair follicles and appendiceal structures do descend into the superficial fascia. Fascia includes all fibrous connective tissue in the body that is not specifically organized, such as tendons and ligaments. Although many regions of the body contain three main types of fascia—superficial, deep, and subserous fascia—the maxillofacial region has no deep fascia. Striated muscle consists of elongated cells covered by an acellular sarcolemma. Bundles of cells are surrounded by the epimysium, which contains vessels and nerves. Facial muscles lay deep to any superficial fascia and superficial to the underlying periosteum.

SKIN PHYSIOLOGY

The epidermis contains a continually regenerating layer of closely packed, keratin-producing squamous cells called the *stratum corneum*. This layer represents the principal barrier to bacteria. The constant desquamation carries away bacteria that accumulate in these cells; thus bacteria normally are limited to the most superficial two to three cell layers.

Skin appendages also provide agents that assist in antimicrobial activities of the skin. The secretory portion of the eccrine sweat glands lies at the dermal-fascial junction with a duct that leads straight to the surface. These glands secrete a hypotonic saline solution containing substances that slightly acidify the skin (pH approximately 5.5) and are of little nutritional value for bacteria. Facial sweat glands are rarely the source of skin infections because of their straight ducts and watery secretions.

Hair follicles are found over most of the maxillofacial region. The follicles are lined with epidermal cells and provide niches in which bacterial colonization can occur.

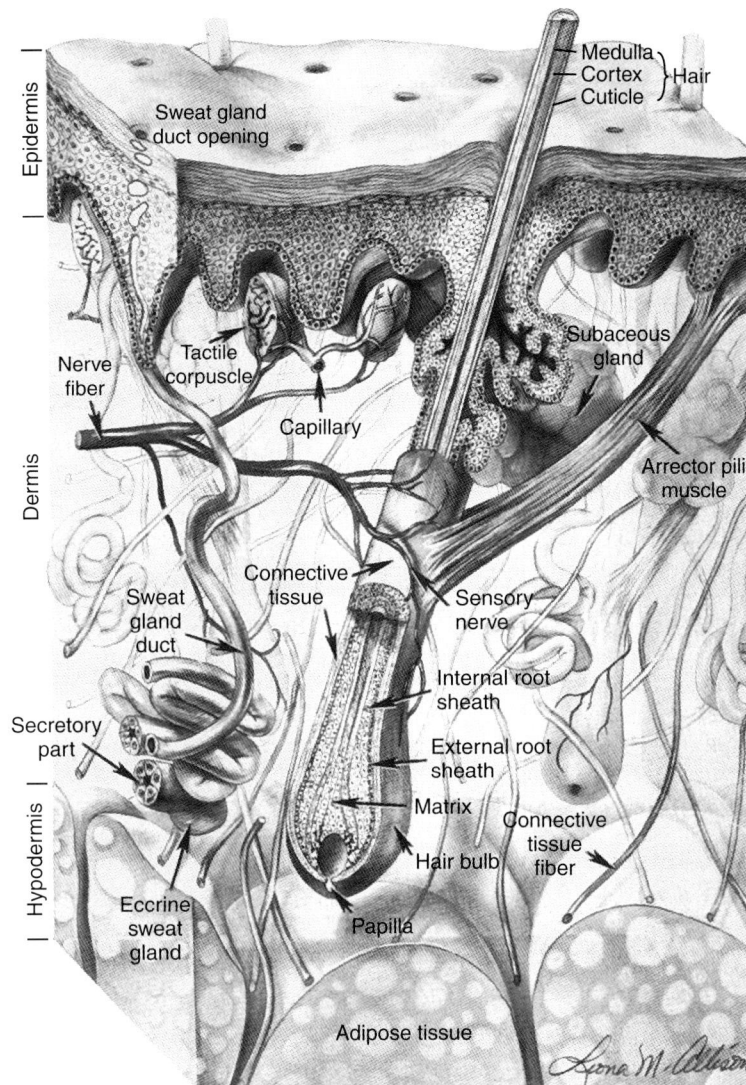

Figure 13-1 Schematic representation of a cross section of facial skin. (From Lesson CR, Leeson TS, Paparo AA: *Textbook of histology,* ed 5, Philadelphia, 1985, WB Saunders.)

Sebaceous glands empty into hair follicles and produce a substance called sebum. Sebum is a mixture of lipids that inhibit streptococci and staphylococci but stimulate diphtheroid growth. Bacteria usually can be found adherent to collections of sebum. In contradistinction to sweat glands, hair follicles are a common site of infection.[4]

SKIN MICROBIOLOGY

The skin of the head and neck carries both resident and transient microbial flora. The large range of numbers of various bacteria found at individual sites is determined by factors such as local anatomy, skin hygiene, environmental exposure, and hormonal variations that alter skin chemistry. Therefore areas such as cheek skin have low bacterial counts because the cheek is a cool and dry location, whereas a warmer and more humid area, such as the anterior nares, normally has a relatively high number of bacteria present.[33]

Transient bacteria are collected from the environment and loosely attached to the skin by sebum or moisture. They tend to be easily lost with hygiene measures and desquamation. Resident flora represent a more stable population, consisting mostly of diphtheroids and staphylococci. These organisms are protected by their location in skin crevices and follicles.[44]

Diphtheroids (genus *Corynebacterium*) are gram-positive pleomorphic rods with a beaded configuration on Gram staining. They may be aerobic or facultative anaerobes. Diphtheroids flourish around sebaceous glands, where they grow on sebum and break it down to form free fatty acids that then inhibit the growth of other bacteria. Diphtheroids rarely cause infections in the maxillofacial region, although they frequently are reported as contaminants during culturing.[4,21]

Staphylococcus epidermidis is the only other common resident skin flora in the head and neck region, but it rarely causes bacterial infections of the face. *Staphylococcus aureus* is a frequent transient bacterium in the maxillofacial region and is the most common single infecting organism in skin. Approximately 10% to 40% of adults are chronic carriers of *S. aureus* in their nasal passages, whereas 100% of recently discharged hospital patients carry this organism.

PATHOGENESIS OF SOFT TISSUE INFECTIONS

Intact skin resists invasion by microbes. Even the application of high concentrations of pathogenic bacteria does not ordinarily cause an infection. Skin infections usually are caused by opportunistic organisms of low pathogenicity that are able to infect tissue because of impaired local host defenses. Several factors, when present, increase the potential for skin infections (Box 13-1).

The number of organisms necessary to create a soft tissue infection varies according to the pathogenicity of the bacteria and the suitability of the local environment for growth. Studies have found that 2×10^9 organisms/mL are necessary to experimentally produce an infection of healthy soft tissue with *S. aureus*. Scrubbing skin and "painting" it with antiseptic solutions decreases resident bacterial counts before incision, thus lowering the inoculum size.[6,49]

Occlusion of the skin surface with materials such as adhesive dressings keeps the surface warm and moist; both factors promote bacterial growth. By limiting the amount of casual mild abrasion to which uncovered skin is naturally subjected, occlusive dressings slow the rate of desquamation, thereby preventing the beneficial shedding of bacteria-coated cells. Dermatological conditions such as atopic eczema also can predispose an area of skin to staphylococcal infections.[6,53]

The presence of nutrients required to promote bacterial growth can lead to creation of larger inoculum sizes. The most common situation occurs when blood is present on the surface and acts as a culture medium for bacteria, especially if it is not allowed to desiccate.

The presence of foreign material (e.g., dirt and grease from the environment or manmade materials such as sutures) dramatically lowers the inoculum size necessary to cause an infection of soft tissue by providing sites se-

questered from natural host immune processes in which bacteria can multiply. The local host immunity primarily depends on the vascularity of a tissue. For this reason, soft tissue infections occur more commonly in the lower extremity than in the face. However, alternative explanations include the pathogenicity of local flora, the likelihood of an area of skin to be injured, and the concentration of the local bacteria. All these factors likely play a role. The most important factor in the pathogenesis of infections of skin and the underlying soft tissues is epidermal integrity. Once a break occurs in the cornified layer of skin, resident and transient bacteria can invade the host. Violations of the epidermis occur by trauma, such as incisions and puncture wounds; removal of hair from follicles; or repeated application and removal of adhesive tape.

MANIFESTATIONS OF SOFT TISSUE INFECTIONS

Several terms are used to describe the lesions of soft tissue disease (Box 13-2). A *macule* is a flat, circumscribed area of abnormal skin color. In infectious processes, macules usually are red as a result of vasodilation or blue-black as a result of tissue infarction. A *papule* is a raised, solid mass less than 1 cm in diameter. Papules are the result of epidermal or dermal hyperplasia or local infiltration. Several infectious exanthems present as maculopapular eruptions (e.g., scarlet fever). Vesicles (<0.5 cm) and bullae (>0.5 cm) are elevated, fluid-filled lesions usually containing serum. Vesicles and bullae can be intraepidermal or subepidermal. A *pustule* is a vesicle containing purulent material. A *crust* is produced by the rupture of a vesicle or pustule, the contents of which then dry. *Ulcerations* are areas in which a break in the continuity of the epithelium exists as a result

---

BOX 13-1

Factors that Increase the Potential for Skin Infections

High concentration of organisms
Occlusion of skin surface, preventing desiccation and desquamation, which help limit colonization
Presence of sufficient and appropriate nutrients
Presence of sufficient foreign or necrotic material
Impaired local host immunity (e.g., decreased vascularity)
Damage of the cornified layer of the epidermis allowing bacterial penetration

---

BOX 13-2

Terms Used for Various Soft Tissue Lesions

Macule	Flat, circumscribed area of abnormal skin color
Papule	Raised, solid mass <1 cm in diameter
Vesicle	Elevated, fluid-filled lesion <0.5 cm in diameter
Bulla	Elevated, fluid-filled lesion >0.5 cm in diameter
Pustule	Vesicle filled with pus
Crust	Desiccated contents of ruptured vesicle or bulla
Ulceration	Any break in epithelial continuity
Scale	Surface accumulation of desquamating epidermis
Nodule	Solid lesion located within the subcutaneous tissue
Cellulitis	Area of red, tender swelling involving the dermis and subcutaneous tissue
Abscess	Accumulation of purulent material

of tissue destruction. A *wheal* is a special form of papule produced by a circumscribed area of edema of the epidermis and dermis. Wheals sometimes are seen at the edges of erysipelas or cellulitis. *Scales* represent accumulations of desquamated keratinaceous epidermis that can be abraded off the skin surface in thin sheets.

Subcutaneous manifestations of infection are less specific than cutaneous signs. *Cellulitis* is an area of red, tender swelling of the dermis and subcutaneous tissues. A *nodule* is a solid lesion that can be palpated and located within the subcutaneous tissue. Nodules usually occur in granulomatous infections. An *abscess* is a localized accumulation of purulent material and, when located in skin, is found in the dermis or subcutaneous tissue. *Gangrene* is necrosis of tissue, including subcutaneous tissue, fascia, and muscle. Blue-black discoloration of the skin may occur if the cutaneous blood supply becomes compromised. *Crepitus* of soft tissues may also occur as a result of the accumulation of gas.[4] Lymph node involvement by infectious processes can lead to node enlargement and tenderness *(lymphadenitis)* in the region draining the primary site of infection.

The soft tissues of the maxillofacial and neck regions can respond to inflammation, triggering insults in a limited number of ways. Therefore recognition that a soft tissue lesion is the result of infection may be difficult. In addition, identification of the infecting agent based on clinical examination alone is impossible in most instances. Cutaneous signs of infection are the most easily recognized, yet they typically are too nonspecific to allow a definitive diagnosis.

PYOGENIC BACTERIAL INFECTIONS

STREPTOCOCCAL INFECTIONS

Scarlet Fever   Scarlet fever can represent a manifestation of either a primary acute systemic infection by strains of *Streptococcus pyogenes* or a secondary reaction to a localized streptococcal infection such as streptococcal pharyngitis or impetigo. Groups C and G streptococci occasionally are isolated from patients with scarlet fever. The rash of scarlet fever is produced by a pyrogenic exotoxin elaborated by bacteriophage-altered streptococci. The rash, which appears about 2 to 4 days after the onset of symptoms of streptococcal infection, causes a generalized erythema and affects the facial region as a generalized flush with a prominent circumoral pallor. The erythema blanches with pressure, and numerous punctate elevations appear on the involved skin, leading to the so-called sandpaper texture. The exanthem of scarlet fever is accompanied by edema, spotty erythema, and petechiae of the soft palate. The tongue may have a white coating that resolves leaving red, swollen papillae (strawberry tongue), which progresses to an uncoated beefy-red appearance (raspberry tongue). The rash lasts 4 to 5 days and then desquamation of the affected skin occurs.[44,61]

The diagnosis of scarlet fever usually is based on the characteristic rash following a sore throat or systemic flulike illness. Confirmatory evidence consists of positive finds of throat culture for streptococci or increasing serum titers of antistreptolysin O antibodies. The differential diagnosis of scarlet fever includes childhood exanthems, infectious mononucleosis, and drug allergy. The management of the rash of scarlet fever consists of control of the streptococcal infection with appropriate antibiotics; penicillin is the drug of choice and a synergistic effect can be achieved by the addition of an aminoglycoside.[26,61]

Streptococcal Impetigo   Streptococcal impetigo (pyoderma) is a rapidly spreading infection of the superficial layers of epidermis. The causative organism usually is β-hemolytic streptococci, although cultures of the lesions also may reveal coagulase-positive staphylococci. The typical lesion begins as thin-walled vesicles or pustules with little erythema. The lesions rapidly progress circumferentially but tend to remain superficial. The fluid-filled lesions soon rupture, leaving oozing wounds and thick, pruritic crusts (Figure 13-2, Plate 31). Erythema appears later, and scarlet fever eventually may appear. Significant regional lymphadenopathy is characteristic, whereas systemic manifestations such as fever and malaise usually are minimal.[44]

Streptococcal impetigo is found primarily in regions with warm, humid climates. The more likely prerequisite for initiating infection is minor trauma, such as repeated scratching of the skin, or poor facial hygiene. Streptococcal impetigo generally occurs in exposed areas of skin, particularly the extremities, and occurs less often on the face. It is most common in children but can affect any age group. Impetigo can spread among individuals, particularly when in close association with each other such as in day care facilities.[33]

Diagnosis of streptococcal impetigo is based on the appearance of the lesions, isolation of *S. pyogenes* from the wound, and elevated serum titers of antideoxyribonuclease B or antihyaluronidase. Antistreptolysin O and anti-NADase titers are of limited value in impetigo because of the usually limited magnitude of their elevation and the time that passes before results become available.[44]

Untreated streptococcal impetigo usually is an indolent, self-limiting disease that causes little patient disability. However, as with other streptococcal infections, acute poststreptococcal glomerulonephritis can occur. Serial urinalyses and monitoring for a decrease in serum C3 levels can help detect this complication.[22]

The treatment of streptococcal impetigo consists of the systemic administration of antibiotics (e.g., penicillin) effective against streptococci. Cultures should be obtained to ensure against the need for β-lactamase–resistant antimicrobial agents. However, prompt treatment of streptococcal infections does not always prevent acute nephritis.[22]

Ecthyma is a form of impetigo in which the bacterial invasion progresses deeper into the skin. The lesions begin as vesicles but eventually form punched-out ulcers with a surrounding violaceous border. The legs of children are affected most frequently, although ecthyma occurs rarely in the maxillofacial region. Streptococci usually are isolated

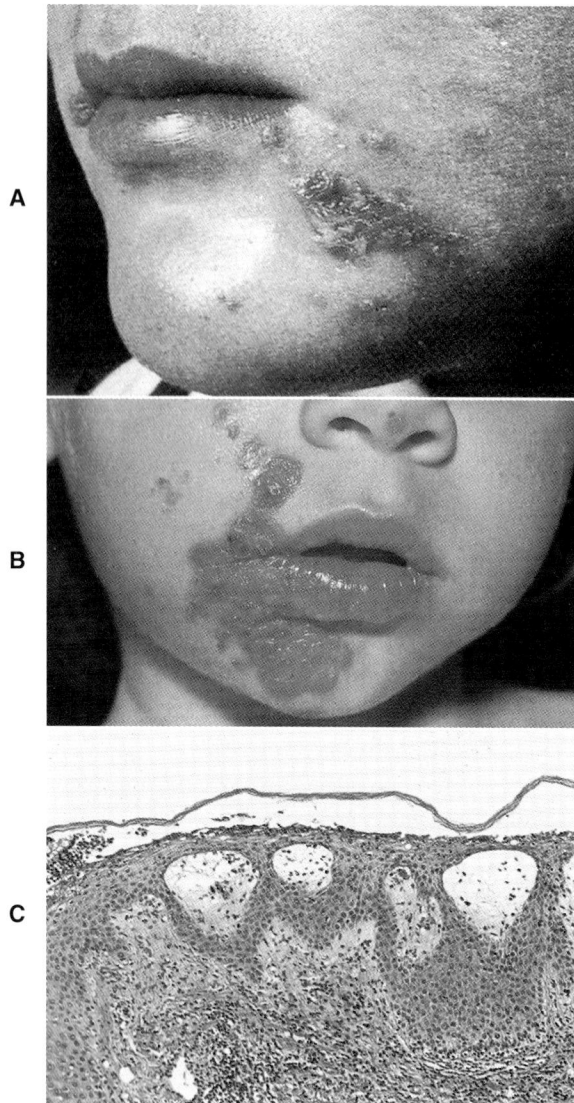

Figure 13-2 A, Streptococcal impetigo: typical presentation of perioral oozing and thickly crusted lesions with erythematous borders. Short-lived vesicles preceded the lesions shown here, but ruptured. (From Lookingbill DP: Principles of clinical diagnosis. In Moschella SL, Hurley HJ, editors: *Dermatology,* ed 3, Philadelphia, 1992, WB Saunders.) **B,** Histopathology of bullous impetigo with subcorneal blister with few neutrophils and acantholytic keratinocytes. (From Rassner G, editor: *Atlas of dermatology,* ed 3, Philadelphia, 1994, Lea & Febiger.) **C,** Histopathology of bullous impetigo with subcorneal blister with few neutrophils and acantholytic keratinocytes. (From Barnhill R, editor: *Textbook of dermatopathology,* New York, 1998, McGraw-Hill.)

from the lesions, although they can be produced by staphylococci. Treatment is the same as for impetigo.[33,57]

Erysipelas   Erysipelas is a superficial cellulitis usually caused by β-hemolytic streptococci that invade the dermis. The affected skin is intensely erythematous, warm, and painful. A well-defined leading edge often is visible (Figure 13-3). As with other streptococcal skin infections, the lesions spread rapidly as a result of hyaluronidase produc-

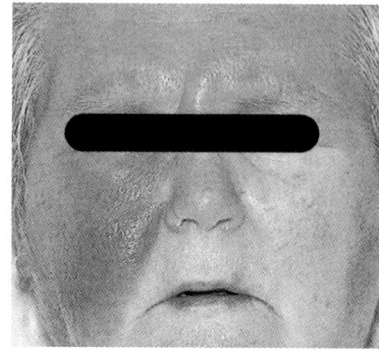

Figure 13-3 Erysipelas with involvement of malar region by intensely erythematous rash that is warm to touch. The leading edge is well defined. (From Cox N, editor: *Diagnostic problems in dermatology,* St Louis, 1998, Mosby.)

tion by the bacteria. Fever, malaise, and regional lymphadenopathy accompany the skin lesion. As the lesions resolve, desquamation of the skin overlying the involved area often occurs.

As with impetigo, the most important etiological factor in erysipelas is skin trauma allowing the introduction of organisms into the dermis. The disease can occur in any region of the body, and although reports of facial erysipelas predominate in the medical literature, surveys show that its most common site of occurrence is the lower leg.[54] The diagnosis of erysipelas is similar to that of impetigo, namely, a characteristic lesion and elevations in appropriate serum antibodies to streptococcal-specific antigens. A sample of the infecting organism for culturing is more difficult to obtain because of the lack of open wounds, but antiseptic preparation of the affected skin along the leading edge followed by the injection and then aspiration of a small amount of sterile normal saline solution may permit culturing of causative organisms.[33,48,54]

If left untreated, erysipelas can progress to a full-thickness cellulitis with deep suppuration and septicemia. Upper neck involvement by erysipelas leads to acute upper airway obstruction.[31] Therefore early diagnosis and aggressive treatment with antibiotics are important. Patients whose disease has been successfully treated may still have residual lymphedema caused by damage to lymphatic vessels. Erysipelas should not be confused with erysipeloid, an uncommon cellulitis caused by *Erysipelothrix rhusiopathiae,* that usually affects the hands.

Staphylococcal Infections Associated with Adnexal Structures   Staphylococcal organisms usually are less invasive than streptococci. However, superficial skin infections are caused more frequently by staphylococci than by streptococci. Facial infections probably are caused by the reservoir of *S. aureus* organisms in the nares of many individuals and an associated lack of β-hemolytic streptococci. An increasing number of staphylococci are becoming methicillin reistant, prompting the need for careful moni-

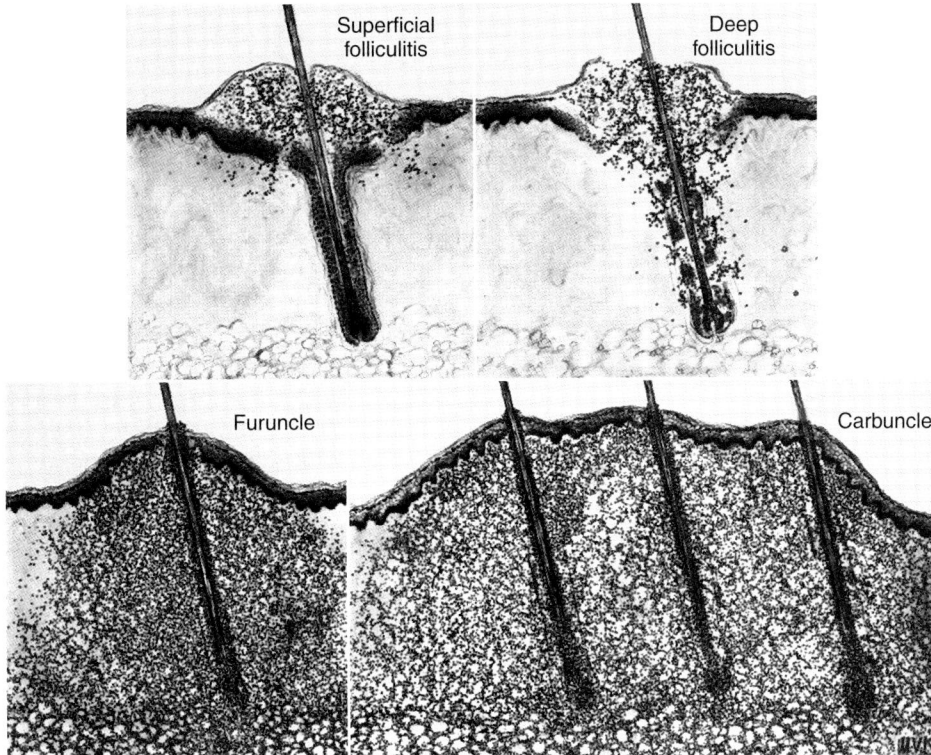

Figure 13-4 Perifollicular staphylococcal infections illustrating the distinction between various perifollicular inflammatory processes. Folliculitis is a well-localized infection generally confined to the hair follicle. A furuncle represents an infection of a single hair follicle in which the inflammation has destroyed the walls of the follicle. A carbuncle represents the coalescence of a group of furuncles. (From Maibach HI, Aly R, Noble W: Bacterial infections of the skin. In Moschella SL, Hurley HJ, editors: *Dermatology,* ed 2, Philadelphia, 1985, WB Saunders.)

toring of patients with staphylococcal infections after antibiotic therapy is initiated.[37]

Most staphylococcal infections of the face are associated with hair follicles. In these conditions the site where a hair exits the follicle or an associated sebaceous gland duct becomes obstructed by debris, allowing the overgrowth of staphylococcal organisms.[1,26,33]

Various terms are used to describe the degree of involvement of hair follicles in inflammatory processes. *Folliculitis* is a localized inflammation of follicles caused by pore obstruction. A *furuncle,* or *boil,* is an abscess of a follicle in which some destruction of the walls of the follicle has occurred. A *carbuncle* forms when a group of furuncles coalesce, and when it spontaneously ruptures, a large necrotic wound remains (Figures 13-4 and 13-5, Plate 32). Finally, a *sycosis* represents a lesion in which the entire depth of a follicle is affected without destruction of the walls of the follicle.[32,46]

Sycosis vulgaris (barbae) is a perifollicular, chronic pustular infection of the bearded region of the face that occurs when staphylococcal organisms infect the hair follicles. The infection begins as an area of erythema and pruritus on the upper lip. Pinhead-sized pustules soon appear, each pierced by a hair. These pustules rupture, leaving an area of erythema that later repustulates. The hair eventually loosens.

The process is spread by repeatedly shaving with the same razor blade or washing with a non-antiseptic soap (Plate 33). Sycosis vulgaris must be differentiated from tinea barbae and pseudofolliculitis barbae. Tinea barbae rarely affects the upper lip, in contrast to sycosis barbae. Pseudofolliculitis barbae is a process of the bearded region that is common in black men, in which short hairs curl back on themselves and grow into the side of the follicle (become ingrown) (Figure 13-6, Plate 33). The ingrown hairs produce pruritic papules and pustules that simulate sycosis vulgaris but require different therapy. Pseudofolliculitis barbae is treated by frequent shaving or allowing the beard hairs to grow long and application of topical corticosteroids until symptoms subside.[11,42]

Sycosis vulgaris is treated by administration of systemic staphylocidal antibiotics, application of hot compresses to the affected area, removal of infected hairs, shaving with a brushless shave cream, and changing razor blades daily. The clinician also may consider long-term application of staphylocidal ointment to the region of the anterior nares in patients who are suspected or proved chronic carriers of *S. aureus* in that location.

Bockhart's folliculitis (impetigo of Bockhart) is a condition similar to sycosis vulgaris but occurs most often in children. This infection is limited to the ostium of hair

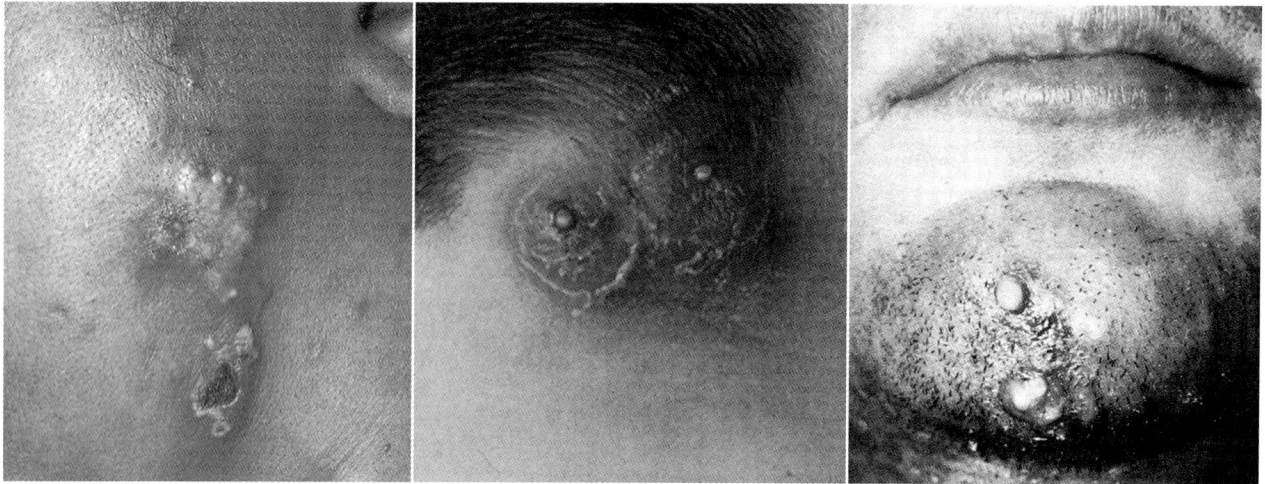

A   **B**   **C**

Figure 13-5 A, Deep pustulation of skin over the parotid gland caused by *Staphylococcus pyoderma*. (From Edwards L, editor: *Dermatology in emergency care*, Edinburgh, 1997, Churchill Livingstone.) **B,** Furuncle on the nape of the neck consisting of a deep pustular nodule. (From Hooper B, editor: *Primary dermatologic care*, St Louis, 1999, Mosby.) **C,** Staphylococcal carbuncle; a group of furuncles involving hair follicles of the chin has coalesced and spontaneously ruptured, leaving a raised, erythematous tender lesion draining purulence. (From Sauer GC: *Manual of skin diseases*, ed 7, Philadelphia, 1996, JB Lippincott.)

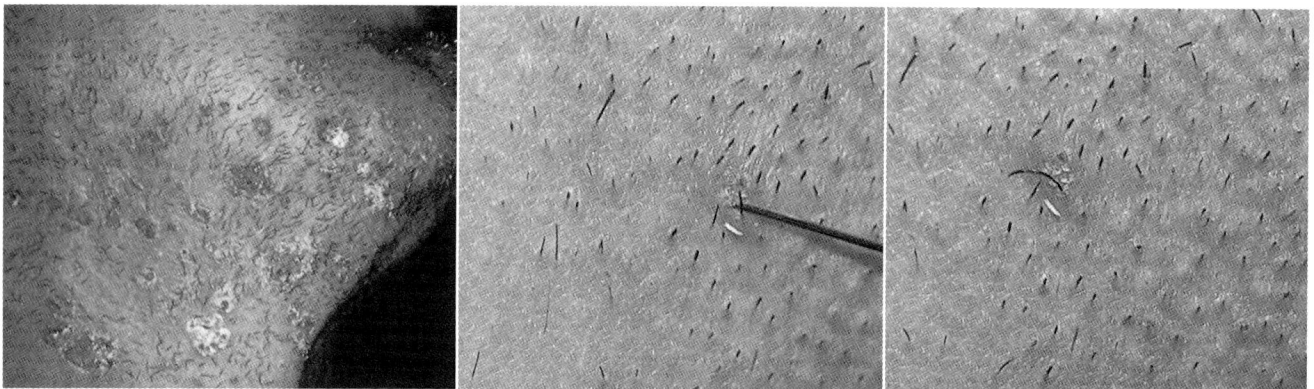

A   **B**   **C**

Figure 13-6 A, Folliculitis in bearded area of face. (From Hall J, editor: *Sauer's manual of skin diseases*, ed 3, Philadelphia, 2000, Lippincott.) **B,** Pseudofolliculitis caused by ingrowing hair. **C,** Hair removed from inflamed adjacent follicle. (*B and C*, From Cox N, editor: *Diagnostic problems in dermatology*, St Louis, 1998, Mosby.)

follicles; therefore it is superficial. It is seen most frequently in the scalp, on the margin of the scalp, the lips, and the extremities. The lesions are yellow pustules with a narrow zone of surrounding erythema (Figure 13-7). Culture of the lesions grows *S. aureus*. The lesions are be self-limited, and cleaning with antiseptic soaps may be the only treatment needed. Resistant infections may warrant the use of systemic antibiotics. Children should be warned not to traumatize the lesions to prevent their spreading.

A stye is a furuncle of an eyelash caused by *S. aureus*. The lesion generally is self-limiting. However, recurrence is possible, and 90% of patients with recurrent styes are found to

be chronic nasal carriers of *S. aureus* and should be treated to eliminate the carrier state.

Folliculitis cheloidalis is another disease commonly attributed to a staphylococcal infection of hair follicles. However, reliable identification of any specific organism associated with the lesions is difficult. Folliculitis cheloidalis is a chronic process involving the formation of pustules in hair follicles in the nape of the neck. The inflammatory reaction stimulates the formation of cheloidal papules (Figure 13-8). Folliculitis cheloidalis occurs most commonly in black males between the ages of 14 and 25 years. Treatment consists of the use of antiseptic soaps.

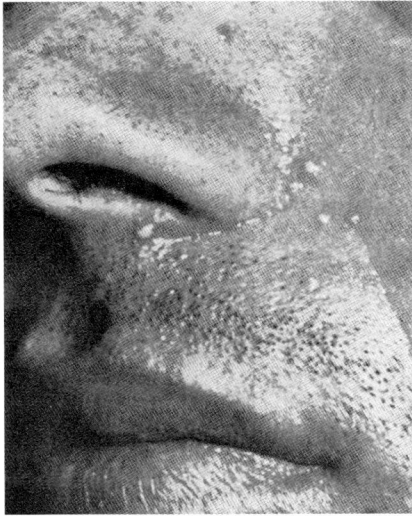

Figure 13-7 Bockhart's folliculitis (impetigo of Bockhart) consists of superficial persistent, yellow pustules with a narrow zone of erythema. Lesions similar to those shown on the upper lip and nasolabial fold also may be present on or near the scalp and on the extremities. (From Arnold HL Jr, Domonkos AN, Odom RB: *Andrew's diseases of the skin,* ed 7, Philadelphia, 1982, WB Saunders.)

Systemic antibiotics may be indicated when inflammation is severe.

Sebaceous cysts (epidermal inclusion cysts) represent intradermal collections of keratinous material caused by proliferation of epithelial cells lying in the dermis. Some patients, especially those with a tendency to acne vulgaris, develop multiple sebaceous cysts that can become infected with staphylococcal organisms. The lesions manifest as tender, discrete, deep nodules with overlying erythema that may form abscesses and eventually rupture. Treatment consists of control of the acne component with tetracyclines, facial cleansers, isotretinoin, and excision of the cysts.[11]

Acne vulgaris, although not known to be caused by an infectious agent, almost always is complicated by secondary infection. The initial event in the onset of an acne lesion is keratinization of the duct of the sebaceous gland. The duct becomes obstructed, causing androgen-stimulated sebaceous gland secretions to accumulate. An inflammatory reaction follows, and bacteria commonly colonize hair follicles, such as *Propionibacterium acnes,* multiplying in the sequestered secretions. This bacterium's propensity for acne lesions probably is related to its production of a lipase that can hydrolyze sebum triglycerides into free fatty acids. Pressure from the secretions can force open the pore, exposing the sebaceous secretions to oxidizing agents in the air and forming an open comedo (blackhead). When the pore is not forced open, the inflammatory process attracts neutrophils and a closed comedo (whitehead) forms. Rupture of the obstructed duct allows the accumulated bacteria and sebaceous secretions to extravasate into the dermis. The subsequent inflammatory reaction typically is intense and

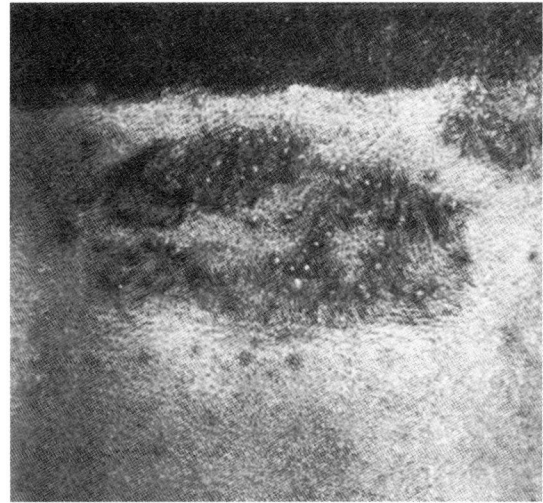

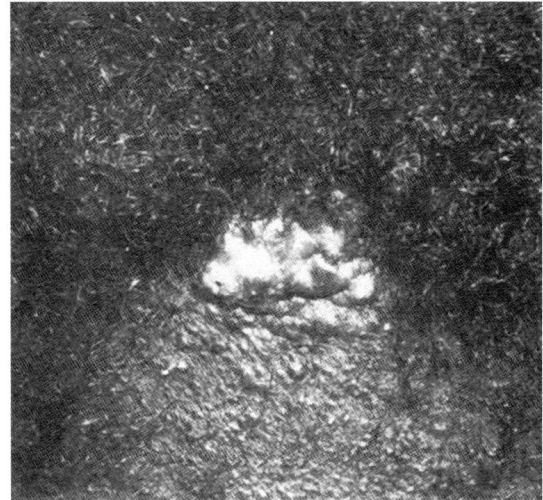

Figure 13-8 Folliculitis cheloidalis commonly occurs on the nape of the neck at the hairline, with either discrete papules **(A)** or coalescence of papules forming a plaque **(B).** (From Rook A, Wilkinson DS, Ebling FJG, editors: *Textbook of dermatology,* ed 3, Oxford, 1979, Blackwell.)

leads to the formation of scar-producing pustules, nodules, and cysts (Figure 13-9).[45]

The lesions of acne vulgaris normally are confined to the face, chest, back, and upper arms, with sparing of the periorbital region. Acne is most common in adolescence and tends to improve or resolve by adulthood. Acne is also a well-recognized feature of Apert's syndrome. The diagnosis of acne vulgaris is based on the presence of characteristic lesions in a typical distribution in the appropriate age group. Acne can also be part of the SAPHO (synovitis, acne, pustulosis palmoplantaris, hyperostosis, and osteitis) syndrome in which acne and osteomyelitis coexist.[50]

Treatments for acne vulgaris have improved greatly in the past two decades. Historically successful therapies such as systemic administration of antibiotics (e.g., tetracycline or minocycline), topical bacteriostatic agents (e.g., benzoyl peroxide), good skin hygiene, and intradermal corticosteroids still have their place.[35] However, the use of tretinoin

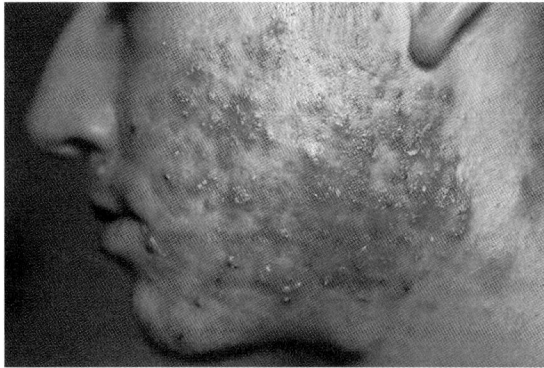

Figure 13-9 Acne vulgaris with comedones, pustules, and intense erythema. Depression represents scarring from previous lesions. (From Helm K, editor: *Atlas of differential diagnosis in dermatology,* Edinburgh, 1998, Churchill Livingstone.)

topically and isotretinoin systemically has revolutionized the treatment for acne resistant to traditional therapies. Tretinoin (Retin-A), a vitamin A derivative, can reduce microcomedo formation and eliminate existing lesions of acne. The drug normalizes follicular keratinization by increasing the turnover of follicular cells and decreases the cohesiveness of those cells shed into the lumen. Factors limiting its use are tretinoin-induced skin irritation and desquamation. Isotretinoin (Accutane), another vitamin A derivative, is used systemically to manage severe or conventional treatment-resistant acne. It decreases sebum secretion, depletes the follicular flora of *P. acnes,* inhibits neutrophil chemotaxis, and reverses the retention follicular hyperkeratosis. The use of isotretinoin is limited by the invariable side effects of mucocutaneous inflammation and desquamation, alopecia, development of pseudotumor cerebri, diffuse skeletal hyperostosis, and retinal malfunction. Isotretinoin-induced laboratory-detected abnormalities include elevation of serum triglyceride levels and liver enzyme concentrations. Because of these adverse effects including psychiatric disturbances, isotretinoin is indicated only in patients with severely problematic acne vulgaris.[4,48] Recent reports have warned of a worldwide trend of increasing resistance of *P. acnes* to antibiotics including tetracyclines, clindamycin, and erythromycin.[52] These findings may explain why many patients experience a lack of or no improvement in their acne during antibiotic therapy.[52]

INFECTIONS UNRELATED TO ADNEXAL STRUCTURES

Staphylococcal Impetigo   Two forms of impetigo caused by staphylococci exist. The epidemic form usually is clinically indistinguishable from streptococcal impetigo and bullous impetigo, which is always caused by *S. aureus.* Epidemic staphylococcal impetigo, like its streptococcal counterpart, appears as a vesicular eruption that progresses to encrustation. Many investigators believe that impetigo always is caused by streptococcal organisms and that staphy-

lococci are involved only secondarily as superinfecting agents. (See the discussion of streptococcal impetigo for the clinical features and management.)

Staphylococcal scalded skin syndrome (SSSS; Ritter's disease) is an unusual but potentially serious soft tissue infection caused by phage group II staphylococci that colonize the epidermis and release an exotoxin known as epidermolysin. The toxin causes the formation of large flaccid bullae. Classically, little erythema exists around the bullae, and both cellulitis and lymphangitis are uncommon. Bullous impetigo represents a localized form of the disease in which bullae are confined to a small area. Systemic SSSS affects most regions of a patient and is most common in neonates and infants. Characteristically, the affected tissue is tender to the touch, which differentiates this disease from other causes of toxic epidermal necrolysis. In the localized and systemic forms of SSSS, the bullae are first filled with clear fluid that becomes purulent. The thin-walled bullae rupture, ooze, and encrustate (Figure 13-10). The widespread desquamation may allow life-threatening dehydration and electrolyte imbalances to occur. A forme fruste of SSSS, termed *scarlatiniform SSSS,* exists in which cutaneous tenderness and desquamation occur without bullae formation.[41,44]

Bullous impetigo is treated with careful hygiene using antiseptic soaps and systemic use of β-lactamase–resistant antibiotics. Patients with SSSS require hospitalization for intravenous hydration, antibiotics, and nursing care. Administration of corticosteroids should be avoided.[43]

Cellulitis   Cellulitis represents a deep extension of infection into tissues underlying the dermis by inoculation of organisms through a wound, spread from adjacent infections, or hematogenous seeding. The involved tissue is erythematous, warm, edematous, and tender (Figure 13-11). The patient usually shows constitutional signs of illness such as fever, chills, and malaise. In the maxillofacial region, *S. pyogenes* is the most common etiological agent in adolescents and adults. However, in children, cellulitis caused by *Streptococcus pneumoniae* or *Haemophilus influenzae* occurs more often. Although the identification of the streptococcal cause of a cellulitic process is difficult on strictly clinical grounds, special efforts should be made to isolate an organism in children because the choice of the proper antibiotic is affected. *H. influenzae* cellulitis tends to occur most commonly in children younger than 2 years of age, but it can appear in older children.[44] Cellulitis in these cases may take on a bluish or purplish hue, suggesting the *H. influenzae* causation. Children with cellulitis that is suspected to be of nonstreptococcal origin require blood cultures and the empirical use of a drug effective against most *H. influenzae* strains. Ampicillin is effective against most *H. influenzae* strains, but recent increases in the number of ampicillin-resistant *H. influenzae* strains warrant the inclusion of chloramphenicol in any empirical regimen. If no suppuration is detectable, the clinician may attempt to inject sterile, bacteriostatic agent–free saline solution into an edge of the affected area and then aspirate the fluid for

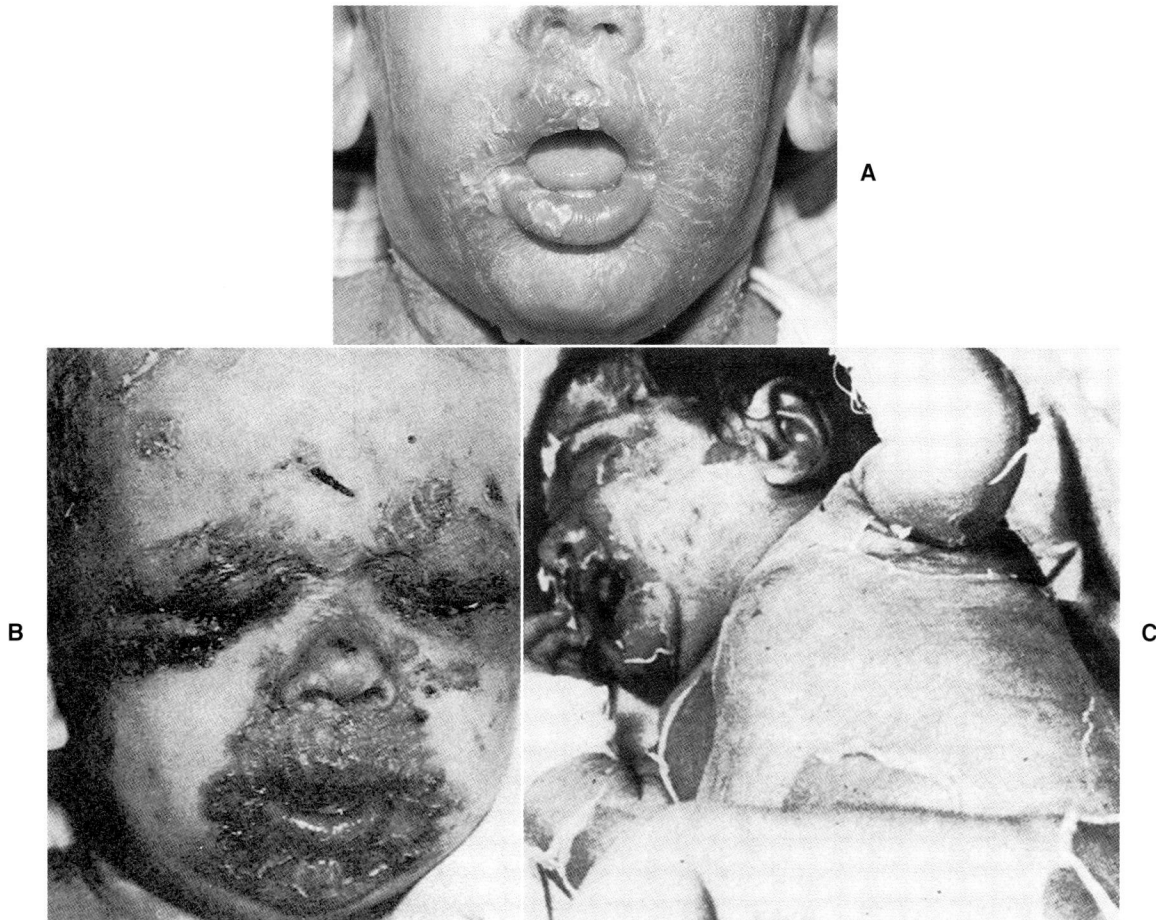

Figure 13-10 A, Perioral region of infant with staphylococcal scalded skin syndrome. The lesions are generally widespread, with the initial formation of thin-walled bullae that rupture, leaving large lesions that ooze serum and pus and encrust. (From Edwards L, editor: *Dermatology in emergency medicine,* Edinburgh, 1997, Churchill Livingstone, 1997.) **B,** A child with facial involvement. (From Weinberg S, Hoekelman RA, editors: Pediatric dermatology for the primary care practitioner, New York, 1978, McGraw-Hill.) **C,** An infant with more generalized lesions that could lead to life-threatening dehydration. (From Weston WL: *Practical pediatric dermatology,* New York, 1979, Little, Brown.)

bacterial identification. Incision and drainage often are necessary for resolution.[4,61]

Necrotizing Fasciitis   Necrotizing fasciitis is an aggressive infection that affects the superficial fascia with undermining of the overlying soft tissues. The process usually occurs in the fascia of the trunk and extremities but can be seen in the maxillofacial region. The disease usually occurs in patients who are chronically debilitated, those with diabetes mellitus, or in patients with small-vessel disease. Various terms, including hospital gangrene, gangrenous erysipelas, and hemolytic streptococcal gangrene, have been used to describe this disorder. Necrotizing fasciitis usually occurs after trauma or surgery when the fascia is inoculated with organisms.

The clinical manifestations usually begin rather quiescently; the affected area becomes swollen and erythematous, and the patient has a low-grade fever. The site deteriorates rapidly with sudden pain, worsening of the erythema

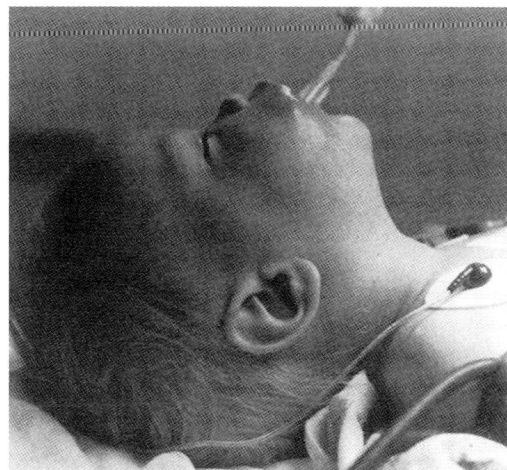

Figure 13-11 *Haemophilus influenzae* cellulitis in a child; the marked buccal swelling is warm, tense, tender to palpation, and erythematous. Bimanual palpation revealed fluctuance that required drainage in addition to antibiotic therapy.

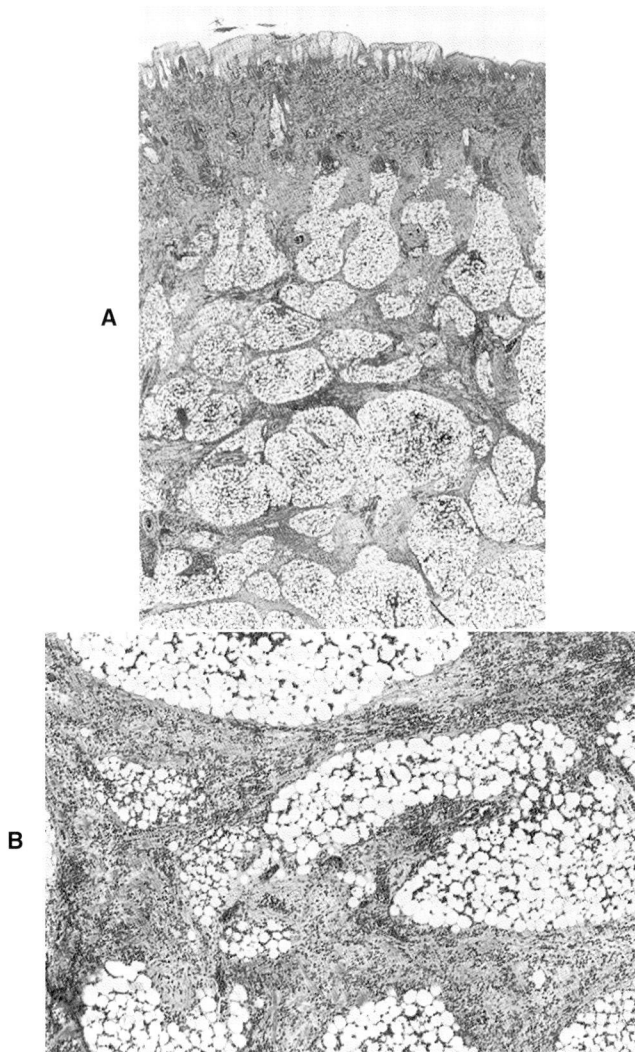

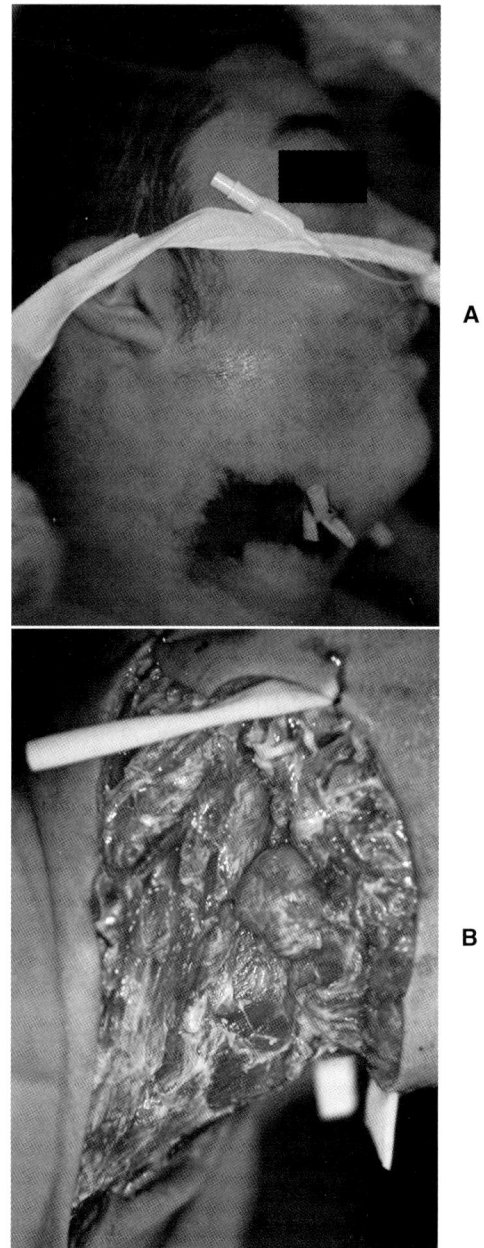

Figure 13-12 A, Histopathology of necrotizing fasciitis with epidermal necrosis and perivascular dermal infiltrate. **B,** Higher-power magnification shows diffuse hemorrhage and mixed inflammatory infiltrate in fibrosing adipose septa and fascia. (From Barnhill R, editor: *Textbook of dermatopathology,* New York, 1998, McGraw-Hill.)

Figure 13-13 A, Necrotizing fasciitis in an otherwise healthy teenage boy a few days after removal of impacted third molars shows dark, blue-black skin in the submandibular region. **B,** Same boy after debridement of involved tissue. (Courtesy Robert Ord and Steve Engroff.)

and edema, and generalized toxicity. As the disease progresses, the pain subsides as cutaneous nerves become necrotic, and anesthesia of the area may occur. The skin overlying the infected fascia becomes dusky with purple mottling. Gas may form under the skin, which may be palpable. If the edges of the affected tissue are probed at this stage, the instrument passes into the plane that the infection is creating between the fascia and the overlying skin. Bullae form as the skin begins to necrose as a result of thrombosis of nutrient vessels as they pass through areas of involved fascia. Frank gangrene of the skin eventually occurs with sloughing of the skin, exposing the underlying necrotizing fascia and subcutaneous fat (Figures 13-12 and 13-13).[29,36,47,51]

Systemic manifestations include signs of sepsis, hemolysis, and intravascular volume depletion. The patient has high fever, tachycardia, apathy, weakness, and nausea. Ane-

mia, jaundice, and hemoglobinuria occur as a result of bacterially induced hemolysis. The patient is hypotensive with decreased skin turgor as a result of fluid losses caused by diaphoresis and extracellular fluid accumulation in the infected site. The overall mortality rate of necrotizing fasciitis is approximately, 30%; however, if the diagnosis is made promptly and treatment is begun early in the disease course, death occurs much more rarely.[19]

Although necrotizing fasciitis historically was thought to be caused by hemolytic streptococci and *S. aureus,* modern culture techniques have revealed that anaerobes usually are present in the wound. In addition, gram-negative bacteria frequently are present; therefore early culturing of areas involved by the infection is important to help guide therapy.[29]

Therapy of necrotizing fasciitis involves management of both the local and systemic problems. Laboratory evaluations of hematocrit, serum electrolyte levels, including calcium, and myoglobin, should be made. Blood for culturing should be obtained before antibiotic therapy is started. A central venous line is helpful to allow determination of intravascular volume and rapid administration of crystalloids. The patient should be taken to the operating suite quickly to begin debridement. Surgery usually involves opening the infected planes widely, resecting frankly necrotic tissue, and packing the area under the undermined skin loosely with gauze. Daily debridements then are started to continue to remove any devitalized tissue.[47] Frozen-section biopsies can assist in guiding resection.[3]

High doses of intravenous antibiotics should be started empirically with agents chosen to cover hemolytic streptococci, staphylococcal organisms, gram-negative bacteria, and anaerobes. A combination of penicillin, clindamycin, and an aminoglycoside, or of penicillin, chloramphenicol, and an aminoglycoside should be effective until the results of culture and sensitivity testing allow a more specific antibiotic regimen.[36] Use of frozen-section biopsy of suspected necrotizing fasciitis is a valuable technique for more rapid diagnosis of this disorder.[56] Some investigators have reported that hyperbaric oxygen treatment has a favorable effect on the diseased tissue.[36] Once the infection has resolved, the overlying skin eventually begins to adhere to the underlying fascia, and any areas of skin loss as a result of gangrene can be grafted temporarily with porcine skin or grafted permanently with meshed autogeneic skin. Punch biopsies to quantitate tissue bacterial counts can be used before grafting; the graft should not proceed until fewer than 10^5 bacteria per gram of tissue exist. Topical sulfadiazine (Sulfadene) can be applied to exposed areas to help clear bacteria.[59]

OTHER NONTRAUMATIC SOFT TISSUE INFECTIONS

ANTHRAX

Anthrax is a serious and potentially fatal disease caused by the gram-positive, aerobic bacteria, *Bacillus anthracis.* This organism naturally exists in soil and on wild and domestic animals, but it is also a potential biological weapon. Anthrax is not a contagious disease; rather it is contracted by contact with *B. anthracis* spores. Contact occurs through open skin wounds, the mucosa of the gastrointestinal tract, or inhalation of spores.

Dermatological lesions of anthrax initially appear as small, pruritic papules that develop 1 to 10 days after contact with spores. Each papule becomes a vesicle surrounded by a ring of erythema and edema. If the vesicle ruptures, it exposes an ulcer that becomes covered with a black eschar (Plate 34). Regional lymphadenopathy also occurs. The disease is rarely life threatening if the lesions are recognized and proper therapy is instituted in a timely manner.[28]

The gastrointestinal form of anthrax can affect the upper or lower gastrointestinal tract, including the pharynx. This form of anthrax is much more serious because of the lower likelihood of early diagnosis, risking progression of the disease process to life-threatening proportions before antibiotic therapy is started. Symptoms of gastrointestinal involvement include sore throat if the pharynx is involved, and nausea, vomiting, anorexia, and fever if other parts of the gastrointestinal tract become infected. Severe abdominal pain and bloody diarrhea occur within 2 to 3 days, and shock and death soon follow.[28]

The most serious form of anthrax occurs when the bacillus spores are inhaled. The spores are dispersed throughout the lungs initiating a multitude of growth sites for the bacteria. The infected pulmonary tissue produces symptoms within 3 to 14 days, and the lung parenchyma is destroyed rapidly, usually leading to death in 1 to 2 days.[13] Unless the presence of spores is recognized very soon after their inhalation and appropriate antibiotic therapy is begun, the process is irreversible in 90% of patients.

Penicillin G is the historic treatment of choice for known or suspected contact with anthrax spores. However, anthrax prepared for use as a weapon can be developed in a form resistant to many antibiotics. The dose of 2 million units intravenously every 2 hours is used for adults known to have anthrax unless penicillin resistance is suspected or penicillin allergy exists. Naturally occurring strains of *B. anthracis* also are typically sensitive to ciprofloxacin, chloramphenicol, erythromycin, and gentamicin. If a patient is believed to have been exposed to anthrax spores, infectious disease specialists and public health officials should be alerted. For patients with known nondermatologic anthrax, supportive therapy with intravenous fluids and ventilatory assistance also are commonly indicated.

CERVICOFACIAL ACTINOMYCOSIS

Although infections caused by actinomycosis rarely are localized to or originate in bone, cervicofacial actinomycosis usually affects soft tissue. The most common causative species of actinomycosis in humans is *Actinomyces israelii,* a gram-positive, non–acid-fast, anaerobic, filamentous bacterium. This organism initiates a chronic granulomatous process with a tendency to form external sinuses. Although *Actinomyces* commonly is detected in the oral flora of healthy individuals, it can become pathological when introduced into deeper tissues by a break in the mucosal barrier.[33]

Clinical manifestations of cervicofacial actinomycosis usually are heralded by the appearance of a hard swelling closely associated with the jaw. As the swelling grows, the enlarging tissues become indurated, and as the process approaches the skin surface a purple discoloration of the overlying skin appears. Over time, abscesses form within the hard swelling and sinus tracts develop to the skin. The drainage from these tracts is seropurulent and quickly crystallizes. Microscopic examination of the exudate reveals characteristic sulfur granules containing large collections of the causative organism. On a hematoxylin-eosin stain, the sulfur granules appear as eosinophilic clubs extending from the center of the actinomycotic colony, helping to differentiate these collections of organisms from other microorganisms. Pain usually is minimal, but trismus develops with involvement of the muscles of mastication. The process generally spreads locally; hematogenous and lymphatic spread are unusual.

A combination of the patient's clinical history and signs, particularly the presence of hard swellings in the maxillofacial region, should suggest cervicofacial actinomycosis in the differential diagnosis in a patient with facial or neck swelling.[39] Anaerobic culture techniques should be used whenever actinomycosis is suspected. In addition, immunofluorescent staining using specific antisera on a smear of the exudate or from a biopsy specimen can be used to confirm the diagnosis more rapidly than awaiting culture results.[40]

Successful therapy for cervicofacial actinomycosis hinges on the combined use of an appropriate antibiotic and surgical management of suppuration. Penicillin, given in large doses over a moderately protracted period, remains the standard treatment. Most recommended regimens begin with a course of intravenous penicillin G, 10 to 20 million units/day for 2 to 6 weeks, followed by several months of oral penicillin V, 2 to 4 g/day. The penicillin G minimal inhibitory concentration (MIC) of all strains of *A. israelii* is 0.03 to 0.5 mg/mL. The attainment of this level of penicillin G given orally may require coadministration of probenecid. Several other antibiotics have easily attained MICs for *A. israelii,* including erythromycin (MIC 0.12 mg/mL) and minocycline and clindamycin (MIC 0.031 mg/mL).[39] Metronidazole, cephalexin, and the semisynthetic penicillins, oxacillin and dicloxacillin, have limited in vitro activity against *A. israelii.*

Surgical intervention often is necessary for the cure of cervicofacial actinomycosis. Purulent accumulations require early drainage, and surgical excision of sinus tracts hastens resolution. Failure of resolution of a soft tissue *A. israelii* infection after appropriate antibiotic therapy should trigger a search for a previously unrecognized collection of purulence.[40]

Nocardial microorganisms can cause infections in the soft tissues of the maxillofacial region. Most maxillofacial soft tissue infections are caused by infections of the underlying bone or hematogenous seeding from primary infections elsewhere in the body. Whereas actinomycosis produces the characteristic signs of induration and fistulization, nocardial infection usually produces cellulitis with subcutaneous abscess formation. The diagnosis is based on culture of purulence. Infection requires treatment by debridement as necessary and systemic sulfa drugs.

TRAUMATIC WOUND INFECTIONS

The maxillofacial region generally is resistant to infections caused by trauma, probably because of the higher degree of vascularity of the tissues in this area relative to other parts of the body. However, the presence of foreign material, impaired host resistance, vascular compromise, or high inoculum level may allow an infection to occur.

Deep puncture wounds are prone to infection because the site cannot drain spontaneously with ease once an infection occurs. The low oxygen environment also permits anaerobic organisms to multiply in an area in which aerobes cannot compete effectively.

Traumatic lacerations generally are less likely to become infected, especially if they are properly debrided and repaired. Cutaneous lacerations of the trunk and extremities usually must be repaired within the first 6 to 8 hours. Otherwise, healing by secondary intention is the best treatment. However, because of the greater resistance to infection, primary repair of lacerations in the head and neck can be accomplished even 24 to 30 hours after their creation without seriously increasing the chance of infection. Patients with infected puncture wounds of the face have erythema and tender induration of the area surrounding the puncture site. An abscess usually soon forms that affects one of the fascial spaces. Infected traumatic lacerations are manifested with erythema and painful induration of the wound. The wound usually dehisces, allowing accumulated purulence to drain.

Treatment of an infected puncture wound consists of the establishment of drainage; this may require excision of the puncture tract. If a repaired laceration becomes infected, sutures should be removed to allow escape of purulence. In either case, once drainage is established, the pus should be sent for aerobic and anaerobic cultures, and administration of systemic antibiotics should begin. The antibiotic for superficial maxillofacial wound infections not in communication with the oral cavity should be effective against β-lactamase–producing *S. aureus*. The clinician may add an antibiotic effective against *Streptococcus viridans* and anaerobes if the wounds are deep or contaminated by oral fluid.

The most effective treatment of infected wounds is prevention through proper debridement techniques, irrigation of wounds with large volumes of fluid under pressure, judicious use of reactive suture materials, and appropriate antibiotics. If large foreign bodies might be buried in the depth of the wound, radiographs of the soft tissues should be obtained to lessen the likelihood of leaving foreign material in the wound.

TETANUS

The bacterium *Clostridium tetani* is a gram-positive, strictly anaerobic rod that is commensal in human and animal gastrointestinal tracts and in soil. When it is inoculated into a wound and local conditions favor its multiplication, *C. tetani* can kill the host organism by causing tetanus within a relatively brief period. Tetanus is caused by the production of a potent neurotoxin, tetanospasmin. This toxin blocks spinal cord inhibitory neurons, producing muscle rigidity. Tetanospasmin is most effective against short motor neurons, such as those that exist in the head and neck, leading to the characteristic early manifestation of tetanus, namely, trismus caused by masseter and medial pterygoid muscle spasm. Other early signs of tetanus include fever, insomnia, irritability, dysphagia, and tremor. Other muscle groups characteristically are affected in more severe cases, including spasm of muscles of facial expression (risus sardonicus) and of spinal muscles (opisthotonos). Muscle spasms usually can be precipitated by stimuli such as noise, bright light, touch, and movement. If the site of inoculation is near the head, cranial nerve palsies occur early, whereas if the infection is in a limb, weakness or paralysis of that limb may be the first sign of *C. tetani* infection.[10] As the disease progresses, other nerves, including those of the autonomic nervous system, are affected with resultant wide variations in blood pressure, cardiac dysrhythmias, and electrolyte abnormalities. Other muscle groups affected include those of the larynx, pharynx, and thorax. In contrast to motor nerves, sensory nerves usually are spared in the beginning. Death is usually a result of respiratory insufficiency, venous thromboembolism, or sympathetic overactivity.[2,8]

The incubation period of *C. tetani* infection ranges from 3 days to 4 weeks. Generally, the longer the incubation period, the better the prognosis. Wounds usually are the site of inoculation; however, in 7% of patients, no obvious entry site can be found. Treatment of tetanus begins with management of any respiratory insufficiency with supplemental oxygen and intubation with mechanical respiratory assistance if necessary; tracheostomy may be necessary.[9] The patient requires cardiac monitoring, insertion of an arterial line for blood pressure monitoring and access for arterial blood gas sampling. Placement of a central venous line assists in intravascular volume assessment and fluid administration. The patient should be protected from unnecessary sensory stimulation; thus a dark, temperature-controlled, quiet environment must be created. Penicillin therapy should be started and human antitetanospasmin antibody administered. Long-acting muscle relaxants are given if the patient's ventilation is assisted. The suspected site of inoculation should be surgically explored and debrided as necessary. Several cases of tetanus that were considered the result of inoculation through the oral mucosa have been reported. This possibility should be considered in a patient with signs of tetanus without an obvious cutaneous wound.[55]

Prevention is the cornerstone of tetanus management (Table 13-1). Childhood immunization against tetanus is practiced widely in North America. Booster injections should be administered every 10 years throughout life. If a wound occurs, the clinician should obtain a reliable history of tetanus immunization. If no history of childhood immunization or recent booster administration is available, the clinician should assume that the patient has no antibody present. In this case a series of three immuniza-

TABLE 13-1

Primary Tetanus Immunization of Infants

DPT at age 2 months, 4 months, 6 months, 18 months, and 5 years
Primary immunization of school age children and adults
    Td: 3 injections, the first followed by the second in 4-8 weeks, and the third following 6-12 months after the second
Booster Td for all individuals having primary immunization, given every 10 years

GUIDELINES FOR TETANUS PROPHYLAXIS				
Immunization History (No. of Doses)	SMALL CLEAN WOUND		ALL OTHER WOUNDS	
	Toxoid	TIG*	Toxoid	TIG*
Uncertain	Yes	No	Yes	Yes
0-1	Yes	No	Yes	Yes
2	Yes	No	Yes	No§
3 or more	No†	No	No‡	No

DPT, Diphtheria, pertussis, and tetanus toxoid vaccines; *Td,* adult type tetanus and diphtheria toxoids.
*250 U human tetanus immune globulin intramuscularly.
†Unless ≥10 years since last booster.
‡Unless ≥5 years since last booster.
§Unless wound >24 hours old.

tion injections should be started to establish active immunity. In addition, tetanus hyperimmune globulin should be administered to provide passive immunity for 4 weeks. If a positive history of childhood immunization is available but more than 5 years has passed since the most recent booster, a booster injection should be given in patients with clean or minimally contaminated wounds. However, if the patient has a wound heavily contaminated with soil, a tetanus booster should be given even if tetanus immunization is up to date. In any case a contaminated wound should be treated with debridement, irrigation, and proper closure.[2,18]

HUMAN BITES

Wounds caused by human bites can be among the most serious from the standpoint of infection. The oral flora has a variety of bacteria; therefore when bacteria from the mouth are inoculated into a wound in the high concentration that is present in oral fluids, infections are common.[24] In general, if a patient sustains a human bite to the maxillofacial region, an anatomical primary repair can be performed. The wound should be irrigated, debrided as necessary, and sutured. Penicillin plus a penicillinase-resistant penicillin or amoxicillin and clavulanic acid should be administered. If infection occurs, it is treated in the same manner as any soft tissue infection, with incision and drainage, debridement, irrigation, and administration of antibiotics; the choice is directed by culture and sensitivity results.[4,25]

ANIMAL BITES

Animal bites to the head and neck can become infected if they are improperly treated but are less likely to be infected than human bites. The most common pathogen responsible for wound infections after cat or dog bites is *Pasteurella multocida.* It is present in approximately 50% of cat bite and 25% of dog bite wound infections.[60] Other organisms commonly present in cat and dog bite infections are *S. aureus,* streptococci, and *Moraxella* and *Neisseria* spp. Anaerobic bacteria frequently are present; the species involved are similar to the anaerobic flora of the human oral cavity.[14,30,60] The oral flora of animals usually is highly sensitive to penicillin. Therefore animal bites can be managed in a similar manner to human bites: debridement, irrigation, suturing, administration of penicillin or a cephalosporin, and tetanus precautions.[38] If *S. aureus* is suspected based on initial wound Gram stain, a second agent such as dicloxacillin should be added if penicillin is used. Alternatively, staphylocidal coverage can be provided using amoxicillin and clavulanic acid. When antibiotics are given for a bite wound that is not infected, antimicrobial administration can be stopped safely within 3 to 5 days. Seven to 14 days is the recommended duration of antibiotic therapy for an infected animal bite.[16,30,62]

RABIES

The most important consideration after an animal bite to the maxillofacial region is whether rabies has been transmitted to the patient. Rabies is a viral infection that causes central nervous system irritation, progressing to total paralysis and death. The virus has an affinity for nerve tissue, traveling along the nerves near the wound to the spinal cord and brain. After an incubation period that can range from 10 days to 1 year, the affected patient manifests symptoms of rabies, which include excitement and increased salivation. The patient soon experiences difficulty in swallowing and speaking. Soon the respiratory system is affected, resulting in death from asphyxia 3 to 10 days after symptoms begin. Once the signs of a rabies infection have occurred, death is almost 100% certain because no effective form of therapy exists.[27]

The chance that an animal bite has transmitted rabies virus varies depending on the animal species involved. Farm livestock, rabbits, and rodents rarely carry rabies; therefore their bites seldom justify anti-rabies treatment. However, bites from unvaccinated domesticated dogs or cats, especially those allowed to roam in rural or semirural areas, should be assumed to have transmitted rabies unless the animal can be monitored closely for 10 days for signs of rabies, such as altered behavior. If the animal shows any signs of disease, it should be destroyed and its brain examined for evidence of rabies infection. Bites from wild animals such as skunks, raccoons, foxes, and other carnivores should be assumed to have transmitted rabies, and antirabies treatment should be initiated immediately. Postexposure prophylaxis for rabies involves providing passive immunity with the administration of human rabies immune globulin, 20 IU/kg, one half of the dose given into the wound and the other half given intramuscularly. At the same time, active immunity should be stimulated by the administration of either human diploid cell vaccine (1 mL intramuscularly on days 1, 3, 7, 14, and 28) or the use of duck embryo vaccine (1 mL intramuscularly twice a day for 7 days, then 1 mL per day for 7 days, followed by 1 mL intramuscularly on days 24 and 34).

Antibody titers should be monitored to ensure that immunization has occurred. Vaccines have proved highly successful. In one series, no cases of rabies occurred after 200,000 courses of the vaccine over a 12-year span (Figure 13-14).[20,27]

OTHER ANIMAL-BORNE INFECTIONS

Cat-Scratch Disease   Cat-scratch disease is another infectious process causing head and neck infection in which an animal acts as the inoculator. The disease usually manifests with chronic lymphadenitis, and cervical lymph nodes are a common site of infection. A history of a cat bite or scratch usually is discovered on careful questioning. Often a few days after receiving the wound a nonpruritic erythematous papule develops at the wound site. Lymph node enlargement out of proportion to the wound size then occurs. The putative agent of cat-scratch disease associated with cats has been identified as *Afipia felis.*[17,25] This gram-negative bacillus can be cultured from affected nodes, but the diagnosis of cat-scratch disease also can be confirmed by meeting at least three of the following four criteria, or when any one of these criteria are met in association with the finding of typical silver-staining bacteria on histopathological sections of lymph nodes:

1. History of contact with cats and presence of a scratch
2. Positive skin test result for cat-scratch disease
3. Negative results on studies for other causes of lymphadenopathy
4. Characteristic histopathological findings in a biopsy specimen

Although cat-scratch disease can affect many organ systems, when it is confined to a cervical node, the course typically is self-limiting with spontaneous resolution in about 6 weeks. Cat-scratch disease also can cause parotitis.[15] Central nervous system involvement, if it occurs, usually develops weeks after the onset of lymphadenopathy. Incision and drainage of accumulated necrotic material when fluctuance appears and supportive therapy usually are sufficient for the management of cat-scratch disease isolated to cervical lymph nodes.

Lyme Disease   Lyme borreliosis is another animal vector–associated infection that can affect the maxillofacial region. It is caused by *Borrelia burgdorferi,* an organism transmitted by certain tick species associated primarily with deer. Erythema migrans, the cutaneous hallmark of Lyme borreliosis, starts at the site of borrelial inoculation by an infected tick. The typical lesion is clear centrally with

Postexposure Rabies Prophylaxis Algorithm

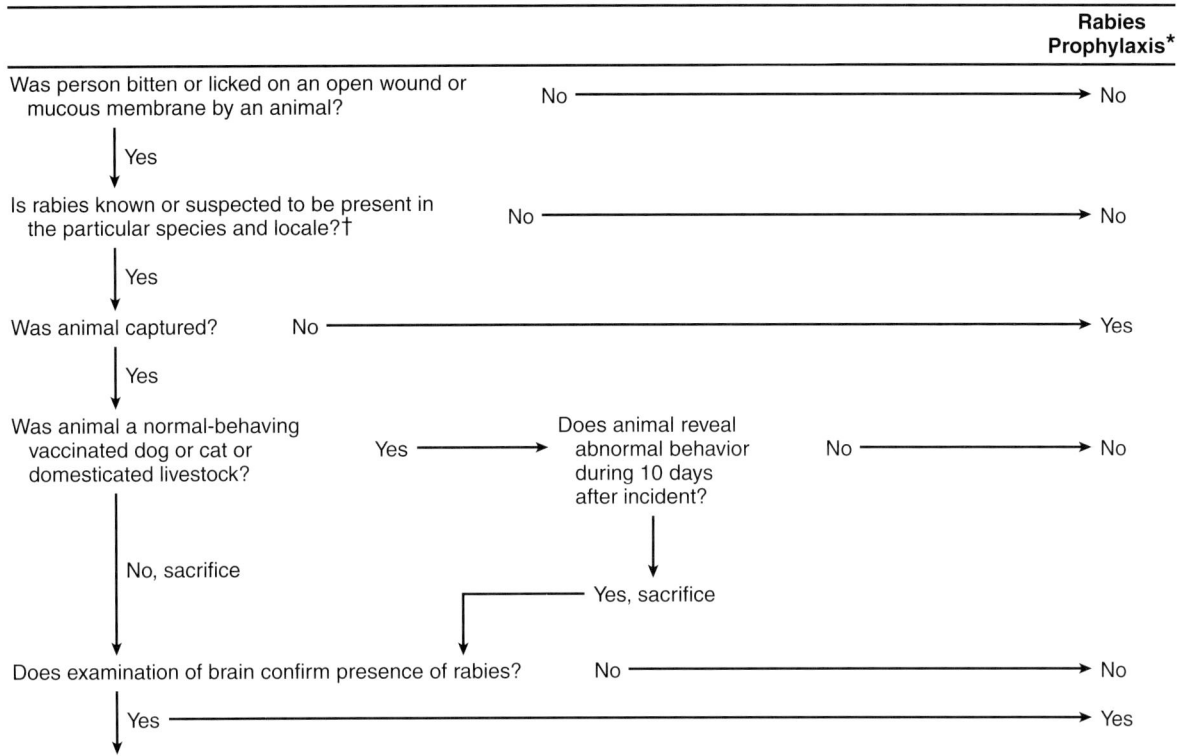

Figure 13-14 Postexposure rabies prophylaxis algorithm.

*Passive immunization using 20 U/kg human rabies immune globulin or 40 U/kg equine antiserum given half into wound and half intramuscularly. Active immunization using human diploid cell vaccine or duck embryo vaccine. Administered intramuscularly as five 2-mL doses on days 1, 3, 7, 14, and 28.

†Commonly rabid: skunk, bat, fox, coyote, raccoon, bobcat, and other carnivores. Occasionally rabid: livestock (check with public health officials in areas), wild dogs and cats. Rarely rabid: squirrels, hamsters, guinea pigs, gerbils, chipmunks, rats, mice, rabbits, vaccinated dogs and cats.

a sharply demarcated peripheral erythematous band. The rash may persist for several weeks and often is accompanied by fever, lethargy, arthralgia, and headache. Although the lower extremity is the most commonly affected site, in children the erythema commonly occurs on the face as an erythematous coloration of the cheek. Other cutaneous manifestations of Lyme disease are acrodermatitis chronica atrophicans and borrelial lymphocytoma. The former is identified by the formation of a blue-red discoloration of the skin followed by atrophy of the involved skin, whereas in the latter blue-red nodules or plaques 1 to 5 cm in diameter develop.[7,34]

Heightened public and professional awareness of Lyme disease has increased the frequency of the proper diagnosis. Usually the diagnosis of erythema migrans can be made on the basis of the clinical appearance. In atypical cases the history of a tick bite at the site of a lesion, the seasonal onset, the nonspecific histopathological findings, and a positive serological test result for *Borrelia* help confirm the diagnosis.

Lyme borreliosis, when discovered early in its clinical course, is treated with tetracycline or penicillin V and supportive therapy for adults, or amoxicillin or penicillin V for children and teenagers in tooth-developing years. About 15% of patients receiving antibiotics for this disease experience a Jarisch-Herxheimer reaction (high fever, generalized erythematous rash, and greater pain) during the first 24 hours after therapy begins. Lyme disease vaccine is available and should be considered for anyone but the very young and elderly persons in susceptible parts of North America.

SEPSIS

Sepsis represents a combination of pathological processes set in motion by the failure of the body to contain a localized infection. The patient with sepsis initially is seen with fever and chills, malaise, weakness, and apathy. However, the most severe manifestation of sepsis is diffuse peripheral vasodilation, which produces septic shock. The vasodilation that occurs during sepsis is believed to be caused by toxins produced by infecting organisms and release of vasoactive substances as the result of the interaction between bacterial products and infected tissues, white blood cells, and platelets. The peripheral vasodilation produces a relative hypovolemia, impairing perfusion of vital organs.

In addition, massive complement activation may predispose patients with sepsis to adult respiratory distress syndrome.[58] Endotoxin released from bacteria also can trigger both the clotting and fibrinolytic systems. Sepsis occurs because of an impaired immune system, a bacterial inoculum size that overwhelms host defenses, or both. The result is often a life-threatening situation. Although septic shock usually is associated with gram-negative bacterial infections, gram-positive bacterial infections can cause the identical problem. Fortunately, clinically significant sepsis rarely is caused by infections in the maxillofacial region for several reasons. These include the usually early diagnosis and treatment of infections in the maxillofacial region, high efficiency of local host defenses in the region compared with other parts of the body, and relative ease of spontaneous external drainage of maxillofacial processes, even those that are untreated. However, sepsis can result from almost any untreated infection of the head and neck and can occur in immunodeficient patients with maxillofacial infections.[5]

The diagnosis of sepsis in a patient with a maxillofacial infection is made based on the presence of systemic manifestations of infection to an extent greater than would be expected from the localized infectious process. Patients with severe sepsis have positive blood culture findings and hemodynamic instability with or without rapidly worsening respiratory distress.[12]

Treatment consists of proper monitoring of vital functions, fluid resuscitation, drainage of accumulated purulence, empirical use of high doses of antibiotics chosen to cover the spectrum of potential pathogens until culture results are available, and supplemental oxygen. Ventilatory support may be required. High doses of corticosteroids frequently are administered, although their use in sepsis is controversial. Intravenous hyperalimentation may be necessary, and vasoactive drugs such as dopamine may be required to maintain adequate blood pressure and vital organ perfusion. Proper treatment of the initial site of infection, including the choice of the appropriate antibiotic and aggressive supportive care, is the key to survival and cure of patients with sepsis.[58]

DIFFERENTIAL DIAGNOSIS OF NECK SWELLING

The appearance of a swelling or swellings in the neck often is accompanied by signs and symptoms of regional disease that usually provide an explanation for the neck mass. This situation most commonly occurs in an oral or pharyngeal infection that produces cervical lymphadenopathy. However, in certain circumstances a neck swelling is the only clinical manifestation of a pathological condition apparent from the historic and physical examination. When this occurs, the clinician should formulate a differential diagnosis from which to work. For neck swellings, narrowing of diagnostic possibilities is assisted by categorizing swellings on the basis of location in the neck and the number of swellings present. A useful method of separating neck locations is classification of position as on the midline or lateral to the midline. Lateral swellings are di-

vided by whether the swelling is solitary or consists of multiple swellings. The diagnostic possibilities for a neck swelling located on the anterior midline of the neck are few. They consist of thyroglossal duct cysts, dermoid cysts, enlarged submental lymph nodes, and enlarged pyramidal lobe of the thyroid gland. Thyroglossal duct cysts arise from epithelial remnants of thyroid anlage. They often first become apparent during or soon after an upper respiratory tract infection, when they commonly expand and become tender to palpation. This mass may move upward when the tongue is protruded and can be located anywhere along the midline from the submental triangle to the cricoid. Aspiration and ultrasonography are useful in confirming the diagnosis. Dermoid cysts also typically occur in the midline, usually in the submental triangle or floor of the mouth. They are filled with fluid and other epidermal products, and aspiration may or may not be diagnostic. The consistency of the neck swelling is doughy compared with the rubbery feel of a thyroglossal duct cyst. Enlargement of dermoids does not closely correlate with respiratory tract infections.

Swellings in the anterior neck midline also can be caused by an enlarged submental node or thyroid disease localized to the pyramidal lobe. Enlargement of a submental node is most likely the result of infected tissues in the mouth or lower lip, particularly if the swelling is tender to palpation. However, the finding of a solitary, firm, enlarged, nontender mass in the midline of the upper neck should be presumed to be a lymph node containing malignant tissue until proven otherwise. Enlargements of the pyramidal lobe of the thyroid appear lower in the neck and can be of inflammatory or neoplastic origin. Thyroid scans and thin-needle biopsy can help confirm this possibility. Carcinomas of the larynx rarely spread to the Delphian node in front of the cricothyroid membrane, causing palpable enlargement. In this case, endoscopic examination of the larynx is necessary.

The list of diagnostic possibilities is much longer for solitary neck swellings located off the anterior midline. The list differs depending on the age of the patient, but in both adults and children enlargement of a single lymph node is the most common cause of a solitary lateral neck swelling. In children the enlarged node usually results from infection but also can be caused by lymphoma. Other relatively common causes of solitary lateral neck swellings in children are branchial cleft cysts and cystic hygroma. Branchial cleft cysts typically arise along the anterior border of the sternocleidomastoid muscle and frequently enlarge during upper respiratory tract infections. Fistulization to the surface can occur but is unusual. Ultrasonography and aspiration help confirm the diagnosis. The same process occurs with cystic hygromas, which can appear anywhere in the lateral neck. Another rare possibility for a solitary lateral neck swelling in children is neuroblastoma.

In adults, other diagnostic possibilities exist, including hemangiomas, lymphangiomas, neurofibromas, lipomas, chemodectomas, and other soft tissue neoplasms. The major two lobes of the thyroid gland sit lateral to the midline, and their enlargement can produce unilateral or bilateral lower neck swellings from inflammatory, metabolic, or neoplastic processes in the thyroid. Submandibular gland swelling to infection, obstruction, or neoplasm can produce a solitary lateral neck swelling and often is accompanied by altered salivary flow from the gland's duct. Sialography or xerography of the suspected gland is helpful in such cases. When a firm, solitary mass occurs in the lateral neck of an adult and is fixed to the surrounding tissue, the clinician must assume that it represents a metastasis from a malignant neoplasm and begin a search for the primary tumor. A final possibility for a solitary lateral neck swelling, particularly if it is bilaterally symmetrical, is that the swelling represents an anatomical variant such as a prominent transverse process of the first cervical vertebra, a large carotid bulb, or physiological hypertrophy of the thyroid gland such as during puberty.

Multiple swellings on the lateral aspect of the neck may represent different diagnostic entities. The most common cause of multiple lateral neck swellings is lymphadenitis caused by an oral or pharyngeal infection. Swellings also can occur in a patient with mononucleosis and other viral infections that cause cervical lymphadenopathy. Other infections causing multiple neck swellings include cervicofacial actinomycosis, nocardiosis, cat-scratch disease, and tuberculosis (scrofula). Neoplastic causes of lateral neck swellings include lymphoma, neurofibroma, and Warthin's tumor.

REFERENCES

1. Abell E: Inflammatory diseases of the epidermal appendages and of cartilage. In Elder DE, Elenitsas R, Jaworsky C, et al: *Lever's histopathology of the skin,* ed 8, Philadelphia, 1997, JB Lippincott.
2. Abrutyn E: Tetanus. In Braunwald E, Fauci A, Kasper DL, et al, editors: *Harrison's principles of internal medicine,* ed 15, New York, 2001, McGraw-Hill.
3. Adreasen TJ, Green SD, Childers BJ: Massive infectious soft-tissue injury: diagnosis and management of necrotizing fasciitis and purpura fulminans, *Plast Reconstr Surg* 107:1025, 2001.
4. Ahrenholz DH, Simmons RL: Infections of the skin and soft tissues. In Howard RJ, Simmons RL, editors: *Surgical infectious diseases,* ed 3, New York, 1995, Appleton-Lange.
5. Altemeier WA, Burke JF, Pruitt BA, et al: The pathophysiology of infection. In Altemeier WA, editor: *Manual on control of infection in surgical patients,* ed 2, Philadelphia, 1984, JB Lippincott.
6. Aly R, Maibach HI: Factors controlling skin bacterial flora. In Aly R, Beutner KR, Maibach HI, editors: *Cutaneous infection and therapy,* New York, 1997, Marcel Dekker.
7. Asbrink E: Cutaneous manifestations of Lyme borreliosis, *Scand J Infect Dis Suppl* 77:44, 1991.
8. Babajews A, Nicholls MW: Tetanus associated with dental sepsis, *Br J Oral Surg* 23:36, 1985.
9. Baronia AK, Singh PK, Dhiman RK: Intractable pharyngeal spasm following tracheal extubation in a patient with undiagnosed tetanus, *Anesthesiology* 75:1111, 1991.
10. Baxter CR: Surgical management of soft tissue infections, *Surg Clin North Am* 52:1483, 1972.
11. Bergfeld WF: Multiple infected sebaceous cysts, *JAMA* 254:2662, 1985.
12. Bevan DR, Pardy BJ: Shock: bleeding disorders. In Dudley HAF, editor: *Hamilton Bailey's emergency surgery,* ed 11, Bristol, 1986, John Wright & Sons.
13. Bortolussi R, Kennedy W: Aerobic gram-positive bacilli. In Armstrong D, Cohen J, editors: *Infectious diseases,* vol 2, London, 1999, Mosby.
14. Brook I: Microbiology of human and animal bite wounds in children, *Pediatr Infect Dis J* 6:29, 1987.
15. Browne R: Cat-scratch disease of the head and neck, *Br J Oral Maxillofac Surg* 23:41, 1985.
16. Callaham M: Prophylactic antibiotics in common dog bite wounds: a controlled study, *Ann Emerg Med* 9:410, 1980.
17. Case records of the Massachusetts General Hospital. Weekly clinicopathological exercises: case 22-1992—a 6½-year-old girl with status epilepticus, cervical lymphadenopathy, pleural effusions, and respiratory distress, *N Engl J Med* 326:1480, 1992.
18. Centers for Disease Control: Diphtheria, tetanus, and pertussis: guidelines for vaccine prophylaxis and other preventative measures, *MMWR Morb Mortal Wkly Rep* 30:392, 1981.
19. Chidzonga MM: Necrotizing fasciitis of the cervical region an AIDS patient, *J Oral Maxillofac Surg* 54:638, 1996.
20. Corey L: Rabies virus and other rhabdoviruses. In Braunwald E, Fauci A, Kasper DL, et al, editors: *Harrison's principles of internal medicine,* ed 15, New York, 2001, McGraw-Hill.
21. Delauney WE, Land WA: *Principles and practice of dermatology,* ed 2, Sydney, 1984, Butterworths.
22. Dillon HC Jr: Streptococcal skin infections and glomerulonephritis. In Hoeprich PD, editor: *Infectious diseases,* ed 4, Philadelphia, 1994, Harper & Row.
23. Eady RA, Leigh IM, Pope FM: Anatomy and organization of human skin. In Champion RH, Burton JL, Burn DA, et al, editors: *Textbook of dermatology,* ed 6, Oxford, 1998, Blackwell.
24. Earley MJ, Bardsley AF: Human bites: a review, *Br J Plast Surg* 37:458, 1984.
25. English CK, Wear DJ, Margileth AM, et al: Cat-scratch disease, *JAMA* 259:1347, 1988.
26. Feingold DS: The changing spectrum of streptococcal and staphylococcal infections. In Aly R, Beutner KR, Maibach HI, editors: *Cutaneous infection and therapy,* New York, 1997, Marcel Dekker.
27. Flanigan TJ, Rippert ET, Nieusma GE: Rabies therapy for animal bites in the head and neck region, *J Oral Maxillofac Surg* 43:704, 1985.
28. Franz DR, Jahrling PB, Friedlander AM, et al: Clinical recognition and management of patients exposed to biological warfare agents, *JAMA* 278:399, 1997.
29. Gaukroger MC: Cervicofacial necrotizing fasciitis, *Br J Oral Maxillofac Surg* 30:111, 1992.
30. Goldstein EJ, Ciron DM: Comparative activities of cefuroxime, amoxicillin-clavulanic acid, ciprofloxacin, enoxacin, and ofloxacin against aerobic and anaerobic bacteria isolated from bite wounds, *Antimicrob Agents Chemother* 32:1143, 1988.
31. Guslits B: Upper airway obstruction due to erysipelas, *Intensive Care Med* 17:370, 1991.
32. Hall JC, editor: *Sauer's manual of skin diseases,* ed 8, Philadelphia, 2000, JB Lippincott.
33. Hay RJ, Adriaans BM: Bacterial infections. In Champion RH, Burton JL, Burn DA, et al, editors: *Textbook of dermatology,* ed 6, Oxford, 1998, Blackwell.

34. Johnson RC: Recent advances in Lyme disease. In Aly R, Beutner KR, Maibach HI, editors: *Cutaneous infection and therapy,* New York, 1997, Marcel Dekker.

35. Katsambas AD, Nicolaidoo E: Acne, perioral dermatitis, flushing, and rosacea: unapproved treatments or indications, *Clin Dermatol* 18:171, 2000.

36. Krespi RP, Lawson W, Blaugrund SM, et al: Massive necrotizing infections of the neck, *Head Neck Surg* 3:475, 1981.

37. Kuroda M, Ohta T, Vchiyama I, et al: Whole genome sequencing of methicillin-resistant *S. aureus, Lancet* 357:1225, 2001.

38. Lackmann G, Draf W, Isselstein G, et al: Surgical treatment of facial dog bite injuries in children, *J Craniomaxillofac Surg* 20:81, 1992.

39. Lerner PI: Actinomyces and Arachnia species. In Mandell GL, Douglas RG Jr, Bennett JE, editors: *Principles and practice of infectious diseases,* ed 5, New York, 2000, Churchill Livingstone.

40. Lerner PI: The lumpy jaw, *Infect Dis Clin North Am* 2:203, 1988.

41. Maibach HI, Aly R: Bacterial infections of the skin. In Moschella SL, Hurley HJ, editors: *Dermatology,* ed 3, Philadelphia, 1992, WB Saunders.

42. Nasemann T, Sauerbrey W, Burgdorf WH: Bacterial infections. In Nasemann T, Sauerbrey W, editors: *Fundamentals of dermatology,* New York, 1983, Springer-Verlag.

43. Odom RB, James WD, Berger TG, editors: *Andrew's diseases of skin,* ed 9, Philadelphia, 2000, WB Saunders.

44. Oumeish I, Oumeish OY, Bataineh O: Acute bacterial skin infections in children, *Clin Dermatol* 18:667, 2000.

45. Plewig G, Kligman AM: *Acne and rosacea,* ed 3, Berlin, 2000, Springer.

46. Quinn PD: Dermatologic infections of the head and neck, *Oral Maxillofac Surg Clin North Am* 3:423, 1991.

47. Rapoport Y, Himelfarb MZ, Zikk D, et al: Cervical necrotizing fasciitis of odontogenic origin, *Oral Surg* 72:15, 1991.

48. Reisner RM: An overview of acne treatment. In Frank SB, editor: *Acne,* New York, 1979, Yorke Medical Books.

49. Roetlinger W, Edgerton MT, Kurtz LD, et al: Role of inoculation site as a determinant of infection in soft tissue wounds, *Am J Surg* 126:354, 1973.

50. Rolden JC, Terheyden H, Dunsche A, et al: Acne with chronic recurrent multifocal osteomyelitis involving the mandible as part of the SAPHO syndrome, *Br J Oral Maxillofac Surg* 39:141, 2001.

51. Roser SM, Chow AW, Brady FA: Necrotizing fasciitis, *J Oral Surg* 35:730, 1977.

52. Ross JI, Snelling AM, Eady EA, et al: Phenotypic and genotypic characterization of antibiotic-resistance *Propionibacterium acnes* isolated from acne patients attending dermatology clinics in Europe, USA, Japan, and Australia, *Br J Dermatol* 144: 339, 2001.

53. Skov L, Olsen JV, Ramm M, et al: Superantigen staphylococcal enterotoxin B induces release of IL-1β in human epidermis, *Acta Derm Venereol* 80:17, 2000.

54. Slade E, Danielson P, Goldberg M: Erysipelas: facial lymphangitis, *J Oral Surg* 35:416, 1977.

55. Smith AT, Drew SJ: Tetanus: a case report and review, *J Oral Maxillofac Surg* 53:77, 1995.

56. Stamenkovic I, Lew PE: Early recognition of potentially fatal necrotizing fasciitis, *N Engl J Med* 310:1689, 1984.

57. Stewart WD, Danto JL, Maddin S: *Dermatology,* ed 4, St Louis, 1978, Mosby.

58. Sugerman HG: Complications of septic shock. In Greenfield LJ, editor: *Complications in surgery and trauma,* ed 2, Philadelphia, 1990, JB Lippincott.

59. Tovi F, Fliss DM, Zirkin HJ: Necrotizing soft-tissue infections in the head and neck: a clinicopathological study, *Laryngoscope* 101:619, 1991.

60. Weber DJ, Wolfson JS, Swartz MN, et al: *Pasteurella multocida* infections, *Medicine* 63:133, 1984.

61. Weston WL: Bacterial infections of the skin. In Weston W: *Practical pediatric dermatology,* ed 2, Boston, 1985, Little, Brown.

62. Wolff K: Management of animal bite injuries of the face: experience with 94 patients, *J Oral Maxillofac Surg* 56:838, 1998.

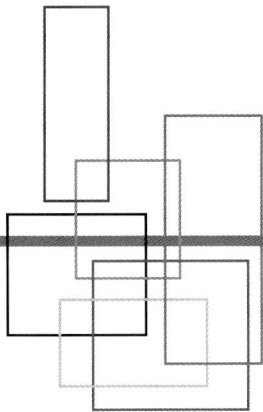

Ear, Nose, and Throat Infections

Eric J. Dierks
George R. Deeb

Infections of the ear, nose, and pharyngeal areas often are encountered by practitioners who care for patients with oral, facial, and neck pathological conditions. Before the availability of penicillin, otolaryngology was referred to as "the specialty of infection" because of constant involvement with infections such as mastoiditis, tonsillopharyngitis, and sinusitis. Clinicians who treat maxillofacial infections must remain up-to-date in their knowledge of common otolaryngological infections to enhance their therapeutic capabilities and optimize outcomes. This chapter discusses infections in the nasal, otic, and pharyngeal regions, including common organisms and the medical and surgical means of treating infections at these sites.

NASAL INFECTIONS

COMMON TYPES OF NASAL INFECTIONS

Furunculosis and Carbunculosis Infections of the hair follicles and sebaceous glands of the nasal lining often begin abruptly. A furuncle is a walled-off abscess that develops in or around a hair follicle. These lesions usually begin as erythematous, firm swellings that rapidly progress, become fluctuant, and drain spontaneously into the nasal vestibule or onto the skin surface. *Staphylococcus aureus* almost always is responsible for this infection because it is commonly among the flora of the nasal cavity.[7] Furuncles that coalesce can form a deeply situated abscess with multiple draining sites referred to as the carbuncle. Pain is associated with both lesions but usually is more severe with carbunculosis.[14]

Treatment is directed at providing drainage. Moist, warm compresses may be applied, and once the area is fluctuant, it should be incised and drained. Antibiotics usually are not needed in patients with intact immune systems but should be considered in immunocompromised hosts. Individuals with recurrent infections may benefit from

prompt intervention with antistaphylococcal antibiotics early in the course of the disease before abscess formation.[7]

Septal Abscess Furuncles or septal hematomas resulting from trauma may lead to septal abscesses. The responsible organism commonly is *S. aureus,* and treatment consists of incision and drainage in addition to appropriate antistaphylococcal antibiotics. A saddle-nose deformity may result from suppurative chondritis and subsequent cartilage erosion.

Paranasal Sinus Infections The functions of the paranasal sinuses are not understood completely. They are involved in nasal respiration, dampening of intranasal pressure, voice resonance, humidification of inspired air, decreasing the weight of the skull, and perhaps some degree of aid in olfaction.[27] At birth the maxillary and frontal sinuses are present, while the sphenoid and frontal sinuses appear by the second to third year of life. Sinus disease is related to several factors: patency of the ostia, function of the cilia, and quality of nasal secretions. Alterations in one or more of these factors may change sinus physiology and lead to sinusitis. Classification of sinusitis in five axes has been proposed with the following criteria: (1) clinical presentation (acute, chronic); (2) anatomical site (frontal, maxillary); (3) responsible organisms (viral, bacterial, fungal); (4) presence of extrasinus involvement (complicated, uncomplicated); and (5) presence of modifying or aggravating factors (immunosuppression, osteomeatal obstruction.[34a]) An example of this analysis is chronic frontal bacterial sinusitis complicated by frontal osteomyelitis and aggravated by chemotherapy.

Acute Sinusitis Acute sinusitis is defined as an inflammatory process persisting in the sinus from 1 day to 4 weeks. The treatment of acute sinusitis primarily is nonsurgical, although some cases involving complications such as orbital involvement may require surgical drainage.

Acute viral sinusitis most often follows viral rhinitis.[27] Viral rhinitis rarely requires treatment and usually is self-limiting. In immunosuppressed patients with persistent cytomegalovirus infections, treatment may be warranted. Viral sinusitis may damage sinus cilia as a result of cilia-toxins and can thereby predispose patients to bacterial infection.

Acute maxillary sinusitis.   The maxillary sinus is a pyramidal structure usually present at birth. The sinus drains into the 2.5-mm diameter ostium in the middle meatus. Accessory ostia often exist, and when present they are located in the infundibulum or the membranous region of the medial sinus wall. The complications of infections of the maxillary sinus usually are not as serious as infections of other sinuses because the sinus is not situated as close to the brain or eye.

The most common organisms responsible for acute maxillary sinusitis are *Streptococcus pneumoniae, Haemophilus influenzae, Moraxella catarrhalis,* and other streptococcal species.[4] Anaerobic pathogens sometimes are isolated during acute infection. Infectious pathogens are similar in children and adults. Nosocomial sinusitis usually is polymicrobial and caused by organisms prevailing at a particular institution.

The most common initial sign of acute sinusitis is pain, which can manifest as nasofacial pain or headache. Other causes of pain should always be considered in the diagnosis. In acute sinusitis, nasal obstruction and discharge are common, in addition to systemic symptoms such as fever, malaise, and lethargy. Acute maxillary sinusitis also may manifest as a numb feeling in the area of the maxillary premolars and molars.

The diagnosis of maxillary sinusitis is made on the basis of history and physical examination and then confirmed by imaging. Anterior rhinoscopy often shows an erythematous and edematous mucosa with streaking of purulent discharge and a meniscus of purulence under the middle turbinate. Facial tenderness may be noted. A complete examination is needed because otitis media and acute sinusitis may coexist. Adult acute maxillary sinusitis usually does not produce facial swelling unless the surrounding bone has been perforated. Facial swelling should alert the clinician to suspect sinus carcinoma with erosion, odontogenic infection, nasolabial cyst infection, or other causes. Transillumination may be performed but is not often reliable. The paranasal sinus computed tomographic (CT) scan series has proved much more useful than the Waters' view or the traditional paranasal sinus plain film series and shows air-fluid levels, thickened mucosa, and complete opacification of the affected sinuses (Figure 14-1). Nasal endoscopy is a useful diagnostic tool and can be performed with the patient under local anesthesia in the clinic or office. Sinus endoscopy, with culture, biopsy, or lavage, may be performed using an antral puncture transfacially or transorally.[18]

Antibiotics are the key to management of maxillary sinusitis and therapy should be started empirically and directed at coverage of gram-positive and gram-negative or-

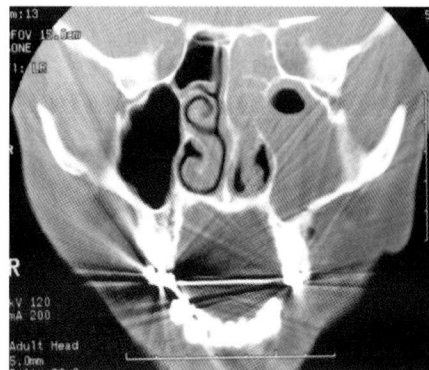

Figure 14-1 Paranasal sinus CT scan showing air-fluid level in left maxillary sinus with opacification of ethmoids.

ganisms. Amoxicillin is a good first choice, but often amoxicillin with clavulanic acid (Augmentin) or ampicillin with sulbactam (Unasyn) is needed because of the increasing resistance to penicillins by *S. pneumoniae.* Second-generation cephalosporins also cover these resistant organisms and may be used. Antibiotic therapy should be continued for 7 days after symptoms have disappeared and often are needed for up to 3 weeks. Topical and systemic decongestants are beneficial to facilitate drainage provided they are not used for more than 3 days. Short-term corticosteroids also can aid in opening normal sinus drainage pathways. Sinus puncture and lavage may speed recovery but should not be performed in the acute phase. The main indication for maxillary sinus irrigation is in treatment of immunocompromised patients with acute sinusitis in which medical management has been unsuccessful. If irrigation is used, the sinus aspirate should be sent for general bacterial culture with testing for fungi, acid-fast bacilli, and anaerobes. The possibility of malignancy should be considered in the presence of unexplained unilateral sinus opacification.[13,17,21,27]

Acute frontal sinusitis.   The frontal sinus usually is present by the second or third year of life and varies greatly in size and shape as it continues to pneumatize into adulthood. The nasofrontal duct drains into the frontoethmoidal recess located in the middle meatus. A rudimentary or absent frontal sinus is noted in 10% to 12% of adults. The mucosa of the frontal sinus may be infected by bacteria; this usually follows viral infection, as in maxillary sinusitis. The microbiology of the frontal sinus is similar to that for the maxillary, and antibiotics should be administered empirically and nasal decongestants prescribed.

The presentation of acute frontal sinusitis begins with a frontal headache above the medial canthus of the eye. The pain is often increased by bending over and may be exacerbated by palpating or tapping over the frontal sinus. Fever with swelling and redness in the eyelid on the affected side are common. The eye is bound on three sides by sinuses; thus periorbital edema may be present with frontal, ethmoid, or maxillary sinusitis.

Physical examination reveals frontal tenderness and intranasal purulence. Extensive disease can produce an os-

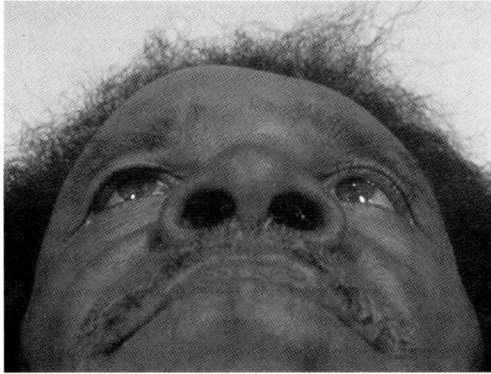

Figure 14-2 Forehead swelling resulting from underlying frontal sinusitis. Pitting edema characteristic of "Pott's puffy tumor" is present.

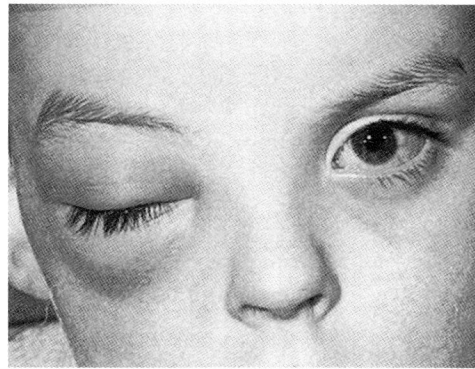

Figure 14-4 Orbital abscess caused by ethmoid sinusitis. (From Becker W, editor: *Atlas of ear, nose and throat diseases*, ed 2, Philadelphia, 1984, WB Saunders.)

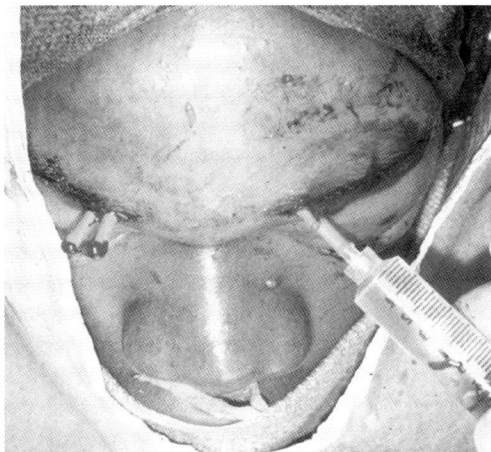

Figure 14-3 Drainage and irrigation of acute frontal sinusitis. Irrigation catheters are left in place for several days.

teomyelitis of the anterior table of the frontal sinus, resulting in a characteristic pitting edema of the forehead termed "Pott's puffy tumor" (Figure 14-2). A CT scan is helpful in establishing the diagnosis without undue delay.

Acute frontal sinusitis requires aggressive treatment and often mandates hospitalization. In severe cases, infection may extend through phlebitic diploic veins and cause epidural and subdural abscess, meningitis, brain abscess, cavernous sinus thrombosis, and death.[30] Drainage of acute frontal sinusitis may be required if the infection does not respond promptly to empirical antistaphylococcal antibiotics. Trephination, irrigation, and drainage can be performed through the thin wall of the anteroinferior aspect of the sinus through a Lynch incision (Figure 14-3).

Acute ethmoid sinusitis.   Acute ethmoid sinusitis usually occurs in combination with other paranasal sinus infections. The microbiology of infections is similar to that of the other sinuses. Patients usually have inner canthal pain on the affected side. Acute infections of the ethmoid sinuses also may produce parietal, occipital, nasal or retroorbital pain. CT scanning is the imaging modality of choice. The ethmoid sinuses are separated from the orbits by the thin lamina papyracea, which has naturally occur-

ring dehiscences through which blood vessels and infection may pass. In the early stages, acute ethmoid sinusitis may be managed medically. Infections in the ethmoid sinuses can lead to periorbital cellulitis or abscess[2] (Figure 14-4). The distinction between orbital abscess and phlegmon may be difficult on CT scanning and surgical drainage may be needed if serial CT scans do not demonstrate improvement. A decline in extraocular movements or visual acuity should mandate consideration of immediate surgical intervention.[2] Drainage usually is best accomplished by an external ethmoidectomy approach, although an endoscopic ethmoidectomy approach also can be used. Patients in whom orbital cellulitis develops should have close follow-up by the surgeon and an ophthalmologist.

Acute sphenoid sinusitis.   Isolated infections of the sphenoid sinus are uncommon and occur in an estimated 1% to 2.7% of cases.[24] Sphenoiditis usually occurs in conjunction with infection in the other paranasal sinuses. Because of the location of the sphenoid, few bacteria or inhaled irritants are carried to the sinus because nasal airflow is directed below the ostia. Secondary infection follows blockage of sinus drainage. The most common initial symptoms are headache, which usually involves the vertex of the skull, followed by visual changes. Cranial nerve abnormalities are encountered in up to 12% of inflammatory cases of isolated sphenoid sinusitis.[24] Antibiotic therapy alone is curative in most cases; however, surgical drainage by endoscopic sphenoidotomy occasionally may be warranted. Both the optic nerve and internal carotid artery course through the lateral wall of the sphenoid sinus and can be covered by only sinus mucosa. Complications include optic nerve compression, blindness, internal carotid artery spasm, intracranial abscesses, meningitis, and cavernous sinus thrombosis.[30]

Chronic Sinusitis   Chronic sinusitis refers to sinusitis of any or all of the paranasal sinuses that has persisted for longer than 3 months. Chronic sinusitis results from undertreated or untreated acute sinusitis. After 3 months the inflammatory process usually has damaged the natural mechanisms that promote sinus drainage, and surgical intervention generally is needed. The abnormal mucosal structure and disruption of function render chronic sinusitis unresponsive or transiently responsive to medical management. With appropriate surgical management the epithelial metaplasia, ciliary defects, congestion of mucous glands, and extensive thickening of the mucous membranes may be reversible. Ventilatory defects in the middle meatus with interruption of normal mucosal clearance lead to persistent inflammation and disruption of frontal, ethmoid, and maxillary clearance. This response often occurs after viral infection and creates an environment conducive to bacterial growth.

Dental diseases such as pulpal infection and periodontal disease sometimes are associated with chronic sinusitis.[9] This type of sinusitis often is referred to as *odontogenic sinusitis* and should be differentiated from routine chronic sinusitis by means of tooth vitality testing, periodontal examination, and elimination of a rhinogenic origin. Dental treatment can be initiated once the focus has been identified.[28] A dental cause of chronic maxillary sinusitis accounts for approximately 12% of cases and may have minimal symptoms. The normal alveolar pneumatization of the maxillary sinus results in a thin layer of bone between the apices of the maxillary premolars and molars and the schneiderian membrane of the sinus floor. The drainage of purulence from the apex of a nonvital maxillary molar or premolar into an otherwise healthy maxillary sinus is carried by the mucociliary blanket to drain through the normal ostium. The patient may report vague discomfort or intermittent maxillary pain that responds transiently to antibiotic therapy. Paranasal sinus CT scanning often demonstrates normal sinus architecture with a slight mucosal thickening around the affected tooth. More severe dental infection initially involves the sinus floor and lateral elements, eventually progressing to total sinus involvement.

The extraction of maxillary molars or premolars can result in the formation of an oroantral fistula; the maxillary first molar is the most commonly implicated tooth. Fistulization commonly produces a condition of chronic maxillary sinusitis with a bacterial flora that includes oral anaerobes. Surgical closure of oroantral fistulas should include adequate maxillary sinus drainage and may include the surgical creation of a nasoantral window. The traditional antrostomy beneath the inferior turbinate is less physiological than the enlargement of the natural ostium beneath the middle turbinate because of the direction of the ciliary beat and the natural movement of the mucociliary blanket tend to bypass surgically created openings.

The presentation of the patient with chronic sinusitis differs from that of acute sinusitis. Pain is not the chief complaint, rather nasal discharge and obstruction. Patients rarely show constitutional or systemic symptoms. A CT scan reveals thickening of the mucosa without air-fluid levels. Persistent mucopurulent discharge is present despite antibiotic therapy. These patients commonly have an allergic history, and control of the allergies can be a critical component of their management.

The microbiology of chronic sinusitis differs from that of acute infection. Aerobic organisms often are present, but anaerobic organisms play the more important role in the pathogenesis of chronic sinusitis. Anaerobic culture is important in determination of the infecting pathogens.[18]

FUNGAL INFECTIONS OF THE SINUSES

Aspergillosis *Aspergillus fumigatus* and *Aspergillus flavus* are the most likely causative agents of aspergillosis.[8] This disease often is classified as allergic, noninvasive, or invasive. Thick, tenacious, dark secretions with calcifications seen on plain film or CT scans are common to all forms. The noninvasive form should be suspected with opacification of the single maxillary sinus. The invasive form may lead to ophthalmoplegia, proptosis, and visual loss with bony destruction of the sinuses evident radiographically. The fungus is difficult to culture, and often antrostomy and biopsy of the tissue are needed. Microscopic examination reveals septate, bifurcating hyphae. Treatment consists of surgery and therapy with amphotericin B.[8,38] At surgery the involved sinuses contain a thick, dark, greasy material that is resistant to irrigation and often requires mechanical removal.

Mucormycosis Mucormycosis in the form of nasal obstruction may be encountered in patients with poorly controlled diabetes or other forms of immunosuppression. The dark or hypoxic appearance of the turbinates, lateral nasal wall, and maxilla may be evident intranasally. The initial findings can be minimal and show only nasal obstruction and turbinate engorgement, but the disease may progress to rhinocerebral and central nervous system mucormycosis. These severe cases show ptosis, ophthalmoplegia, and facial and trigeminal nerve dysfunction. The diagnosis is confirmed by identification of pathological organisms with methenamine silver staining. The treatment of mucormycosis requires a combined approach. Wide surgical debridement including maxillectomy and orbital exenteration often is needed. Strict diabetic control and treatment of immunocompromised states also are necessary. High-dose amphotericin B therapy usually is indicated.

COMPLICATIONS OF ACUTE OR CHRONIC SINUSITIS

Mucocele Mucoceles are expansile, cystic lesions occurring as complications of chronic sinus inflammation, trauma, surgery, or tumor; the common factor is obstruction of sinus drainage. All paranasal sinuses can be affected, but the frontal sinus is involved most frequently. These lesions are slow growing and usually cause symptoms by the destruction of surrounding bone and displacement of anatomical structures. Radiographs reveals the smooth, rounded enlargement of a sinus cavity or an air cell. The walls are thin and often barely discernible (Figure 14-5). Mucoceles of the frontoethmoidal complex are

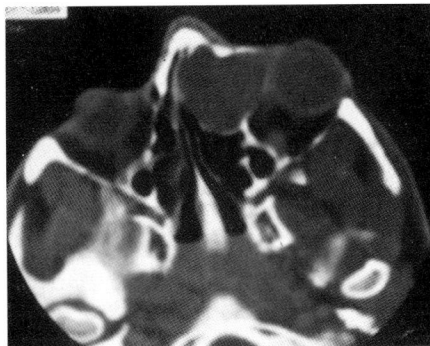

Figure 14-5 CT scan demonstrating anterior ethmoidal mucocele.

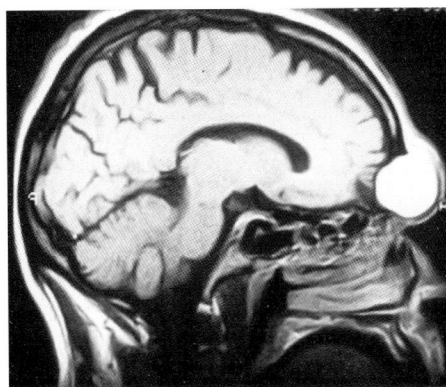

Figure 14-6 Magnetic resonance image demonstrating frontal mucocele.

the most significant. The bone of the anterior table can become thinned and destroyed (Figure 14-6), and the patient often has a history of headache, frontal mass, proptosis, or diplopia (Figure 14-7). Secondary infection of a mucocele results in a mucopyocele. Ethmoid mucoceles can be drained endoscopically, and if permanent drainage is established, the mucocele usually slowly recedes. Frontal mucoceles commonly require surgical excision with management of the frontal sinus by means of either cranialization or obliteration using fat or other materials.

Orbital Complications   Because the eye and orbit are surrounded on three sides by the paranasal sinuses, an inflammatory process in any of the sinuses can spread readily to the orbit. Orbital complications are most common with frontal and ethmoidal sinusitis. Lid edema is the first sign of the orbital involvement, and if the inflammatory process is anterior to the orbital septum, it is referred to as a *periorbital cellulitis or abscess*. A periorbital abscess can progress quickly to diffuse orbital cellulitis or formation of an orbital abscess. In the late stages of cellulitis, patients may have decreased extraocular movements. If an orbital abscess is formed, the patient will have proptosis, oph-

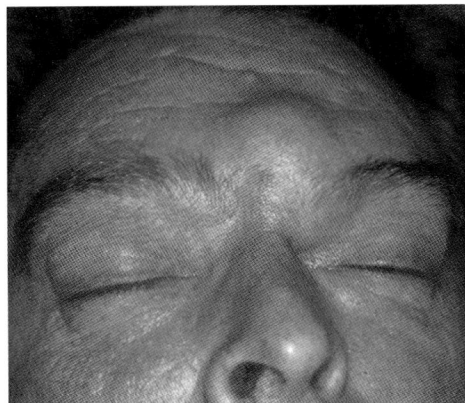

Figure 14-7 Frontal bulge produced by mucocele of frontal sinus that has destroyed anterior table. The mass is depressible but pitting edema is not present.

thalmoplegia, and decreased visual acuity. Abscess formation sometimes leads to cavernous sinus thrombosis. Patients should be hospitalized and intravenous antibiotic therapy started early in the disease process. If signs have not begun to reverse in 24 to 48 hours, surgical intervention is indicated.[2,27,28,30] Drainage generally is performed by incisions in the eyelids.

EAR INFECTIONS

EXTERNAL NONCANAL EAR INFECTIONS

The external ear includes the auricle, projecting laterally from the head, and the external auditory canal, leading medially to the tympanic membrane. The external ear is located above the rest of the body as an evolutionary strategy to optimize interaction with the environment.

Furunculosis and Carbunculosis   Similar to the diseases mentioned with nasal infections, furuncles and carbuncles are caused by staphylococcal and other gram-positive infections of the hair follicles. These lesions often start as pustules, progress to abscess formation, and frequently drain spontaneously. Their location is usually at the junction of the concha and canal skin. Coalescence of multiple pustules leads to carbunculosis.[6,12]

Therapy is similar to that for nasal disease: application of warm packs, and incision and drainage for formed abscesses. Supplemental topical and systemic antibiotics also may be used.

Perichondritis and Chondritis   Perichondritis and chondritis are caused by inflammation of the perichondrium and cartilage of the ear. The common causes are trauma or surgical manipulation of the ear. Initially the skin is pruritic, and later the overlying skin becomes crusted and may weep serous or purulent exudate. The organism usually responsible is *Pseudomonas aeruginosa*, but often secondary gram-positive infections occur. Once infection has become established, control can be difficult because the blood supply of the cartilage of the ear is poor.

Treatment should begin with antipseudomonal drugs, often in combination with gram-positive coverage if secondary infection is suspected. The disease typically requires parenteral antibiotics and surgical intervention. Knowledge of ear anatomy is crucial because surgical debridement can result in significant deformity.

Relapsing Polychondritis   The exact cause of this rare disease is unknown, although it is considered autoimmune. It can mimic a chronic infection, but no purulence exists. Multiple cartilaginous tissues such as ear, larynx, trachea, bronchi, and nose also may be affected. The disorder is relapsing and remitting, and may be accompanied by fever, anemia, erythema, swelling and pain. Nasal saddling, ear deformities, and respiratory tract obstruction may ensue. Tissue biopsy shows inflammation, cartilage destruction, and fibrous tissue replacement.[31]

Oral corticosteroids such as prednisone are the primary treatment. An antibiotic may be prescribed if infectious complications occur. Surgical debridement of necrotic cartilage and drainage may be needed. Often esthetic procedures are warranted to correct resulting deformity of affected structures. Progressive tracheal stenosis may require tracheostomy.

INFECTIONS OF THE EXTERNAL AUDITORY CANAL

The external canal is an S-shaped structure lying between the auricle and the tympanic membrane with an osseous inner part and the cartilaginous outer part. The skin of the external canal has many hair follicles and apocrine glands that act as defense mechanisms against infection and foreign bodies. The normal ear flora usually includes staphylococci, micrococci, and corynebacteria with occasional gram-negative organisms.

Acute Otitis Externa   Otitis externa is an infection of the external ear canal. This infection usually appears during hot and humid weather, and appears in acute and chronic forms (Figure 14-8). Often referred to as "swimmer's ear," this infection usually follows removal of the protective lipid layer of the canal, which allows bacteria to enter the pilosebaceous unit. Removal of the lipid layer may result from excessive cleansing, trauma, or swimming. Pain or itching in the canal usually are the initial symptoms; as the infection progresses pain increases as the periosteal tissues of the canal are lifted off the bone. Later in the disease process a purulent discharge begins, and the preauricular and postauricular tissues become swollen and erythematous. The pathogens usually responsible are *P. aeruginosa*, *Proteus mirabilis*, streptococci, staphylococci, and other gram-negative bacilli. Treatment may be divided into four broad categories: (1) frequent cleaning; (2) administration of appropriate antibiotics using otic drops and systemic

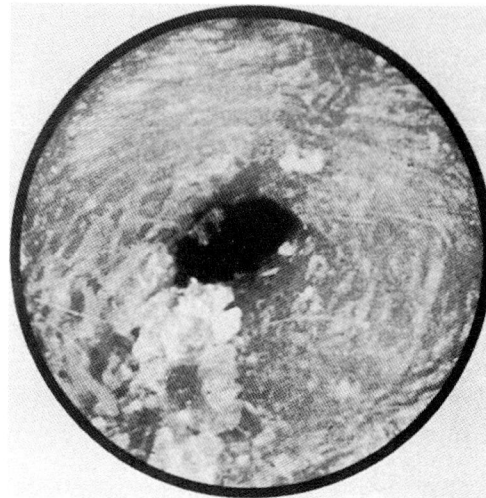

Figure 14-8 Chronic otitis externa results in thickened canal skin. (From Becker W, editor: *Atlas of ear, nose and throat diseases,* ed 2, Philadelphia, 1984, WB Saunders.)

antibiotics; (3) treatment of associated pain and inflammation; and (4) prevention of further infections.[33]

The external canal must be cleansed and all infectious debris removed by suctioning. These procedures are performed most easily with the use of an office microscope and microsuction. The patient is treated with a topical drop containing polymyxin, neomycin, gentamicin, or a floxin antibiotic. A topical steroid such as hydrocortisone may be useful for edema and inflammation and helps reduce discomfort. Moderate disease may necessitate placement of an otic wick to ensure transport of the topical medication into the entire external canal, and severe disease can require intravenous antibiotics for 10 to 14 days.[16]

Chronic Otitis Externa   The chronic form of otitis externa usually begins as pruritus rather than pain. The longstanding infection may cause hyperkeratosis, acanthosis, and epithelial exfoliation. Flakes of desquamated dry skin often are seen in the canal. Gram-negative bacilli such as *P. mirabilis* regularly are implicated. Treatment consists of repeated cleansing and instillation of antibiotics and steroids. Triamcinolone (Kenalog) or dexamethasone (Decadron) ophthalmic drops may be used with antibiotics. If the disease progresses to canal obliteration, surgical intervention may be needed to restore canal patency.[16]

Necrotizing External Otitis   Necrotizing external otitis, a nonneoplastic condition also referred to as *malignant otitis externa,* can be a potentially lethal infection involving osteomyelitis of the skull base. The disease almost always occurs in elderly patients with diabetes and usually is caused by *P. aeruginosa.* Other causative pathogens include *P. mirabilis, A. fumigatus, Proteus* and *Klebsiella* spp., and staphylococci. Other immunocompromised states, such as human immunodeficiency virus and chemotherapy for malignancy, also may predispose patients to this serious infection.

The disease usually begins with minor trauma affecting the external canal and progresses into the soft tissue at the cartilaginous-osseous junction of the canal. The infection then spreads to the cartilage and temporal bone, commonly producing early facial paralysis. Continued progression causes osteomyelitis of the skull base, with palsies of cranial nerves X, XI, and XII, meningitis, sigmoid sinus thrombosis, brain abscess, and death.

Physical examination usually reveals a characteristic polyp of granulation tissue in the external canal at the junction of the bony and cartilaginous elements of the canal. The area surrounding the temporomandibular joint and skin of the canal are tender, and surrounding tissues are erythematous, indurated, and often macerated. Purulence is common.

Aggressive treatment with serial cleansing of the external auditory canal and administration of intravenous antibiotics, such as antipseudomonal coverage and third-generation cephalosporins, are indicated. Surgical debridement and medical treatment are needed. Magnetic resonance imaging and CT scans are helpful for defining disease extension and planning surgical resection.[29,32,41]

Bullous External Otitis   Bullous external otitis is a painful condition caused by vesicular formation in the bony portion of the external canal. Often the vesicles are red as a result of hemorrhage; then the disease is termed *hemorrhagic bullous otitis externa.* The vesicles rupture, and bloody or serous discharge appears in the canal. The vesicles should not be ruptured intentionally because secondary infection may ensue. *Mycoplasma* and *Pseudomonas* spp. are among the causative organisms, and otic drops should be prescribed. Packing of the canal may prolong the disease process.

Herpes Simplex   Herpes simplex vesicular inflammation of the external canal is caused by herpes simplex virus type 1. In infants and children the disease may be subclinical on first exposure and only manifest with fever, pain and adenopathy. On secondary expose and in elderly patients with previous exposure, the lesions begin with burning erythema followed by vesicle formation. The vesicles eventually crust and heal completely within 3 weeks. Lesions may recur and often are preceded by stress, sun and wind exposure, and trauma.

The treatment of the disease is symptomatic because it is self-limiting. Patients may benefit from antiviral therapy if initiated early in the disease process with agents such as acyclovir.

Herpes Zoster   Varicella-zoster is another virus that affects the external canal. Patients initially experience burning pain followed by vesicle formation. This infection often occurs after a period of stress, sun exposure, or surgery, and has been described after mandibular anesthetic blocks. As in herpes simplex virus type 1 infections, the vesicles coalesce and rupture forming crusts. Herpes zoster vesicles may cause ulcers and scar formation. This disease follows a dermatomal pattern after a prior outbreak of chickenpox because the virus then resides in the nerve ganglia. When reactivated the virus spreads through the nerve fibers from the dorsal root to the skin.[26,44]

If the disease involves the geniculate ganglion of the facial nerve, rash and vesicles form on the uvula, palate, tongue, auricle, and ear canal. Jaw pain may accompany symptoms. The facial nerve can become nonfunctional, and with accompanying disturbances of hearing and the vestibular system it is referred to as the Ramsay Hunt syndrome (herpes zoster oticus).[44]

Treatment is supportive, with topical application of a drying agent such as hydrogen peroxide for crusts. Application of bacitracin ointment may prevent superinfection. Acyclovir, famciclovir, and valacyclovir ameliorate herpetic infections, especially herpes zoster oticus, particularly when administered early in the disease course. Famciclovir reduces postherpetic neuralgia but must be used with caution in patients with decreased liver function because it causes an elevation in hepatic enzyme levels. Immunocompromised patients may require more aggressive treatment.[25]

MIDDLE EAR INFECTIONS

The middle ear is an air-filled space that houses the ossicles. It is separated from the external ear by the tympanic membrane and communicates with the pharynx through a narrow auditory or eustachian tube. Eustachian tube dysfunction is the basic underlying cause of middle ear infectious diseases.

The eustachian tube connects the middle ear and mastoid air cells to the nasopharynx. The tube is shorter in children than in adults. In adults it measures 30 to 40 mm and lies at an approximately 45-degree angle. The angle in children is more horizontal, and most growth in tube length occurs before 6 years of age. The posterior portion of the tube is osseous, and the anterior two thirds are membranous and cartilaginous. A narrowed isthmus is located between the proximal and distal parts.

The mucosal lining of the tube is continuous with that of the nasopharynx and middle ear and is characterized as respiratory epithelium. Mucous glands predominate at the nasopharyngeal orifice; a change to a mixture of goblet columnar and ciliated cells occurs near the tympanum.

The eustachian tube functions as the pressure regulator or ventilator of the middle ear to equilibrate gas pressure in the middle ear with atmospheric pressure in the pharynx. The tube protects the middle ear from effusions, which can produce conductive hearing loss. The tube normally is closed and dilates during swallowing, yawning, and sneezing through the action of the tensor veli palatini, thereby allowing equalization of middle ear and atmospheric pressures.

Mucous flow is directed at the nasopharynx by the mucociliary system of the eustachian tube and middle ear mucus membrane. This flow prevents accumulation of secretions. The mucus contains muramidase, secretory immunoglobulin A, enzymes, and opsonins. These materials are swept from the middle ear mastoid complex to the nasopharynx. The clearance depends on normal atmospheric pressure and oxygen tension in the ear. In the healthy state the middle ear and mastoid complex are protected from unwanted nasopharyngeal secretions by the anatomy of the eustachian tube system and the middle ear gas cushion.

Otitis Media   Otitis media is the single most common diagnosis reported in pediatric offices. Otitis media and its various subtypes (acute, acute otitis media without effusion, chronic, chronic with perforation and drainage, and serous otitis media) account for more than 25 million physician visits annually by children younger than 15 years of age.

Acute Otitis Media   Acute otitis media produces clinical signs and symptoms of infection including pain, fever, decreased hearing, redness, and altered anatomical appearance on otoscopic examination (Figure 14-9). It is a benign, self-limited infection of the middle ear cavity involving the deep surface of the tympanic membrane. The area is lined with respiratory mucosa that extends slightly into the mastoid cavity and possibly down into the eustachian tube but does not involve the cochlea or the external ear canal. Many risk factors exist, including male gender, absence of breast-feeding, cigarette smoking, and immunodeficiency. The single largest cause for acute otitis media is viral respiratory infection with adenovirus influenza and respiratory syncytial virus. Bacterial organisms are usually the same as in other respiratory tract bacterial infections with pneumococci, *H. influenza, M. catarrhalis,* group A, β-hemolytic streptococci, and occasionally staphylococci. Most clinicians still use oral β-lactam antibiotics such as amoxicillin as their empirical treatment for acute otitis media. The 10-day course of the relatively high dose of antibiotics similar to that for sinusitis is recommended. Many clinicians favor

second-generation cephalosporins because some have been shown to be effective against both β-lactamase–producing strains and intermediate resistant pneumococci. Penicillin with a β-lactamase inhibitor such as clavulanic acid or an enhanced-generation macrolide such as clarithromycin or azithromycin also may be used.[1,19,20] Myringotomy for acute otitis media is performed only in instances of complications such as facial nerve paralysis or in some patients who are immunocompromised.

Serous Otitis Media   Serous otitis media is known as *otitis media with effusion.* This clinical condition is defined as the presence of fluid in the middle ear without clinical signs or symptoms of active infection. The disease may encompass the spectrum of disorders sharing the presence of fluid or effusion in the middle ear as a common denominator. The presence of fluid in the middle ear produces a conductive hearing loss, and this fluid may serve as a culture medium for bacteria. The use of decongestants and antihistamines occasionally is effective; however, little evidence supports a significant beneficial role. Systemic steroids have been studied with mixed results, and their use is questioned. The Valsalva maneuver may relieve negative pressure in the middle ear if the patient can perform it successfully. Surgical treatment with myringotomy with or without insertion of ventilating tubes may be reserved for patients in whom the condition becomes chronic and disturbing.[19]

Chronic Otitis Media with Perforation   Chronic otitis media exists when a perforation in the pars tensa of the tympanic membrane has been presence for more than 6 weeks. Intermittent drainage of pus may exude through the perforation, preventing its closure, or the perforation may remain dry (Figure 14-10). A variable degree of conductive hearing loss may be present. An intermittent, low-grade chronic infection usually follows an incompletely

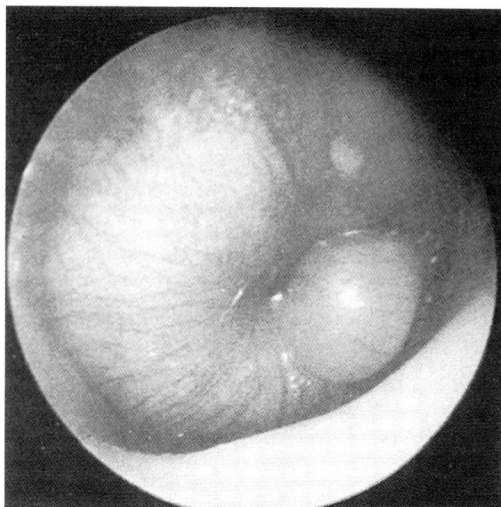

Figure 14-9 Acute otitis media. Bulging tympanic membrane precedes impending rupture. (From Chole RA: *Color atlas of ear disease,* New York, 1982, Appleton-Century-Crofts.)

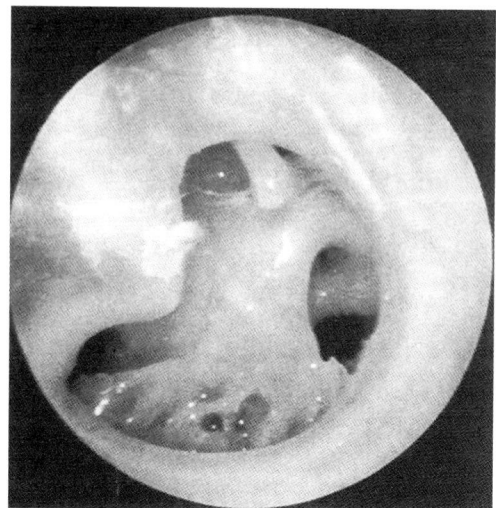

Figure 14-10 Subtotal tympanic membrane perforation. (From Chole RA: *Color atlas of ear disease,* New York, 1982, Appleton-Century-Crofts.)

treated acute otitis media episode where pressure and ischemia cause the rupture of the tympanic membrane and eustachian tube dysfunction persists. This condition formerly was common and is still common in many developing third-world countries where chronic otorrhea is a frequent finding during childhood. The untreated ear has been called the "safe" ear because drainage has been established and minimal complications are found. Decreased hearing and risk of other complications such as scarring and cholesteatoma formation occur if the infection is treated improperly. Chronic otitis media with perforation can be treated with otic antibiotic drops, such as used for otitis externa, for 3 weeks and has improved the condition in almost 80% of patients. Debris should be suctioned under direct vision. The perforated tympanic membrane can be reconstructed surgically by tympanoplasty (myringoplasty) using fat or fascial grafting.[19]

Chronic Otitis Media without Perforation   Definition of chronic otitis media without perforation is difficult; many consider it the continuum between acute otitis media and serous otitis media. An acute ear infection with symptoms for more than 3 weeks is an acceptable definition. Some authors reserve the diagnosis of chronic otitis for disease that persists for more than 3 months. Atypical organisms such as fungi, *Pseudomonas,* and anaerobes are not unusual in this condition. Complications such as cholesteatoma and granulation tissue formation are frequent and occur without surgery. Many surgeons believe that surgery is the treatment of choice for this condition with insertion of tympanostomy tubes.[19,20]

Complications of Otitis Media   The complications of otitis media may be divided into intratemporal and intracranial complications. Intratemporal complications include hearing loss, vestibular dysfunction, mastoiditis, petrositis, facial paralysis, labyrinthitis, atelectasis of the middle ear, adhesive otitis media, cholesteatoma (Figure 14-11), cho-

lesterol granuloma, tympanosclerosis, ossicular fixation, ossicular discontinuity, and external otitis. Intracranial complications include meningitis, extradural abscess, subdural empyema, focal otic encephalitis, brain abscess, dural sinus thrombosis, and otic hydrocephalus.[3,32]

INNER EAR INFECTIONS

The inner ear consists of the cochlea, labyrinth, and semicircular canals. The inner ear often is referred to as the labyrinth and is situated medial to the middle ear. This neuromembranous structure lies within the petrous bone. The perilymphatic or periotic spaces within the temporal bone are the osseous labyrinth and the complex neuromembranous portion referred to as the otic labyrinth. The space between the osseous and membranous labyrinth is the perilymphatic space. This perilymph-filled space communicates with the subarachnoid space through the cochlear aqueduct. The osseous labyrinth contains three semicircular canals and two and a half turns of cochlea. The vestibule houses the ampullated ends of the semicircular canals, utricle, and saccule. The vestibule is an enlarged portion of the labyrinth that receives both ends of each semicircular duct. The utricle and another large part of the membranous labyrinth, the saccule, lay in close association in the larger chamber of the perilymphatic space, the vestibule. The endolymphatic duct and sac are part of the membranous labyrinth. These structures in the membranous labyrinth contain endolymph.

The sense organ of the ear is the cochlea, which is triangular in cross section and attached to the osseous spiral lamina. From its attachment the cochlear duct extends across the bony labyrinth and separates the scala vestibuli from the scala tympani except at the cochlear apex. The oval and round windows are the communication between middle ear and labyrinth.

Labyrinthitis   A variety of organisms may be responsible for inflammatory inner ear disorders characterized as labyrinthitis. These disorders often are associated with hearing loss or systemic diseases. These disorders may be subdivided into six major groups.

Serous Labyrinthitis   Serous labyrinthitis usually is an inner ear inflammation caused by a nearby infection or surgery. This aseptic condition may develop from upper respiratory tract infections, inner ear surgery, or serous otitis media. Patients have mild to severe vertigo, nausea and vomiting, and, more rarely, hearing loss.[37] The diagnosis can be made with caloric testing that reveals the hypoactive response on the affected side. This self-limiting disease usually lasts for 4 to 6 weeks and is treated symptomatically.

Suppurative Labyrinthitis   Exudative infections of the middle ear often occur as the consequence of bacterial meningitis, suppurative otitis media, or chronic middle ear disease. These conditions may cause severe damage to the inner ear that results in absent or near absent caloric response and profound sensorineural hearing loss. The

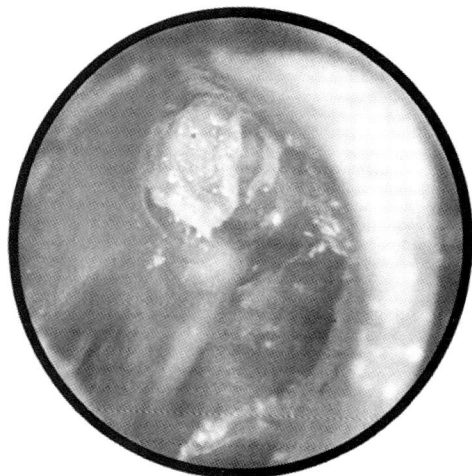

Figure 14-11 Early pars flaccida cholesteatoma. (From Becker W, editor: *Atlas of ear, nose and throat diseases,* ed 2, Philadelphia, 1984, WB Saunders.)

purulence in the middle ear requires prompt surgical drainage, and treatment with antibiotics as indicated. Anaerobic pathogens often are found after otitis media.[11] The organisms implicated most often as a result of bacterial meningitis are *H. influenzae, Neisseria meningitidis,* and *S. pneumoniae.*

Labyrinthine Fistula Labyrinthitis   Labyrinthine fistula labyrinthitis is the result of a fistula between the contaminated middle ear and the inner ear. The fistula usually occurs in the oval or round window, or through the erosion of bone from a cholesteatoma. Testing for fistula formation is accomplished by application of positive and negative pressure in the external auditory canal with the pneumatic otoscope. This action creates vertigo and nystagmus in the presence of the fistula. The treatment for this condition is surgical repair of the fistula.

Toxic Labyrinthitis   Ototoxic drugs may cause sensorineural hearing loss and tinnitus. The most common drugs include aminoglycoside antibiotics, high-dose aspirin, intravenous erythromycin, and ethacrynic acid. The potential for sensorineural hearing loss and tinnitus should be considered in use of these agents, in addition to vestibular and hearing testing to avoid complications.

Varicella-Zoster Labyrinthitis   The varicella-zoster virus is a member of the herpes virus family, a deoxyribonucleic acid virus family that includes herpes simplex types 1 and 2, cytomegalovirus, and Epstein-Barr virus. Herpes zoster oticus (Ramsay Hunt syndrome) develops when latent virus is reactivated and consists of variable facial nerve paralysis, sensorineural hearing loss, and vertigo in association with the painful vesicular rash. Other findings in the inner ear include atrophy of cochlear neurons and the sensorineural elements of the vestibular labyrinth. A history of previous chickenpox and presence of the vesicular rash are required to diagnose herpes zoster oticus. Varying degrees of hearing loss develop in approximately 6.5 % of patients with Ramsay Hunt syndrome. Steroids and acyclovir have been used to treat these infections.[44]

Luetic Labyrinthitis   *Treponema pallidum* is the causative agent in syphilis infections. Patients with the congenital or acquired forms may develop sensorineural hearing loss, episodic vertigo, and a sensation of fullness in the ears. Congenital syphilis in its early form usually is fatal. The first sign of late congenital syphilis may be sensorineural hearing loss that is generally bilateral, symmetrical, and begins during childhood. In 50% of these patients the hearing loss appears suddenly between the ages of 25 and 35 years, progresses at a variable rate, and often is associated with vertigo and tinnitus. Rarely does sensorineural hearing loss occur in acquired primary syphilis; it more often occurs in the secondary and tertiary form of the disease. Patients who develop cochleovestibular symptoms with late acquired syphilis have symptoms similar to those of patients with the congenital form of the disease. Vertigo

occurs more frequently and the hearing loss may be so asymmetrical that is appears unilateral. Once luetic labyrinthitis is suspected, the diagnosis should be confirmed by laboratory testing. Serological tests for nonspecific reagins include the rapid plasma reagin and the Venereal Disease Research Laboratory tests. Specific antibody tests include the fluorescent treponemal antibody, absorbed, *T. palladium* immobilization, and microhemagglutination assay for *T. palladium* antibodies tests. The treatment for syphilis is long-term administration of penicillin or ampicillin.[7]

Autoimmune Inner Ear Disease   The concept of sensorineural hearing loss induced by an autoimmune process has gained acceptance since the late 1970s. Progressive sensorineural hearing loss occurs with this condition. Whether sudden hearing loss occurs with this disease process is debatable, but immunological activity in the cochlea is supported by a growing body of evidence. The process usually starts by affecting one ear and the hearing loss usually progresses slowly over several years, although rapid progression of hearing loss over hours has been reported. Histological examination shows vasculitis, the hallmark of autoimmune diseases. Patients may have elevated erythrocyte sedimentation rates and antinuclear antibody results and positive findings on lymphocyte inhibition assay. In addition, patients may have another form of autoimmune disorder such as rheumatoid arthritis, ulcerative colitis, or Hashimoto's disease. Steroids and cyclophosphamide have been used for treatment, often with good response.[22]

THROAT INFECTIONS

THE OROPHARYNX AND NASOPHARYNX

The oropharynx is continuous with the oral cavity through the fauces or oral pharyngeal isthmus and is lined with stratified squamous epithelium. The fauces ("faucial pillars") extend from the posterior border of the soft palate superiorly, to the palatine arches laterally, and the dorsum of the tongue. The lateral wall of the passageway of the fauces houses the palatine tonsils. The anterior lingual tonsils, lateral palatine tonsils, and pharyngeal tonsils or adenoids superiorly form Waldeyer's tonsillar ring.

The nasopharynx is contiguous with the nasal cavities. The floor of the nasopharynx is the soft palate and the roof is the nasopharyngeal mucosa, which overlies the base of the skull and slopes posteriorly to form the posterior wall. The eustachian tubes are prominent on the lateral surface of the nasopharynx. The nasopharynx is covered by stratified squamous epithelium.

Pharyngitis   Pharyngitis is the common inflammatory process of the mucosal and submucosal structures of the throat. Infection may or may not be a component of the disease. The pharynx is the common chamber of the respiratory and digestive tracts. It is usually 12 to 14 cm in length and is the musculomembranous tube that extends from the base of the skull and the back of the nose and mouth to the level of the sixth cervical vertebra where it joins the esophagus. The mucosa in the upper pharynx is covered with pseudostratified ciliated respiratory epithelium, whereas the mucosa in the lower pharynx is covered with stratified squamous epithelium. Many infectious causes of pharyngitis may affect the epipharynx, nasopharynx, oropharynx, and hypopharynx.

Streptococcal Pharyngitis　The most frequent pathogenic microorganism implicated with pharyngitis is group A β-hemolytic streptococcus. *S. pneumoniae* and group C streptococci also can cause pharyngitis. Patients usually have a severe sore throat, difficulty swallowing, malaise, and fever. Physical examination typically reveals erythema of the involved mucosa with a mucopurulent exudate that may streak and appear confluent over the tonsils and pharyngeal walls. Cervical lymphadenopathy occurs frequently. The diagnosis is established by throat culture, although a rapid streptococcal screening test can help guide empiric therapy.

Treatment of streptococcal pharyngitis is by oral or intravenous penicillin. Patients allergic to penicillin can be treated with erythromycin or cephalosporins. Complications of streptococcal infections include rheumatic fever, rheumatic heart disease, and acute poststreptococcal glomerulonephritis.[4,34]

Scarlet fever is an acute streptococcal pharyngotonsillitis accompanied by skin rash. The rash usually appears on the second day of illness on the chest and trunk and then spreads over the entire body except the face, palms, and soles. Another characteristic finding is strawberry tongue, which appears as a red, mottled appearance on the dorsum.

Staphylococcal Pharyngitis　Mucosal erythema and edema with localized pustules in the tonsils and mucopurulent drainage are associated with pharyngitis caused by either *Staphylococcus aureus* or *salivarius*. These staphylococcal infections can be treated with staphylocidal penicillin, erythromycin, or cephalosporin antibiotics based on culture findings.[4,34]

Diphtherial Pharyngitis　Corynebacteria are gram-positive, nonfilamentous rods that formerly were a common cause of pharyngitis. Only a few hundred cases occur per year in the United States because of nearly universal immunization. Diphtheroids gain access to the host through the nose and mouth, and after the short incubation period of 2 to 4 days produce exotoxins that cause localized tissue necrosis. The necrosis produces a gray-black pseudomembrane that adheres firmly to the underlying tissue.[34] The extension of this membrane to the nasopharynx and larynx lead to respiratory obstruction, requiring tracheotomy. Antitoxin remains the only specific method of treatment.

Gonococcal Pharyngitis　*Neisseria gonorrhoeae* is an important cause of pharyngitis among the sexually transmit-ted diseases. This gram-negative diplococcus causes an infection that produces no initial symptoms, but patients may have sore throat, tonsillar hypertrophy, or cervical adenopathy. Cultures prepared on chocolate agar are diagnostic. The organism affects the mucosal surface and glandular tissue, causing ulceration and polymorphonuclear neutrophil infiltrate with exudative pharyngitis.[34] Treatment with penicillin, tetracycline, cephalosporins, or quinolones, dictated by results of cultures and sensitivity testing, is effective.

Acute Tonsillitis　The palatine tonsils (usually referred to as the "tonsils") are paired, ovoid-shaped masses located in the oropharynx on the lateral walls. The deep surface of the palatine tonsil is attached to the fascia overlying the superior constrictor muscle. The palatine tonsils may extend inferiorly to become continuous with the lingual tonsillar tissue at the base of the tongue.

Group A β-hemolytic streptococcus is the most often implicated bacterial organism in acute tonsillitis. A host of other bacteria both aerobic and anaerobic also have a role in acute tonsillitis.[36] Groups B, C, and G streptococci; *H. influenzae; S. pneumoniae; M. catarrhalis; S. aureus;* and *Bacteroides, Peptococcus,* and *Actinomyces* spp. have been implicated. Viruses cultured from tonsils include Epstein-Barr, adenovirus, influenza virus types A and B, herpes simplex, and parainfluenza virus.

No single pathogenesis exists for tonsillitis; however, viral infection with secondary bacterial invasion is widely accepted. Infections in the tonsils may be classified as acute, recurrent acute, and chronic.

Patients with acute tonsillitis complain of sore throat, odynophagia, fever, and malaise. Physical examination reveals inflamed, enlarged tonsils that are erythematous with a localized, nonconfluent exudate. Not all signs are present in every patient. The disease usually is self-limiting with a course of 7 to 10 days. Bacterial tonsillitis can occur alone or as an infection superimposed on viral tonsillitis. Acute lingual tonsillitis is rare and results from similar causative agents. Patients have inflamed lingual tonsils on indirect mirror examination or fiberoptic nasopharyngoscopy.

The differential diagnosis of acute palatine tonsil infection is varied, and culture and laboratory tests may help eliminate mononucleosis, gonococcal pharyngitis, Vincent's angina, and diphtheria. Vincent's angina is caused by fusiform bacteria and spirochetes and may be accompanied by necrotizing stomatitis. Throat cultures should be obtained in the evaluation of such patients and are often geared toward elimination of group A β-hemolytic streptococcus as the source. Unfortunately, cultures may be misleading and some patients are chronic carriers.

Treatment is directed toward identification of the causative pathogen, and penicillin is the drug of choice. The presence of β-lactam–producing organisms is increasing, and treatment with amoxicillin-clavulante (Augmentin) often is indicated. A 10-day course of an oral antibiotic is standard, and supportive care with analgesics and fluids is given if clinically indicated.[4,34,36,39]

Peritonsillar Abscess A potential complication of acute tonsillitis of the palatine tonsils is peritonsillar abscess. The peritonsillar abscess (quinsy) develops between the medial surface of the superior constrictor of the pharynx and the tonsil. The condition usually is unilateral, and the patient relates a history of sore throat that has progressed to increased pain, odynophagia, significant trismus, and dysphonia or "hot potato" voice. In extreme infections, patients cannot tolerate their own secretions and may experience airway compromise. Physical examination often is difficult because of trismus but demonstrates a bulging mass in the superior aspect of the tonsillar fossa, deviating the uvula to the opposite side (Figure 14-12). This finding helps differentiate peritonsillar abscess from an abscess of the lateral parapharyngeal space, which lies on the lateral side of the superior constrictor muscle. Drainage by 18-gauge needle aspiration in the lateral soft palate adjacent to the superior pole of the tonsil can be performed with the patient under local anesthesia. If purulence is encountered, needle aspiration produces immediate relief, but aspiration must often be repeated within 1 to 2 days. Antibiotic therapy is begun; those who are unable to swallow liquids merit overnight hospital admission. A single dose of a corticosteroid often is added to speed the patient's ability to resume oral alimentation. In selected cases, tonsillectomy also may be performed at the time of infection (quinsy tonsillectomy) to drain the infection. The occurrence of one episode of peritonsillar abscess does not mandate tonsillectomy because recurrence rates are low in patients with no history of repeated episodes of tonsillitis.[4,34-36,39]

Chronic Tonsillitis Chronic tonsillitis can be identified with chronic sore throat, malodorous breath, excessive tonsillar debris, peritonsillar erythema, and persistent cervical adenopathy. The disease results from recurrent bouts of acute tonsillitis and the presence of chronic sore throat in the absence of acute infection. The bacteriology of this disease varies from that of acute tonsillitis, and surgical specimens reveal mixed aerobes and anaerobes. Medical management usually fails to eradicate the disease, and tonsillectomy is the recommended therapy, within certain guidelines. Recurrent infections mandating tonsillectomy are defined variably as from four to seven episodes in 1 year, five episodes for 2 consecutive years, or three episodes per year for 3 consecutive years.[36]

Tonsilloliths are whitish, focal accumulations of bacterial debris within the crypts of the tonsils and frequently cause chronic halitosis. Gentle irrigation with a dental hygiene irrigating device can assist removal of foul-smelling accretions.

LARYNX

The thyroid cartilage and cricoid cartilages are the major structural elements of the larynx. Overlying the structure of the skeletal framework are the infrahyoid muscles, including the paired sternothyroid, sternohyoid, omohyoid, and thyrohyoid muscles. This framework helps prevent airway collapse and serves as attachment for laryngeal muscles, ligaments, and membranes. The epiglottis is formed of fibroelastic cartilage and has multiple perforations that allow free access of lymphatic drainage and spread of infection. The larynx functions in air passage, airway protection, and phonation; therefore characteristic signs and symptoms of disease consist of pain, cough, hoarseness, stridor, aspiration, and dysphagia.

Acute Laryngitis The term *laryngitis* refers to any acute or chronic, infectious or noninfectious, localized or systemic inflammatory process that involves the larynx. The clinical presentation depends on the underlying cause, amount of tissue swelling, region of the larynx involved, and patient age.

Acute laryngitis usually is the result of viral infection. Patients have low-grade fever, mild dysphonia, cough, or rhinitis. Rhinovirus, parainfluenza virus, respiratory syncytial virus, and adenovirus are implicated most often. Diagnosis is based on history and symptoms. Examination reveals erythematous and edematous laryngeal mucosa with normal vocal cord mobility.

Common viral laryngitis is self-limiting; treatment usually consists of hydration, humidification, antipyretics, and decongestants. Antibiotics are indicated if secondary bacterial infection is present.[40] With the increasing incidence of human immunodeficiency virus infection, syphilis and tuberculosis of the larynx are more common chronic infections causing laryngitis.[23]

Acute Epiglottitis in Children Acute epiglottitis is a life-threatening infection of the larynx that affects the epiglottis and other supraglottic structures, including the arytenoids and aryepiglottic folds. The disorder usually is caused by *H. influenza* type B and is a medical emergency because of the possibility of airway obstruction and death. Children between 2 and 6 years initially have fever, sore throat, and inspiratory stridor. As the supraglottic structures become increasingly inflamed, these children appear frightened and ill, and sit in an upright, sniffing position. They may be unable to handle

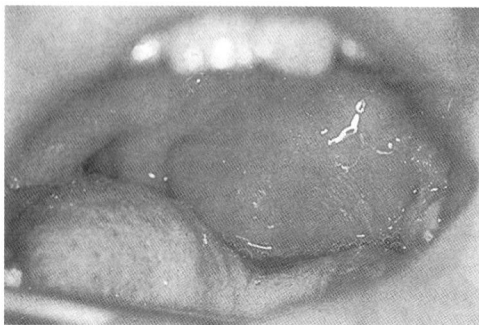

Figure 14-12 Peritonsillar abscess with displacement of uvula. (From Becker W, editor: *Atlas of ear, nose and throat diseases,* ed 2, Philadelphia, 1984, WB Saunders.)

their own secretions; therefore drooling commonly occurs.

Rapid diagnosis is based on history and clinical findings; however, bedside pharyngeal or laryngeal examination is not recommended because it may precipitate airway obstruction. Lateral soft tissue radiographs may reveal the classic but nonspecific "thumb sign" of the edematous epiglottis (Figure 14-13). Treatment should not be delayed to obtain radiographs in a child with threatening airway obstruction.

Children with acute epiglottitis should be treated expeditiously in the operating room to establish the diagnosis and secure the airway. The child with suspected epiglottitis should be accompanied by a surgeon capable of tracheotomy and an anesthesiologist at all times. The patient should be orally intubated while under controlled inhalation anesthesia. Direct laryngoscopy reveals the cherry-red, swollen epiglottis. The endotracheal tube then may be converted to the nasotracheal tube or tracheotomy. In settings without a skilled pediatric anesthesiologist, tracheotomy may be preferred, although in most children oral or nasal intubation is successful.

Antimicrobial therapy is directed against *H. influenzae.* Extubation can be performed when the edema has subsided enough to allow for an air leak around the endotracheal tube. The *H. influenzae* type b vaccine has been available since 1988 and has resulted in the dramatic decrease in the incidence of the disease; however, *H. influenzae* remains the leading cause of epiglottitis. β-Hemolytic streptococci and staphylococci also may cause supraglottics.

The mortality rate for acute supraglottics remains high despite modern advances in airway management. Prompt diagnosis is essential in differentiating the illness from croup.[4,10,34,42]

Acute Epiglottitis in Adults   Supraglottitis in adults is becoming more common, probably as the result of immunization of children against *H. influenzae.* The average patient age is between 42 and 47 years, and the incidence is approximately 1:100,000 per year. The symptoms include severe sore throat, fever, painful dysphagia, and shortness of breath. Lymphadenopathy, drooling, neck tenderness, and hoarseness are common physical signs. A variety of organisms have been implicated; the most common pathogen is *H. influenzae,* although to the lesser degree that in children. β-Hemolytic *Streptococcus, S. aureus,* and *Streptococcus pyogenes* are other common organisms. The diagnosis in adults is based on history and physical examination and may be made by indirect laryngeal examination or flexible fiberoptic nasopharyngoscopy after proper precautions have been taken. Careful monitoring in an intensive care unit with airway intervention equipment readily available is acceptable treatment in the adult. In some cases a precipitous decrease in airway patency may prompt emergency intubation or tracheotomy. Antibiotic coverage is similar to that for the pediatric age group until cultures are obtained, and corticosteroids may be helpful.[4,5,34,42]

Acute Laryngotracheitis (Croup)   Croup is a common viral infection that usually affects children younger than 5 years of age and lasts from 3 to 7 days. The disease is more common in the winter months and has a 2:1 male/female ratio. Multiple viruses have been implicated, but parainfluenza-1 is the most common viral agent. Parainfluenza-2, rhinovirus, and respiratory syncytial virus also may be causative organisms.

Children develop viral upper respiratory tract infection followed by the classic barky or croupy cough. This classic cough is nonproductive and worsens at night. In severe cases, airway obstruction and exhaustion may lead to total airway obstruction. The diagnosis is made on the basis of history, physical examination, and the classic "steeple sign" on the lateral neck film caused by subglottic narrowing (Figure 14-14).

Treatment is directed at reduction of edema, thinning of secretions by intensive humidification, and hydration.

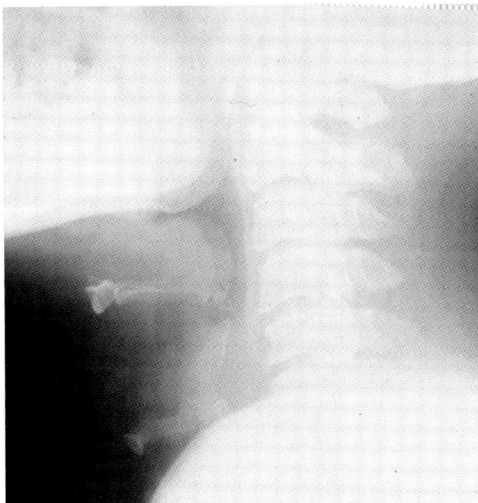

Figure 14-13 "Thumb sign" of epiglottis seen on lateral neck radiograph.

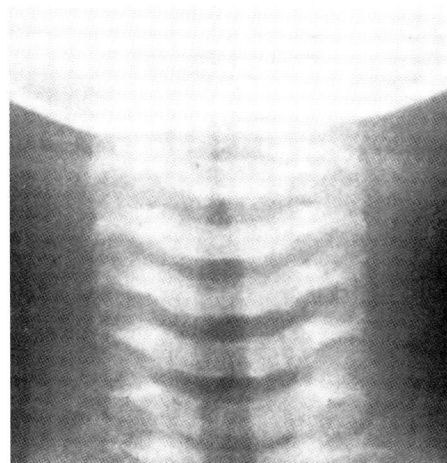

Figure 14-14 "Steeple sign" of croup seen on posteroanterior neck radiograph.

Aerosolized epinephrine and high-dose steroids should be used to prevent further progression of the edema. Intubation or tracheotomy may be required to secure the airway and allow pulmonary toilet in severe cases with airway obstruction. Secondary bacterial infection by staphylococci and pneumococci may necessitate antibiotic treatment.[4,10]

Laryngotracheal Diphtheria   Outbreaks of laryngeal diphtheria are uncommon in most parts of the world because of effective immunization; however, outbreaks have been reported in eastern Europe as a result of low immunization rates. The infection is caused by *Corynebacterium diphtheria* and usually affects the larynx, pharynx, and tonsils. The disease usually affects children older than 6 years and causes gray-green, plaquelike pseudomembranous exudate over the affected structures. The exudate is difficult to dislodge and may cause bleeding and airway obstruction. Tracheotomy often is performed, and treatment is directed toward elimination of the disease with erythromycin, penicillin, and antitoxin.[4]

Herpes Laryngitis   Herpes laryngitis is caused by the herpes simplex virus and is a self-limiting infection of the larynx. Like most herpetic infections the disease is characterized by vesicular eruption with subsequent ulceration of supraglottic mucosa. The treatment is supportive and palliative and no significant sequelae usually occur.[43]

REFERENCES

1. Aronovitz GH: Antimicrobial therapy of acute otitis media: review of treatment recommendations, *Clin Ther* 22:29, 2000.
2. Berenholz L, Kessler T, Shlomkovitz N, et al: Superior ophthalmic vein thrombosis: complication of ethmoidal rhinosinusitis, *Arch Otolaryngol Head Neck Surg* 124:95, 1998.
3. Bluestone CD: Clinical course, complications and sequelae of acute otitis media, *Pediatr Infect Dis J* 19:37, 2000.
4. Brook I: Microbiology of common infections in the upper respiratory tract, *Prim Care* 25:633, 1998.
5. Carey MJ: Epiglottitis in adults, *Am J Emerg Med* 14:421, 1996.
6. Chan KL, Soo G, van Hasselt CA: Furunculosis, *Ear Nose Throat J* 76:126, 1997.
7. Chan YM, Adams DA, Kerr AG: Syphilitic labyrinthitis: an update, *J Laryngol Otol* 109:719, 1995.
8. Clancy CJ, Nguyen MH: Invasive sinus aspergillosis in apparently immunocompetent hosts, *J Infect* 37:229, 1998.
9. Connor SE, Chavda SV, Pahor AL: Computed tomography evidence of dental restoration as aetiological factor for maxillary sinusitis, *J Laryngol Otol* 114:510, 2000.
10. Cressman WR, Myer CM: Diagnosis and management of croup and epiglottitis, *Pediatr Clin North Am* 41:265, 1994.
11. Egelund E, Bak-Pedersen K: Suppurative labyrinthitis caused by anaerobic bacteria, *J Laryngol Otol* 108:413, 1994.
12. Eley CD, Gan VN: Picture of the mouth. Folliculitis, furunculosis, and carbuncles, *Arch Pediatr Adolesc Med* 151:625, 1997.
13. Executive summary: antimicrobial treatment guidelines for acute bacterial rhinosinusitis, *Otolaryngol Head Neck Surg* 123(suppl):S1, 2000.
14. Gidley PW, Ghorayeb BY, Stiernberg CM: Contemporary management of deep neck space infections, *Otolaryngol Head Neck Surg* 116:16, 1997.
15. Gurr PA, Evans K, Dewey FM, et al: Otomycosis: the detection of fungi in ears by immunofluorescence microscopy, *Clin Otolaryngol* 22:275, 1997.
16. Hannley MT, Denneny JC, Holzer SS: Use of ototopical antibiotics in treating 3 common ear diseases, *Otolaryngol Head Neck Surg* 122:934, 2000.
17. Hickner JM: Antibiotics for acute maxillary sinusitis in adults, *J Fam Pract* 46:281, 1998.
18. Jiang RS, Hsu CY, Jang JW: Bacteriology of the maxillary and ethmoid sinuses in chronic sinusitis, *J Laryngol Otol* 112:845, 1998.
19. Jung TTK, Hanson JB: Classification of otitis media and surgical principles, *Otolaryngol Clin North Am* 32:369, 1999.
20. Karver SB: Otitis media, *Prim Care* 25:619, 1998.
21. Kennedy DW, Senior BA: Endoscopic sinus surgery: a review, *Prim Care* 25:703, 1998.
22. Kumar BN, Walsh RM, Wilson PS, et al: Sensorineural hearing loss and ulcerative colitis, *J Laryngol Otol* 111:277, 1997.
23. Lacy PD, Alderson DJ, Parker AJ: Late congenital syphilis of the larynx and pharynx presenting at endotracheal intubation, *J Laryngol Otol* 108:688, 1994.
24. Lawson W, Reino AJ: Isolated sphenoid sinus disease: an analysis of 132 cases, *Laryngoscope* 107:1590, 1997.
25. Lucente FE: Impact of the acquired immunodeficiency syndrome epidemic on the practice of laryngology, *Ann Otol Rhinolaryngol Suppl* 161:1, 1993.
26. Maini S, Preece M: Herpes zoster oticus following mandibular block, *J Laryngol Otol* 114:212, 2000.
27. Maltinski G: Nasal disorders and sinusitis, *Prim Care* 25:663, 1998.
28. Mehra P, Caiazzo A, Bestgen S: Odontogenic sinusitis causing orbital cellulitis, *J Am Dent Assoc* 130:1086, 1999.
29. Midwinter KI, Gill KS, Spencer JA, et al: Osteomyelitis of the temporomandibular joint in patients with malignant otitis externa, *J Laryngol Otol* 113:451, 1999.
30. Mortimore S, Wormald PJ: Management of acute complicated sinusitis: a 5-year review, *Otolaryngol Head Neck Surg* 121:639, 1999.
31. O'Connor Reina C, Garcia Iriarte MT, Barron Reyes FJ, et al: When is the biopsy justified in the case of relapsing polychondritis? *J Laryngol Otol* 113:663, 1999.
32. Osma U, Cureoglu S, Hosoglu S: The complications of chronic otitis media: report of 93 cases, *J Laryngol Otol* 114:97, 2000.
33. Pedersen HB, Rosborg J: Necrotizing external otitis: aminoglycoside and beta-lactam antibiotic treatment combined with surgical treatment, *Clin Otolaryngol* 22:271, 1997.
34. Perkins A: An approach to diagnosing the acute sore throat, *Am Fam Phys* 55:131, 1997.
34a. Pinheiro AD, Facer GW, Kern EB: Sinusitis. In Bailey BJ, Cahoun KH, editors: *Head and neck surgery–otolaryngology*, ed 2, Philadelphia, 1998, Lippincott-Raven.
35. Raut VV, Yung MW: Peritonsillar abscess: the rationale for interval tonsillectomy, *Ear Nose Throat J* 79:206, 2000.
36. Richardson MA: Sore throat, tonsillitis, and adenoiditis, *Med Clin North Am* 83:75, 1999.

37. Ryu JH: Vestibular neuritis: an overview using the classical case, *Acta Otolaryngol Suppl* 503:25, 1993.

38. Schubert MS: Medical treatment of allergic fungal sinusitis, *Ann Allergy Asthma Immunol* 85:90, 2000.

39. Scott PM, Loftus WK, Kew J, et al: Diagnosis of peritonsillar infections: the prospective study of ultrasound, computerized tomography and clinical diagnosis, *J Laryngol Otol* 113:229, 1999.

40. Spiegel JR, Hawkshaw M, Markiewicz T, et al: Acute laryngitis, *Ear Nose Throat J* 79:488, 2000.

41. Subburaman N, Chaurasia MK: Skull base osteomyelitis interpreted as malignancy, *J Laryngol Otol* 113:775, 1999.

42. Valdepena GH, Wald ER, Rose E, et al: Epiglottitis and *Haemophilus influenzae* immunization: the Pittsburgh experience—a five year review, *Pediatrics* 96:424, 1995.

43. Vrabec JT, Molina CP, West B: Herpes simplex viral laryngitis, *Ann Otol Rhinol Laryngol* 109:611, 2000.

44. Wackym PA: Molecular temporal bone pathology: II. Ramsay Hunt syndrome (herpes zoster oticus), *Laryngoscope* 107:1165, 1997.

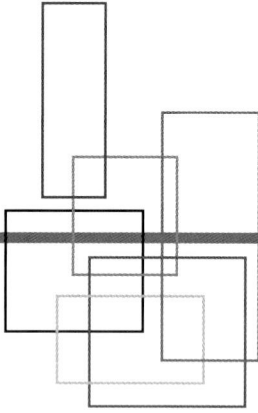

Ophthalmic Considerations in Oral and Maxillofacial Infections

Iftach Yassur
Marc J. Hirschbein
James W. Karesh

The eye and orbit frequently are affected by inflammatory and infectious processes seen by those who perform facial surgery. The anatomical proximity and the common blood supply and drainage system make the orbit susceptible to infectious processes in the soft tissue of the face, paranasal sinuses, nose, teeth, gingiva, and nasopharynx. Bacterial, viral, or fungal infections can affect the eye and orbit by direct spread of the pathogen or alteration of the blood supply and venous or lymphatic drainage. The ophthalmic symptoms and signs may be the earliest manifestations of an infectious process at an adjacent location or may be a sign of progression of the preliminary infection. Infections of the upper respiratory tract mucous membranes also may involve the conjunctiva and cornea, with ophthalmic manifestations the most severe. Infections of the conjunctiva may spread to regional lymph nodes and cause symptoms remote from the eye. Embolic spread of infections of oral and facial origin may cause severe eye infections and even blindness. Finally, scarring and destruction of tissue caused by infections of the face and sinuses can result in severe ocular problems. Surgeons who treat infections of areas adjacent to the eye must be aware of the ophthalmic manifestations of maxillofacial infections to prevent the potentially blinding or even lethal complications.

ANATOMICAL CONSIDERATIONS

The orbit is a pear-shaped structure that tapers posteriorly; the walls are composed of seven bones. At its entrance the orbit is approximately 35 mm vertically and 40 mm horizontally. Behind the rim the diameter of the orbit first widens and then gradually narrows toward the apex. The orbit is composed of four walls: inferior, superior, medial, and lateral. The distance from the rim to the apex at the inferior wall is approximately 45 mm.

Several openings exist in the orbital walls. The optic foramen transmits the optic nerve, ophthalmic artery, and sympathetic fibers from the carotid plexus. The superior orbital fissure transmits the superior and inferior ophthalmic veins; oculomotor, trochlear, and abducens nerves; and branches of the ophthalmic division of the trigeminal nerve. The inferior orbital fissure transmits branches of the maxillary division of the trigeminal nerve and venous connections between the orbit and pterygoid fossa. Small foramina transmit the anterior and posterior ethmoidal neurovascular complex.

All air sinuses share a bony wall with the orbit. The frontal sinus above, the maxillary sinus below, the ethmoidal sinus medially, and the sphenoid sinus at the apical area all have a common wall with the orbit. This close relationship renders the orbit prone to infections originating from the sinuses.

In addition to anatomical proximity, several other factors predispose the orbit to the spread of sinus infection. The walls of the orbit are extremely thin and congenital dehiscence is often present. Openings often occur at the junction of the anterior and middle third of the thin lamina papyracea or over its posterior third. Dehiscence behind the supraorbital notch of the superior wall or at the ethmoidomaxillary suture of the inferior wall also may be present. These areas of dehiscence add to the preexisting foramina in the orbital walls through which blood vessels and nerves enter the orbit.[32] As a result, pus and transudate may rupture into the subperiosteal space of the orbit. This process is exacerbated by the increased pressure in the sinuses that is present in acute sinusitis. The apex of the orbit is exposed to the same process when the sphenoid sinus is involved. The periorbita is loosely attached to the bone except at the orbital rim, the apex of the orbit, and along suture lines; therefore the periorbita can be elevated easily from the bone by collections of pus originating in the sinuses. A large amount of pus can cross the subperiosteal space into the deep orbit and accumulate as a subperiosteal abscess.

The orbit is a relatively closed compartment with limited compliance formed by a complex structure of bones, fibrous septa, and ligaments. Thus even a small amount of additional volume (an abscess, edema, or inflammation) can cause a significant increase in orbital pressure that can compromise the blood supply to vital structures in the orbit. The orbital septum is a thin, fibrous, nonelastic sheet that is a continuation of the periorbita. It originates from the orbital rim as the arcus marginalis and inserts into the levator aponeurosis. Inferiorly, it inserts in the area of the inferior tarsus. The tarsal plates are connected to the bones by the fibrous medial and lateral canthal ligaments. These limit the anterior compliance, contributing to the orbit's function as a closed compartment.

The lateral extensions of the sheaths of the extraocular muscles, the intermuscular septa, extend from one rectus muscle to the next and from the insertions of the muscles to their origins at the annulus of Zinn posteriorly. The fascia between the rectus muscles posteriorly in the orbit is thin and often incomplete, which allows easy extension between the extraconal and intraconal orbital spaces.

The communication between the vascular system of the orbit and sinuses is another factor predisposing the orbit to spread of sinus infection. Valves are absent in the orbital veins. This network forms a rich venous plexus of free communications predisposing the orbit to hematogenous transmission of infection. In the presence of acute sinusitis with increased pressure in the sinuses, reversal of flow through the anterior and posterior ethmoidal vessels provides a route for hematogenous transmission of the infection. Hematogenous spread also occurs from the soft tissue of the face, nose, nasopharynx, pharynx, and lids. The superior ophthalmic vein receives tributaries from the angular vein, nasofrontal veins, and vessels originating from the ophthalmic artery. The inferior ophthalmic vein drains blood from the areas of the orbital floor, medial wall, and lower lid

EXAMINATION OF THE EYE, ORBIT, AND VISUAL PATHWAY

A basic clinical examination of the eye and orbit should be part of the routine examination in head and neck infections. Non-ophthalmologists can easily gain valuable information regarding orbital and intracranial extension of the infection using a step-by-step evaluation of the eye. Ophthalmic consultation may be indicated in selected cases to complete the examination. If visual loss is present, time may be a critical factor in preventing permanent visual loss.

External Examination The external examination of the eye provides valuable information regarding orbital and intracranial processes. First, the position of the eye is evaluated in all three dimensions. Proptosis (exophthalmos or

anterior displacement of the globe) or enophthalmos (posterior displacement of the globe) is evaluated with a Hertel exophthalmometer. Tilting the patient's head backward and comparing the position of the eye on both sides by looking from above or below is an additional option (Figure 15-1). The eye also is evaluated for hypoglobus (eye displaced inferiorly) or hyperglobus (eye displaced superiorly) and lateral or medial displacement of the globe. Next, the lid and skin are examined for swelling, edema, erythema, or signs of trauma to the skin. Pressure may be applied to the lids for evaluation of orbital pressure (by gauging the ease of orbital "retropulsion").

Vision Vision (far and near distance) is examined with the patient's best optical correction whenever possible. Vision is one of the most important early indicators of optic nerve damage but also may be affected by many other factors. Tearing, irritation, discharge, surface disease and other corneal problems, change in refraction caused by pressure on the globe or metabolic problems, vitreous opacities, and retinal problems are some causes of decreased vision. Color vision is a more sensitive indicator for optic nerve damage. The Ishihara color test should be performed whenever possible. Red saturation test is a less sensitive test that compares the red saturation between both eyes and should be performed whenever the Ishihara color test is unavailable. Patients with nerve damage may describe the red color seen in the affected side as washed-out red or brown.

Visual Fields Visual fields are important signs of optic nerve damage and sometimes can help to localize the site of nerve injury. Computerized visual fields are more accurate but usually are impractical in a disabled or ill patient. Confrontation visual fields should be performed in all patients at the bedside.

Extraocular Movements Extraocular movements are assessed in all directions of gaze for signs of nerve damage or mechanical restriction. The lid level is evaluated for ptosis, and the levator muscle excursion also is assessed. When ocular movement is limited, forced duction testing may be applied to differentiate mechanical restriction from nerve paresis.

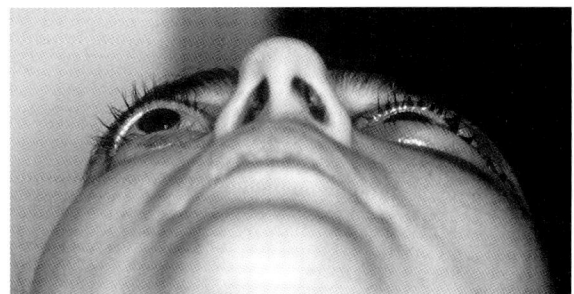

Figure 15-1 Exophthalmos or enophthalmos becomes evident when the head is tilted back and the eyes are observed from below (or above). In this case, right exophthalmos is seen.

Pupillary Reaction   Pupillary reaction may be the only method to assess optic nerve dysfunction in noncooperative patients such as infants or unconscious patients. In the setting of orbital infection, every pupillary abnormality should first be attributed to damage of the ipsilateral optic nerve or oculomotor nerve. When a history of trauma is evident, damage to the iris sphincter or globe also may change the size and shape of the pupil. Corneal or vitreal opacities do not cause pupillary abnormalities. Also, optic nerve damage on one side does not cause mydriasis (dilation) on the same side but causes an abnormal pupillary reaction to light if the affected side is tested. Mydriasis usually indicates damage to the parasympathetic fibers of the ipsilateral oculomotor nerve.

The most valuable test to detect significant optic nerve dysfunction is the swinging flashlight test (the relative afferent pupillary defect). A bright light is alternately swung from eye to eye. If a relative difference in light transmission exists between the left and right optic nerve (because of nerve damage), the pupils constrict in reaction to light when shined into the healthy eye; when the light is shined into the eye with nerve damage, the pupils dilate relative to their previous constricted condition. This finding verifies that one optic nerve transmits less light than the contralateral one.

Ophthalmoscopy   Ophthalmoscopy with a direct or indirect ophthalmoscope is necessary to complete a thorough eye examination. Possible findings include venous stasis manifesting as dilated, tortuous veins with or without retinal hemorrhages, or central or branch retinal artery occlusion seen as narrowing of the retinal arteries with edema of the nerve fiber layer and a cherry red spot appearance. Optic nerve ischemia may manifest as a swollen optic disc with or without surrounding flame-shaped hemorrhages and soft exudates. Choroidal folds may be seen with an orbital mass pushing the globe from behind. Septic emboli to the retina are seen as hemorrhages with a white center and vitreous opacities. A slit-lamp examination should be performed in any case of corneal opacity, red eye, photophobia, or vision loss.

Optic nerve evaluation includes vision testing, color vision testing, assessment of the visual fields, pupillary reaction, and direct visualization of the optic nerve head. Imaging also may reveal nerve compression, nerve stretching, or thickening of the nerve. In the setting of an acute event, abnormality in any of these test findings may indicate an ophthalmic emergency and consultation is warranted.

CONTIGUOUS SPREAD OF MAXILLOFACIAL INFECTIONS

In the ocular conditions listed in the following sections, the source of the preliminary infection can be an adjacent head and neck site, and the eye is affected only secondarily.

BACTERIOLOGY

The organisms responsible for orbital infections of contiguous spread are the same organisms that comprise the

---

BOX 15-1

Predominant Normal Flora at Various Sites

Body Site	Microbial Flora
Conjunctiva	*Staphylococcus epidermidis*
	Aerobic and anaerobic diphtheroids
Nose and nasopharynx	*S. epidermidis*
	Staphylococcus aureus
	Streptococcus spp.
Mouth and oropharynx	*S. epidermidis*, non–group A streptococci, *Streptococcus pneumoniae*, *Streptococcus mitis*, *Streptococcus salivarius*, nonpathogenic *Neisseria*, *Haemophilus*, *Veillonella*, *Bacteroides*, *Fusobacterium*, *Treponema*, *Lactobacillus*, yeasts

normal flora of the sinuses, nose, oropharynx, and conjunctiva (Box 15-1). Their frequency varies according to patient age, geographical location, and whether the orbit or preseptal tissue is involved. Anaerobic organisms are present in the upper respiratory tract flora and are frequent with odontogenic and sinus infections. Mixed infections also are common.

CLASSIFICATION OF ORBITAL INFECTIONS

Orbital infections are classified into five stages that generally represent degrees of severity.

Stage 1: preseptal cellulitis. Infection is confined to the lids and periocular soft tissue anterior to the orbital septum. The orbit may be inflamed secondarily but is not directly infected.
Stage 2: orbital cellulitis with proptosis, limitations in movements, and possible optic nerve compromise.
Stage 3: orbital cellulitis with a subperiosteal abscess.
Stage 4: orbital cellulitis with a true orbital abscess within the orbital fat.
Stage 5: retroorbital spread of the infection into the cavernous sinus or brain.

PRESEPTAL CELLULITIS

Preseptal cellulitis is defined as superficial cellulitis of the lids and periorbita anterior to the orbital septum. The orbital structures posterior to the septum are not infected but may be secondarily inflamed. If the infection spreads posterior to the septum, the condition is termed *orbital cellulitis.*

Causes   Preseptal cellulitis occurs from three primary sources:

1. Preseptal cellulitis as a result of paranasal sinusitis. This type of infection usually occurs in children and represents the majority of periorbital cellulitis cases.

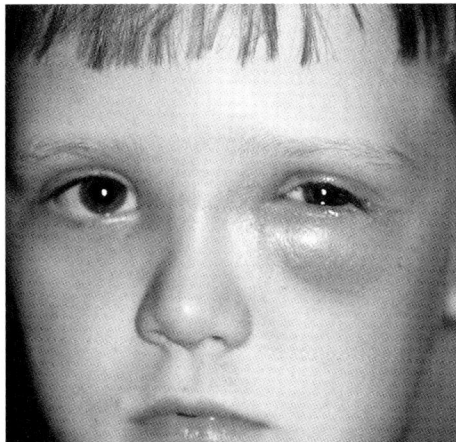

Figure 15-2 Preseptal cellulitis caused by dacryocystitis in a young child.

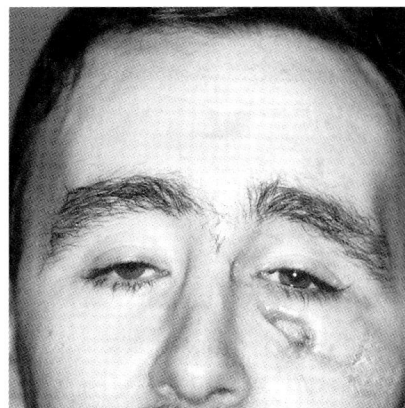

Figure 15-3 An extruding plate in a patient with previous surgery for facial fracture.

The bacteria are present mainly in the sinuses, whereas the periorbital swelling is mostly the result of secondary inflammation and venous congestion.[4,62] Blood cultures usually are sterile.

2. Preseptal cellulitis related to upper respiratory tract infections. In this group of young children (<5 years of age), preseptal cellulitis occurs after bacteremic spread from a primary focus such as otitis media or pneumonia. Blood cultures frequently yield positive findings. The condition may be associated with meningitis, and progression to orbital cellulitis is more common. In many instances, affected children have a history of recent upper respiratory tract infection. *Haemophilus influenzae* is a less significant pathogen today but was the primary pathogen in patients younger than 4 years before the availability of vaccination.

3. Preseptal cellulitis as a result of direct inoculation. In these children a history of trauma to the skin, lid insect bite, dacryocystitis, conjunctivitis or chalazion usually is present and bacteremia is usually absent (Figure 15-2). An extruding plate or screw from previous maxillofacial surgery also can serve as the source of the infection in preseptal or even orbital cellulitis (Figure 15-3).

Symptom and Signs   Patients with preseptal cellulitis often have a brief history of painless or tender swelling of the eyelids. The eyelid is characteristically erythematous and edematous and may show signs of trauma, an insect bite, or a chalazion that induced the cellulitis. Signs and symptoms of sinusitis or upper respiratory tract infection may be present.

Fever is present in more than half of patients but is a nonspecific sign. The eyelid may be painful to palpation. The spread of the infection usually is confined to the lid (by the attachment of orbital septum to the arcus marginalis). Sometimes the infectious agent may be diagnosed clinically. *H. influenzae* typically produces nonsuppurative preseptal cellulitis with a purplish discoloration and sharp

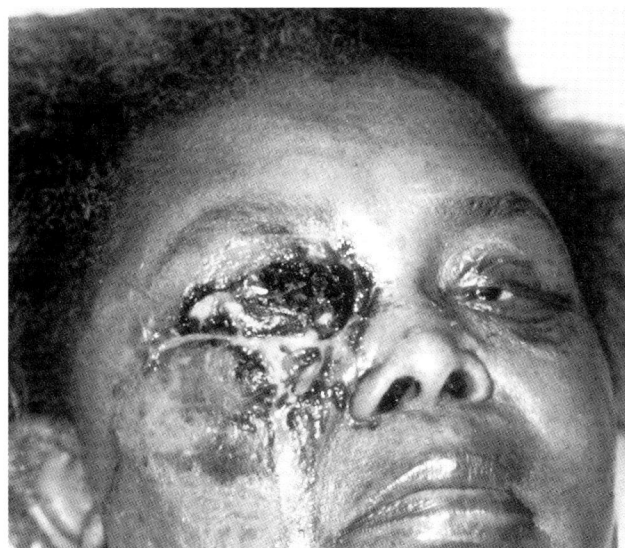

Figure 15-4 Necotizing fasciitis as a result of dacryocystorhinostomy surgery. Cultures grew group A β-hemolytic *Streptococcus*.

margins. Group A β-hemolytic streptococci may produce necrotizing cellulitis of the lids (Figure 15-4). Chemosis may occur as a result of edema caused by the inflammation. Proptosis, limited eye movement, and optic nerve dysfunction typically are not present and are considered signs of orbital cellulitis. Extraocular movements, proptosis, vision and color vision testing, determination of visual fields by confrontation, and tests for pupillary function therefore are important to differentiate preseptal cellulitis from orbital cellulitis.

Laboratory Tests and Imaging   Complete blood cell count, blood cultures, and computed tomographic (CT) scans of the orbits and sinuses are recommended in all cases. Cultures from the skin, sinuses, conjunctiva, nasopharynx, and cerebrospinal fluid usually are not indicated. CT scanning should be preformed using thin sections with axial and coronal views to exclude orbital cellulitis or a subperiosteal abscess. CT scanning demonstrates edema of the lids and periorbital soft tissue without orbital involvement in patients with oroseptal cellulitis. The sinuses may show evidence of acute or chronic sinusitis. Consultation with an otolaryngologist usually is advised if concurrent sinusitis or abscess formation is present.

Management After blood tests and nasal cultures are obtained, most patients with preseptal cellulitis are admitted for broad-spectrum parenteral antibiotic treatment. Most adult patients may be treated on an outpatient basis with an oral antibiotic and close monitoring. A CT scan should be obtained if any orbital involvement is suspected and if sinuses are the suspected source of infection. The antibiotic agent depends on patient age and infection site. Treatment may later be modified according to culture results and clinical response. Amoxicillin-clavulanate (Augmentin, 875 mg twice daily) is appropriate for empiric therapy. Close monitoring for signs of orbital involvement should be performed at least once a day.

ORBITAL CELLULITIS AND ABSCESS

Orbital cellulitis implies active infection of the retroseptal soft tissue of the orbit. The preseptal soft tissue also may be infected or secondarily inflamed. Orbital cellulitis is a serious condition that should be quickly diagnosed and treated to prevent associated morbidity and mortality.

The sinuses are the source of infection in 85% of cases.[60] The frequency of orbital complications from sinus infection ranges from 0.5% to 3.9%.[32] Children younger than 9 years of age represent 68% of cases; only 17% of cases occur in patients older than 15 years.[59]

Causes Orbital cellulitis is associated with paranasal sinusitis in 85% of cases. The ethmoid and maxillary sinuses are present from birth and are responsible for 57% to 75% of orbital cellulitis cases of sinus origin.[21,35] The frontal sinus is absent at birth and begins to develop at age 5 to 7 years. After its development the frontal sinus plays an equally significant role.[28,50] The sphenoid sinus is present at birth, but its clinical significance only occurs at more advanced ages. The proximity of the sphenoid sinus to the orbital apex produces clinical signs at an early stage.

Approximately 15% of orbital cellulitis occurs from other head and neck sources. Spread of the infection from contiguous dacryocystitis or preseptal cellulitis is a well-recognized cause of orbital cellulitis. Endophthalmitis may be complicated by orbital cellulitis, but this rarely occurs because the sclera acts as an effective barrier to extraocular spread of bacterial infections. Odontogenic infections, maxillary osteomyelitis, and dental work (specifically, dental extraction) are also well-known sources of orbital infection.[2,18,34] Trauma can cause orbital cellulitis by direct inoculation of the infection, promoting infection around a foreign body, or providing the normal flora of the nose and sinuses a direct route of entrance when a fracture is present.[32] Finally, the orbit may be

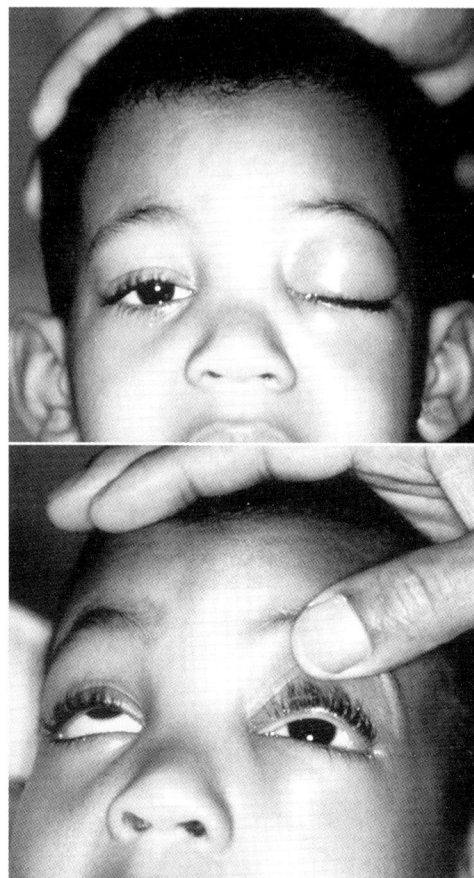

Figure 15-5 A, Orbital cellulitis manifests as swollen erythematous lids. **B,** Orbital cellulitis characterized by limited ocular movement, confirming the presence of an orbital process.

infected secondarily by hematogenous seeding of the infection from a remote source.

The organism presumed responsible for orbital cellulitis depends on patient age and cause of the infection. In children, most common organisms include *Staphylococcus aureus, Streptococcus* spp., and anaerobes. In adults, *S. aureus, Escherichia coli, Streptococcus pneumoniae,* and anaerobes are the most common organisms responsible for orbital cellulitis.[70] *H. influenzae* is a pathogen that occurs much less frequently in children since the development of the vaccination. Anaerobes are common with human or animal bites.

Symptoms and Signs Orbital cellulitis typically begins with painful swelling of the eyelid that is also erythematous and warm to the touch (Figure 15-5). Conjunctival chemosis is more common than preseptal cellulitis and usually is more severe, occasionally prolapsing through the orbital fissure (Figure 15-6). Lid swelling may be minimal in sphenoid sinusitis, which may manifest as a posterior orbital cellulitis and orbital apex syndrome. The classic signs that clinically distinguish orbital cellulitis from preseptal cellulitis include proptosis, limitation of ocular movements, pupillary dysfunction, and signs of optic nerve damage (decreased visual acuity, visual field loss,

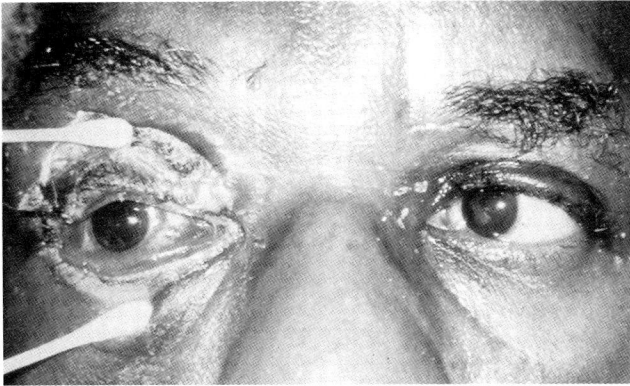

Figure 15-6 Orbital cellulitis is characterized by discharge, conjunctival chemosis, and proptosis.

problems with color vision, relative afferent papillary defect, and rarely optic nerve swelling demonstrated by funduscopy). Proptosis may be prominent enough to cause severe corneal exposure. The globe also may be displaced because of a subperiosteal or an orbital abscess. A dilated or nonreactive pupil is the result of damage to the oculomotor nerve or ciliary ganglion. Limited ocular movements may result from damage to the third, fourth, or sixth cranial nerves or mechanical restriction caused by muscle swelling or an abscess.

Signs of optic nerve decompensation are the result of increased orbital pressure with compression and stretching of the optic nerve caused by the anterior displacement of the globe (Figure 15-7). As the pressure within the orbit exceeds the perfusion pressure, ischemia to the optic nerve or the retina may result with permanent damage and even blindness. This represents an ophthalmic emergency that should be immediately addressed. Funduscopic examination may show signs of venous stasis, central retinal occlusion, optic nerve head edema, or choroidal folds. In rare cases the infection itself causes direct damage to the nerve tissue or septic thrombosis of the orbital vessels (usually with mucormycosis infection).

Systemic signs are nonspecific and cannot be used to differentiate orbital from preseptal cellulitis. These include fever, headache, leukocytosis, and bacteremia. Symptoms and signs of the condition that led to the development of orbital cellulitis (sinusitis, cellulitis, dental or ear infection, and trauma) also may be present.

Differential Diagnosis Orbital cellulitis should be distinguished from several conditions that appear in a similar manner. Preseptal cellulitis looks similar but does not include proptosis, ocular motility problems, optic nerve dysfunction, or pupillary abnormalities. A subperiosteal or orbital abscess is a radiologic diagnosis that cannot be based entirely on clinical grounds. Clues to the development of an abscess include globe displacement (by the mass effect of the abscess), limited ocular motility, insufficient response to antibiotic treatment, or worsening of local signs despite adequate treatment.

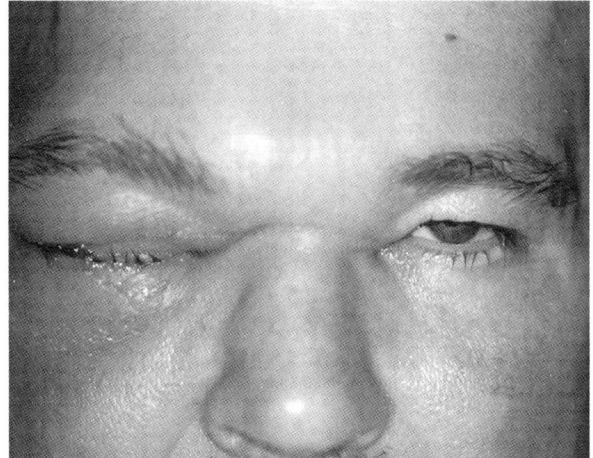
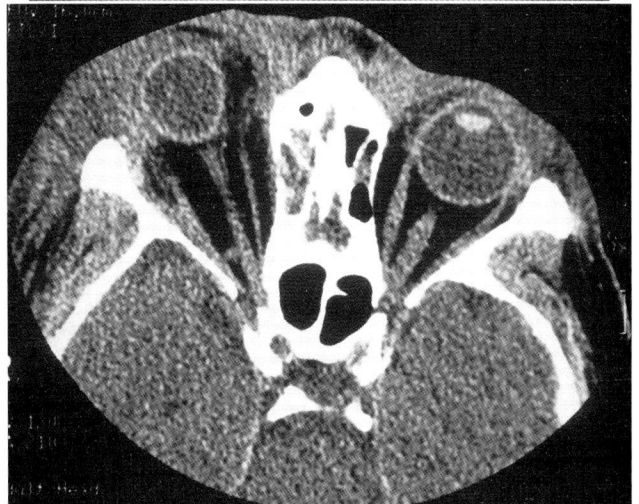
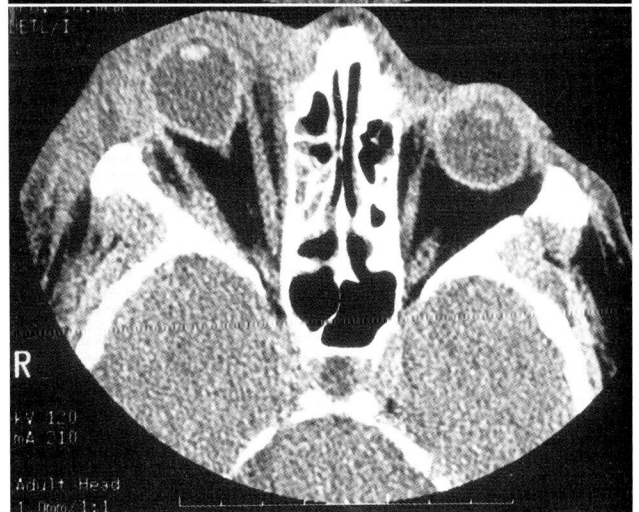

Figure 15-7 A, Orbital cellulitis in a middle-aged man with severe orbital cellulitis and swelling of the brow and temporal areas. The lids are very tense and painful. Complete ophthalmoplegia was present. **B,** CT scan of the same patient demonstrating the "stretched" optic nerve. **C,** CT scan shows severe proptosis and tenting of the posterior sclera. The optic nerve cannot stretch any farther, which causes tethering of the anteriorly displaced globe at the insertion of the optic nerve and distortion of the posterior sclera.

Cavernous sinus thrombosis may be present with the same signs and symptoms and sometimes can be differentiated from orbital cellulitis only by neuroimaging. Findings suggestive of cavernous sinus thrombosis include ophthalmoplegia disproportionate to the amount of proptosis, severe systemic findings, signs of central nervous system impairment, and bilateral involvement. Findings suggestive of orbital cellulitis include ocular adnexal tenderness and loss of vision.

Other conditions that may mimic orbital cellulitis are idiopathic orbital inflammation (orbital pseudotumor [Figure 15-8, *A*]), other inflammatory conditions (e.g., thyroid orbitopathy [Figure 15-8, *B*] and Wegener's granulomatosis [Figure 15-8, *C*]), orbital tumors with acute presentations (ruptured orbital dermoid cyst, lymphangioma, lymphoma, rhabdomyosarcoma [Figure 15-8, *D* and *E*]), orbital trauma or organic foreign bodies, acute carotid cavernous fistula (Figure 15-8, *F*), fungal orbital cellulitis (mucormycosis and aspergillosis), and rarely viral infections such as herpes zoster ophthalmicus.[61] During acute stages these conditions may be easily confused with orbital cellulitis.

Imaging   Routine imaging of every patient with an orbital infection is prudent. CT is the preferred method for

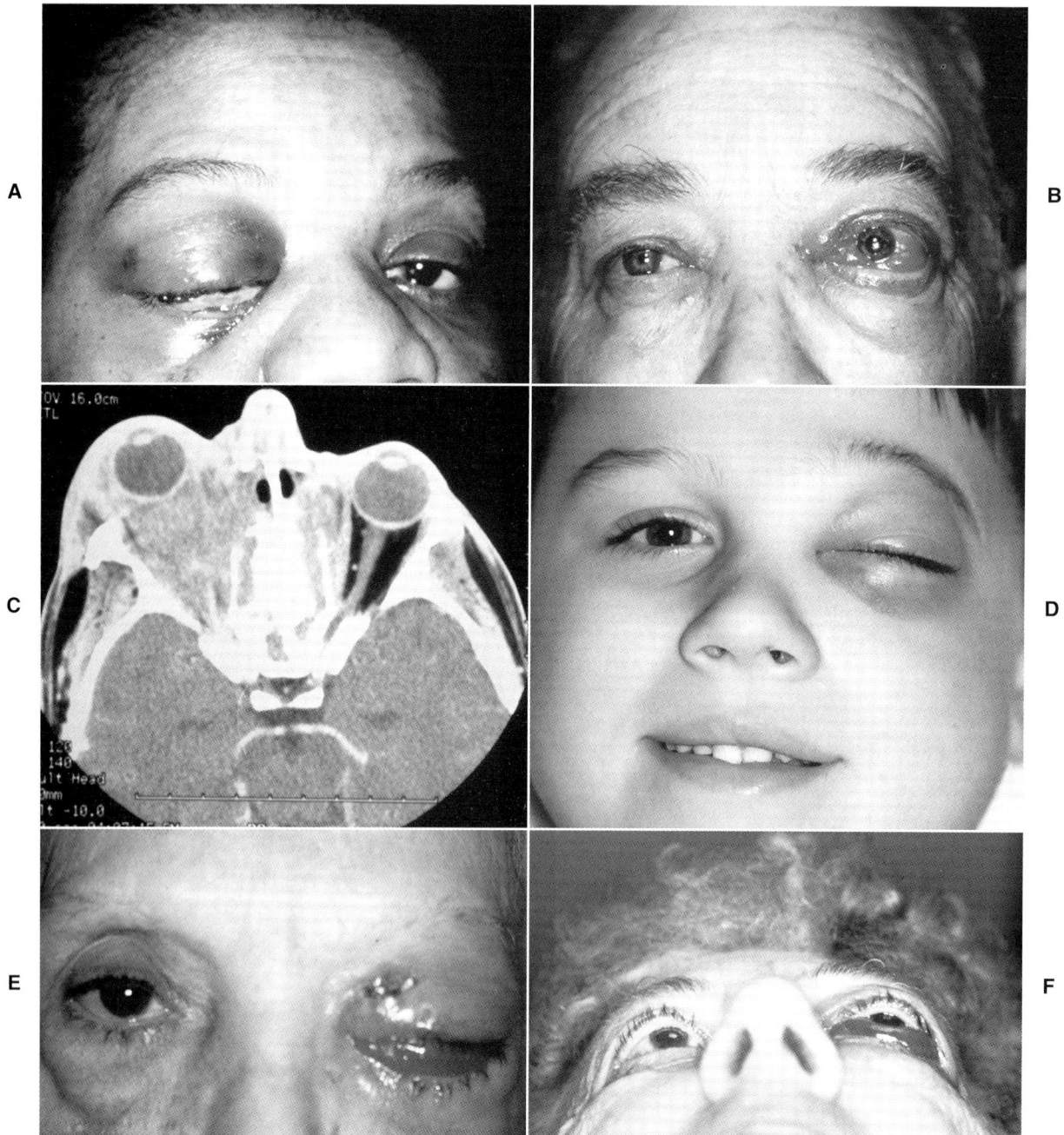

Figure 15-8 Conditions simulating orbital cellulitis. **A,** Idiopathic orbital inflammation. **B,** Thyroid orbitopathy. **C,** CT scan of a patient with Wegener's granulomatosis. **D,** A child with lymphangioma. **E,** Orbital lymphoma. **F,** Acute carotid cavernous fistula.

orbital imaging, but ultrasonography and magnetic resonance imaging (MRI) are indicted in specific conditions.

CT scanning should be performed with axial and coronal thin cuts (2 to 4 mm). CT's advantages include its capability to demonstrate the orbit, bones, sinuses, and brain, and its cost-effectiveness. With orbital cellulitis the eye may be proptotic and the orbital fat more intense compared with the other side (Figure 15-9). The extraocular muscles usually are normal but may be thickened. CT scanning can identify a subperiosteal abscess that is demonstrated as a convexity in the orbital periosteum with lower intensity than bone (Figure 15-10). CT usually cannot determine whether the subperiosteal fluid is pus, transudate, or blood. An orbital abscess is demonstrated as a mass with the peripheral ring enhanced with contrast. CT often can-

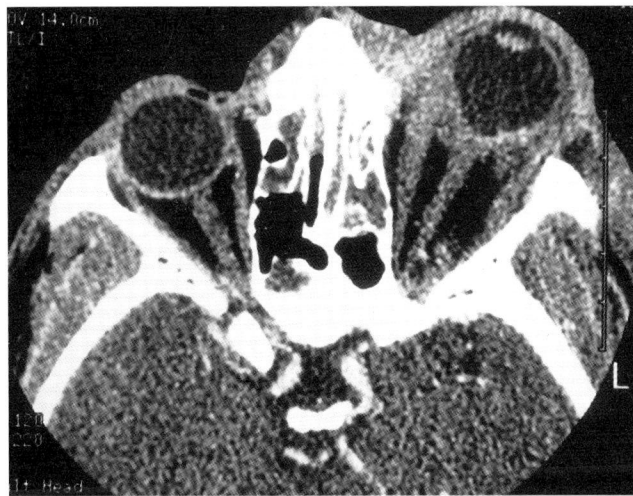

Figure 15-9 CT scan of a patient with orbital cellulitis demonstrating proptosis, ethmoid sinusitis, tenting of the posterior sclera, and increased intensity of the orbital fat on the left side.

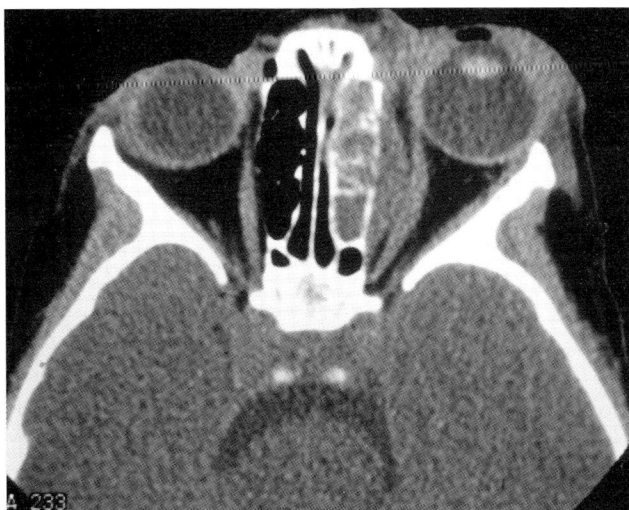

Figure 15-10 Subperiosteal abscess: CT scan of the orbits shows left ethmoidal sinusitis with collection of subperiosteal fluid along the medial wall. The displacement of the medial rectus muscle is caused by the mass effect.

not demonstrate an organic foreign body and is less accurate than MRI in demonstrating lesions in the area of the cavernous sinus.

MRI may show the soft tissue in preseptal cellulitis better than CT scanning and is superior to CT in demonstrating the cavernous sinus, orbital abscess, and organic foreign bodies. However, MRI is more expensive than CT, does not demonstrate the bones as well, and therefore has a limited role in orbital infections.

Ultrasonography provides better resolution than CT and performs well in demonstrating subperiosteal or orbital abscess in the anterior two thirds of the orbit.[37] Ultrasonography also is the most sensitive tool to demonstrate an organic foreign body. However, it has limited penetration and cannot image the posterior third of the orbit or the sinuses and therefore is seldom used.

Treatment The following management is recommended for all patients with orbital infections:

1. Hospital admission. Orbital infection is a potentially lethal infection that can cause rapid deterioration in a patient's condition, especially in small children. Close observation in a hospital setting is always recommended.
2. Performance of blood cultures and blood cell counts. Conjunctival and nasal cultures have limited value. A CT scan of the orbit and sinuses should be performed with thin axial and coronal cuts. Scans should be repeated to follow the patient's progress if no improvement occurs within 48 hours.
3. Initiation of intravenous broad-spectrum antimicrobial treatment. Current antibiotic recommendations include cefotaxime (50 mg/kg q6h IV) or ceftriaxone (50 mg/kg q6h IV). If anaerobic infection is suspected, clindamycin (40 mg/kg/day IV in three divided doses) may be added to the regimen. Treatment may be modified according to the culture result. Intravenous treatment is given for 10 to 14 days followed by oral treatment for a total of 3 weeks of antibiotics. Consultation with an infectious disease specialist is advisable.
4. Daily follow-up of the patient's general condition and vital signs, white blood cell count, lid edema, exophthalmometry, visual acuity, color vision, confrontation visual fields, ocular movements, and pupillary reaction.
5. Ancillary treatment, including pain control, nasal decongestants, warm compresses, and head elevation to reduce swelling.

Several points merit special attention. If no improvement is evident within 48 hours of appropriate treatment or worsening occurs, the clinician should repeat imaging to look for an abscess, a cavernous sinus thrombosis, or a brain abscess. The antibiotic coverage should be reevaluated and cultures repeated. Biopsy sampling of the nose or sinuses should be considered to rule out mucormycosis and other atypical pathological conditions.

Treatment of a subperiosteal abscess is controversial. In the past, immediate drainage of all abscesses was recommended. In recent years, several authors demonstrated that medical treatment of a subperiosteal abscess as a result of sinusitis is effective and can replace surgery in children younger than 6 years of age.[27,28,54,58] However, all authors agree that a subperiosteal abscess that does not respond to medical treatment should be drained surgically.[27,28,54,58] Drainage may be performed by a transcutaneous or transconjunctival approach; or more recently through the nose using an endoscope. Drainage of the infected sinus or an odontogenic abscess sometimes is sufficient and precludes the need for entry to the orbit.

Clinical information regarding the role of steroids in the treatment of orbital cellulitis is limited. Many clinicians routinely use steroids in cases of orbital cellulitis; 1 mg/kg of prednisone starting 24 hours after initiation of antibiotic is an appropriate dose. Inflammation with edema as a result of infection plays a major role in the development of ocular complications because of its effect on intraorbital pressure. Steroids significantly reduce the intraorbital pressure and lid edema and are safe when given simultaneously with antibiotics.

Signs of optic nerve dysfunction represent a medical emergency. Irreversible damage to neural tissue may begin minutes after signs of visual loss are present. Elevated intraorbital pressure with optic nerve compression is the main problem in most cases. The orbital content cannot expand to the sides because the orbital walls are bony and noncompliant. The canthal tendons and orbital septum limit the forward displacement of the orbital contents. Emergency lateral canthotomy and cantholysis may allow forward movement of the orbital contents and thus cause reduction in the orbital pressure. The procedure can be done at the bedside with minimal instrumentation and preparation, but this approach often is inadequate and the patient should be taken to the operating room for additional decompression. If CT scanning clearly demonstrates an orbital or subperiosteal abscess, it can be drained through a transcutaneous or an endoscopic approach. If no drainable abscess exists, bony decompression is the only option to save vision. Transnasal endoscopic medial wall decompression is preferred in these patients because the edema usually is so severe that a cutaneous or transconjunctival approach is technically difficult. Removal of the bone is not sufficient to achieve decompression. The periosteum (periorbita) also is noncompliant and if it is not opened widely, the intraorbital pressure remains elevated. Once the periorbita is opened, the orbital fat can be seen prolapsing into the sinus. This should be the endpoint of the procedure.

Complications   Complications of orbital cellulitis include cavernous sinus thrombosis, meningitis, subdural, dural and brain abscesses, carotid occlusion, and death. These complications are rare with the improvement of antibiotic regimens and imaging techniques, but all have been reported.* Ocular complications include permanent

visual loss, limitation in ocular movements, diplopia, severe corneal exposure with development of corneal ulcers, corneal scars, and even corneal perforation. Scleral rupture as a result of elevated intraocular and orbital pressure also has been reported.[23] Deformities in the lid and enophthalmos are potential complications in surgical cases.

INVASIVE FUNGAL ORBITAL INFECTIONS

Invasive fungal orbital cellulitis is the most acutely fatal fungal infection in humans. It almost always occurs as part of an extensive infectious process involving the sinuses and adjustment structures. The most common pathogens causing this infection are members of the family Mucoraceae *(Rhizopus, Mucor, and Absidia),* and the infection is referred to as *rhinoorbital-cerebral mucormycosis* (ROCM). *Aspergillus* spp. also are reported as pathogens causing orbital cellulitis and are difficult to differentiate from mucormycosis, especially in patients with an underlying systemic condition.

Underlying Conditions   ROCM almost exclusively affects patients with well-recognized immunological or metabolic abnormalities, but rare cases have been reported in healthy individuals.[5,22,36,57] The major predisposing factor for development of ROCM is diabetes mellitus, accounting for more than 60% of cases in most series.[71] Patients with uncontrolled diabetes with hyperglycemia and ketoacidosis have an especially high risk of developing ROCM. Renal disease (primarily renal failure and renal transplantation) is responsible for as many as 14% of cases.[71] An association between desferoxamine therapy for iron or aluminum excess also has been described in patients with renal failure and other conditions.[63] Another group of patients at risk for developing ROCM includes patients with malignancy (especially hematological malignancies), leukopenia, those receiving corticosteroid therapy or immunosuppressive drugs, and recently, those infected with human immunodeficiency virus.[44] An extensive list of other conditions has been associated with ROCM, including infectious disease (tuberculosis, typhoid fever, hepatitis, amebic dysentery, and viral myocarditis), autoimmune diseases (lupus erythematosus, polyarthritis nodosa, sarcoidosis), chronic systemic diseases (hepatic failure, cirrhosis, aplastic anemia, Fanconi's anemia, kwashiorkor), and acute conditions (trauma, severe burns, dehydration, diarrhea).[71]

Several reasons have been suggested for the increased frequency of mucormycosis in these inpatients. The use of antibiotics, steroids, immunosuppressive and antineoplastic drugs, along with the increased longevity of patients who are debilitated, have been identified as a few of the predisposing factors.[68]

Pathogenesis   Classic ROCM is believed to be spread by aerosol transmission of spores and typically begins in the nasal or oral mucosa. From the paranasal sinuses, ROCM spreads into the orbits or cranial cavity, a process greatly facilitated by the organism's propensity to invade blood

*References 8, 12, 17, 21, 23, 28, 32, 35, 53, 54, 60.

vessels, notably arteries, and to propagate within vessel walls and lumens. Ischemic infarctions of the tissue normally supplied by the affected vessels become superimposed on septic necrosis. Orbital symptoms result from ischemia to the cranial nerves of the orbit and orbital content. Blindness results from occlusion of the central retinal artery or ischemia to the optic nerve. Death occurs from disease extension into the brain and fungal invasion of cerebral arteries leading to occlusions, rupture, and hemorrhage.[22,33]

Initial Signs and Symptoms   Recognition of the early signs and symptoms in ROCM is important in initiation of early treatment and thus offers the patient a better chance of survival. The black eschar on the skin or mucosa that is so suggestive of mucormycosis is found at presentation only in one fifth of patients and therefore is not a reliable early indicator. Signs and symptoms at presentation include fever (44%), nasal mucosal ulceration (38%), periorbital and facial swelling (34%), decreased vision (30%), ophthalmoplegia (29%), sinusitis (22%), headache (25%), facial pain (22%), and change in mental status (22%).[71]

Ophthalmic Signs and Symptoms   Orbital signs are the result of ischemic necrosis of the intraorbital cranial nerves, orbital blood vessels, and orbital content. With full-blown disease, ophthalmic signs and symptoms include external ophthalmoplegia (67%) and often total ophthalmoplegia. Other signs include vision loss (65%), proptosis (64%), periorbital edema (43%), internal ophthalmoplegia (40%), afferent pupillary defect (38%), trigeminal hypoesthesia (28%), and less frequently, chemosis, central retinal artery occlusion, periorbital pain, periorbital necrosis, orbital abscess, and optic disc edema.[71] Characteristic presentations include unilateral orbital apex syndrome with pain or signs of orbital cellulitis associated with early vision loss caused by central retinal artery occlusion.

Nonocular Signs and Symptoms   Necrosis of nasal (48%) or oral (32%) mucosa is the most common finding in patients with full-blown disease. Palatal lesions account for most of the oral lesions. Necrotic lesions typically are dark red to black and bleed minimally during biopsy (ischemic necrosis). Sinusitis is present in 79% of patients. Fever, mental status changes, facial swelling, and pain are present in approximately one third of patients. Less common signs include facial numbness, facial paralysis, facial necrosis, nasal discharge, epistaxis, reduced hearing, hemiplegia, and internal carotid occlusion.

Diagnosis   Early diagnosis is important in the management of ROCM; therefore a high index of clinical suspicion is required. ROCM should be suspected in every patient who is at risk of developing ROCM or who has orbital signs or symptoms suggestive of nasal or sinus disease. A thorough clinical examination of the mouth, nose, and sinuses is vital. Biopsies of every suspected lesion

should be performed to confirm the diagnosis. Because ROCM has been reported in healthy individuals and as the initial sign in some patients unaware of any underlying disease, the possibility of ROCM should be considered in all patients, irrespective of immune status, in the following clinical situations: orbital cellulitis unresponsive to antibiotics, mixed cranial nerve palsies, and retinal or orbital infarction. Distinction of orbital mucormycosis from bacterial orbital cellulitis or cavernous sinus thrombosis sometimes is difficult. Early visual loss and retinal artery occlusion favor a diagnosis of ROCM over bacterial cavernous sinus thrombosis, in which blindness is a much later finding.[8,36,42,46]

Imaging   Imaging studies with CT or MRI of the orbits, sinuses, and brain should be obtained to determine the presence of sinus disease and the extent of the disease. CT scans typically demonstrate mucosal thickening without air-fluid levels. Bone destruction is a late manifestation and can lead to spread of the infection into the pterygoid or infratemporal fossa or parapharyngeal space.[24] The orbital cellulitis caused by mucormycosis is indistinguishable from other kinds of orbital cellulitis. The intracranial extension appears as low-density masses with variable peripheral enhancement.

MRI may show hyperintense signals from the thickened mucosa on proton density and T2-weighted images. Orbital fat invasion and soft tissue of the face is seen best with proton density–weighted images. Absence of flow void in the orbital and cranial vessels may be demonstrated and reflects the septic thrombosis in the arteries.[55]

Biopsy   Biopsy specimens should be sent for fresh tissue preparation, frozen sections, and permanent sections. Fresh tissue specimens should be inoculated directly onto the culture media to avoid excessive specimen chopping or grinding, which can damage the hyphae and render the fungi nonviable, resulting in false-negative culture findings.[15,31] For diagnosis of mucormycosis, large branching, nonseptate hyphae should be identified in the tissue specimen on hematoxylin-eosin staining or methenamine silver staining. Fresh tissue preparation uses 10% or 20% potassium hydroxide. Septal fungal hyphae of relatively uniform width are diagnostic of aspergillosis. Multiple biopsies and biopsy of the transitional zone between necrotic and normal tissue are recommended to increase the biopsy yield. If biopsy of only the necrotic tissue is performed, the fungus may not be identified. The presence of blood vessels in the biopsy specimen also helps to increase the yield of the test.

Treatment   Proper treatment for mucormycosis requires early diagnosis, reversal of the underlying condition (when possible), aggressive local surgical debridement, and intravenous amphotericin B therapy. Control of diabetic ketoacidosis, hyperglycemia, or other metabolic acidosis and discontinuation of steroids or other immunosuppressive drugs can establish a better immune state and improve the chance of survival.

Wide surgical excision of all necrotic tissue is critical for survival. Ideally, tissue should be removed until normal bleeding is encountered. The delivery of antifungal therapy is dependent on normal perfusion; therefore all necrotic tissue should be removed. This is not always possible because infection can invade dura and brain tissue. In addition to conventional surgical debridement, endoscopic sinus approaches in the management of mucormycosis have been reported.[3]

Invasion of the orbit poses a difficult dilemma to the surgeon. Exenteration (complete removal of the eye and orbital content) may be lifesaving by decreasing the total fungal load even after intracranial extension of the infection, but patients (and surgeons) are reluctant to undergo exenteration. Exenteration should be considered for a blind, immobile eye. Exenteration may be deferred in a seeing eye unless extensive fungal invasion of the orbit can be demonstrated. No controlled studies exist, but reports of survival without exenteration do exist.[43] Some authors recommend frozen section–guided surgical debridement to avoid wide exenteration.[45]

Intravenous amphotericin B is the treatment of choice for mucormycosis. Amphotericin B therapy should be initiated gradually in an increasing dosage. A single daily dose of up to 0.7 to 1.0 mg/kg is recommended if tolerated. Liposomal amphotericin may result in increased efficacy. Amphotericin B encapsulated in liposomes significantly decreases toxicity, allowing administration of higher dosages. Liposomal encapsulation appears to enhance delivery to fungi, infected organs, and phagocytes. Some authors report excellent results by adding daily amphotericin irrigation and packing of affected orbit and sinuses (1 mg/mL).[43] This likely aids the delivery of amphotericin B to poorly perfused infected and necrotic tissue.

Several small studies demonstrated increased survival using hyperbaric oxygen therapy in addition to conventional therapy, but the role of this treatment is still uncertain. Despite many advances in diagnosis and treatment, individuals with ROCM still have a high mortality rate that varies from 15% to 34%, but this is a significant improvement compared with reports from 1961 when the mortality rate was 88%.[8,20]

SEPTIC CAVERNOUS SINUS THROMBOSIS

Cavernous sinus thrombosis may occur as a complication of infectious and noninfectious processes. The infectious type is also called septic cavernous sinus thrombosis. This condition is a serious, life-threatening state with a mortality rate of up to 30%.[17]

Causes   Areas drained by the cavernous sinus include the orbit, paranasal sinuses, anterior mouth, and middle portion of the face. Several infectious processes predispose a patient to develop cavernous sinus thrombosis, including infections of the soft tissue of the face (especially the middle third). They are the most common foci associated with this serious complication.[17,29] The infection spreads to the cav-

ernous sinus through the pterygoid plexus or superficially through the facial and ophthalmic veins. Gram-positive organisms (specifically *S. aureus*) are usually the pathogens in this setting.[66,67] Acute or chronic ethmoid or sphenoid sinusitis is another common cause of cavernous sinus thrombosis.[12,38,64] Gram-positive organisms (*S. aureus* and streptococci) are more common with acute sinusitis, whereas gram-negative rods, coagulase-negative staphylococci, Aspergilli, and Mucoraceae are more common with chronic sinusitis resulting in cavernous sinus thrombosis.[39]

Dental infections cause approximately 10% of septic cavernous sinus thrombosis. Maxillary teeth usually are the infectious source, and streptococci, fusobacteria, and *Bacteroides* spp. are the common pathogens.[53]

Dissemination of orbital cellulitis is another potential source of cavernous sinus thrombosis. Although the superior ophthalmic vein drains directly into the cavernous sinus, orbital cellulitis rarely progresses to involve this structure.[56] Otitis media once was considered a common cause of cavernous sinus thrombosis but is a rare cause since the availability of antibiotics.

Symptoms and Signs   Cavernous sinus thrombosis is a severe disease with local and systemic signs. It usually starts as a unilateral process but later may progress to the contralateral side. The patient appears toxic and may have headache, nausea, giddiness, vomiting, and somnolence. Fever usually is present. If the disease progresses, signs of meningitis or brain abscess may occur. Associated signs of sinusitis orbital cellulitis and suppurative gingivitis may be present. Leukocytosis usually is present, and the organism often can be isolated from the blood.

Local congestive ocular signs usually are present. Chemosis and proptosis occur in almost all cases. Eyelid edema, particularly of the upper lid, is prominent. The upper lid may be swollen and ptotic and may obscure the ophthalmoplegia. The abducens nerve, which is the only nerve that runs in the cavernous sinus cavity and not in the wall, usually is affected first. Involvement of the oculomotor, trochlear, and sensory trigeminal nerve soon follows. The increasing venous stasis within the orbit causes edema and mechanical restrictions of extraocular movement that add to the paralytic ophthalmoplegia. Funduscopic examination may reveal venous dilation of the retinal vessels, but retinal hemorrhages usually are absent.

Visual loss is uncommon but may result from central retinal artery occlusion, ophthalmic vein occlusion, thrombosis of the carotid artery, or ischemic optic neuropathy. In some cases, septic cavernous sinus thrombosis may have a more chronic course and manifest with fewer signs of congestion. Chronic sphenoid sinusitis is present in most cases; an isolated abducens paresis is the most common neurological sign.

Cavernous sinus thrombosis, orbital apex syndrome, superior orbital fissure syndrome, and superior ophthalmic vein thrombosis are four entities with significant clinical overlap. *Superior orbital fissure syndrome* refers to a process (infection, inflammation, tumor, trauma, vascular) that af-

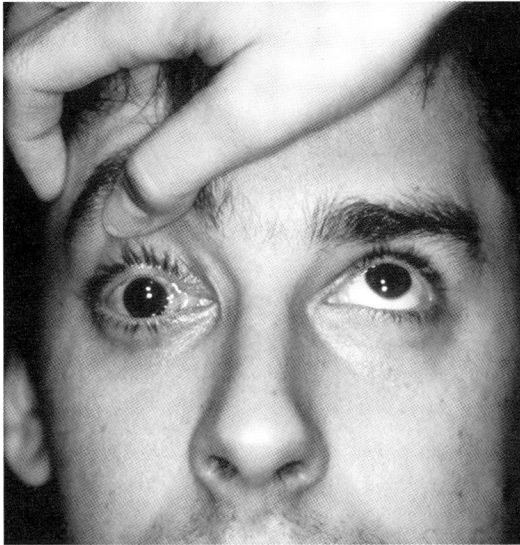

Figure 15-11 Orbital apex syndrome characterized by ptosis, complete ophthalmoplegia, decreased vision, and a nonreactive dilated pupil on the right.

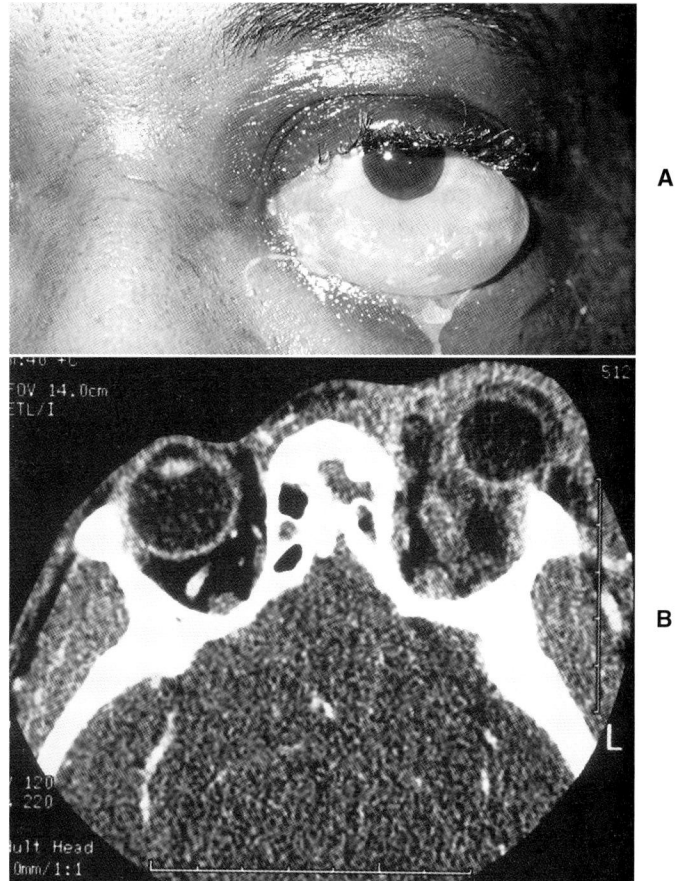

A

B

Figure 15-12 A, Superior ophthalmic vein thrombosis in a young male patient who initially had left proptosis ophthalmoplegia and severe conjunctival chemosis. **B,** Orbital CT scans of the same patient with contrast media. The superior ophthalmic vein on the right shows contrast media and normal diameter. A dilated superior ophthalmic vein with absence of contrast media is demonstrated on the left.

fects all three branches of the ophthalmic (first) division of the trigeminal nerve, the sympathetic nerves of the eye, and one or more of the cranial nerves that move the eye or eyelid (oculomotor, trochlear, and abducens nerves). Proptosis is usually present. *Orbital apex syndrome* is similar to that of the superior orbital fissure but the optic nerve also is involved (Figure 15-11). *Superior ophthalmic vein thrombosis* appears similar, but the superior ophthalmic vein also is involved and signs of congestion are more prominent (Figure 15-12).

Because of the anatomical proximity of the orbital apex, superior orbital fissure, and cavernous sinus, every process that affects the area—infectious or otherwise—may spread rapidly between these anatomical locations. Although some clinical and radiological characteristics may distinguish these syndromes, the differentiation has little clinical importance. Sphenocavernous syndrome was proposed as a collective term to describe all these syndromes. Although the infection in all cases is treated similarly, two special treatment considerations are important. (1) Whenever signs of optic nerve impairment are present, rapid intervention is needed. (2) When thrombosis is present in the superior ophthalmic vein or cavernous sinus, anticoagulant treatment should be considered.

Orbital cellulitis and cavernous sinus thrombosis can have similar signs and symptoms, and differentiation between them sometimes is impossible on clinical bases alone. Findings suggestive of cavernous sinus thrombosis include bilateral disease, ophthalmoplegia disproportionate to the amount of proptosis, severe systemic findings, and signs of central nervous system impairment. Findings suggestive of orbital cellulitis or apex syndrome include ocular adnexal tenderness and loss of vision. Neuroimaging with CT, MRI, or magnetic resonance angiography may help distinguish these entities.

Management A combination of intravenous antibiotics, anticoagulants, and surgery is the optimal treatment for septic cavernous sinus thrombosis. Wide spectrum intravenous antimicrobial treatment is indicated as an initial treatment in all cases. An infectious disease specialist should be consulted. Antibiotic therapy may be altered after preliminary culture results. Parenteral administration of antibiotics should be continued until clinical improvement is evident. Oral antibiotic therapy then may be initiated for a total course of 3 weeks. Anticoagulant therapy with heparin ideally is started early in the disease course if no contraindications exist. The primary site of infection may require early drainage, especially when acute sinusitis is the cause of the infection. Transnasal endoscopy is the preferred approach. Exploration of the cavernous sinus itself is rarely indicated.

Prognosis Before the antibiotic era, all cases of cavernous sinus thrombosis resulted in death. The mortality rate since the availability of antibiotic treatment is approximately 30%. Half of all survivors have morbid sequelae, including sensory visual impairment, diplopia, and neurotrophic keratitis (as a result of sensory deficiency).

DACRYOCYSTITIS

Dacryocystitis is a bacterial infection of the lacrimal sac and the adjacent soft tissue that usually is associated with complete obstruction of the lower lacrimal drainage system. Chronic tear stasis and retention leads to secondary infection with bacteria. The obstruction is at the level of the lacrimal sac, the nasolacrimal duct (NLD; most common type), or the nose. NLD obstruction is classified into congenial NLD obstruction, primary acquired NLD obstruction, and secondary NLD obstruction. Secondary causes include midface trauma involving the NLD, surgical trauma to the NLD or sac, granulomatous processes of the lacrimal sac (primarily sarcoidosis or Wegener's granulomatosis), tumors of the lacrimal sac, nasal polyps, nasal mucosal scarring, deviation of the nasal septum, allergies, and infections of the nasal mucosa. Ectopic teeth have been reported as a cause of NLD obstruction.[1]

Organisms isolated from patients with dacryocystitis resemble those of the normal conjunctival flora. A single organism is present in most cases, but mixed infection is responsible for at least one third of cases. Gram-positive organisms (primarily *Staphylococcus epidermidis* and *S. aureus*) are the most common pathogens. Gram-negative organisms and streptococci also are common and have a higher incidence in chronic dacryocystitis. Anaerobic organisms are recovered from 7% to 11% of isolates, and fungal infections represent less than 5% of cases.[9,13,30]

Symptoms, Signs, and Diagnosis   Dacryocystitis begins as an acute painful swelling in the medial canthal area (Figure 15-13, *A*). Most of the lacrimal sac is located inferior to the medial canthal tendon; therefore the swelling is more prominent at the most medial aspect of the lower lid. Purulent discharge from the eye and tearing may be present. A fistula to the skin may develop over the infected sac (Figure 15-13, *B*). In chronic dacryocystitis, intermittent swelling, tearing, and discharge from the eye are present. Systemic signs usually are absent unless the disease has progressed to preseptal or orbital cellulitis.

In the acute phase the diagnosis of dacryocystitis is made on the basis of clinical findings. Painful swelling occurs at the anatomical area of the lacrimal sac (inferior to the medial canthal tendon) with or without mucopurulent discharge from the eye. Pus may be regurgitated from the puncti when pressure is applied to the sac, but this is painful and usually not necessary to make the diagnosis. In the more chronic phase when pain and swelling are absent, this test is more useful. The material that is pushed out the sac in chronic dacryocystitis is mucoid or mucopurulent. Irrigation and probing of the canalicular system is not recommended until resolution of the acute infection. Irrigation sometimes is necessary to demonstrate obstruction of the NLD in the more chronic stage. When

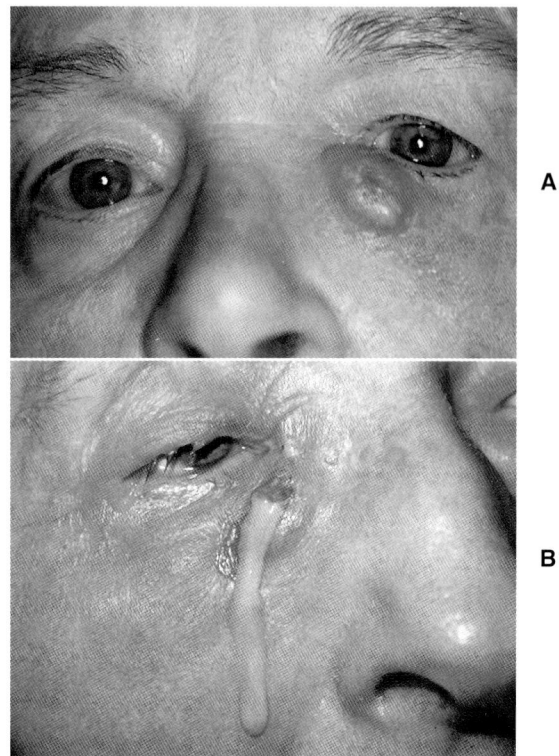

Figure 15-13 A, Acute dacryocystitis. **B,** A fistula from the infected lacrimal sac to the skin with drainage of pus.

tearing is the main symptom a complete ophthalmic evaluation is necessary because NLD obstruction is only one of numerous causes of tearing.

Treatment   Acute dacryocystitis should be treated with systemic antibiotics. Oral antibiotic therapy is of value in most cases, but in more severe infections parenteral antibiotics are necessary. Topical treatments with antibiotic drops and ointments have limited value. If a large abscess is present or when the infection is localized to a point, incision and drainage of the abscess is indicated. The material drained should be sent for culturing and Gram staining, and the incision should be left open to heal by secondary intention. Warm compresses may be applied to the area.

A surgical procedure should always be performed after the acute phase if necessary. Recurrence of acute dacryocystitis is likely without surgical bypass of the obstruction. The surgical procedure of choice depends on the patient's age and cause of infection. In congenital NLD obstruction, irrigation and probing of the lower lacrimal system with or without placement of silicone tubes is performed. In adult patients with complete obstruction a dacryocystorhinostomy is the procedure of choice. Dacryocystectomy (excision of the lacrimal sac) may be preformed at the bedside in patients who are poor surgical candidates.

Periorbital cellulitis often complicates the course of acute dacryocystitis. Complications such as orbital cellulitis, cavernous sinus thrombosis, or brain abscess rarely occur.[52]

ALLERGIC FUNGAL SINUSITIS

Allergic fungal sinusitis is characterized by recurrent sinusitis, eosinophilia, and increased immunoglobulin E level. Patients are typically immunocompetent, young, and have a history of asthma and nasal polyposis.[10,35] Allergic fungal sinusitis accounts for 7% of patients with chronic sinusitis.[41] *Aspergillus* spp. once were considered the most common pathogen, but recent studies have shown that dematiaceous fungi *(Bipolaris, Exserohilum, Curvularia, Alternaria)* are more common.[7,14,48]

Symptoms and Signs   Orbital signs have been reported in 17% of patients with allergic fungal sinusitis and are the result of sinus cavity expansion or extension of the inflammatory processes beyond the boundaries of the sinuses.[14] The fungal infection itself is a noninvasive process as opposed to invasive fungal infection in patients who are immunocompromised.

Ocular symptoms in allergic fungal sinusitis include diplopia, proptosis, droopy eyelid, epiphora, and periorbital swelling. Anecdotal cases of visual loss also have been reported in the literature.[9a,12a]

Diagnosis   Recognition of allergic fungal sinusitis and differentiation from chronic bacterial sinusitis and other forms of fungal sinusitis is important because the treatments and prognoses for these disorders vary significantly. Preoperative diagnosis is based on clinical suspicion. A history of asthma in immunocompetent patient, an elevated total immunoglobulin E level, a positive result of a skin test or radioallergosorbent test to fungal antigens, unilateral predominance, and the presence of nasal polyps are all clues to the diagnosis. Imaging studies show certain characteristic findings. On CT scan, allergic fungal sinusitis appears as soft tissue lesion with heterogeneous opacification of the sinuses. Serpiginous areas of increased attenuation typically present in the sinus are considered ferromagnetic elements from fungi. Bone erosion is common. On MRI scans the T1-weighted images reveal a lesion that is isointense or slightly hypointense, and on T2-weighted images the lesion is significantly hypointense.[7] The lesion enhances with contrast agents. Pathological examination uniformly reveals eosinophilic mucus without fungal invasion into soft tissue; fungi are always identified on fungal smear. Culture results usually are positive.[7]

Treatment   Surgical debridement of the involved sinus is recommended. Treatment with drainage alone commonly results in recurrence. Treatment with systemic and local steroids for 3 to 6 months is recommended to prevent recurrence. Orbital symptoms always respond to this treatment, and orbital surgery is not indicated.[11]

SIMULTANEOUS INFECTIONS OF THE EYE, HEAD, AND NECK

With simultaneous infections the eye is primarily infected with a pathogen that also affects other sites in the head and neck. Patients usually are first seen by an ophthalmologist but occasionally may be seen initially by other surgeons who should recognize the ophthalmic condition and treat it appropriately in conjunction with the ophthalmologist.

PHARYNGEAL CONJUNCTIVAL FEVER

Pharyngeal conjunctival fever is a common contagious ocular adenoviral infection consisting of pharyngitis, fever, and nonpurulent follicular conjunctivitis. The usual cause is adenovirus type 3. The disease primarily affects children between 4 and 9 years of age. The follicular conjunctivitis usually is bilateral and a preauricular lymph node is present. Subconjunctival hemorrhages may be present and corneal involvement is rare. The infection usually resolves spontaneously within 1 to 3 weeks.

CONJUNCTIVITIS ASSOCIATED WITH POSITIVE LYMPH NODE FINDINGS

The medial conjunctiva drains to the submandibular lymph nodes, whereas the lateral conjunctiva drains to the preauricular lymph nodes. These lymph nodes may become enlarged and painful during the course of a conjunctival infection. Infectious conjunctivitis infections that commonly affect a lymph node include adenovirus conjunctivitis (epidemic keratoconjunctivitis), herpes simplex keratoconjunctivitis, chlamydial conjunctivitis, and gonococcal conjunctivitis. In all these infections the lymph node is tender to palpation but usually remains small. The diagnosis is made on the basis of clinical and laboratory findings. Gonococci infection and herpes simplex conjunctivitis are important because both may cause vision-threatening complications.

PARINAUD'S OCULOGLANDULAR CONJUNCTIVITIS

Parinaud's oculoglandular conjunctivitis a unilateral, granulomatous conjunctivitis associated with an ipsilateral, visible, preauricular, or submandibular lymph node. Fever or other systemic signs may or may not be present. The lymph node may progress to suppuration. The condition is self-limiting and usually resolves within several weeks.

Parinaud's oculoglandular conjunctivitis has no specific origin. A variety of infectious agents may cause this syndrome, but the most common, and the first described by Parinaud, is cat-scratch disease. In cat-scratch disease, most patients have a history of exposure to a cat and a skin or other mucous membrane lesion is present. Unilateral conjunctivitis develops 1 to 2 weeks after exposure. The typical conjunctival lesion is a granulomatous nodule surrounded by follicles on the palpebral conjunctiva of the upper or lower lid. Regional lymphadenopathy is present in all cases of cat-scratch disease. The node is firm, nontender, and may be as large a golf ball. Progression to suppuration occurs in 10% of cases. When systemic signs are present, they usually are mild. The course is benign with spontaneous recovery within 2 to 3 months. The diagnosis is suspected in a patient with typical clinical findings and an appropriate history. Laboratory tests to support the diagnosis include serological tests for *Bartonella henselae,* skin tests (Hanger-Rose test), conjunctival biopsy demonstrating a granuloma with epithelioid cells with or without the gram-negative bacilli, and lately, a positive conjunctival culture result. Treatment with erythromycin, doxycycline, trimethoprim and sulfamethoxazole, rifampin, or ciprofloxacin usually is effective, although the disease is self-limited and spontaneously resolves. Aspiration of the lymph node is indicated only if pain is severe or material is needed for skin testing. Other bacterial infections that may cause similar signs and are considered part of Parinaud's ocular glandular syndrome include tularemia and tuberculosis.[26]

HERPES ZOSTER OPHTHALMICUS

Herpes zoster infections of the eye may occur as part of chickenpox during childhood but usually are very mild at that stage. Infections that develop through reactivation of the virus in older individuals or immunocompromised patients with eye involvement are dangerous because they can cause significant ocular morbidity. Zoster manifests as painful vesicular dermatitis localized to a dermatome supplied by a spinal or cranial sensory ganglion. When the ophthalmic branch of the trigeminal nerve is affected, the condition is termed *herpes zoster ophthalmicus* (regardless of whether the eye is involved). The eye is affected in 70% of cases of herpes zoster ophthalmicus and should always be examined by an ophthalmologist even if no symptoms are present. Every part of the eye may be involved in the infection. Cellulitis, keratitis, scleritis, anterior and posterior uveitis, acute retinal necrosis, optic neuritis, orbital cellulitis, and orbital apex syndrome are well-known complications of herpes zoster (Figure 15-14, *A*). Even when the eye is not affected, the secondary scarring of the skin can cause severe ocular complications. These include cicatricial ectropion, trichiasis, and lid retraction with severe corneal exposure (Figure 15-14, *B*). Tearing, chronic conjunctivitis, ocular irritation, and postherpetic neuralgia can be major problems in addition to the cosmetic appearance. Oral acyclovir therapy decreases the severity and duration of most ocular symptoms. Acyclovir treatment (800 mg five times a day for 10 days starting 72 hours from the beginning of skin lesions) should be initiated whenever possible. Steroid eye drops may be given in selected cases. Oral steroid therapy may prevent postherpetic neuralgia. Surgery to the eyelids sometimes is necessary to correct ectropion and lid retraction.

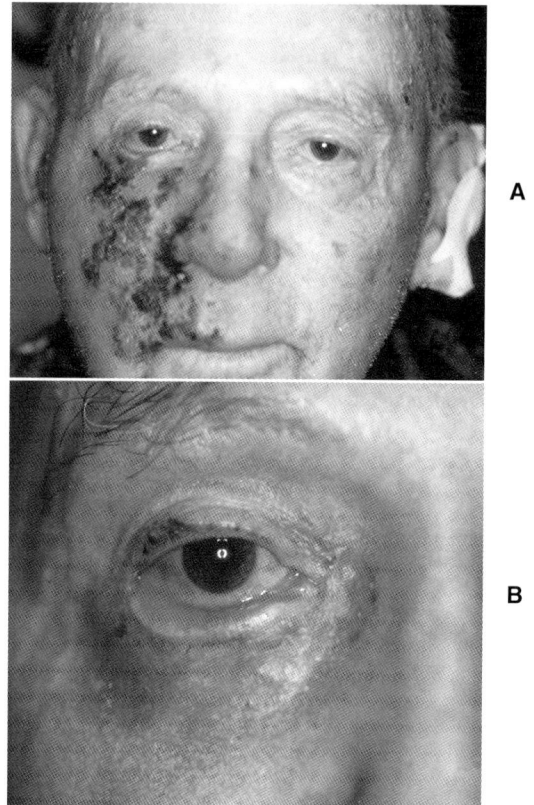

Figure 15-14 A, Herpes zoster ophthalmicus with secondary bacterial infection in the distribution of the second branch of the trigeminal nerve. The eyeball itself is involved only minimally. **B,** The same patient after 1 month has cicatricial ectropion and lid retraction caused by scarring of the skin.

Endogenous (Embolic) Endophthalmitis   Endophthalmitis is a vision-threatening infection of the posterior segment of the retina and vitreous. Most cases of endophthalmitis occur after surgery, trauma, or as an extension of an uncontrolled corneal infection. Orbital processes only anecdotally can cause endophthalmitis because the sclera is a natural barrier for infections. Hematogenic spread of an infection to the posterior pole is termed *endogenous endophthalmitis.* It is an uncommon occurrence, and candidal sepsis is the most common pathogen. Dental infections and procedures also have been reported as a cause of endogenous endophthalmitis.[40,49,51]

Endogenous endophthalmitis manifests with decreased vision, pain, and typical retinal findings. If endogenous endophthalmitis is not recognized early, panophthalmitis (diffused ocular infection) may result with loss of the eye. Preliminary funduscopic findings may include hemorrhages with a white center termed *Roth's spots.* Vitreous opacity above the infected area occurs next and is followed by clouding of the entire vitreous body. The anterior chamber may be affected with hypopyon (a layer of white blood cells in the anterior chamber) and corneal precipitates. The conjunctiva usually is injected, and in later stages pain may be prominent (Figure 15-15).

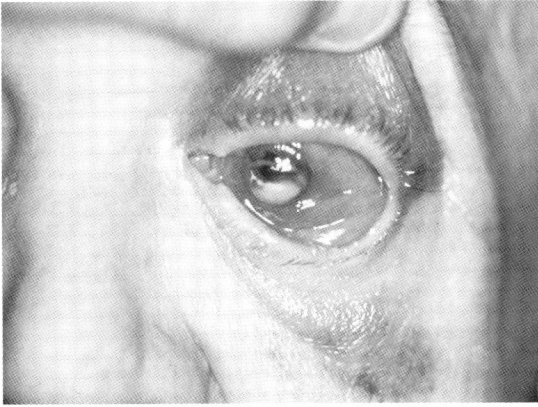

Figure 15-15 Endophthalmitis with lid swelling, conjunctival injection, and a large hypopyon.

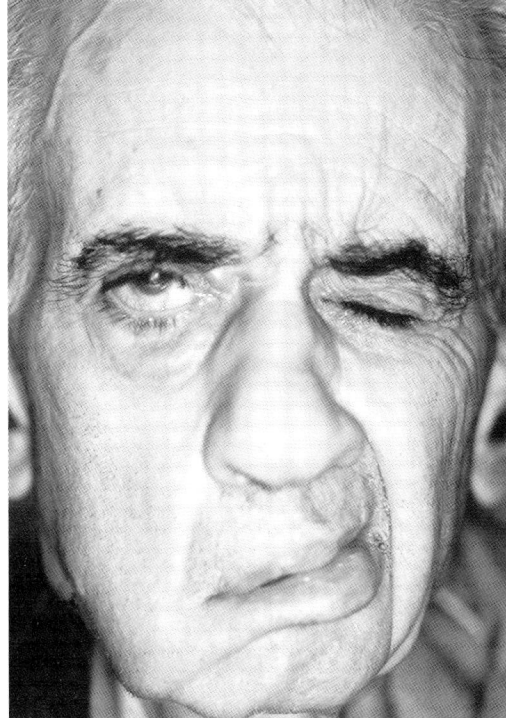

Figure 15-16 A patient with facial nerve palsy and inability to completely close the eye (lagophthalmos). Bell's phenomenon was absent; exposure keratitis is present of the lower third of the cornea.

Early diagnosis and treatment are essential. Every effort should be made to isolate the pathogen from the blood or the primary site. A vitreous tap or vitrectomy usually is performed to identify the organism. Systemic antibiotic treatment is given in endogenous endophthalmitis, but penetration of antibiotic from the blood to the eye is limited. Injection of antibiotics into the vitreous is standard treatment. Controversy exists regarding the necessity and timing of steroid treatment to limit intraocular inflammation and scarring. If the infection cannot be controlled, evisceration (removal of the intraocular content) is indicated. The scleral shell is not removed to prevent posterior spread of the infection. Some surgeons prefer enucleation of the entire eye (including the sclera) because of the risk of sympathetic ophthalmia. Some routinely place an orbital implant at the time of the primary evisceration to compensate for volume loss, whereas others defer placement of an orbital implant at the time of the primary procedure.

OTHER OCULAR COMPLICATIONS OF MAXILLOFACIAL INFECTIONS

EXPOSURE KERATOPATHY, NEUROTROPHIC KERATOPATHY, AND CORNEAL ULCERS

Corneal conditions often occur in hospitalized, severely ill patients with central nervous system involvement, individuals with paralysis of the trigeminal or facial nerve, and patients with proptosis or lid problems.

Exposure Keratopathy Exposure keratopathy (corneal exposure) is characterized by punctate epithelial keratopathy that usually affects the inferior third of the cornea. Large epithelial breaks and defects may result and progress to deeper ulceration, melting, and perforation of the cornea. Alternatively, chronic exposure may lead to corneal scarring and loss of vision. The epithelial defect may predispose the cornea to bacterial infections and endoph-

thalmitis. Pain, foreign body sensation, photophobia, tearing, and blurred vision are the most common symptoms.

Common causes of exposure include seventh nerve palsy, proptosis, lid retraction, and ectropion. Many of these conditions may result from infections of the head and neck.

Examination begins with observation of the spontaneous blink and forced lid closure. Lagophthalmos (inability to completely close the eye) is evaluated (Figure 15-16). The Bell's phenomenon, upward movement of the eye when the lids are closed, is an important protective mechanism of the cornea. In some individuals this reflex is absent and leads to corneal exposure if lagophthalmos is present. Whenever possible a complete ophthalmic examination, including slit-lamp examination, should be performed because the early findings may be seen only with the slit lamp. An inflamed eye, conjunctival injection, irregularity of the light reflex, and any opacity of the cornea is looked for meticulously. Fluorescent dye should be used to detect an epithelial defect.

Treatment of the preliminary cause combined with frequent uses of artificial tears, ointments, or taping of the lids is initiated. In more severe cases, surgical narrowing of the palpebral fissure by tarsorrhaphy, tightening of the lower lid, or elevation of the lower lid and entire cheek with a midfacial or suborbicularis oculi fat lift may be performed. Dynamic solutions include implantation of a gold weight in the upper lid or implantation of a lid spring.

Neurotrophic Keratopathy   *Neurotrophic keratopathy* is a term reserved for keratopathy that results from trigeminal damage. Common causative infections are herpes simplex keratitis or herpes zoster ophthalmicus. Other causes include trauma, tumors, and vascular causes. The damage to the corneal sensation interferes with the blink reflex but also changes tear osmolarity and the ability of the cornea to secrete factors necessary for repair of a corneal defect. The symptoms, signs, and treatment are similar to those for exposure keratitis. Some cases are so severe that complete closure of the eye is needed.

Both neurotrophic and exposure keratitis predispose the eye to secondary bacterial infection and development of an infectious corneal ulcer (Figure 15-17). Certain pathogens such as *Pseudomonas* and *Pneumococcus* are particularly aggressive and may invade deep into the cornea, penetrate the anterior chamber, and cause panophthalmitis with loss of the eye. Pain, photophobia, lid swelling, erythema, and mucopurulent discharge are important clues. An ophthalmologist should be consulted immediately for any white spot on the cornea regardless of size. Local antibiotic drops penetrate the cornea in high concentrations and are the optimal treatment in early stages. Cycloplegic drops for relief of pain and photophobia and local steroids may be required. If the infection spreads into the eye, treatment as described for endophthalmitis is needed.

LID RETRACTION AND CICATRICIAL ECTROPION

Cicatricial ectropion and lid retraction occurs as the result of vertical shortening or scarring of the anterior lamella of the lid (skin, orbicularis muscle, or septum). Ectropion of the lower lid is more common than upper lid ectropion. Even a small amount of vertical shortening can cause severe symptoms in the lower lid; especially if a component of horizontal laxity also exists. Several conditions can result in scarring of the anterior lamella and lead to cicatricial ectropion. Some are related to infections of the skin,

mainly herpes zoster or herpes simplex skin infections (see Figure 15-14, *A*).

Symptoms can be divided into three major groups: tearing, ocular irritation, and cosmetic disturbance. Tearing is multifactorial in origin. The ectropion moves the punctum away from the tear lake and interferes with normal tear drainage. Reflex tearing caused by exposure further contribute to epiphora.

Chronic irritation, burning, stinging, foreign body sensation, mucous discharge, pain, photophobia, and blurry vision are common symptoms resulting from exposure of the conjunctiva and cornea and inadequate spread of the tear film by the ectropic lid. Keratinization or edema of the exposed conjunctiva may contribute to these complaints. The patient also may be bothered by the appearance of the red, inflamed, and thickened lid margin.

Cicatricial skin changes are assessed first by observation and then by pulling the lower lid upward with the examiner's finger. In the absence of cicatricial changes the lower lid should easily reach the level of the superior limbus. Vertical shortening also can be demonstrated by asking the patient to open the mouth. When cicatricial changes are present, the lid will pull away from the eye with this maneuver.

When symptoms are mild, symptomatic treatment includes lubrication drops and ointments. In more severe cases, surgery is needed. Scar lysis and Z-plasty may be adequate in selected cases, but usually a skin flap or graft is needed to lengthen the anterior lamella (Figure 15-18).

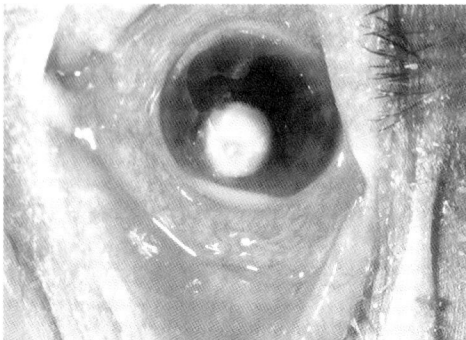

Figure 15-17 A round corneal ulcer with a small hypopyon in the anterior chamber.

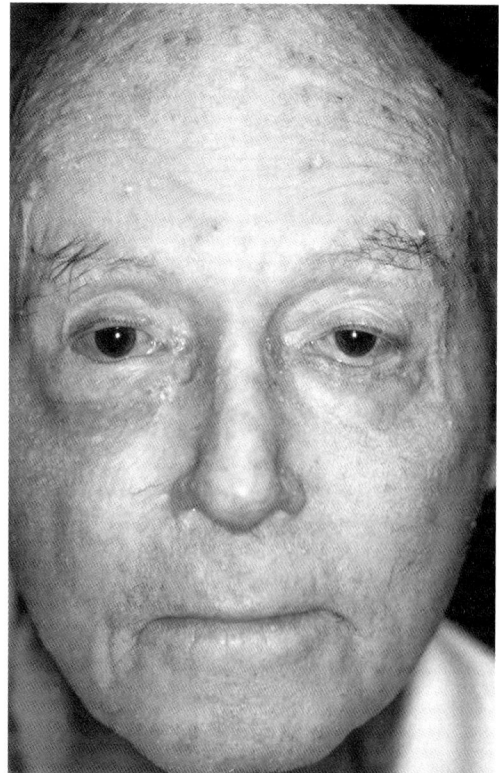

Figure 15-18 The right eye of the same patient in Figure 15-14 after correction with a full-thickness skin graft from the retroauricular area to the lower lid.

POSTSTREPTOCOCCAL UVEITIS

Poststreptococcal bilateral anterior uveitis develops after streptococcal pharyngitis as part of the poststreptococcal syndrome. The inflammation is sterile and considered an autoimmune reaction between streptococcus-sensitized lymphocytes and host tissue because of "molecular mimicry." Common manifestations of poststreptococcal syndrome include acute rheumatic fever, reactive arthritis, and acute glomerulonephritis. Only recently uveitis was described as a sign of poststreptococcal syndrome.[6] Symptoms may include photophobia, ocular redness, and blurred vision after an episode of streptococcal pharyngitis. Slit-lamp examination may demonstrate signs of inflammation in the anterior chamber of the eye (flare and cells in the anterior chamber and keratic precipitates on the corneal endothelium). Elevated titers of antistreptolysin O and isolation of the organism from the pharynx support the diagnosis. Treatment with steroid eye drops and cycloplegia is effective. Penicillin prophylaxis and tonsillectomy can reduce the frequency and severity of attacks in recurrent cases.[47]

SILENT SINUS SYNDROME

Silent sinus syndrome is a spontaneous development of unilateral enophthalmos and hypoglobus associated with an ipsilateral small maxillary sinus and maxillary sinus bone thinning. This condition is rare; only case reports and small series have been reported in the literature.[16,19,25,65,69] Silent sinus syndrome usually develops in the third and fourth decades and affects both sexes. The patient has no history of trauma or other destructive bone process and usually has no symptoms before the development of ocular signs. A history of sinus disease, sometimes many years before presentation, is reported by one third of patients. The condition may develop over a period of days to months and is not painful.

The cause of silent sinus syndrome remains speculative. Several theories have been suggested, but none has been proved. Chronic sinusitis with associated obstruction of the ostium is believed to be the cause of this condition by some authors.[23,65] According to this theory the chronic inflammation in the sinus wall causes absorption of the sinus walls and collapse of the orbital floor. Negative pressures within the sinus or collapse of a pseudocyst were proposed as alternative mechanisms for the development of this syndrome.

Surgery with standard reconstruction of the orbital floor is the treatment if enophthalmos or hypoglobus are significant.

REFERENCES

1. Alexanderakis G, Hubbell RN, Aitken PA: Nasolacrimal duct obstruction secondary to ectopic teeth, *Ophthalmology* 107: 189, 2000.
2. Allan BP, Egbert MA, Myall RW: Orbital abscess of odontogenic origin: case report and review of the literature, *Int J Oral Maxillofac Surg* 20:268, 1991.
3. Avet PP, Kline LB, Sillers MJ: Endoscopic sinus surgery in the management of mucormycosis, *J Neuroophthalmol* 19:56, 1999.
4. Barone SR, Aiuto LT: Periorbital and orbital cellulitis in the *Haemophilus influenzae* vaccine era, *J Pediatr Ophthalmol Strabismus* 34:293, 1997.
5. Baum JL: Rhino-orbital mucormycosis occurring in an otherwise apparently healthy individual, *Am J Ophthalmol* 63:335, 1967.
6. Benjamin A, Tufail A, Holland GN: Uveitis as the only clinical manifestation of poststreptococcal syndrome, *Am J Ophthalmol* 123:258, 1997.
7. Bent JP 3rd, Kuhn FA: Diagnosis of allergic fungal sinusitis, *Otolaryngol Head Neck Surg* 111:580, 1994.
8. Bray WH, Giangiacomo J, Ide CH: Orbital apex syndrome, *Surv Ophthalmol* 32:136, 1987.
9. Brook I, Frazier EH: Aerobic and anaerobic microbiology of dacryocystitis, *Am J Ophthalmol* 125:552, 1998.
9a. Carter KD, Graham SM, Carpenter KM: Ophthalmic manifestations of allergic fungal sinusitis, *Am J Ophthalmol* 127: 189, 1999.
10. Chang WJ, Shields CL, Shields JA, et al: Bilateral orbital involvement with massive allergic fungal sinusitis, *Arch Ophthalmol* 114:767, 1996.
11. Chang WJ, Tse DT, Bressler KL, et al: Diagnosis and management of allergic fungal sinusitis with orbital involvement, *Ophthal Plast Reconstr Surg* 16:72, 2000.
12. Clifford-Jones RE, Ellis CJ, Stevens JM, et al: Cavernous sinus thrombosis, *J Neurol Neurosurg Psychiatry* 45:1092, 1982.
13. Coden DJ, Hornblass A, Haas BD: Clinical bacteriology of dacryocystitis in adults, *Ophthal Plast Reconstr Surg* 9:125, 1993.
14. Cody DT 2nd, Neel HB 3rd, Ferreiro JA, et al: Allergic fungal sinusitis: the Mayo Clinic experience, *Laryngoscope* 104:1074, 1994.
15. Cook BA, White CB, Blaney SM, et al: Survival after isolated cerebral mucormycosis, *Am J Pediatr Hematol Oncol* 11:330, 1989.
16. Davidson JK, Soparkar CN, Williams JB, et al: Negative sinus pressure and normal predisease imaging in silent sinus syndrome, *Arch Ophthalmol* 117:1653, 1999.
17. DiNubile MJ: Septic thrombosis of the cavernous sinuses, *Arch Neurol* 45:567, 1988.
17a. Dunlop IS, Billson FA: Visual failure in allergic *Aspergillus* sinusitis: case report, *Br J Ophthalmol* 72:127, 1988.
18. el-Toukhy E, Szal M, Levine MR, et al: Osteomyelitis of the orbit, *Ophthal Plast Reconstr Surg* 13:68, 1997.
19. Eto RT, House JM: Enophthalmos, a sequela of maxillary sinusitis, *AJNR Am J Neuroradiol* 16(4 suppl):939, 1995.
20. Fairley C, Sullivan TJ, Bartley P, et al: Survival after rhino-orbital-cerebral mucormycosis in an immunocompetent patient, *Ophthalmology* 107:555, 2000.
21. Fearon B, Edmonds B, Bird R: Orbital-facial complications of sinusitis in children, *Laryngoscope* 89(6 Pt 1):947, 1979.
22. Ferry AP, Abedi S: Diagnosis and management of rhino-orbitocerebral mucormycosis (phycomycosis): a report of 16 personally observed cases, *Ophthalmology* 90:1096, 1983.
23. Forstot SL, Ellis PP: Nontraumatic rupture of the globe secondary to orbital cellulitis, *Am J Ophthalmol* 88:262, 1979.
24. Gamba JL, Woodruff WW, Djang WT, et al: Craniofacial mucormycosis: assessment with CT, *Radiology* 160:207, 1986.
25. Gillman GS, Schaitkin BM, May M: Asymptomatic enophthalmos: the silent sinus syndrome, *Am J Rhinol* 13:459, 1999.

26. Grando D, Sullivan LJ, Flexman JP, et al: *Bartonella henselae* associated with Parinaud's oculoglandular syndrome, *Clin Infect Dis* 28:1156, 1999.

27. Greenberg MF, Pollard ZF: Medical treatment of pediatric subperiosteal orbital abscess secondary to sinusitis, *J AAPOS* 2:351, 1998.

28. Harris GJ: Subperiosteal abscess of the orbit, *Arch Ophthalmol* 101:751, 1983.

29. Harbour RC, Trobe JD, Ballinger WE: Septic cavernous sinus thrombosis associated with gingivitis and parapharyngeal abscess, *Arch Ophthalmol* 102:94, 1984.

30. Hartikainen J, Lehtonen OP, Saari KM: Bacteriology of lacrimal duct obstruction in adults, *Br J Ophthalmol* 81:37, 1997.

31. Holland J: Emerging zygomycoses of humans, *Curr Top Med Mycol* 8:27, 1997.

32. Hornblass A, Herschorn BJ, Stern K, et al: Orbital abscess, *Surv Ophthalmol* 29:169, 1984.

33. Hussain S, Salahuddin N, Ahmad I, et al: Rhinocerebral invasive mycosis, *Eur J Radiol* 20:151, 1995.

34. Hovinga J, Christiaans BJ: Odontogenic infection leading to orbital cellulitis as a complication of fracture of the zygomatic bone, *J Craniomaxillofac Surg* 15:254, 1987.

35. Jarrett WH 2d, Gutman FA: Ocular complications of infection in the paranasal sinuses, *Arch Ophthalmol* 81:683, 1969.

36. Johnson EV, Kline LB, Julian BA, et al: Bilateral cavernous sinus thrombosis due to mucormycosis, *Arch Ophthalmol* 106:1089, 1988.

37. Kaplan DM, Briscoe D, Gatot A, et al: The use of standardized orbital ultrasound in the diagnosis of sinus induced infections of the orbit in children: a preliminary report, *Int J Pediatr Otorhinolaryngol* 48:155, 1999.

38. Karlin RJ, Robinson WA: Septic cavernous sinus thrombosis, *Ann Emerg Med* 13:449, 1984.

39. Katz BJ: Lesions produced by infections and inflammations of the central nervous system. In Miller NR, Newman NJ, editors: *Walsh and Hoyt's clinical neuro-ophthalmology,* vol 4, ed 5, Baltimore, 1998, Williams & Williams.

40. Kilmartin DJ, Barry P: Recurrent septic retinal emboli following dental surgery, *Br J Ophthalmol* 80:1111, 1996.

41. Klapper SR, Lee AG, Patrinely JR, et al: Orbital involvement in allergic fungal sinusitis, *Ophthalmology* 104:2094, 1997.

42. Kline MW: Mucormycosis in children, *Pediatr Infect Dis* 4:672, 1985.

43. Kohn R, Hepler R: Management of limited rhino-orbital mucormycosis without exenteration, *Ophthalmology* 92:1440, 1985.

44. Kronish JW, Johnson TE, Gilberg SM, et al: Orbital infections in patients with human immunodeficiency virus infection, *Ophthalmology* 103:1483, 1996.

45. Langford JD, McCartney DL, Wang RC: Frozen section–guided surgical debridement for management of rhino-orbital mucormycosis, *Am J Ophthalmol* 124:265, 1997.

46. Lehrer RI, Howard DH, Sypherd PS, et al: Mucormycosis, *Ann Intern Med* 93:93, 1980.

47. Leiba H, Barash J, Pollack A: Poststreptococcal uveitis, *Am J Ophthalmol* 126:317, 1998.

48. Manning SC, Schaefer SD, Close LG, et al: Culture-positive allergic fungal sinusitis, *Arch Otolaryngol Head Neck Surg* 117:174, 1991.

49. May DR, Peyman GA, Raichand M, et al: Metastatic *Peptostreptococcus intermedius* endophthalmitis after a dental procedure, *Am J Ophthalmol* 85(5 Pt 1):662, 1978.

50. Morgan PR, Morrison WV: Complications of frontal and ethmoid sinusitis, *Laryngoscope* 90:661, 1980.

51. Nightingale JM, Simpson AJ, Towler HM, et al: Fungal feeding-line infections: beware the eyes and teeth, *J R Soc Med* 88:258, 1995.

52. Ntountas I, Morschbacher R, Pratt D, et al: An orbital abscess secondary to acute dacryocystitis, *Ophthalmic Surg Lasers* 28:758, 1997.

53. Ogundiya DA, Keith DA, Mirowski J: Cavernous sinus thrombosis and blindness as complications of an odontogenic infection: report of a case and review of literature, *J Oral Maxillofac Surg* 47:1317, 1989.

54. Pereira KD, Mitchell RB, Younis RT, et al: Management of medial subperiosteal abscess of the orbit in children: a 5-year experience, *Int J Pediatr Otorhinolaryngol* 38:247, 1997.

55. Press GA, Weindling SM, Hesselink JR, et al: Rhinocerebral mucormycosis: MR manifestations, *J Comput Assist Tomogr* 12:744, 1988.

56. Price CD, Hameroff SB, Richards RD: Cavernous sinus thrombosis and orbital cellulitis, *South Med J* 64:1243, 1971.

57. Radner AB, Witt MD, Edwards JE Jr: Acute invasive rhinocerebral zygomycosis in an otherwise healthy patient: case report and review, *Clin Infect Dis* 20:163, 1995.

58. Rubin SE, Rubin LG, Zito J, Goldstein MN, et al: Medical management of orbital subperiosteal abscess in children, *J Pediatr Ophthalmol Strabismus* 26:21, 1989.

59. Schramm VL Jr, Curtin HD, Kennerdell JS: Evaluation of orbital cellulitis and results of treatment, *Laryngoscope* 92(7 Pt 1):732, 1982.

60. Schramm VL, Myers EN, Kennerdell JS: Orbital complications of acute sinusitis: evaluation, management, and outcome, *Otolaryngology* 86:221, 1978.

61. Seedat RY, Hamilton PD, de Jager LP, et al: Orbital rhabdomyosarcoma presenting as an apparent orbital subperiosteal abscess, *Int J Pediatr Otorhinolaryngol* 52:177, 2000.

62. Shapiro ED, Wald ER, Brozanski BA: Periorbital cellulitis and paranasal sinusitis: a reappraisal, *Pediatr Infect Dis* 1:91, 1982.

63. Slade MP, McNab AA: Fatal mucormycosis therapy associated with desferoxamine, *Am J Ophthalmol* 112:594, 1991.

64. Sofferman RA: Cavernous sinus thrombophlebitis secondary to sphenoid sinusitis, *Laryngoscope* 93:797, 1983.

65. Soparkar CN, Patrinely JR, Cuaycong MJ, et al: The silent sinus syndrome: a cause of spontaneous enophthalmos, *Ophthalmology* 101:772, 1994.

66. Southwick FS, Richardson EP Jr, Swartz MN: Septic thrombosis of the dural venous sinuses, *Medicine* 65:82, 1986.

67. Tveteras K, Kristensen S, Dommerby H: Septic cavernous and lateral sinus thrombosis: modern diagnostic principles, *J Laryngol Otol* 102:877, 1988.

68. Wieden MA, Steinbronn KK, Padhye AA, et al: Zygomycosis caused by *Apophysomyces elegans, J Clin Microbiol* 22:522, 1985.

69. Wilkins RB, Kulwin DR: Spontaneous enophthalmos associated with chronic maxillary sinusitis, *Ophthalmology* 88:981, 1981.

70. Wulc AE: Orbital infections. In Tasman W, Jaeger EA editor: *Duane's clinical ophthalmology,* vol 2, Philadelphia, 1997, Lippincott-Raven.

71. Yohai RA, Bullock JD, Aziz AA, et al: Survival factors in rhino-orbital-cerebral mucormycosis, *Surv Ophthalmol* 39:3, 1994.

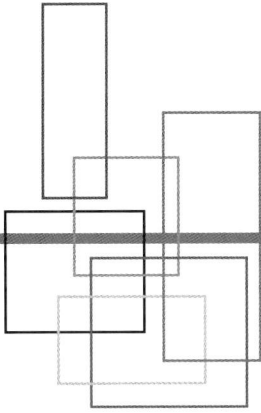

Neurological Considerations in Oral and Maxillofacial Infections

Richard H. Simon

Oral and maxillofacial surgeons treat infections that anatomically are closely related to the central nervous system (CNS). Fortunately, these infections usually are localized and do not involve the skull or its contents. However, occasionally patients with neurological involvement require the clinician to assess the gravity and urgency of the problem.

NEUROLOGICAL EXAMINATION

An index of suspicion, a carefully developed history, and the presence of constitutional signs and symptoms of infection stratify the clinical interpretation of neurological signs.

HEADACHE

Headache is a common and nonspecific symptom that often is of extracranial origin. Headache can vary widely in degrees of severity with any intracranial space-occupying mass, including edema alone. Headache also is associated with meningeal irritation alone from subarachnoid blood, infection, or aseptic inflammation.

LEVEL OF CONSCIOUSNESS

Alteration in the level of consciousness is a sensitive warning of increased intracranial pressure. Although the usual alteration is progressive somnolence, other manifestations, such as confusion or disorientation, exist. After pharmacological causes and hypoxia and electrolyte imbalances have been excluded, the surgeon must eliminate intracranial hypertension as the cause of altered level of consciousness.

MENINGEAL IRRITATION

Irritation of any part of the meninges can lead to headache, stiff neck and photophobia (meningismus), malaise, and nausea. The dura readily transmits symptoms of meningeal irritation; even a disk stretching the dura at a low lumbar level can cause signs of irritation.

CRANIAL NERVE DYSFUNCTION

Cranial nerve involvement in infection is not common but worrisome. Cranial nerve function may be impaired by inflammation, stretching (injury), compression (mass or shift), or encasement (granuloma, tumor). Careful cranial nerve assessment sometimes can provide early identification and localization of disease.

Anosmia cannot be identified unless function of the first nerve is tested specifically. Testing of first nerve function often is overlooked, yet anosmia can be a common concomitant symptom of chronic sinusitis and trauma.

Hearing loss in infection usually is conductive as a result of otitis media. Neurosensory hearing loss from direct involvement of the eighth nerve more frequently occurs with seventh nerve involvement and other posterior fossa signs. Third nerve dysfunction (oculomotor paresis with pupillary paralysis) generally does not occur in isolation, but instead with nerves IV, V, and VI related to disturbances of the posterior orbit or cavernous sinus. Occasionally paralysis of ocular movements may be muscular, not neurological, in origin. Mucormycosis typically causes only muscular paralysis. Although a herniating brain can cause an ipsilateral paresis of the third nerve, the so-called uncal herniation syndrome, a patient with impending herniation likely will have an impaired level of consciousness with a contralateral hemiparesis.

Some classic syndromes associated with inflammatory disease involve groups of cranial nerves.

Tolosa-Hunt Syndrome Tolosa-Hunt syndrome is caused by a granuloma at the orbital apex and superior orbital fissure that results in painful ophthalmoplegia and loss of the first division of the fifth nerve. Granulomatous diseases can implicate any (and sometimes many) of the cranial nerves, including the optic nerves.

Cavernous Sinus Syndrome   Cavernous sinus syndrome is caused by septic thrombosis of the cavernous sinus. It manifests as loss of the first and second divisions of the fifth cranial nerve with complete ophthalmoplegia.[2] Blindness also may occur.

Angle Syndrome   Angle syndrome usually results from a mass that affects the fifth, seventh, and eighth cranial nerves in the cerebellopontine angle.

Gradenigo's Syndrome   Gradenigo's syndrome is caused by fifth and sixth cranial nerve dysfunction. It initially causes pain, occasioned by an inflammatory or infectious process in the petrous apex. Ear drainage almost invariably occurs (Figure 16-1).

MOTOR PARESIS

Motor weakness is important in localization of contralateral motor system involvement in disease. Weakness alone does not pinpoint the precise location in the tract, except when considered with cranial nerve dysfunction or other signs. Motor loss is not specific in distinguishing among diseases. If neurological function is impaired, careful examination generally allows localization of the lesion to the tract or system and sometimes to a specific location. The neurological examination seldom can be used to differentiate among diseases, especially specific brain infections. Tumor, injury, and demyelinating disease all may have identical initial symptoms, as can encephalitis, abscess, or empyema.

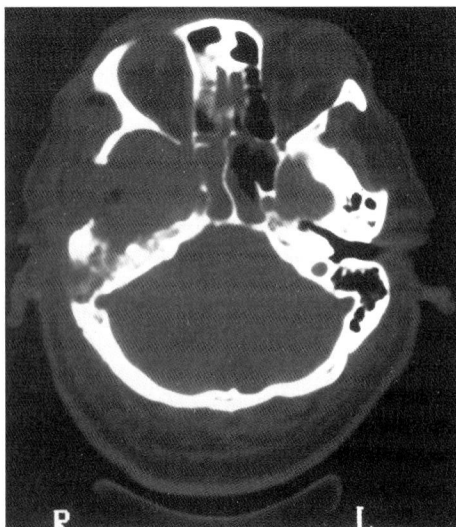

Figure 16-1 Mastoiditis extension into the petrous bone. The bony cortex of the petrous bone is dissolved in the area where the fifth nerve would pass over the petrous ridge into Meckel's cave. This patient had Gradenigo's syndrome.

SPECIAL ASPECTS OF BRAIN INFECTIONS

Special anatomical and physiological aspects of the brain and its environment must be considered when infection exists. The particular anatomy of the brain helps to establish a barrier to infection; conversely, the environment enveloping the brain exposes it to special risks of infection and renders it recalcitrant to many common forms of treatment. The microanatomy differs from other organ systems in a manner that directly relates to infection.

PROTECTIVE FACTORS

The brain is enveloped by layers of protection. Beneath the scalp the resilient and highly vascularized galea aponeurotica yields slowly and heals quickly. The skull is thick in most areas; fracture through the skull is difficult other than by extraordinary force. The dura matter, a tough, thick, watertight membrane, envelops the brain. Finally, the pia mater forms an adherent "body stocking" over the brain, providing another elastic investment. Few vascular channels lead into the brain.

Arterial vascular entry routes to the brain must be along the carotids or vertebral basilar system, or through branches of the external carotid (such as the middle meningeal artery) or the posterior cervical artery to the meninges. The only remaining access to the brain is by structures passing through the foramen magnum, including the spinal fluid, or the cranial nerves.

EXPOSURE FACTORS

Several emissary veins in the retrofacial and scalp regions pass through the diploic spaces connecting the dural sinuses and extracranial veins. These veins have no valves to check backflow and retrograde propagation of thrombi or sepsis. Because of the absence of these valves, phlebitis of the emissary veins is a common mechanism of spread of infection to the brain. Other vulnerable points include the fovea ethmoidalis, lamina cribriforma, and thin posterior wall of the frontal sinuses.

Unlike other organ systems the brain has no lymph nodes or channels through which infectious agents can pass in and out of the brain. The nearest approximation to a brain lymphatic system consists of the Virchow-Robin spaces. Virchow-Robin spaces are potential perivascular spaces through which histiocytes and microglial cells may slip. Although the brain does not possess a strong mesodermal "sense," these phagocytic cells are the exception.

PATHOGEN HABITAT IN THE BRAIN REGION

The base of the brain is surrounded by cavities colonized with a variety of potential pathogens. When infection reaches one of these cavities, the organism that normally colonizes the cavity can become an active pathogen. In addition, the uncolonized mastoid cells and middle ear, when infected, may assume a similar role.

Bacteria that colonize the nasal and oral cavities are mixed aerobic and anaerobic species. *Peptostreptococcus, Fusobacterium,* and *Bacteroides* spp. are the most common anaerobes. The aerobic organisms are *Staphylococcus, Streptococcus, Haemophilus,* and *Diplococcus pneumoniae.* The same organisms and aerobic streptococci are present in the sinuses. The sinuses also are frequently colonized by the fungi *Cryptococcus, Histoplasma, Aspergillus,* and *Phycomycetes.*[20] In the nasopharynx, particularly in the tonsillar crypts, the higher bacteria *Nocardia* and *Actinomyces* may be found in addition to the usual flora. Herpes simplex virus II may be found in the vault of the nose. The middle ear normally is not colonized. Contamination from the nasopharynx through the eustachian tube by *Staphylococcus, Streptococcus,* and *D. pneumoniae* may cause meningitis if a spinal fluid leak involves the mastoid area.

FACTORS THAT PROTECT AND EXPOSE THE BRAIN

Certain features of the brain that normally provide protection may become liabilities when infection occurs.

Blood-Brain Barrier The concept of the blood-brain barrier was described in 1931 when Goldmann injected a vital dye intravenously into a white rat and noticed that although the tissues stained with the methylene blue, the brain did not. Some "barrier" prevented percolation of large molecules into the brain tissue. Characterization of the blood-brain barrier developed over many years. The barrier now is defined as a physiological phenomenon rather than a structural one. Tight junctions in the capillary endothelium of the vessels in the brain prevent leakage of large molecules. No fenestrations exist through which these molecules can pass as in other capillary beds. Thus the blood-brain barrier is not a barrier in the sense of a physical object, but rather a unique ultrastructure of tight junctions between capillary endothelial cells in the absence of fenestrations. These features are not found elsewhere in capillary systems. Breach of this barrier requires physical disruption of the capillary or loosening of the tight junctions so that the capillary may "leak" like a normal capillary. The only other path across the barrier is through the barrier, which requires lipid solubility.

Immunological Privilege The presence of the blood-brain barrier and the brain's lack of lymphatic channels have created concern that the standard responses of immunity, particularly cell-mediated responses, do not operate in the brain. Early work demonstrated that transplanted tumors grew rapidly within the brain, apparently unchecked by host immune responses. This finding has been confirmed in certain experimental animals. Accordingly, the brain is considered "immunologically privileged." In view of new information regarding graft rejection and demonstrated induction of immune responses,

Apuzzo and Mitchell[1] have suggested that the concept of "partial privilege" is more realistic and that the "rigid concept" requires revision.

Cerebrospinal Fluid The spinal fluid provides direct access to the brain. Neutrophils, even in an immunologically competent host, cannot swim. Bacteria can gain a foothold and extend to the leptomeninges. Brain neutrophils find and neutralize invading pathogens only after stabilization of the bacteria on the surface of the meninges. Normal spinal fluid does not contain opsonins and complement to combat specific infection.[11] As a consequence, after contamination the spinal fluid is a breeding ground until the complement and opsonin systems become operational. However, the spinal fluid acts as a natural barrier to viruses.[21]

PATHWAYS TO THE NERVOUS SYSTEM

Brain infection depends on the virulence of the pathogen, size of the inoculum, and host resistance. Borges[4] suggested a mathematical formula relating these three factors. Nevertheless, unless virulence or the inoculum size is extraordinary, necrosis, ischemia, or injury must be present for infection to occur. This theory relates best to parenchymal infections, particularly brain abscess, but may not apply to other situations. Host resistance is a significant factor in most nervous system infections.

ROUTES OF INFECTION

Hematogenous Spread The arterial emboli that pass into the brain usually cause brain abscess. Necrosis, ischemia, or injury may be necessary for the infection to obtain a foothold. However, septic emboli from heart valves can cause brain abscess without any recognized premorbid disturbances in the brain. The embolus itself may lodge in a capillary, causing local infarction and thus generating the requisite breach in the blood-brain barrier necessary for infection.

Thrombophlebitis The usual route of septic phlebitis is from the facial area. With classic cavernous sinus thrombosis, septic thrombus originates in the pterygoid plexus or propagates backward along veins from the nose and upper lip that drain into the cavernous sinus. Sagittal sinus thrombosis usually is associated with generalized sepsis and dehydration rather than facial infection. Development of phlebitis from scalp infections is possible because the emissary veins have no valves. With petrous apicitis, thrombophlebitis of the petrosal sinus or the petrosal veins is not unusual. The petrous apex may become inflamed from the mastoid area or along the dura from the sphenoid sinus.

Because of the limited number of drainage routes from the brain, thrombotic occlusion of larger veins can result in venous hypertension with subsequent infarction. The aftermath can be as disastrous as an arterial infarction.

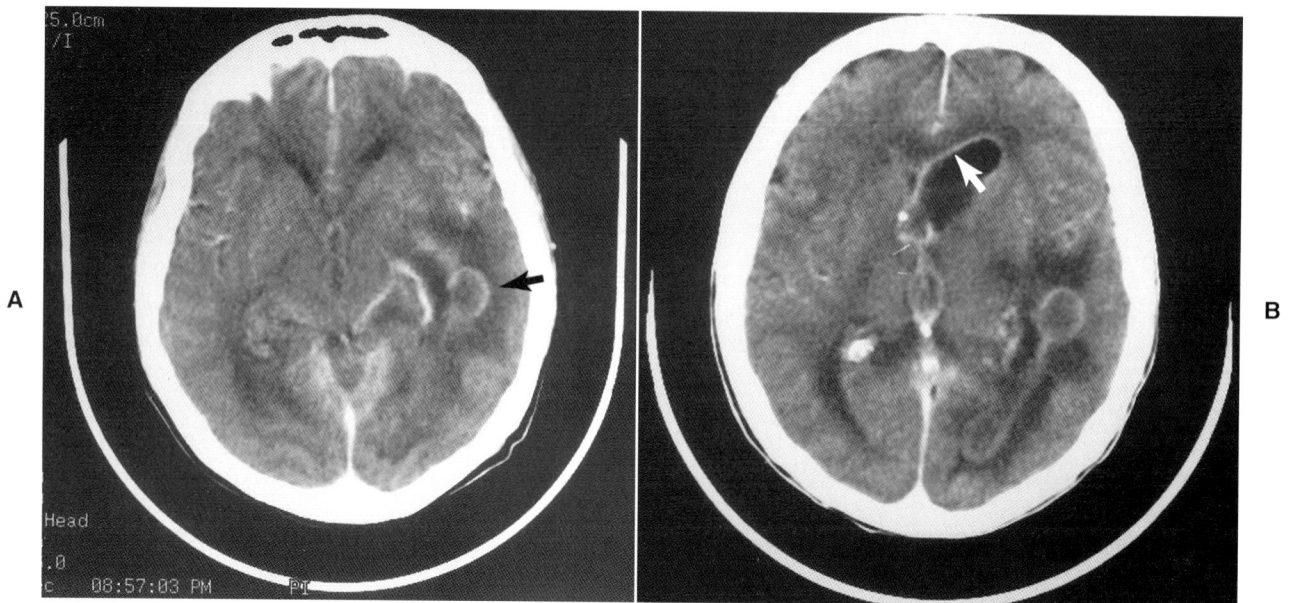

Figure 16-2 A, An abscess *(arrow)* close to the temporal horn when ependymitis already is present. **B,** The abscess has ruptured into the ventricle with resultant fulminant ventriculitis. The ventriculitis encases the temporal horn and involves the left frontal horn *(white arrow)* with focal hydrocephalus.

Meningitis   Meningitis may progress from contamination of the spinal fluid or directly from the pachymeninx. When infection begins in the spinal fluid, it initially affects the leptomeninges. Leptomeningitis then may cause local inflammation of the brain—cerebritis—and may cause infarction. The bacteria also may lodge in the meninges through hematogenous spread because the arteries to the brain are suspended in the pia arachnoid, and the arteries to the meninges are in the dura mater itself. Depending on whether the pathogens enter through an internal or an external route, either leptomeningitis or pachymeningitis occurs first.

The delay between infection of the spinal fluid and release of complement and opsonins and neutrophil mobilization represents a vulnerable period for the spinal fluid, especially in an immunocompromised host whose immune system cannot mobilize neutrophils. Whenever the dura is disrupted, meningitis is a possibility. This possibility exists not only with open fractures of the calvarium, but more commonly with basilar fractures. Basilar fractures frequently remains unrecognized while spinal fluid leaks into the mastoid air cells or frontal or ethmoid sinuses. This direct route allows colonization of a sinus or an air cell. Penetrating wounds similarly allow access but carry the additional problem of disruption and contamination of the brain and meninges.

Cranial Nerves   Herpes simplex virus enters the nervous system along the first cranial nerve.

Osteomyelitis   Osteomyelitis of the skull does not cause neurological problems unless the inflammation affects a foramen in the base of the skull through which a cranial

nerve passes. However, osteomyelitis may affect the extradural space by thrombophlebitis of the diploic veins.[2] Chronic osteomyelitis leads directly to contamination, infection, and ultimately, suppuration in the space between the bone and the dura, which results in an epidural abscess. When the infection crosses the dura to enter the space between the dura and pia arachnoid and forms pus, the abscess is called a *subdural empyema*. If the infection inflames the arachnoid, meningitis results.

Ventricular Seeding   Primary ventricular infection is rare, although septic emboli can lodge in the choroid plexus, leading to an evident primary intraventricular abscess. Fulminant ventriculitis after rupture of an abscess into the ventricle is another possibility (Figure 16-2). However, ventriculitis is common when ventricular shunts are used. Shunts frequently are colonized with *Staphylococcus epidermidis,* a common skin contaminant, or with *Propionibacterium acnes.*[9]

DIAGNOSIS OF INFECTION

Two difficulties are encountered in imaging infections of the brain: (1) distinguishing images of brain infection from those of normal brain tissue, and (2) distinguishing abnormal images resulting from infection from images that are abnormal because of other disease processes.

DIAGNOSTIC TOOLS

Computed Tomographic Scanning   The computed tomographic (CT) scan maps the x-ray attenuation coefficients of various small, cross-sectional areas in a cross-

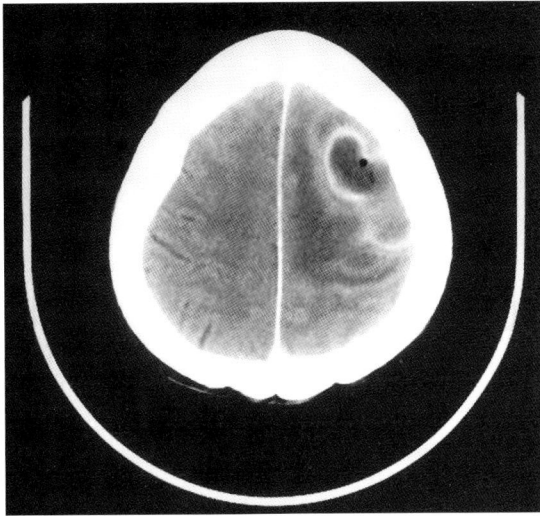

Figure 16-3 CT scan shows classic changes associated with an abscess. The area of edema around the abscess is marked by a decreased attenuation coefficient. The capsule strongly enhances with contrast. The capsule without contrast (not pictured) also has a high attenuation coefficient. Hypodense pus is present inside the abscess capsule, and the bubble of gas was formed by the anaerobic organism.

sectional slice of brain anatomy. Attenuation coefficients of infected material do not differ from those of normal brain. The sensitivity of this technique relies on the identification of attenuation coefficients that are abnormal because of consequences of infection. For example, infected parenchyma causes reactive changes in the brain. The inflammatory change has an attenuation coefficient consistent with edematous brain (Figure 16-3). Capsular reactive gliosis around an abscess produces a high attenuation coefficient that enhances with contrast. Pus itself produces an attenuation coefficient that ranges from isodense to hypodense. Thus with respect to the attenuation coefficient, the CT scan answers the question of whether fluid levels are present.

Because the CT scan images anatomical features, it provides other invaluable information: mass effect and shifts of normal structures. Mass effects can assist in the detection of occult infections, particularly when another pathological condition is not suspected. The bone level and window thresholds on the CT scan provide valuable information regarding osteomyelitis of the calvarium, sinuses, and petrous bones. Sinus infections and fluid levels also are well visualized in this window.

Magnetic Resonance Imaging Magnetic resonance imaging (MRI) relies on relaxation constants of protons, the predominant atom in the water composing the brain and its enveloping structures. Because the relaxation properties of these protons depend not only on the location of the proton but also on the interaction with its milieu (i.e., its spin lattice interaction), differences in the signal intensity can be detected with various acquisition sequences. Identical tissues can yield different signals depending on

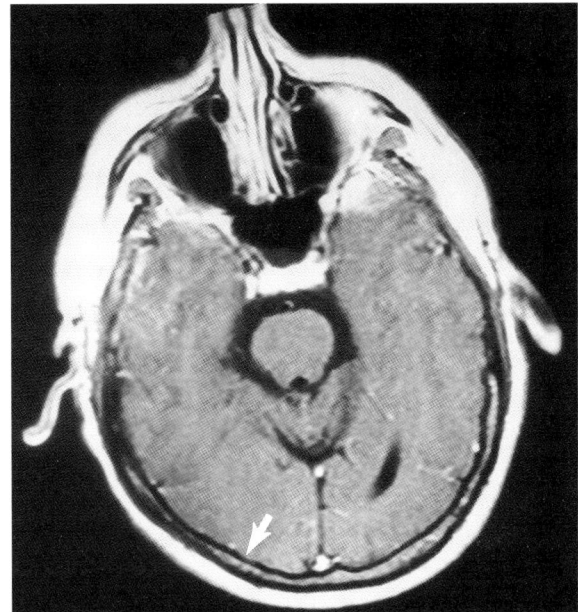

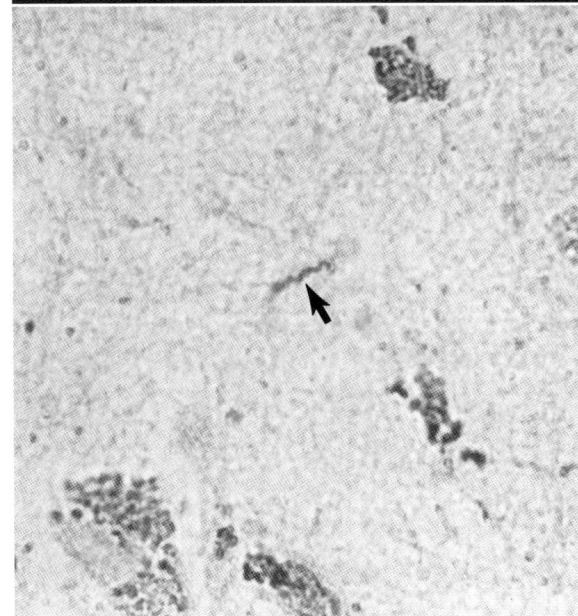

Figure 16-4 A, Hyperintense signal of Lyme meningitis *(arrow).* MRI is useful for imaging meningitis. **B,** The meningitis shown in **A** was caused by the spirochete *Borrelia burgdorferi (arrow).*

the location within the magnetized tissue mass. Thus the MRI sometimes can "see" infection, unlike the CT scan. Meningeal inflammation in the early stages of meningitis can be detected by an increase in the MRI signal (Figure 16-4). Similarly, the paramagnetic contrast agent gadolinium is helpful in delineating areas of increased perfusion and blood-brain barrier leakage associated with infection (Figures 16-5 and 16-6).

Ultrasonography Ultrasonography is most specific for determining gas-fluid or solid-fluid interfaces from which the echoes are reflected. As a result the ultrasonic image of an abscess can be dramatic. Because ultrasonography cannot penetrate adult bone, it is clinically relevant only in

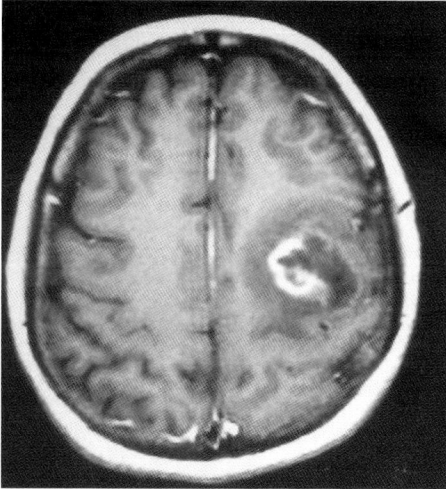

Figure 16-5 Striking gadolinium contrast enhancement outlines the capsule of the abscess on this T1-weighted image.

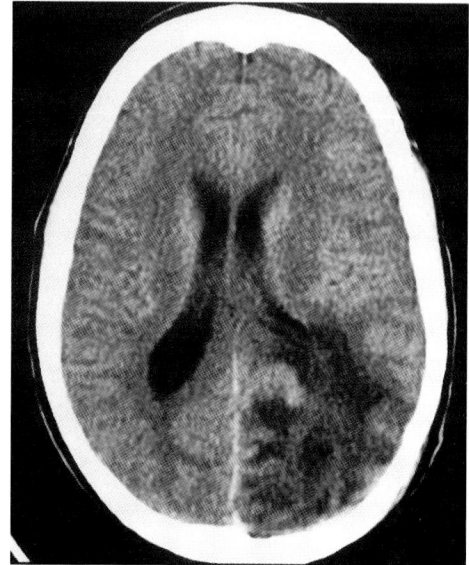

Figure 16-7 Non–constrast-enhanced CT scan of bacterial abscess caused by *Pseudomonas aeruginosa;* the scan was obtained at approximately day 5. Cerebritis and early capsule formation are evident.

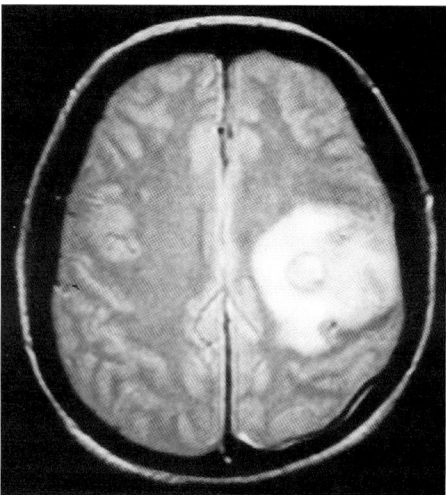

Figure 16-6 T2 weighting of the same abscess shown in Figure 16-5. On the first echo of T2 weighting the capsule is seen as hypointense. Strong signal intensity corresponds to the white matter involvement, shown as a hypointense signal in Figure 16-5.

neonates, if an opening in the bone already exists, or for intraoperative localization.

Radionuclide Scan   Radionuclide scanning, previously overshadowed by more back-projection imaging techniques, now is used more frequently. With the availability of radioisotopes specific for certain pathological processes, radionuclide scanning plays a greater role in diagnosis of infections. For example, in the diagnosis of early cerebritis, gallium can distinguish cerebritis caused by edema from that caused by other disease processes. Similarly, a new role for thallium chloride is being studied. Thallium

avidity is a characteristic of hypermetabolic cells and dividing cells. Thallium avidity may assist in distinguishing tumor from abscess as the cause of a ring-enhancing mass, particularly in the context of a subtraction scan sensitive to blood flow. Technetium bone uptake in osteomyelitis is a reliable diagnostic method. The anticipated results from imaging of infected brain depend on the character, stage, and extent of the pathophysiological process. For example, Britt and Enzmann[5] described the histopathology of an abscess as characterized by early cerebritis. Edema is present on the outer zone with a polymorphonuclear leukocyte infiltration and a nidus of organisms, which may be embedded in necrosis (Figure 16-7). By the end of the first week (the late stage of cerebritis), the center of necrosis increases, a fibroblast border and neovascular channels form, and astrocytes are present (Figure 16-8). In both cases the edema surrounds the lesion; however, in early cerebritis the lesion is seen poorly. All imaging modalities would be sensitive to late cerebritis. At the end of the second week the capsule begins to form, creating a thickened rim with decreased edema. The area of actual necrosis is smaller. After 2 weeks in the late capsule formation stage, the necrotic center is much smaller and a dense collagenase capsule encircles the lesion. Contrast enhances the striking neovascularity around the capsule; without contrast the capsule still appears dense because of the reactive gliosis.

Lumbar Puncture   Lumbar puncture remains the "gold standard" for diagnosis of meningitis. Various algorithms specify use of spinal fluid findings (independent of culture) in categorization of fungal, bacterial, and viral (aseptic) meningitis.[20] Characteristically, bacterial meningitides

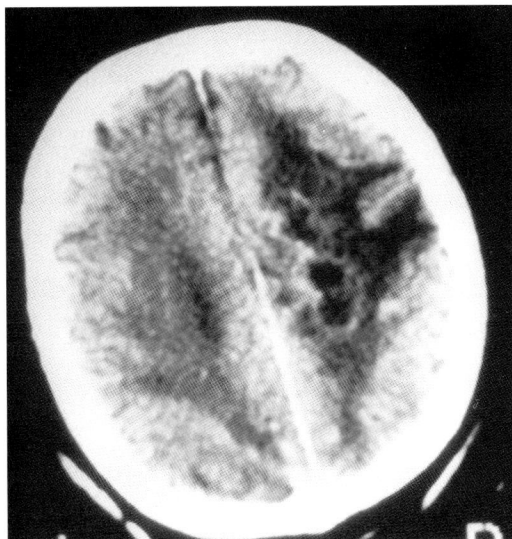

Figure 16-8 Late-stage cerebritis. Although the cerebritis is dramatic, the capsule of the abscess can be defined clearly on this contrast-enhanced scan. This abscess was caused by the fungus *Aspergillus*. The patient was undergoing long-term steroid therapy for a dermatological condition.

have reduced glucose content (hypoglycorrhachia), elevated protein levels, increased polymorphonuclear cell counts (pleocytosis), and demonstrate bacteria on Gram stain. Chronic meningitides such as tuberculous meningitis have similar findings, but organisms rarely are seen. Spirochete infections (e.g., Lyme disease) have a low-grade lymphocytic pleocytosis, whereas other *Borrelia* infections (relapsing fever) have much higher white blood cell counts in spinal fluid. Viruses cause mild pleocytosis that almost always is lymphocytic but seldom involves reduced spinal fluid glucose level and no organisms on Gram stain.

Specific serological tests of spinal fluid can detect several pathogens, particularly nonbacterial ones. Most bacteria can be cultured except tuberculosis, leprosy, or *Actinomyces*, all of which are difficult to culture.

Lumbar puncture is limited by two factors: risk of physical harm and failure to establish a diagnosis. Although lumbar puncture is the test of choice for meningitis, in the presence of an intracranial mass such as an abscess, it carries significant risk of serious harm from shift caused by decompressing the spinal fluid pressure at the base of the brain. A safer approach uses CT or MRI scanning before lumbar puncture to exclude a mass lesion. The potential for recovery of material for culture by lumbar puncture may be limited. In many nongranulomatous abscesses the spinal fluid is not necessarily contaminated by the organism; furthermore, no products of the inflammatory response are necessarily noted in the spinal fluid. Typically, bacterial brain abscesses have no abnormal cerebrospinal fluid (CSF) findings. Even some granulomas, such as tuberculoma, are unlikely to yield abnormal CSF findings. In such cases, biopsy or excisional biopsy is necessary. In some

cases of nongranulomatous cerebral abscess the requisite biopsy (i.e., culture) can be accomplished in the form of a curative excision.

The development of image-directed stereotaxic surgery has allowed access to small and deep subcortical lesions that previously could not be drained safely. Stereotaxic surgery allows the placement of catheters for drainage and irrigation. More superficial lesions, particularly those that are encapsulated, usually are treated by excisional biopsy.

THE FACIAL SURGEON AND BRAIN INFECTION

TRAUMA

Direct bone infection resulting in an epidural abscess is one of the most likely infectious consequences of an open skull fracture. Controversy exists regarding the management of open skull fractures, particularly if they are depressed. Early approaches emphasized mandatory, rapid, and aggressive debridement. More recent treatment protocols advocate surgical nihilism with complete management by wound closure and antibiotics. Entrapped hair, dirt, grease, bacteria, or other foreign particles thrive in the extradural space and can lead to extradural abscess. If the dura is torn, as usually occurs with a basilar fracture, meningitis is more likely. The organisms causing meningitis are the normal flora of the paranasal sinuses or the middle ear; *D. pneumoniae* is the most probable, followed by *Streptococcus* spp. and *H. influenzae*.

CSF fistula is one consequence of basilar fracture, or fracture with spinal fluid leak. CSF fistulas may open weeks to months after the original injury. The presentation is subtle; they often are confused with rhinorrhea or serous otitis. CSF fistulas are responsible for many recurrences of pneumococcal meningitis.

Penetrating wounds can lead to brain abscess or ventriculitis. The offending agent in the penetrating wound can be the bony sequestrum, devitalized bits of skin, devitalized brain, or the missile itself. In high-velocity wounds the amount of devitalized brain is substantial; the area of devitalization is related to the kinetic energy of the missile, which, in turn, is related to the square of the velocity. Although removal of bone and debridement of devitalized brain has been the standard treatment, newer antibiotics have prompted a surgically nihilistic approach. The bony sequestrum is not likely to cause infection unless wound dehiscence occurs.[19]

ORAL AND FACIAL SURGERY

The specific risk of infection depends on the surgical area, nature of the surgery, organisms endogenous to the area, and host resistance. The decision regarding administration of prophylactic antibiotics is important to the oral and maxillofacial surgeon, particularly in procedures on a contaminated operating field. Opinion regarding antibiotic

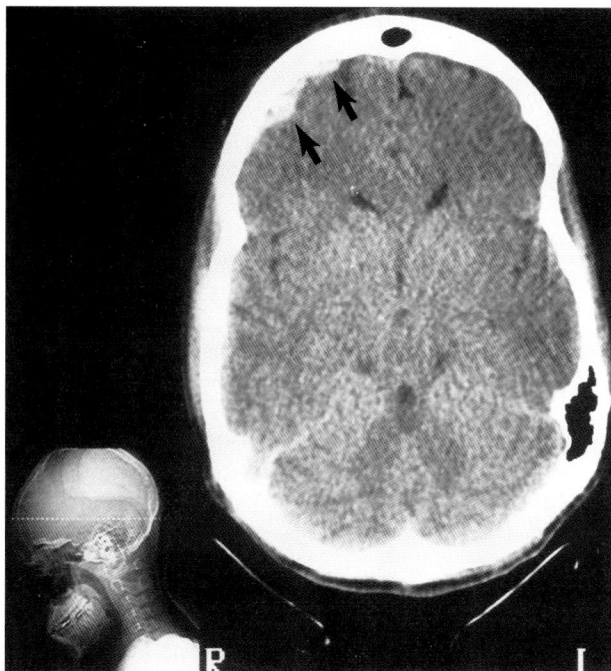

Figure 16-9 Arrows indicate an epidural abscess in a young boy after a fractured skull through the frontal sinus.

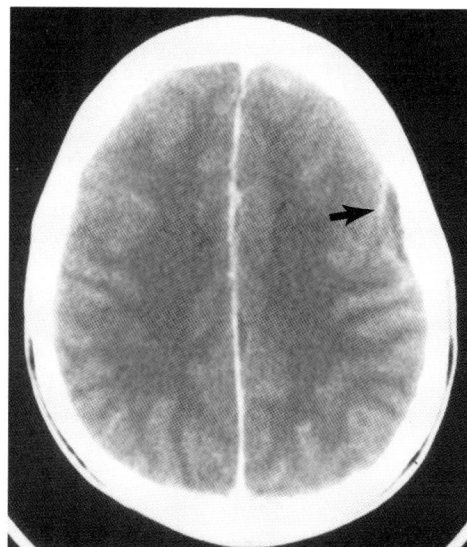

Figure 16-10 Subdural empyema appears similar to a subdural hematoma (see Figure 16-9).

use has varied. Current protocols are more aggressive on the use of prophylactic drugs, although differences in outcome remain unknown. Although the possible reduction of infection by prophylactic antibiotics has been known for the past 20 years, development of resistants organism is a danger. Conversely, if a foreign body (shunt, plate, implant, screw) is to be placed during surgery, the argument for use of prophylactic antibiotics is strong.

FACIAL SOFT TISSUE, BONE, AND SINUS INFECTIONS

Pericranial infections that infect the brain usually develop from chronic osteomyelitis (with subsequent involvement of the dural structures) or, more commonly, from thrombophlebitis. After surgery in these regions, routes of direct spread are most likely.

The archetypal pericranial infection is the diseased sinus. The acutely infected frontal, ethmoidal, or sphenoidal sinus infects the brain by phlebitis of the emissary veins or by passage through the fovea ethmoidalis. Similarly, phlebitis causes spread of infection from acutely infected mastoid or petrous bones. Acute maxillary sinusitis indirectly affects the brain by ascending to the ethmoid or frontal sinus or spreading posteriorly to the sphenoid sinus.

Untreated sinusitis leads to chronic osteomyelitis, which then seeds the meningeal coverings of the brain. This local meningitis leads to an aggregation of pus in the extradural space (the epidural abscess) or penetrates the dura to form an abscess between the dura and the arachnoid, the so-called subdural empyema (Figures 16-9 and 16-10). The causative organisms usually are mixed aerobes and anaerobes.

Dural sinus thrombosis may follow maxillofacial infections. Even today, classic cavernous sinus thrombosis is a dreaded disease with a substantial mortality rate. It results from infections of the maxillofacial region with origins in the pterygoid or pharyngeal plexus or skin and soft tissues drained by the angular vein. Infections of the sphenoid sinus can cause thrombosis of the cavernous sinus, presumably by phlebitis of the emissary veins (Figure 16-11).

TRANSORAL APPROACHES TO THE ODONTOID AND CLIVUS

The atlas, axis, and anterior lower clivus may be reached through a transoropalatal approach.[13] Although this approach commonly is used for access to the anterior spinal elements, it can be used to treat certain tumors. Wound dehiscence is the most common complication.[10] Fang and Ong[10] emphasized the importance of closure; osteomyelitis, meningitis, and death have been associated with dehiscence. Nervous system infection occurs directly through the incision rather than by ascent through the usual pathways.

MEDICAL PREDISPOSITION

Prudent surgeons realize the importance of a careful history; certain medical conditions predispose the patient to certain types of brain infection. For example, a patient with a septal defect of the heart is susceptible to brain abscess, specifically with microaerophilic streptococci. Another important factor is the presence of a ventricular shunt. Although primary ventriculitis may be rare, secondary infection of a ventricular shunt is a genuine concern; pro-

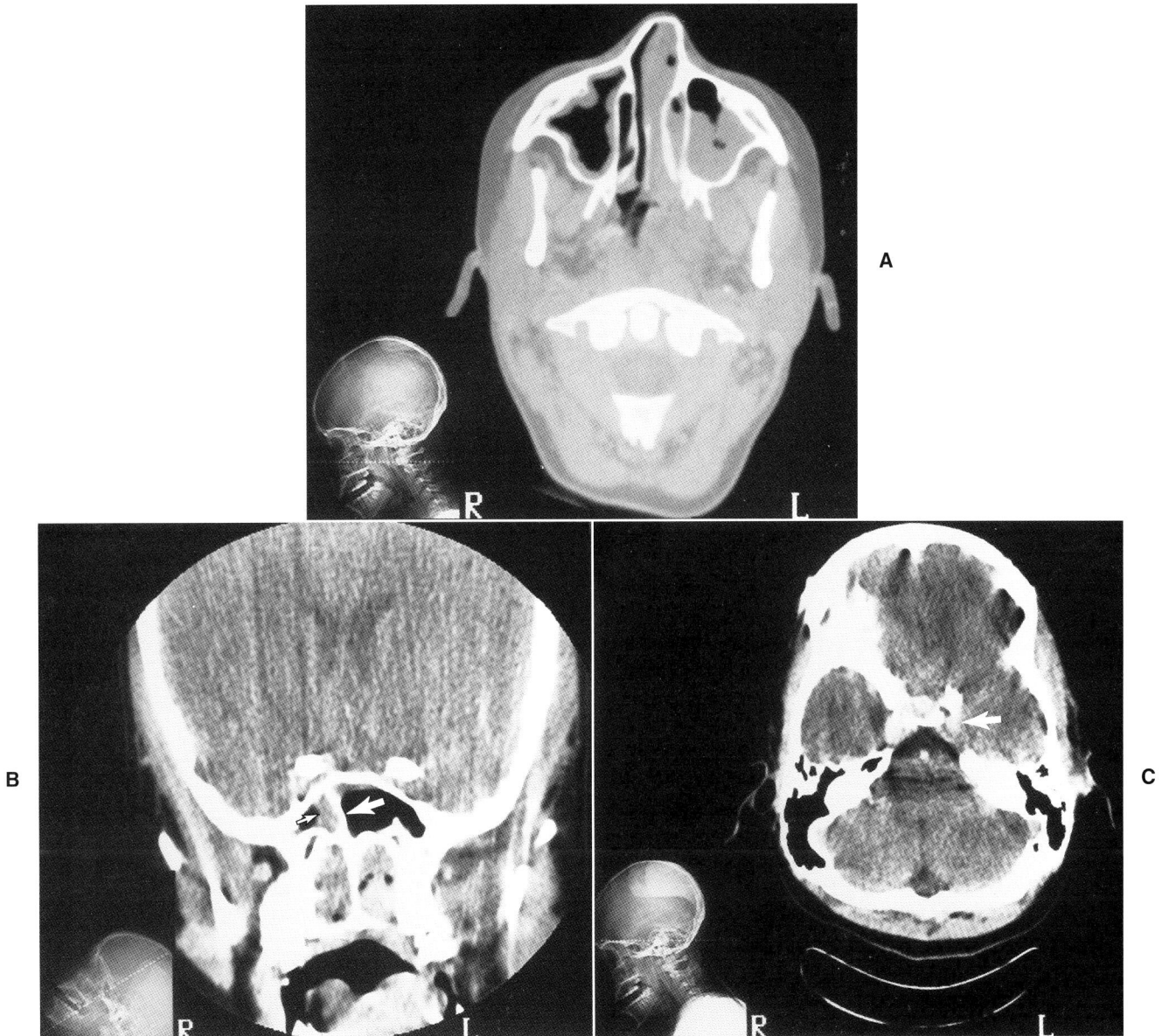

Figure 16-11 A, This patient with aplastic anemia was severely immunocompromised and had just undergone bone marrow transplantation. Maxillary sinusitis is evident. The causative organism was the fungus *Phycomycetes* (mucormycosis). **B,** Attendant sphenoid sinusitis is evident in this coronal section *(arrow)*. **C,** After contrast enhancement the right cavernous sinus *(arrow)* has a rim of medial opacity. This patient had ophthalmoplegia, proptosis, and hemifacial anesthesia on the left side. This cavernous sinus thrombosis probably was acquired by direct extension from the sphenoid sinusitis shown in **B.**

phylactic antibiotics should be used when surgery through a contaminated area is performed in a patient with a ventricular shunt. Certain environmental and endemic predispositions exist to specific infections. Lyme disease often is manifest as meningitis with malaise and fever of unknown origin. This possibility should be considered when forming a differential diagnosis. Although the concern might be most compelling if the patient lives in a location inhabited by many deer, and particularly in southern Connecticut, Lyme disease can occur wherever ticks carry the organism *Borrelia burgdorferi.*

IMMUNOCOMPROMISED HOSTS

Immune compromise is defined by disturbance in cell-mediated or humoral immunity or by decreased granulocyte function. Hall[12] lists the following immunocompromised conditions: leukemias, lymphomas, and myelomas; aplastic anemia; sarcoma and carcinoma; intravenous drug abuse; acquired immunodeficiency syndrome (AIDS); severe trauma; brain tumor; pregnancy; diabetes; alcoholism; and immunosuppressive therapy.

The failure of granulocyte function allows normally nonpathogenic enteric gram-negative rods to become pathogenic. Similarly, the fungi *Aspergillus, Cryptococcus,* and *Mucor,* which are also endogenous organisms, become pathogenic. When cell-mediated immunity is disturbed, *Nocardia* organisms may become pathogenic. The parasite *Toxoplasma* has a distinct advantage in this situation; it is the archetypal AIDS-related brain infection. Meningitis commonly follows the loss of humoral immunity.

Patients with severe diabetes have a higher incidence of infections with mucormycosis.[17] In general, patients treated with steroids or who are immunodepressed are susceptible to overgrowth of endogenous *Actinomyces* (normal flora) or the fungus *Aspergillus.*[14] Those with AIDS commonly are infected by the protozoan *Toxoplasma,* JC polyoma virus, or both organisms.

ASCENDING MIDFACE INFECTION

Infections of the face usually gain access to the brain through the ethmoid, sphenoid, or frontal sinus. Therefore surgeons should be aware of the danger from infections arising elsewhere that may ascend to affect these sinuses. A typical sequence might begin with an odontogenic infection, or infection in the buccal sulcus or anywhere in the mouth or pharynx. These sources can affect the nervous system primarily, but primary infection is not likely.[16] However, the potential increases if infection ascends to the maxillary sinus. At this point, periorbital edema, but not necessarily cellulitis, may represent a reaction to the sinusitis. Once the infection ascends to the ethmoid, concern increases that orbital swelling represents true cellulitis as a consequence of ethmoidal self-decompression through the lamina papyracea.

The patient usually has fever, headache (from the sinusitis), and proptosis. Eye movements are full despite proptosis. The emissary veins can transmit the infection retrograde to the dura. Alternatively, the infection may pass through the fovea ethmoidalis (Figure 16-12). If either transmission occurs, the first true neurological signs appear: worsening headache, meningismus, and possibly altered level of consciousness. Once the infection has reached this stage, several paths of infection are possible: meningitis alone or progression to abscess.

If the infection passes retrograde to the pterygoid plexus, septic phlebitis of the larger facial veins can occur. The retrograde infection continues until the cavernous sinus is involved. Infection of the cavernous sinus by small vessels from the sphenoid sinus also is possible. Cavernous sinus thrombosis leads to unilateral ophthalmoplegia and sensory loss in the first and second divisions of the fifth cranial nerve. Blindness also may occur.

Large-vein phlebitis does not always involve the cavernous sinus; septic thrombosis of the sagittal sinus is a devastating complication that results in severely elevated intracranial pressure, quadriparesis, and often death.

In summary, involvement of the maxillary sinuses should prompt serious concern. Ascending infection into

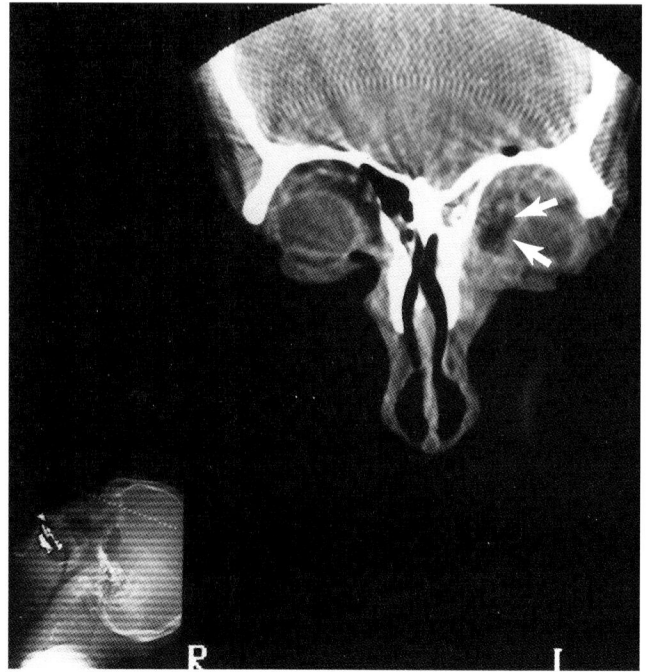

Figure 16-12 Classic ascending midface infection. In this case the sinusitis has extended into the ethmoid; orbital involvement with a frank orbital abscess is present *(arrows)*. The gas bubble is a tell-tale sign that the infection has passed though the fovea ethmoidalis to the intracranial structures.

the ethmoid or sphenoid sinus should trigger an aggressive response, with antibiotics, drainage of the sinuses, and increased vigilance for early neurological signs.

MANAGEMENT

Infections are treated by antimicrobial agents and, if appropriate, by surgical drainage with or without debridement.

MEDICAL MANAGEMENT

Medical management of brain infection is straightforward: identification of an organism; choice of an antibiotic of proper sensitivity; and facilitation of the breach of the blood-brain barrier, either through its lipophilicity or breaks in the barrier. The blood-brain barrier, when intact, is an efficient barrier. Only small or lipid-soluble molecules can pass through the barrier. Successful treatment of brain infections often depends on disruption of the integrity of the blood-brain barrier so that tissue levels of antimicrobials can be established. Chloramphenicol, a classic drug that is both small in molecular size and lipophilic, is used to treat infections when the blood-brain barrier is intact. Metronidazole and rifampin, because of their molecular size and solubility, characteristically can generate high brain tissue levels.

Most antimicrobials rely on a breach of the blood-brain barrier, and because of a low brain tissue/serum concentration ratio, high doses must be used. These drugs often are given in concentrations eightfold to thirtyfold above the minimum bactericidal concentration. Low protein binding and ionization at a physiological pH also contribute to a drug's effectiveness.

Antibiotic treatment is complicated further by the so-called partial privilege of the CNS. Because immunoglobulin and complement concentrations in the subarachnoid space are reduced, bactericidal rather than bacteriostatic doses must be used. For example, the only effective drug to date for treatment of certain fungal infections is amphotericin B. Drugs such as amphotericin (which is a large molecule) require such high serum concentrations to establish brain tissue levels that nephrotoxicity sometimes cannot be avoided.[22]

Penicillin G crosses the blood-brain barrier poorly but can be given in massive doses; thus it is still an excellent drug for the treatment of bacterial meningitis. Chloramphenicol, which is a small molecule, lipophilic, and dissociates at neutral pH, is an ideal drug. Unfortunately, its marrow toxicity vitiates its otherwise useful qualities. Amoxicillin-clavulanate and other β-lactamase–resistant drugs cross the blood-brain barrier poorly but are likely to cross at the time of breach in the barrier. Metronidazole can cross the barrier to counter a wide range of organisms, including some protozoans.

SURGICAL MANAGEMENT

Surgical management difficulties occur because the infection is in a closed space. Ideally, spaces containing pus should be drained openly; this is a basic principle of surgery. In many neurosurgical situations, however, open drainage may be unreasonable and unfeasible. The infection may not be reachable, it may not be sufficiently contained to drain, or drainage may be more dangerous than closed treatment.

TREATMENT OF SPECIFIC INFECTIONS

Meningitis The treatment of meningitis depends on the causative organisms. Penicillin should be given until identification of the organisms is possible. For children, ampicillin and chloramphenicol should be given to treat *Haemophilus* infection.[7] Third-generation cephalosporins should be used if the responsible organism is considered gram-negative.

Brain Abscess Surgery is the preferred treatment modality for brain abscess. In some situations, abscess can be managed without surgery. Mampalam and Rosenblum[15] treated 17 of 102 patients with abscess medically. Others have reported similar experiences; as early as 1978 Berg et al.[3] treated four patients medically with cure. Earlier reports showed poor outcome; presumably the difference is attributable to the advent of CT scanning. Patients who are good candidates for medical treatment are those in poor preoperative condition (i.e., bad candidates for

surgery) or those who have excellent neurological status and small abscesses. Unfortunately, medical treatment vitiates proper identification of the organism and determination of antibiotic sensitivities.

Drainage and total excision are among the surgical options. Excision is favored when the abscess has a thick capsule, is superficial, and is located on a neurologically "silent" area. With the ready availability of stereotaxic surgery the drainage of abscesses is simplified and can be done with the patient under local anesthesia. Drainage may be the only option for treatment of multiple or deep subcortical abscesses.[8] Drainage and total excision provide identical outcomes.

Osteomyelitis, Epidural Abscess, and Subdural Empyema Few reports of surgery for osteomyelitis of the skull exist, and current consensus is that radical debridement provides the best result.[6] The only choice for epidural abscess is surgical management with debridement of osteomyelitic bone. At the time of drainage the full extent of involvement of osteomyelitis may not be known. Subsequent debridement may be necessary. No studies with good outcomes from medical management of epidural abscess have been reported.

Occasionally infection spares the epidural space and lodges in the potential space between the dura and arachnoid. A subdural hematoma may become secondarily infected. As may occur with a subdural hematoma, the abscess may dissect into the potential space to cover an entire hemisphere. Pathak et al.[18] reviewed medical treatment of subdural empyema and presented reports of cases successfully treated with antibiotics alone.

Cavernous Sinus Thrombosis The elements of septic sinus thrombosis include dehydration and blood hyperviscosity. Accordingly, treatment includes hydration and administration of antibiotics. Thrombectomy is not indicated. Anticoagulant treatment is controversial.

ACQUIRED IMMUNODEFICIENCY SYNDROME

The management of patients with AIDS poses new considerations. Patients with AIDS may have concomitant multiple infections or sequential infections with different agents. Typically a patient infected with human immunodeficiency virus may initially have an enhancing lesion on CT scan. This lesion could be progressive multifocal leukoencephalopathy (the aftermath of infection with JC virus) or lymphoma, both of which are not treated surgically. Conversely, the lesion could be mycobacterial or fungal abscess or toxoplasmosis abscess, all of which are treated surgically. One algorithm suggests biopsy of the first lesion and treatment of others based on the biopsy results. Another approach first treats toxoplasmosis medically with subsequent biopsy if no response occurs within a prescribed period (approximately 2 weeks).

REFERENCES

1. Apuzzo MLJ, Mitchell MS: Immunological aspect of intrinsic glial tumors, *J Neurosurg* 55:1, 1981.
2. Baker AS: Role of anaerobic bacteria in sinusitis and its complications, *Ann Otol Rhinol Laryngol (Suppl)* 154:17, 1991.
3. Berg B, Franklin G, Cuneo R, et al: Nonsurgical cure of brain abscess: early diagnosis and follow-up with computerized tomography, *Ann Neurol* 3:474, 1978.
4. Borges LF: Host defenses, *Neurosurg Clin North Am* 3:275, 1992.
5. Britt RH, Enzmann DR: Clinical stages of human brain abscesses on serial CT scans after contrast infusion: computerized tomographic, neuropathological, and clinical correlations, *J Neurosurg* 59:972, 1983.
6. Bullit E, Lehman RAW: Osteomyelitis of the skull, *Surg Neurol* 11:163, 1979.
7. Durack DT, Perfect JR: Acute bacterial meningitis. In Wilkins RH, Rengachery SS, editors: *Neurosurgery,* New York, 1985, McGraw-Hill.
8. Dyste GN, Hitchon PW, Menezes AH, et al: Stereotaxic surgery in the treatment of multiple brain abscesses, *J Neurosurg* 69:188, 1988.
9. Everett ED, Eichoff T, Simon RH: Cerebrospinal fluid shunt infections with anaerobic diphtheroids (*Propionibacterium* sp.), *J Neurosurg* 44:580, 1976.
10. Fang HSY, Ong GB: Direct anterior approach to the upper cervical spine, *J Bone Joint Surg* 44A:1588, 1962.
11. Garvey G: Current concepts of bacterial infections of the central nervous system: bacterial meningitis and bacterial brain abscess, *J Neurosurg* 59:735, 1983.
12. Hall WA: Neurosurgical infections in the compromised host, *Infect Neurol Surg* 3:435, 1992.
13. Harris JP, Godin MS, Krekorian TD, et al: The transoropalatal approach to the atlantoaxial-clival region: considerations for the head and neck surgeon, *Laryngoscope* 99:467, 1989.
14. Lad SD, Chandy MJ: Cranio-facial actinomycosis, *Br J Neurosurg* 5:451, 1988.
15. Mampalam TJ, Rosenblum ML: Trends in the management of bacterial brain abscesses: a review of 102 cases over 17 years, *Neurosurgery* 23:451, 1988.
16. Marks PV, Patel KS, Mee EW: Multiple brain abscesses secondary to dental caries and severe periodontal disease, *Br J Oral Maxillofac Surg* 26:244, 1988.
17. Meyers BR, Wormser G, Hirschman SZ, et al: Rhinocerebral mucormycosis: premortem diagnosis and therapy, *Arch Intern Med* 139:557, 1979.
18. Pathak A, Sharma BS, Mathuriya SN, et al: Controversies in the management of subdural empyema: a study of 41 cases with review of literature, *Acta Neurochir* 102:25, 1990.
19. Taha JM, Haddad FS, Brown JA: Intracranial infection after missile injuries to the brain: report of 30 cases from the Lebanese conflict, *Neurosurgery* 29:864, 1991.
20. Wald ER: Infective agents in the central nervous system, *Infect Neurol Surg* 3:259, 1992.
21. Weiner LP, Fleming JO: Viral infections of the nervous system, *J Neurosurg* 61:207, 1984.
22. Young RF, Gade G, Grinnel V: Surgical treatment for fungal infections in the central nervous system, *J Neurosurg* 63:371, 1985.

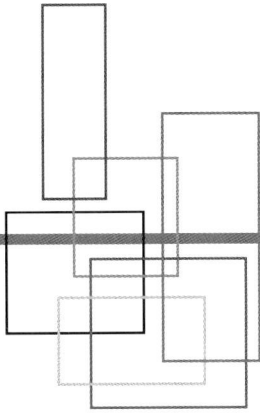

Infection in the Maxillofacial Trauma Patient

Richard H. Haug
Leon A. Assael

Infection is a primary concern in the care of patients who have sustained maxillofacial trauma. Infection may be the outcome of the primary injury or subsequent treatment. It may result in failure of wound healing, systemic sepsis, and fracture nonunion and often results in prolonged hospitalization and additional surgery. The results of infection in the trauma patient may produce irretrievable damage to the patient, including disfigurement, dysfunction, and death. Minor infections also may severely compromise the quality of clinical results in the management of maxillofacial trauma (Figure 17-1).

Even when the final outcome is favorable, the occurrence of an infection is always a source of distress to the patient, the patient's family, and the surgeon. Therefore the prevention of infection is central to all elements of maxillofacial trauma care. No procedure or therapy may be advocated if it increases the risk of infection. Maneuvers, medication, or procedures that appear to decrease the risk of infection always attract attention and are incorporated into clinical practice when their benefit is demonstrated.

PATHOPHYSIOLOGY OF INFECTION IN MAXILLOFACIAL TRAUMA

GENERAL

Infection results from the presence of pathogenic organisms and the alteration of the homeostatic relationship between individuals and their environment. Nothing alters homeostasis more suddenly than acute trauma. An understanding of the key elements of altered homeostasis in trauma is necessary to assess and mitigate infection risk and to subsequently manage an infection.

After trauma is sustained, the major organ systems are mobilized to respond to increased demands. These responses are designed to retain cardiopulmonary function,

preserve the perfusion and nutrition of the brain and splanchnic bed, initiate and modulate the inflammatory process, and retain physical flight and defense abilities.

CARDIOVASCULAR RESPONSE

The initial cardiopulmonary response to trauma is primarily sympathomimetic. Tachycardia, increased peripheral arteriolar tone, and elevated blood pressure result. A decrease in skin temperature, decreased perfusion, and hypoxia can result in a diminished host response to cutaneous pathogens. Arteriolar constriction in wound sites generally is temporary and sustained primarily until initial hemostasis is complete. Rebound vasodilation occurs in wound sites within several hours and is modulated primarily by the inflammatory process. Tissue edema and hematological response cause sluggish arteriolar blood flow in the hours after injury.

In hypovolemic shock the decrease in peripheral perfusion and temperature is even more profound and sustained. This change occurs to preserve core temperature and perfusion. Local vessel injury may be caused by laceration or concussion. Thrombosis of the associated vessels results in locally hypoxic or necrotic tissue that is more susceptible to the invasion of organisms.

PULMONARY RESPONSE

The initial pulmonary response to trauma includes tachypnea with a decrease in serum carbon dioxide. Compensatory respiratory alkalosis occurs, which partially balances the metabolic acidosis of tissue injury and tissue hypoxia. For the patient who has survived the initial days after trauma, the greatest systemic threat to the wounds sustained is pneumonia. The decrease in partial pressure of oxygen in peripheral tissues caused by pneumonia increases

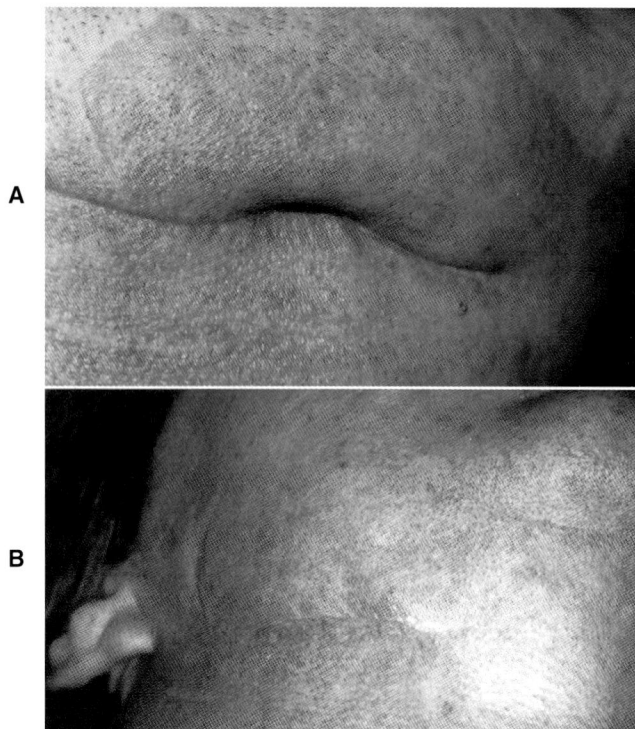

Figure 17-1 A, An unsightly scar developed from this chronically infected and draining mandibular fracture. **B,** The same patient after removal of loose and infected hardware, enucleation of the sinus tract, and scar revision.

the likelihood of wound infection. Because of hypoxia the risk of systemic sepsis increases. In trauma patients the most frequent cause of death after admission is infection, and the most frequent infection is pneumonia.[28]

Immobility and a posttraumatic catabolic state also contribute to the risk of aspiration and pneumonia.[80] In maxillofacial trauma, upper airway obstruction, supine positioning, alcohol ingestion, bleeding, and intermaxillary fixation increase the risk of aspiration. Patients requiring ventilators, tracheostomy, or blood transfusion, or those with associated rib injuries are more likely to develop pneumonia after trauma.

Maintaining oxygen transport in the injured and septic patient is essential because oxygen requirements of major organs such as the liver are increased up to 72%.[24] Supplemental oxygen, the early and sustained use of ventilators, blood transfusion, and all other means of maintaining oxygen transport are essential to a favorable outcome in these patients.

ENDOCRINE AND METABOLIC RESPONSE

The major endocrine responses in the trauma patient are designed to produce the stress response and maintain homeostasis after an external assault. Elevation of circulating catecholamine levels is the earliest response that results in positive chronotropic and inotropic cardiovascular responses, peripheral vasoconstriction, and elevated serum glucose. Activation of the renin-angiotensin system and in-

creased levels of antidiuretic hormone decrease urine production to preserve intravascular volume. Cortisol levels increase to modulate the inflammatory response, elevate serum glucose, and mobilize the production of usable energy. These hormonal responses make patients less susceptible to infection because these mechanisms enhance physiological activity.

Glycogenolysis, proteinolysis, and the production of fatty acids from fat sustain hypermetabolism of 25% to 100% over preinjury needs.[27] This may result in ketosis, fluid loss, and substantial weight loss, with or without loss of muscle mass in the days after injury. Unfortunately, these systems may fail as a result of preexisting disease or the overwhelming of available hormonal and metabolic homeostatic mechanisms in the hours and days after injury. Nutritional support with enteral or parenteral nutrition, hydration, and oxygenation are key elements in preventing organ failure and permitting healing in the trauma patient.[6,10]

WOUND RESPONSE

Cutaneous Injury   The skin and mucosa are essential barriers to the entry of pathogenic organisms into the underlying connective tissue and organs. The integument normally is exposed to bacteria only to the depth of the adnexa. Lacerations result in the activation of host defense mechanisms. Because of the systemic response to injury, patients with major injuries are more susceptible to wound infection than individuals with local trauma.[15,22,31] Oral and cutaneous injuries expose the underlying tissues of the skin to oral microflora and the oral mucosa to skin microflora. Host defenses unique to these sites are less able to defend against bacteria from remote sites. For example, a wound infection of the neck may be far more severe if driven by an oral anaerobe compared with skin microflora.

Muscle Injury   Myonecrosis of muscle results when concussion, maceration, or avulsion occurs.[79] The risk of myonecrosis is increased after a period of hypovolemic shock or when associated burns are present. Muscle infection is frequent when a contaminated wound sustains myonecrosis. Anaerobic bacteria are the most likely pathogens in muscle infection. Although virtually any anaerobic pathogen may cause myonecrosis, the most notable are *Clostridium perfringens* and *Clostridium tetani* (Figure 17-2). Muscle injury, muscle hypoxia, and subsequent infection may produce rhabdomyolysis and myoglobinemia. Myoglobinemia and myoglobinuria may produce acute renal failure. Maintenance of oxygenation, hydration, wound perfusion, and judicious use of wound compression may mitigate rhabdomyolysis.

Gas Gangrene and Other Necrotic Wound Infections

C. perfringens is the prototypical organism in gas gangrene. In this situation, gas-producing bacteria are associated with a foul-smelling, hypoxic, necrotic wound. The infection progresses rapidly along fascial planes. The loss of tissue, including overlying skin, is a frequent occurrence.

Although classically associated with *C. perfringens,* many

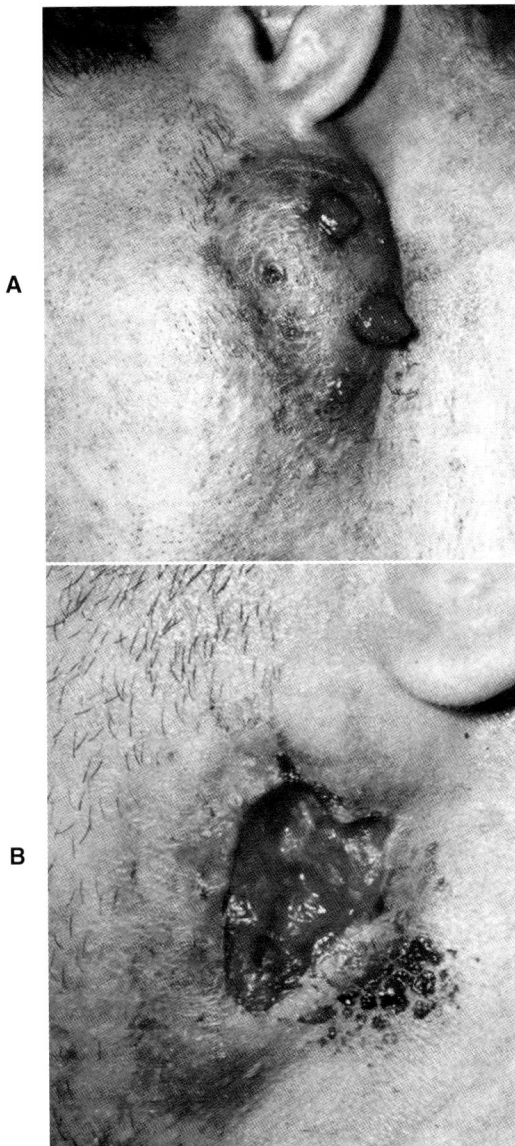

Figure 17-2 This necrotizing wound infection **(A)** resulted in sloughing of the preauricular area **(B).**

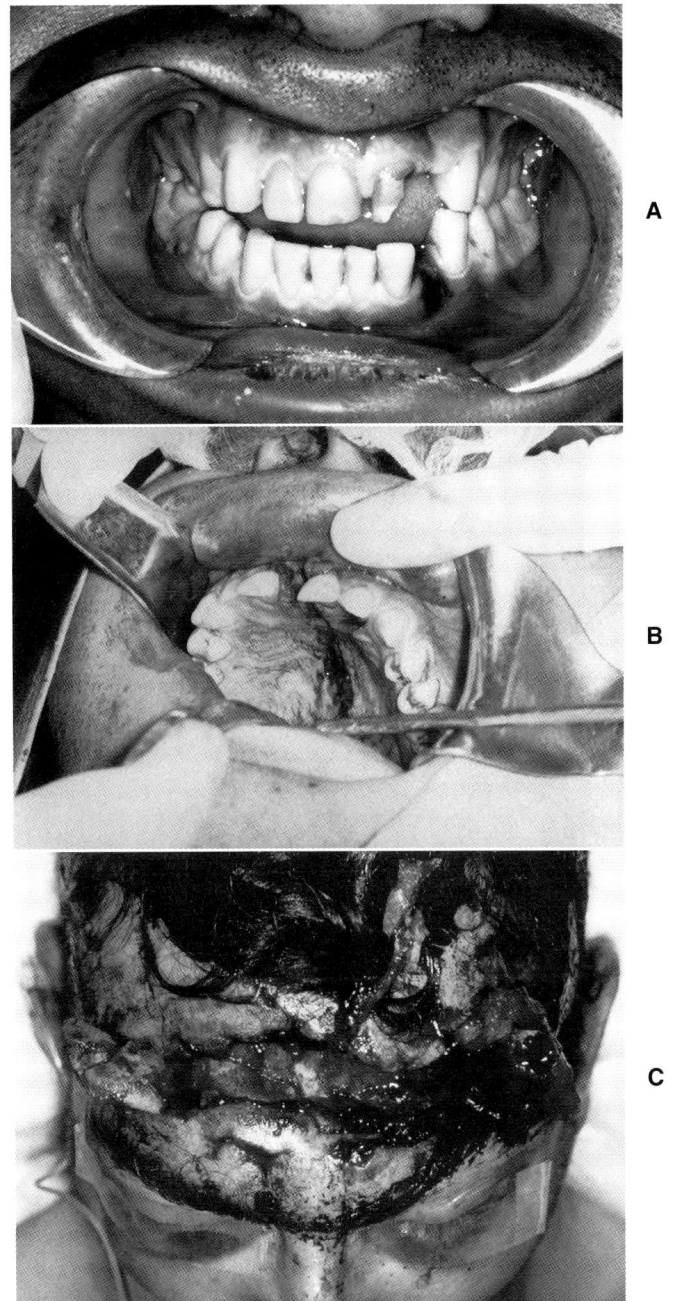

Figure 17-3 Compound fractures. A fracture can communicate with the external environment through a tooth crypt **(A),** or an overlying mucosal wound **(B).** The central nervous system also may communicate with the skin, frontal sinus, and nasal cavity **(C).**

pathogenic bacteria may cause necrotic wound infections in the maxillofacial region (see Figure 17-2). The early signs of necrotic wound infection are severe pain, gas production, mottling, darkening of wound edges, and sepsis.

Although *C. perfringens* infection rarely occurs in the face, when it is found it may cause tissue mottling, severe muscle necrosis, gas production, and a rapid life-threatening toxemia known as *gas gangrene*. Because the organism is normal in feces, the entry into the wound may be the result of exposure to soil or secondary wound contamination.

Gas gangrene is frequent in war injuries. The increased incidence may occur because of the sharply decreased number of organisms necessary to cause disease when the organism is combined with normal soil; therefore prompt and thorough cleansing of wounds may be the best means of preventing gas gangrene.[79] In addition, because *C. perfringens* typically is sensitive to penicillin, penicillin is an excellent choice to assist in infection prevention when road

and dirt injuries occur. These methods have reduced the incidence of gas gangrene sharply in war-related trauma. The incidence of clostridial myositis (in U.S. casualties) was 5% in World War I, 0.7% in World War II, and 0.08% during the Korean War.[26]

Fracture Considerations Fractures in the dentate segment and those communicating with the sinuses usually are considered compound fractures. Compound fractures are initially contaminated with the organisms present at the site of injury (Figure 17-3). In the oral cavity this can include the entire spectrum of oral flora present. These include bacteria such as *Streptococcus, Provetella, Neisseria, Klebsiella, Eikenella, Bacteroides, Haemophilus,* and *Corynebacterium* species and aerophilic fungi such as *Candida albicans.*[86] Contamination from the skin includes preexisting organisms such as *Staphylococcus epidermidis, Staphylococcus aureus,* and environmentally acquired organisms. Road-, water-, and soil-associated injuries may be contaminated with fecal and saprophytic organisms.

The bacterial contamination of compound fractures in the mandible results in a higher infection rate in these locations. Infection of closed subcondylar and ramus fractures is very rare. Mandibular angle fractures associated with third molar teeth have the highest infection rate: as high as 24% and even higher in patients with preexisting pericoronitis.[3,9] Edentulous fractures demonstrate a lower infection rate than fractures in dentate segments.[4]

Teeth in the Line of Fracture   Because of the higher infection rate in compound fractures of the dentate seg-

ment, removal of all teeth in the fracture site has been advocated.[75] However, no difference in infection rate has been shown in clinical studies comparing the removal of teeth versus allowing teeth to remain in the fracture site.[4,5,42,81] Completely mobile teeth in the fracture site may be considered for removal because micromotion causes the continued percolation of pathogenic bacteria. Teeth in the fracture site with preexisting periapical or periodontal infection also should be considered for removal because the generation of pathological organisms from a previously infected tooth would likely increase the risk of infection.

The presence of partially erupted third molars carries the greatest risk for the development of infection in the fracture site regardless of tooth removal.[5,74] A 1990 survey of surgeons revealed that nonmobile teeth are not routinely removed from the line of fracture. The survey also indicated that early treatment and preservation of teeth (including impacted teeth) resulted in a lower incidence of infection.[81]

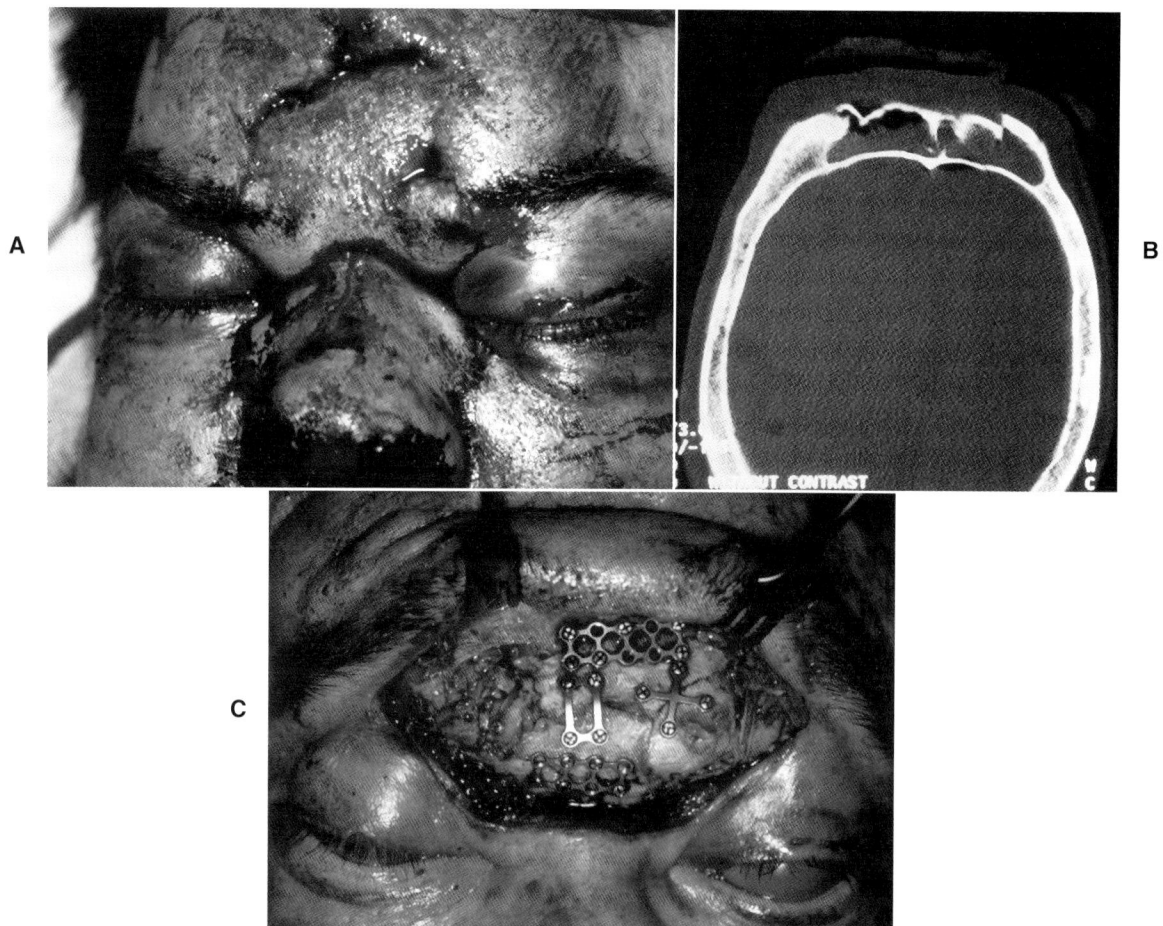

Figure 17-4 Highly comminuted fractures demand special attention to underlying bone stability to ensure that both soft and hard tissue heals uneventfully. Titanium plates, screws, and mesh are invaluable in accomplishing this goal. This patient sustained a significant frontal sinus, supraorbital rim, and nasoorbitalethmoid fracture that communicated with the external environment through a degloving laceration **(A).** The nature of the injury is documented with computed tomography **(B).** The fracture was approached through the existing laceration and stabilized with multiple titanium plates and screws **(C).**

Unstable Fractures Unstable fractures have a higher infection rate because bacteria can continue to invade the fracture site during motion.[82] Also, the maturation of new blood vessels is disrupted by motion. Hemorrhage and increased inflammation in the fracture site cause increased bacterial counts. Healing of lacerations is delayed when associated fractures are not stabilized. This increases the risk of infection with hospital-acquired organisms.

When motion occurs in a fracture site, callus organization is delayed and the orientation of the callus may not result in a bridging callus. Reorientation of the callus may result in a pseudoarthrosis with resorption and eburnation of the bone ends.[82] This pseudarthrosis invariably is colonized with bacteria in compound fractures of the maxillofacial bones.[82] A mixed bacterial flora with many gram-negative saprophytic organisms is frequent when necrotic bone is present in the fracture site.

Comminuted Fractures Comminuted fractures are more prone to infection than simple fractures (Figure 17-4). The loss of blood supply to fractured segments makes them more susceptible to bacterial growth. Because of the vascular compromise, prophylactic antibiotics are less able to penetrate the comminuted site.

Comminuted fractures usually are the result of higher-energy injury associated with greater collateral damage. If the fracture is the result of a penetrating wound, pathogenic bacteria have been seeded both deeply and widely through the injured tissues. These factors combine to make comminuted fractures a high risk for infection.[8,50]

Central Nervous System Injury Associated central nervous system (CNS) injury sharply increases the risk of infection in patients with maxillofacial trauma. Gram-negative pneumonia is the greatest risk, with early appearance at an average of 3 days after injury.[43] Wound infection in the maxillofacial site more frequently contains nosocomial gram-negative organisms such as *Serratia* and *Pseudomonas* spp. in patients with a head injury because these patients frequently are located in intensive care units. Nosocomial infection associated with these species is especially frequent around tracheostomy sites and open wounds of the head and neck. Another emerging pathogen that has colonized intensive care units is methicillin-resistant *S. aureus*. Thus appropriate universal barrier precautions and hand washing after treatment of each patient are important in patients with CNS injury.

Exposure of the CNS to the organisms of the nose, sinuses, mastoid, skin, and ear is common in maxillofacial trauma. Exposure is frequent in upper midface and cranial base fractures. Rarely a mandibular fracture may produce CNS involvement. Prevention of postinjury meningitis or brain abscess requires maintenance of positive intracranial pressure to prevent pneumoencephalocele. Intubation is preferable over laryngeal mask airway or bag-valve-mask ventilation in the patient with CNS injury. Prevention of infection of the CNS also depends on prophylactic antibiotics. Early surgical management to eliminate the communication with other structures often is indicated, but such management generally is not applicable when cranial base and cribriform plate fractures have occurred. In these instances, early reduction of fractures is beneficial. Cerebrospinal fluid leaks infrequently persist beyond the initial fracture treatment.[60]

GENERAL CONSIDERATIONS IN THE MANAGEMENT AND PREVENTION OF INFECTION IN THE PATIENT WITH MAXILLOFACIAL TRAUMA

Some considerations in the management of the patient with maxillofacial trauma have been identified as effective in the elimination and prevention of infection. Many of these practices have remained unchanged for decades.[65] Although listed as one comprehensive group, each individual activity or principle cannot be applied to every situation. Individual activities or principles should be considered separately and applied as appropriate to specific clinical circumstances.

APPROPRIATE SYSTEMATIC HISTORY AND CLINICAL EXAMINATION

As with any patient the care of the maxillofacial trauma victim begins with an assessment of the patient's history and a clinical examination. The portion of the history important for the trauma victim with a traumatic wound that is infected or could become infected includes an assessment of predisposing medical illnesses, compromised host defenses, presence of prostheses, and identification of the hallmarks of infection. Although medical illnesses that predispose the patient to infection and compromised host defense mechanisms are discussed in detail in another chapter, a general list is provided (see Chapter 24). Predisposing conditions include diabetes mellitus or immune system compromise, ethanol abuse, use of chemotherapeutic agents or steroids, very young or old age, and presence of devices such as prosthetic joints and heart valves, and cardiac, urological, or neurological stents and shunts.[10,15,24,31,56] Other important historical points are the mechanism of injury, environment surrounding the victim, and time since injury. For instance, animal bites (especially those that include puncture wounds) and farm injuries (or those that have occurred in soil or free-standing water) are particularly prone to infection and should be noted.[16,40] Attacks with instruments or by individuals suspected of being contaminated with blood-borne pathogens should be identified. In addition, the time since injury should be recorded.

The systematic clinical examination should include the Advanced Trauma Life Support primary and secondary survey and focus on hallmarks of infection and their extent and duration. This includes obvious local signs of infection such as edema, erythema, tenderness and warmth, and the systemic responses to infection such as an elevated temperature, respiratory rate, pulse rate, and serum white blood cell count.[67] Occult injuries that are newly discovered are a frequent cause of infection and sepsis. Bacteremia without an identified source is frequent (21% in polytrauma patients).[19]

IMAGING EVALUATION

The imaging examination may include several modalities directed at various forms of injury and types of infection. Plane radiography effectively identifies many facial fractures (60% of mandible fractures) and foreign bodies.[21] Although the panoramic radiograph is the most effective image in the evaluation of mandibular injury (92%), it is less effective in identification of foreign bodies and infection.[21] One of the most effective images in the assessment of both trauma (especially midfacial and upper facial) and infection is computed tomography. By alteration of the image window, the hard and soft tissues, cellulitis, abscesses, and various foreign bodies may be identified. Glass, shrapnel, wood, and plastic foreign bodies may be identified routinely using computed tomography with the appropriate window.

Other imaging techniques also are effective in the identification of foreign bodies and the evaluation of infection (Figure 17-5). These include xeroradiography, ultrasonography, and magnetic resonance imaging. Xerora-

diography, the technology developed for mammography, is particularly effective in identifying nonradiopaque foreign bodies. Ultrasonography is useful in the assessment of fluid collections and is rapidly becoming a modality effective in the identification of infection. Magnetic resonance imaging may be the most effective tool in evaluating soft tissues and can be used to confirm the presence of a foreign body or infection.

FOCUSED WOUND EXAMINATION

The examination of the local wound includes an assessment of the condition of both the soft and hard tissues. In addition to completing the diagnosis and classifying the injury, the presence or absence of an infection, foreign body, or both should be confirmed or refuted. The condition of the injured soft tissue and the soft tissues overlying the injured bone should be assessed for quality (i.e., necrosis, vascularity, contamination) and quantity (i.e., avulsion). In an animal attack, all punctures should be identified and explored. Contamination by various forms of debris (i.e., soil, vegetation, feces, or chemicals) should be noted.

CULTURE OF WOUND WITH GRAM STAIN AND ANTIBIOTIC SUSCEPTIBILITY

If purulence is identified, or contamination suspected, wound sampling is an important adjunct. The purulence or contaminated tissues may be cultured for anaerobic and aerobic bacteria in addition to other types of microorganisms (see Chapter 3). The cultures should be tested for antibiotic susceptibility. Gram staining of the purulence or contaminated tissues is important in directing the initial course of antibiotic therapy.

HEMOSTASIS

The initial management of the wound should provide hemostasis to prevent development of a hematoma. Bacteria multiply rapidly in fresh clotted blood. Residual blood in a wound multiplies the risk of infection. Incision and removal of a hematoma are considered more frequently for a traumatic wound than for a surgically created clean incision in the maxillofacial region.

A bacterially invaded hematoma undergoes liquefaction and abscess formation. This process usually occurs 3 to 5 days after initial trauma. Drainage of the hematoma alone at this point may cause severe or prolonged hemorrhage resulting from eroded vessels in the abscess site. Therefore, incision and drainage should be performed under controlled operating room conditions so that open treatment and careful attention to hemostasis may be achieved.[40,64]

IRRIGATION AND FOREIGN BODY REMOVAL

A lower infection rate has been demonstrated with appropriate foreign body removal in facial injuries.[51] Jet lavage may be used to remove soil and other wound debris.[14,36]

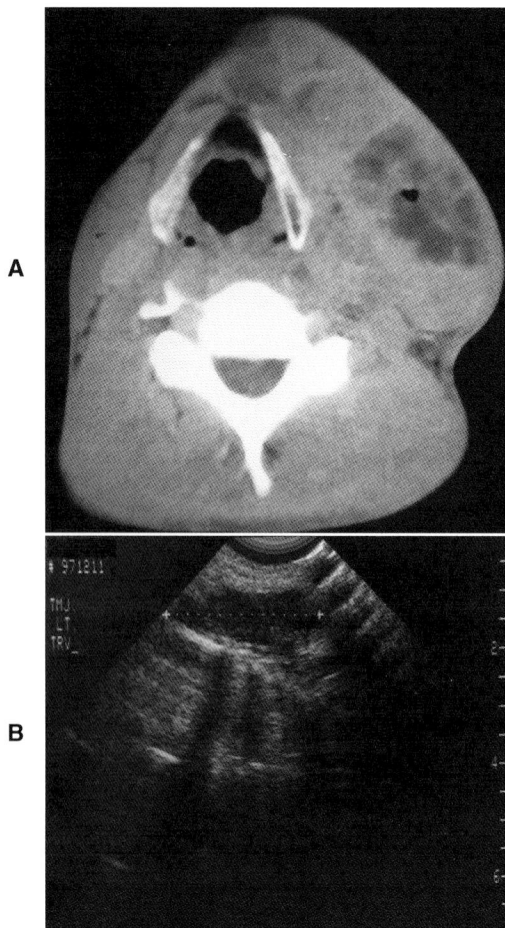

Figure 17-5 Computed tomography **(A)**, magnetic resonance imaging, xeroradiography, and ultrasonography **(B)** are invaluable aids in confirming the resonance of an infection.

Sterile isotonic solutions such as normal saline solution are currently the ideal irrigants for this purpose.[14] If the clinical or imaging examination reveals a foreign body, it should be removed before or during definitive repair of the injury. Removal may be accomplished with the patient under regional or general anesthesia. Although irrigation with saline and antibiotic solutions has been identified as effective in the prevention or reduction of infection, so has the use of antimicrobial skin preparation agents.[14,36,63] Povidone-iodine solution has been identified as the closest to an ideal antimicrobial skin preparation agent for the maxillofacial region. Surgical scrubbing cleansers should be avoided because the alcohol in tincture and the detergent in scrub can cause corneal chemical ulceration. For these same reasons, hexachlorophene preparations also should be avoided. Povidone-iodine solution may be used as an irrigant for both lacerations and puncture wounds. However, all of the povidone-iodine solution should be rinsed from the wound at the end of the procedure with normal saline solution because povidone-iodine can cause soft tissue fibrosis.[63]

Consideration should be given to the use of antibiotics in the saline solution lavage. Except in patients with allergy or sensitization, irrigation of lacerations with antibiotic solutions just before suturing is beneficial. In one prospective, double-blind study in which 5% solution of sodium benzyl penicillin was used with saline solution to irrigate lacerations, early infection decreased from 22% to 6% and late infection from 9% to 1%.[59] Benzalkonium chloride also has been reported effective in the elimination or reduction of viruses in the wound when used as an irrigant. This finding is a important in treatment of animal bites, especially punctures.

CONSERVATIVE DEBRIDEMENT OF NECROTIC TISSUE

Debridement of the wound to decrease bacterial counts and remove necrotic tissue should be accomplished without compromising the blood supply. Vasoconstriction from the infiltration of local anesthesia with epinephrine may decrease the blood supply sufficiently to make the wound more prone to infection. Hence, the use of local anesthetic block techniques may be considered for wound closure.

DRAIN PLACEMENT BEFORE OR DURING DEFINITIVE REPAIR

Many lacerated, contused tissues do not respond to the usual hemostatic measures reserved for surgical wounds. In addition, they usually are contaminated with pathogenic bacteria. Therefore wound drainage is an essential feature in the treatment of many traumatic injuries. The higher the risk of infection, the more likely that wound drainage will be beneficial. Both active and passive drains may be used effectively.

Passive drainage, such as that provided by a Penrose drain, is effective for soft tissue wounds and assists in the evacuation of hematoma or seroma collections. Active drainage, such as that provided by a suction-activated device, is more effective in the elimination of dead space collections than passive drains, but negative pressure also has the potential disadvantage of drawing contaminants into the wound. Wide-bore rubber catheters may be used passively or actively. They also may be used to provide intermittent irrigation and attached to suction.

ABSOLUTE RIGID FIXATION OR IMMOBILIZATION OF FRACTURES

An essential principle in the management of facial fractures is the application of sufficient fixation of the fractured bones to permit undisturbed healing under stable conditions.[6,8,25,54,78] Instability of fractures and resulting motion causes the tearing of juvenile blood vessels invading the injured site. This causes repeated hemorrhage, bacterial growth, the formation of granulation tissue, and the inhibition of collagen formation. Instability of contaminated fractures often results in cellulitis, suppuration, eburnation of the fracture ends, and a nonunion pseudarthrosis. Healing under stable conditions permits bridging of the fracture with maturing blood vessels, effective migration of fibroblasts, early appearance of woven bone, and functional union of the fracture ends.[82] Current rigid internal fixation systems provide the stability necessary to achieve these goals.

An additional advantage of rigid internal fixation of fractures is early return to function. This includes improved nutrition, improved mobility, and improved speech. The value of early function extends beyond the injured site, as the risk of associated multiple trauma complications, such as pneumonia, decreases when the patient's functional behavior is restored.[80]

DEFINITIVE SOFT TISSUE WOUND REPAIR

If possible, early closure (within 12 hours of injury) of soft tissue injury should be attempted. Within this time frame the inflammatory process has not yet compromised the wound margins enough to warrant significant wound margin revision. A layered closure directed at precise anatomical reconstruction is the goal. With the use of resorbable sutures such as gut, resorption is achieved through the inflammatory process or hydrolysis. An already inflamed (or infected) wound may compromise both the integrity of the suture material and wound closure. Consideration should be given, whenever possible, to the use of sutures that induce the least inflammation and are less likely to harbor bacteria. Fewer, smaller, and nonbraided sutures are preferred. 4-0 Monocryl (Johnson and Johnson, Princeton, NJ) for deep tissues and 6-0 monofilament nylon for skin are good choices for wound closure.

Restoration of tensile strength across the wound margin is delayed in traumatic wounds because of contusion, edema, and bacterial contamination. Closure under tension results in early wound breakdown because of these cofactors. If the wound cannot be closed without tension, delayed wound closure should be considered. Open packing with or without moist normal saline solution dressings may be a necessary alternative.

Failure to close a traumatic wound in layers results in dead space. Hemorrhage and subsequent breakdown of an infected wound are likely in the presence of contused tissues. Restoration of each structure to its preinjury position also assists in the elimination of dead space. Under certain conditions during the management of patients with maxillofacial trauma and infection, a primary layered closure becomes impossible. Maneuvers such as open packing or wound pexing are particularly effective for visibly contaminated wounds with multiple foreign bodies (i.e., gravel or soil) that cannot be removed at the time of initial surgery, or in situations in which soft tissue is absent or cannot be closed primarily without tension. Other procedures that may assist the definitive repair of soft tissues include local, regional, or free flaps, especially when soft tissues are absent.

ANTIBIOTIC THERAPY

General Considerations   Antibiotic therapy is perhaps the most important consideration in the management of the maxillofacial trauma victim with an infection or the potential to develop one. The victim invariably is contaminated with an array of microorganisms from both the host and external environment.[35] Aside from numerous unknown organisms that exist in the victim's surrounding environment, normal flora of the skin, mouth, nose and accessory sinuses may be introduced into the wound.[3] For the mouth alone, more than 42 individual microorganisms have been identified in the healthy patient and for those with gingivitis, caries or periodontitis, more than 190.[40]

The use of antibiotics in patients with facial fractures has reduced the incidence of infection. In one randomized, prospective clinical trial of antibiotic use in facial fractures, cefazolin therapy started 1 hour before open reduction surgery reduced the infection rate from 42% to 9%.[20] Current therapy for contaminated wounds requires that antibiotics be started as soon as the patient is seen with an injury and are continued at least through the perioperative phase. Soft tissue injuries also demand the early administration of antibiotics. In a prospective, double-blind study of 64 patients with intraoral lacerations, the use of penicillin reduced the incidence of infection from 19% to 0% when noncompliant patients were excluded.[87]

Animal bites are contaminated with all of the same bacteria as human bites but also may include *Pasteurella multocida* or a variety of organisms that cause zoonotic diseases.* These are diseases that occur in humans by bacteria of an animal's normal flora. Examples include the Psittacosis-lymphogranuloma group, which causes cat-scratch fever, *Streptobacillus moniliformis* or Spirillum minus, which causes rat-bite fever, and *Yersinia pestis,* which causes the plague.[1,23,38]

Antibiotic therapy in animal bites is not the same as for other lacerations.[1,38] Clindamycin and erythromycin are particularly poor choices because they do not eliminate *Pasteurella multocida.*[17,30,40,85] Penicillin or amoxicillin are good choices with the exception of poor activity against *S. aureus.* Because of this, amoxicillin with clavulanic acid (Augmentin) has become a favored choice for prophylactic therapy or empirical management of infected bites.[33,40]

Human bites become infected with even greater frequency than animal bites. Common organisms in human bites include *Streptococcus viridans, Bacteroides* spp., *Peptostreptococcus, Fusobacterium nucleatum,* and *Eikenella corrodens.*[11,17,32,33,40] Some *Bacteroides* spp. are resistant to penicillin and are β-lactamase positive.[17] For humans, as for animals, amoxicillin with clavulanic acid is a good choice.[40]

Prophylactic Antibiotics   Principles of prophylactic antibiotic therapy as defined by Peterson[66] should be considered when deciding on its use in the patient with maxillofacial trauma.

Does the Patient Have a Significant Risk of Infection?
Maxillofacial trauma patients with lacerations, abrasions, burns, puncture wounds, macerated contusions, penetrating injuries, dentoalveolar injury, or compound fractures have a significant risk for infection. Closed fractures, such as subcondylar fractures and simple contusions, often do not have a significant risk of infection. The consequences of infection also must be assessed. Will a potential infection resolve without consequence, or will it cause failure in healing, scarring, and subsequent functional deficits?

Has the Appropriate Antibiotic Been Selected?
For intraoral wounds, penicillin provides excellent bactericidal coverage. Facial wound prophylaxis should preserve the penicillin spectrum while adding coverage against penicillinase-producing *S. aureus.* A first-generation cephalosporin or clindamycin works well. As noted previously, bites, burns, and other special wounds need individual considerations as to antibiotic selection.

Debate persists regarding the selection of an antibiotic in patients with cerebrospinal fluid leaks.[57] Although patients are at risk for the development of meningitis from local flora, the ability of antibiotic therapy to prevent its occurrence is debated. The extended use of antibiotics may promote the development of meningitis with resistant organisms. Prevention of meningitis with early use of antibiotics has been reported and remains common practice.[57,60,89] Because facial trauma patients with cerebrospinal fluid leaks generally require antibiotics for their facial fractures, withholding of all antibiotics rarely occurs. Antibiotics associated with the highest concentrations in cerebrospinal fluid are the penicillins (especially ticarcillin, piperacillin, nafcillin, and ampicillin, in descending order), the cephalosporins (especially cefuroxime and ceftazidime), and chloramphenicol.

Is the Antibiotic Level Appropriate?   Initial use of parenteral antibiotics is recommended when the risk of infection is high and the penetration of the drug to the target

---

*References 2, 11, 17, 22, 40, 64, 85.

site is encumbered. As a practical matter, most inpatients receive high intravenous doses of prophylactic antibiotics. With a decided shift from inpatient to outpatient management for all patients (including patients with trauma), enteral antibiotics have become a necessary instrument in the traumatologist's armamentarium. The antibiotic

should be chosen based on the type of injury and suspected contaminants (Table 17-1).

Is the Timing of the Antibiotic Correct? Immediate use of the correct antibiotic represents the optimal means of limiting the incidence of infection. Although only some

TABLE 17-1

Suggested Antibiotic Therapy for the Maxillofacial Trauma Patient

Wound Type	Intraoperative Intravenous*	Postoperative Topical	Postoperative Enteral*
Abrasions	Unnecessary	Bacitracin zinc (500 U/g) bid Polymyxin B (5000 U/g) bid Neomycin sulfate (3.5 mg/g) bid	Unnecessary
Contusions and hematomas	Unnecessary	Unnecessary	Cephalexin Adults: 500 mg q6h Children: 25-50 mg/kg/d in 4 equal divided doses
Punctures	Unnecessary	Unnecessary	Penicillin V or amoxicillin with clavulanic acid Adults: 500 mg q6h Children: 15-50 mg/kg in equal divided doses q6h
Simple lacerations	Unnecessary	Bacitracin zinc (500 U/g) bid Polymyxin B (5000 U/g) bid Neomycin sulfate (3.5 mg/g) bid	Unnecessary
Complex lacerations	Cefazolin Adults: 0.5-1.5 g/q4-12h Children: 25-50 mg/kg/d in 4 equal divided doses	Bacitracin zinc (500 U/g) bid Polymyxin B (5000 U/g) bid Neomycin sulfate (3.5 mg/g) bid	Cephalexin Adults: 500 mg q6h Children: 25-50 mg/kg/d in 4 equal divided doses
Soft tissue avulsions	Cefazolin Adults: 0.5-1.5 g/q4-12h Children: 25-50 mg/kg/d in 4 equal divided doses	Bacitracin zinc (500 U/g) bid Polymyxin B (5000 U/g) bid Neomycin sulfate (3.5 mg/g) bid	Cephalexin Adults: 500 mg q6h Children: 25-50 mg/kg/d in 4 equal divided doses
Burns	Cefazolin 0.5-1.5 Adults: g/q4-12h Children: 25-50 mg/kg/d in 4 equal divided doses	Bacitracin zinc (500 U/g) bid Polymyxin B (5000 U/g) bid Neomycin sulfate (3.5 mg/g) bid	Cephalexin Adults: 500 mg q6h Children: 25-50 mg/kg/d in 4 equal divided doses
Mandibular fractures	Aqueous penicillin G,* 2 million units	Unnecessary	Penicillin V, 500 mg*
Maxillary fractures	Aqueous penicillin G,* 2 million units for oral contaminants; or cefazolin Adults: 0.5-1.5 g/q4-12h Children: 25-50 mg/kg/d in 4 equal divided doses, for cutaneous contaminants	Unnecessary	Penicillin V Adults: 500 mg q6h Children: 15-50 mg/kg in equal divided doses q6h or Cephalexin Adults: 500 mg q6h Children: 25-50 mg/kg/d in 4 equal divided doses
Craniofacial fractures	Cefazolin Adults: 0.5-1.5 g/q4-12h Children: 25-50 mg/kg/d in 4 equal divided doses	Unnecessary	Cephalexin Adults: 500 mg q6h Children: 25-50 mg/kg/d in 4 equal divided doses
Suspected intracranial contamination	Nafcillin 2-6 g q6h,† gentamicin 3-5 mg/kg/d in 3 equal divided doses (adults)	Bacitracin zinc (500 U/g) bid Polymyxin B (5000 U/g) bid Neomycin sulfate (3.5 mg/g) bid	Cephalexin Adults: 500 mg q6h Children: 25-50 mg/kg/d in 4 equal divided doses

*For adult patients with suspected allergy to penicillins or cephalosporins, clindamycin, 150 to 900 mg q8h intravenously, or 0.15 to 0.45 g q6h enterally, are effective alternatives.
†For adult patients with suspected allergy to nafcillin, vancomycin, 1.0 g q12h intravenously, is an effective alternative.

TABLE 17-2

Summary Guide to Tetanus Prophylaxis in Routine Wound Management, 1991

History of Adsorbed Tetanus Toxoid (Doses)	CLEAN, MINOR WOUNDS		ALL OTHER WOUNDS*	
	Td†	TIG	Td†	TIG
Unknown or <3	Yes	No	Yes	Yes
≥3‡	No§	No	No‖	No

From Recommendations of the Immunization Practices Advisory Committee (ACIP). Diptheria, Tetanus, and Pertussis: Recommendations for vaccine use and other preventative measures, *MMWR Morb Mortal Wkly Rep* 40(RR-10):21, 1991.
Td, Tetanus-diphtheria toxoid; *TIG,* tetanus immunoglobulin.
*Such as, but not limited to, wounds contaminated with dirt, feces, soil, and saliva; puncture wounds; avulsions; and wounds resulting from missiles, crushing, burns, and frostbite.
†For children <7 years old; diphtheria-pertussis-tetanus (DPT) (diphtheria-tetanus if pertussis vaccine is contraindicated) is preferred to tetanus toxoid alone. For persons ≥7 years of age, Td is preferred to tetanus toxoid alone.
‡If only three doses of *fluid* toxoid have been received, then a fourth dose of toxoid, preferably an adsorbed toxoid, should be given.
§Yes, if >10 years since last dose.
‖Yes, if >5 years since last dose. (More frequent boosters are not needed and can accentuate side effects.)

emergency medical services begin antibiotic therapy in the field, nearly all patients can receive their first dose of parenteral antibiotics while still in the emergency department.

Is the Shortest Effective Duration of the Antibiotic Being Used? The extended use of prophylactic antibiotics days and weeks after open reduction of facial fractures has become a more frequent practice. Advocates of this method explain that the continued production of pathogenic organisms and the inability to provide an occlusive dressing in the oral cavity requires the extended use of antibiotics. Detractors of the extended use of prophylactic antibiotics suggest that the risk of the development of clinical infection with resistant organisms outweighs the benefit of continued therapy. In related clinical practice (orthognathic surgery), no practical difference has been observed with these differing clinical practices.

Immunization Tetanus prophylaxis should be considered for all wounds that are complex or contaminated (Table 17-2).[70] All crush injuries and animal bites that are partial crush injuries fall into this category, in addition to those wounds exposed to earth-borne contaminants or free-standing water.[70] *C. tetani,* a gram-positive spore-forming anaerobic bacillus, is the causative organism in the devastating posttraumatic infection tetanus. Nearly complete immunization of the U.S. population has made tetanus a rare disease in the United States.[70] Because of immigration and lapses in the immunization program, tetanus may be more common in future years.

Tetanus occurs as the result of wound contamination with the causative organism. *C. tetani* thrives in a necrotic and anaerobic environment.[18] Hence, appropriate wound debridement, cleansing, oxygenation, and antibiotic use all contribute to the prevention of tetanus. An antibiotic, such as penicillin or a cephalosporin, active against *C. tetani* should be administered.

Essentially any common maxillofacial injury can harbor tetanus organisms. Immunization is the most important feature in the prevention of tetanus. Therefore every patient with maxillofacial trauma must be confirmed to have effective immunization as recommended by the Centers for Disease Control, National Center for Prevention Services, Division of Immunization (CDC, NCP) (see Table 17-2). If the immunization schedule was not met, is outdated, or cannot be confirmed, tetanus toxoid or immunoglobulin should be administered according to the CDC, NCP.[70] Active immunization with tetanus toxoid within the last 10 years is effective in preventing tetanus. If such immunization in the last 10 years cannot be confirmed, a 0.5-mL dose of tetanus toxoid is recommended for active immunization. If no previous history of immunization exists, then passive immunization with hyperimmune human tetanus globulin and 0.5 mL of tetanus toxoid is given.[70]

Although tetanus is commonly perceived as a systemic ailment, local forms of the disease have been reported. Two thirds of cases with head and neck symptoms (cephalic tetanus) progress to generalized tetanus.[18] Maxillofacial symptoms of cephalic tetanus include trismus with facial pain, spasms of the muscles of mastication and facial expression (risus sardonicus), nuchal rigidity, and nystagmus.

Rabies should be considered a possible pathogen in all animal bites.[13,40] If the animal is domestic, a veterinarian must rule out the presence of rabies through observation over a 10-day period. If the animal is wild and of a species such as raccoons, skunks, foxes, and bats, it must be captured for evaluation of rabies antibody or, if not captured, the patient must receive postexposure prophylaxis.[13,40,50,69] In the United States, domestic animal populations are widely immunized. Postexposure prophylaxis, although uncomfortable, is highly effective in preventing rabies (Table 17-3).[69] Treating animal bites without appropriate attention to these procedures is contraindicated because rabies is nearly always fatal.

PREVENTION OF SECONDARY CONTAMINATION OF WOUNDS AND CATHETERS

Nosocomial infection of wounds continues to be a substantial problem despite significant efforts in education. The essential features in preventing nosocomial wound or catheter infection are the following[19]:

1. Universal barrier precautions
2. Hand washing between patients
3. Use of sterile gloves, instruments, scissors, and so forth for dressing changes

TABLE 17-3		

Rabies Postexposure Prophylaxis Schedule, United States, 1999

Vaccination Status	Treatment	Regimen*
Not previously vaccinated	Wound cleansing	All postexposure prophylaxis should begin with immediate thorough cleansing of all wounds with soap and water. If available, a virucidal agent such as povidone-iodine solution should be used to irrigate the wounds.
	RIG	Administer 20 IU/kg body weight. If anatomically feasible, *the full dose* should be infiltrated around the wounds and any remaining volume should be administered IM ay an anatomical site distant from vaccine administration. Also, RIG should not be administered in the same syringe as vaccine. Because RIG might partially suppress active production of antibody, no more than the recommended dose should be given.
	Vaccine	Administer HDCV, RVA, or PCEC 1.0 mL, IM (deltoid area†), one each on days 0,‡ 3, 7, 14, and 28.
Previously vaccinated§	Wound cleansing	All postexposure prophylaxis should begin with immediate thorough cleansing of all wounds with soap and water. If available, a virucidal agent such as povidone-iodine solution should be used to irrigate the wounds.
	RIG	RIG should *not* be administered.
	Vaccine	Administer HDCV, RVA, or PCEC 1.0 mL, IM (deltoid area†), one each on days 0‡ and 3.

From Recommendations of the Immunization Practices Advisory Committee (ACIP). Human Rabies Prevention—United States, 1999, *MMWR Morb Mortal Wkly Rep* 48(RR-1):12, 1999.
RIG, Rabies immune globulin; *HDCV,* human diploid cell vaccine; *IM,* intramuscular; *RVA,* rabies vaccine adsorbed; *PCEC,* purified chick embryo vaccine.
*These regimens are applicable for all age groups, including children.
†The deltoid area is the only acceptable site of vaccination for adults and older children. For younger children, the outer aspect of the thigh may be used. Vaccine should never be administered in the gluteal area.
‡Day 0 is the day the first dose of vaccine is administered.
§Any person with a history of preexposure vaccination with HDCV, RVA or PCEC; before exposure prophylaxis with HDCV, RVA or PCEC; or previous vaccination with any other type of rabies vaccine and a documented history of antibody response to the prior vaccination.

4. Use of sterile occlusive dressings when practical
5. Optimal management of catheter insertion sites
6. Frequent changing of catheter access sites (at least every 48 hours)
7. Attention to current hospital-acquired infections at institution
8. Use of only well-focused antibiotic therapy to decrease emergence of resistant organisms

PATIENTS WITH MAXILLOFACIAL TRAUMA WITH INFECTED INJURIES

SOFT TISSUE INJURIES

Patients who initially have an infected soft tissue injury usually are seen days after the original traumatic episode, with either a puncture wound, hematoma, foreign body, contaminated wound, or with compromised host defenses. Clinicians must obtain an accurate history, conduct a focused wound examination, and promptly initiate treatment before the infection spreads to adjacent tissues or results in local morbidity.

Perioral Infection The perioral region is particularly resistant to the development of infection. When a patient has a posttraumatic infection in this area, puncture wounds, the presence of foreign bodies, or both conditions

should be suspected. Appropriate imaging should be performed to confirm or refute the presence of a foreign body. Incision, drainage, culture, sensitivity, irrigation, and foreign body removal should be performed. The placement of a drain during definitive repair and administration of appropriate antibiotics based on culture and susceptibility results are suggested. Penicillin remains the empirical prophylactic antibiotic of choice in the treatment of intraoral infections.[83]

Perinasal Infections Perinasal posttraumatic infection management should focus on the presence of an infected hematoma, including that of the nasal septum and antra, in addition to the possibility of underlying osseous injury. Failure to manage this form of infection could jeopardize the blood supply and thus health of the perinasal cartilaginous structures. A focused clinical and imaging examination confirms the diagnosis. Acute sinusitis should be managed with antibiotic therapy, antrostomy, and antral lavage. Incision, drainage, culture, sensitivity, irrigation, and strict attention to the elimination of dead space provide the best management of an infected hematoma. Dead space management may be accomplished with Doyle airway splints (Xomed-Treace, Jacksonville, FL) and nasal packing for 4 days. Toxic shock has been associated with packs left in place longer. A pressure dressing is applicable to external nares injury. Amoxicillin with clavulanic acid (for those patients who are not allergic) is often the initial drug used in the management of infections suspected to have been caused by nasal or accessory sinus flora. Definitive antibiotic selection is based on the results of culture and susceptibility.

Periauricular Infection The focus of management of periauricular infection is much the same as for perinasal injury. An infected subchondral hematoma could compromise the integrity of the auricular cartilage. Incision, drainage, culture, sensitivity, irrigation, and strict attention to the elimination of dead space are indicated.[71] Dead space elimination may be accomplished with loose Kerlex (Kendall Healthcare Products Co., Mansfield, MA) gauze and a Glasscock ear dressing (Oto-Med. Inc, Lake Havasu, AZ) after definitive wound closure. Antibiotic therapy should be based on the results of the Gram stain and culture results (Figure 17-6). Cephalosporins offer an excellent choice as an empirical prophylactic antibiotic. For patients with a periauricular infection days to weeks subsequent to the traumatic episode, *Pseudomonas* spp. should be considered. Under these circumstances, imipenem and cilastatin (250 to 1000 mg q6 to 8h), meropenem (1.0 g

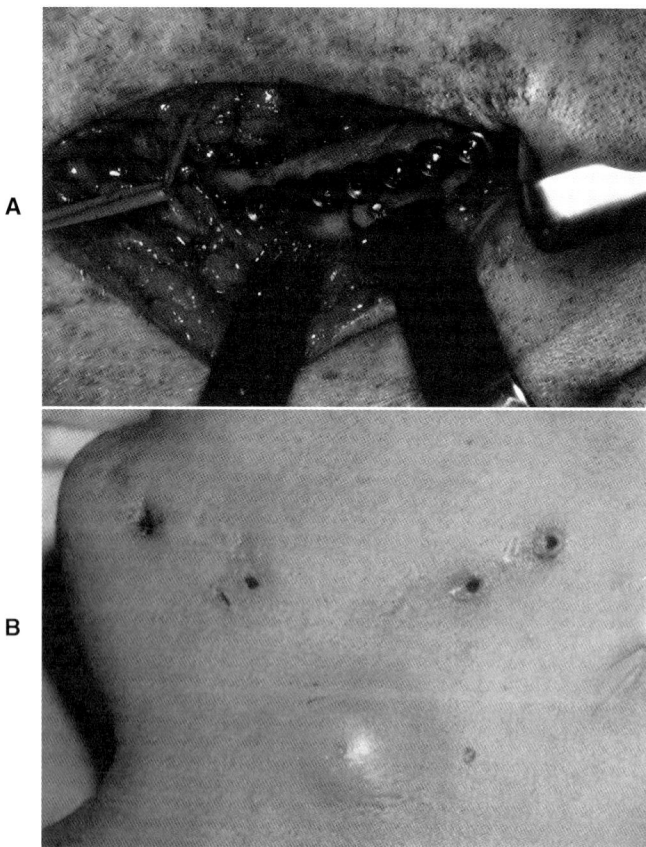

Figure 17-6 The infected mandibular fracture **(A)** is best treated with absolute immobilization. Locking reconstruction plates are the best alternative **(B)**. They act as internal, external fixators and do not depend on compression of the plate/screw/bone system for stability. The race between buccal plate resorption and osseous healing is eliminated.

q8h), or ciprofloxacin (400 mg q12h) should be considered for intravenous administration for adults.

Periorbital Infection A posttraumatic periorbital infection most likely is the result of a fracture, foreign body, or hematoma.[62] Computed tomography should be used to determine whether a foreign body is present and may help localize any infection and identify underlying osseous injury. A postseptal infection should elicit concern, and the assistance of an ophthalmologist is appropriate. Intraorbital potential spaces include subperiosteal, peripheral (bounded by the rectus muscles, membrane and septum), central (within the muscle cone and Tenon's capsule), and between Tenon's capsule and the globe. The presence of concomitant osseous injury should be verified or refuted. Once the location of the infection has been determined, it may be drained with attention to osseous injury and foreign body removal if necessary.

Facial Infection Posttraumatic infection of the nonspecialized soft tissues of the face should focus on both the identification of an infected hematoma and the presence of a foreign body. Management should include appropriate imaging, to confirm or refute the presence of a foreign body, with subsequent incision, drainage, culture, sensitivity, and irrigation. The placement of a drain, whether passive or active, before or during definitive wound repair should be considered. The cephalosporins are effective empirical prophylactic antibiotics in the management of infections in this area.

Scalp Infection Posttraumatic infection of the scalp should focus on the prevention of intracranial extension. The pathways for transmission include direct extension through the cranium or metastasis through emissary veins. Attention should be directed to detection of an underlying cranial fracture and its treatment.[41] Simple soft tissue infections require incision, drainage, culture, sensitivity, irrigation, and placement of a drain. The cephalosporins (intravenous or enteral) are an excellent choice for empirical prophylactic antibiotic therapy. If extension to the central nervous system is suspected, then nafcillin (2 to 6 g IV q6h) and gentamicin (3 to 5 mg/kg/d in three equal divided doses) should be considered for adults during hospitalization.[41]

OSSEOUS INJURIES

Mandible Fractures Significant progress has been made during the past decade in the management of skeletal injury, specifically because of advances in rigid internal fixation. Although implanted plates and screws previously were considered to act as foreign bodies and were contraindicated in the treatment of infected mandibular fractures, current practice demonstrates stable fracture fixation is desirable (see Figure 17-6).* In managing a patient

---

*References 25, 29, 45, 47, 54, 78.

with an infected mandibular fracture, the cause of the infection must be determined in addition to the type of mandibular fracture (Box 17-1).[12] If the infection is related to a pathological condition affecting a tooth, the tooth should be removed. Whether an infected hematoma or abscess, the incision that provides access to the site of fracture will also provide drainage. Obtaining a culture with Gram stain followed by sensitivity testing helps guide antibiotic therapy. Penicillin remains the antibiotic of choice in the management of infections of odontogenic origin (see Table 17-1). If infection resulting from cutaneous contaminants is suspected, then the cephalosporins are excellent choices. The application of absolute rigid immobilization ensures fracture site stability without the percolation of microorganisms associated with other means of fixation.[29,54] The placement of a drain should be considered.[54]

Midfacial Fractures   Patients occasionally have infected midfacial fractures.[39] Many of the principles for rigid internal fixation of the mandible may be applied to the midfacial skeleton. The cause of the initial infection should be identified. Contaminants should be considered from odontogenic sources and from the remainder of the mouth, in addition to the nasal cavity and accessory sinuses.[39] Aspiration with Gram stain, culture, and sensitivity help direct antibiotic therapy. Incisions providing access for fracture immobilization also provide drainage. After the application of rigid internal fixation, copious irrigation reduces the concentration of bacteria to nonpathogenic concentrations. Drains with or without sinusotomy rarely are necessary. Intravenous administration of

cephalosporins is effective during hospital admission and the perioperative phase (see Table 17-1).

Craniofacial Fractures   Craniofacial fractures that involve the neurocranium and associated sinuses pose a significant problem when infection is present.[89] The greatest concern is the development of meningitis or other central neurological infection. When the brain has been injured or exposed, neurosurgical considerations are the overriding priority. Maintenance of normal intracranial pressure and restoration of integrity in fracture sites are essential. Antibiotic management with intravenous nafcillin (2 to 6 g IV q6h) and gentamicin (3 to 5 mg/kg/d in three equal divided doses) should be considered for these adult patients. For other craniofacial fractures without exposure of the central nervous system, management is the same as for midfacial injury; cephalosporins are the preferred agent.

PREVENTION OF INFECTION AFTER MAXILLOFACIAL TRAUMA

SOFT TISSUE INJURIES

Surgical repair performed before development of wound desiccation, bacterial growth, morbid edema, and decreased tissue perfusion offers the best opportunity for success without infection. Treatment usually is required within the first hours (14 to 24 hours) after injury.[73] Delaying surgical repair for several days often is necessary because of the patient's general status and serious edema. Under these circumstances, prophylactic antibiotics, occlusive dressings, and open packing are among the measures that can assist in preventing infection (Box 17-2).

Abrasions   Deep abrasions beyond the dermis or epidermis should be managed in the same manner as an avulsion (see later text discussion). Simple superficial abrasions should be cleansed with an antimicrobial cleansing agent, such as povidone-iodine solution (Box 17-3).[34,63] All foreign debris should be removed, which sometimes requires a scrub brush and some form of local or regional anesthesia. Once debrided and cleansed, the abrasion should be irrigated with normal saline solution, dried, and dressed with an antimicrobial ointment.[11,41,68] Because *S. epidermidis* and *S. aureus* are indigenous skin flora, bacitracin zinc ointment (500 U/g), polymixin B ointment (5000 U/g), and neomycin sulfate ointment (3.5 mg/g) are effective (see Table 17-1).

Contusions and Hematomas   A hematoma may indicate a more serious underlying injury.[41] If self-limiting and without evidence of concomitant underlying injury, simple observation is acceptable, because most hematomas resolve.[41,68] Aspiration of a nonexpansile hematoma frequently results in an infection where no infection previously existed. In addition, the gelatinous nature of the congealed hematoma is difficult, if not impossible, to

---

BOX 17-1

Management Considerations for Patients with Infected Fractures

- Conduct appropriate generalized history and clinical examination
- Obtain appropriate imaging evaluation (may include radiographs or computed tomographs)
- Conduct focused fracture examination
- Culture wound with Gram stain and for antibiotic susceptibility
- Irrigate with saline solution/povidone-iodine solution/saline solution (consider benzalkonium chloride for contamination with viruses, e.g., animal bites)
- Perform conservative debridement of necrotic tissue
- Examine for presence of foreign bodies and remove if present
- Consider incision and drain placement before or during definitive repair
- Treat with absolute rigid fixation or immobilization
- Consider antibiotic regimen based on Gram stain and culture results

---

B O X 17-2

Management Considerations for Patients with Infected Soft Tissue Injuries

Conduct appropriate generalized history and clinical examination

Obtain appropriate imaging evaluation (may include radiographs, computed tomographs, magnetic resonance images, and ultrasonography)

Conduct focused wound examination

Culture wound with Gram stain and for antibiotic sensitivity

Achieve hemostasis

Irrigate with saline solution/povidone-iodine solution/saline solution (consider benzalkonium chloride for contamination with viruses, e.g., animal bites)

Perform conservative debridement of necrotic tissue

Examine for presence of foreign bodies and remove if present

Consider drain placement before or during definitive repair

Perform definitive wound repair

Perform adjunctive procedures if indicated (e.g., wound pexing, open packing)

Consider antibiotic regimen based on Gram stain and culture results

Consider immunization (e.g., tetanus prophylaxis for crush injuries, rabies prophylaxis for animal bites)

B O X 17-3

Infection Prevention Measures for Patients with Soft Tissue Injuries

Conduct appropriate generalized history and clinical examination

Obtain appropriate imaging evaluation (may include radiographs, computed tomographs, magnetic resonance images, and ultrasonography)

Conduct focused wound examination

Achieve hemostasis

Irrigate with saline/povidone-iodine solution/saline (consider benzalkonium chloride for contamination with viruses, e.g., animal bites)

Perform conservative debridement of necrotic tissue

Examine for the presence of foreign bodies and remove if present

Eliminate dead space during definitive repair

Consider prophylactic antibiotics for compromised hosts or patients with implanted materials

Consider immunization (e.g., tetanus prophylaxis for crush injuries, rabies prophylaxis for animal bites)

Perform adjunctive procedures if indicated (e.g., local or regional flaps)

---

extract with needle aspiration. If the hematoma is expanding and an open exploration and control of hemorrhage is required, antibiotic therapy directed at Staphylococcus spp. should be considered.[41] Cephalexin (500 mg PO every 6 hours for adults, 25 to 50 mg/kg/d in four equal doses for children) is effective enterally as a choice for prophylaxis.

Simple Lacerations Simple lacerations should be repaired without shaving, if possible, because a relationship has been found between shaving and higher rates of infection.* Depilatories are associated with allergic responses. Hair can be clipped, the wound explored, hemorrhage controlled, and then irrigated with copious amounts of saline solution. After saline solution irrigation, povidone-iodine solution irrigation and repeated saline solution irrigation (because residual povidone-iodine has been shown to cause fibrosis), definitive wound repair may proceed.[34,63] A topical antimicrobial ointment, as described for treatment of abrasions, should be applied to the wound. If the wound is clean and not contaminated, systemic antibiotic therapy is unnecessary.[52]

Complex Lacerations Complex lacerations include those that are (1) excessive in length (>10 cm), (2) stellate, (3) associated with areas of contamination or necrosis, present more than 12 hours after injury,(4) include a vital structure (as the eyes, auricle, nasal cartilages or salivary glands), or (5) those that occur with underlying osseous injury.[41,68] Because of their inherent complexity, these injuries may be best managed in the operating room with the patient under general anesthesia. Facial or scalp hair may be considered for removal under these conditions so that hair remnants or particles do not become entrapped within the wound. Removal of hair with "barber's shears" is acceptable.[41] Irrigation with copious amounts of saline solution removes clots, foreign debris, and necrotic tissue and assists in identification of hemorrhagic vessels. Alcohol may then be used to remove oils from the skin to enhance the cleansing nature of povidone-iodine solution.[34,63] Layered closure should be undertaken, with consideration to the management of dead space. This may be accomplished with passive or active drains with or without pressure dressings. The wound may be dressed with an antimicrobial ointment as outlined in previous sections. The intraoperative adminis-

---

*References 2, 23, 41, 68, 71, 77.

A   **B**   **C**

D   **E**

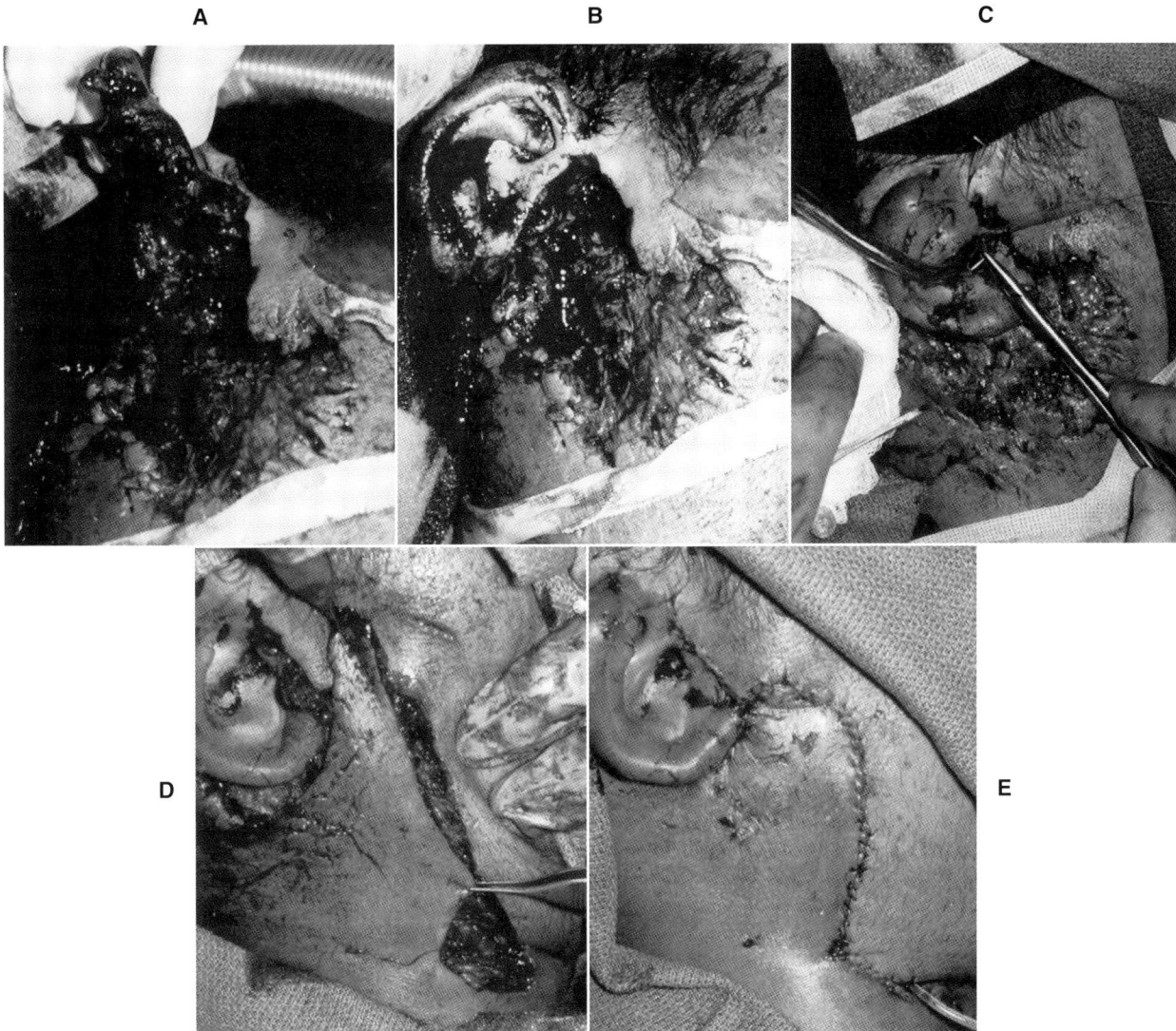

Figure 17-7 A and **B,** Multiple general considerations for the prevention of soft tissue infection were applied to this grossly contaminated, subtotally avulsed ear with partial adjacent cutaneous avulsion. The wound was irrigated with normal saline solution, hemostasis was achieved, the wound was cleansed with povidone-iodine solution, and irrigated again. **C,** Primary layered closure of the external auditory canal and auricle was accomplished. **D,** A local flap was advanced to replace the avulsed tissue. Dead space was then eliminated with the assistance of a suction drain. **E,** After appropriate antibiotic therapy and local wound care, a desirable result was achieved.

tration of intravenous antibiotics such as cephazolin (0.5 to 1.5 g q4 to 12h for adults, 25 to 50 mg/kg/d in four equal divided doses for children) helps to prevent infections caused by *Staphylococcus* spp. and anaerobes. Enteral cephalexin (500 mg q6h for adults and 25 to 50 mg/kg/d in four equal doses for children) for a 5- to 10-day post-operative course is effective.

Soft Tissue Avulsion   The management considerations for soft tissue avulsions vary according to the location, depth, and surface area of the missing tissue.[41,68] A variety of surgical techniques including secondary intention, skin grafts, advancement, rotational or transpositional flaps, and microvascular grafts may be considered. For simple secondary intention, dressing with topical antimicrobial ointments is effective.[41] For any graft or flap techniques, intraoperative and postoperative intravenous antibiotic therapy as described for complex lacerations is important, because the accumulation of 10^5 bacteria per gram of tissue at the graft site causes graft failure.[41,68] Intravenous clindamycin sulfate (900 mg) or cephazolin sodium (2 g) administered preoperatively and every 8 hours postoperatively for a total of 24 hours has been shown to be equally effective in the reduction of postoperative flap reconstruction wound infection.[49] Elimination of dead space is important for graft survival and infection prevention (Figure 17-7).

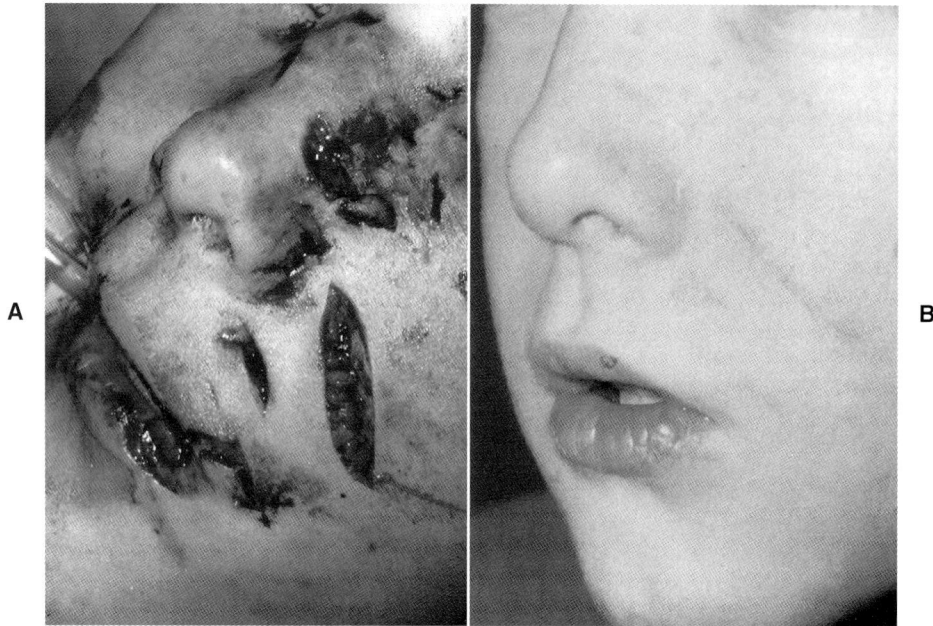

Figure 17-8 Wounds may become contaminated in a number of different ways. **A,** Multiple punctures and lacerations were associated with this dog bite injury that was contaminated by the normal oral flora of the animal. **B,** After wound cleansing, irrigation, primary closure, tetanus immunization, and appropriate antibiotic therapy, a desirable result was achieved.

Puncture Wounds Simple puncture wounds may be treated by irrigation alone, permitting the wound to remain open, and observing it at 2 days, 1 week, and 1-month intervals postoperatively. Irrigation should include saline solution first, then povidone-iodine solution, followed by saline solution again.[73] Bacitracin sulfate (50,000 U in 1000 mL of normal saline solution) also is effective. A Teflon angiocatheter may be used to to reach the depth of the puncture. An alternative method of treatment is to convert the puncture to a laceration by using a No. 11 scalpel at the depth of the puncture and incising in opposite directions. The puncture can then be managed as a simple laceration (Figure 17-8).

If an animal (especially a cat) has caused the puncture, antibiotic therapy should be considered.[11,40] Penicillin or amoxicillin with clavulanic acid (500 mg PO q6h for adults, and 15 to 50 mg/kg/d in four equal doses for children) should be considered in addition to tetanus prophylaxis. Rabies prophylaxis should be administered for bites incurred by animal suspected as harboring the virus.[40] If a zoonotic disease develops, the appropriate antimicrobial agent should be administered.[40]

Burns Second-degree superficial burns may be treated by washing with an antimicrobial cleansing agent such as povidone-iodine solution and dressing with silver sulfadiazine 1% cream (Silvadene). Third-degree burns without osseous involvement may be managed initially as for minor superficial burns.[87] Topical antimicrobial ointments applied liberally twice a day may replace Silvadene (Figure

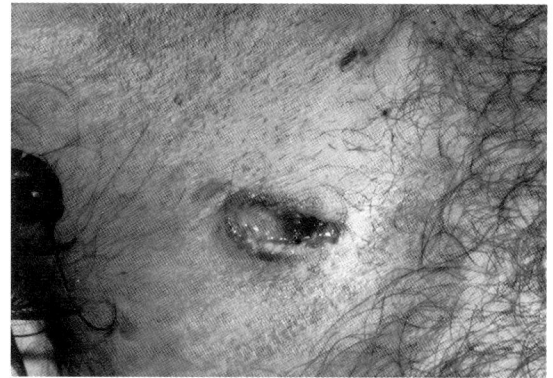

Figure 17-9 The burn associated with this small-caliber entrance wound was treated with irrigation and topical antibiotic ointment.

17-9). Wet-to-dry mesh gauze dressings may be applied for 2 weeks to aid debridement of superficial necrotic skin and maintain moisture. More significant injuries should be managed as an avulsive injury.

Burns produce tissue injury beyond the visible margins of the wound,[44] especially in electrical burns and burns associated with blast injuries. These burns are prone to secondary infection because of the deepithelialized surface and the presence of deep muscle damage that accompanies such an injury. High levels of parenteral antibiotics are necessary to penetrate these compromised tissues (see Table 17-1). In patients with severe burns, infection is the cause of most deaths. Careful and frequent debridement of necrotic tissue, the use of Silvadene superficially, and appropriate parenteral antibiotic therapy (cephalosporin as a first-line agent) helps to control the weeping suppurative surface that occurs in most electrical burns. Early coverage of burns with skin grafts also controls the incidence of late infection.

Contaminated Injuries Environmental contaminants can include such organisms as *C. tetani* or *Actinomyces* spp. from the soil, or *E. coli* from free-standing water. Grossly contaminated soft tissue injuries require a careful history to assess the type and form of contaminant. A culture of the suspected contaminant or contaminated tissue helps determine appropriate antimicrobial management. When soil, excrement, free-standing water, or multiple foreign bodies (i.e., gravel, glass) are suspected, these injuries are best treated with the patient under a general anesthetic in the sterile environment of the operating room. Pulsatile irrigation is particularly useful in eliminating pathological concentrations of bacteria while removing foreign matter. Tetanus prophylaxis must be considered for these injuries.

Many water-borne pathogens can produce wound infection when a laceration or compound fracture has been sustained. Fresh-water contamination, particularly in brackish water, has caused *Aeromonas hydrophila* infection.[48] This aerobic gram-negative rod may cause severe facial cellulitis and myonecrosis. Enteric organisms such as *E. coli* also frequently contaminate wounds exposed to coastal seawater. Injuries contaminated with soil also are particularly susceptible to infection.[58] A high incidence of infection after farm machine injuries has been reported.[16] Predominant organisms in these injuries include gram-negative enteric organisms, group D *Streptococcus,* and anaerobes. Appropriate prophylactic antibiotics should be considered when a wound has been exposed to water- or earth-borne pathogens. The choice of antibiotic for these situations is problematic because of the inherent resistance to antibiotics by these organisms and the ability to transmit this resistance to other organisms. The appropriate choice is based on culture and susceptibility results. The most likely agent is a penicillin drug with β-lactamase resistance.

Mandibular Fractures The prevention of infection during the management of mandibular fractures requires consideration of the anatomical location of the fracture and the magnitude and form of contamination (Box 17-4). For the closed management of injuries such as ascending ramus or condylar fractures, no special concerns should be offered. For compound injuries exposed to the oral environment (by laceration or tooth crypt), prophylactic antibiotic therapy directed at oral contaminants should be considered. These injuries may include angle, body, symphysis, and alveolar fractures. Intraoperative intravenous administration of aqueous crystalline benzyl penicillin provides effective prophylactic antibiotic for these injuries (see Table 17-1). If exposed to the skin, the use of prophylactic antibi-

BOX 17-4

Infection Prevention Measures for Patients with Fractures

Conduct appropriate generalized history and clinical examination
Obtain appropriate imaging evaluation (may include radiographs or computed tomographs)
Conduct focused fracture examination
Irrigate with saline solution/povidone-iodine solution/saline solution
Examine for the presence of foreign bodies and remove if present
Ensure absolute rigid fixation or immobilization
Consider prophylactic antibiotics (especially for compromised hosts or patients with implanted materials)

otics directed at cutaneous contaminants should be considered; cephalosporins are a good choice in such cases. Reduction of facial fractures through clean surgical wounds also results in the risk of incisional cellulitis. In these cases, *S. aureus* is a suspected contaminant and antibiotic coverage should be provided before, during, and after open reduction. Analysis of the organisms associated with wound infection after head and neck surgery also reveals other aerobes (91%), anaerobes (74%), and fungi (48%).[75] In one case-controlled trial the use of cefazolin sodium 1 hour preoperatively and one dose 8 hours postoperatively reduced the incidence of infection postoperatively from 42.2% to 8.9% compared with patients treated without antibiotics.[20] All other general principles regarding fracture management should be considered (see Box 17-4).

Titanium plates and screws are the most effective fixation modality (Figure 17-10). They are not associated with any greater incidence of postoperative infection than other fixation methods and may be left intentionally as permanent implants. For patients with multiple medical illnesses, host compromise, or multiple systems injuries, early repair should be considered. In one case-controlled trial, early (within 48 hours) operative repair of facial injuries for patients with multiple trauma resulted in no infections, whereas for delayed repair, the infection rate was 5%.[88] Patients without multiple medical illnesses, polytrauma, or host compromise may be treated on an outpatient basis with enteral antibiotics.

Midfacial Fractures The management of midfacial fractures should be similar to that for mandibular fractures in timing and technique, with the added concern for nasal and accessory sinus contaminants. The prophylactic use of the penicillins is warranted when the oral environment is considered to have the highest potential for contamination. Cephalosporins should be considered if the skin is considered the most threatening contaminant. Amoxicillin with clavulanic acid is the prophylactic agent of choice when nasal or accessory sinus contaminants are

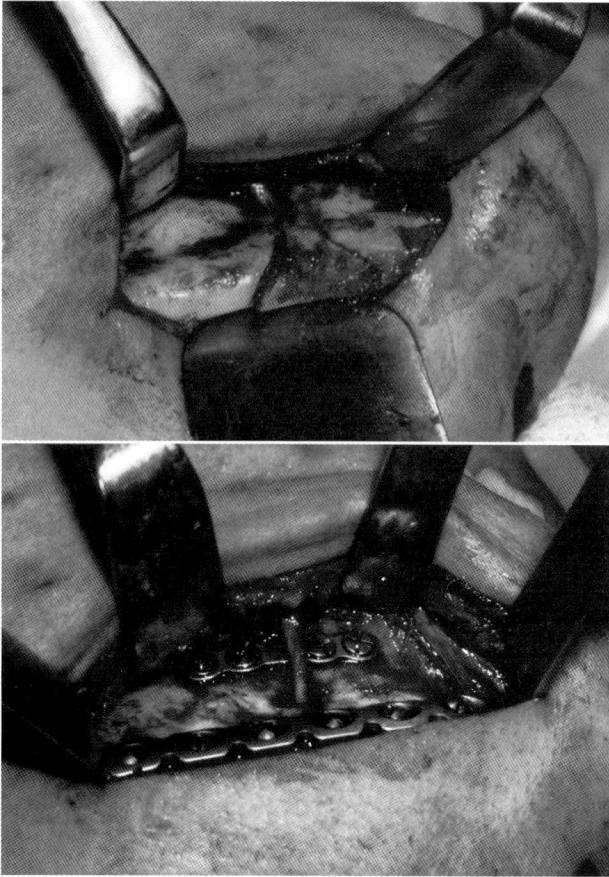

Figure 17-10 Titanium plates and screws are effective in the reconstruction of mandibular injury without concern for an increased incidence of infection compared with other means of stabilization.

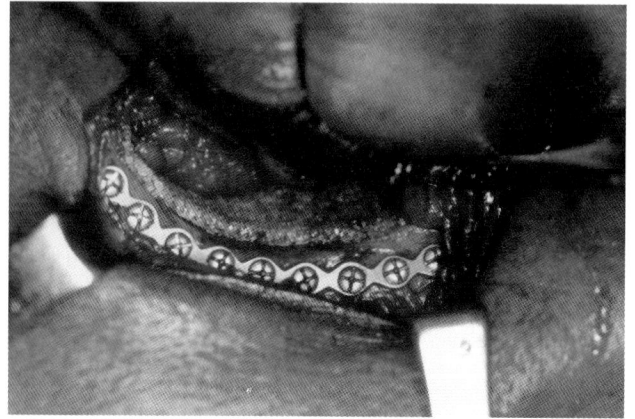

Figure 17-11 High-density polytetrafluoroethylene sheets are valuable in supporting the globe and isolating it from the nasal cavity and paranasal sinuses from the orbit.

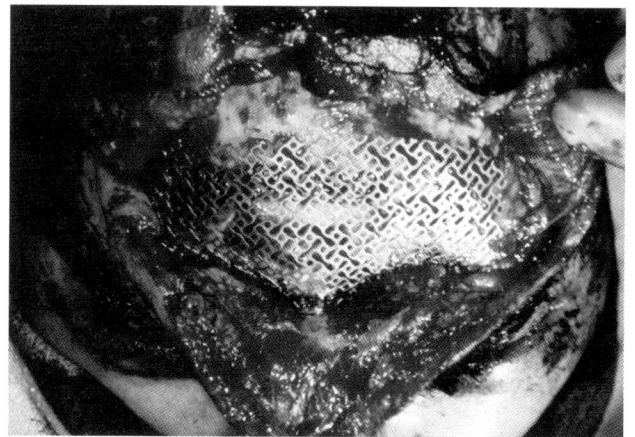

Figure 17-12 Titanium mesh is an excellent modality for reconstruction of the craniomaxillofacial skeleton without adding concern for infection. The mesh may be placed directly adjacent to the dura or used to repair the frontal sinus.

suspected. Titanium plates and screws are favored for fixation of midface fractures as for mandible fractures. The various forms of titanium mesh and screen effectively support compromised bone or replace absent bone without increasing the incidence of infection or nonunion. This advantage also applies to porous high-density polytetrafluoroethylene (Medpore, Porex Surgical, Athens, GA) (Figure 17-11).[88] When used to support the orbital floor and isolate the nasal cavity and accessory sinuses, these alloplasts are effective and of no more concern for development of infection than any other biomaterial.

Craniofacial Fractures   Management principles for craniofacial fractures are similar to those for midfacial fractures with addition emphasis on protection of the brain and remainder of the CNS. For visibly contaminated craniofacial fractures, or those in which the brain is exposed, the clinician should consider prophylactic use of intravenous nafcillin (2 to 6 g IV q6h) and gentamicin (3 to 5 mg/kg/d in three equal divided doses) in adult patients. If communication is not suspected and the fracture is not considered contaminated, many neurosurgeons choose not to use prophylactic antibiotics. Their rationale is that should an infection develop, the chance of growth of an

organism resistant to conventional antibiotic therapy is lessened. The use of titanium plates and screws has proved a favorable modality for craniofacial reconstruction. Titanium mesh and screen also is effective in the reconstruction of voids in cranial bone and may be applied immediately adjacent to the dura (Figure 17-12).

MANAGEMENT OF POSTOPERATIVE INFECTIONS

HOST FACTORS

Host factors in the development of postoperative infection include medical and social risk factors. Medical risk factors include human immunodeficiency syndrome (HIV), diabetes mellitus, pulmonary problems, renal failure, cancer, nutritional deficiencies, and use of immunosuppressive medications[31] (see Chapter 24). Social risk factors include noncompliance, intravenous drug use, alcoholism,

BOX **17-5**

Management of Postoperative Infections

Obtain appropriate generalized history and clinical examination
Conduct appropriate imaging evaluation (may include radiographs, computed tomographs, magnetic resonance images, and ultrasonography)
Conduct wound examination focused on fracture mobility with or without the presence of foreign bodies
Perform incision and drainage
Culture wound with Gram stain and for antibiotic susceptibility
Irrigate with saline solution/povidone-iodine solution/saline solution
Debride necrotic tissue
Ensure absolute rigid fixation or immobilization
Remove loose or broken hardware and/or foreign bodies if present
Place drain
Consider open packing
Initiate antibiotic regimen based on Gram stain and culture results

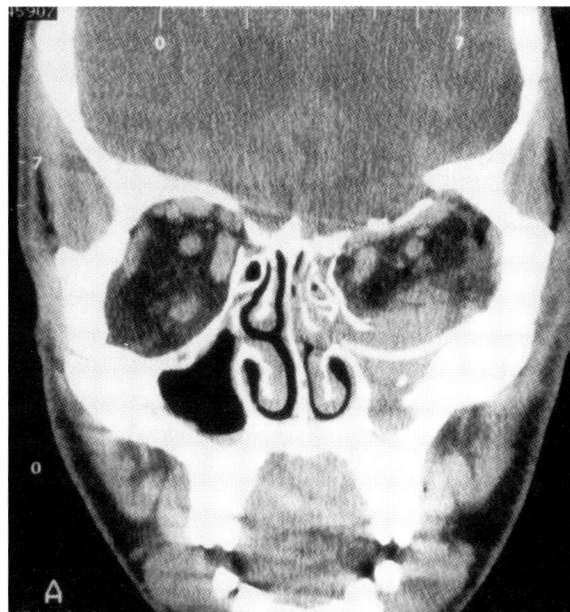

Figure 17-13 Infection may develop even years after placement of an alloplast (polytetrafluoroethylene orbital floor).

and smoking. HIV, diabetes mellitus, renal failure, cancer, and the use of immunosuppressive drugs; all are associated with a diminished ability to resist infection.[15,22,56] Pulmonary insufficiency and low levels of inspired oxygen delay soft tissue healing.[53] Smoking has been shown to cause significant morbidity associated with the healing of soft tissue surgery.[72] The interference with normal bone metabolism and development of infection in chronic alcohol abusers has been well established. Alcohol abuse results in hypocalcemia, hypercalciuria, diminished levels of vitamin D metabolites, low levels of osteocalcin, and suppressed function of osteoblasts.[15] Thus patients who are alcoholics are at a higher risk for the development of infected nonunions.

Intravenous drug use has been associated with the development of respiratory ailments including lung abscesses, bacterial pneumonia, pneumonitis, and fibrosis. In addition to pulmonary infections, endocarditis, osteomyelitis, and cutaneous infections affect the intravenous drug abuser. Malabsorption, malnourishment, acquired immunodeficiency syndrome, and hepatitis complete the clinical profile of these patients; each predisposes the patient to infection. Management of both medical and social risk factors must occur concurrently with the treatment of infection and for those patients who develop a postoperative infection.

Fracture Management   Infection after the treatment of facial fractures is caused by pathogenic organisms in the fracture site and a site with sustained susceptibility to infection (Box 17-5). The persistence of susceptibility to infection in the operative site is usually the result of failure to

achieve functional stability of the fractures or failure to prevent mobility of the fracture site. Additional factors include the continued communication of the fracture site with the external environment, compromised nutrition, catabolic state, decreased blood supply to the fracture site, damage to vital associated structures such as salivary glands, or the continued presence of foreign bodies.

Treatment of infection after fracture management includes careful analysis of the causes and addressing each cause individually. Surgical management of infected maxillofacial fractures must include assurance of fracture stability.[46] Stability is best achieved through absolute rigid internal fixation with titanium plates and screws (see Figure 17-10).[54] Hardware in place at the time of infection should be inspected closely and removed only if it is loose.[7] Alloplasts in infected sites (such as those that support or isolate the orbital contents) usually should be removed, and secondary reconstruction should be planned after the acute infection has been controlled (Figure 17-13).

If internal fixation devices loosen or break, they should be removed. New, preferably locking, hardware should be placed in nonadjacent, noninfected bone of good quality.[38,46] Screws placed in infected bone loosen early with suppuration. In addition to clinical evaluation and the presence of intact periosteum over the planned hardware site, differential bone scanning with technetium, indium, and gallium can be helpful in determining the extent to which infection has invaded the adjacent bone. This information assists in planning the location of screws remote from the infected site.

The immediate use of bone grafts in infected fractures has gained popularity.[37,61,83] This practice carries a high risk of failure in the presence of acute cellulitis. When infection has become chronic and clinical evidence indicates no extension of the infection beyond the pseudoarthrosis, the fracture site may be excised and bone grafting may be successfully accomplished with rigid internal fixation. Supportive therapy, including antibiotics, should complement the procedure.

Osteomyelitis is a term that has been frequently and inaccurately associated with fracture reconstruction by rigid internal fixation hardware.[42,55] Loose hardware with an underlying bone resorption usually is the result of avascular necrosis under the hardware or a chronic foreign body granuloma. Histopathological examination reveals an accumulation of particulate matter from the hardware within the soft tissues and a foreign body giant cell reaction. Osteomyelitis is an infective condition of the bone involving the medullary cavity, haversian systems, and adjacent cortex.[55] Documentation of this infection requires a bone biopsy that identifies microorganisms within lacunae, or positive bone culture results. History and clinical examination confirmed by radiographic scans, cultures and microscopic examination complete the diagnosis. [99m]Tc and ^{111}In effectively localize the inflamed tissues, and this combined technique is highly sensitive for detection of osteomyelitis.[55] Treatment includes debridement of necrotic or granulomatous bone, rigid internal fixation,

and long-term antibiotic therapy directed at isolates from bone or blood culture (Figure 17-14). Aqueous crystalline penicillin G (2 million units q4h) and metronidazole (500 mg q6h) intravenously preoperatively and throughout hospitalization are effective. Clindamycin (600 mg q6h) is the alternative for those patients who are allergic to penicillin or metronidazole. Intravenous antibiotics may be continued for 12 weeks through an indwelling catheter and visiting nurse service. Some authors report success with the use of enteral antibiotics 4 to 6 weeks postoperatively.[55]

Soft Tissue Management   Management of postoperative soft tissue infection should focus on the possibility of the presence of an infected hematoma or previously undetected foreign body. An appropriate imaging examination should be performed to confirm or refute the presence of a foreign body.[62] Incision, drainage, culture, sensitivity, irrigation, and foreign body removal (if present) should be performed. The placement of a drain and administration of appropriate antibiotics are recommended. Medical risk factors should be addressed with the appropriate medical management and consultation, whereas social risk factors should be eliminated or addressed with counseling. Antibiotic therapy should be based on the results of the Gram stain and culture.

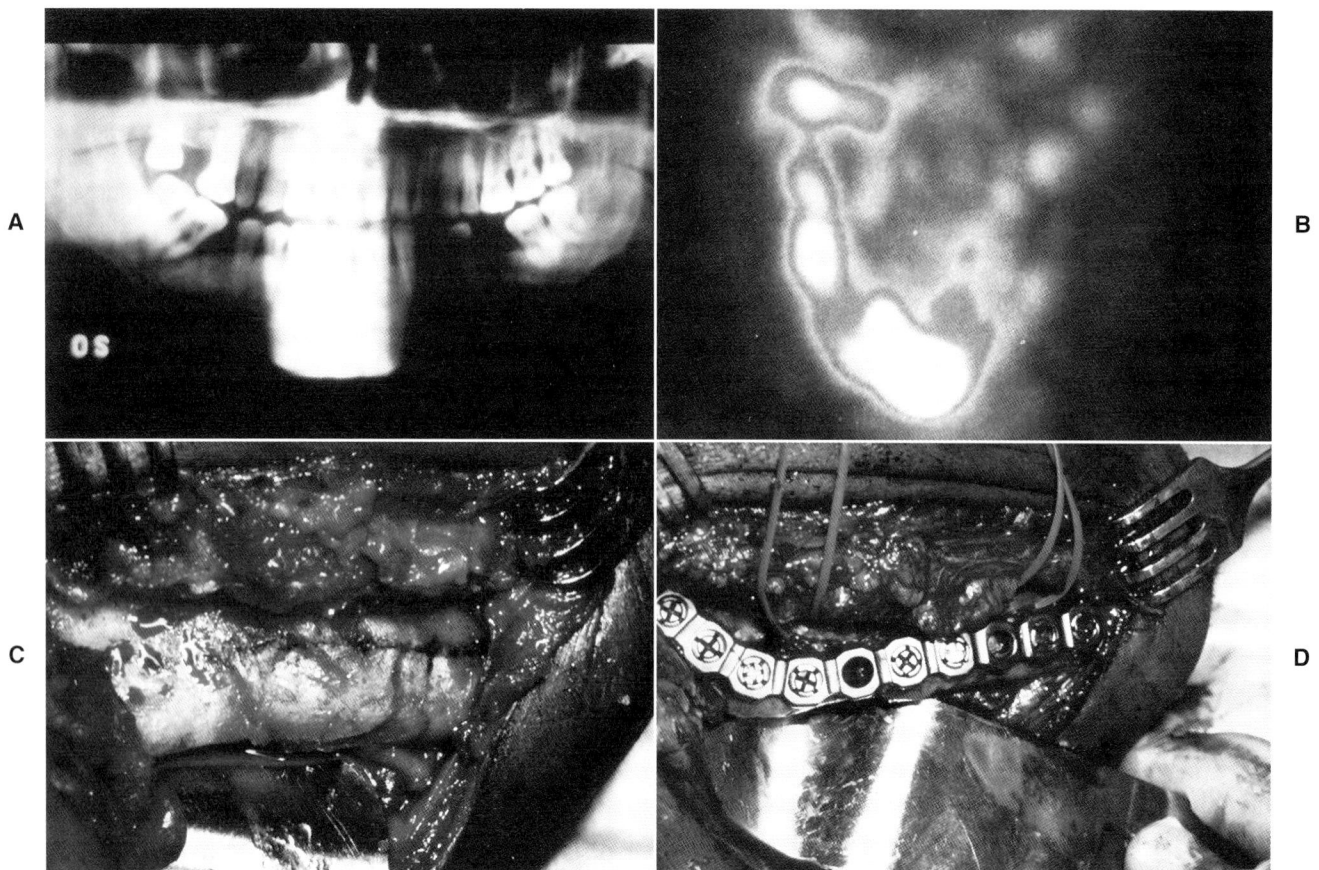

Figure 17-14 Late development of nonunion and osteomyelitis is noted in this panoramic radiograph **(A)** and confirmed with the digitized technetium scan **(B).** This entity is best managed by debridement to viable bone, removal of sequestra or other foreign bodies **(C),** and application of a locking plate **(D)** before closure and long-term antibiotic therapy.

REFERENCES

1. Aghababian RV, Conte JE Jr: Mammalian bite wounds, *Ann Emerg Med* 9:79, 1980.
2. Alexander J, Fischer J, Boyajian M, et al: The influence of hair removal methods on wound infections, *Arch Surg* 118:347, 1983.
3. Alpert B: Complications in the treatment of facial trauma, *Oral Maxillofac Surg Clin North Am* 2:171, 1990.
4. Amaratunga N: A comparative study of the clinical aspects of edentulous and dentulous mandibular fractures, *J Oral Maxillofac Surg* 46:3, 1988.
5. Amaratunga N: The effect of teeth in the line of mandibular fractures on healing, *J Oral Maxillofac Surg* 45:312, 1987.
6. Ardary W: Prospective clinical evaluation of the use of compression plates and screws in the management of mandible fractures, *J Oral Maxillofac Surg* 47:1150, 1989.
7. Assael L: Complications of rigid internal fixation of the facial skeleton, *Oral Maxillofac Surg Clin North Am* 2:615, 1990.
8. Assael L, Friedrich J: Results in rigid internal fixation of comminuted mandible fractures, *J Oral Maxillofac Surg* 475:119, 1989.
9. Assael L, Hammon K: A comparison of rigid internal fixation with wire osteosynthesis of mandibular fractures, *Case reports and outlines of scientific sessions,* Chicago, Ill, 1987, American Association of Oral and Maxillofacial Surgeons.
10. Baue A: Nutrition and metabolism in sepsis, *Surg Clin North Am* 71:549, 1991.
11. Baker MD, Moore SE: Human bites in children: a six year experience, *Am J Dis Child* 141:1285, 1987.
12. Beckers HL: Treatment of initially infected mandibular fractures with bone plates, *J Oral Surg* 37:310, 1979.
13. Bernhard K, Fishbein D: Rabies virus. In Mandel G, Douglas R, Bennett J, editors: *Principles and practice of infectious diseases,* ed 3, New York, 1990, Churchill Livingstone.
14. Betts NJ, Cocolis PK, Beanland D: Using pulsatile pressure saline/antibiotic irrigation before reduction and fixation of mandibular fractures: literature review and report of two cases, *Compend Contin Educ Dent* 17:871, 1996.
15. Bikle DD: Effects of alcohol abuse on bone, *Comp Ther* 14:16, 1988.
16. Brennen S: Infection after farm related injuries in children and adolescents, *Am J Dis Child* 144:710, 1990.
17. Brook I: Microbiology of human and animal bites in children, *Pediatr Infect Dis J* 6:29, 1987.
18. Burgess J, Wambaugh G, Koczarski M: Reviewing cephalic tetanus, *J Am Dent Assoc* 123:67, 1992.
19. Caplan E, Hoyt N: Infection surveillance and control in the severely traumatized patient, *Am J Med* 70:638, 1981.
20. Chayra GA, Meador LR, Laskin DM: Comparison of panoramic and standard radiographs for the diagnosis of mandibular fractures, *J Oral Maxillofacial Surg* 44:677, 1986.
21. Chole RA, Yee J: Antibiotic prophylaxis for facial fractures. A prospective, randomized clinical trial, *Arch Otolaryngol Head Neck Surg* 113:1055, 1987.
22. Cook H, Peoples J, Paden M: Management of the oral surgery patient addicted to heroin, *J Oral Maxillofac Surg* 47:281, 1989.
23. Cruse P, Foord R: A five year prospective study of 23,649 surgical wounds, *Arch Surg* 107:206, 1983.
24. Dahn M: Hepatic parenchymal oxygen tension following injury and sepsis, *Arch Surg* 125:441, 1990.
25. Dodson T, Perrott D: Fixation of mandible fractures: a comparative analysis of rigid fixation and standard fixation techniques, *J Oral Maxillofac Surg* 48:362, 1990.
26. Fackler M: Wound ballistics misconceptions, *JAMA* 259:2730, 1990.
27. Faist E: Immunologic aspects of shock, trauma, and sepsis, *Compl Surg* 10:37, 1991.
28. Fife D: Infection as a cause of death in motor vehicle trauma, *Am J Surg* 155:278, 1988.
29. Fischer-Brandies E, Dielert E: The infected mandibular fracture, *Arch Orthop Trauma Surg* 103:337, 1984.
30. Fridrich KL, Partnoy BE, Zeitler DL: Prospective analysis of antibiotic prophylaxis for orthognathic surgery, *Int J Adult Orthodon Orthognath Surg* 9:129, 1994.
31. Gavin LA: Perioperative management of the diabetic patient, *Endocrinol Metabol Clin North Am* 21:457, 1992.
32. Goldstein E, Citron D, Finegold S: Role of anaerobic bacteria in bite wound infection, *Rev Infect Dis* 6(Suppl 1):S177, 1984.
33. Goldstein E: Bites. In Mandel G, Douglas R, Bennett J, et al, editors: *Principles and practice of infectious diseases,* ed 3, New York, 1990, Churchill Livingstone.
34. Gravett A, Sterner S, Clinton JE, et al: A trial of povidone-iodine in the prevention of infection in sutured lacerations, *Ann Emerg Med* 16:167, 1987.
35. Greenberg RN, James RB, Marnier RL, et al: Microbiologic antibiotic aspects of infections in the oral and maxillofacial region, *J Oral Surg* 37:873, 1979.
36. Gross A, Bhaskar S, Cutright D: The effect of pulsating water jet lavage on experimental contaminated wounds, *J Oral Surg* 29:187, 1971.
37. Gruss J, Mac Kinnon S, Kassel EE, et al: The role of primary bone grafting in complex craniomaxillofacial trauma, *Plast Reconstr Surg* 75:17, 1985.
38. Haug RH: Retention of asymptomatic bone plates used for orthognathic surgery and facial fractures, *J Oral Maxillofac Surg* 54:611, 1996.
39. Haug RH, Adams JM, Jordan RB: A comparison of the morbidity associated with maxillary fractures treated by maxillomandibular and rigid internal fixation, *Oral Surg Oral Med Oral Pathol* 80:629, 1995.
40. Haug RH, Morgan JP 3rd: Management of scalp injuries, *Oral Maxillofac Surg Clin North Am* 10:597, 1998.
41. Haug RH, Morgan JP: Management of human and animal bites. In Fonseca RJ, Walker RV, Betts NJ, et al, editors: *Oral and maxillofacial trauma,* Philadelphia, 1997, WB Saunders.
42. Haug RH, Schwimmer A: Fibrous union of the mandible: a review of 27 patients, *J Oral Maxillofac Surg* 52:832, 1994.
43. Helling T, Evans L, Fowler DL, et al: Infectious complications in patients with severe head injury, *J Trauma* 28:1575; 1988.
44. Hirschfeld J, Assael L: Conservative management of electrical burns of the lips of children, *J Oral Maxillofac Surg* 42:197, 1984.
45. Hoffman W, Barton R: Rigid internal fixation vs. traditional techniques for the treatment of mandible fractures, *J Trauma* 30:1032, 1990.
46. Iizuka T, Lindquist C, Hallikaien D, et al: Infection after rigid fixation of mandibular fractures: a clinical and radiologic study, *J Oral Maxillofac Surg* 49:585, 1991.
47. Johansson B, Krekmanov L, Thomsson M: Miniplate osteosynthesis of infected mandibular fractures, *J Craniomaxillofac Surg* 16:22, 1988.
48. Johnson D, Kuzmik M, Chorazy C: Aeromonas infection following facial injury, *J Oral Maxillofac Surg* 44:563, 1986.
49. Johnson JT, Wagner RL, Schuller DE, et al: Prophylactic antibiotics for head and neck surgery with flap reconstruction, *Arch Otolaryngol Head Neck Surg* 118:488, 1992.

50. Kaplan M, Kaprowski H: Rabies, *Sci Am* 242:120, 1980.

51. Kelly J, editor: *Management of war injuries to the jaws and related structures,* Washington, DC, 1976, US Government Printing Office.

52. Knapp JF: Updates in wound management for the pediatrician, *Pediatr Clin North Am* 46:1201, 1999.

53. Knighton DR, Silver IA, Hunt TK: Regulation of wound healing angiogenesis: effect of oxygen gradient and impaired oxygen concentrations, *Surgery* 90:262, 1981.

54. Koury M, Ellis E 3rd: Rigid internal fixation for the treatment of infected mandibular fractures, *J Oral and Maxillofac Surg* 50:434, 1992.

55. Koury ME, Perrott DH, Kaban LB: The use of rigid fixation in mandibular fractures complicated by osteomyelitis, *J Oral Maxillofac Surg* 52:1114, 1994.

56. Laitinen K, Lamberg-Allardt C, Tuninen R, et al: Bone mineral density and abstention-induced change in bone and mineral metabolism in non-cirrhotic alcoholics, *Am J Med* 93:642, 1992.

57. Leech P, Paterson A: Conservative and operative management for cerebrospinal fluid leakage after closed head injury, *Lancet* 1:1013, 1973.

58. Lieblich S, Topazian RG: Infection in the patient with maxillofacial trauma. In Fonseca R J, Walker RV, editors: *Oral and maxillofacial trauma,* Philadelphia, 1991, WB Saunders.

59. Lindsey D, Nava C, Marti, M: Effectiveness of penicillin irrigation in control of infection in sutured lacerations, *J Trauma* 22:186, 1982.

60. MacGee E, Cauthen H, Brackett C, et al: Meningitis following acute traumatic cerebrospinal fistula, *J Neurosurg* 33:312, 1970.

61. Manson P, Crawley W, Yaremchuck MJ, et al: Midface fractures: Advantages of immediate extended open reduction and bone grafting, *Plast Reconstr Surg* 6:1, 1985.

62. Michon J, Liu D: Intraorbital foreign bodies, *Semin Ophthalmol* 9:193, 1999.

63. Morgan JP 3rd, Haug RH, Kosman JW: Antimicrobial skin preparations for the maxillofacial region, *J Oral Maxillofac Surg* 54:89, 1996.

64. Morgan JP 3rd, Haug RH, Murphy MT: Management of facial dog bite injuries, *J Oral Maxillofac Surg* 53:435, 1995.

65. *NATO Handbook: emergency war surgery,* Washington, DC, 1975, US Government Printing Office.

66. Peterson L: Antibiotic prophylaxis against wound infection in oral and maxillofacial surgery, *J Oral Maxillofac Surg* 48:617, 1990.

67. Procter C: Infection and trauma: An overview. In Kirby R, Brown D, editors: *Anesthesia for trauma,* Boston, 1987, Little, Brown.

68. Punjabi AP, Haug RH, Jordan RB: Management of injuries to the auricle, *J Oral Maxillofac Surg* 55:732, 1997.

69. Recommendations of the Immunization Practices Advisory Committee (ACIP). Human Rabies Prevention—United States, 1999, *MMWR Morb Mortal Wkly Rep* 48(RR-1):12, 1999.

70. Recommendations of the Immunization Practices Advisory Committee (ACIP). Diptheria, tetanus, and pertussis: recommendations for vaccine use and other preventative measures, *MMWR Morb Mortal Wkly Rep* 40(RR-10):21, 1991.

71. Reed BR, Clark AF: Cutaneous tissue repair: practical implications of current knowledge II, *J Am Acad Dermatol* 13:919, 1985.

72. Reifkohl R, Wolfe JA, Cox EB, et al: Association between cutaneous occlusive vascular disease, cigarette smoking, and skin slough after rhytidectomy, *Plast Reconstr Surg* 77:592, 1986.

73. Robson MC, Lea C, Dalton J: Quantitative bacteriology and delayed wound closure, *Surg Forum* 19:501, 1968.

74. Rubin J, Johnson J, Killeen R, et al: Bacteriologic analysis of wound infection following major head and neck surgery, *Arch Otolaryngol* 114:969, 1988.

75. Rubin PA, Bilyk JR, Slone JW: Orbital reconstruction using porous polyethylene sheets, *Ophthalmology* 101:1692, 1994.

76. Rubin M, Koll T, Sadoff RS, et al: Morbidity associated with incompletely erupted third molars in the line of mandibular fractures, *J Oral Maxillofac Surg* 48:1045, 1990.

77. Seropian R, Reynolds B: Wound infections after perioperative depilatory versus razor preparation, *Am J Surg* 121:251, 1971.

78. Schiel H, Hammer, Ehrenfeld M, et al: Therapy of infected mandibular fractures, *Fortschr Kiefer Gesichtschir* 41:170, 1996.

79. Schwarz M: Myositis. In Mandel G, Douglas R, Bennett J, editors: *Principles and practice of infectious diseases,* ed 3, New York, 1990, Churchill Livingstone.

80. Seibel R, LaDuca J, Hassett J, et al: Blunt multiple trauma (ISS36) femur traction and the pulmonary failure-septic state, *Ann Surg* 202:283, 1985.

81. Shetty V, Freymiller E: Teeth in the line of fracture: a review, *J Oral Maxillofac Surg* 47:1303, 1990.

82. Spiessl B: *Internal fixation of the mandible,* Berlin, 1989, Springer Verlag.

83. Stanley R, Schwartz M: Immediate reconstruction of contaminated central craniofacial injuries with free autogenous grafts, *Laryngoscope* 99:1011, 1989.

84. Steele M, Sainsbury C, Robinson WA, et al: Prophylactic penicillin for intraoral wounds, *Ann Emerg Med* 18:847, 1989.

85. Stevens D, Higbee J, Oberhofer T: Antibiotic susceptibility of human isolates of *Pasteurella multocida, Antimicrob Agents Chemother* 16:322, 1979.

86. Storoe W, Haug RH, Lillich TT: The changing face of odontogenic infections, *J Oral Maxillofac Surg* 59:739, 2001.

87. Ward H, Ahrenholz DH, Crandall H, et al: Primary closure of wounds in burned tissue: experimental and clinical study, *J Trauma* 25:125, 1985.

88. Weider L, Hughes K, Ciarochi J, et al: Early versus delayed repair of facial fractures in the multiply injured patient, *Am Surg* 65:790, 1990.

89. Young RF, Lawner PM: Perioperative prophylaxis for prevention of postoperative neurosurgical infections: a randomized clinical trial, *J Neurosurg* 66:701, 1987.

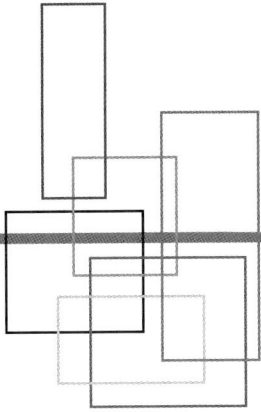

Microbiological Considerations with Dental Implants

Stuart E. Lieblich
Joseph F. Piecuch

The restoration of the dental structures with endosseous implants has arguably been one of the defining advances in dentistry over the past 30 years. The success of implants once was considered impossible to predict, but today implants are placed routinely in dental practice with excellent success rates. The ability of titanium to form a direct attachment to living bone led to the term *osseointegration,* coined by Branemark, to describe this bone-metal fusion.[12] Other materials such as hydroxyapatite and various treatments of titanium surfaces more recently have emerged as potential ways to decrease the time needed to obtain osseointegration, increase success rates, or achieve both these goals.[26]

This chapter reviews issues associated with prevention of infection in surgical implant placement. The factors known to cause infection, the putative bacteria involved, and the means to control infection once it occurs also are reviewed. Two types of implant infections are identified. One affects the apical region similar to a periapical lesion around teeth; the other is periimplantitis. As with any surgical procedure, the potential for serious and even life-threatening infections can occur in surgical implant placement. The surgeon therefore must appreciate these potential infections and treat them appropriately should an infection occur.

PROPHYLAXIS AND SURGICAL PREPARATION

Implant placement for the restoration of teeth, partial edentulous segments, and entire dental arches now is considered routine patient care. The benefits of implants and their ability to restore form and function for a patient have led to their widespread use in clinical practice. However, as noted in the orthopedic literature, a dental implant must survive in a potentially contaminated field.[19]

As with any foreign body, the amount of bacteria necessary to create an infection around an implant is substantially less than in a clean surgical wound. For example, the placement of a suture reduces the amount of bacteria necessary to create a wound infection by a factor of 1000. In addition, the placement of an intraoral endosseous implant is complicated by the initial bacterial load present at the time of surgery and the continued bombardment of the tissue-to-implant bond by bacteria throughout the lifespan of the fixture.[33]

Endosseous implants also are placed in extraoral sites for the restoration of craniofacial defects. Other types of implants are placed transcutaneously into the oral cavity; thus resistance to infection by both skin and intraoral bacteria is necessary. The majority of implants are successful and are placed without complication. However, the development of infection may lead to loss of the implant and the surrounding bone, teeth, and nerves with extension into adjacent spaces. The practitioner placing implants must be aware of these risks, practice appropriate techniques to minimize the chance of infection, and be prepared to intervene rapidly if an infection occurs.

Most authors recommend the administration of prophylactic antibiotics in conjunction with implant surgery.[56,57] As with any type of antibiotic administration the most important dose for the patient is before the initiation of the surgical procedure. The decision to continue antibiotic therapy postoperatively has not been reviewed in controlled studies. Certain patient situations such as complex grafting or preexisting compromise of the immune system may dictate an empirical decision to continue antibiotics for 5 to 7 days.

Gynther et al.[24] studied the response of patients who received 1 g of penicillin preoperatively and every 8 hours thereafter for 10 days compared with a group that did not receive any antibiotics. They found no difference in the survival of implants in patients who did not receive any antibiotics before or after surgery. They also reported no difference in the frequency of infections between the two groups. Despite these findings, most other authors and protocols suggest the use of perioperative antibiotics.[56,57] Dent et al.[18] verified the use of antibiotics and showed a failure rate of 2.6% with presurgical antibiotics and 4.0% without antibiotics.

The actual surgical procedure described by Branemark[10] and promulgated in the original protocols taught worldwide used a full surgical patient draping technique. This practice originated through Dr. Branemark's training as an orthopedic surgeon. Kraut[31] has discussed the controversy regarding the necessity of full surgical draping in a known contaminated field. Newer implant surgical protocols recommended by other implant companies do not specifically promote the use of full surgical draping (Dentsply/Implant Division, Encino, CA). The use of full surgical preparation may increase the "awareness" of the surgical team to maintain asepsis as much as possible with the understanding that the procedures are being performed in a contaminated field. However, surgically "clean" procedures using sterile instruments and gloves are acceptable as a minimum preparation.

Two major classifications exist for implants: endosseous and transosseous fixtures. Endosseous implants typically are placed intraorally into the maxilla, mandible, or zygoma. Occasionally endosseous implants may be placed extraorally to support prosthetic ears, eyes, or other facial structures. Transosseous implants, such as the Small staple implant (Linvatec, Largo, FL) and Boskar transmandibular implant (TMI Incorporated, Jacksonville, FL) are placed through a submental incision. The antibiotic regimen for these two types differs and is outlined in Box 18-1.

The decision regarding antibiotic management also is dictated by the patient's condition. Certain medical conditions such as diabetes may increase the risk of implant failures, although outcomes in patients with compromised immune systems have not been studied directly. Other host factors, such as cigarette smoking, increase the risk of implant failures but not necessarily because of infection.

Chlorhexidene gluconate rinses (e.g., Peridex, Perioguard) are recommended for use immediately preoperatively and continued for 5 to 7 days postoperatively. With the use of chlorhexidene the rate of complications resulting from infection was reduced from 8.7% to 4.1%.[28] This supplements patients' use of saline solution rinses because often their oral hygiene regimen is negatively affected because of surgical site discomfort.

Before placement of an implant the clinician must survey the surgical site clinically and radiographically to ascertain that no residual infection is present in the bone. Adjacent teeth should be evaluated for the presence of an occult periapical lesion, which could infect the implant.[54] This evaluation is critical because many patients who have implant procedures are partially dentate, in contrast of the fully edentulous patients in Branemark's original treatment groups. Most protocols recommend waiting at least

---

BOX 18-1

Antibiotic Administration for Implant Surgery

Intraoral endosseous implants (routine)
   Penicillin V 2.0 g PO, then 500 mg qid for 5-7 days, or clindamycin 600 mg PO, then 300 mg tid for 5-7 days
Intraoral endosseous implants (entering maxillary sinus)
   Amoxicillin 2.0 g PO, then 500 mg qid for 5-7 days or clindamycin 600 mg PO, then 300 mg tid for 5-7 days
Intraoral implants with extensive local grafting
   Penicillin V 2.0 g plus metronidazole 500 mg PO, then penicillin V 500 mg qid and metronidazole 250 mg bid, or clindamycin 600 mg PO, then 300 mg PO tid
Intraoral endosseous implants with sinus grafting
   Augmentin 875 mg PO, then 875 mg bid for 5-7 days, or clindamycin 600 mg PO then 300 mg tid for 5-7 days, or clarithromycin 500 mg PO then 500 mg bid for 5-7 days
Transosseous implants (with skin and intraoral communication)
   Augmentin 875 mg PO, then 875 mg bid for 5-7 days, or penicillin V 2.0 g and metronidazole 500 mg PO, then penicillin V 500 mg qid and metronidazole 250 mg bid, or clindamycin 600 mg PO, then 300 mg PO tid
Extraoral implants
   Cephalexin 1.0 g, then 500 mg qid for 5-7 days, or cephazolin 1.0 g IV, then cephalexin 500 mg qid for 5-7 days, or clarithromycin 500 mg, then 500 mg bid

---

2 to 3 months after the removal of a tooth before insertion of an implant. That period should allow resolution of any residual infection in the bone and intact soft tissue coverage over the planned surgical site.

Infection adjacent to an implant site is a potential source of implant infection. The surgical site should be radiographed carefully before surgery to determine whether adjacent teeth are infected. Ideally, any active endodontic lesions adjacent to the implant site should be treated before endosseous implant placement.[53] Endodontically involved teeth typically represent a mixed flora infection. The most common organisms are *Propionibacterium acnes, Staphylococcus epidermidis, Streptococcus intermedius, Wolinella recta,* and *Porphyromonas* and *Prevotella* sp.[52] These bacteria, when harbored in teeth or the periapical regions adjacent to an implant site, can contaminate the newly placed implant. The natural dentition also may be a source of bacteria, which have been implicated in implant infections.[48] Reduction of plaque and overt bacterial contamination should be accomplished in presurgical hygiene visits.

The placement of an immediate implant into an extraction socket is controversial. Many authors advocate waiting a period of months after the removal of a tooth to ensure any residual infection has cleared and early bone healing has been initiated.[2] Others recommend immediate placement if the extraction can be done atraumatically and no preexisting infection is present.[22] Yet another group proposes that implants may even be placed into infected tooth sockets.[42] Novaes[42] has published a protocol for infected sites that includes initiation of antibiotic therapy 24 to 48 hours before surgery, thorough debridement and irrigation of the socket, and continuation of antibiotic therapy for 10 days after surgery. The results have not been confirmed by others, and thus this protocol is controversial.

Recalcitrant periodontal disease (defined as one that has not responded to conventional periodontal therapy and continues to cause loss of periodontal attachment around teeth) has not been shown to reduce implant survival if the teeth are extracted first.[41] In fact, two important periodontal pathogens, *Actinobacillus actinomycetemcomitans* and *Porphyromonas gingivalis,* are not found around implants of patients with previous periodontal disease who have had all their teeth extracted.[17] However, the microbiology of the periimplant region differs in patients with periodontal disease who are only partially edentulous with the persistence of organisms known to be periodontal pathogens.[7]

OVERVIEW OF IMPLANT INFECTIONS

Although the nonintegrated implant initially may appear as localized bacterial infection, it often is unclear whether the infection caused the failure to integrate or the infection is a result of the mobility of the implant and the presence of a connective tissue encapsulation. Reports regarding the causes of failures of implants include factors such as increased load (especially during the healing phase), heat generated during the surgery, local contamination of the implant site, and host factors.[20] Because implant failures are not frequent, with 5-year success of more than 90% for most systems, control for all variables is difficult. Animal models may provide indications of which factors lead to infection and eventual loss.

The microbiological findings differ significantly in the gingival tissues of healthy and failing implants. In unsuccessful implants with mobility, pain, and bleeding, a large proportion of organisms were gram-negative anaerobic rods (*Bacteroides* spp.) and *Fusobacterium* spp.[4] In contrast, healthy implant sites had predominately coccoid cells without the presence of spirochetes.[39] Other species identified in failing implants, including *A. actinomycetemcomitans, P. gingivalis,* and *Prevotella intermedia,* were detected by deoxyribonucleic acid probes.[34] The identification of the bacterial contamination of failing implants therefore assists in the choice of antibiotic management. In testing the microbial sensitivity to antibiotics in failing implants, Sbordone et al.[51] noted penicillin G and amoxicillin have greater activity than clindamycin, amoxicillin-clavulanate, and the combination of amoxicillin and metronidazole against the putative organisms isolated.

In addition to local bacteria surrounding an implant,

the surfaces of contaminated implants are coated with a biofilm.[16] Biofilms develop on inert and even living tissues releasing antigens and reacting with the local tissues. Although the antibiotic treatment may reverse the symptoms, unless the biofilm is removed surgically, the symptoms will persist.[57]

The source of bacteria may be from the endogenous population of oral bacteria. The implant and its various components can harbor bacteria once inserted into the oral cavity. The space between the abutment and implant and the internal aspect of the fixture act as reservoirs for bacteria.[43]

Celletti et al.[13] studied intentionally overloaded osseointegrated implants in a baboon model to determine the role of hyperfunction as a cause of implant failure. Although they found failures of components and fractures of implants in some cases, the loss of integration or crestal bone loss with secondary infection did not occur.

The surface of an implant may predispose it to development of infection. Many authors report the increased roughness may provide isolation of the bacteria from the systemic circulation to remove them. Polished metal cylinders required 40 times more bacterial inoculum than porous implants to create infection.[15] The concerns with hydroxyapatite implants are that they may be predisposed to bacterial contamination progressing to loss of or failure of osseointegration.[27] Although hydroxyapatite reportedly increases the success and speed of osseointegration,[30] the potential for increased bacterial contamination has changed its use. Previous implants with hydroxyapatite attached to the gingival surface have now been replaced with a polished titanium collar to reduce the risk of periimplantitis (Figure 18-1).

EARLY IMPLANT INFECTIONS

After implant placement the raising of a subperiosteal flap with development of a hematoma can create a nidus for bacterial growth. Patients may have vestibular fullness that creates difficulty with the seating of the prosthesis. If the patient has been taking antibiotics, the presence of a penicillin-resistant bacterium such as *Prevotella* may be suspected. The addition of metronidazole should eliminate the infection. The use of the provisional prosthesis may need to be delayed an additional week. Early infections rarely require surgical drainage.

The transmission of a load to a submerged implant may lead to loosening of the cover screw from the internal aspect of the implant. This process usually creates an opening in the overlying mucosa, causing a localized superficial infection (Figure 18-2). A sinus tract also may be present. Reopening the incision and reseating the cover screw may resolve the local infection. In persistent cases of localized drainage, exposing the implant completely to the oral cavity by the placement of a longer healing abutment resolves these localized infections. This maneuver is indicated only if the implant is solidly placed in bone at the initial surgery without the use of an associated graft.

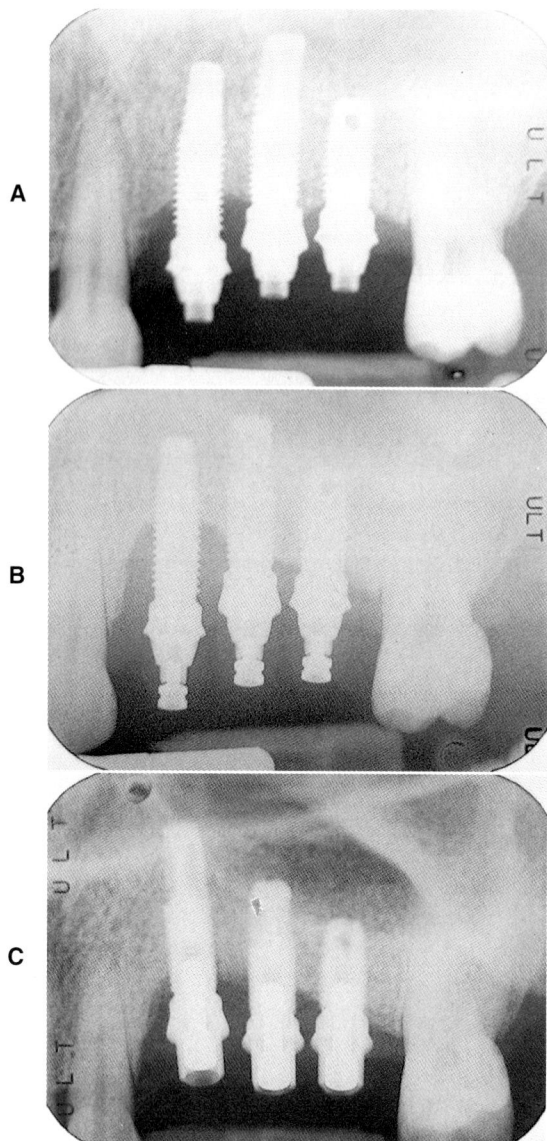

Figure 18-1 **A,** Bone level at final abutment placement. The anterior implant is a hydroxyapatite-coated implant. **B,** Bone level 4 months after abutment placement. Constant drainage from the anterior hydroxyapatite implant causing bone loss was uncontrolled with two surgical debridement procedures that included the placement of a local tetracycline delivery system. **C,** Anterior hydroxyapatite implant removed with a trephine and replaced with a solid titanium fixture.

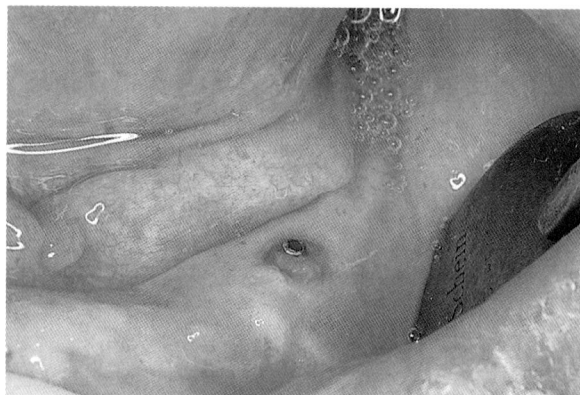

Figure 18-2 Local infection resulting from loosening of a cover screw from forces transmitted to it by an overlying removable prosthesis. This infection will clear with reseating of the cover screw or alternatively placing a longer healing abutment to keep the site open and easier to clean. Antibiotics generally are not needed unless an adjacent space infection has occurred.

Early implant failures may lead to spontaneous exfoliation of the fixture from the osteotomy site. The patient may notice sudden inflammation and pain at the surgical site, followed by immediate relief with the spontaneous loss of the implant. This type of implant failure typically is the result of an acute infection that resolves with the loss of the implant. Further treatment with antibiotics is unnecessary if no other spaces are affected by the infection. A new implant, usually of a wider diameter, may be placed after 4 to 8 weeks.

Implants that compromise adjacent teeth may lead to development of an acute infection (Figure 18-3). Iatrogenic devitalization of a tooth adjacent to an implant site may create a periapical infection. This infection can then spread to involve the adjacent implants in the region, leading to their loss. Optimally, at least 3 mm of bone should separate the implant from a tooth to reduce this risk of local vascular compromise to an adjacent apex of a tooth. However, the surgeon must be aware that because of the length of the implant and angulation of insertion, the apical end of the implant may impinge on adjacent structures even though adequate space is present at the initial bone penetration site. In addition, a "plaque front" has been shown to move laterally 2 mm to affect adjacent teeth through an infrabony pocket.[58] It is likely that an implant within 2 mm of a periodontal pocket also could be adversely affected.

APICAL IMPLANTITIS

A unique type of infection associated with the apical region of an implant has been described (Figure 18-4). It has some characteristics of an endodontic infection because it localizes to the apical region of the implant and initial symptoms of pain and fistula formation are common.[45] The spread of infection within the medullary bone can create pressure on the inferior alveolar nerve causing paresthesia and dysesthesia. In other cases the finding is noted coincidentally as an asymptomatic radiolucency on a radiograph.

The bone around the apical end of the newly placed implant may become compromised during the surgical procedure, permitting the buildup of heat. The lack of irrigation to the apical end of the drill may cause heat formation, which may be exacerbated if the drills are dull or excessive pressure is used. Gentle pressure and removing the bur every 15 to 20 seconds is recommended to clear any bone fragments from the drill flutes.[14] Compression of the bone and vascular compromise at the apex also may

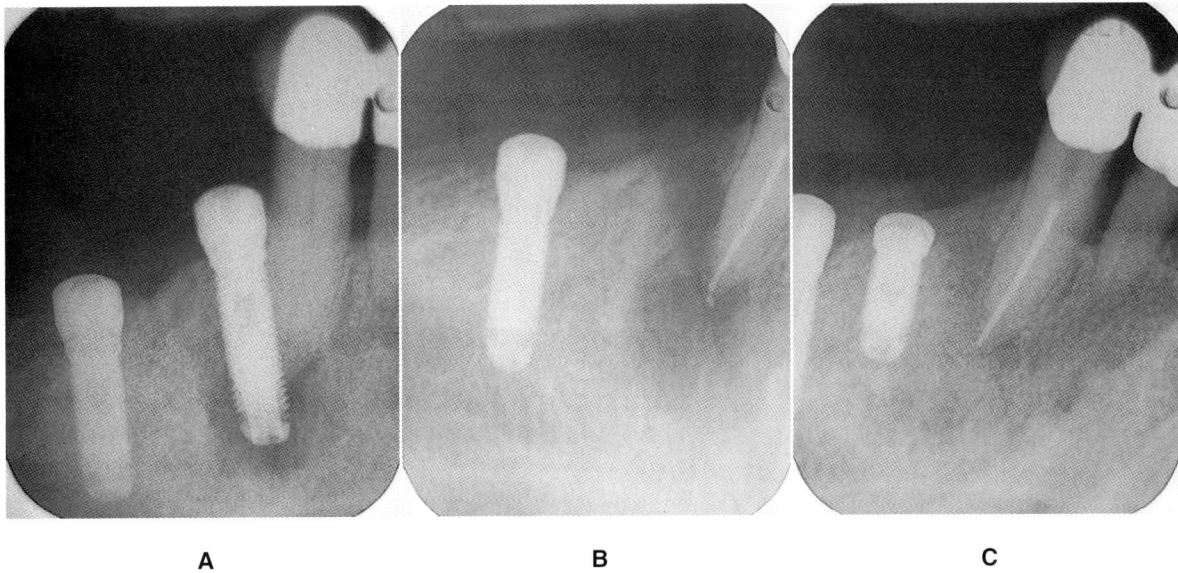

A   **B**   **C**

Figure 18-3 A, Fixture placement in close proximity of the apex of an adjacent tooth causing an iatrogenic infection of the tooth and implant. **B,** Subsequent infection required endodontic treatment of the tooth and removal of the grossly infected implant. **C,** After waiting 3 months, resolution of the infection is demonstrated radiographically. Replacement of a new implant at an appropriate distance from the tooth permitted a successful completion of the case.

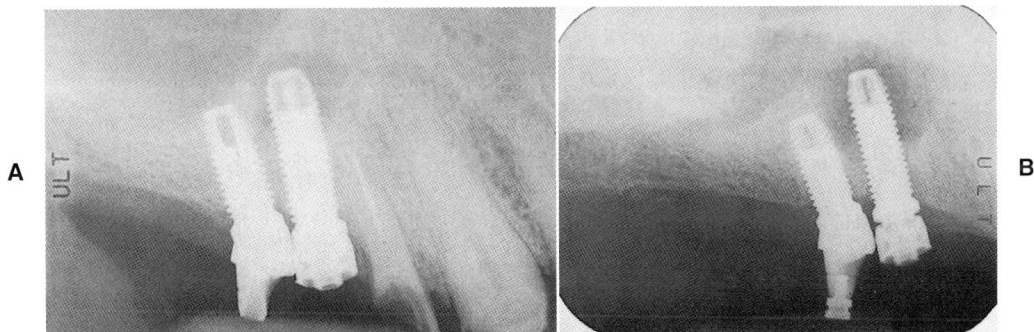

A   **B**

Figure 18-4 A, Film at abutment placement shows the beginning of a periapical lesion at the apex of the anterior implant. **B,** Despite extraction of the adjacent tooth, the area continues to enlarge 4 years later. Although clinically stable, the patient had chronic pain and drainage, requiring removal of the implant.

occur as a result of the biomechanics of achieving primary implant stabilization. The devitalized bone may sequester forming a nidus for bacterial contamination. Other potential causes and sources for formation of periapical implant infection are listed in Box 18-2.

The study of implants with apical infections that are removed shows extensive bacterial contamination, often in the apical vents or antirotational holes that are present in certain implant designs. The adjacent bone shows a histological pattern consistent with localized suppurative osteomyelitis.[44] As expected from the extent of bone involvement, attempts to treat this type of infection solely with antibiotics have been unsuccessful.[52]

McAllister et al.[36] described a surgical procedure to treat this type of infection. The procedure involves thorough

---

BOX 18-2

Causes of Implant Periapical Lesion

Contamination of the implant surface
Fenestration of the vestibular bone
Bone overheating during surgery
Excessive tightening of the implant with compression of the apical bone chips
Presence of preexisting bone pathology
Overloading of the implant
Poor quality of the bone site

Adapted from Piatelli A, Scarano A, Balleri P, et al: Clinical and histologic evaluation of an active "Implant periapical lesion": a case report, *Int J Oral Maxillofac Implants* 13:713, 1998.

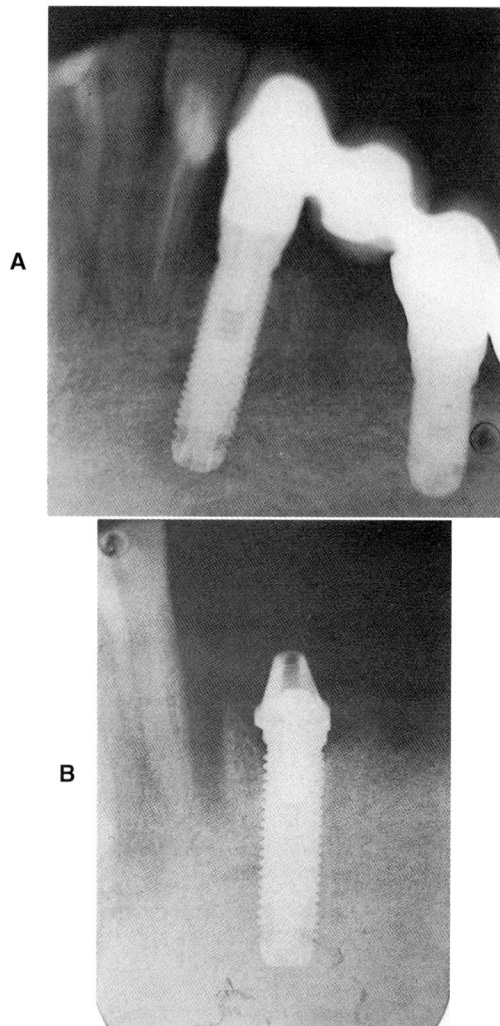

Figure 18-5 A, "Periapical lesion" associated with apical end of implant. A chronic sinus tract was noted in mucobuccal fold. **B,** Treatment by surgical debridement, tetracycline powder, and extraction of the adjacent mobile, endodontically treated incisor.

curettage of the apical region of all granulation tissue, which should be done with a titanium or plastic scaler to reduce the potential for implant damage. Resection of the exposed portion of the implant may be necessary if a large section is exposed and without bone coverage. Resection of the apical third also may remove the antirotational hole, which may continue to harbor bacteria and is mechanically difficult to thoroughly debride. Tetracycline powder is placed into the defect, left for 3 to 5 minutes, and then irrigated. This process further debrides and identifies soft tissue remnants resulting from the cauterization effect of the acid environment it creates. The defect is filled with freeze-dried demineralized bone, autogenous bone, or alloplastic material (Figure 18-5). A membrane may be placed over the defect and the patient prescribed antibiotics for a 10-day course. Balshi et al.[5] reviewed three options for surgical approach of the apex of infected mandibular implants: an intraoral transmandibular approach, a periosteal dissection, and an extraoral approach in selected cases.[5]

PERIIMPLANTITIS

The marginal tissues around implants have been of interest since osseointegrated implants were developed. The effect of plaque and bacterial contamination on the bone-implant junction initially was studied in the fully edentulous population. Adell et al.[3] found that gingivitis around implants could occur with or without the presence of plaque, leading to the conclusion that the attachment and periodontal problems around implants are different than teeth. In contrast to teeth the periodontal attachment to the implant abutment at the gingival level differs significantly. The collagen fibers from cementum are oriented in a perpendicular arrangement from the tooth forming a direct attachment. The collagen fibers around implants are oriented parallel to the implant surface and without evidence of a direct attachment to the smooth titanium surface.[9] *Periimplantitis* has become the accepted term to describe the diseased attachment state around implants.[38] However, the presence of plaque and bacteria do not always lead to the progression of periimplantitis.[21] Host susceptibility and other variables must occur in addition to the bacterial contamination.

Many authors report anecdotally that the presence of keratinized tissue is critical around implants.[59] The theory is that the periimplant area is at a greater risk of breakdown because the attachment of soft tissues to the implant abutment is of a different nature than around natural teeth. The benefit of immobile tissue around implants may preserve the integrity of the connective tissue attachment at the gingival margin. However, the benefits of a keratinized border around the abutment in reducing the effect of periimplantitis has been shown only around hydroxyapatite implants and titanium plasma-sprayed implants.[25,59]

Clinical classifications of periimplant complications have been divided into various groups. Meffert[37] used the terminology "ailing, failing and failed" to describe implants in progressive stages of infection. "Ailing" implants have bone loss with pocket formation. "Failing" implants have bone loss irrespective of therapy, bleeding on probing, and a purulent exudate. "Failed" implants have mobility, a dull sound on percussion, and periimplant radiolucency. According to Meffert's classification system, implants that are ailing or failing may be able to be treated and maintained. Failed implants with frank mobility require removal.

Periimplantitis is defined as the pathological changes confined to the surrounding hard and soft tissues adjacent to the implant. It is differentiated from periimplant mucositis, which is a reversible inflammatory change in the soft tissue surrounding the implant. Periimplant mucositis is analogous to gingivitis and is primarily an inflammatory disorder caused by plaque accumulation.[46] Once normal oral hygiene resumes, the mucositis resolves with no permanent changes or bone loss.

Periimplantitis has been documented and its accepted cause is the detrimental effect of anaerobic bacteria on the periimplant tissue health. Various studies support this theory, including an experimental induction in humans and

Evidence for a Bacterial Cause of Periimplantitis

Experimentally induced periimplant mucositis: plaque accumulation leads to periimplant mucositis

Distinct differences in microflora of successful versus failing implants

No shift in microflora over time in successful implants

Transmission of periodontal pathogens from residual teeth to implants

Reduction of periimplant microflora with resultant improvement in symptoms with therapy

Induction of periimplantitis by placement of plaque-retentive ligatures in animals

Increased bone resorption in edentulous implant in patients with poor oral hygiene compared with those with good hygiene

Adapted from Mombelli A, Lang NP: The diagnosis and treatment of periimplantitis, *Periodontol 2000* 17:63, 1998.

development of an animal model of periimplantitis.[6,46] The evidence for a bacterial cause is summarized in Box 18-3.

Periimplantitis begins with bone loss at the coronal portion of the implant that progresses and is associated with a purulent exudate. The apical end of the implant maintains its osseointegration; therefore the implant is not mobile until the final stage of periimplantitis. The clinical diagnosis includes increased probing depths, patient reports of pain, spontaneous bleeding, and radiographic evidence of bone loss. Diagnostic markers such as interleukin-1β, proteases, glycosaminoglycan, and prostaglandin E_2 levels may provide predictive information of ongoing periimplantitis that has not developed clinical manifestations.[29]

The microbiology of failing implants is composed of various species of bacteria. The typical periodontal pathogens (*P. gingivalis, P intermedia,* and *A. actinomycetemcomitans*) are found in approximately half the cases of periimplantitis. Other microorganisms such as enteric bacteria and *Staphylococcus* and *Candida* spp. also are found frequently around compromised implants.[50] These organisms typically are not associated with odontogenic periodontal disease states. Therefore antimicrobial therapy should be directed by culture and sensitivity testing. Periimplantitis has an overall frequency of 5% to 10%, although rates of specific implant systems cannot be compared because of differences in reported diagnostic criteria.[38]

As periimplantitis persists, additional attachment is lost. Bone levels decrease and eventually may lead to the loss of integration. Periodontal probing is useful to determine whether bleeding on probing is present or if suppuration is found. Actual pocket depths are not as indicative of the disease in contrast with teeth. However, increasing pocket depths over time are indications of the progression. Radiographic evidence of additional bone loss requires well-positioned parallel films. Digital radiography often provides a more sensitive indication of bone loss.

Certain types of implants may be more susceptible to periimplantitis based on the type of implant surface.[55] Hydroxyapatite-coated implants can harbor bacteria as a result of surface roughness creating localized tissue reactions.[27] These reactions can persist and lead to implant loss. Wolinsky[61] reported that certain species of bacteria such as *Actinomyces viscosus; Fusobacterium* sp., and *Peptostreptococcous prevotti* may preferentially adhere to hydroxyapatite causing the increased propensity for periimplantitis around these fixtures.

The initial goal of treatment of periimplantitis is to confirm that all the components are seated on the implant fixture. Abutments with internal hexes may become offset and create a gap trapping bacteria leading to a fistula. Loose components also may cause a localized tissue infection. After components are removed, the stability of the fixture is checked to ensure that the tissue response is not caused by a failed implant.

Therapy of periimplantitis is performed by subgingival debridement and removal of calculus. Calculus is not as adherent to titanium and is removed with graphite or plastic scalers to avoid damage to the implant surface. More extensive cases of attachment loss require open flap procedures and pocket reduction surgery. Tetracycline powder placed into the defect has been shown to be effective as a topical means to suppress putative periodontal pathogens in the periimplant defect.[40] Irrigation with chlorhexidine gluconate subgingivally should be done in the office and the patient instructed for continuation of therapy at home. Antibiotic therapy often is instituted. Some authors recommend guided tissue regeneration procedures with membrane placement.[28] However, the placement of membrane into an area of infection often leads to complications of secondary infection of the membrane and failure to restore bone height.[26] The use of autogenous bone blocks to treat the bone defects successfully has been described by Behneke et al.[8] Their protocol includes debridement of soft tissues without touching the implant and air abrasion of the implant surface. Autogenous block grafts were harvested from either the retromolar or symphysis region of the mandible. The blocks were stabilized against the implant with bone screws, and fibrin glue was used to retain bone chips to fill the residual defect. Their long-term successful treatment of 23 of 25 fixtures over a 6-month time interval makes this one of the most successful protocols to be studied prospectively.

The propensity of hydroxyapatite implants to retain bacteria often requires special management to remove the coating. This can be accomplished with the use of an ultrasonic scaler and decontamination with citric acid solutions. The tissue height then is reduced to permit easier access for hygiene.

An analogous situation to periimplantitis is associated with endosseous implants placed for craniofacial reconstruction (Figure 18-6, Plates 35 and 36). Localized infections can form in the soft tissue surrounding the implants. The frequency of these infections is high, with 15% to 20% of patients experiencing an infection at some point.[1]

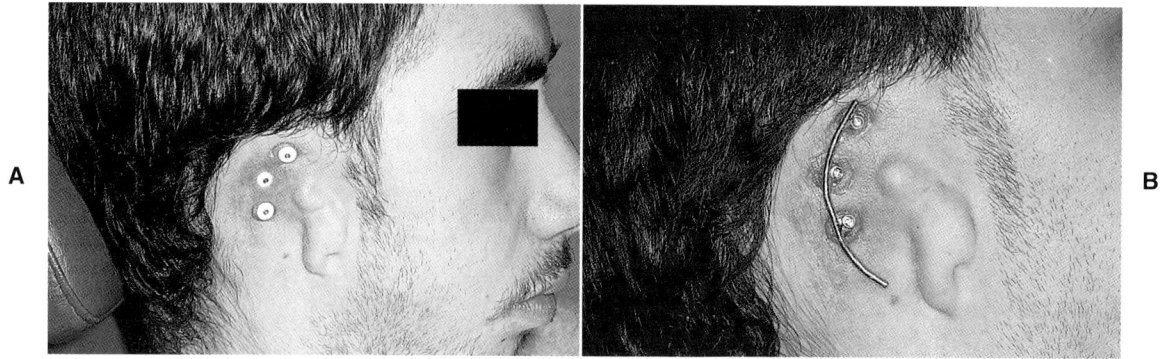

Figure 18-6 A, Local tissue infection after external implants for an ear prosthesis. Cultures grew methicillin-resistant *Staphylococcus epidermidis,* demonstrating the need for sensitivity testing. The overhanging plastic healing caps further impeded this patient's ability to perform adequate hygiene around the fixtures. **B,** Resolution of the infection with appropriate antibiotics, local cleansing, and placement of the final bar prosthesis, which facilitated hygiene.

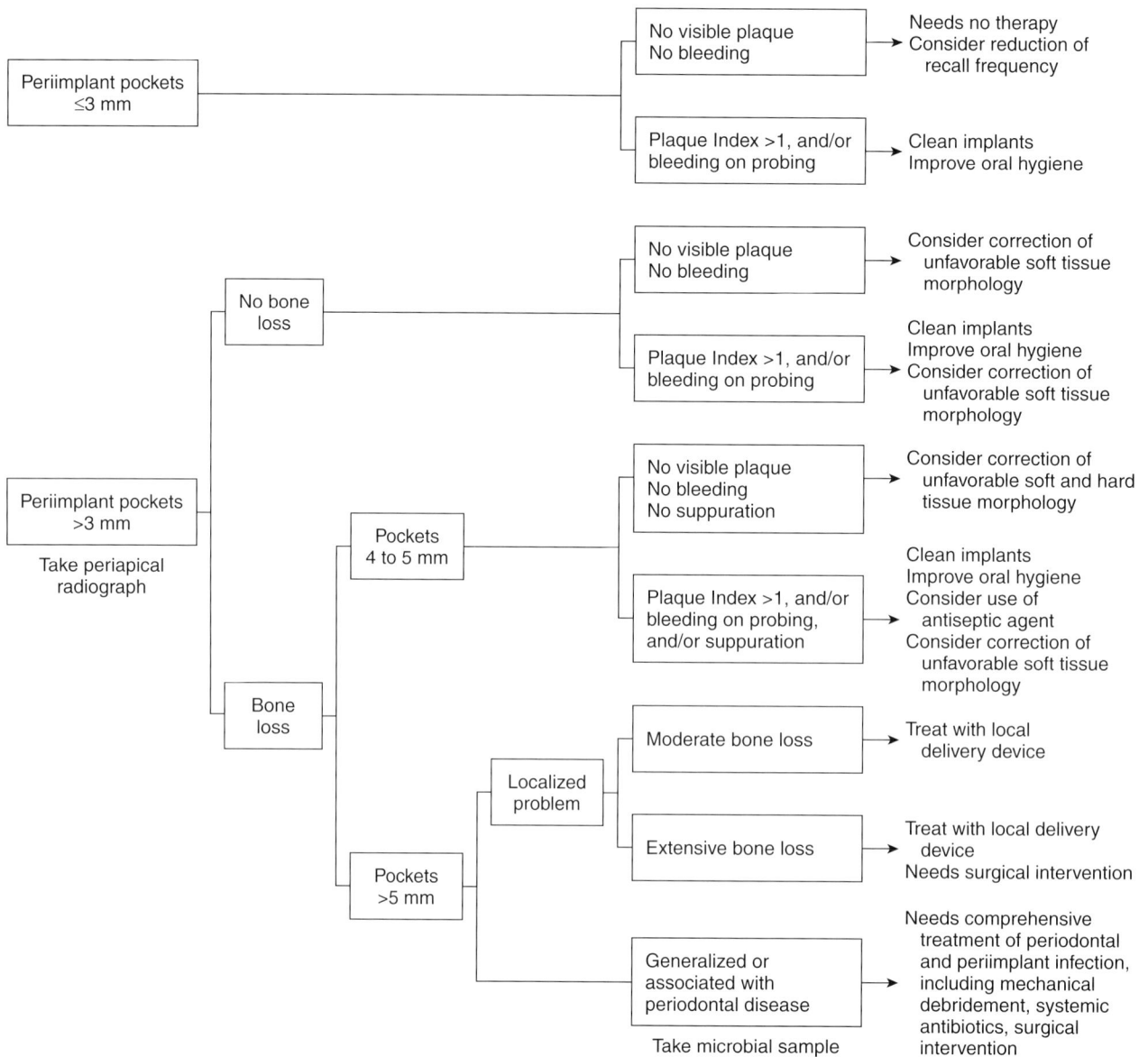

Figure 18-7 Decision process for periimplant diagnosis. The initial assessment includes periimplant probing, evaluation of oral hygiene, and bleeding tendency of the periimplant tissues. (From Mombelli A, Lang NP: The diagnosis and treatment of peri-implantitis, *Periodont 2000* 17:63, 1998.)

Sebaceous crusting acts in a manner similar to calculus, causing a local tissue inflammation and creating a potential nidus for bacterial infection. Most of these infections are associated with *S. aureus* with additional reports implicating *Streptococcus* spp. and other gram-negative bacilli. As with intraoral implants, the development of an infection of the soft tissues does not always lead to failure of osseointegration. However, the pain and erythema associated with the infection are problematic.

A site-specific relationship exists in the success of craniofacial implants. In general, the endosseous fixtures placed in the mastoid and temporal bone for ear reconstruction and hearing aids have a higher success rate than orbital implants.[49] The loss of orbital implants is related to a higher infection rate and exposure of the implant flange. The proximity of these implants to the nasal cavity and its native bacteria may account for the increased infection rate.

To improve the patient's ability to perform adequate hygiene, the dermal tissues are thinned as much as possible at the time of surgery. This also removes local skin appendages and reduces the mobility of the tissue around the implant that are critical to reducing local reactions.[11] Patients benefit from an extension of the abutment and reduction of overhangs to facilitate hygiene.

When managing the infections associated with craniofacial implants, attention is directed at improving hygiene with daily removal of all sebaceous crusting by the patient. Antimicrobial therapy is initiated based on culture and sensitivity testing. Additional benefits of topical therapy with mupirocin (Bactoban) or oxytetracycline-hydrocortisone (Terra-Cortril) help resolve the infection. The placement of palatal tissue free grafts around the abutments of craniofacial implants also has been suggested as a means to prevent the chronic infection.[47] This tissue has a higher degree of keratinization and reduces the mobility around the implant site.

The potential for yeast infections, especially under facial prostheses that create a warm, moist environment ideal for fungal growth, must be considered. Abu-Serriah et al.[1] found yeasts associated with ear prosthesis implants but not with bone-anchored hearing aids in the same region. Yeasts that are not part of the normal microflora of skin may be opportunistic with the removal of normal coagulase-negative *Staphylococci* caused by antibiotic therapy. The most commonly isolated yeast is *Candida parapsilosis,* which is a known pathogen of endocarditis, ocular and dermal infections, and arthritis.[56]

A protocol for managing periimplantitis is provided in Figure 18-7. The surgical treatment is a necessary adjunct to the need for home care and frequent office visits.

OTHER INFECTIONS ASSOCIATED WITH IMPLANT SURGERY

The reflection of a local flap and insertion of an implant may lead to severe infection in rare cases. The surgeon must be aware of the potential space involvement and urgently treat infections of the maxillofacial region should they occur. Because the implant is a persistent foreign

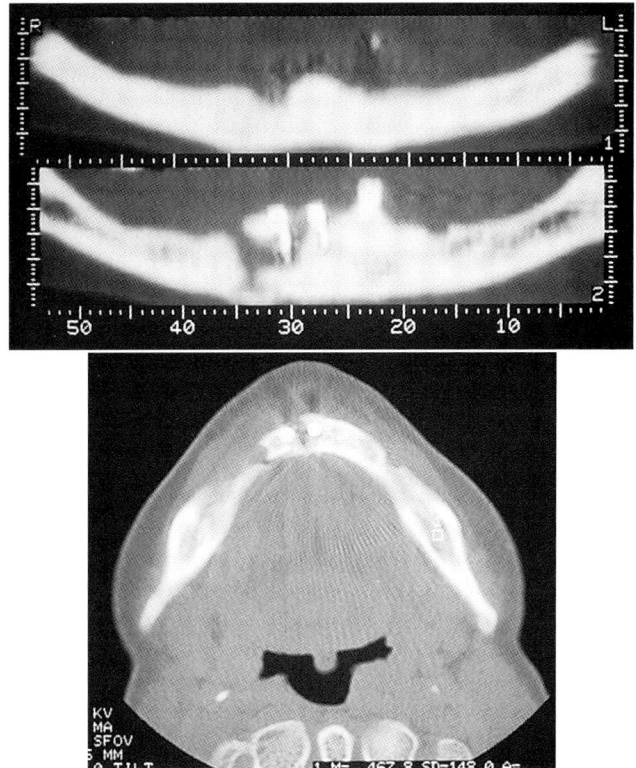

Figure 18-8 Sequestrum and involucrum formation resulting from infected implants. Fixtures were left in place despite severe infection for 2 months in an attempt to preserve the implants. Pathological fracture and need for discontinuity bone grafting resulted. (Courtesy Morton H. Goldberg, Hartford, CT.)

body, it should be removed once an infection has spread from the local area adjacent to the fixture. The area around the implant should be explored and necrotic bone removed. Specimens of bone and soft tissue are sent for culture and sensitivity testing.

Serious infections have been reported during attempts to maintain a fixture in cases of spreading infection. Descending necrotizing fasciitis has been reported as a consequence of implant surgery.[35] A severe infection can develop into osteomyelitis with pathological fracture of the mandible, as shown in Figure 18-8. An attempt was made to manage the infection with oral penicillin. After definitive treatment, including removal of the implants, necrotic bone, and stabilization of the pathological fractures, the primary organism identified was a strain of *S. aureus* resistant to penicillin.

The placement of implants creates a site susceptible to the distant spread of osteomyelitis. Goldberg[23] noted a case of *Klebsiella* osteomyelitis that occurred 1 month after a severe urinary tract infection. Enteric rods such as these are not associated with failing implants.[39] The isolates from the bone in this case were consistent with the bacteria cultured from the urinary tract, with the same sensitivity profile. Therefore the osteomyelitis was caused by blood-borne spread of the organism. The infection did not resolve until the implants were removed, the necrotic bone debrided, and the appropriate antibiotics administered.

REFERENCES

1. Abu-Serriah MM, Bagg J, McGowan DA, et al: The microflora associated with extra-oral endosseous craniofacial implants: a cross-sectional study, *Int J Oral Maxillofac Surg* 29:344, 2000.
2. Adell R, Lekholm U, Rockler B, et al: A 15-year study of osseointegrated implants in the treatment of the edentulous jaw, *Int J Oral Surg* 10:387, 1981.
3. Adell R, Lekholm U, Rocker B, et al: Marginal tissue reactions at osseointegrated titanium fixtures (I). A 3-year longitudinal prospective study, *Int J Oral Maxillofac Surg* 15:39, 1986.
4. Augthun M, Conrads G: Microbial findings of deep peri-implant bone defects, *Int J Oral Maxillofac Implants* 12:106, 1997.
5. Balshi TJ, Pappas CE, Wolfinger GJ, et al: Management of an abscess around the apex of a mandibular root form implant: clinical report, *Implant Dent* 3:81, 1994.
6. Baron M, Haas R, Dortbudak O, et al: Experimentally induced peri-implantitis: a review of different treatment methods described in the literature, *Int J Oral Maxillofac Implants* 15:533, 2000.
7. Becker W, Becker BE, Newman MG, et al: Clinical and microbiological findings that may contribute to dental implant failure, *Int J Oral Maxillofac Implants* 5:31, 1990.
8. Behneke A, Behneke N, d'Hoedt B: Treatment of peri-implantitis defects with autogenous bone grafts: six-month to 3-year results of a prospective study in 17 patients, *Int J Oral Maxillofac Implants* 15:125, 2000.
9. Berglundh T, Lindhe J, Ericsson I, et al: The soft tissue barrier at implants and teeth, *Clin Oral Impl Res* 1:8, 1991.
10. Branemark PI: *Manual: jawbone anchored bridge,* Gothenburg, Sweden, 1987, Institute for Biotechnology.
11. Branemark PI, Albrektsson T: Titanium implants permanently penetrating human skin, *Scand J Plast Reconstr Surg* 16:17, 1982.
12. Branemark PI, Breine U, Adell R, et al: Intra-osseous anchorage of dental prosthesis. I. Experimental studies, *Scand J Plast Reconstr Surg* 3:81, 1969.
13. Celletti R, Pameijer CH, Brachchetti G, et al: Histologic evaluation of osseointegrated implants restored in nonaxial functional occlusion with preangled abutments, *Int J Periodontics Restorative Dent* 15:563, 1995.
14. Clarizio LF: Peri-implant infections, *Atlas Oral Maxillofac Surg Clin North Am* 8:35, 2000.
15. Cordero J, Munuera L, Folgueira MD: The influence of the chemical composition and surface of the implant on infection, *Injury* 27(Suppl 3):SC34, 1996.
16. Costerton JW, Stewart PS, Greenberg EP: Bacterial biofilms: a common cause of persistant infections, *Science* 284:1318, 1999.
17. Danser MM, van Winlelhoff AJ, van der Velden U: Periodontal bacteria colonizing oral mucous membranes in edentulous patients wearing dental implants, *J Periodontol* 68:209, 1997.
18. Dent CD, Olson JW, Farish SE, et al: The influence of preoperative antibiotics on success of endosseous implants up to and including stage II surgery: a study of 2,641 implants, *J Oral Maxillofac Surg* 55:19, 1997.
19. Drake DR, Paul J, Keller JC: Primary bacterial colonization of implant surfaces, *Int J Oral Maxillofac Implants* 14:226, 1999.
20. Eckert SE, Meraw SJ, Cal E, et al: Analysis of incidence and associated factors with fractured implants: a retrospective study, *Int J Oral Maxillofac Implants* 15: 662, 2000.
21. Ericsson I, Berglundh T, Marinello C, et al: Long-standing plaque and gingivitis at implants and teeth in the dog, *Clin Oral Implants Res* 3:99, 1992.
22. Gelb DA: Immediate implant surgery: three-year retrospective evaluation of 50 consecutive cases, *Int J Oral Maxillofac Implants* 8:388, 1993.
23. Goldberg MH: Personal communication, July 2000.
24. Gynther GW, Kondell PA, Moberg LE, et al: Dental implant installation without antibiotic prophylaxis, *Oral Surg* 85:509, 1998.
25. Hanisch O, Cortella CA, Boskovic MM, et al: Experimental breakdown around hydroxyapatite-coated implants, *J Periodontol* 68:59, 1997.
26. Hurzler MB, Quinones CR, Schupback P, et al: Treatment of peri-implantitis using guided bone regeneration and bone grafts, alone or in combination, in beagle dogs. Part 2: histologic findings, *Int J Oral Maxillofac Implants* 12:168, 1997.
27. Johnson BW: HA coated dental implants: long-term consequences, *J Calif Dent Assoc* 20:33, 1992.
28. Jovanovic SA: Diagnosis and treatment of peri-implant disease, *Curr Opin Periodontol* 194, 1994.
29. Kao RT, Curtis DA, Murray PA: Diagnosis and management of peri-implant disease, *J Calif Dent Assoc* 25:872, 1997.
30. Kent JN, Block MS, Finger IM, et al: Biointegrated hydroxylapatite-coated dental implants: 5-year clinical observations, *J Am Dent Assoc* 121:138, 1990.
31. Kraut RA: Clean operating conditions for the placement of intraoral implants, *J Oral Maxillofac Surg* 54:1337, 1996.
32. Lambert PM, Morris HF, Ochi S: The influence of 0.12% chlorhexidine digluconate rinses on the incidence of infectious complications and implant success, *J Oral Maxillofac Surg* 55(12 suppl 5):25, 1997.
33. Lee KH, Maiden MF, Tanner AC, et al: Microbiota of successful osseointegrated dental implants, *J Periodontol* 70:131, 1999.
34. Leonhart A, Renvert S, Dahlen G: Microbial findings at failing implants, *Clin Oral Implant Res* 10:339, 1999.
35. Li KK, Vavares MA, Meara JG: Descending necrotizing mediastinitis: a complication of dental implant surgery, *Head Neck* 18:192, 1996.
36. McAllister B, Masters D, Meffert R: Treatment of implants demonstrating periapical radiolucencies, *Pract Periodontics Aesthet Dent* 4:37, 1992.
37. Meffert RM: How to treat ailing and failing implants, *Implant Dent* 1:25, 1992.
38. Mombelli A, Lang NP: The diagnosis and treatment of peri-implantitis, *Periodontol 2000* 17:63, 1998.
39. Mombelli A, van Oosten AC, Schurch E, et al: The microbiota associated with successful or failing osseointegrated titanium implants, *Oral Microbiol Immunol* 2:145, 1987.
40. Muller E, Gonzalez YM, Andreana S: Treatment of peri-implantitis: longitudinal clinical and microbiological findings: a case report, *Implant Dent* 8:247, 1999.
41. Nevins M, Langer B: The successful use of osseointegrated implants for the treatment of the recalcitrant periodontal patient, *J Periodontol* 66:150, 1995.
42. Novaes AB: Immediate implants placed into infected sites: a clinical report, *Int J Oral Maxillofac Implants* 10:609, 1995.
43. Orsini G, Fanali S, Scarano A, et al: Tissue reactions, fluids and bacterial infiltration in implants retrieved at autopsy: a case report, *Int J Oral Maxillofac Implants* 15:283, 2000.
44. Piatelli A, Scarano A, Balleri P, et al: Clinical and histologic evaluation of an active "implant periapical lesion": a case report, *Int J Oral Maxillofac Implants* 13:713, 1998.

45. Piatelli A, Scarano A, Piatelli M: Abscess formation around the apex of a maxillary root form implant: clinical and microscopical aspects: a case report, *J Periodontol* 66:899, 1995.

46. Pontoriero R, Tonelli MP, Carnevale G, et al: Experimentally induced peri-mucositis: a clinical study in humans, *Clin Oral Implants Res* 5:254, 1994.

47. Powers MP: Personal communication, Cleveland, Ohio, February 2000.

48. Quirynen M, Listgarten MA: The distribution of bacterial morphotypes around natural teeth and titanium implants ad modem Branemark, *Clin Oral Implant Res* 1:8, 1990.

49. Roumanas E, Nishimura RD, Beumer J, et al: Craniofacial defects and osseointegrated implants: six year follow-up report on the success rates of craniofacial implants at UCLA, *Int J Oral Maxillofac Implant* 9:579, 1994.

50. Salcetti JM, Moriarty JD, Cooper LF, et al: The clinical, microbial, and host response characteristics of the failing implant, *Int J Oral Maxillofac Implants* 12:32, 1997.

51. Sbordone L, Barone A, Ramaglia L, et al: Antimicrobial susceptibility of periodontopathic bacteria associated with failing implants, *J Periodontol* 66:69, 1995.

52. Shaffer MD, Juruaz DA, Haggerty PC: The effect of periradicular endodontic pathosis on the apical region of adjacent implants, *Oral Surg* 86:578, 1998.

53. Sussman HI, Moss SS: Localized osteomyelitis secondary to endodontic-implant pathosis. A case report, *J Periodontol* 64:306, 1993.

54. Takeshita F, Iyama S, Ayukawa Y, et al: Abscess formation around a hydroxyapatite-coated implant placed into the extraction socket with autogenous bone graft: a histological study using light microscopy, image processing, and confocal laser scanning microscopy, *J Periodontol* 68:299, 1997.

55. Tillmanns HWS, Hermann JS, Cagna DR, et al: Evaluation of three different dental implants in ligature-induced peri-implantitis in the beagle dog. Part 1. Clinical evaluation, *Int J Oral Maxillofac Implants* 12:611, 1997.

56. Topazian RG: The basis of antiobiotic prophylaxis. In Worthington P, Branemark P-I, editors: *Advanced osseointegration surgery,* Chicago, 1992, Quintessence.

57. Trieger N: Antibiotics and anti-inflammatory agents in dental implantology, *Implant Dent* 8:343, 1999.

58. Waerhaug J: The infrabony pocket and its relationship to trauma from occlusion and subgingival plaque, *J Periodontol* 50:355, 1979.

59. Warrer K, Buser D, Lang NP, et al: Plaque-induced peri-implantitis in the presence or absence of keratinized mucosa: an experimental study in monkeys, *Clin Oral Implants Res* 6:131, 1995.

60. Weems JJ: *Candidia parasilosis:* epidemiology, pathogenicity, clinical manifestation and antimicrobial susceptibility, *Clin Infect Dis* 14:756, 1992.

61. Wolinsky L, deCamargo P, Erard J, et al: A study of *in vivo* attachment of *Streptococcous sanguis* and *Actinomyces viscosus* to saliva treated titanium, *Int J Oral Maxillofac Implants* 4:27, 1989.

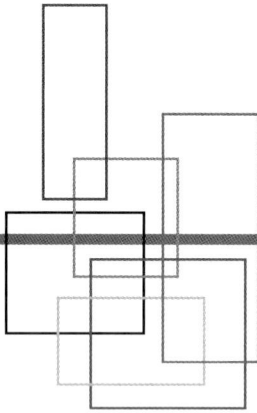

Esthetic Facial Surgery and Infections

John R. Werther

Experience with infection after facial esthetic surgery is limited because of a low incidence. Relatively few clinical reports have been written on the subject. Compared with patients undergoing functional surgery, the tolerance of patients for postoperative infection is lower in elective surgery and even less in esthetic surgery.

The treatment of infection after facial cosmetic surgery generally is the same as for any other facial surgical procedure. Specifically, the wound is opened and drainage is established, the causative agent is cultured, and presumptive broad-spectrum antimicrobial agents are administered until culture and sensitivity results are available, failure of improvement in the patient's condition, or both dictate a change in therapeutic agents or technique.

The use of prophylactic antibiotics is controversial because most facial esthetic surgery is performed in a clean or clean-contaminated field and historically is associated with very low rates of infection. Given the highly emotional atmosphere associated with infection in the patient who has undergone facial esthetic surgery, prompt, aggressive management is indicated. Empathic support and close supervision by both the physician and staff, direct acknowledgment of the problem, and a clear-cut plan of action are indicated.[36,37] Patients are less likely to institute legal action if they perceive that the physician cares about their problem.[13] Frequent office visits and consultation with and referral to other specialists, if necessary, can help ensure that the problem is identified early and managed appropriately. Complete, accurate records and photographs aid in documentation of the problem and are useful to the surgeon in reconstructing the events that have occurred.

BLEPHAROPLASTY

The abundant blood supply to the eyelids confers resistance to infection and necrosis after surgery; thus, as expected, infections after blepharoplasty are rare. Although minor wound separation and epithelial cyst or granuloma

formation account for the majority of minor infections after blepharoplasty, orbital abscess and blindness also have been reported.[24,28]

Minor wound separation can result from inadequate suturing technique or patient manipulation of the incision line in the early postoperative period and result in superficial wound infection (Figure 19-1, Plates 37 through 39). Gentle wound care and lubrication of the wound with a thin layer of topical antibiotic ointment usually resolves this problem. The affected eyelid typically is tighter following healing after an infection but in most cases does not require revision surgery. Inclusion cysts or granulomas caused by entrapped suture, eyelashes, or surgical debris are best treated expectantly. If they persist, they can be unroofed with a scalpel, the point of a 22- or 25-gauge needle, or electrocautery unit and be removed.

Mycobacterial infection after blepharoplasty was reported by Kevitch and Guyuron[16] in a nurse employed in a nursing home. Bilateral localized eyelid abscesses developed 1 month after blepharoplasty that required 10 months of antibiotic therapy for resolution. The authors hypothesize that exposure to debilitated patients while providing nursing home care and the patient's compromised anatomy (i.e., a unilateral Jones tube) increased the risk for acquiring this infection.

Patients with orbital cellulitis typically have moderate to severe pain, eyelid swelling, intense erythema, conjunctival injection and chemosis, and orbital or ocular motility disturbance. Rees et al.[28] described a patient with a postseptal orbital cellulitis that occurred 5 days after an uncomplicated blepharoplasty. The diagnosis was made on the basis of clinical findings and confirmed with ultrasonography. In this case, administration of intravenous antibiotics and application of warm compresses resolved the infection. Incision and drainage may be necessary depending on the patient's clinical progress.

Although blindness after blepharoplasty usually is associated with intraconal hemorrhage, in 1979 Morgan[24]

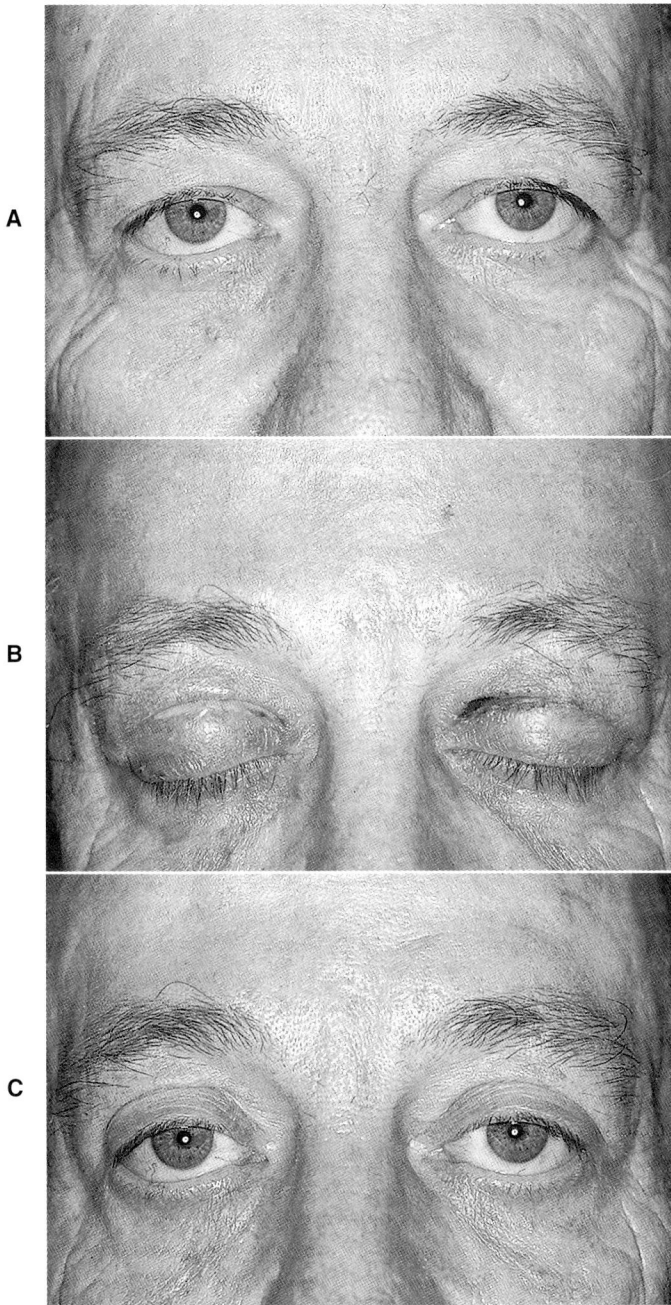

Figure 19-1 A patient with a previous mid-forehead lift is prepared for forehead dermabrasion and bilateral upper lid blepharoplasty for dermatochalasis and scar camouflage. **A,** Before surgery. **B,** Five days after surgery. The patient had rubbed his incisions and created a wound separation with superficial infection, which was treated with gentle wound care and antibiotic ointment. **C,** Nine months after surgery.

described a patient in whom orbital cellulitis developed 3 days after blepharoplasty that resulted in blindness. Loss of vision in this case was ascribed to extreme orbital edema with secondary compression of the retinal artery. Regardless of the cause, surgeons who perform blepharoplasties should have an established protocol for managing blindness after blepharoplasty. Timely management is crucial because the retina can tolerate only approximately 90 min-

utes of vascular occlusion before severe visual impairment results.[12] Severe pain, loss of vision, increased intraocular pressure, proptosis, and ophthalmoplegia are consistent with impending blindness. An emergency ophthalmology consultation should be obtained, but initial evaluation and treatment must not be delayed. The goal of treatment is decompression of the orbit and provision for drainage of the infection. Medical decompression can be initiated with intravenous acetazolamide and mannitol. Surgical intervention, including lateral canthotomy with cantholysis, orbitotomy, and anterior chamber paracentesis, may be necessary.

RHINOPLASTY

Among facial esthetic surgical procedures, nasoseptal surgery has one of the highest risks of infection—approximately 3% overall.[13,32] Infection after purely esthetic rhinoplasty occurs less frequently. How-ever, devastating infections, including toxic shock syndrome,[10,14,18,34] necrotizing fasciitis, cavernous sinus thrombosis, and brain abscess, have been described.[6,18,19] Antibiotic prophylaxis in nasal surgery has been proposed because the nose is a contaminated field. However, no clear evidence exists of a decrease in the incidence of infection after nasal surgery when prophylactic antibiotics have been used. Although many surgeons use prophylactic antibiotics for cosmetic and reconstructive nasal surgery, this practice is controversial. Meyers[22] recommended administration of antibiotics in the following circumstances: (1) active infection at the operative site, (2) use of nasal packing for more than 24 hours, (3) presence of hematoma, (4) use of alloplastic implants, and (5) host immunocompromise or immunosuppression.

Most intracranial complications are traumatic in origin and follow manipulation of the skull base in nasal and sinus surgery.[18,33] When deviated segments of the perpendicular plate of the ethmoid or vomer are to be removed during septorhinoplasty, a scissor or back-action forceps should be used first to create the desired horizontal fracture plane. If the entire ethmoid is rocked to create the fracture, a crack in the cribriform plate can occur leading to cerebrospinal fluid (CSF) leak, pneumocephalus, and intracranial infection. If a CSF leak is noted intraoperatively, immediate neurosurgical consultation is indicated. Most CSF leaks noted during surgery resolve spontaneously within 10 to 14 days if the patient is treated with bed rest and head elevation. The decision to use antibiotics in the absence of overt infection and CSF leak is controversial. Lumbar drainage or surgical exploration may be necessary to control a persistent leak and decrease the risk of infection.

Unless a culture is performed before surgery, it is not possible to determine whether the patient has nasal carriage of *Staphylococcus aureus*. Carriers of *S. aureus* are at risk of toxic shock syndrome after surgery. Prophylactic antibiotics do not eliminate the risk of toxic shock syndrome in susceptible individuals.[15,18] Similarly, avoidance of nasal packing does not entirely eliminate the risk of toxic

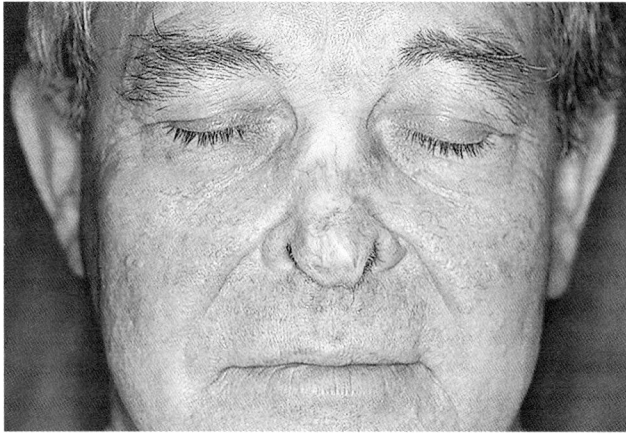

Figure 19-2 This patient had undergone carbon dioxide laser treatment of rhinophyma elsewhere approximately 5 years earlier. The skin–soft tissue envelope over the nose is densely scarred. This patient would be a poor candidate for alloplastic nasal augmentation because of scarring, hypovascularity, and decreased resistance to infection.

Figure 19-3 This patient had previously fractured and lacerated his nose and was prepared for nasal reconstructive surgery. **A,** Before surgery, with visible nasal left lateral scar. **B,** Endonasal nasal harvest of deflected septal cartilage. **C,** Planned position of cartilage for dorsal augmentation. The graft subsequently was divided longitudinally and the halves were glued together with a thin layer of n-butyl histocryl as a two-layer stack graft to elevate the dorsum. The patient was treated with a cephalosporin antibiotic before and for 5 days after surgery. **D,** At 17 days after surgery the infected area was drained manually, the material was cultured, and the patient started amoxicillin-clavulanate therapy for presumed staphylococcal infection. **E,** Frontal view at 21 days after surgery. The cultures from the dorsum and nasal septum grew *Enterobacter,* which was resistant to amoxicillin-clavulanate and cephalosporin antibiotic therapy. Based on sensitivities and incomplete response to empirical antibiotic therapy, the patient's antibiotic regimen was changed to ofloxacin and the infection resolved completely. **F,** Oblique view at 21 days after surgery. **G,** At 3 months after surgery the original scar has widened and will likely require revision. Dorsal augmentation has been maintained despite infection.

shock syndrome in susceptible individuals.[38] In many cases the onset of symptoms is nonspecific. Generalized malaise, with or without nausea, may be among the first signs of infection. Sudden-onset fever, nausea, vomiting, diarrhea, rash, and myalgia 3 to 5 days after surgery are hallmarks of toxic shock syndrome. As with any patient with sepsis, patients with toxic shock syndrome can become profoundly hypotensive and typically are volume depleted. They require immediate hospitalization for intravenous fluid resuscitation, broad-spectrum intravenous antibiotic coverage, removal of any nasal packing, culture, and Gram stain. An infectious disease consultation is indicated in most cases because of the life-threatening nature of this infection.

Selection criteria for alloplastic implants are based primarily on biophysical and chemical properties and ease of clinical use. The principal materials used in esthetic nasal and facial surgery are silicone, polyethylene, and polytetrafluoroethylene. Silicone polymer implants are used most commonly worldwide, primarily because of their popularity in Asia. Silicone implants are smooth, inert, hydrophobic, and highly resistant to degradation. The smooth surface contributes to the risk of capsular contracture and the concomitant risk of disfigurement. The lack of soft tissue in-growth increases the risk of late infection by hematogenous bacterial seeding. Frank exposure of a silicone implant invariably leads to progressive infection and mandates removal. Polytetrafluoroethylene implants are extremely stable. With a pore size of 10 to 30 μm, minimal soft tissue in-growth and capsule formation occur. Polytetrafluoroethylene has good early resistance to infection but, like silicone, usually must be removed if it becomes exposed. Polyethylene implants have much larger pore size (150 to 250 μm) and consequently substantially greater soft tissue in-growth. Porosity of the material allows for antibiotic impregnation, but the value of this property on infection resistance is unknown.

The use of alloplastic implants in nasal reconstruction is controversial. It generally is accepted that patients with previous trauma, severe scarring, or loss of blood supply resulting from radiation should not undergo alloplastic reconstruction of the nose, but some surgeons use alloplasts successfully. (Figures 19-2 and 19-3, Plates 40 through 47). A recent animal study comparing polyethylene and polytetrafluoroethylene implants challenges the concept that adverse outcomes with alloplastic dorsal augmentation are related strictly to soft tissue thinning over rhinion.[30] The authors showed that both polytetrafluoroethylene and polyethylene implants became infected if inoculated with pathogens at the time of initial surgical implantation. This finding confirms the traditional teaching of minimal, careful handling of the alloplastic implant during surgery, and the need for perioperative administration of antibiotics. Once the tissue around the implants healed, however, the polyethylene implants were significantly more resistant to infection than polytetrafluoroethylene implants. Although the polytetrafluoroethylene implants had minimal capsule formation and soft tissue in-growth after initial healing, the polyethylene implants generated a thicker, more densely invested fibrovascular capsule, which protected the implant from late infection. A follow-up clinical patient study revealed similar findings with regard to infection[29]; the authors noted that when removal of polyethylene implants was required (2%), no difficulty with soft tissue dissection for retrieval was encountered. These results should be repeated by other investigators but indicate that the accepted teaching of avoidance of alloplastic nasal implants may be modified under certain conditions.

FACELIFT

The incidence of infection after facelift surgery is low, typically less than 1%.[3-5,17,20] In the largest series reported to date,[17] 11 (0.18%) of 6166 consecutive patients undergoing

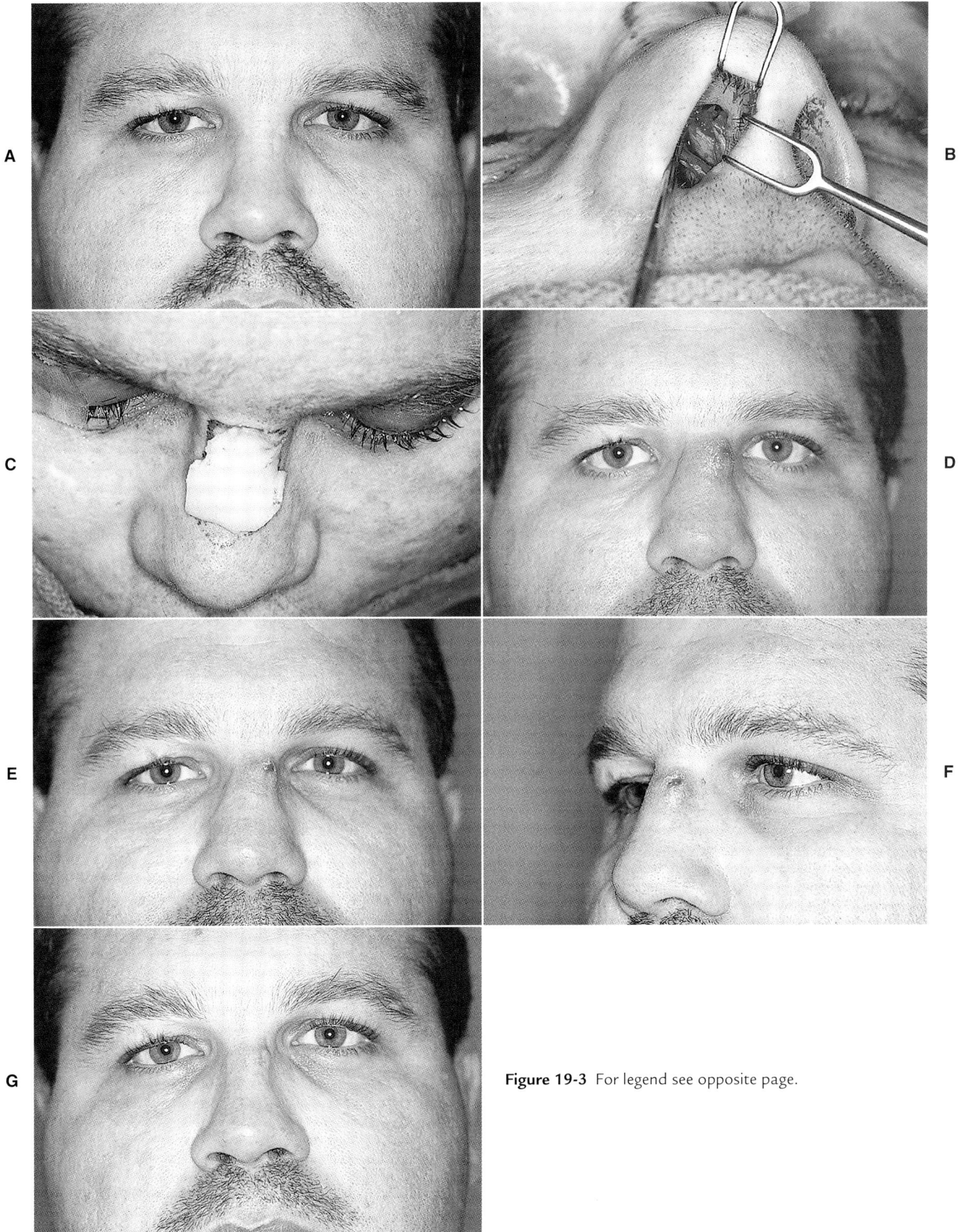

Figure 19-3 For legend see opposite page.

facelift developed infection requiring hospital readmission. Two of the 11 patients had a superficial skin-flap rhytidectomy, and the remaining nine patients had a superficial musculoaponeurotic system (SMAS) elevation procedure. All patients underwent at least one concurrent procedure including blepharoplasty and liposuction, but none had rhinoplasty simultaneously. Four of the 11 patients received prophylactic antibiotics and seven did not. Only one patient smoked. The patients were readmitted between 4 and 30 days after surgery; eight patients were admitted between the fifth and seventh days after surgery. *Staphylococcus* and *Streptococcus* spp. caused early infections, and gram-negative infections predominated in late-onset infections. In six of the 11 patients, Mersilene (Ethicon Inc., Somerville, NJ) suture was used for the SMAS suspension, and all suture abscess complications were isolated to the side of infection. The ipsilateral permanent sutures not removed during initial abscess treatment required removal in the surgeon's office after resolution of the initial infection. No clinically recognizable hematomas developed in any patient before infection. The authors could not demonstrate a clear-cut pattern with respect to past medical history, perioperative antibiotics, surgical equipment, complexity of surgical dissection, or drains as the cause of infection after rhytidectomy. All patients were considered good candidates for surgery, and perioperative antibiotic use depended on the surgeon's routine. Because of the low infection rate the authors believed that no imperative exists for individual surgeons to change their routine use or nonuse of perioperative antibiotics. In a follow-up letter to the editor, the authors replied, "We do not recommend the use of perioperative antibiotics for clean cases."[39]

A recent survey study of facelift procedures found similar results regarding the rate of infection.[20] Specifically, the reported rate of infection requiring hospitalization after rhytidectomy was less than 0.1%. In the survey, 72% of the surgeons used perioperative antibiotics. A significant difference in antibiotic use existed among surgeons and depended on the length of practice experience. For surgeons with less than 5 years of practice experience, perioperative antibiotics were administered to 90% of patients. For those with more than 20 years of experience, perioperative antibiotics were used in 8% of cases. No noted difference in incidence of infection after surgery was demonstrated.

The incidence of infection after esthetic surgery probably is higher in patients with diabetes or other medical conditions that predispose them to infection, but few data exist. Extrapolating from other experience, most surgeons would choose to use prophylactic antibiotics in this setting. Surgeons who operate on patients with such conditions must use their judgment regarding use of prophylactic antibiotics before facelift surgery.

SKIN RESURFACING

Resurfacing of the skin by chemical peel, dermabrasion, or laser energy constitutes a clean-contaminated procedure. Despite the unproven efficacy of antifungal and antibacterial prophylaxis,[35] many surgeons use antibiotic and antifungal agents in the perioperative period.[9] Most cutaneous bacterial and fungal infections can be prevented and treated by proper wound care, including frequent wound cleansing and application of noncontaminated bland emollients.[7] The most common bacterial pathogens include *Staphylococcus* and *Streptococcus* spp. and *Pseudomonas aeruginosa.* The most common fungal agent is *Candida albicans.* Occlusive dressings accelerate healing and decrease discomfort after skin resurfacing. However, the risk of bacterial and fungal infection is increased when occlusive dressings are used, particularly if they are used more than 2 consecutive days. In such circumstances, antibiotic prophylaxis with cephalexin or ciprofloxacin and antifungal prophylaxis with ketoconazole or fluconazole should be considered.

Differential diagnosis among bacterial, fungal, or viral infection after skin resurfacing can be challenging, even for experienced clinicians, because epithelial landmarks are removed and the initial symptoms of pain and burning frequently are nonspecific. When infection occurs, it should be treated empirically. Choice of antibiotic is based on the examination and analysis of the Gram stain and is refined based on culture results and the patient's clinical response to therapy. The initial coverage with broad-spectrum agents may include amoxicillin plus clavulanate (875 mg) or ciprofloxacin (750 mg bid). The fungal infection can be treated with ketoconazole (400 mg per day) or fluconazole (200 mg per day).

In contrast to potential bacterial and fungal infection, infection caused by herpes simplex virus (HSV) or reactivation of the virus is a clear risk. The risk is highest for patients undergoing full-face or perioral skin resurfacing and those with a history of prior HSV infection. Prophylactic antiviral therapy is indicated even for patients with no history of HSV infection. HSV outbreak has been reported in 2% to 7% of patients undergoing resurfacing despite prophylactic antiviral therapy.[2,23,25] Symptoms include pain ranging from tingling to intense discomfort, burning, and discharge from the affected area. Urgent treatment is indicated because disseminated infection can result in severe and permanent facial scarring. The most common antiviral prophylaxis regimens include acyclovir (400 mg five times per day), valacyclovir (500 mg bid), or famciclovir (500 mg bid) beginning the day before or the day of surgery and continuing for 7 to 10 days until complete reepithelialization occurs.[3,9] Valacyclovir and famciclovir offer significant therapeutic advantage because patient compliance is much better with twice-daily dosing compared with medications requiring five administrations per day. If an outbreak of herpetic infection occurs despite prophylactic therapy, options include increasing the original prophylactic agent to the maximum dose (acyclovir, 800 mg five times per day; valacyclovir, 500 mg tid; or famciclovir, 500 mg tid) or changing to the maximum dose of an alternative agent. Obagi and Bridenstine[26] reported total effectiveness in prevention of herpetic outbreak with valacyclovir (1000 mg once daily started the morning of surgery and continued for at least 15 days after surgery). They recommend continuing coverage to the fifteenth postoperative day based on case reports and experience with herpetic outbreak beyond 12 days. Any infection that does not respond to oral medication and wound care may require hospitalization for intravenous therapy.

OTOPLASTY

Infection after otoplasty has been reported in approximately 2% of cases. Infection usually occurs between the third and fifth day after surgery and is marked by a sharp increase in pain on the affected side or sides that respond poorly, if at all, to narcotics.[1,31] Distinction between hematoma and infection usually is not possible on the basis of history alone. Prompt removal of the dressing and inspection of the wound is mandatory. Whereas a localized hematoma is treated by drainage and through-and-through mattress suture approximation of the skin flaps to prevent fluid reaccumulation, mild cellulitis is treated by opening the wound in the affected area and culturing any material that is expressed. Gram stain analysis of the material can be performed quickly and aids initial antibiotic selection. Application of warm saline solution compresses, topical antibiotic ointment, and empirical maximum-dose oral antibiotic therapy is indicated. The most common bacterial pathogens associated with infection after otoplasty are *S. aureus, Escherichia coli,* and *P. aeruginosa.* Pending culture results, initial oral antibiotic therapy options include ciprofloxacin (750 mg po bid) or amoxicillin plus clavulanate (850 to 1000 mg po bid). Patients with progressive or unresponsive infection, severe cellulitis, abscess, or perichondritis should be treated with intravenous antibiotics until culture results are available.

If the infection resolves rapidly, maintenance of the permanent sutures used for the otoplasty procedure may be possible. Monofilament sutures trap fewer bacteria and therefore, at least theoretically, are more likely than braided sutures to be maintained after infection. However, when ongoing infection does not resolve with antibiotics, removal of most, if not all, of the permanent sutures may be necessary. Persistent perichondritis may require one or more operative drainage and debridement procedures to control infection and prevent progression to necrosis. The patient should be advised that unfavorable appearance may result and that delayed revision surgery likely will be necessary to improve the outcome. (Treatment of malignant external otitis is discussed in detail in Chapter 14.)

GENIOPLASTY

Infection can occur after transoral or transcutaneous access to the bony chin during surgery. The risk of infection after genioplasty is approximately 2% to 6%.[8,11] Higher rates of infection have been reported when alloplastic implants[11] or fillers are used, when the chin button is com-

pletely degloved of its soft tissue envelope for large advancement, and when the chin is multiply segmented for maximal advancement.[21] Whereas the submental approach can be completed in a sterile fashion, transoral incisions are at least clean-contaminated; thus prophylactic antibiotics are indicated.[27] Localized infection after genioplasty surgery, usually via exposure of deep sutures used to reapproximate the mentalis muscle, may respond to antibiotic treatment and local measures. However, if infection persists or progresses or an alloplastic implant becomes exposed, it must be removed. Typically an infected osseous genioplasty site breaks down with opening of both the mucosal and muscular periosteal layers. Obviously, necrotic material should be removed and the area packed open to allow for resolution of the infection. Often removal of the hardware is not necessary, particularly if it is stable. The wound typically heals well by secondary intention with minimal effect on the lip and external chin appearance.

REFERENCES

1. Adamson PA, Strecker HD: Otoplasty techniques, *Facial Plast Surg* 11:284, 1995.
2. Alster TS, Nanni CA: Famciclovir prophylaxis of herpes simplex virus reactivation after laser skin resurfacing, *Dermatol Surg* 25:242, 1999.
3. Alster TS, Lupton JR: Treatment of complications of laser skin resurfacing, *Arch Facial Plast Surg* 2:279, 2000.
4. Baker DC: Complications of cervicofacial rhytidectomy, *Clin Plast Surg* 10:543, 1983.
5. Baker TJ, Gordon GL: Complications of rhytidectomy, *Plast Reconstr Surg* 40:31, 1967.
6. Casaubon JN, Dion MA, Labrisseau A: Septic cavernous sinus thrombosis after rhinoplasty, *Plast Reconstr Surg* 59:119, 1977.
7. Christian MM, Behroozan DS, Moy RL: The late infections following full-face CO_2 laser resurfacing and occlusive dressing use, *Dermatol Surg* 26:32, 2000.
8. Dann JJ, Epker BM: Proplast genioplasty: a retrospective study with treatment recommendations, *Angle Orthod* 47:173, 1977.
9. Demas PN, Bridenstine JB: Diagnosis and treatment of postoperative complications after skin resurfacing, *J Oral Maxillofac Surg* 57:837, 1999.
10. Fairbanks DNF: Complications of nasal packing, *Arch Otolaryngol Head Neck Surg* 94:412, 1986.
11. Guyuron B, Raszewski RL: A critical comparison of osteoplastic and alloplastic augmentation genioplasty, *Aesthetic Plast Surg* 14:199, 1990.
12. Hayreh SS, Kolder AG, Weingeist TA: A central retinal artery occlusion and retinal tolerance time, *Ophthalmology* 87:75, 1980.
13. Hickson GB, Clayton EW, Entman SS, et al: Obstetricians prior malpractice experience and patient's satisfaction with care, *JAMA* 272:1583, 1994.
14. Jacobson JA, Kasworm EM: Toxic shock syndrome after nasal surgery, *Arch Otolaryngol Head Neck Surg* 112:329, 1986.
15. Jacobson JA, Stevens MH, Kasworm EM: Evaluation of single-dose cefazolin prophylaxis for toxic shock syndrome, *Arch Otolaryngol Head Neck Surg* 114:326, 1988.

16. Kevitch R, Guyuron B: Mycobacterial infection following blepharoplasty, *Aesthetic Plast Surg* 15:229, 1991.

17. Leroy JL, Rees TD, Nolan WB III: Infections requiring hospital readmission following facelift surgery: incidence, treatment, and sequelae, *Plast Reconstr Surg* 93:533, 1994.

18. Maniglia AJ: Fatal and major complications secondary to nasal and sinus surgery, *Laryngoscope* 99:276, 1989.

19. Maniglia AJ, Goodwin J, Arnold JE: Intracranial abscesses secondary to nasal, sinus and orbital infection in adults and children, *Arch Otolaryngol Head Neck Surg* 15:1424, 1989.

20. Matarraso A, Elkwood A, Rankin M, et al: National plastic surgery survey: facelift technique and complications, *Plast Reconstr Surg* 106:1185, 2000.

21. Mercuri LG, Laskin DM: Avascular necrosis after anterior horizontal augmentation genioplasty, *J Oral Surg* 35:296, 1977.

22. Meyers AD: Prophylactic antibiotics in nasal surgery, *Arch Otolaryngol Head Neck Surg* 116:1125, 1990.

23. Monheit GD: Facial resurfacing may trigger the herpes simplex virus, *Cosmetic Dermatol* 8:9, 1995.

24. Morgan SC: Orbital cellulitis and blindness following a blepharoplasty, *Plast Reconstr Surg* 64:823, 1979.

25. Nanni CA, Alster TS: Complications of carbon dioxide laser resurfacing, *Dermatol Surg* 24:315, 1998.

26. Obagi S, Bridenstine JB: Skin resurfacing. In Piecuch JF, editor: *Oral and maxillofacial surgery knowledge update,* vol III, Chicago, Ill, 2001, American Association of Oral and Maxillofacial Surgery.

27. Peterson LJ: Antibiotic prophylaxis against wound infections in oral and maxillofacial surgery, *J Oral Maxillofac Surg* 48:617, 1990.

28. Rees TD, Craig SM, Fisher Y: Orbital abscess following blepharoplasty (case report), *Plast Reconstr Surg* 73:126, 1984.

29. Romo T, Sclafani AP, Sabini P: Use of porous high-density polyethylene in revision rhinoplasty and in the platyrrhine nose, *Aesthetic Plast Surg* 22:211, 1998.

30. Sclafani AP, Regan JT, Cox AJ, et al: Clinical and histologic response of subcutaneous expanded polytetrafluoroethylene (Gore-Tex) and porous high-density polyethylene (Medpor) implants to acute and early infection, *Arch Otolaryngol Head Neck Surg* 123:328, 1997.

31. Spira M: Reduction otoplasty. In Goldwyn RM, editor: *The unfavorable result in plastic surgery: avoidance and treatment,* ed 2, vol I, Boston, 1984, Little Brown.

32. Teichgraeber JF, Riley WB, Parks DH: Nasal surgery complications, *Plast Reconstr Surg* 85:527, 1990.

33. Teichgraeber JF, Russo RC: Treatment of nasal surgery complications, *Ann Plast Surg* 30:80, 1993.

34. Thomas SW, Baird IM, Frazier, RD: Toxic shock syndrome following submucous resection and rhinoplasty, *JAMA* 247:2402, 1982.

35. Walia S, Alster TS: Laser resurfacing infection rate with and without prophylactic antibiotics, *Dermatol Surg* 25:857, 1999.

36. Wright MR: Management of patient dissatisfaction with results of cosmetic procedures, *Arch Otolaryngol Head Neck Surg* 106:466, 1980.

37. Wright MR: The male aesthetic patient, *Arch Otolaryngol Head Neck Surg* 113:724, 1987.

38. Younis RT, Lazar RH: Delayed toxic shock syndrome after functional endonasal sinus surgery, *Arch Otolaryngol Head Neck Surg* 122:83, 1996.

39. Nolan WB: Infection after face lift, *Plast Reconstr Surg* 95:599, 1995 (letter reply).

Identification, Management, and Prevention of Infections After Head and Neck Surgery

Remy H. Blanchaert, Jr.

Head and neck surgery is a multispecialty discipline challenged by an array of tumors affecting the structures of the head and neck. The majority of these tumors require entrance into a contaminated site in the course of their surgical extirpation and reconstruction. This particular aspect of head and neck surgery causes significant concern regarding postoperative surgical wound sepsis or wound infection. Currently the accepted rate of infection in such cases is approximately 20% when appropriate antibiotic prophylaxis is administered.[15] This rate is markedly better than the 84% noted in the past without the administration of prophylactic antibiotics.

Head and neck surgery includes surgical ablation of tumors and reconstruction of the resulting defect. Benign and malignant tumors are encountered. Malignancies require sizable resection margins and therefore result in large, difficult, three-dimensional deformities prone to salivary leakage and fistula formation. Many malignant tumors require preoperative or postoperative radiotherapy, chemotherapy, or both modalities, and surgeons must consider the potential effects of these treatments on wound healing. Many tumors are massive and limit nutritional intake and therefore compromise normal wound healing.

Flap reconstruction is common in tumor resection cases; in the head and neck region, microvascular free tissue transfer offers several advantages over traditional pedicled myocutaneous flaps. These advantages include single-stage definitive surgery, improved function, improved cosmesis, and fewer flap-related complications. Therefore free flaps now are common in head and neck surgery. The most common causes for late failure of a free flap are wound infection and salivary fistula formation.[76]

This chapter presents techniques to identify and manage infections after maxillofacial tumor ablation and facial reconstruction. The microbiology of established postoperative infection in clean-contaminated head and neck surgical wounds is presented as the baseline of knowledge for the remainder of the chapter. Published attempts to predict surgical site infections are assessed. This information allows comparison of personal practice outcomes with those reported in the literature and identifies areas for modification to reduce infection rates.

The chapter also provides ready reference to the literature and standard of practice regarding the use of antimicrobial prophylaxis in head and neck surgery. Guidelines are provided for the development of an evidence-based antimicrobial prophylaxis protocol. The extensive review of literature relevant to the use of prophylactic antibiotics in head and neck surgery provides the basis for later recommendations. The chapter also presents an algorithm for the development of a standard protocol for wound infection prevention and assessment of outcomes.

SURGICAL WOUND CATEGORIES

A clean wound is one in which the surgical site can be prepared thoroughly and one with no contamination of the area by communication with a site colonized by bacteria. In head and neck surgery, common clean surgical operations are thyroidectomy, parotidectomy, and isolated neck dissection. Clean-contaminated wounds are the most frequent wound classification in head and neck surgery. This category includes procedures that are started in an uninfected environment and proceed to incorporate entry into a contaminated (colonized) environment. Common examples include tracheostomy, in-continuity neck dissection and/or resection with or without flap reconstruction, and laryngectomy. Contaminated surgical procedures have extensive soilage, such as in unprepared distal bowel surgery, a major break in sterile technique, or the presence of acute, nonpurulent inflammation. Wounds are categorized as dirty if they are infected or the result of contaminating trauma.[60] Expected infection rates using the National Research Council (NRC) classification are clean (<2%), clean-contaminated (5% to 15%), contaminated (15% to 30%), and dirty (>30%).[61] The National Nosocomial Infection Surveillance (NNIS) program has developed a surgical wound risk index.[22] This system considers the patient's American Society of Anesthesiologists (ASA) classification and duration of surgery in addition to the NRC wound classification. According to this system, any patient with medium or high risk based on the NNIS index should receive prophylactic antibiotics.

MICROBIOLOGY OF FLORA IN ESTABLISHED POSTOPERATIVE WOUND INFECTIONS

The most valuable information regarding the causative organisms in postoperative wound infection after head and neck surgery is derived from a review of the bacteriological profile of organisms isolated from infections incurred during prospective randomized trials of the most common prophylactic antibiotic therapy regimens. Clayman et al.[16] reported the culture and sensitivity results of 43 wound infections in 212 patients who were randomly assigned to receive either ampicillin-sulbactam (1.5 g) or clindamycin (600 mg). The protocol ordered the administration of the appropriate antibiotic 1 hour before surgery and then every 6 hours for an additional 8 doses (48-hour therapy). Forty-three (20%) of the patients developed wound infection; 55 bacterial isolates were recovered from 34 of these patients. The infections were frequently polymicrobial, consistent with previously reported data.[3,4,13,48,80] The ampicillin-sulbactam group accounted for 14 (13.3%) infections, and in the clindamycin group 29 (27.1%) patients had postoperative wound infections. The most common isolates identified were *Eikenella corrodens, Escherichia coli,* coagulase-negative *Staphylococcus,* and *Bacteroides, Enterobacter,* and *Fusobacterium* spp. Streptococci, *Klebsiella pneumoniae,* and *Haemophilus* and *Proteus* spp. were less common isolates (Table 20-1). *E. corrodens, E. coli,* and *Haemophilus parainfluenzae* were resistant to clindamycin, and some isolates of *Pseudomonas* spp. were resistant to ampicillin-sulbactam.[79] *S. aureus* and *Enterococcus* spp. demonstrated resistance to both antibiotics. A major criticism of this study was the prophylactic dose of antibiotic selected. Clindamycin usually is used in higher doses of 900 mg, whereas only a 600-mg dose was administered in this study.

Performance of dental extractions during tumor ablation procedures affects the incidence of wound infections. Removal of teeth as a result of periodontal disease or caries adds risk to the patient undergoing head and neck surgery, particularly in relation to the development of anaerobic wound infection. In one study a significant difference in the presence of anaerobic isolates from postoperative wound infections was evident.[16] Anaerobic isolates were obtained from 9 (36%) of 25 patients who had undergone simultaneous dental extraction compared with only 1 (3%)

TABLE 20-1

Common Isolates Identified in Postoperative Wound Infections

Type of Organism	Incidence (%)
Aerobic	
Gram-positive	
Coagulase-negative *Staphylococcus* spp.	5
Streptococcus (non–group A)	2
Gram-negative	
Eikenella corrodens	8
Escherichia coli	5
Pseudomonas aeruginosa	4
Klebsiella spp.	3
Anaerobic	
Gram-negative	
Bacteroides	5
Fusobacterium	4
Haemophilus parainfluenzae	2

From Clayman GL, Raad II, Hankins PD, et al: Bacteriologic profile of surgical infection after antibiotic prophylaxis, *Head Neck* 15:526, 1993.

of 30 patients in whom no dental extractions were performed at the time of head and neck surgery. Thus the poor state of the dentition requiring extraction, not the mere presence of teeth, may increase the inoculum of anaerobic organisms within the surgical wound. This factor is relevant because dental extractions commonly are performed after tumor ablation and before flap reconstruction, causing surgical wound contamination. Therefore in cases requiring dental extraction because of advanced periodontal disease or caries, the recommended dosage of antibiotic prophylaxis may require an increase to the level used for treatment of odontogenic infection (ampicillin-sulbactam, 3.0 g; clindamycin, 900 mg). In the absence of patient sensitivity to penicillin, the ampicillin-sulbactam regimen may be the more appropriate therapy.

RISK PREDICTION FOR POSTOPERATIVE WOUND INFECTION

Surgical wound infections develop because several specific determinants jointly overwhelm the hosts' response. Meakins[56] defines the infecting organism, local response, and host defense as the three major determinants in development of postoperative wound infections. His analysis states that infection seldom results from an abnormality in only one of these three factors. This concept can be adapted easily for patients undergoing head and neck surgery. Bumpous and Johnson[15] expanded on this concept and promote preoperative assessment of patient tumor and treatment factors to develop an organized wound infection prevention protocol. Patient factors include nutritional assessment and understanding the effect of co-

TABLE **20-2**

Antibiotic Prophylaxis Regimens

Antibiotic	Dose/Interval*
Ampicillin-sulbactam	1.5 g q6h
Clindamycin	900 mg q6h
Cefazolin	2 g q8h
Cefazolin plus metronidazole	Cefazolin 2 g q8h and metronidazole 500 mg q8h

*Parenteral antibiotic therapy is instituted before skin incision and maintained for at least 24 hours, but not more than 48 hours.

morbid conditions. Tumor stage also has a significant effect on the incidence of wound infection. Important treatment factors include preoperative radiation therapy or chemotherapy, previous head and neck surgery (especially tracheostomy), and operative time.

The NNIS system was developed in response to the deficiencies of the index developed during the Study on the Efficacy of Nosocomial Infection Control (SENIC).[22,33] The NNIS index uses the ASA classification,[50] duration of surgery, and the NRC wound classification to determine risk of wound infection. The NNIS index selects any ASA 3, 4, or 5 classification as one point for scoring in the index. Surgical operating time is also a scoring point. The average times for surgical procedures performed as part of the NNIS were calculated, and the seventy-fifth percentile was determined as a cut point defining normal and long duration of surgery. Any procedure longer than the cut time (<4 hours for head and neck surgery) is considered a scoring point in the index. The standard definitions of wound classification are defined by the NRC.[60] Any wound classified as contaminated or dirty was considered a scoring point in the index.

Notable improvement was observed in the stratification of risk of wound infection with the NNIS index method. ASA classification alone was at least as good as traditional (NRC) wound classification in prediction of wound infection; however, the combination of all three factors showed considerable improvement in the prediction of wound infection. Wound infections in the study ranged from 1.5% to 13%. The presence of each risk factor resulted in a near doubling of the risk of significant wound infection.[22] The NNIS index also was an excellent predictor of infection of all sites (e.g., pulmonary, line sepsis). Therefore the index provides an appropriate method of assessing the overall risk of complications after surgery. Given the incidence with which patients undergoing head and neck surgery are classified as ASA class 3 and the long duration of most procedures required for tumor ablation and reconstruction, the high rate (20%) of infectious wound complications is not surprising.

Prediction of wound complications in surgical patients is important in institution of antibiotic prophylaxis during the perioperative period (Table 20-2), surgical modifications (reinforcement of suture lines in oral and oropha-

ryngeal sites), and increased suspicion during wound surveillance throughout the postoperative period. Early identification of wound complications and early definitive management are valuable.[27]

PATIENT FACTORS

Approximately 20% of patients with head and neck malignancies have some degree of malnutrition. Most clinicians agree that poor nutritional status impairs wound healing. However, a simple, accurate determination of the presence and degree of malnutrition is difficult.[42] Temporal wasting, poor skin turgor, and anthropometric measurements provide clinical clues of malnutrition. Anthropometric measurements are cumbersome and time consuming and therefore not readily available or applicable. The preoperative laboratory investigation of protein levels is more useful clinically. Serum albumin levels less than 3.5 g/dL have been correlated with increased risk of wound infection.[10] Some believe that total protein and albumin levels are ineffective indicators because of their long half-life.[10,66] Determinations of prealbumin and transferrin levels are readily available, clinically useful laboratory tests. Standard blood test profiles may contain total protein levels but are unlikely to report these other parameters unless specifically ordered. Complex nutritional analyses have been used to demonstrate correlation of postoperative wound infection and poor nutritional status.[10,66] These tests are impractical from a clinical point of view because of the time and data required for their computation.

Treatment of malnutrition in patients undergoing head and neck surgery likely has a positive effect on their perioperative course. Snyderman et al.[71] demonstrated in a prospective, randomized, double-blind study that an immune-enhancing nutritional formula (Impact) was superior to traditional tube feeding.[71] These data showed a statistically significant decrease rate of infection (all sites) in the test subjects given the immune-enhancing formula.

Comorbid medical conditions have been studied to determine their effect on wound healing and complication rates. The most commonly reported comorbid conditions include diabetes mellitus, atherosclerosis, tobacco use, alcohol abuse, corticosteroid use, and acquired immunodeficiency syndrome.[10,14,17,18] The microangiopathy of diabetes potentially results in decreased wound oxygen and nutrient delivery. Hyperglycemia decreases leukocyte function. Some studies have shown that diabetes mellitus results in a tendency toward an increase in postoperative wound infection.[10,39] Other authors report no effect.[14] A prospective study showed that increasing degrees of tobacco and alcohol use and the presence of one or more comorbid conditions significantly increased the risk of postoperative wound infection.[18]

TUMOR FACTORS

Head and neck malignancies are staged in a standardized manner by description of tumor (T) stage, node involvement

(N) stage, and the presence or absence of metastases (M). Although this method is standardized in general format, the specifics of the three major components vary based on tumor location (e.g., oral cavity, larynx, parotid). The higher the stage in each patient the greater is the tumor burden. Tumor burden has been correlated directly with the development of postoperative wound infection.* Whether the correlation is related to underlying consequences of tumor burden, such as poor nutrition as a result of odynophagia and difficulties with deglutition, impaired immune function, and depression, is unknown. All these factors may decrease a patient's immune response to the bacterial insult received during clean-contaminated head and neck surgery.

TREATMENT FACTORS

Several treatment variables may contribute to the incidence of postoperative wound infection after head and neck surgery. Literature reports focus on preoperative radiation therapy, preoperative chemotherapy, previous head and neck surgery (especially tracheostomy), and duration of operation.

Radiation therapy is implicated as a possible increased risk factor because of its known effects on non-tumor tissue, but the literature provides no evidence of such an association. Numerous studies have reported that prior radiation therapy resulted in no increase in the rate of wound infection even in cases requiring microvascular free flaps.† However, universal agreement exists that infections in patients who received preoperative radiotherapy are more difficult to manage than in patients who had no radiotherapy. Cole et al.[18] reported that chemotherapy did not increase perioperative wound infection. However, other studies found statistical significance in the relationship between preoperative chemotherapy and wound sepsis.[20,63]

Many surgeons believe that previous head and neck surgery results in increased risk of infection. A retrospective evaluation of wound infections after head and neck surgery reported a statistically significant increase in infections in patients with prior tracheostomy.[21] This finding is supported by a recent prospective multivariate study that identified tracheostomy as an independent risk factor.[63] However, other prospective multivariate analyses have failed to demonstrate a statistically significant difference.[14,18] Of the potential treatment factors outlined as possible risks of increased wound infection, only duration of surgery (clean-contaminated) has been shown unequivocally to correlate significantly with the development of wound sepsis.[18,56]

PROPHYLAXIS

Antibiotic prophylaxis can decrease the incidence of wound complications after surgical procedures. In the majority of cases the organisms responsible for surgical wound infections originate from the patients themselves. A prophylactic antibiotic should be chosen on the basis of its activity against endogenous flora at the surgical site, drug toxicity, and drug cost (factors listed in order of weighting).[54] The decision to use a prophylactic antibiotic or antibiotic regimen requires an understanding of the risks of developing a wound infection for which prophylaxis has been shown to be preventive, and with minimal costs or injury to the patient, compared with the effects of infection.

The use of antibiotic prophylaxis in clean surgery of the head and neck is debatable. Some authors report the incidence of wound infection in clean surgery of the head and neck as less than 2% and therefore recommend against prophylaxis.[46] This rate is consistent with data from the NNIS system.[22] However, contrary data provided in a cost analysis study of clean head and neck surgery found a wound infection rate of 10% without antibiotic prophylaxis versus 3% with antibiotics.[7] This study showed an increased cost per patient of $36,000 (1992 dollars) related to the wound infection. The cost of just a single wound infection was greater than the costs of prophylactic antibiotic administration to the entire study population.

Historically prophylaxis has been recommended for clean-contaminated head and neck surgery. Infection rates as high as 80% have been reported in such cases when no antimicrobial prophylaxis was administered. Antibiotic use has produced infection rates approaching 20%.*

ORAL CAVITY DECONTAMINATION

Intraoperative bacterial contamination of the neck wound in contaminated head and neck surgery may be the most important variable in the development of wound infection. Saliva contamination of the wound is the most common cause of orocutaneous fistulas. Resection of the operative site closure under tension, difficulty of insetting myocutaneous flaps, and the effect of gravity or pull on pedicled flaps have been suggested as the most common mechanisms of late saliva contamination of the wound. Such contamination commonly results in wound infection.[30,72] Studies confirm that the organisms normally present in saliva are the organisms most commonly implicated in the polymicrobial infections accompanying clean-contaminated head and neck surgery.[67,68,75]

Use of topical antibiotics traditionally has been a part of the perioperative antibiotic regimen of colorectal surgeons. Such therapy markedly decreases surgical wound infection in distal bowel surgery.[19,24,62] Experimental models formed the basis for clinical use of combined parenteral and topical antimicrobial agents.[5,28] The same theories are applicable to clean-contaminated head and neck surgery. Clindamycin used to form a mouthwash (1.5 g of clindamycin elixir in 60 mL of sterile water) to decontaminate the oral cavity reduced both aerobic and anaerobic organisms

---

*References 10, 14, 17, 18, 39, 42, 63.
†References 14, 17, 18, 39, 40, 42, 51, 63, 66, 74.

*References 15, 45, 65, 66, 73, 74.

of the normal oropharyngeal flora for up to 8 hours with dramatic effect for 4 hours.[25,32,52] Topical antibiotic prophylaxis was studied in multiple forms in a trial comparing parenteral clindamycin, 1 day of topical clindamycin, 5 days of topical clindamycin, and 1 day of topical amoxicillin-clavulanate plus parenteral ticarcillin-clavulanate. All topical regimens more effectively reduced the number of bacteria from neck wound cultures than the parenteral regimens. These authors have studied the clinical effectiveness of a 24-hour oral topical regimen in preventing postoperative wound sepsis in patients undergoing laryngectomy.[32] Further evidence is available regarding the utility of oral cavity decontamination with povidone-iodine. Redleaf and Bauer[64] studied the value of oral cavity decontamination with povidone-iodine solution in clean-contaminated head and neck surgery and found a significant decrease in wound complications in the treatment group. Topical wound irrigation also was beneficial when clindamycin (900 mg/L normal saline solution) was used but not when piperacillin-sulbactam (3.375 g/L normal saline solution) was administered.[32,70]

Evidence supports the routine use of topical antimicrobial prophylaxis in clean-contaminated head and neck surgery. Topical wound irrigation and oral antimicrobial rinse provide head and neck surgeons with meaningful additions to standard antibiotic prophylaxis. Sensitivity to penicillin within a population favors the use of the clindamycin regimens instead of penicillin or cephalosporin. Chlorhexidine mouth rinse is an appropriate addition to the armamentarium.*

ANTIBIOTIC SELECTION

Clinical investigations have been conducted for years to determine the most appropriate antibiotic or antibiotic combination, and the most appropriate duration of therapy.† The number of such studies and the various antibiotics and protocols used for antimicrobial therapy require significant study to identify meaningful data applicable outside the particular studies. Using standard meta-analysis techniques, Velanovich[78] studied the majority of the earlier studies that met standard criteria. The analysis revealed that the antibiotics chosen produced a relative difference in infection rates from placebo alone of 44%. A slight improved outcome of 8% favored use of multiple antibiotics versus single-antibiotic prophylaxis. A 4% difference in favor of multiple-day regimens of antibiotic therapy was demonstrated over single-day therapy.

Antibiotic selection should focus on the premise that the majority of wound infections after head and neck surgery are the result of saliva contamination of the wound.[1] Reports describe the typical polymicrobial nature of such infections.[13,16,68] Two particular regimens of antibiotic therapy have proved superior: ampicillin-

sulbactam and clindamycin. The presence of clindamycin in maxillofacial tissues after administration of a standard dose maintains a concentration greater than the minimal inhibitory concentration for those organisms to which the tissues are likely to be exposed.[58] The ampicillin-sulbactam combination may have increased efficacy when tooth extraction for periodontal disease or advanced caries is required in conjunction with head and neck surgery.[58] Twenty-four–hour therapy appears to be equally efficacious compared with multiday regimens.* No relevant data exist to support the use of prophylactic antibiotics for more than 48 hours.

POSTOPERATIVE INFECTION

RECOGNITION AND GRADING OF WOUND INFECTION

Erythema and edema commonly are present during the normal healing process after head and neck cancer surgery. Considerable differences exist regarding the criteria for wound infection. The presence of purulent drainage clearly represents a wound infection. To assist researchers and clinicians in standardization of wound infection management, Johnson et al.[43] developed a useful wound grading scale (Table 20-3). This system is more acceptable and user-friendly than the Centers for Disease Control Surgical Site Infection Definition as modified and reported by Horan et al. in 1992.[37]

The time to the recognition of a wound infection provides clues regarding the origin of the clinical problem. Early (<3 days) infections usually result from inadequate oral seal or early breakdown of the oral closure. Friedman et al.[27] elegantly showed that early (within 48 hours) fever greater than 101.5° F highly correlated with salivary leak at the oral or oropharyngeal closure site. Infections that occur later than 5 days after surgery probably result from fistula formation or late oral wound breakdown. Wound

---

*References 11, 15, 26, 43, 59, 75.

TABLE 20-3

Grading Scale for Postsurgical Head and Neck Wounds

Grade*	Definition
0	Normal healing
1	Erythema around suture line limited to 1 cm
2	1-5 cm of erythema
3	More than 5 cm of erythema
4	Purulent drainage
5	Orocutaneous fistula

From Johnson JT, Myers EN, Thearle PB, et al: Antimicrobial prophylaxis for contaminated head and neck surgery, *Laryngoscope* 94:46, 1984.
*Grades 4 and 5 are considered clinically significant.

---

*References 15, 45, 65, 66, 73, 74.
†References 2, 6, 11, 23, 26, 41, 43, 44, 47, 48, 49, 57, 59, 69, 75, 77.

infections that develop between these two time frames without evidence of continued wound saliva contamination result from failed antibiotic prophylaxis. Becker[1] studied drain effluent after clean-contaminated head and neck surgery and demonstrated that 100% of drains contained aerobic organisms and 8% contained anaerobic organisms. Despite these rates of contamination the series infection rate was only 13%.

MANAGEMENT OF INFECTED WOUNDS

The clinical appearance of the surgical wound, character of the drain effluent, and systemic status of the patient are the major criteria used to diagnose a postoperative wound infection. The effect of wound infection on hospital stay, treatment cost, and clinical outcomes is considerable. Early intervention is vital to decreasing the morbidity of this common complication. Standardized wound assessments should be made on a daily basis using the previously outlined clinical criteria. A frothy appearance of the drain output on shaking is characteristic of ongoing saliva contamination of the wound and a strong predictor for the development of a fistula.[42,55] Drain effluent also can be easily tested for the presence of amylase. The clinical characteristics of the case and the method of oral or pharyngeal wound closure are equally important in increasing suspicion of salivary contamination. Fever is a common clinical sign of infection, as are tachycardia and hemodynamic instability. The clinician must determine whether the source of these alterations in homeostasis is a noninfectious cause such as alcohol withdrawal or related to the surgical site itself. Non-wound sites of infection also must be considered (e.g., pulmonary, urinary tract).

When the diagnosis of postoperative wound infection has been made, appropriate interventions are tailored to the specific characteristics of each case. Routine culture and sensitivity testing are required in all cases. The wound infection usually includes organisms that are resistant to the perioperative prophylaxis regimen, especially with protocols that use β-lactam antibiotics.[29] The empiric antibiotic selection used after obtaining cultures but before the availability of the sensitivity report should reflect local (hospital-specific) rates of resistance and patterns of infection. The common flora of wound infection after head and neck surgery is well established (see Microbiology of Flora in Established Postoperative Wound Infections). The antibiotic selection should be reassessed as the results of culture and sensitivity become available.[39,42]

The airway should be protected from soilage from adjacent sites of infection by adequate surgical drainage and inflation of the tracheotomy tube cuff. Failure to inflate the cuff may allow aspiration of infectious material and result in the development of pulmonary infection.[15,40] Aggressive management of the patient's nutritional status requires more attention in cases of postoperative head and neck wound infection.[10,15,39,56]

Many forms of appropriate surgical drainage of the

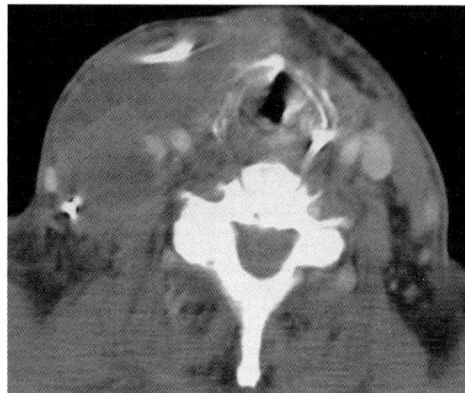

Figure 20-1 CT scan demonstrates hematoma collection within the neck dissection. The drain is seen within the body of the hematoma.

wound infection are available. Few wound infections after head and neck surgery should be drained at the bedside. The majority of wound infections should be drained in the operating room to ensure complete drainage, permit exploration of all contiguous sites containing infection, and allow an assessment of the potential sources of contamination such as salivary leak at sites of primary closure or flap margins. Wide access and direct visualization are the only means to ensure complete drainage. Computed tomographic (CT) scans can assist in location of loci of infection but are not helpful in all cases (Figure 20-1).

Necrotic tissues require immediate debridement. Pedicled myocutaneous flaps differ markedly from free tissue transfers in their tendency to experience marginal necrosis. Conversely, well-designed free flaps generally are alive or dead. Neither of these reconstructions tolerates the presence of continued saliva contamination or wound infection (Figure 20-2, Plates 48 and 49). The infected head and neck wound should be irrigated with copious amounts of physiological saline solution. Wound care is started with noncytotoxic plain-gauze dressing materials and the use of physiological saline solution or nontoxic topical antimicrobials such as 0.25% acetic acid or clindamycin irrigation solution. Materials and solutions that cause cellular injury such as iodoform gauze and providone-iodine solution should be avoided.

Continued wound management depends on several variables. Specifically, the closure of salivary leaks, carotid artery protection, and the presence or absence of alloplastic materials (metal plates) must be considered. Any salivary contamination of the neck must be stopped. The patient should have no oral intake, and efforts to seal or close the fistula should be instituted immediately if possible. Often additional procedures such as myocutaneous flaps or free flaps are required to achieve an oral or oropharyngeal seal. Early fibrosis of the wound margins caused by the inflammatory process prevents sufficient mobilization to allow secondary closure. The carotid artery is intolerant of continued salivary contamination or exposure to the out-

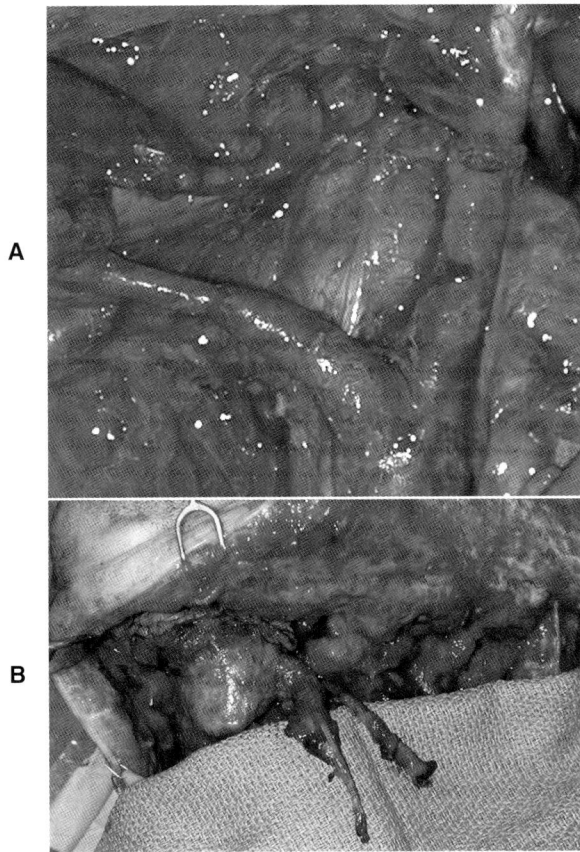

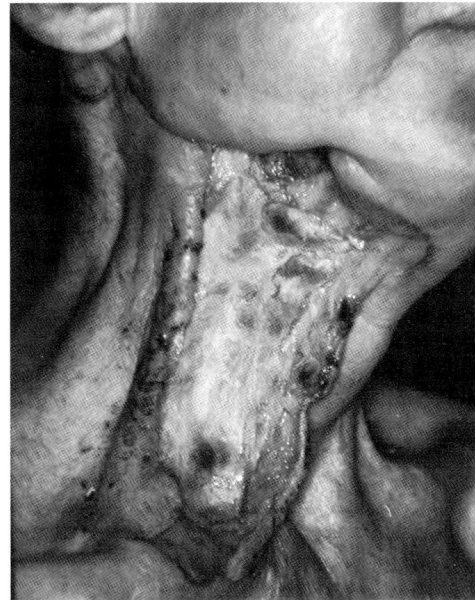

Figure 20-3 This patient had previous surgery and radiation treatment. An orocutaneous fistula developed as a result of the breakdown of the oral closure. The patient subsequently lost a sizable portion of the cervical skin flaps. The wound demonstrates the effect of the application of iodoform gauze (toxic) to the wound bed. The gauze essentially fixed the tissue, preventing healing and risking the integrity of the carotid arterial wall.

Figure 20-2 **A,** A free radial forearm flap microvascular anastomosis demonstrates the skeletonization of the flap vascular pedicle and recipient vessels required to complete the microvascular anastomosis. Such isolation of the vascular pedicle decreases resistance to the insults of wound infections and salivary fistulas. **B,** Salivary contamination of a wound after composite resection, neck dissection, and free radial forearm flap reconstruction. The cephalic vein is thrombosed (distended; clot is visible at site of transection) without compromise of the radial artery (collapsed) and the compromise of the flap. The adjacent tissues demonstrate fibrosis and a white-gray film caused by exposure to saliva.

REOPERATION IN A PREVIOUSLY INFECTED FIELD

Literature reports provide little useful information with regard to reoperation in previously infected sites. The surgeon must maximize use of clinical examination, imaging, antibiotic prophylaxis, clinical site preparation, and vascularized tissue to achieve success in these difficult cases. All available data must be considered to determine that the risk-benefit relationship favors success before proceeding with surgery.

Clinical examination provides signs of acceptable levels of contamination by the presence of granulation tissue throughout the wound or resolution of previously evident induration of the wound. If hardware remains at the site of the previous infection, the surgeon should be particularly suspicious of localized areas of contamination sufficient to interfere with further surgical goals. Imaging (CT scan or magnetic resonance imaging [MRI]) also is helpful in identification of localized sites of continued inflammatory processes deep within the wound. Review of previous culture and sensitivity results and antibiotic exposure histories guide the prophylactic use of antibiotic therapy at the time of reoperation.

Reconstructive procedures are elective and therefore require a different system of evaluation in the setting of prior wound infection. The need for additional ablative surgery or closure of a fistula represents a different clinical circumstance. Delay and aggressive systemic support can optimize patient resistance to infection and resolve

side environment (Figure 20-3). Closure of fistulas and carotid artery coverage are urgent considerations because of the catastrophic consequences of carotid artery rupture (massive blood loss, stroke, death). Any small amount of bleeding in a neck containing an exposed carotid artery should be considered an indication of premonitory bleeding; therefore immediate action is required.[15,39,42]

Management of wounds containing exposed hardware requires careful consideration. In the majority of cases, maintenance of the hardware in acute setting is preferred to assist in support of the airway and deglutition; the wound is managed by dressing changes and healing by secondary intention. Many authors agree that surgical flap coverage of infected wounds must be considered whenever carotid artery exposure, skin flap necrosis, large tissue defect requiring more than 6 weeks of healing by secondary intention for resolution, or prior radiation injury exists.[15,17,39,40,42] the acute effects of the inflammatory process from the prior infection. Recovery from fibrosis is determined easily by direct clinical palpation and is an excellent indicator of a general healthy state within the wound. In the alternate situation requiring urgent additional surgery, the clinician can augment the health of the wound through careful debridement and wound dressings, hyperbaric oxygen therapy, aggressive nutritional support, salivary diversion, and use of vascularized tissue at the time of surgery. The surgeon should anticipate that complete closure of skin-platysma flaps might not be possible in reoperation during the early period after wound infection because of the fibrosis and contracture of the wound. Vascularized muscle flaps (free or pedicled) used to close the fistula or manage the additional surgical defect readily accept skin grafting.

Surgeons treat patients referred for primary bone graft failures as a result of infection after excision of benign tumors of the mandible resulting in oral contamination of the graft. Komisar et al.[53] documented the poor reliability of this technique and advocate its abandonment. However, clinicians cite the minimal complication with transoral bone grafting in preparation for implant surgery as justification for the continued practice of primary bone grafting after mandibular reconstruction. This practice represents a misinterpretation of clinical data. The amount of dissection, and therefore tissue injury, dead space, and contamination are markedly greater in primary major reconstructive bone grafting of the mandible compared with sinus lifts or onlay augmentation. Contemporary management principles of mandibular reconstruction have been described.[8] In the author's opinion the only reliable primary mandibular reconstruction after ablative surgery that results in a composite defect is a free vascularized tissue transfer. Urken et al.[76] reported excellent success with free tissue transfer reconstruction of the mandible in the primary setting.

INFLUENCE OF WOUND INFECTION ON RECURRENCE

Published reports reveal an increased risk of recurrence and death in patients with head and neck cancer who develop postoperative wound infections.[31,38] A 3.2-times increased risk of recurrence and 2.4-times increase in death was reported in one study.[31] Whether the effect on outcome is a result of the infection or if the infection and altered outcome are a result of inherent abnormalities in immune response within the host is undetermined.

COST OF WOUND INFECTION

Surgical wound infections represent an annual rate of approximately 24% of all nosocomial infections (approximately 500,000).[34] The major costs related to surgical wound infection that can be calculated are related directly to increased length of hospital stay. Although no appropriate study has been performed for clean-contaminated

head and neck surgery, the effect can be appreciated by evaluation of studies on this topic in relation to open heart surgery. Length of stay after open heart surgery increased by 20 days as a result of postoperative wound infection.[12] Approximately 15% of the hospital bill is related directly to the infection itself. In addition, if systemic bacteremia and sepsis develop, the charges can increase up to 3.5-fold the normal costs.[35] Up to 95% of the costs related to the wound infection are borne by the facility.[36] With increasingly narrow profit margins the difference can result in a net loss to the hospital.[9]

Although these data are not related directly to head and neck surgery, the principles do apply. All preventive measures should be conducted in cases of postsurgical wound infection in head and neck surgery to improve patient outcome and decrease cost.

SUMMARY

The use of prophylactic antibiotics in head and neck surgery is well supported. Prophylactic antibiotics always should be considered in clean-contaminated surgery. The decision to use antimicrobial prophylaxis in clean surgery must be made by the individual surgeon. However, evidence supports the use of perioperative antibiotics in clean surgery when all variables are considered. The most important predictors of perioperative wound infection are duration of surgery and presence of comorbid conditions (ASA classification).

The development of a standardized antibiotic prophylaxis protocol prevents simple dosing errors or errors of omission and allows meaningful objective assessment of clinical outcomes. A comprehensive protocol includes oral decontamination, parenteral antibiotics, antibiotic irrigation, attention to tension-free wound closure supported by appropriate flap selection, use of closed suction drains, careful daily wound monitoring, early detection of salivary leak or fistula, and assessment of clinical outcomes with attention to antibiotic sensitivities. Each service performing clean-contaminated surgery should carefully investigate possible causes of increased infection rates whenever an interval assessment indicated an incidence greater than 20%. All efforts should be made to shorten surgical time because of its significant effect on wound infection index. Nutritional support of the head and neck surgical patient should begin as soon as possible.

Oral decontamination should be accomplished with any of the available agents intended for this purpose. The clindamycin elixir–saline solution mouthwash may be the most physiological combination for the oral tissues, and the use of preoperative oral rinse can be supplemented with oral lavage just before tumor resection. Because the majority of oral and oropharynx cancers are resected after neck dissection, the time from preoperative mouthrinse to oral incision could exceed the 4 hours of maximum effectiveness. Other solutions, such as providone-iodine and chlorhexidine oral rinse, may harm tissue if left in contact with nonintact mucosa. If these solutions are used before resection, any residual solution should be removed completely before resection.

Parenteral antibiotic therapy is instituted before skin incision and maintained for no longer than 48 hours. Appropriate antibiotics for clean-contaminated head and neck surgery are ampicillin-sulbactam (1.5 g q6h), clindamycin (900 mg q6h), cefazolin (2 g q8h), and metronidazole (500 mg q8h). The ampicillin-sulbactam regimen may be better when periodontally diseased or grossly carious teeth are extracted simultaneously.

Neck wounds become contaminated during resection and flap reconstruction and require copious irrigation to decrease the bacterial contamination below the level likely to produce a wound infection. Irrigation with clindamycin (900 mg in 1 L of normal saline solution) significantly improves wound infection rates. This simple addition to standard therapies should be considered part of the antimicrobial prophylaxis regimen.

Reconstruction of tumor defects must be accomplished in a manner that maximizes patient function, minimizes deformity and alteration of esthetics, and supports the isolation of the neck from the continued assault of the oraloropharynx environment. Microvascular free tissue transfer accomplishes these goals. Free flaps should be used whenever their benefit outweighs the morbidity of the procedure and the patient is a physiologically acceptable candidate. Previous radiotherapy or prior surgical site infection dictate the use of free flaps to limit the incidence of postoperative wound infection. Careful attention to the closure of mucosal defects that are appropriately managed by primary closure (pharynx in laryngectomy) should be standard practice. Reinforcement with a second layer of closure is recommended. Closed suction wound drainage is imperative in head and neck surgery.

Daily wound monitoring is required. Considerable experience is required to distinguish alterations in normal wound healing from the normal erythema and induration of these wounds. Standardized recording of the wound classification should be conducted every 24 hours during hospitalization. Drain output must be evaluated carefully for the presence of saliva. Any detected salivary leak demands immediate attention. The morbidity of salivary contamination of the wound, microvascular anastomosis, and great vessels outweighs any morbidity of reexploration and correction and requires immediate management. The identification of purulence drainage requires an operating room environment to provide a sterile environment and obtain cultures, drain the wound, and initiate any necessary debridement. Bedside incision and drainage should be undertaken with great caution.

Assessment of wound infection outcomes is critical in the appropriate management of a head and neck surgical service just as routine surveillance of margins and clinical outcome is undertaken. When the wound infection rate significantly exceeds that reported in the published literature, careful evaluation and alteration of the service protocol are warranted. Surgeons should consult hospital epidemiologists for assistance.

REFERENCES

1. Becker G: Ineffectiveness of closed suction drainage cultures in the prediction of bacteriologic findings in wound infection in patients undergoing contaminated head and neck cancer surgery, *Otolaryngol Head Neck Surg* 93:743, 1985.
2. Becker GD, Parell GJ: Cefazolin prophylaxis in head and neck cancer surgery, *Ann Otol Rhinol Laryngol* 88:183, 1979.
3. Becker GD, Welch WD: Quantitative bacteriology of intraoperative wound tissue in contaminated surgery, *Head Neck* 12:293, 1990.
4. Becker GD, Welch WD: Quantitative bacteriology of closed-suction drainage in contaminated surgery, *Laryngoscope* 100:205, 1990.
5. Bergamini TM, Lamont PM, Cheadte WG, et al: Combined topical and systemic antibiotic prophylaxis in experimental wound infection, *Am J Surg* 147:753, 1984.
6. Bhathena HM, Kavarana NM: Prophylactic antibiotics administration in head and neck cancer surgery with major flap reconstruction: 1-day cefoperazone versus 5 day cefotaxime, *Acta Chir Plast* 40:36, 1998.
7. Blair EA, Johnson JT, Wagner RL, et al: Cost analysis of antibiotic prophylaxis in clean head and neck surgery, *Arch Otolaryngol Head Neck Surg* 121:269, 1995.
8. Blanchaert RH: Contemporary principles of surgical reconstruction of the oral cavity. In Ord RA, Blanchaert RH, editors: *Oral cancer; the dentist's role in diagnosis, management, rehabilitation and prevention*, Chicago, 2000, Quintessence.
9. Boyce JM, Potter-Bynoe G, Dziobek L, et al: Hospital reimbursement patterns among patients with surgical wound infections following open heart surgery, *Infect Control Hosp Epidemiol* 11:89, 1990.
10. Boyd J, Maves M: Malnutrition from cancer. In Gates G, editor: *Current therapy in otolaryngology–head and neck surgery*, ed 5, St Louis, 1994, Mosby.
11. Brand B, Johnson JT, Meyers EN, et al: Prophylactic antibiotics in contaminated head and neck surgery, *Otolaryngol Head Neck Surg* 90:315, 1982.
12. Bremmelgaard A, Raahave D, Beier-Holgersen, et al: Computer-aided surveillance of surgical infections and identification of risk factors, *J Hosp Infect* 13:1, 1989.
13. Brook I, Hirokawa R: Microbiology of wound infection after head and neck cancer surgery, *Ann Otol Rhinol Laryngol* 98:323, 1989.
14. Brown B, Johnson J, Wagner R: Etiologic factors in head and neck wound infections, *Laryngoscope* 97:587, 1987.
15. Bumpous JM, Johnson JT: The infected wound and its management, *Otolaryngol Clin North Am* 28:987, 1995.
16. Clayman GL, Raad II, Hankins PD, et al: Bacteriologic profile of surgical infection after antibiotic prophylaxis, *Head Neck* 15:526, 1993.
17. Clayman G, Weber R: Pharyngocutaneous fistulae. In Gates G, editor: *Current therapy in otolaryngology–head and neck surgery*, ed 5, St Louis, 1994, Mosby.
18. Cole R, Robbins K, Cohen JI, et al: A predictive model for wound sepsis in oncologic surgery of the head and neck, *Otolaryngol Head Neck Surg* 96:165, 1987.
19. Condon RE, Bartlett JG, Greenlee H, et al: Efficacy of oral and systemic antibiotic prophylaxis in colorectal operations, *Arch Surg* 118:496, 1983.
20. Corey J, Caldarelli D, Hutchinson J, et al: Surgical complications in patients with head and neck cancer receiving chemotherapy, *Ann Otolaryngol Head Neck Surg* 112:437, 1986.

21. Coskun H, Erisen L, Basut O: Factors affecting wound infection rates in head and neck surgery, *Otolaryngol Head Neck Surg* 123:328, 2000.
22. Culver DH, Horan TC, Gaynes RP, et al: Surgical wound infection rates by wound class, operative procedure and patient risk index, *Am J Med* 91(suppl):152, 1991.
23. Dor P, Klastersky J: Prophylactic antibiotics in oral, pharyngeal, and laryngeal surgery for cancer: a double-blind study, *Laryngoscope* 83:1992, 1973.
24. Edmondson HT, Rissing JP: Prophylactic antibiotics in colon surgery, *Arch Surg* 118:227, 1983.
25. Elledge ES, Whiddon RG, Fraker JT, et al: The effects of topical oral clindamycin antibiotic rinses on the bacterial content of saliva of healthy human subjects, *Otolaryngol Head Neck Surg* 105:836, 1991.
26. Fee WE, Glenn M, Handen C, et al: One day vs. two days of prophylactic antibiotics in patients undergoing major head and neck surgery, *Laryngoscope* 94:612, 1984.
27. Friedman M, Venkatesan TK, Yakovlev A, et al: Early detection and treatment of postoperative pharyngocutaneous fistula, *Otolaryngol Head Neck Surg* 121:378, 1999.
28. Galland RB, Heine KJ, Trachtenberg LS, et al: Reduction of surgical wound infection rates in contaminated wounds treated with antiseptics combined with systemic antibiotics: an experimental study, *Surgery* 91:329, 1982.
29. Garibaldi RA, Cushing D: Risk factors for postoperative infection, *Am J Med* 91(suppl 3B):158S, 1991.
30. Grandis JR, Johnson JT: Antibiotics in head and neck oncology, *Curr Opin Otolaryngol Head Neck Surg* 3:84, 1995.
31. Grandis J, Snyderman C, Johnson J, et al: Postoperative wound infection: a poor prognostic sign for patients with head and neck cancer, *Cancer* 70:166, 1992.
32. Grandis JR, Vickers RM, Rihs JD, et al: The efficacy of topical antibiotic prophylaxis for contaminated head and neck surgery, *Laryngoscope* 104:719, 1994.
33. Haley RW, Culver DH, Morgan WM, et al: Identifying patients at high risk of surgical wound infection: a simple multivariate index of patient susceptibility and wound contamination, *Am J Epidemiol* 121:206, 1985.
34. Haley RW, Culver DH, White JW, et al: The nationwide nosocomial infection rate: a new need for vital statistics, *Am J Epidemiol* 121:159, 1985.
35. Haley RW, Schaberg DR, Crossley KB, et al: Extra charges and prolongation of stay attributable to nosocomial infections: a prospective inter-hospital comparison, *Am J Med* 70:51, 1981.
36. Haley RW, White JW, Culver DH, et al: The financial incentive for hospital to prevent nosocomial infection under the prospective payment system: an empirical determination from a nationally representative sample, *JAMA* 257:1611, 1987.
37. Horan TC, Gaynes RP, Martone WJ, et al: CDC definitions of nosocomial surgical site infections, 1992; a modification of CDC definitions of surgical wound infections, *Am J Infect Control* 20:271, 1992.
38. Jackson B, Rice D: Wound infections and recurrence in head and neck cancer, *Otolaryngol Head Neck Surg* 102:331, 1990.
39. Johnson J: Postoperative infection. In Eisle D, editor: *Complications in head and neck surgery,* St Louis, 1993, Mosby.
40. Johnson JT, Bloomer WD: Effect of prior radiotherapy on postsurgical wound infection, *Head Neck* 11:132, 1989.
41. Johnson JT, Kachman K, Wagner RL, et al: Comparison of ampicillin/sulbactam versus clindamycin in the prevention of infection in patients undergoing head and neck surgery, *Head Neck* 19:367, 1997.
42. Johnson J, Meyers E: Management of complications of therapeutic intervention. In Suen J, Meyers E, editors: *Cancer of the head and neck, ed 2,* New York, 1989, Churchill Livingstone.
43. Johnson JT, Myers EN, Thearle PB, et al: Antimicrobial prophylaxis for contaminated head and neck surgery, *Laryngoscope* 94:46, 1984.
44. Johnson JT, Schuller DE, Silver F, et al: Antibiotic prophylaxis in high-risk head and neck surgery: one day vs. five day therapy, *Otolaryngol Head Neck Surg* 95:554, 1986.
45. Johnson JT, Wagner RI, Schuller DE, et al: Prophylactic antibiotics for head and neck surgery with flap reconstruction, *Arch Otolaryngol Head Neck Surg* 118:488, 1992.
46. Johnson JT, Yu VL: Role of aerobic gram-negative rods, anaerobes, and fungi in wound infections after head and neck surgery: implications for antimicrobial prophylaxis, *Head Neck* 11:27, 1989.
47. Johnson JT, Yu VL, Meyers EN, et al: Efficacy of two third-generation cephalosporins in prophylaxis for head and neck surgery, *Arch Otolaryngol Head Neck Surg* 110:224, 1984.
48. Johnson JT, Yu VL, Meyers EN, et al: An assessment of the need for gram-negative bacterial coverage in antibiotic prophylaxis for oncological head and neck surgery, *J Infect Dis* 155:332, 1987.
49. Johnson JT, Yu VL, Meyers EN, et al: Cefazolin vs. moxalactam? A double-blind randomized trial of cephalosporins in head and neck surgery, *Arch Otolaryngol Head Neck* 112:151, 1986.
50. Keats AS: The ASA classification of physical status: a recapitulation, *Anesthesiology* 49:732, 1978.
51. Kiener J, Hoffman W, Mathes S: Influence of radiotherapy on microvascular reconstruction in the head and neck region, *Am J Surg* 162:404, 1991.
52. Kirchner JC, Edberg SC, Saasaki CT: The use of topical oral antibiotics in head and neck prophylaxis: is it justified? *Laryngoscope* 98:26, 1988.
53. Komisar A, Warman, Danziger E: A critical analysis of immediate and delayed mandibular reconstruction using A-O plates, *Arch Otolaryngol Head Neck Surg* 115:830, 1989.
54. Ludwig KA, Carlson MA, Condon RE: Prophylactic antibiotics in surgery, *Ann Rev Med* 44:385, 1993.
55. Martin R, Fielder C, Dorman E: Prediction and prevention of fistulae after major head and neck surgery: a preliminary report, *Aust N Z J Surg* 58:488, 1992.
56. Meakins J: Guidelines for prevention of surgical site infection. In Holcroft JW, Meakins JL, Harkin AH, et al, editors: *Care of the surgical patient,* New York, 1994, Scientific American.
57. Mombelli G, Coppens L, Dor P, et al: Antibiotic prophylaxis in surgery for head and neck cancer: comparative study of short and prolonged administration of carbenicillin, *J Antimicrob Chemother* 7:665, 1981.
58. Mueller AC, Henkel KO, Neuman J: Perioperative antibiotic prophylaxis in maxillofacial surgery: penetration of clindamycin into various tissues, *J Craniomaxillofac Surg* 27:172, 1999.
59. Mustafa E, Tahsin A: Cefotaxime prophylaxis in major non-contaminated head and neck surgery: one-day versus seven-day therapy, *J Laryngol Otol* 107:30, 1993.

60. National Research Council: Postoperative wound infections: the influence of ultraviolet radiation of the operating room and of various other factors, *Ann Surg* 2 (suppl):1, 1964.

61. Nichols RL: Surgical wound infection, *Am J Med* 91(suppl): 54, 1991.

62. Nichols RL, Condon RE, Gorbach SL, et al: Efficacy of preoperative antimicrobial preparation of the bowel, *Ann Surg* 176:227, 1972.

63. Penel N, Lefebvre D, Bournier C: Risk factors for wound infection in head and neck cancer surgery: a prospective study, *Head Neck* 23:447, 2001.

64. Redleaf MI, Bauer CA: Topical antiseptic mouthwash in oncological surgery of the oral cavity and oropharynx, *J Laryngol Otol* 109:973, 1994.

65. Robbins KT, Byers RM, Cole R, et al: Wound prophylaxis with metronidazole in head and neck surgical oncology, *Laryngoscope* 98:803, 1986.

66. Robbins K, Favrot S, Hanna D, et al: Risk of wound infection in patients with head and neck cancer, *Head Neck* 12:143, 1990.

67. Rodrigo JP, Alvarez JC, Gomez JR, et al: Comparison of three prophylactic antibiotic regimens in clean-contaminated head and neck surgery, *Head Neck* 19:188, 1997.

68. Rubin J, Johnson JT, Wagner RL, et al: Bacteriologic analysis of wound infection following major head and neck surgery, *Arch Otolaryngol Head Neck Surg* 114:969, 1988.

69. Shapiro M: Prophylaxis in otolaryngologic surgery and neurosurgery: a critical review, *Rev Infect Dis* 13(suppl):858, 1991.

70. Simons JP, Johnson JT, Yu VL, et al: The role of topical antibiotic prophylaxis in patients undergoing contaminated head and neck surgery with flap reconstruction, *Laryngoscope* 111:329, 2001.

71. Snyderman CH, Kachman K, Molseed L, et al: Reduced postoperative infections with an immune-enhancing nutritional supplement, *Laryngoscope* 109:915, 1999.

72. Soylu L, Kiroglu M, Aydogan B, et al: Pharyngocutaneous fistula following laryngectomy, *Head Neck* 20:22, 1998.

73. Strauss M, Saccogna PW, Allphin AL: Cephazolin and metronidazole prophylaxis in head and neck surgery, *J Laryngol Otol* 111:631, 1997.

74. Tabet J, Johnson J: Wound infection in head and neck surgery: prophylaxis, etiology, and management, *J Otolaryngol* 19:197, 1990.

75. Tandon DA, Bahadur S, Laldina HC, et al: Role of prophylactic antibiotics in surgery for advanced head and neck cancer, *J Laryngol Otol* 106:621, 1992.

76. Urken ML, Buchbinder D, Costantino PD, et al: Oromandibular reconstruction using microvascular composite flaps, report of 210 cases, *Arch Otolaryngol Head Neck Surg* 124:46, 1998.

77. Van Laethem Y, Lagast H, Klasssstersky J: Anaerobic infections in cancer patients: comparison between therapy oriented strictly at anaerobes or both anaerobes and aerobes, *J Antimicrob Chemother* 10(suppl A):137, 1982.

78. Velanovich V: A meta-analysis of prophylactic antibiotics in head and neck surgery, *Plast Reconstr Surg* 87:429, 1991.

79. Weber RS, Raad I, Frankenthaler RA, et al: Ampicillin/sulbactam vs. clindamycin in head and neck oncologic surgery: the need for gram negative coverage, *Arch Otolaryngol Head Neck Surg* 118:1159, 1992.

80. Weber RS: Wound infection in head and neck surgery: implications for perioperative antibiotic treatment, *Ear Nose Throat* 76:790, 1997.

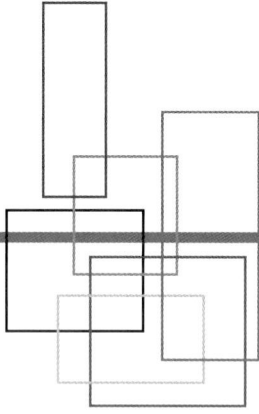

Pediatric Maxillofacial Infections

Jeffrey Kingsbury
David M. Shafer
Brett A. Weyman

Although many of the tenets of treating maxillofacial infections in adults also apply to pediatric patients, important differences in younger patients must be considered. The challenge of pediatric care is the recognition and treatment of unique anatomical and physiological conditions that occur in growing and relatively vulnerable patients. Treatment may be complicated by their small physical size, sometimes subtle anatomical differences, unique physiological responses, emotional immaturity, and difficulty in obtaining an accurate history. However, the basic principles of the treatment of infections must be followed: consideration of host factors (health history, immunological status, systemic illnesses), accurate anatomical diagnosis, early incision and drainage, identification of causative organisms, and sensitivity-based selection of antimicrobial therapy. Constant vigilance and preciseness of care are required for successful outcomes. Fortunately, the resilience of children is remarkable, and a favorable outcome is likely when their conditions are managed appropriately.

The pediatric patient is a unique host in cases of infectious processes of the head and neck. Accurate diagnosis and aggressive treatment are the mainstays of all pediatric conditions, particularly infections of the head and neck. A thorough physical examination and the most accurate history that can be obtained are critical.[3] The inability of many children to effectively communicate the history of their present illness and the increased likelihood of referral to a maxillofacial surgeon without a known diagnosis present treatment challenges. The source of facial infection in children is never clearly identified in 50% of cases.[5] Therefore the surgeon must use the knowledge of anatomy and likely primary sources and then couple them with the differential diagnosis for pain, swelling, trismus, lethargy, alteration of vital signs, and so on. The rapidity with which a primary source can be identified and empirical therapy initiated often is critical.[1,4,11] Identification of the most likely source includes consideration of the dentition, oropharyngeal mucosa and tonsillar regions, overlying skin, paranasal sinuses, ears, and salivary glands.

As with all patients, historical information is important. With pediatric patients, this information should be obtained from both the child and the primary caregiver when possible. The history should include the patient's age and gender, duration of symptoms, recent changes in severity of symptoms, and the other standard components of a health history. For example, a fast-developing, aggressive infection is suggestive of *H. influenzae* infection, whereas a more slowly developing infection may indicate an odontogenic source. A series of queries regarding systemic symptoms also is helpful. Has the child been febrile (if not, have any antipyretics been given which might mask fever), lethargic, had a change in personality, or loss of appetite? Is there any recent history of trauma to the maxillofacial area, including insect bites, bruises, and so forth? Is there a known history of sinus disease, upper respiratory tract infections, or otitis media? Certain clues are helpful. Statistically a temperature greater than 38.5° C (101.5° F) suggests cellulitis and bacteremia of nonodontogenic origin.[4]

Laboratory testing often provides little information in patients with maxillofacial infections.[13] However, in some patients it can provide critical information and assistance in tracking the patient's progress. If the diagnosis is questioned or if outpatient care versus inpatient care is a concern, a complete blood cell count (CBC) with differential and an electrolyte panel should be ordered. In more seriously ill patients a comprehensive chemistry profile, coagulation profile, and renal function tests may be appropriate. Radiographic imaging should be used when needed to support a clinical diagnosis, delineate the specifics of surgical management, or determine the extent and spread of disease. However, overreliance on imaging studies in formulating a working diagnosis can waste valuable time and resources.

Children are much more susceptible to volume depletion as a result of dehydration and become toxic much faster than adults.[12,13] A child with a maxillofacial infection requires a thorough physical examination, including accurate assessment of vital signs, intraoral assessment, and clinical evaluation of swallowing, vision, and intranasal examination. Does the child appear active and alert, or lethargic and irritable? Are the mucous membranes moist or dry? Temperature at or above 38.5° C (101.5° F) suggests bacteremia and is an important criterion in consideration of hospital admission. Rapid pulse or hypotension suggests volume depletion caused by dehydration and may indicate vasodilation as a result of sepsis warranting inpatient management. A child often does not exhibit tachycardia until dehydration is severe; thus a normal pulse does not preclude the possibility of volume depletion. Normal pediatric vital signs and hematological values are shown in Table 21-1. Dehydration is an important consideration in the evaluation of ill children because of differences in renal function relative to adults. Children produce nearly 65% more urine than adults when calculated on a milliliter per kilogram per day basis and become depleted more easily. Dehydrated patients tend to be lethargic with rapid, open-mouth breathing. The skin is warm and dry. If intravascular volume is depleted, the extremities feel cool. Skin turgor should be evaluated; if immediate return to resting position after tenting of the skin does not occur, dehydration should be suspected. In neonates the fontanel should be inspected and any sunken appearance noted carefully.

Physiological crystalloid solution usually is used for fluid resuscitation in dehydrated children, and serum electrolyte levels must be monitored regularly. Fluid deficits should be calculated as accurately as possible and replaced over 3 to 4 hours with Ringer's lactate solution. Combined with ongoing maintenance fluid, the patient may receive up to 10 mL/kg per hour for the first few hours. Urine output and electrolyte levels should be checked regularly.

Children require nearly twice the amount of maintenance fluid, calculated on a milligram per kilogram per hour basis, than adults would need. Children require 2 to 4 mL/kg per hour, whereas neonates and infants may require 4 to 6 mL/kg per hour depending on the respiratory rate, ambient temperature, and environmental humidity.

ANATOMICAL CLASSIFICATION

The specific anatomical location of an infection is an important clinical clue to diagnosis and treatment.[3-5,11] This chapter reviews certain infections with particular clinical relevance in children. Anatomical location of maxillofacial infections in children can be divided into upper and lower face infections. This division is helpful from an anatomical standpoint of management and potential complications. Upper and lower face infections have unique clinical patterns and statistically have distinct differences in terms of causes and microbiological flora (Table 21-2 and Box 21-1).

UPPER FACE INFECTIONS

Upper face infections are defined as localized infections or those originating from anatomical structures of the

TABLE 21-1

Normal Pediatric Vital Signs and Hematological Values

	PEDIATRIC STANDARD VALUE			
Age	Respiration Rate (breaths/min)	Heart Rate (beats/min)	Blood Pressure (Systolic; mm Hg)	Average Weight (kg)
6 mo	22-36	110-150	75-105	6
2 yr	22-28	90-130	88-112	12
6 yr	18-24	82-118	92-108	20
9 yr	18-22	80-105	102-118	30
12 yr	18-22	68-102	105-125	40
Adult	12-16	65-80	110-140	68

					WBC COUNT			
						DIFFERENTIAL		
Age	Hemoglobin (g/100 mL)	Hematocrit (%)	Total	PMN (mm³)	L	E	M	Platelet Count (mm³)
6 mo-6 yr	10.5-14.0	33-42	6,000-15,000	45	48	2	5	150,000-300,000
7 yr-12 yr	11.0-16.0	34-40	4,500-13,500	55	38	2	5	150,000-300,000
Adult	(F) 12-16 (M) 14-18	37-50	5,000-10,000	55	35	3	7	150,000-300,000

From Gross RD: Oral surgery for the adolescent patient. In Castaldi CR, Brass GA: *Dentistry for the adolescent,* Philadelphia, 1980, WB Saunders.
L, Lymphocytes; *E,* eosinophils; *M,* monocytes.

TABLE 21-2

Characteristics of Upper and Lower Facial Infections

Variable	Upper Face	Lower Face
Age	Young (≤4 years)	Older (≥5 years)
Common source	Unknown	Odontogenic
Microbiology	Highly variable	Less variable
Empirical therapy	Antibiotic (cefuroxime)	Antibiotic—penicillin, (clindamycin if severe), drainage
Treatment outcome	Favorable	Unfavorable

Adapted from Dodson TB, Kaban LB: Diagnosis and management of pediatric facial infections, *Oral Maxillofac Surg Clin North Am* 6:13, 1994.

BOX 21-1

Organisms Isolated from Pediatric Head and Neck Infections

Upper Face	Lower Face (in Order of Frequency)
Staphylococcus aureus*†	*S. aureus*
Staphylococcus epidermidis*	*S. viridans*
Streptococcus viridans*	β-Hemolytic *Streptococcus*
Mixed oral flora*	*S. epidermidis*
Haemophilus influenzae*	Mixed oral flora
Haemophilus parainfluenzae*	Anaerobic gram-negative
Streptococcus pneumoniae	rods
β-Hemolytic *Streptococcus*	
Gram-positive rods	
Adenovirus or herpesvirus	
Pseudomonas†	
Escherichia coli†	
Enterobacter spp.†	

From Dodson TB, Perrott DH, Kaban LB: Pediatric maxillofacial infections: a retrospective study of 113 patients. Presented at the 70th Annual Meeting of the American Association of Oral and Maxillofacial Surgeons, Boston, September 29-October 2, 1988.
*These organisms represent 75% of the positive cultures in upper face infections.
†Penicillin-resistant organisms: 10 of 11 *S. aureus,* all *Pseudomonas, Enterobacter* spp., and *E. coli.*

upper face, including the sinuses, skin, maxillary teeth, and the orbits and lacrimal apparatus (Figure 21-1).[11] Buccal space infections are classified as upper face infections unless the origin is a lower facial structure.[11] Patients with upper face infections often complain of pain, swelling, fever, and difficulty with oral intake. Differentiating between odontogenic causes and sinus origin is aided by historical information. Has there been any recent maxillary toothache, or does the child have a history of upper respiratory tract problems or chronic sinus drainage and nasal discharge? Is there any recent history of trauma, including insect bites? The age of the child

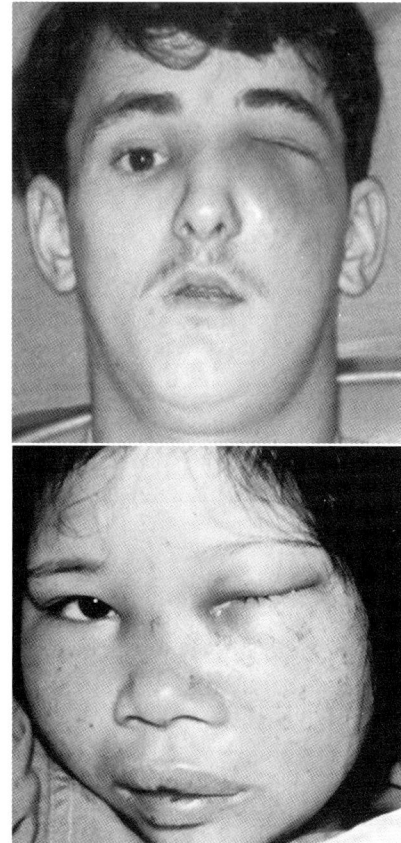

Figure 21-1 Differential diagnosis of upper face infections. **A,** Dacryocystitis with minimal involvement of nasolabial fold. **B,** Odontogenic cellulitis. The nasolabial fold is effaced.

may be helpful. Studies by Dodson et al.[5] indicated that upper face infections of nonodontogenic origin were more common in children 5 years or younger than in children age 6 to 12 years. An obvious exception are children with "milk bottle" caries. These upper face infections had a higher incidence of culture of *H. influenzae* and *Staphylococcus aureus.*

Physical examination findings may show little difference despite the cause of infection. Swelling and pain on palpation of the affected area are hallmarks. Erythema is usually present (*H. influenzae* cellulitis classically is violaceous). The eyelids may be affected with resultant edema or cellulitis. Intraoral examination may disclose swelling of the buccal sulcus; and if the cause is odontogenic, caries may be grossly visible. If the cause is maxillary sinusitis, many teeth may be sensitive to percussion, including the surrounding gingival tissue. When palpated from outside the mouth, the anterior maxilla frequently is very tender. Transillumination of the sinus may be helpful in older children.

A panoramic radiograph is useful for demonstration of dental pathological conditions and fluid in the maxillary sinus. An upright Waters' view visualizes the maxillary, ethmoid, and frontal sinuses. Computed tomography (CT) scans are useful in more serious infections when disease may be more extensive or in planning operative treatment

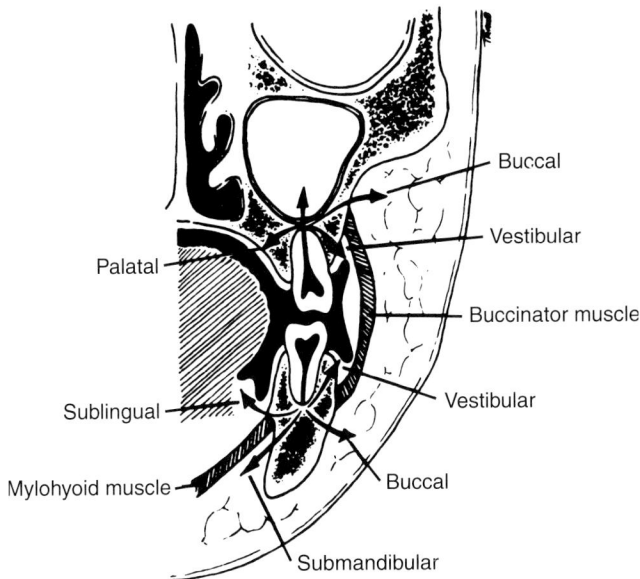

Figure 21-2 Potential routes of spread of infection.

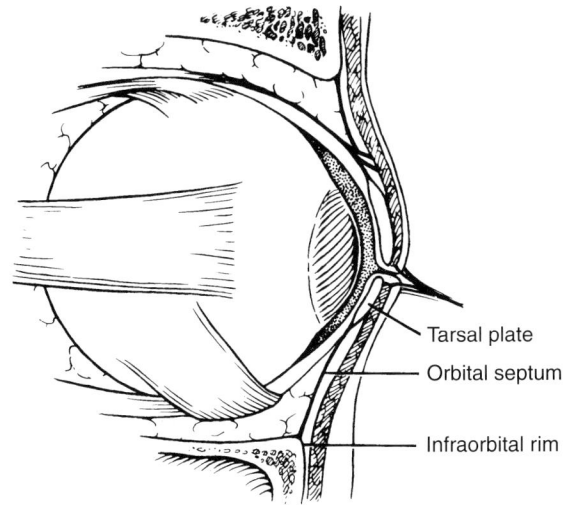

Figure 21-3 Lateral diagrammatic view of the orbit. (From Kaban LB: *Pediatric oral and maxillofacial surgery,* Philadelphia, 1990, WB Saunders.)

to ensure drainage of all involved spaces. An anatomical approach to evaluation of maxillofacial infections also aids understanding the routes of infection spread through tissue planes of the upper and lower face (Figure 21-2).

Oral and maxillofacial surgeons are familiar with treating odontogenic infection. The anatomical path of spread is the same as for other causes. In the era of common antibiotic use, the most serious complications of infections of the upper face are rare. They include cavernous sinus thrombosis (or meningitis or intracranial abscess) with or without blindness. Cavernous sinus thrombosis results from spread of infection along tissue planes into the orbit or central nervous system or through the valveless facial and angular veins. Infections that affect the orbit are defined by their relationship to the orbital septum. The orbital septum separates the eyelids from the orbital contents (Figure 21-3). Preseptal cellulitis involves tissue superficial to the septum, whereas orbital cellulitis involves tissue deep to the septum. Postseptal cellulitis is characterized by proptosis, chemosis, pain with extraocular muscle function, and changes in visual acuity. True orbital cellulitis is rare in children. Studies have determined that only 2 of 39 patients studied had true orbital cellulitis.[14] The other 37 had preseptal cellulitis. However, recognition of the signs associated with true orbital cellulitis is important in evaluation of cellulitis of the upper face because orbital cellulitis is a true ophthalmological emergency (see Chapter 15).

Cavernous sinus thrombosis shares many symptoms with orbital cellulitis. In addition, loss of consensual pupillary response to light occurs with decreased sensitivity in the ipsilateral first division of the trigeminal nerve. Orbital cellulitis and cavernous sinus thrombosis are rare in children. However, meningitis is a relatively common sequela of serious upper face infections. Positive cerebrospinal fluid culture findings have been reported in as many as 10% to 15% of children with facial cellulitis and bacteremia.[10]

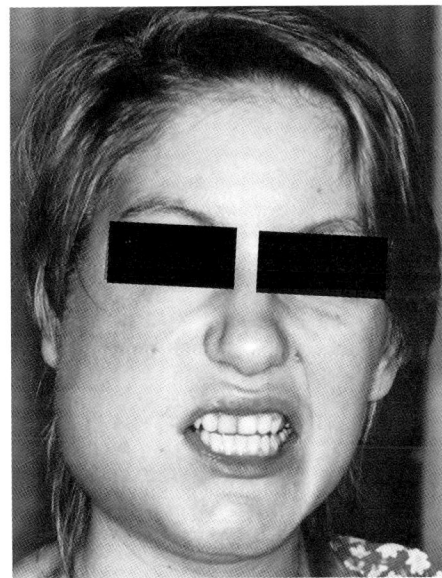

Figure 21-4 Severe trismus associated with masticator space infection. The masseter muscle overlying the deep space infection is bulging and the patient is unable to open her mouth.

LOWER FACE INFECTIONS

Individuals with infections of the lower face usually have pain, swelling, and trismus (Figure 21-4). Because of the anatomical relationships illustrated in Figure 21-2, these infections can travel in several different directions depending on the precise location of the source in the lower face. The most important hallmark of infections involving the masticator space is trismus. Infections that involve the buccal or masseteric space cause prominent swelling of the cheek. Rarely these infections ascend to involve the eyelids. An infection medial to the mandibular ramus often

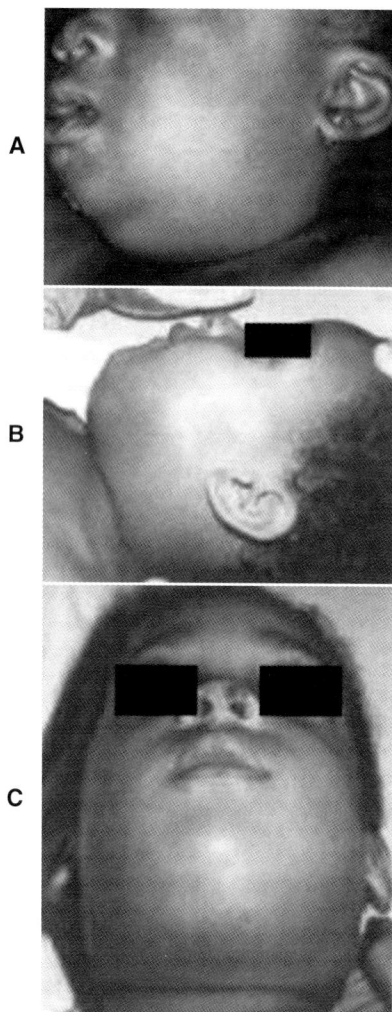

Figure 21-5 Ludwig's angina. **A,** Cellulitis arising from a mandibular tooth affects the floor of the mouth and neck. **B,** Diffuse inflammation of submandibular and sublingual spaces occurs most often in young adults with odontogenic infections. **C,** Severe neck pain, swelling, fever, malaise, and dysphagia can compromise airway. (Courtesy Richard E. Hall, SUNY at Buffalo.)

spreads to the infratemporal fossa and produces swelling in the lateral pharyngeal wall, pterygomandibular raphe, and soft palate. Often little or no extraoral swelling is present. The hallmarks of this type of infection are pain and trismus.

Infection of the submandibular space manifests as extraoral swelling below the inferior border of the mandible. If the sublingual space is affected, the tongue is painful and elevated. If the sublingual and submandibular spaces are involved bilaterally, Ludwig's angina exists (Figure 21-5).

The common sources of infection in the lower face are teeth, skin, lymph nodes, salivary glands, burns, trauma, and insect bites. Dodson et al.[5] reported that odontogenic infection is the most common diagnosis in children with lower facial swelling. Secondarily infected cervical lymph nodes are common in children with a history of repeated urinary tract infections with generalized adenopathy.

Infections of the lower face often produce the most serious, life-threatening sequelae that oral and facial surgeons routinely encounter. Mandibular molars can be the source of infections that spread medially and posteriorly into the infratemporal fossa, or laterally and posteriorly into the buccal space. If the spread is medial, it can cause sublingual or submandibular spread depending on its location as superior or inferior to the mylohyoid muscle. The same process applies for premolars and anterior teeth, which may involve the sublingual or submental areas.

The principles of treatment are the same: accurate diagnosis, appropriate antibiotic therapy, and adequate surgical drainage. The most important emergency consideration in evaluating a patient with lower face infection is the status of the airway. The swelling that may exist in the upper airway is considerable with potential for airway occlusion. When coupled with trismus and tongue elevation, the swelling creates an uncertain situation. If the status of the airway is doubtful, soft tissue neck films and CT scans of the neck may be helpful. In management of children with edema of the upper airway, careful observation of their breathing and ability to swallow are helpful. If the child is sitting forward in the "sniffing" position or drooling because of inability to swallow his or her own secretions, a dire situation is pending. Close monitoring may allow surgical management of the infection with elective intubation rather than an emergency tracheotomy.[10,11]

ODONTOGENIC INFECTIONS

Despite the tremendous advances in dental care in Western society, odontogenic infections remain a serious problem of dental practice.[15] Many of the factors regarding diagnosis, treatment, and complications of odontogenic and other bacterial infections are discussed in detail in other chapters. As noted previously, the systemic considerations in the evaluation of children are important, as are some local factors that may affect the course of their disease. Differences in medication dosages exist and are summarized in Table 21-3.

Because of the growing dimensions of the facial structures, the height of muscle attachments on the alveolar process differs in children, which leads to a tendency for children to develop cutaneous fistulas as a result of odontogenic infections (Figure 21-6). Recognition of this difference is important; therefore the clinician should search diligently for odontogenic causes of such lesions. Failure to recognize the dental origin of these problems results in delays and unnecessary surgical procedures. In addition, the developing permanent tooth buds in the growing child may be jeopardized by the development of intraosseous abscess cavities in the jaws. Odontogenic infections in children tend to occur in children older than 5 years of age and usually manifest as infections of the lower face.

The bones of developing children are less dense than adult bones. The marrow space also is much wider. Because of these differences, bacterial infections may face

TABLE 21-3

Pediatric Medication Dosages (in mg/kg/d or mg/kg)*

Drug	BODY WEIGHT <2000 kg		BODY WEIGHT >2000 kg		
	0-7 Days Old	8-28 Days Old	0-7 Days Old	8-28 Days Old	>28 Days Old
Aminoglycosides (IV or IM)					
Amikacin	7.5 q18-24h	7.5 q12h	10 q12h	10 q12h	10 q8h
Gentamicin/tobramycin	2.5 q18-24h	2.5 q12h	2.5 q12h	2.5 q12h	2.5 q8h
Aztreonam (IV)	30 q12h	30 q8h	30 q8h	30 q6h	30 q6h
Cephalosporins					
Cefaclor					20-40 mg divided tid
Cefadroxil					30 divided bid (maximum 2 g/d)
Cefazolin	20 q12h	20 q12h	20 q12h	20 q8h	25-100 divided q8h
Cefepime					150 divided q8h
Cefixime					8 as qd or divided bid
Cefotaxime	50 q12h	50 q8h	50 q12h	50 q8h	50 q8h (75 q6h for meningitis)
Cefoxitin			20 q12h		80-160 divided q6h
Cefpodoxime					10 divided bid (maximum 800 mg/d)
Cefprozil					30 divided bid (maximum 1 g/d)
Ceftazidime	50 q12h	50 q8h	33 q8h	50 q8h	50 q8h
Ceftibuten					4.5 bid
Ceftizoxime					33-66 18h
Ceftriaxone	50 qd	50 qd	50 qd	75 qd	100 qd
Cefuroxime					75-150 (200-240 for meningitis) divided q8h (IV) 10-15 bid (maximum 1-2 g/d) (PO)
Cephalexin					25-50 divided 4 ×/d (maximum 4 g/d)
Loracarbef					15-30 divided bid (maximum 0.8 g/d)
Chloramphenicol (IV)					12.5-25 q6h (maximum 2-4 g/d)
Clindamycin					15-40 divided q6-8h (IV) 10-20 divided 3-4 ×/d (PO)
Ciprofloxacin (PO)†					20-30 divided bid (maximum 1.5 g/d)
Imipenem (IV)					10-15 q6h (maximum 2 g/d)
Macrolides					
Erythromycin (IV, PO)	10 q12h	10 q8h	10 q12h	13 q8h	10 q6h
Azithromycin (PO)					10-12 day 1, then 5/d
Clarithromycin (PO)					7.5 divided bid (maximum 1 g/d)
Meropenem (IV)					60-120 divided q8h
Metronidazole (IV, PO)	15 q24h	7.5 q12h	7.5 q12h	15 q12h	30 divided 6-12 h
Penicillins					
Ampicillin	50 q12h	50 q8h	50 q8h	50 q6h	50 q6h
Ampicillin-sulbactam					100-300 divided q6h
Amoxicillin (PO)					25-50 divided tid
Amoxicillin-clavulanate (PO)					For 875/125 formulation: 45 divided bid
Cloxacillin					50-100 divided 4 ×/d
Dicloxacillin					25-50 divided 4 ×/d
Mezlocillin	75 q12h	75 q8h	75 q12h	75 q8h	75 q6h

Adapted from Gilbert DN, Moellering RC Jr, Sande MA: *The Sanford guide to antimicrobial therapy,* ed 30, Vienna, Va, Antimicrobial Therapy Inc, 2000.
TMP/SMX, Trimethoprim-sulfamethoxazole; UTI, urinary tract infection.
*May need higher doses in patients with meningitis.
†With exception of cystic fibrosis, not approved for use in patients younger than 18 years.

Continued

416   *Oral and Maxillofacial Infections*

TABLE 21-3

Pediatric Medication Dosages (in mg/kg/d or mg/kg)—cont'd

Drug	BODY WEIGHT <2000 kg		BODY WEIGHT >2000 kg		
	0-7 Days Old	8-28 Days Old	0-7 Days Old	8-28 Days Old	>28 Days Old
Nafcillin (IV)	50 q12h	50 q8h	50 q8h	50 q6h	50 q6h
Oxacillin (IV)	50 q12h	50 q8h	50 q8h	50 q6h	50 q6h
Piperacillin (IV)					100-300 divided q4-6h
Piperacillin/tazobactam (IV)					100-300 divided q4-6h
Ticarcillin (IV)	75 q12h	75 q8h	75 q8h	75 q6h	75 q6h
Ticarcillin/clavulanate	75 q12h	75 q8h	75 q8h	75 q6h	75 q6h
Penicillin G (IV)	50,000 u q12h	75,000 u q8h	50,000 u q8h	50,000 u q6h	33,000 u q4h
Penicillin G procaine (IM)					25,000-50,000 u
Penicillin V					25-50 divided 3-4 ×/d
Rifampin (PO)			10, single dose	20, single dose	20, single dose
Sulfisoxazole (PO)				120-150	
TMP/SMX (PO, IV) UTI: 8-12 TMP component (divided bid) *Pneumocystis:* 20 TMP component divided 4 ×/d					
Tetracycline (PO) (≥8 years)					20-50 divided 4 ×/d
Doxycycline (PO, IV) (≥8 years)					2-4 divided bid
Vancomycin (IV)					40-60 divided q6h

TMP/SMX, Trimethoprim-sulfamethoxazole; *UTI,* urinary tract infection.

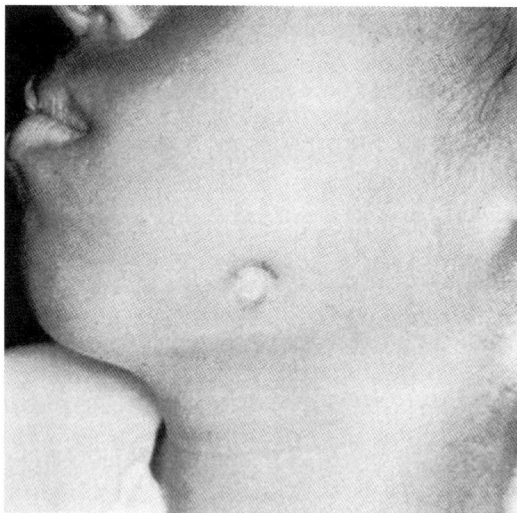

Figure 21-6 Facial fistula associated with an abscess of the lower first molar tooth in an 8-year-old patient.

less resistance to spread through osseous tissue in children. If infections are not treated promptly and aggressively, they may lead to common osteomyelitis or proliferative osteomyelitis (Garré's sclerosing osteomyelitis (Figure 21-7). Garré's sclerosing osteomyelitis occurs primarily in children and young adults and is characterized by "onion skinning" of the cortex on radiographs. It usually results from a carious first molar, although cases with no dental origin have been reported.[15] When no dental disease exists,

biopsy should be performed. The differential diagnosis should include Ewing's sarcoma, osteosarcoma, and cortical hyperostosis (Caffey's disease). Treatment of Garré's sclerosing osteomyelitis focuses on removal of the source of inflammation; antibiotics are not required unless signs of active infection are present. The organisms most commonly cultured are *S. aureus* and *Staphylococcus epidermidis.* If the infection involves the condylar growth area, significant growth deformities may develop.

Another type of osteomyelitis found in infants is infantile osteomyelitis (Figure 21-8). This disease is not common; however, when present serious deformities may develop if it is not recognized and promptly treated. Infantile osteomyelitis usually occurs during the first few weeks of life and frequently affects the maxilla. Before the era of antibiotic therapy the mortality rate for this disease was 25% to 30%.[15] Hematogenous spread or perinatal trauma to the gingiva (suctioning at birth) are considered possible causes. The maxillary sinus or suckling from contaminated nipples may also be causative factors.[15] These children often have upper facial cellulitis centered about the orbit and a history of irritability and lethargy at initial presentation. They may also have fever, anorexia, emesis, and dehydration. Intraoral examination usually reveals a swollen maxilla, both buccally and palatally, most prominent in the posterior. Fluctuance and fistulas may be present in the alveolar mucosa.

The causative agent usually is *S. aureus,* although streptococci also are frequently cultured. Treatment should be

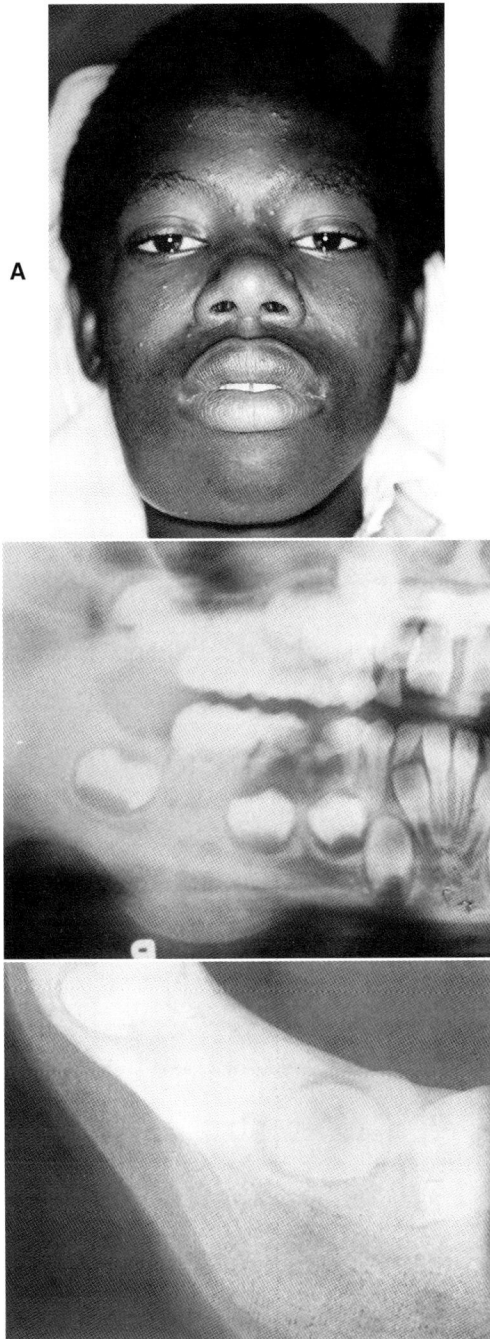

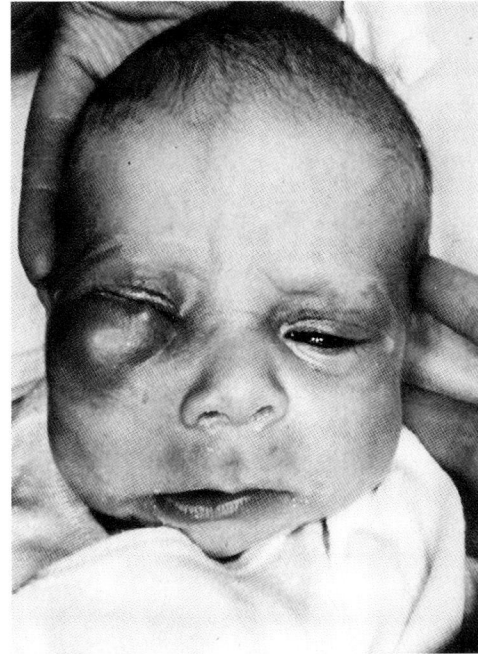

Figure 21-8 A 3-week-old infant with osteomyelitis of the newborn of unknown origin. This infection was treated successfully with penicillin. (Courtesy M. Michael Cohen, Sr.)

as indicated by sensitivity studies. These therapies usually are effective. A conservative approach to sequestrectomy is advisable because of possible damage to the tooth buds.

OTHER BACTERIAL INFECTIONS

Several common nonodontogenic bacterial causes of facial cellulitis are possible in children. In children younger than 5 years of age the majority of serious facial infections are nonodontogenic.[11] However, because of the diagnostic issues discussed previously, many patients are seen by the dental or facial surgeon for primary evaluation.

Haemophilus influenzae   The differential diagnosis of cellulitis of the upper face in any child younger than 5 years should include *H. influenzae* (Figure 21-9). *H. influenzae* infection may occur as an extension from the paranasal sinuses or by hematogenous spread as a result of bacteremia. Cellulitis caused by *H. influenzae* occurs in the maxillofacial region in 75% of all diagnosed cases.[10] It typically occurs with upper respiratory tract infections. In past studies, approximately 10% of 83 children with severe *H. influenzae* respiratory infection developed facial cellulitis and 1% subsequently developed orbital cellulitis. Cellulitis caused by this organism is diffuse, tender, and indurated. It usually extends unilaterally from the orbit to the mandible and has a distinct violaceous color. *H. influenzae* can progress to fatal meningitis, osteomyelitis, septic arthritis, and epiglottitis. Therefore it requires prompt aggressive treatment. Incision, drainage, and culture and sensitivity studies are critical. Empirical therapy should assume ampicillin resistance, but amoxicillin-clavulanate (Augmentin) is an appropriate choice. In more severe cases, ampicillin-

Figure 21-7 A, Facial deformity caused by Garré's sclerosing osteomyelitis in an 8-year-old boy. Apical infection associated with the primary molars was the apparent cause. **B,** Panographic film shows marked periosteal reaction. **C,** Occlusal film showing the "onion skin" appearance of the newly formed bone. (Courtesy Larry J. Peterson.)

prompt and aggressive. Complications of this infection include permanent optic damage, neurological complications, extension into the dural sinuses, loss of tooth buds, and permanent deformation of the maxilla.

Treatment of infantile osteomyelitis includes incision and drainage and treatment with intravenous penicillin and a penicillinase-resistant penicillin. Repeated culture specimens are appropriate with the antibiotic regimen adjusted

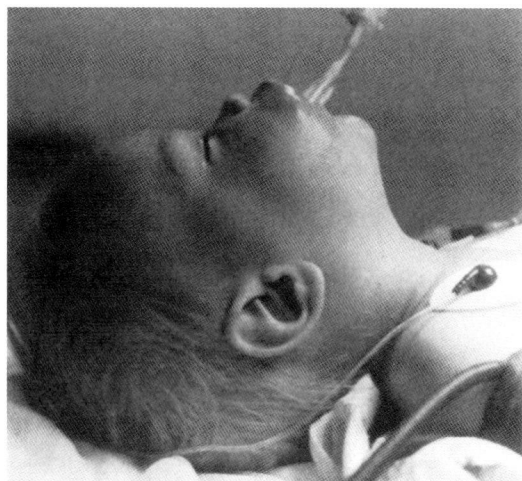

Figure 21-9 *Haemophilus influenzae* cellulitis. The child has marked buccal swelling that is warm, tender to palpation, and erythematous. Bimanual palpation revealed fluctuance requiring drainage and antibiotic therapy.

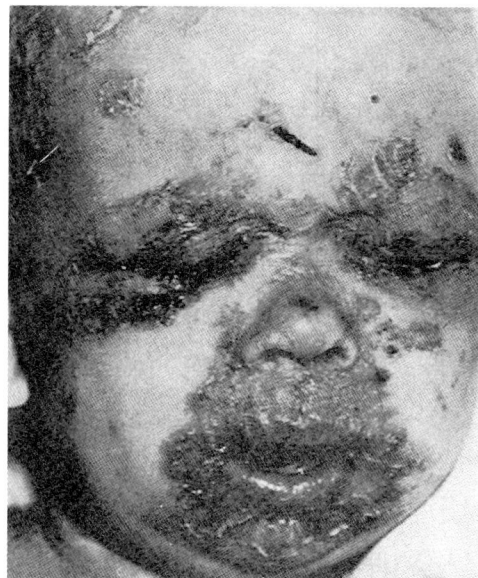

Figure 21-10 Staphylococcal scalded skin syndrome. (From Weinberg S, Hoekelman RA, editors: *Pediatric dermatology for the primary care practitioner,* New York, 1978, McGraw-Hill.)

sulbactam (Unasyn) or trimethoprim-sulfamethoxazole should be started.[6-8] Recent changes as a result of the availability of *H. influenzae* type B vaccine should be considered. In 1985 the vaccine was approved for use in children older than 2 years of age, which proved ineffective because most severe cases occur in children younger than 2 years. In 1990 the first vaccine became available for children younger than 2 years old. This vaccine resulted in a dramatic decrease in the incidence of disease caused by *H. influenzae* type B organisms. Most infections now are caused by nontypable strains of the disease.[10]

IMPETIGO

Streptococcal Impetigo   Although impetigo can occur in any age group, it is most common in children. It tends to occur in warm, humid climates and often is believed to be associated with mosquito bites. No direct evidence of inoculation by the mosquito has been demonstrated, and the disease most likely occurs by scratching of the affected skin. Impetigo is a rapidly spreading streptococcal infection of the superficial layer of the epidermis. It generally is caused by β-hemolytic streptococci, although cultures also may grow coagulase-positive staphylococci.[9,15] This disease typically manifests as thin, friable vesicles with minimal surrounding erythema. The lesions are intensely pruritic, which may lead to scratching and secondary infection in children. Erythema appears later in the disease and may lead to scarlet fever.[15] Noticeable regional lymphadenopathy is present, but constitutional symptoms such as fever and lethargy are minimal. The diagnosis is made on the basis of the unique appearance of the lesions and isolation of *Streptococcus pyogenes* from the wound. Untreated streptococcal impetigo is an indolent, self-limiting disease.

However, as with other streptococcal infections, poststreptococcal glomerulonephritis can occur; serial urinalyses are useful for monitoring. Treatment consists of systemic administration of antibiotics; culture of the wound should be checked for β-lactamase resistance.

Staphylococcal Impetigo   Many investigators believe that impetigo always is caused by streptococcal organisms, and that staphylococcal organisms are involved as secondary superinfecting agents.[15] In the pediatric population, staphylococcal scalded skin syndrome is an unusual but potentially serious infection (Figure 21-10). This infection occurs when phage group II staphylococci colonize the epidermis and release an exotoxin known as epidermolysin. The toxin causes formation of large bullae, which are filled with clear fluid that turns purulent. Little surrounding erythema is present. These bullae rupture, and widespread desquamation can cause life-threatening dehydration and electrolyte imbalances. This disease should be treated with careful hygiene, β-lactamase–resistant antibiotics, and patients with staphylococcal scalded skin syndrome require hospitalization for intravenous fluid replacement and nursing care (see Chapter 13).

NOMA

Noma is known also as gangrenous stomatitis and cancrum oris. It is an acute, fulminating, gangrenous process of oral and facial tissues usually seen children who are debilitated and malnourished (Figure 21-11). The term *noma* is derived from Greek and means "to devour."[15] Noma occurs usually in the presence of famine, persistent poverty, prison conditions, and with outbreaks of febrile diseases.

Noma is characterized by a rapid progressive course. It

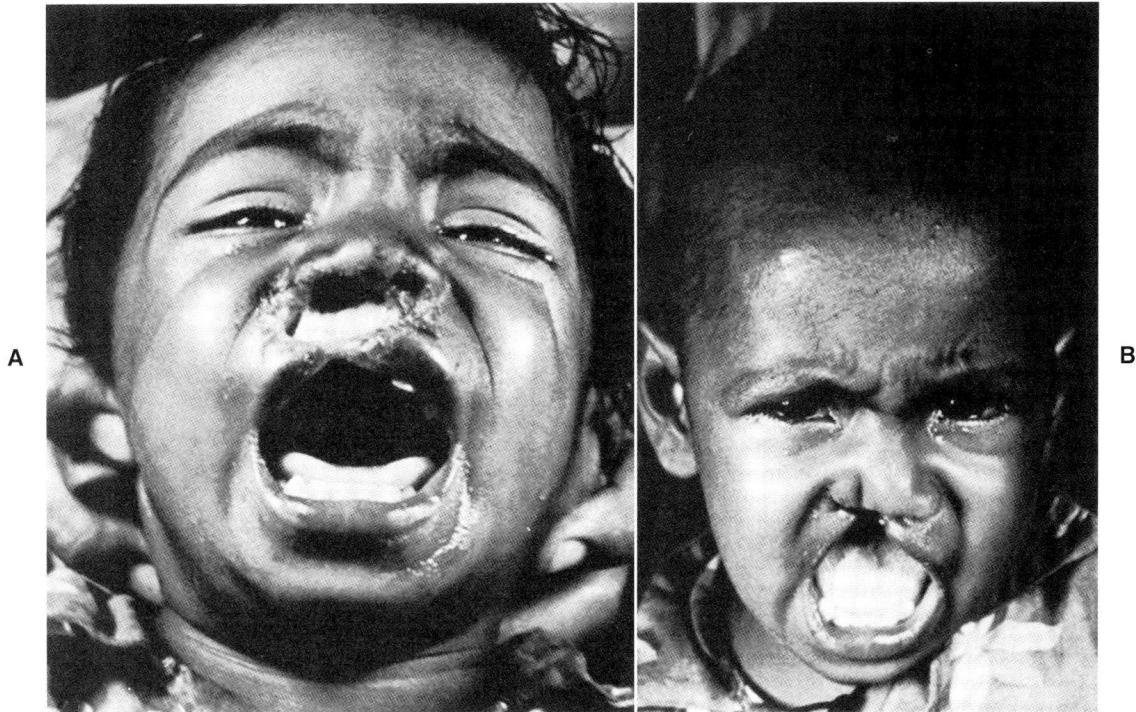

Figure 21-11 A, Marked necrosis of the soft tissues of the upper lip and anterior maxilla in a 4-year-old child with noma. Correction of the nutritional status and antibiotic therapy arrested the advance of the disease. **B,** Facial deformity resulting from noma. The necrotic anterior portion of the maxilla sloughed after 2 weeks of treatment and produced the defect shown.

begins as a small, painful vesicle or red spot on the attached gingiva in the premolar region of the mandible or maxilla. A necrotic ulcer rapidly forms and extends outward, causing painful cellulitis of the lips and cheek. The disease is noted for causing fever, fetid odor, hypersalivation, leukocytosis, and purulent oral discharge. Rapid progression occurs, with sloughing of associated soft tissues, exposing underlying bone, teeth, and deeper soft tissue. Microbiological study of the disease has shown that *Pseudomonas aeruginosa, Borrelia vincentii, Fusobacterium nucleatum*, and *Prevotella melaninogenicus* can be cultured from the wound.

Treatment involves correction of underlying nutritional deficiency, establishment of fluid and electrolyte balance, and administration of antibiotics. Penicillin is the drug of choice and should be administered in high doses. Blood transfusions are indicated in children with severe anemia. Local wound irrigation with saline solution and conservative removal of necrotic debris also are necessary. Treatment with caustic agents or aggressive excision is not indicated (see Chapter 22).

Erysipelas and Necrotizing Fasciitis Erysipelas is superficial cellulitis caused by β-hemolytic streptococci that invade the dermis. The skin becomes intensely erythematous, in contrast to impetigo. Necrotizing fasciitis is an aggressive infection that involves the superficial fascia and causes necrosis of the overlying tissue. Historically, it was believed to be caused by β-hemolytic streptococci.[15] Its ori-

gin now is accepted as polymicrobial. Both diseases can occur in children but have no unique propensity for them. The appropriate therapy is covered elsewhere in the text (see Chapter 13).

Ear, Nose, and Throat Infections Ear, nose, and throat infections are discussed in Chapter 14. *H. influenzae* sinusitis is a significant concern in pediatric patients. Otitis, pharyngitis, epiglottitis, tonsillitis, and peritonsillar abscess are all obvious concerns in the pediatric population and are discussed elsewhere, as are the numerous other types of bacterial infections of the maxillofacial region that can occur in pediatric patients but have no special predilection for affecting them.

VIRAL INFECTIONS

DNA VIRUSES

Herpesviruses Herpesviruses include herpes simplex 1 (HSV1) and 2 (HSV2), varicella-zoster, cytomegalovirus, and Epstein-Barr virus. These viruses produce a variety of manifestations, including those seen in maxillofacial problems in children.

The most common oral manifestation of HSV is acute herpetic gingivostomatitis, which is a systemic illness with oral lesions. It primarily affects children younger than 5 years.[15] The virus enters the body through the oral mucosa and has a short incubation period. Early in the disease the patient experiences cervical lymphadenopathy, tender oral mucosa, and is febrile. Vesicles then form on the tongue and buccal mucosa that rupture and cause painful ulcers. The gingiva is edematous and has a characteristic bright red gingival margin. These lesions last 1 to 2 weeks. After the initial infection subsides, the virus becomes latent and causes recurrent herpes labialis. Laboratory tests that confirm the presence of herpetic intranuclear inclusion bodies are the Tzanck smear or Giemsa stain. Treatment consists of orally administered acyclovir (15 mg/kg five times a day for 1 week) and supportive therapy with anesthetic mouth rinses to relieve discomfort. Antibiotics sometimes are used to control secondary infection by oral flora.

Epstein-Barr virus was first observed as an infectant of cells derived from Burkitt's lymphoma, an endemic illness of children in Africa. It is also the suspected causative agent of infectious mononucleosis. Infectious mononucleosis is the most common clinically evident Epstein-Barr virus infection in the United States. It is a self-limiting disease of children and young adults but occasionally causes serious complications. The incubation period is 4 to 7 weeks, followed by a prodromal phase of 3 to 5 days. This phase is characterized by headache, lethargy, and anorexia. Nausea, emesis, photophobia, and myalgia also may occur. Sore throat and dysphagia are the most common symptoms and those with oral relevance. Clinically this process often resembles exudative pharyngotonsillitis with cervical lymphadenopathy. Diagnosis is based on clinical symptoms and the serum heterophile antibody (Monospot) test, which has an accuracy rate of approximately 90%.[15] Treatment is mainly supportive.

The significance of EBV outside the United States is its association with Burkitt's lymphoma. Burkitt's lymphoma is the leading cause of lymphoma in children in Africa and is considered endemic there.[10] Often the initial symptom is a lesion in the mandible or maxilla. The prognosis for Burkitt's lymphoma is fair. Treatment consists of aggressive chemotherapy.

Varicella-zoster virus is the causative agent in chickenpox and shingles. In the pediatric population, chickenpox is the more significant concern. Although chickenpox develops classically on the trunk, oral lesions do develop. The oral lesion is very painful and primarily treated on a supportive basis. A vaccine is now available for this disease.

Adenovirus is important because it can cause pharyngoconjunctivitis in infants and children. Adenovirus characteristically occurs in the summer months and often is diagnosed based on the unique constellation of symptoms (pharyngitis and conjunctivitis) and a history of recent exposure to a contaminated swimming pool. Treatment is supportive therapy.

RIBONUCLEIC ACID VIRUSES

Paramyxoviruses   Measles (rubeola) is a common viral disease with high morbidity in children. Vaccination is common today and has greatly diminished the incidence. Patients with measles often have a transient illness characterized by fever and vomiting followed by a 2-week period of apparent good health. The next symptoms are characteristic white spots on an erythematous base on the oral mucosa; these are known as Koplik's spots. Fever develops and a rash begins on the forehead and spreads over the rest of the body. Complications can include otitis, bronchopneumonia, croup, myocarditis, and encephalitis. Treatment is symptomatic and antibiotics are used to treat secondary infections.

Mumps (parotitis) is another common paramyxovirus. The mumps vaccine should be part of the routine pediatric immunization schedule. Initial exposure occurs in the respiratory epithelium. The virus proliferates and moves to the cervical lymph nodes and enters the bloodstream, where it involves the salivary glands. The testes, ovaries, heart, kidneys, and central nervous system also can be affected.[15] Onset of the disease is sudden and is characterized by pain, fever, headache, and swelling of the salivary glands. The swelling usually is bilateral but may not be symmetrical. The salivary duct openings are inflamed and edematous. Treatment is mainly supportive. However, because orchitis is the most frequent complication, immunoglobulin therapy may be useful in postpubertal male patients.

Picornaviruses   Coxsackievirus infections are divided into groups A (23 types) and B (at least 6 types). Coxsackieviruses cause numerous diseases; of these, herpangina and hand-foot-mouth disease have significant oral lesions.

Herpangina usually affects young children; the viruses are transmitted by close contact, fomites, or fecal contamination. The incubation period is approximately 5 days, and the onset of symptoms is sudden. Patients have fever, dysphagia, sore throat, emesis, and abdominal pain. Small gray papules appear on the palate, tongue, pharynx, and tonsils but rarely are present on the buccal mucosa and gingiva. Symptoms usually last 3 to 5 days, and the temperature may be as high as 104° F. Treatment is supportive and complete recovery usually occurs.

Hand-foot-and-mouth disease occurs mainly in children but may occur in adults. A maculopapular rash forms on the hands and feet, which may develop into vesicles. The oral lesions form on the cheeks, hard and soft palate, tongue, pharynx, and mucobuccal fold. The disease lasts several days; treatment is symptomatic.

Rubella (German measles) is a mild disease and resembles a milder form of rubeola. Rubella is dangerous because it can cause congenital defects in a fetus if the mother is infected during pregnancy. Congenital abnormalities have been reported in up to 75% of fetuses infected during the first trimester. Rubella typically manifests as a macular rash on the face, followed by migration of the rash onto the trunk and extremities. Serological testing is the most reliable diagnostic technique.

Acquired immunodeficiency syndrome has no predilection for children. However, it affects children in the same risk groups as adults and should be considered when historical information places a child in a risk category.

MYCOTIC AND PROTOZOAL INFECTIONS

Mycotic Infections Candidiasis can be a local infection of the skin or mucosa or a systemic illness, caused primarily by *Candida albicans*. The disseminated, systemic form of the disease has a high mortality rate.[13,15] The greatest predisposing factor is lowered host resistance, which may occur in immunosuppressive diseases, immunosuppressive therapy, vitamin deficiencies, or other systemic illnesses. The most common manifestation in children is oral thrush. These oral lesions can develop in an apparently healthy infant shortly after birth. The lesions are white and flaky, and the surrounding mucosa is erythematous. Treatment with nystatin and improved hygiene are recommended.

Histoplasmosis is caused by a yeastlike fungus, *Histoplasma capsulatum*. A rare form of disseminated disease occurs in infants. This form of the disease has a rapid, fatal course and may appear with granulomatous lesions on the lips, buccal mucosa, palate, and tongue.[2,15] Diagnosis is based on clinical appearance and microscopy.

Phycomycosis, also known as mucormycosis, is an opportunistic fungal disease that typically occurs in individuals with severely impaired immunological resistance. The classic presentation of this disease is orbital cellulitis in a patient with acidotic diabetes mellitus.[15] It is cause by *Rhizopus oryzae*.[7] Phycomycosis is accompanied by unilateral headache, epistaxis, red-black necrotic appearance of nasal mucosa, and, in some cases, necrotic lesions of the palate. Treatment focuses on control of underlying disease, excision of necrotic tissue, and chemotherapy with amphotericin B.

Protozoal Infections Amoebic meningoencephalitis (Naegleria) is associated with children swimming in freshwater lakes and ponds. The organism is found throughout the United States and other parts of the world. This disease usually occurs in the summer months, and the amoeba enters the cribriform plate through the nasal mucosa. Symptoms include epistaxis, severe frontal headache, lethargy, and fever. The disease usually is fatal within 96 to 120 hours of the onset of symptoms.[2] The disease is treated with amphotericin B but usually is recognized too late to prevent death (Table 21-4).

TABLE 21-4

Lymphadenitis in Children

Primary Disease	Involved Node or Nodes	Node Characteristics
Acute Unilateral Adenitis		
Pharyngitis or tonsillitis	Jugulodigastric	
Periapical dental abscess	Submandibular	
Impetigo of the face	Submental or submandibular	Pyogenic, tender
Infected acne	Submental or submandibular	
Otitis externa	Preauricular	
Acute Bilateral Adenitis		
Nonspecific viral pharyngitis	Cervical	
Herpes simplex	Submandibular or submental	
Gingivostomatitis involving gingiva and		Nonpyogenic, tender
buccal mucosa		
Group A streptococcal infection	Cervical	
Infectious mononucleosis	Cervical or generalized	
Diphtheria	Cervical	Pyogenic, tender
Tularemia	Varies with site of infection	
Subacute Adenitis		
Cat-scratch disease	Varies with site of injury	
Infection with atypical	Submandibular	Granulomatous, mildly tender
mycobacteria		
Cervical Node Cancers		
Reticulum cell sarcoma		
Leukemia	Cervical or generalized	Firm to hard, nontender
Hodgkin's disease		
Lymphosarcoma		
Primary nasopharyngeal tumors	Cervical	Firm to hard, nontender
(e.g., rhabdomyosarcoma)		
Thyroid cancer		

From Schmitt BD: Pediatrics: cervical adenopathy in children, *Postgrad Med* 60:251, 1976.

SUMMARY

Diagnosis and management of diseases in children is a complex process. Maxillofacial infections are no exception. An accurate history, thorough physical examination, and astute laboratory testing do not always ensure a definitive diagnosis. However, maxillofacial surgeons can rely on the available statistical evidence and approach the diagnosis and treatment of maxillofacial infections in children armed with certain information. The statistical evidence of considering anatomical location and patient age as critical information in determining diagnosis, initial therapy, and prognosis has been clearly demonstrated. This ability to improve the efficiency with which a definitive diagnosis is made, coupled with an in-depth knowledge of specific disease management, create a rational approach to treatment of infections in children. Close follow-up is an important factor in successful treatment of infections in children. Children's conditions improve and deteriorate much faster than in adults, and clinicians must be prepared for either eventuality.

REFERENCES

1. Barkin RM: Facial and periorbital cellulitis in children, *J Emerg Med* 1:195, 1984.
2. Brown HW, Neva FA: *Basic clinical parasitology,* Norwalk, Conn, 1983, Appleton-Century-Crofts.
3. Dodson TB, Barton JA, Kaban LB: Predictors of outcome in children hospitalized with maxillofacial infections: a linear logistic model, *J Oral Maxillofac Surg* 49:838, 1991.
4. Dodson TB, Kaban LB: Diagnosis and management of pediatric facial infections, *Oral Maxillofac Surg Clin North Am* 6:13, 1994.
5. Dodson TB, Perrott DH, Kaban LB: Pediatric maxillofacial infections: a retrospective study of 113 patients, *J Oral Maxillofac Surg* 47:327, 1989.
6. Fleisher G, Heeger P, Topf P: *Haemophilus influenzae* cellulitis, *Am J Emerg Med* 3:274, 1983.
7. Gilbert DN, Moellering RC Jr, Sande MA: *The Sanford guide to antimicrobial therapy,* ed 30, Vienna, Va, Antimicrobial Therapy Inc, 2000.
8. Goldberg M: Antibiotics: old friends and new acquaintances, *Oral Maxillofac Surg Clin North Am* 13:15, 2001.
9. Israele V, Nelson JD: Periorbital and orbital cellulitis, *Pediatr Infect Dis J* 6:404, 1987.
10. Johnson JT, Yu VL: *Infectious diseases and antimicrobial therapy of the ears, nose and throat,* Philadelphia, 1997, WB Saunders.
11. Kaban LB: *Pediatric oral and maxillofacial surgery,* Philadelphia, 1990, WB Saunders.
12. Sabiston DC Jr: *Sabiston's essentials of surgery,* Philadelphia, 1987, WB Saunders.
13. Schwartz SI: *Principles of surgery,* New York, 1989, McGraw-Hill.
14. Smith TF, O'Day D, Wright PF: Clinical implications of preseptal (periorbital) cellulitis in childhood, *Pediatrics* 62:1006, 1978.
15. Topazian RG, Goldberg MH: *Oral and maxillofacial infections,* ed 3, Philadelphia, 1993, WB Saunders.

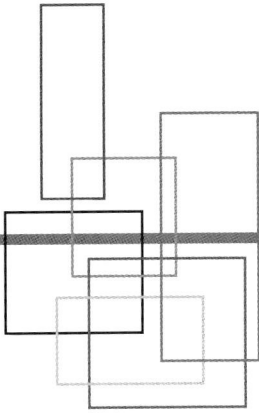

Uncommon Inflammatory Conditions and Infections of the Orofacial Region

Richard G. Topazian

This chapter discusses uncommon problems that are not presented elsewhere in this book or are of sufficient importance to the practitioner to warrant additional emphasis.

PATHOGENIC FUNGI WITH MAXILLOFACIAL MANIFESTATIONS

Most fungi are saprophytes and rarely cause human disease. However, fungal diseases may occur when defense mechanisms are compromised because of an underlying disease or the action of immunosuppressive drugs. Prolonged antibiotic treatment, long-term steroid therapy, immunosuppressive and antimetabolic drugs, immunodeficiency disease, chronic alcoholism, drug abuse, hematopoietic neoplasms, and diabetes may predispose an individual to fungal diseases. Fungal diseases also may occur in apparently healthy individuals who have received a large or persistent inoculum. Of 100,000 species of fungi, approximately 20 are known to cause systemic infection, 20 are regularly isolated from cutaneous infections, and 12 are associated with severe subcutaneous disease. Many opportunistic species cause disease in patients who are medically compromised.

Among the diseases caused by pathogenic or opportunistic fungi are the systemic mycoses. Two diseases caused by opportunistic fungi that are seen with increasing frequency are aspergillosis and mucormycosis (zygomycosis, phycomycosis).

ASPERGILLOSIS

Aspergillosis is caused by members of the genus *Aspergillus,* a ubiquitous mold present in soil, decaying vegetation, and all types of organic debris. Because its spores can be airborne, it is a common laboratory contaminant. Three species, *Aspergillus fumigatus, Aspergillus niger*, and *Aspergillus flavus*, account for most instances of human infections. It occurs in apparently healthy individuals, although increasingly it is seen in patients who are immunocompromised or chronically debilitated, particularly patients with cancer.[12,41]

The disease is characterized by granulomatous inflammation with lesions of the skin, external ear, nasal sinuses, orbit, eye, bronchi, lungs, and occasionally other organs, including the brain. Unlike other fungal diseases, aspergillosis often occurs without predisposing factors, although it can be seen in medically compromised patients.

The three general categories of clinical aspergillosis are allergic, colonizing, and invasive. Invasive aspergillosis may be disseminated and occurs most often in patients with an underlying disease such as leukemia, lymphoma, or alcoholic cirrhosis, and in patients being treated with steroids, antibiotics, or immunosuppressive or cytotoxic drugs. Dissemination results from disruption of the normal flora, an abnormal inflammatory response, lowered resistance caused by debilitating disease or drugs, and a point of entry for the fungus.

Nasoorbital (sinoorbital) aspergillosis is important to oral and maxillofacial surgeons and others involved in the diagnosis and treatment of lesions in this region. The fungus may occur primarily in the maxilla and orbit or may be derived from respiratory secretions in patients with pulmonary aspergillosis. Sinusitis may allow this saprophytic organism to become sufficiently established to elicit a granulomatous response.

Nasoorbital aspergillosis generally is characterized by an aspergilloma of the sinus that may involve the orbit and its contents and the brain. The presenting symptoms are sinusitis that has not responded to conventional medical or surgical measures or sinusitis associated with swelling of the orbital soft tissues, causing unilateral proptosis. A malodorous nasal discharge may be present, and the turbinates may be swollen and gangrenous. Occasionally blindness occurs.

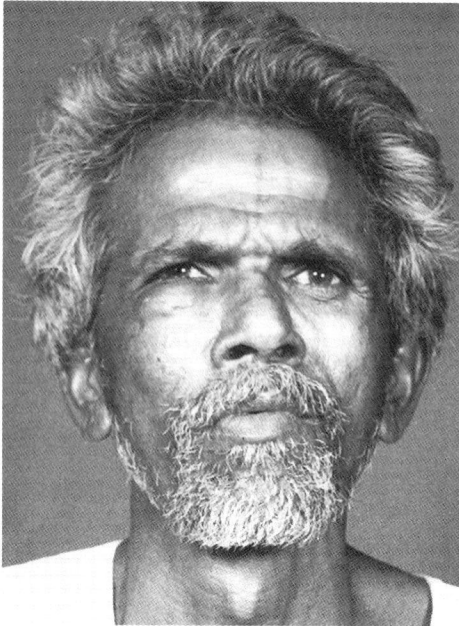

Figure 22-1 Aspergillosis manifested as a firm swelling of 3 years' duration in a 50-year-old farmer. Radiographs showed opacity of the right maxillary sinus and bone destruction of the sinus walls. A chest radiograph suggested pulmonary aspergillosis, but this could not be confirmed by biopsy because the patient refused to have the procedure. Biopsy of the maxillary lesion was consistent with the diagnosis of aspergillosis.

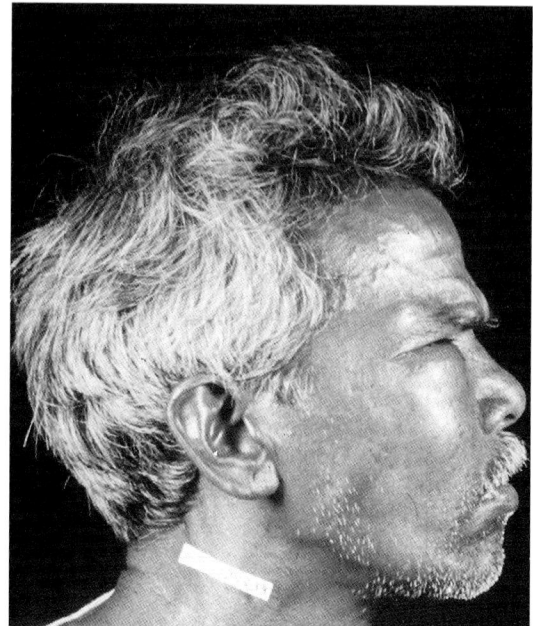

Figure 22-2 Lateral view of patient in Figure 22-1 shows swelling.

A review of 17 patients with paranasal aspergillosis showed 15 patients with proptosis, 8 with ethmoidal mucosal swelling, 8 with maxillary mucosal swelling, and 2 with both ethmoidal and maxillary mucosal swelling.[33] Endonasal granulomas and polyps were seldom present, and loss of vision occurred in approximately 12% of the patients studied. The facial lesions typically were firm and painless, and the duration of the disease ranged from 4 months to 10 years. A significant minority of patients with chronic invasive sinus aspergillosis have diabetes, use alcohol excessively, or have acquired immunodeficiency syndrome (AIDS).[9]

Radiographically ethmoidal, antral, and ethmoidoantral forms of aspergillosis are found (Figures 22-1 through 22-5), and bone may or may not be involved (see Figure 22-5). The differential diagnosis includes suppurative sinusitis, malignancy of the sinus, and other types of fungal disease such as rhinocerebral mucormycosis. Culture of specimens produces the typical conidiophore and spore chains. Microscopic examination of frozen paraffin sections of *Aspergillus* reveals hyphae 3 to 12 μm thick with distinct cross septa at intervals (Figures 22-6 and 22-7).[10] Erlichman and Trieger[16] described a facial form of aspergillosis in a patient receiving immunosuppressant drugs caused by *A. fumigatus* and characterized by submental space swelling and abscess formation. (See Chapters 3 and 11 for a detailed discussion of culture and identification techniques and a description of typical fungal diseases.)

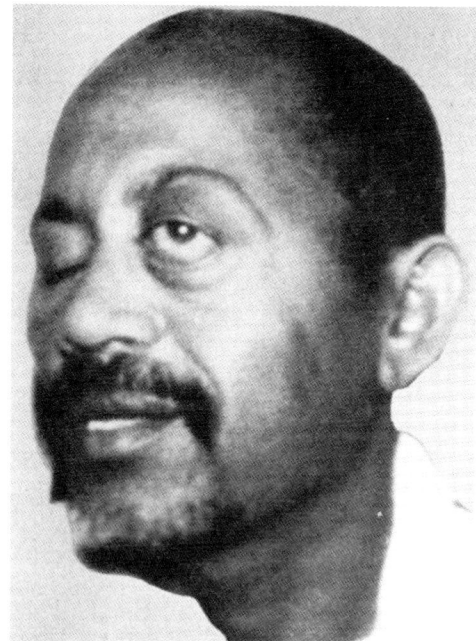

Figure 22-3 Left proptosis caused by advanced maxillary sinus aspergillosis. (From Mahgoub ES, Osman AA: Primary aspergilloma of paranasal sinuses in the Sudan: a review of seventeen cases, *Br J Surg* 56:132, 1969.)

Treatment The preferred treatment for aspergillosis consists of surgical excision, adjunctive antifungal therapy, and supportive care. If untreated, the disease is almost always fatal.[10] As much of the lesion should be removed as possible without damaging vital structures. The surgical opening should be large enough to allow continued drainage. Accordingly, the Caldwell-Luc approach is used

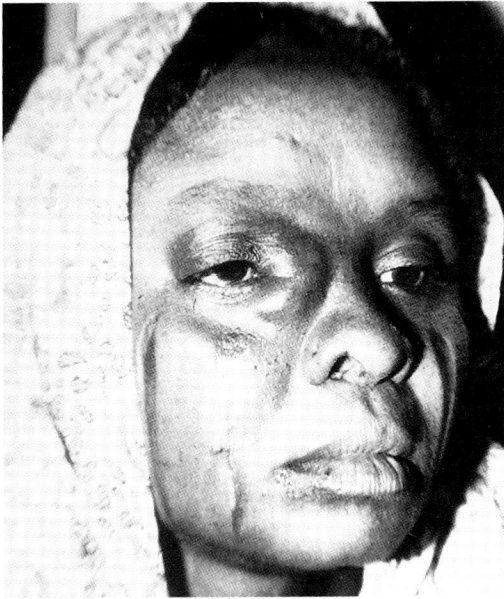

Figure 22-4 Right ethmoidal aspergilloma with proptosis and characteristic swelling of the medial canthal region. (From Mahgoub ES, Osman AA: Primary aspergilloma of paranasal sinuses in the Sudan: a review of seventeen cases, *Br J Surg* 56:132, 1969.)

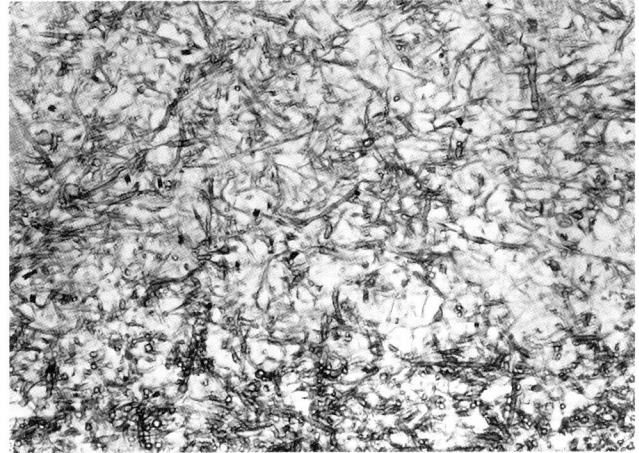

Figure 22-6 Biopsy of soft tissue mass shows segments of septate lyphae consistent with aspergillosis, some of which are cut at right angles so that they resemble spores. (×360, Gomori's methamine silver stain.) (Courtesy S. Roser, New York, NY.)

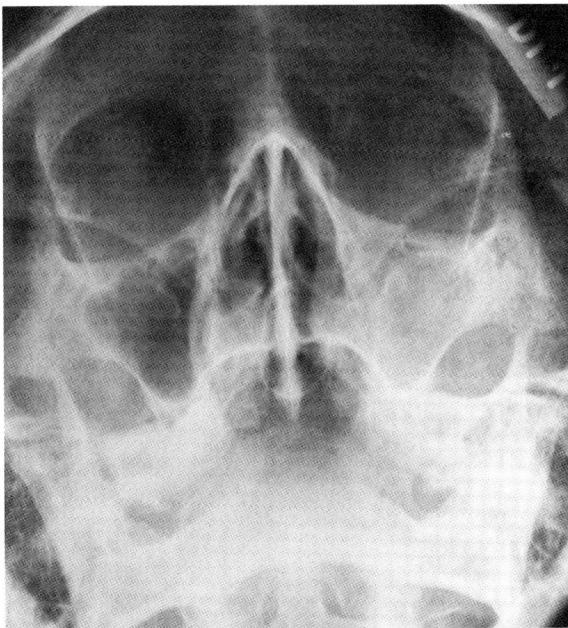

Figure 22-5 Opacity of the left maxillary sinus in a 55-year-old woman with aspergillosis. (Courtesy S. Roser, New York, NY.)

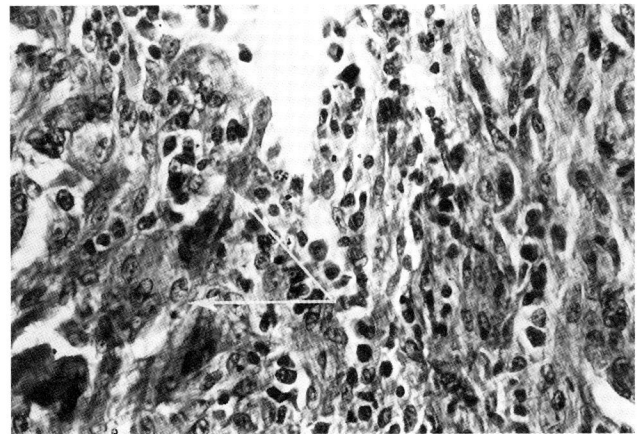

Figure 22-7 High-power view of a granulomatous lesion composed of fibrous tissue infiltrated by lymphocytes and giant cells containing elongated septate fungal filaments *(arrows)* that are consistent with aspergillosis. (Periodic acid–Schiff stain.)

for maxillary sinus disease to permit the wide removal of the medial antral wall. A radical ethmoidectomy is used when the ethmoid sinuses are involved. Medicated packs may be placed loosely in surgical defects for the initial postoperative period, but they should be removed within several days to permit drainage. Broad-spectrum antifun-

gal therapy alone is not effective for nasoorbital aspergillosis. However, it is valuable as an adjunct to surgery. Intravenous amphotericin B is the drug of choice for invasive disease; however, when the lung or paranasal sinuses are affected, the drug is not effective as the sole therapy but should be combined with surgery.[4] Flucytosine with amphotericin B is no more effective than amphotericin B alone according to some studies.[13] A combination of flucytosine and rifampin has been used successfully in a patient with orbital aspergillosis.[52] The prognosis for recovery is good, and cures have been achieved with surgery alone. When amphotericin B is used, a daily dose of 0.8 to 1.5 mg/kg per day or up to double that dose given every other day for a minimum total dose of 2.5 to 3.0 g should be administered to adult patients. This treatment extends for 6 to 8 weeks, and close monitoring for possible side effects is required.[21] Amphotericin B therapy is described more fully subsequently. Inhalation of a nystatin mist may be useful in the treatment of pulmonary aspergillosis.

RHINOCEREBRAL MUCORMYCOSIS (ZYGOMYCOSIS, PHYCOMYCOSIS)

Mucormycosis is an uncommon, acute fungal disease with a high mortality rate. It occurs in rhinocerebral, pulmonary, cutaneous, gastrointestinal, central nervous system, and disseminated forms.[18,46] Rhinocerebral mucormycosis is the type that most frequently involves the structures of the head. The fungus is widespread and occurs in soil, in manure, on vegetables and fruits, and as bread mold. It is a common laboratory contaminant. The disease in humans is caused by the genera *Mucor, Rhizopus,* and *Absidia* rather than by *Mucor* alone.

The rhinocerebral form of the disease occurs predominantly in dehydrated and acidotic patients, particularly in patients with poorly controlled diabetes, patients with leukemia, and occasionally in patients with kidney transplants.[24,25,34] It occurs in children who have become dehydrated from vomiting and diarrhea, in individuals with renal disease, in those undergoing dialysis, and in association with corticosteroid or cytotoxic therapy in patients with hematological neoplasms.

The patient initially has signs and symptoms primarily in the intraoral, facial, orbital, paranasal sinus, or cerebral regions. Symptoms referable to these areas in patients who are dehydrated and acidotic warrant a high index of suspicion. Because of its lethal nature, rhinocerebral mucormycosis must be recognized early and treated aggressively. Death can occur within several days of the onset of symptoms even when appropriate treatment has been instituted.

Clinical Features   In a comprehensive article, Schwartz et al.[43] reviewed 99 cases. Among 70 patients, palatal ulceration was present in 39%, facial swelling in 34%, facial discoloration in 20%, facial necrosis in 14%, nasal eschar or ulceration in 47%, proptosis in 66%, periorbital edema in 61%, and ptosis in 40%. Eighty percent of the patients had diabetes, and patient ages ranged from 2 months to 76 years (Figures 22-8 through 22-11). The disease can affect the mandible alone or the mandible and maxilla in the same patient.[5,15]

Pillsbury and Fischer[40] reviewed 13 cases and found facial swelling, intranasal necrosis, lethargy, fever, and headache in all patients. Decreased vision was present in 92%, dehydration in 85%, acidosis in 77%, and facial nerve

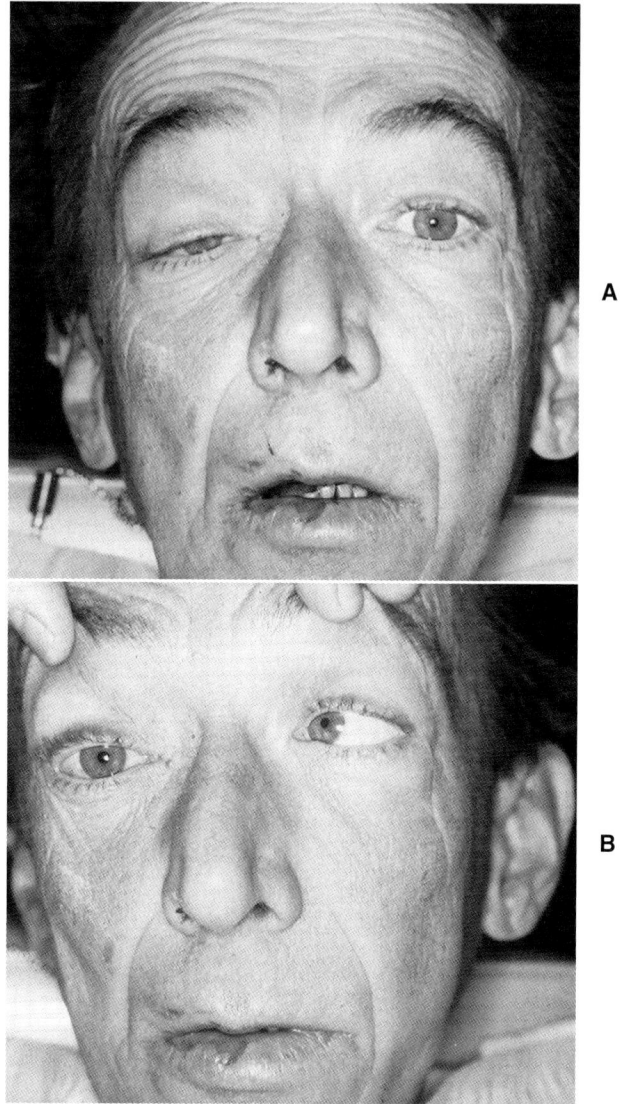

Figure 22-8 A, Necrotic area of the right palate and proven mucormycosis in a 48-year-old man with ketoacidosis with fasting blood glucose level of 420 mg/100 mL. Maxillary posterior teeth had been extracted because of right facial pain of 18 months' duration. A sanguineous discharge from the right nostril had been present for 1 month. Internal and external ophthalmoplegia was present with corneal anesthesia but with no pupillary dilation. Right-sided ptosis was the most obvious sign of disease. **B,** Paralysis of right lateral rectus muscle (cranial nerve VI) demonstrated when attempt was made to direct the right eye laterally. (From Berger CL, Disque FC, Topazian RG: Rhinocerebral mucormycosis: diagnosis and treatment, *Oral Surg* 40:27, 1975.)

palsy in 77%. Other investigators have reported that the palate or alveolar process is affected in 66% of patients. The prognosis is better when orbital signs are not present.[30] The most constant findings are facial pain and headache.

Pathogenesis   Mucormycosis probably is initiated in the susceptible individual by the inhalation of spores into the nasal passages. The fungi invade arteries, causing thrombosis with central extension, ischemia, and dry gangrene of the affected structures. As the disease progresses from the nose to the orbit and skull, the patient may become

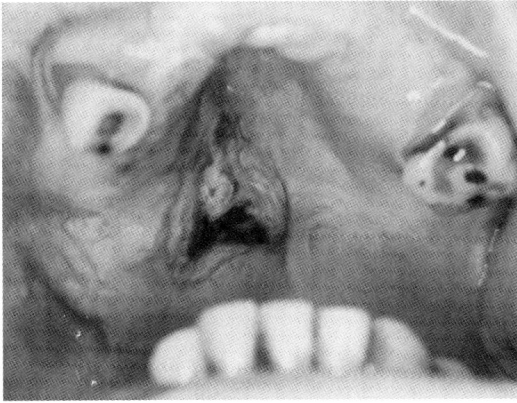

Figure 22-9 Characteristic necrotic area on the palate associated with thrombosis of the sphenopalatine artery. Necrosis of the nasal turbinates also may be seen in mucormycosis. (From Berger CL, Disque FC, Topazian RG: Rhinocerebral mucormycosis: diagnosis and treatment, *Oral Surg* 40:27, 1975.)

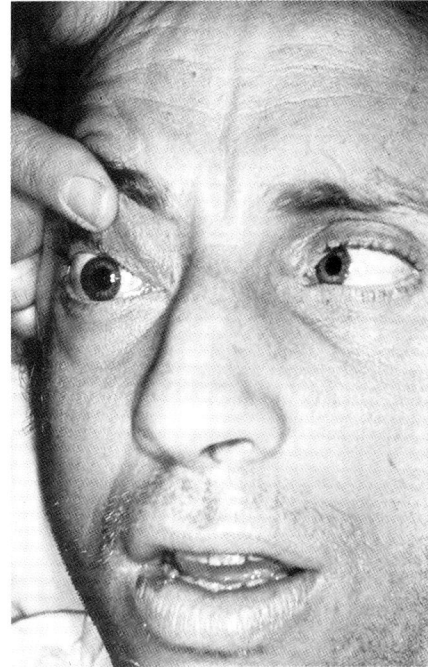

Figure 22-11 Dilated and fixed right pupil and weakness of the right lateral rectus muscle in a 33-year-old man with diabetic ketoacidosis. Cranial nerves III, IV, V, and VI were affected. The right palate and alveolar process showed signs of gangrenous necrosis. The patient developed left hemiplegia and became comatose. He was treated with insulin, amphotericin B, and antibiotics. After a prolonged hospitalization, he recovered and subsequently was discharged. (From Tabachnick TT, Levine B: Mucormycosis of the craniofacial structures, *J Oral Surg* 33:164, 1975.)

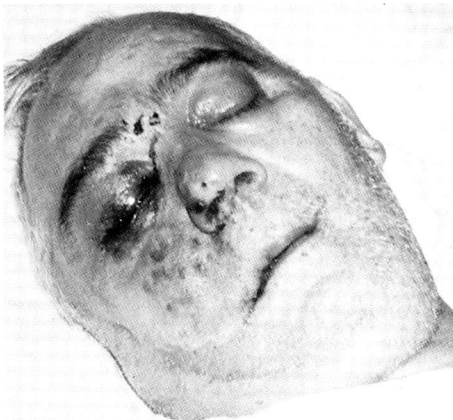

Figure 22-10 Orbital cellulitis and ecchymosis of the right side of the face were prominent signs of rhinocerebral mucormycosis in this 63-year-old patient with diabetes whose blood glucose level at admission was 590 mg/100 mL and whose urinary acetone level was 3+. A maxillary third molar had been extracted for facial pain 5 days earlier. The patient had been admitted to the hospital because of worsening facial pain but became comatose and died 1 day after admission despite intensive treatment. Marked gangrenous necrosis was present on the right palate and alveolar process. (From Eilderton TE: Fatal postextraction cerebral mucormycosis in an unknown diabetic, *J Oral Surg* 32:297, 1974.)

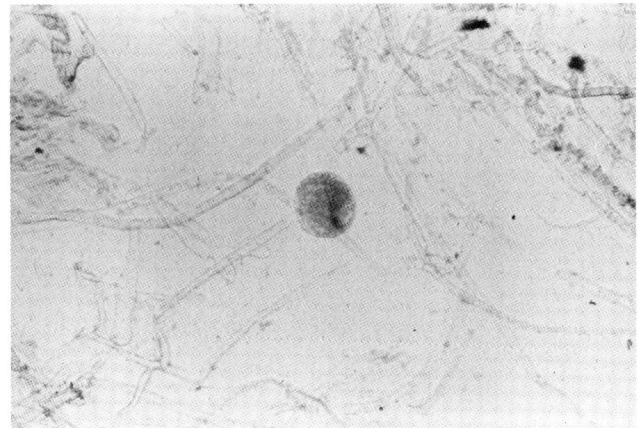

Figure 22-12 Microscopic appearance of mucormycosis, with long, broad, branching, nonseptate hyphae with terminal globose sporangia.

confused, obtunded, and comatose.[14,19] Orbital signs and symptoms result from vascular compromise of the orbital contents caused by thrombosis of the ethmoid arteries with central extension through the sphenopalatine artery. When the apex of the orbit is affected, the organisms extend through the lateral wall of the cavernous sinus and involve the internal carotid artery with resultant cerebral ischemia and brain infarction.

Microscopically the fungus consists of wide, uneven, nonseptate, branching hyphae 6 to 50 μm wide with long sporangiophores (Figures 22-12 and 22-13). It grows in 2 to 9 days on Sabouraud's agar and must be distinguished from *Aspergillus,* which is smaller and septate, with more

acute branching than *Rhizopus* and *Mucor.* Direct examination and culture of scraping and biopsy specimens are necessary for diagnosis.

Differential Diagnosis   When the cerebral and orbital features predominate, the differential diagnosis includes meningitis, superior orbital syndrome, cavernous sinus

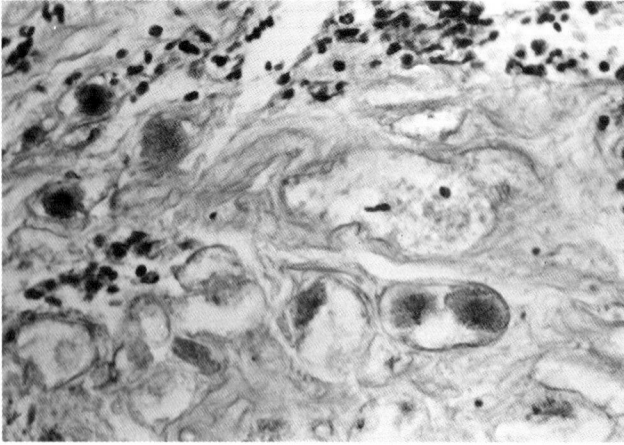

Figure 22-13 Sporangia of mucormycosis present in necrotic palatal tissue.

thrombosis, diabetic polyneuritis, retrobulbar tumor, and retroorbital abscess. Other fungal diseases, particularly aspergillosis, must be distinguished from rhinocerebral mucormycosis because the sites and predisposing causes for both diseases are similar. Necrosis and sloughing of facial soft tissues suggestive of noma rarely occur.

Paralysis of cranial nerves III, IV, and VI is common and causes external and internal ophthalmoplegia. Cranial nerves V and VII are affected in approximately one third of cases, resulting in corneal anesthesia and pupillary dilation. Loss of vision also may occur. The disease usually is unilateral. Orbital cellulitis from other causes should be distinguished from mucormycosis (see Chapter 15).

On examination a fetid, purulosanguineous exudate commonly is seen on the nasal mucosa. The nasal turbinates become dark and necrotic. Palatal involvement begins as a unilateral, gray necrotic area overlying the distribution of the sphenopalatine artery, particularly the anterior (greater) palatine branch. The alveolar processes and the anterior maxilla also may become necrotic because of nasopalatine artery involvement.

The nose is the most common site of initiation of this form of the disease and is associated with direct extension to the paranasal sinuses, orbit, and cranial cavity. Odontalgia and extraction of maxillary teeth have been associated with the onset of acute symptoms. Whether the toothache is the inciting cause or the result of sinus disease remains unclear. In some cases with orbital involvement, no clinical evidence of sinus or nasal disease exists.

Treatment   Early recognition of symptoms and institution of vigorous surgical and medical therapy are essential in the proper management of mucormycosis. Rapid correction of dehydration and acidosis and administration of insulin in patients with diabetes are required. Alternative treatment for the primary disease should be considered in patients receiving antibiotics, immunosuppressive agents, or antineoplastic drugs. Amphotericin B (Fungizone) is the antifungal agent of choice (daily dosage 1.0 to 1.5 mg/kg per day), although isolates may be resistant in vitro. Am-

photericin B is fungistatic in patient serum 48 hours after alternate-day doses of 1.0 mg/kg and can be given intravenously by one of several regimens. Generally a total dose of 2 to 4 g should be given over 6 to 12 weeks. Administration of small doses over a long interval minimizes toxicity and undesirable side effects.

Initially a test dose of 1 mg in 50 to 150 mL of 5% dextrose in water is given intravenously over 20 to 30 minutes with careful monitoring for side effects, particularly chills, fever, phlebitis, renal damage, and anaphylaxis. On the second day the patient is given 0.25 mg/kg in 500 mL of 5% dextrose in water over 2 to 6 hours. The dose is increased daily in increments of 5 mg until the daily dose of 0.6 mg/kg is achieved. If minor side effects such as headache, nausea, vomiting, and fever occur during the first few days or weeks, the drug may be given on alternate days at a dose of 1.0 to 1.2 mg/kg. Although creatinine clearance has been advocated as an excellent means of monitoring toxicity, if the blood urea nitrogen level exceeds 40 mg/100 mL or the serum creatinine level exceeds 3.0 mg/100 mL, consideration should be given to temporarily decreasing the dosage. Flucytosine given with amphotericin B offers no advantage over amphotericin B alone.[13]

Surgical treatment to remove necrotic material and establish drainage of all involved sinuses is essential. Accordingly, nasal septectomy, sphenoid sinusotomy, the Lynch operation (exposure of the frontal sinus through the frontal sinus floor through the orbit), intranasal ethmoidectomy, Caldwell-Luc operation with large nasal antrostomy, and partial palatectomy often are required (Figure 22-14). Irrigation of the antrum with amphotericin B solutions has been advocated in the past but has not proved effective. Orbital exenteration is necessary if vision has been lost.

Hyperbaric oxygen has been used as an adjunct to aggressive surgical debridement, amphotericin B, and control of the underlying predisposing conditions. Hyperbaric oxygen is fungistatic in vitro and reduces tissue hypoxia and acidosis.[18]

Prognosis   Long-term survival ranges from 50 to 85% in patients treated with surgery and amphotericin B. Variable recovery of cranial nerve function has been reported.

■ CASE REPORT ■

A 48-year-old man was admitted to a hospital medical service with severe pain and anesthesia of the right side of the face. Eighteen months earlier the patient had severe toothaches in the maxillary right quadrant. Extraction of the maxillary right premolars and first molar did not relieve the pain. Diabetes mellitus had been diagnosed 1 year before admission, and the patient was following an American Diabetic Association diet and taking chlorpropamide (Diabinese), 250 mg three times per day. Follow-up was erratic because of poor cooperation by the patient. A bloody nasal discharge was noted 1 month before admission. The patient's physician started antibiotic and analgesic therapy. Over the next several days the areas innervated by the right

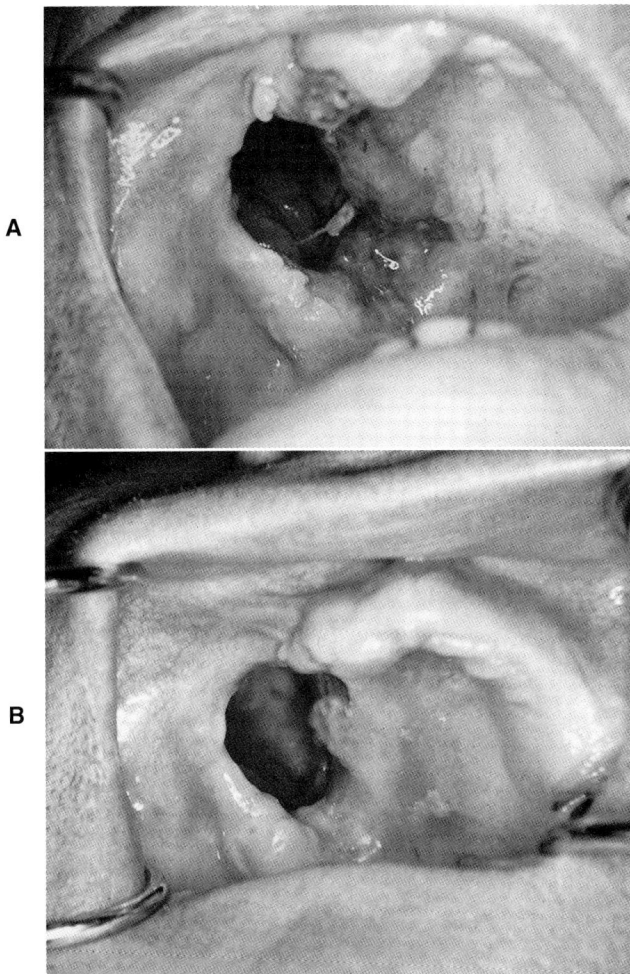

Figure 22-14 A, Result of partial palatectomy in a patient with mucormycosis. Organisms were found in the sphenopalatine artery (see Figure 22-9). **B,** Site of palatectomy 2 years after surgery. The defect was obturated initially by a complete denture and subsequently was closed surgically.

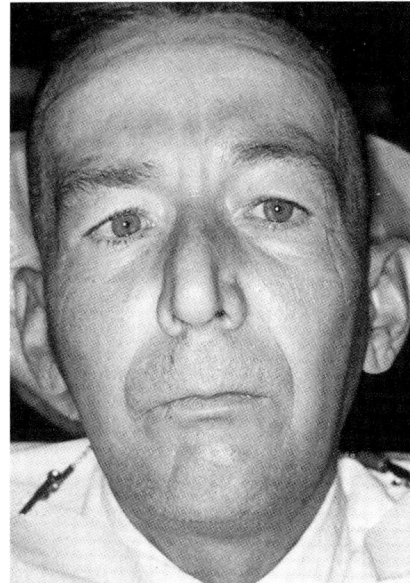

Figure 22-15 Follow-up photograph of patient in Figure 22-8, *A* 2 years after successful treatment of mucormycosis with amphotericin B, control of diabetes, and partial palatectomy. Third cranial nerve function had returned.

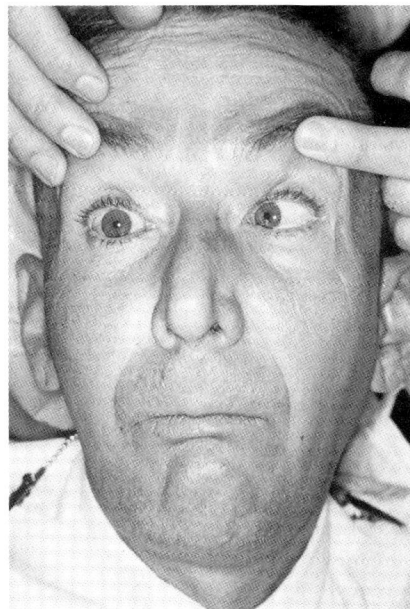

Figure 22-16 Persistent paralysis of the right lateral rectus muscle (cranial nerve VI) 2 years after treatment of mucormycosis (see Figure 22-8, *B*).

frontal, maxillary, and mandibular nerves exhibited paresthesia. During the week before admission, analgesics were less effective in controlling pain and the patient was referred to the hospital for treatment.

Examination revealed total right ophthalmoplegia, ptosis, decreased vision of the right eye, and a necrotic area of the hard palate (see Figures 22-8 and 22-9). The differential diagnosis included carcinoma of the palate, carcinoma of the maxillary antrum, and rhinocerebral mucormycosis.

The patient was admitted to the hospital with mild ketoacidosis. Laboratory findings at admission included hemoglobin, 13.2 g/100 mL; hematocrit, 42%; white blood cell count, 7500/mm³; and fasting blood glucose concentration, 420 mg/100 mL. Radiographic examination revealed considerable membrane thickening and an air-fluid level in the right maxillary antrum. Biopsy of the palatal ulceration was performed, and a diagnosis of rhinocerebral mucormycosis was made (see Figure 22-13).

The patient received amphotericin B for 4 weeks. The dosage was increased until a daily dose of 1 mg/kg was reached. Surgical therapy included excision of the necrotic area of the hard palate and a right partial palatectomy. The surgical site healed well, and a prosthesis was inserted (see Figure 22-14, *B*).

The patient was discharged 2 months after admission and was seen as an outpatient 1 year later. He was in good health, and the diabetes was well controlled. The right eye ptosis resolved completely, but the patient had not regained function of the ipsilateral fourth and sixth cranial nerves[3] (Figures 22-15 and 22-16).

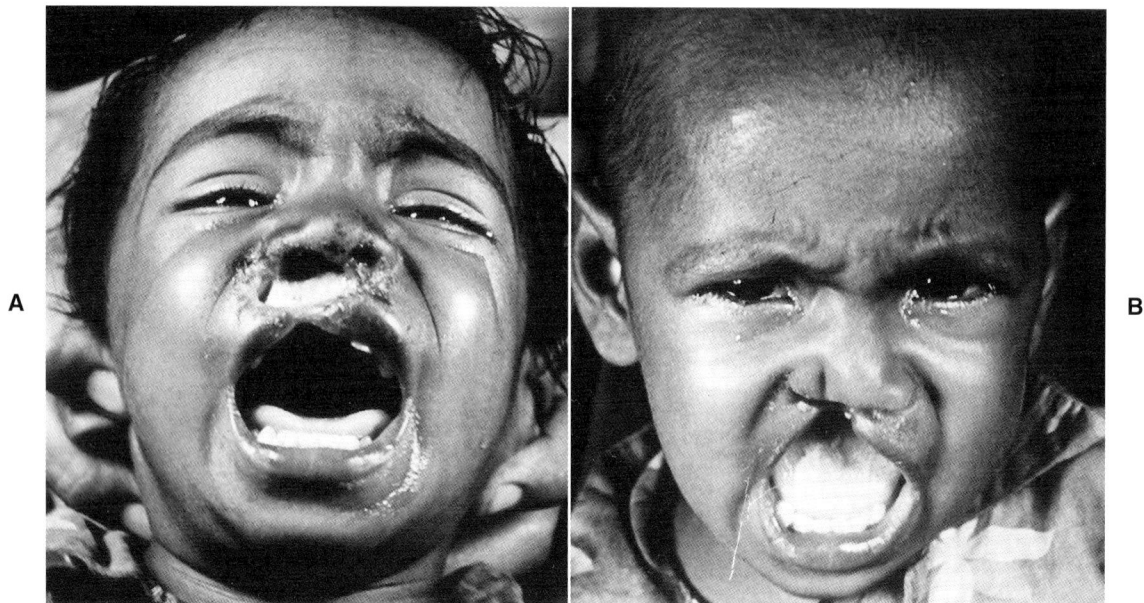

Figure 22-17 A, Marked necrosis of the soft tissues of the upper lip and anterior maxilla in a 4-year-old child with noma. Correction of the nutritional status and antibiotic therapy arrested the progression of the disease. **B,** Facial deformity resulting from noma. The necrotic anterior portion of the maxilla sloughed after 2 weeks of treatment producing the defect shown.

NOMA AND NOMALIKE LESIONS

Noma, also known as gangrenous stomatitis and cancrum oris, is an acute, fulminating, toxic, progressive gangrenous process of the oral and facial tissues that usually is seen in children who are debilitated and poorly nourished. Early recognition, correction of predisposing factors, and the use of antibiotics have reduced the mortality from a range of 75 to 90% in the preantibiotic era to approximately 10% today.

Noma usually occurs in the presence of malnutrition and dehydration. Conditions favorable to the development of noma include famine, persistent poverty, prison camp life, and epidemics of measles, typhoid, and other febrile diseases. Noma has been described as a worldwide scourge with a global incidence of 140,000 cases.[6] In developed countries, however, a nomalike condition occurs in patients with blood dyscrasias or leukemias, and treatment is similar to that for classic noma. Although it has been recognized since antiquity, reports of the disease in the United States and in Europe first appeared in the seventeenth century.

CHARACTERISTICS OF NOMA

Clinical Features   Noma is characterized by a rapid, progressive course beginning as a small, painful, red spot or vesicle on the attached gingiva in the premolar-molar region of the mandible. A necrotic ulcer rapidly forms and exposes underlying bone. Stomatitis develops as the lesion extends outward in a conelike fashion, causing painful cellulitis of

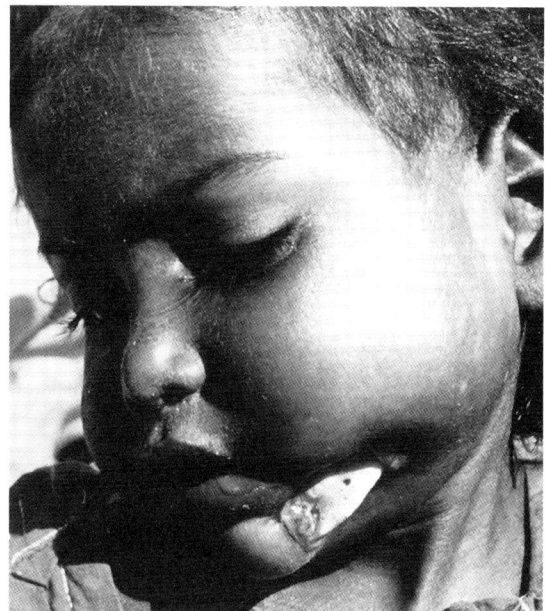

Figure 22-18 Exposure of the left side of the mandible in an 8-year-old child with noma.

the lips and cheeks. Marked salivation, fetid odor, hyperpyrexia, dehydration, leukocytosis, and a purulent oral discharge are prominent. Overlying skin becomes inflamed, edematous, dark, and necrotic. Within a short period, sloughing of soft tissues occurs, exposing underlying bone, teeth, and deeper soft tissues (Figures 22-17 and 22-18). Secondary hemorrhage is rare. The process may be arrested at any stage, particularly if treatment is instituted. If the patient's general physical condition continues to deteriorate, death usually results from pneumonia, septicemia, or persistent diarrhea.[32]

Tempest[47] reviewed the causes of cancrum oris and noted that it is primarily a disease of children younger than 10 years; 75% of cases occur in children between the ages of 2 and 5 years. Only 3 of 250 cases occurred in adults. He confirmed that febrile diseases and malnutrition are important predisposing factors. The most common predisposing diseases, in descending order of frequency, are measles, scarlet fever, typhoid, whooping cough, typhus, syphilis, tuberculosis, and leukemia. Kala-azar, kwashiorkor, and magnesium deficiency also are considered important predisposing factors.[7]

Associated gangrenous lesions in the anal region, scrotum, scalp, umbilicus, and eyelids have been noted in low-weight, ill, premature babies.[20] *Pseudomonas aeruginosa* has been cultured from these lesions, and the disease has been considered a result of *P. aeruginosa* septicemia. In a study by Ghosal et al.,[20] all but 2 of 48 affected children died within 1 to 3 days after onset of the disease despite treatment. The course of the disease was so rapid that the typical slough often was absent.

Microbiology and Pathogenesis   The fusospirochetal organisms *Borrelia vincentii* and *Fusobacterium nucleatum* (*Fusiformis fusiformis* or *Bacillus fusiformis*) consistently are cultured from noma lesions. *Prevotella melaninogenicus* also may be present. Biopsy of tissue shows a mat of predominantly gram-negative, threadlike bacteria that cannot be identified positively. *Fusobacterium necrophorum*, a pathogen primarily associated with animal disease, may have important causative and animal transmission implications.[17]

Uohara and Knapp[51] suggested that a distinct pattern of progression characterizes noma. It is initiated by acute necrotizing ulcerative gingivitis (ANUG) that leads to acute necrotizing ulcerative mucositis (Vincent's angina). Under the influence of local and systemic factors, gangrenous stomatitis, agranulocytic ulcerations, and deep necrotizing fusospirochetal infections eventually occur. Areas of gangrene result from vascular thrombosis, causing a typical bluish or purple discoloration. Sloughing of soft tissues and exposure and devitalization of underlying bone and teeth ultimately occur.

Differential Diagnosis   In its fully developed state, few diseases can be confused with cancrum oris. The patient's age, history of febrile illness, debilitated appearance, and the presence of classic signs and symptoms clearly indicate the diagnosis.

Treatment   Treatment involves control of the underlying disease, correction of nutritional deficiencies, establishment of fluid and electrolyte balance, and adminis-

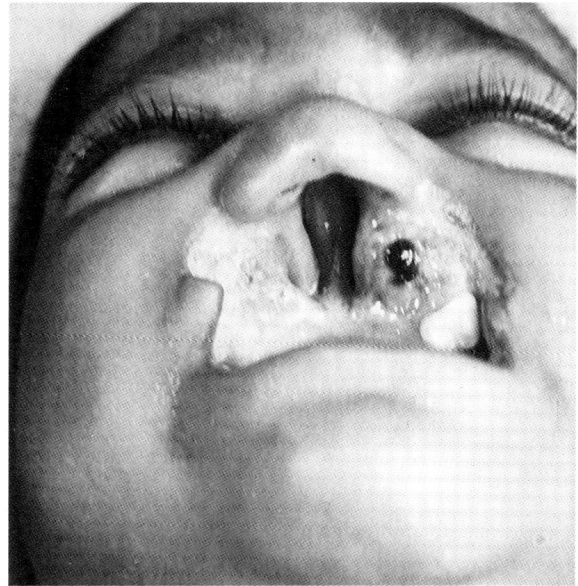

Figure 22-19 The anterior portion of the maxilla in a child with noma immediately after removal of the loose bone segment. A bed of granulation tissue and a large nasal fistula are visible.

tration of antibiotics. Penicillin is the drug of choice and initially should be given intravenously in high doses. Blood transfusions may be indicated in children with severe anemia. Local irrigation with saline solution and gentle removal of necrotic debris improve hygiene and speed resolution. Aggressive treatment with caustics, cautery, or wide excision should be avoided. After the patient's defenses have been restored and assisted with antibiotics, the inflammatory process regresses. Loose teeth and sequestra may be removed, but saucerization should be avoided. A bed of granulation tissue develops beneath sequestra and permits subsequent healing by secondary intention (Figure 22-19). If large orocutaneous defects exist, fluid leakage may be controlled initially by packing with saline solution–soaked or petroleum jelly gauze.

In the ensuing 3 to 6 months, significant quantities of scar tissue can develop that cause serious deformity and require subsequent corrective surgery (Figure 22-20; see Figures 22-17, *B;* 22-18; and 22-19). Major problems include facial deformity, persistent saliva loss through orocutaneous fistulas, trismus, facial asymmetry, and maldevelopment. Treatment of such deformities has been well described by Adolph et al.[2] and Tempest[47] and generally requires the use of local and distant flaps. One-stage reconstruction has been especially useful when scheduling of multiple procedures is difficult.[8]

True (intraarticular) ankylosis is uncommon after cancrum oris. In 229 cases of intraarticular ankylosis of the mandible from a variety of causes, cancrum oris was not found as the cause in a single instance reported by Topazian.[49,50] However, in another study, 3 of 22 patients did show true ankylosis of the temporomandibular joint (TMJ)

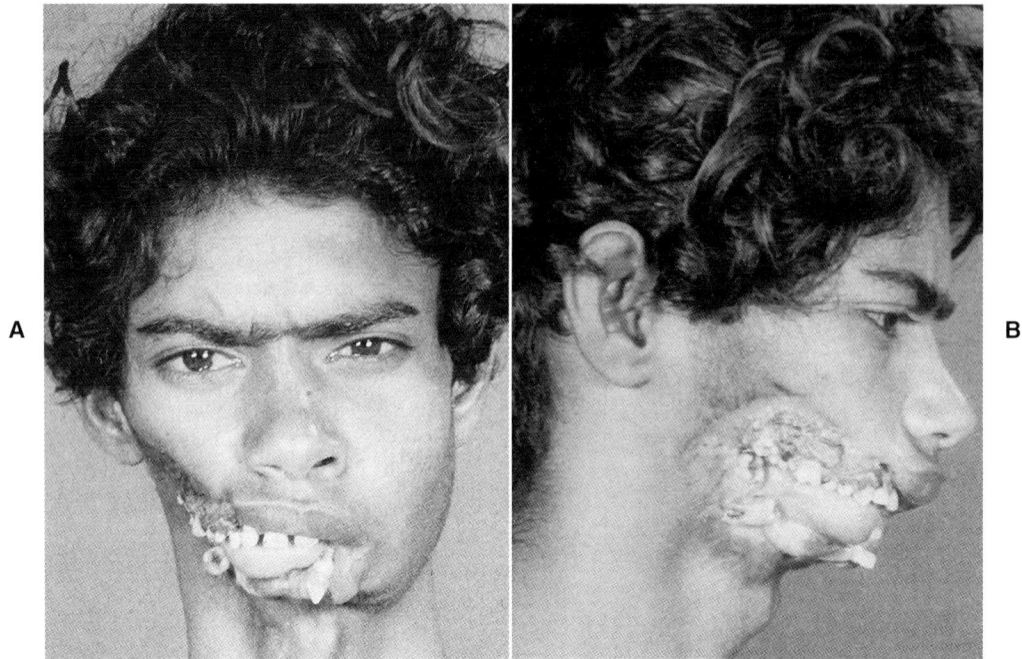

Figure 22-20 Sequelae of noma present a challenge for reconstruction.

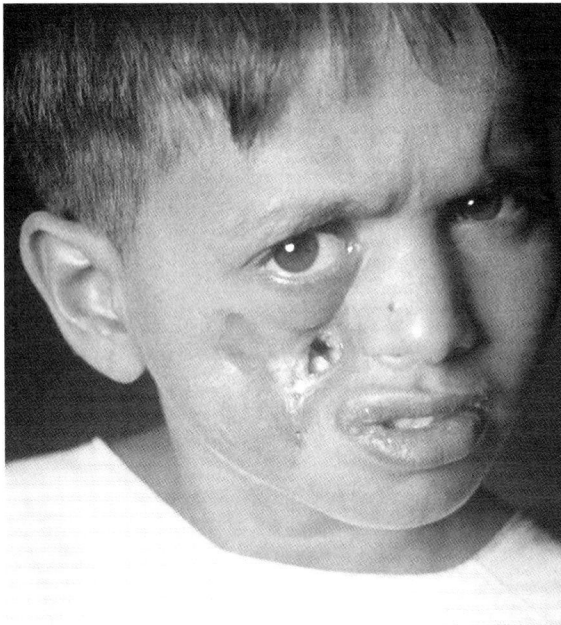

Figure 22-21 Extraarticular ankylosis subsequent to scarring of noma.

and other bone changes after cancrum oris.[26] Although intraarticular ankylosis is infrequent, false or extraarticular ankylosis is common and results from the scarring of the soft tissues of the jaws (Figure 22-21). Correction of trismus by forceful opening brisement generally is ineffective; however, excision of scar tissue between the jaws followed by grafting and possibly coronoidectomy frequently is suc-

cessful in rehabilitation of patients with noma-induced trismus.[38]

Nomalike Lesions   Individuals with compromised defenses are susceptible to a variety of infections, including pathogenic fungal lesions. In adults, nomalike conditions have been associated with chronic lymphatic leukemia, agranulocytosis, use of cytotoxic drugs, and systemic diseases such as kala-azar, tuberculosis, leprosy, and syphilis.[28] Nomalike lesions differ from true noma in that they usually occur in adults rather than in children, the predisposing cause is not a febrile disease or malnutrition, the inflammatory reaction in the surrounding soft tissues is absent, and the condition progresses slowly. The condition responds to correction of the underlying disease, antibiotic therapy, and improvement of nutritional status. If feasible, discontinuation or reduction of the dosage of cytotoxic drugs and steroids is helpful.

CAT-SCRATCH DISEASE

Cat-scratch disease is a self-limiting, benign illness characterized by malaise, inflammation of solitary lymph nodes, low-grade fever, headache, and development of a papule at the site of a cat bite or scratch, with regional lymph node involvement in approximately two thirds of patients. The disease is caused by infection with organisms of the species *Bartonella,* nearly always *Bartonella henselae* with occasional cases caused by *Afipia felis.*[45] Also known as benign lymphoreticulosis, benign inoculation lymphoreticulosis, and nonbacterial regional lymphadenitis, cat-scratch disease is common yet not generally reported because of its benign course.

CHARACTERISTICS

Because cervical and preauricular nodes are enlarged in many patients, lymph node diseases should be included in the differential diagnosis. When an illness resembles cat-scratch disease but is atypical in certain respects, the nature of the lymphadenopathy should be investigated further. Atypical manifestations include central nervous system disease, particularly encephalitis, erythema nodosum, thrombocytopenic purpura, erythema annulare, papulovesicular eruptions, maculopapular rashes, and Parinaud's oculoglandular disease. The differential diagnosis should include lymphogranuloma venereum, tularemia, tuberculosis, infectious mononucleosis, brucellosis, coccidioidomycosis, and other unilateral neck swellings.[11,23] Criteria necessary for diagnosis of cat-scratch disease include lymphadenopathy, presence of an inoculation site, absence of clinical and laboratory evidence of another disease, and history of contact with a cat.

Clinical Findings   The characteristic finding of cat-scratch disease in a child or young adolescent is a single, tender lymph node in the region draining the site of a cat scratch or bite that develops 2 to 8 weeks after injury. The lesion at the site of inoculation persists for weeks after injury. The enlarged node is variable in size (Figure 22-22), and occasionally bilateral or generalized nodal disease may occur. Multiple-node involvement is believed to be the result of a midline site or two separate sites of inoculation.[9] The nodes are tender and tend to suppurate.

The order of frequency of nodal involvement is axillary, cervical, preauricular, submandibular, epitrochlear, femoral, inguinal, and subclavicular.[25] Pain is not a prominent feature, but a low-grade fever, headache, and malaise usually are present. A history of contact with cats, particularly kittens, is usually noted, and papule formation usually occurs from 3 to 30 days after inoculation. The painful node develops approximately 2 weeks later. A flu-like syndrome of fever, malaise, anorexia, headache, and elevated temperature may be observed for several days. Patients with human immunodeficiency virus may develop skin lesions from which the cat-scratch bacillus has been demonstrated.[21]

Because of concern for potential transmission of hepatitis viruses, human immunodeficiency virus, and prions even from well-screened sources, skin testing currently is not often used. Diagnosis is based on clinical findings.[9]

Treatment and Prognosis   Within 2 months the disease usually has run its course, as seen by an absence of malaise and nodal regression. Recurrence of nodal tenderness has been reported for periods as long as 2 years. Fluctuant nodes should be aspirated. Incision and drainage should

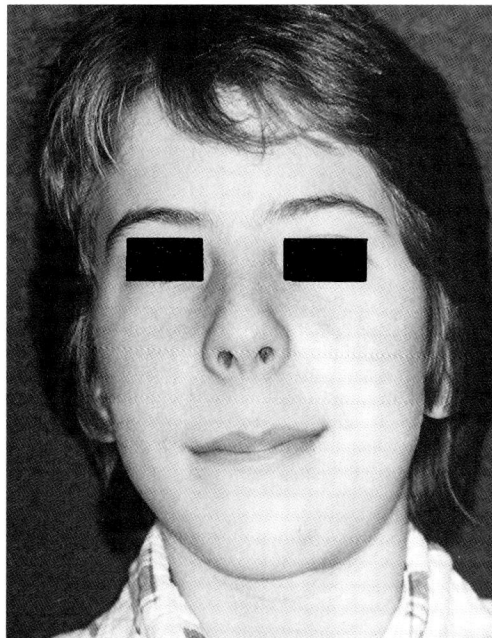

Figure 22-22 A 14-year-old patient with a 4 × 5-cm, slightly tender mass in the left submental region. One week before the onset of symptoms, his hand was scratched at home by one of numerous pet cats. Because of a lack of other positive findings, he was tested with cat-scratch skin test antigen and had a positive reaction. (From Gross BD, Case D: Cat-scratch disease, *Oral Surg* 43:698, 1977.)

be avoided because of the possibility of fistula formation. If a large node persists, it should be removed to confirm a positive skin test diagnosis or to exclude malignant disease. Antibiotics apparently do not affect the course of the disease, although erythromycin or doxycycline have been used in treatment. In 15% of cases, atypical pneumonia, acute encephalopathy sometimes terminating in death, and Parinaud's oculoglandular syndrome occur.

Parinaud's Oculoglandular Syndrome   Parinaud's oculoglandular syndrome is the most common ocular manifestation of cat-scratch fever. In 15% to 17% of patients with cat-scratch disease, unilateral conjunctivitis with a single palpebral conjunctival polypoid granulomata is found with preauricular lymphadenopathy.[10,44] Preauricular lymphadenopathy, conjunctivitis, and fever characterize this disease. Patients are only mildly ill and generally completely recover. The granulomatous area of the conjunctiva commonly is polypoid in configuration, measures 0.5 to 2.0 cm in diameter, and has an irregular nonerythematous border (Figure 22-23).

Preauricular nodes invariably are affected, and 50% of patients have cervical node involvement.[29] The disease is self-limiting but may be treated with erythromycin or doxycycline with or without rifampin.[7] The granulomatous lesions should not be surgically removed because they regress spontaneously.[9,22]

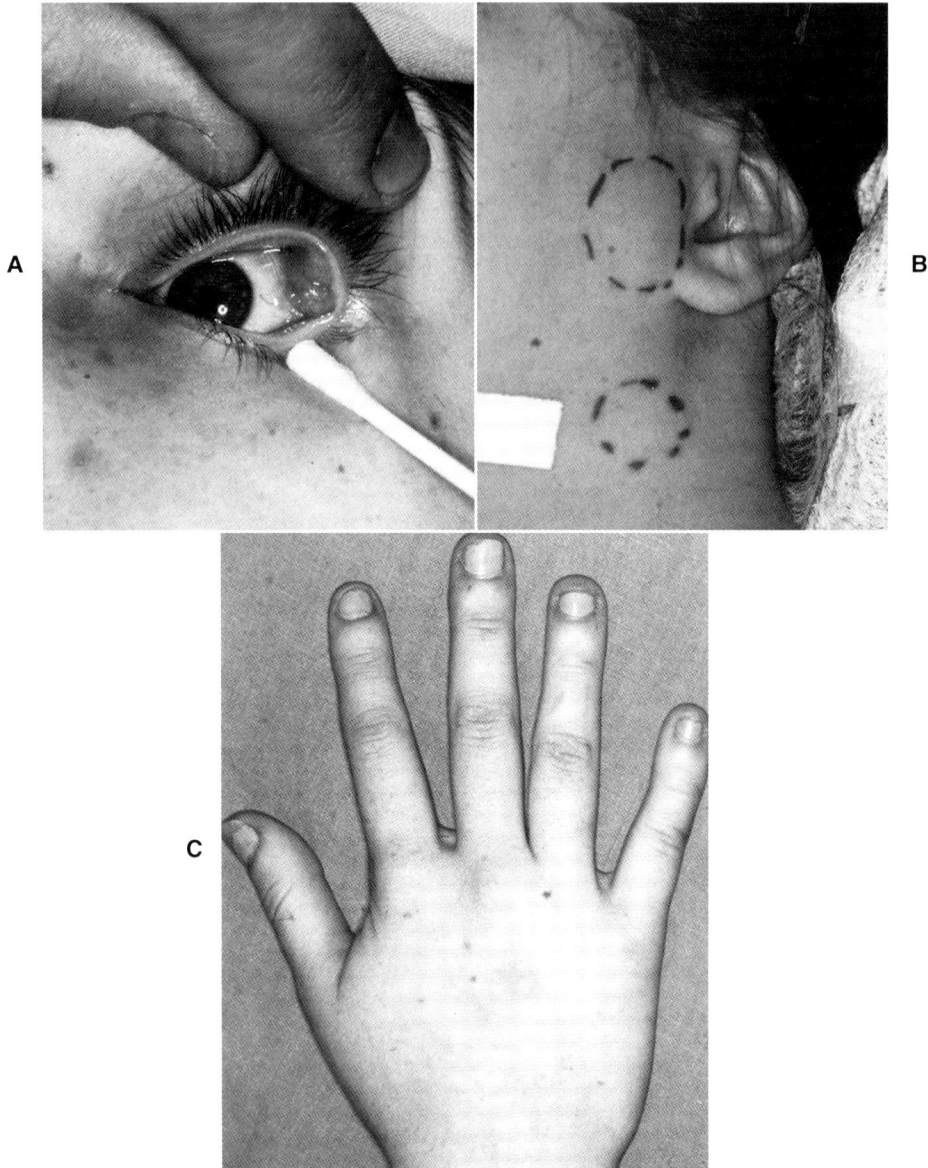

Figure 22-23 A, Granulomatous lesion of the left conjunctiva in a 13-year-old girl with Parinaud's oculoglandular syndrome and a 2-week history of low-grade fever, malaise, and anorexia. The patient had regular and frequent contact with cats and dogs. **B,** Two tender preauricular nodes were present that were rubbery in consistency and freely mobile. **C,** The dorsal surface of the hands demonstrated numerous puncture and scratch marks. (From Loftus MJH, Sweeney G, Nemarich A, et al: Parinaud's oculoglandular syndrome, *J Oral Surg* 38:218, 1980.)

ERYSIPELAS: FACIAL LYMPHANGITIS

CHARACTERISTICS

Erysipelas is a rapidly spreading, distinctive type of superficial cellulitis of the skin, caused by streptococci, with prominent lymphatic involvement and with a predilection for the skin of the face and scalp (Figure 22-24). On the face it is characterized by edema and erythema. It should be distinguished from cellulitis caused by trauma, odontogenic infections, streptococcal pneumonia, staphylococcal infections, furunculosis, and atopic dermatitis. Erysipelas dif-

fers from cellulitis by its raised, well-defined margins.[37] Onset usually is abrupt. Although uncommon, erysipelas should be included in the differential diagnosis of acute facial swelling.

The lesion generally affects infants, children, and the elderly. It is limited to the superficial layers of the skin and is characteristically warm, tender, painful, indurated, and erythematous. The swelling is raised with sharply demarcated borders and scalloped edges. It is distinctly pink to deep red and thereby distinguishable from staphylococcal infections. Constitutional signs and symptoms include

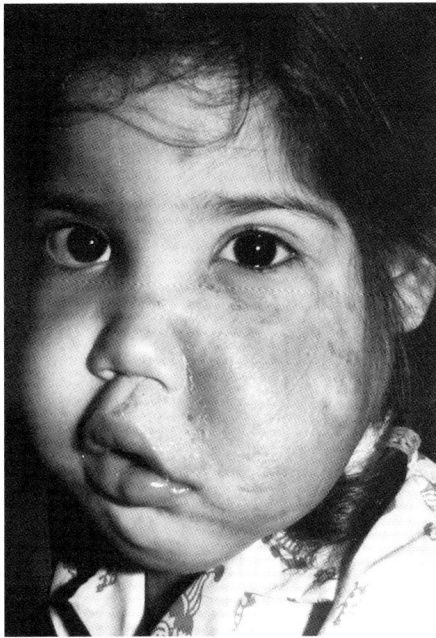

Figure 22-24 Erysipelas in a 2-year-old child. The lesion has a characteristic pink to deep red color, with sharply demarcated and scalloped borders. (From Slade E, Danielson P, Goldberg M: Erysipelas: facial lymphangitis, *J Oral Surg* 35:416, 1977.)

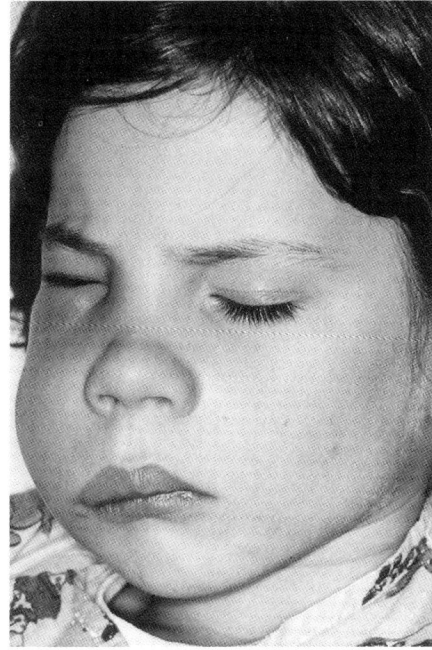

Figure 22-25 Marked cellulitis of the face in a 7-year-old boy whose blood cultures grew both *H. influenzae* and streptococcal organisms of the viridans group. The color and distribution of the cellulitis were typical of *H. influenzae* cellulitis.

fever (104° F to 105° F) and regional lymphadenopathy. The lesion reaches its maximum extent by 3 to 5 days and leaves a desquamated surface after regression.

Erysipelas is caused by group A β-hemolytic streptococci after bacterial invasion of facial abrasions, lacerations, or punctures. Colonization of lymphatic channels produces diffuse lymphangitis. Erysipelas also has been reported after tooth extraction.

Treatment Before the discovery of antibiotics, the mortality rate for erysipelas was approximately 10% to 20%, with death resulting from streptococcal septicemia, particularly in infants, the elderly, and the debilitated. Currently treatment consists of the penicillin-resistant semisynthetic penicillins, nafcillin or oxicillin (2.0 g q4h IV). If symptoms are not severe, doxycycline (500 mg q6h PO) or cefazolin (1.0 g q8h IV) is recommended.[21] Antibiotic therapy usually results in a rapid resolution.

HAEMOPHILUS INFLUENZAE CELLULITIS

Haemophilus influenzae cellulitis must be considered in the differential diagnosis of any swelling of the cheek or periorbital region, particularly in children between the ages of 3 months and 3 years, regardless of sex. It typically appears as facial cellulitis in association with influenza, and its frequency is increasing.

Among 83 children with severe *H. influenzae* infection, 10% had facial cellulitis and 1% had orbital cellulitis.[48] *H. influenzae* cellulitis occasionally occurs after soft tissue injury of the cheek or face and begins with a diffuse cel-

lulitis that extends unilaterally from the mandible to the orbit (Figure 22-25); the cellulitis is indurated, tender, and has a distinctive purple-blue or purple-red color. Symptoms develop slightly before or shortly after a short, febrile, nonspecific, upper respiratory tract infection. The white blood cell count and temperature are elevated, and blood culture results usually are positive. *H. influenzae* type B commonly is cultured from blood or cellulitis aspirate. Infection spreads by a hematogenous route to the cheek from the nasopharynx, maxillary sinus, or middle ear. Some children develop other septic foci (meningitis) because of the accompanying bacteremia.[35]

■ CASE REPORT

A 7-year-old boy had facial cellulitis of odontogenic origin and a 1-week history of an upper respiratory tract infection. No evidence of facial or cheek abrasion was present (Figure 22-25). *H. influenzae* and streptococcal organisms of the viridans group were cultured from the cellulitis. Subsequent incision and drainage, extraction of the involved tooth, and administration of parenteral and oral penicillin resulted in rapid resolution of the condition. Although *H. influenzae* may have been a contaminant, the cellulitis strongly resembled that of infantile *H. influenzae*.

An association between *H. influenzae* cellulitis and ipsilateral otitis media has been reported. The organism can be cultured from the ear, and involvement of the cheek can be explained by lymphatic spread.[36] This lesion must be distinguished from the more common cellulitis of *Streptococcus pyogenes*, which usually produces elevated borders and is uniformly red. It also must be distinguished from the less common cellulitis caused by *Streptococcus pneumoniae* (*Diplococcus pneumoniae*), which also can cause blue-purple cellulitis.

Treatment   Because *H. influenzae* bacteremia may progress to fatal meningitis and osteomyelitis, septic arthritis, and epiglottitis, it should be treated vigorously. Ampicillin has been the drug of choice for the treatment of *H. influenzae* infections. Recently, however, an increasing number of *H. influenzae* type B infections have been resistant to ampicillin. Therefore trimethoprim-sulfamethoxazole is recommended for upper respiratory tract infections and bronchitis; a variety of other antibiotics are suggested as alternatives. For *H. influenzae* infection, meningitis, epiglottitis, arthritis, and other serious infections, cefotaxime (2.0 g q8h IV) plus gentamicin (2 mg/kg, first dose, then 1.7 mg/kg q8h) is recommended as the drug of first choice.[21]

INFECTIOUS ARTHRITIS OF THE TEMPOROMANDIBULAR JOINT

Arthritis of the TMJ may be traumatic, degenerative, rheumatoid, or infectious. Infectious arthritis is the least common. It should be recognized and treated promptly to prevent destruction and consolidation of the joint with subsequent ankylosis.[42] In the growing individual, infectious arthritis of the joint affects growth of the mandible and may result in hypoplasia of the involved side of the mandible with facial asymmetry, micrognathia, and inability to open the mouth (Figure 22- 26).[49]

Organisms may reach the joint by instrumentation, by laceration, through the bloodstream, by direct extension, or by blunt trauma that predisposes the joint to infection.[1,27,31] Almost any organism can cause infectious arthritis, but it generally is caused by staphylococci, streptococci, and occasionally gonococci. Infectious arthritis has been reported after pneumonia, gonorrhea, tuberculosis, syphilis, meningitis, subacute bacterial endocarditis, septic sore throat, scarlet fever, osteomyelitis, typhoid, measles, infected wounds, peritonsillar abscess, otitis media, mastoiditis, furunculosis, infected burns, pyelitis, and sinusitis. Scarlet fever and typhoid fever may result in septicemia that can affect any joint and lead to otitis media or mastoiditis, which can involve the joint by direct extension. In addition, TMJ arthritis may result from direct extension of temporal or condylar osteomyelitis or from soft tissue abscesses.[50]

Study of the causes of intraarticular (true) ankylosis of the TMJ showed that 25 (57%) of 44 patients and 87 (47%) of 185 patients, respectively, had infectious arthritis preceding ankylosis.[49,50] Infectious arthritis usually is suppurative, whereas that associated with scarlet fever, dysentery, and other acute febrile illnesses is nonsuppurative.

Clinical and Radiographic Findings   Infectious arthritis is characterized by the sudden onset of chills, fever,

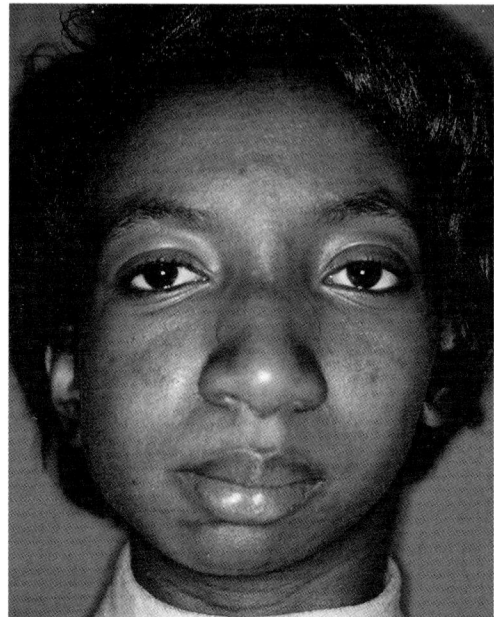

Figure 22-26 In this growing child, ankylosis resulted in hypoplasia of the mandible on the right side and inability to open the mouth because of fibrous or bony adhesions of the condyle to the glenoid fossa alone, or to the zygomatic arch and skull base. In this patient the right joint is affected with flatness of the face on the left with deviation of the chin to the affected side as the mandible continues to grow on the unaffected side.

swelling over the joint, and tenderness of the joint to palpation. Movement of the jaw is painful. Although early conventional radiographs may not disclose abnormalities, destructive changes often are seen later. Early panographic or computed tomographic images of the joint show separation of the articular surfaces caused by accumulation of fluid or pus. Positive bone scan findings, although not specific for septic arthritis, suggest inflammation. These results and clinical findings confirm joint involvement.

Treatment   Treatment is directed at overcoming the infection as early as possible to minimize joint destruction and subsequent fibrous or bony ankylosis and other complications, such as temporal bone osteomyelitis and intracranial abscesses.[39] Whenever possible, antibiotic therapy should be based on culture results. The joint should be aspirated under sterile conditions, and Gram stain performed. Aerobic and anaerobic cultures should be obtained for sensitivity testing. Empirical therapy should begin immediately, directed at a broad spectrum of organisms because of the numerous potential sources of infection. Distant loci of infection should be identified and treated.[4] Antibiotics recommended are clindamycin (600 mg IV every 6 hours), ampicillin-sulbactam (Unasyn, 3 g IV every 6 hours), or cefazolin (1.5 g every 6 hours). These drugs should be administered for 1 week followed by oral administration for an additional 3 weeks. When methacillin-resistant *S. aureus* is suspected or cultured, vancomycin is recommended (15 mg/kg q12h IV; 125 mg q6h PO).[12]

Formal incision and drainage seldom is necessary, but repeated aspiration with a 20-gauge needle is advised until cultures are sterile. Arthroscopy has been used to confirm the diagnosis of suppurative arthritis of the TMJ, for lavage with saline solution and antibiotic solutions, and for direct monitoring of convalescence.[27,31] Warm preauricular soaks, analgesics, and adequate fluid and food intake are important supportive measures.

The patient should consume a liquid or soft diet in the early stages of the disease. Resting the joint is desirable initially. After infection has subsided, joint function is encouraged to prevent ankylosis.

REFERENCES

1. Abubaker AO: Differential diagnosis of arthritis of the temporomandibular joint, *Oral Maxillofac Surg Clin North Am* 7:1, 1995.
2. Adolph HP, Yugueros P, Woods JE: Noma: a review, *Ann Plast Surg* 37:657, 1996.
3. Berger CJ, Disque FC, Topazian RG: Rhinocerebral mucormycosis: diagnosis and treatment, *Oral Surg* 40:27, 1975.
4. Bounds GA, Hopkins R, Sugar A: Septic arthritis of the temporomandibular joint: a problematic diagnosis, *Br J Oral Maxillofac Surg* 25:61, 1987.
5. Brown OE, Finn R: Mucormycosis of the mandible, *J Oral Maxillofac Surg* 44:132, 1986.
6. Bourgeois DM, Leclercq MH: The World Health initiative on noma, *Oral Dis* 5:172, 1999.
7. Caddell JL: Magnesium in the therapy of orofacial lesions of severe protein-calorie malnutrition, *Br J Surg* 56:826, 1969.
8. Dean JA, Mcgee W: One-stage reconstruction for defects caused by cancrum oris, *Ann Plast Surg* 38:29, 1997.
9. Denning D: *Aspergillus* species. In Mandell GL, Bennett JE, Dolin R, editors: *Mandell, Douglas and Bennett's principles and practice of infectious disease*, ed 5, Philadelphia, 2000, Churchill Livingstone.
10. Denning DW: Therapeutic outcome of invasive aspergillosis, *Clin Infect Dis* 23:608, 1996.
11. Donlon WC, Jacobsen PL: An unusual submandibular mass-cat-scratch disease: report of case, *J Am Dent Assoc* 109:581, 1984.
12. Dreizen S, Bodey GP, McCredie KB, et al: Orofacial aspergillosis in acute leukemia, *Oral Surg* 59:499, 1985.
13. Drugs for treatment of fungal infections, *Med Lett Drugs Ther* 32:58, 1990.
14. Eilderton TE: Fatal postextraction cerebral mucormycosis in an unknown diabetic, *J Oral Surg* 32:297, 1974.
15. Eisenberg L, Wood T, Boles R: Mucormycosis, *Laryngoscope* 87:347, 1977.
16. Erlichman MC, Trieger N: Aspergillosis infection in a patient receiving immunosuppressive drugs, *J Oral Surg* 36:978, 1978.
17. Falker WA Jr, Enwonwu CO, Idigbe EO: Microbiological understandings and mysteries of noma (cancrum oris), *Oral Dis* 5:150, 1999.
18. Ferguson BJ: Mucormycosis of the nose and paranasal sinuses, *Otolaryngol Clin North Am* 33:349, 2000.
19. Ferguson BJ, Mitchell TG, Moon R, et al: Adjunctive hyperbaric oxygen for treatment of rhinocerebral mucormycosis, *Rev Infect Dis* 10:551, 1988.
20. Ghosal SP, Sen Gupta PC, Mukherjee AK, et al: Noma neonatorum: its aetiopathogenesis, *Lancet* 2:289, 1978.
21. Gilbert DN, Moellering RC Jr, Sande MA: *The Sanford guide to antimicrobial therapy 2000*, ed 30, Hyde Park, Vt, 2000, Antimicrobial Therapy, Inc.
22. Heroman WM, McCurley WS: Cat scratch disease, *Otolaryngol Clin North Am* 15:649, 1982.
23. Kalter SS: Cat scratch disease, *Int J Dermatol* 17:656, 1978.
24. Kavanagh KT, Hughes WT, Parham CM, et al: Fungal sinusitis in immunocompromised children with neoplasms, *Ann Otol Rhinol Laryngol* 100:331, 1991.
25. Korbitz BC: Systemic cat scratch disease, *Rocky Mt Med J* 709:23, 1973.
26. Lagundoye SB, Oluwasanmi JO: Radiologic examination of trismus as a complication of cancrum oris, *Oral Surg* 39:812, 1975.
27. Leighty SM, Sprach DH, Myall RWT, et al: Septic arthritis of the temporomandibular joint: review of the literature and report of two cases in children, *Int J Oral Maxillofac Surg* 22:292, 1993.
28. Limongelli WA, Clark MS, Williams AC: Noma-like lesion in a patient with chronic lymphocytic leukemia, *Oral Surg* 41:40, 1976.
29. Loftus MJ, Sweeney G, Nemarich A, et al: Parinaud's oculoglandular syndrome, *J Oral Surg* 38:218, 1980.
30. Maniglia AJ, Mintz DH, Novak S: Cephalic phycomycosis: a report of eight cases, *Laryngoscope* 92:755, 1982.
31. McCain JP, Zabiegalski NA, Levine RL: Joint infection as a complication of temporomandibular joint arthroscopy: a case report, *J Oral Maxillofac Surg* 51:1389, 1993.
32. Menenzes DM: The etiology and effects of cancrum oris in children, *J Dent Child* 43:92, 1976.
33. Milosev B, el-Mahgoub S, Aal OA, et al: Primary aspergilloma of paranasal sinuses in the Sudan: a review of seventeen cases, *Br J Surg* 56:132, 1969.
34. Morduchowicz G, Shmueli D, Shapira Z, et al: Rhinocerebral mucormycosis in renal transplant recipients: report of three cases and review of the literature, *Rev Infect Dis* 8:441, 1986.
35. Moxon ER, Murphy TF: *Hemophilus influenzae*. In Mandell GL, Bennett JE, Dolin R, editors: *Mandell, Douglas and Bennett's principles and practice of infectious disease*, ed 5, Philadelphia, 2000, Churchill Livingstone.
36. Nelson JD, Ginsburg CM: A hypothesis on the pathogenesis of *Hemophilus influenzae* buccal cellulitis, *J Pediatr* 88:709, 1976.
37. Ochs MW, Dolwick MF: Facial erysipelas: report of a case and review of the literature, *J Oral Maxillofac Surg* 49:1116, 1991.
38. Oiuwasanmi JO, Lagundoye SB, Akinyemi OO: Ankylosis of the mandible from cancrum oris, *Plast Reconstr Surg* 57:342, 1976.
39. Piecuch JF, Lieblich SE: Anatomy and pathology of the temporomandibular joint. In Peterson LJ, editor: *Principles of oral and maxillofacial surgery*, Philadelphia, 1992, JB Lippincott.
40. Pillsbury HC, Fischer ND: Rhinocerebral mucormycosis, *Arch Otolaryngol* 103:600, 1977.
41. Romett JL, Newman RK: Aspergillosis of the nose and paranasal sinuses, *Laryngoscope* 92:764, 1982.
42. Sarnat BG, Laskin DM: *The temporomandibular joint*, ed 3, Springfield, Ill, 1980, Charles C Thomas.
43. Schwartz JN, Donnelly EH, Klintworth GK: Ocular and orbital phycomycosis, *Surv Ophthalmol* 22:3, 1977.
44. Shoham N, Miron D, Rax R, et al: Familial Parinaud oculoglandular syndrome in cat-scratch disease, *Harefuah* 138:1034, 2000.

45. Slater LN, Welch DF: *Bartonella* species, including cat-scratch disease. In Mandell GL, Bennett JE, Dolin R, editors: *Mandell, Douglas and Bennett's principles and practice of infectious disease,* ed 5, Philadelphia, 2000, Churchill Livingstone.

46. Sugar AM: Agents of mucormycosis and related species. In Mandell GL, Bennett JE, Dolin R, editors: *Mandell, Douglas and Bennett's principles and practice of infectious disease,* ed 5, Philadelphia, 2000, Churchill Livingstone.

47. Tempest MN: Cancrum oris, *Br J Surg* 53:949, 1966.

48. Todd JK, Bruhn FW: Severe *Hemophilus influenzae* infections, *Am J Dis Child* 129:607, 1975.

49. Topazian RG, Simon GT, Selvapandian AJ: Ankylosis of the temporomandibular joint, *Indian J Surg* 23:69, 1961.

50. Topazian RG: Etiology of ankylosis of the temporomandibular joint: analysis of forty-four cases, *J Oral Surg* 22:227, 1964.

51. Uohara GI, Knapp MJH: Oral fusospirochetosis and associated lesions, *Oral Surg* 24:113, 1967.

52. Yu VL, Wagner GE, Shadomy S: Sino-orbital aspergillosis treated with combination of antifungal therapy, *JAMA* 244:814, 1980.

Anesthetic Considerations in Orofacial Infections

Jeffrey D. Bennett
Thomas R. Flynn

Few situations present the surgeon a more challenging situation than the anesthetic and airway management of the patient with an infection of the oromaxillofacial region. The infection and its associated edema can distort the normal anatomical structures compromising the integrity of the respiratory tree. On one extreme, such patients may initially have an acute or a potentially impending airway obstruction. The complexity of managing the care of these patients pertains not only to the actual difficulty in securing the airway but also to the decision as to whether the patient requires elective artificial control of the airway. In simpler situations the primary concern is control of profound pain, which facilitates incision and drainage. The efficacy of local anesthesia may be impaired as a result of infection. In addition, access for the administration of the local anesthetic may be compromised by trismus and attempts to avoid inserting the needle through an infected region.

This chapter focuses on the anesthetic and airway considerations in orofacial infections, progressing from problems with local anesthesia to the physical evaluation and triage of patients with airway compromise. A discussion of the latter presents an approach to the compromised airway divided into various stages including airway assessment, anesthetic induction and intubation techniques, and extubation criteria.

IMPORTANCE OF THE AIRWAY IN MAXILLOFACIAL INFECTIONS

Patients with head or neck fascial space infections present a potentially complex and emergency situation. The primary concern is that almost all fascial space infections of the orofacial region are adjacent to the airway. The lateral pharyngeal and retropharyngeal spaces are separated from the pharynx by only the thin layers of the

pharyngeal constrictor muscles. Peritonsillar space infections are separated by only mucosa from the oropharynx.[61] Spontaneous or iatrogenic disruption of the mucosa can contaminate the lower airway. An infection of the submandibular or sublingual space results in a superior and posterior displacement of the tongue. Cleavage planes exist within the base of the tongue that allow sublingual and submandibular infections to pass posteriorly toward the epiglottis.[52] Many infections of these spaces are associated with epiglottitis (Figure 23-1). The submasseteric, pterygomandibular (masticator space infections), lateral pharyngeal, and infratemporal spaces

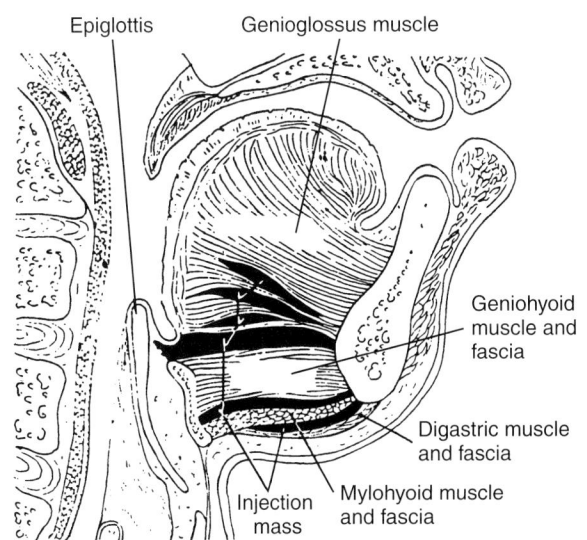

Figure 23-1 Cleavage planes in the tongue, floor of the mouth, and submandibular space, which allow extension of submandibular and sublingual space infections to cause epiglottitis. (From Grodinsky M: Ludwig's angina: an anatomical and clinical study with review of the literature, *Surgery* 5:678, 1939.)

are bordered by muscles of mastication. Infections of these spaces cause trismus. Furthermore, fascial spaces are continuous with each other and an infective process is dynamic. Clinicians always should be concerned that the infection will continue to expand beyond the boundaries detected on initial examination. In summary, fascial space infections often result in morbidity and mortality by impeding airway access and causing bronchopneumonia as a result of aspiration of infected material.[118]

AIRWAY EXAMINATION

INITIAL AIRWAY ASSESSMENT

The initial survey of the patient should occur within the first minute and must assess whether the patient is in respiratory distress and therefore in an imminent, life-threatening condition. This survey consists of a gross observation of the patient's ventilatory and oxygenation status. The clinician should observe the patient's ability to move air into and out of the respiratory passages. The astute clinician also may look for subtle changes, such as irritability and agitation, that may be early signs of hypoxia. As hypoxia worsens, it may progress to deteriorating levels of altered consciousness, ultimately resulting in unconsciousness.

The adequacy of oxygenation may be inferred by assessing the patient's oxygen saturation from pulse oximetry. The actual oxygen saturation value provides more clinical meaning if the initial value is obtained before supplemental oxygen is administered. An initial value of 97% or greater generally indicates respiratory sufficiency. A baseline oxygen saturation of less than 97% requires further evaluation. The decreased oxygen saturation may be related to an underlying medical condition. An oxygen saturation of less than 94% or a diminishing trend suggests the need for more urgent airway intervention. Although pulse oximetry provides insight into the patient's oxygenation, it is limited in the information presented. Once supplemental oxygen is administered, satisfactory oxygen saturation may provide a false sense of security.

If the patient has a total or near-total airway obstruction, definitive treatment is required immediately. In the complete absence of inspired oxygen, brain damage begins within 4 to 6 minutes.[41] The urgency of the situation may preclude obtaining a complete history detailing the patient's systemic diseases. Once the airway is secured, the surgical team can resume the process of obtaining a detailed history.

HISTORY

If the patient is not in acute respiratory distress, the surgeon can conduct a more orderly history and physical examination. One of the purposes of this examination is to determine the potential for airway compromise and collect the appropriate data to establish a treatment plan. In addition to questions pertaining to the patient's present condition, the history should identify systemic diseases that may affect the patient's care. For example, a patient with chronic cardiac or pulmonary disease may have little reserve and therefore be more susceptible to the deleterious effects of airway compromise than an otherwise healthy patient. The patient also may demonstrate greater hemodynamic fluctuations associated with the stress of securing the airway.

When obtaining the history of the present condition, the surgeon should inquire about the time of onset and the progression of symptoms. A condition that appeared suddenly or progressed rapidly over the past few hours requires more urgent attention than one that increased gradually over several days. Additional inquiries should be made regarding dyspnea, dysphagia, or dysphonia, all of which suggest involvement of the upper airway. Further investigation is important to grade the severity of the situation once these complaints are registered. Patients who allow themselves to be placed in a semisupine or supine position generally are not in acute respiratory distress. Alternatively, as the supraglottic and pharyngeal airway becomes more edematous, the patient may assume the "sniffing" position. This is an upright position with the neck flexed and the head extended (held forward). Because patients who are in respiratory distress will seek a position that optimizes airway patency, they frequently insist on remaining in the upright position. The clinician also may inquire about the patient's ability to sleep the previous night. A history of dyspnea and inability to sleep in the supine position the previous night should raise concern. Many patients complain of dysphagia as a result of affected muscles of mastication, lingual swelling, or pharyngeal swelling. However, these patients usually demonstrate no drooling. Although the complaint should not go unnoticed, the ability to handle secretions demonstrates a level of airway patency. Alternatively, if the patient is unable to handle secretions, this finding may be associated with a more significant narrowing of the airway or lingual involvement (potentially requiring more urgent attention). Pain on speaking or a change in the character of a patient's voice is an important clue to the site of airway involvement. The latter may be unrecognized by the patient. Therefore the surgeon should be inquisitive about a perceived abnormality. A coarse or hoarse voice suggests progression of the infection to the level of the glottis, whereas a muffling of the voice is characteristic of supraglottic or pharyngeal space involvement.[94,96]

An additional factor is patient maturity. Children and mentally impaired patients pose a unique challenge. These individuals may lack the ability to cooperate. Techniques selected for the typical adult patient for safety purposes may need to be foregone because they require a degree of patient cooperation, such as awake intubations.

PHYSICAL EXAMINATION

Several components of physical examination are pertinent to the airway and anesthetic management of the patient.

These include (1) limited ability to extend and flex the neck, (2) limited interincisal opening, (3) edematous, displaced, or immobile tongue, (4) decreased airway space, (5) distorted anatomy, (6) skeletal deformity of the maxillofacial complex, and (7) risk of aspiration.[82]

As the practitioner inspects for pathological conditions associated with the infection, he or she also should note congenital conditions that may predispose the patient to difficulty in airway manipulation if artificial airway support is required. Areas of erythema may be the first sign of an expanding infection, especially when the erythema extends along the anterior aspect of the neck. If erythema is noted, the patient's voice should be assessed. Asymmetries are suggestive of edema in one or more of the deep fascial spaces. Deviation of the thyroid cartilage or trachea is an ominous sign. The patient should demonstrate the ability to flex and extend the neck. Limitation may indicate a deep fascial space infection. Regardless of its cause, infection may affect the ability to secure the airway artificially. As the head and neck are inspected, the clinician should simultaneously palpate for tenderness, induration, or fluctuance, and differentiate between abscess and cellulitis. Areas of tenderness suggest deep fascial space involvement. One example is tenderness above the zygomatic arch, which may indicate the presence of an infratemporal space infection. This finding should alert the clinician to the potential development of trismus (if not already present) and airway restriction at the level of the soft palate.

The patient should be asked to open the mouth widely to evaluate the severity of trismus. Normal incisal opening should be at least 3.5 cm. Decreased opening compromises the ability to satisfactorily perform laryngoscopy and visualize the glottis.[96,120] A significant decrease in interincisal opening also impairs the surgeon's ability to inspect the soft palate and pharynx. This inspection should not be dismissed because of its associated discomfort (Figure 23-2).

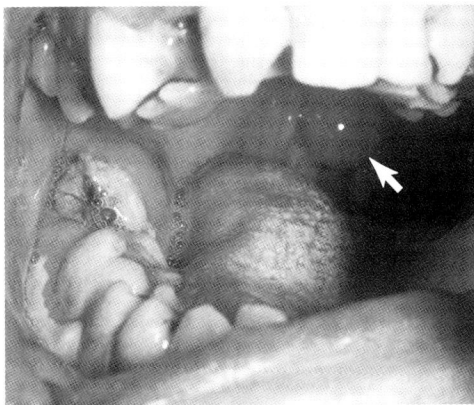

Figure 23-2 Pterygomandibular space abscess. In this case the ability to photograph the distended anterior tonsillar pillar and the edematous and displaced uvula *(arrow)* was aided by a displaced fracture of the mandibular angle. (From Flynn TR, Topazian RG: Infections of the oral cavity. In Waite DE, editor: *Textbook of practical oral and maxillofacial surgery,* ed 3, Philadelphia, 1987, Lea and Febiger.)

The surgeon also must thoroughly inspect the floor of mouth in addition to the edema and mobility of the tongue. Unless ankyloglossia is present, a patient should be able to protrude the tongue past the vermilion border of the upper lip. The patient also should be able to close the mouth into maximal intercuspation without discomfort in the tongue or floor of mouth. The surgeon should look for purulent drainage or areas in which the infection is pointing and drainage may occur as a result of iatrogenic manipulation. Both pose a risk for aspiration during airway intubation.

DIAGNOSTIC TESTS

Radiographic imaging can help define the extent of the infection and any distortion of the airway. Historically, soft tissue radiographs of the neck taken in the lateral and posteroanterior positions demonstrate airway shadows. They can be helpful in distinguishing deep space infection involving the airway from more superficial infection. Computed tomography (CT) has advanced over the past several years. It is fast, and the information obtained demonstrates the specific areas of airway involvement from the nasopharynx to the glottis. Except for the patient in acute or imminent respiratory distress requiring immediate airway management, the CT scan should be a component of the evaluation and provides information pertinent to airway management. An exception to obtaining a CT scan is that not all hospitals have 24-hour, in-house CT technicians. The delay in waiting for the study may have deleterious results. Soft tissue images may be beneficial in these situations, although some disagreement exists; if the patient needs urgent treatment, the soft tissue radiographs can be deferred because they may provide no information beyond that obtained with the clinical examination. However, if the CT study can be obtained expediently, it provides invaluable information and is recommended. The emergency department may establish a protocol of contacting the radiology technician at the same time as the surgical consultation is requested when a patient comes to the emergency department with a severe oral or facial swelling.

Soft tissue swelling and trismus impair the surgeon's ability to inspect the airway, and radiographs do not provide a clear view of the airway. Fiberoptic examination allows direct inspection of the airway. Endoscopy also provides details of the glottis that otherwise would not be obtainable.

CRITERIA FOR ASSESSMENT OF AIRWAY COMPROMISE

Many methods have been proposed to predict the success of laryngoscopy and intubation.[2,30,82] These methods should be simple and rapidly performable. The Mallampati test assesses the airway based on the ability to visualize the faucial pillars and uvula when the mouth is wide open, the tongue maximally protruded, and neck extended forward. The more the base of the tongue conceals the faucial pillars and the uvula, the greater the difficulty in intubation.[82] The thyromental distance is a measurement from the prominence of the thyroid cartilage to the menton with the neck in full extension. A distance less than 6 cm may predict difficulty with visualizing the larynx. Alignment of the three axes of the airway also optimizes direct laryngoscopy. The occiput is elevated approximately 10 cm above the shoulder blades and the neck is hyperextended. Inability to achieve appropriate positioning has been associated with failed intubations. Interincisal opening was noted as one of five predictors of difficult intubation.[120]

The Mallampati and thyromental distance tests, when used individually, lack sensitivity and specificity.[9,42,92,119] However, combining the information from more than one test increases the ability to predict a difficult intubation. Frerk[45] suggested that all preoperative patients undergo the Mallampati and thyromental distance tests to significantly decrease the false-positive rate. However, in assessment of a patient with significant orofacial infection, missing difficult intubations is more problematic than an artificially high false-positive rate. Karkouti et al.[68] suggested assessment of mouth opening, chin protrusion, and atlantooccipital extension. They predict that only 3 (0.15%) difficult intubations would be missed among every 1000 cases in which the incidence of difficult intubations would be 2%. The Mallampati classification better correlates the prediction of difficult laryngoscopy with the extremes of the classification scheme.[100] A 93% correlation with the inability to visualize the glottis adequately on laryngoscopy has been reported with a grade IV Mallampati classification.[82] Although these tests have limitations, they may provide an objective indication of suspected difficult intubation in patients with infection.

Although many tests address difficulty with intubation, they do not directly address the potential difficulty with mask ventilation.[95] Soft tissue swelling can result in posterior displacement of the tongue and pharyngeal soft tissues. Although the patient may not be in distress while awake, the soft tissues may collapse after the administration of sedative medication or supine positioning. Soft tissue swelling also may distort the anatomy so that a satisfactory mask fit cannot be achieved.

The onset of acute infection and the need for urgent airway intervention is not planned. Therefore the patient frequently has not fasted for the appropriate period. Concerns regarding a full stomach, with increased gastric contents and acidity, relate to the potential risk of gastric aspiration in the patient who is anesthetized before intubation. Anesthetic induction compounds the complexity of the situation and must be considered in airway management. For the patient whose airway does not require emergency intubation, the clinician should consider delayed surgical intervention and the risk of gastric aspiration associated with anesthetic induction. However, gastric emptying is delayed or arrested as a result of multiple factors including pain, anxiety, or both. Fortunately, many patients with significant infection have limited their oral intake because of their physical inability to eat.

AIRWAY MANAGEMENT STRATEGIES

TRIAGE

The goal of triage is to classify patients into various categories identifying the urgency and immediacy of treatment. Brown and Satloff[23] suggest three categories: (1) occult impending respiratory distress, (2) obvious respiratory distress, and (3) total or nearly total airway obstruction. They defined the patient with occult impending respiratory distress as being at risk for airway difficulties after they are medicated or manipulated. Patients in this category initially may have one of four distinctly different patterns of potential airway compromise. A patient may have a mild or moderate supraglottic or lateral pharyngeal infection for which he or she has compensated by muscular effort. The administration of sedative medication may result in sufficient muscular relaxation so that the patient no longer compensates and airway patency is compromised. Airway compromise may not resolve with simple elevation of the chin. An example of a patient in this category would be one with trismus but no severe swelling impinging directly on the airway. The administration of sedative medication does not resolve the trismus and thus access to the airway is limited. This creates a potential problem because the patient now may have depressed respirations and an unprotected airway that cannot be secured easily. Another problem exists when a patient is sedated and an incision and drainage is performed. The proximity of the surgical site and the quantity of purulent discharge could result in aspiration. The last type of patient in this category may have a moderate infection with no overt signs of respiratory distress. Although the patient demonstrates no signs of respiratory distress, the potential for development of distress exists. The infection (e.g., cellulitis associated with a salivary gland infection) does not require immediate surgical intervention. However, observation is required and pharmacological techniques to minimize reactive airway edema should be considered.

The patient with obvious respiratory distress is defined as initially having stridor, labored breathing, intercostal retractions, and tracheal tug.[23] Although they are alert, these patients may be fatigued. However, their ventilation barely maintains adequate oxygenation. Such situations are urgent because near or total airway obstruction may result from further fatigue or sedation.

Total or Near-Total Airway Obstruction   Patients with total or near-total airway obstruction have hypoxia, hypercarbia, and delirium and may be unconscious. Patients in this category should be identified during the primary survey and require immediate establishment of a patent airway. The most certain and rapid technique to artificially secure the airway is required. The initial intervention to relieve upper airway obstruction should be delivery of positive-pressure ventilation by mask with 100% oxygen, which may require a two-person technique in which one individual holds the mask against the patient's face forming an airtight seal while the other individual compresses the bag. The gentle insertion of an artificial airway facilitates mask ventilation. The clinician should remain cognizant of the urgency of the situation. If the ventilation attempt fails, laryngoscopy and intubation under direct vision should be attempted. This attempt requires optimal patient positioning and selection of the most appropriate laryngoscope blade. Optimal external laryngeal manipulation should be used.[16] Laryngoscopy may traumatize the pharyngeal mucosa resulting in drainage from an abscess, which may soil the lower airway. Although this may be considered a relative contraindication, the alternative is a surgical airway with potential complications associated with the infection. Laryngoscopy may be the most appropriate first choice, although in some situations its use is contraindicated. If laryngoscopy and intubation fail, immediate creation of a surgical airway is required. The need for a surgical airway should be determined before airway manipulation. Then the patient should be positioned properly and the anatomical structures appropriately outlined on the patient to facilitate the surgical procedure. A surgical airway may entail a cricothyrotomy or a tracheotomy; surgical details of these procedures are discussed later in the chapter. If a surgical airway cannot be achieved, a needle cricothyrotomy can be used as a temporary lifesaving measure. High-frequency jet ventilation may provide greater protection against aspiration than percutaneous transtracheal ventilation, yet neither provides protection comparable to a cuffed endotracheal or tracheostomy tube.

CORTICOSTEROIDS IN AIRWAY MANAGEMENT

Inflammation increases dilation and permeability contributing to an exudation into the tissue. Macrophages and leukocytes within the tissues promote cell breakdown. Enzymes from cell breakdown cause cell destruction and propagation of the inflammation. In the patient with an infection the inflammation may be caused by the infective process or be the result of the surgical incision and drainage of the infection. The inflammation is a reactive process that may extend beyond the boundaries of the infection. Regardless of the causes of inflammation the consequence is airway edema with resultant airway narrowing.

Corticosteroids suppress the inflammatory response of disease regardless of the cause. They prevent or suppress capillary dilation and permeability, leukocyte migration, and phagocytosis, which results in less cellular destruction and swelling. Corticosteroids are used as adjunctive therapy in the management of various infective processes including central nervous system bacterial infections, laryngotracheitis, and epiglottitis.* Literature reports spanning more than four decades disagree about the value of steroid administration. Some studies demon-

strate therapeutic efficacy, whereas others show no beneficial effect of administration of steroids. The diagnostic criteria and methodological standards used in several of these studies may have contributed to the equivocal findings. Regardless of the lack of therapeutic efficacy the risks associated with short-term administration of a corticosteroid are minimal.[57] None of the studies reported a statistical difference in the rate of bacterial complications in patients receiving corticosteroids compared with placebo. The use of corticosteroids pertaining to their use in reducing postextubation stridor and swelling has been studied.[8,17,60] The literature also is inconclusive on this topic.

Corticosteroids have been used extensively in facial surgery to reduce postoperative edema.[4,47,87] However, few reports have addressed the use of corticosteroids in the management of orofacial infections.[11] Studies of the administration of corticosteroids in the management of laryngotracheitis show that optimal results are obtained with high doses of drug administered early in the course of the disease.[11] Recommended doses in the adult patient should exceed the equivalent of 100 mg of hydrocortisone administered intravenously every 8 to 12 hours for the first 24 hours. Dexamethasone, methylprednisolone, or hydrocortisone in appropriate doses also should be effective. Because literature reports are inconclusive, the routine use of corticosteroids during infections cannot be recommended. However, their use should be considered to avoid the need for intubation or decrease the duration of intubation.

In summary, the administration of corticosteroids as adjunctive therapy in management of orofacial infections is controversial. The concerns of immunosuppression and dissemination of the infection always must be balanced against the antiinflammatory benefits of steroids.

PATIENT AGE

For many situations in which significant orofacial infection compromises the airway, the preferred method of airway control requires that the patient be sedated but not unconscious. This goal is achievable in most adults and adolescents. However, young children, children with special needs, or adults with mental impairments may not understand or cooperate with an awake-sedated technique.[117] These situations dictate consideration of one of the following techniques: (1) premedication with oral midazolam or ketamine-midazolam, (2) intramuscular administration of ketamine with or without a benzodiazepine and anticholinergic agent, or (3) induction of general anesthesia with halothane or sevoflurane. Intravenous access is established once the patient is sedated or asleep. Neither oral nor intramuscular ketamine is recommended for the patient with a compromised airway. However, ketamine administered intravenously in slow incremental doses may be advantageous in establishing an appropriate anesthetic state to facilitate airway manipulation and intubation of the airway.

---

*References 33, 40, 56, 58, 67, 73, 75, 109, 111.

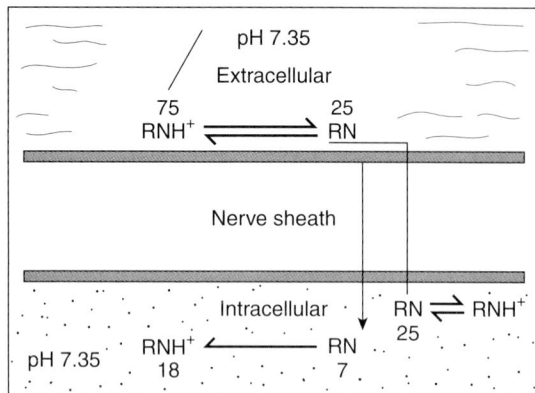

Figure 23-3 Dissociation of a local anesthetic at normal tissue pH. (From Malamed SF: *Handbook of local anesthesia*, ed 4, St Louis, 1997, Mosby.)

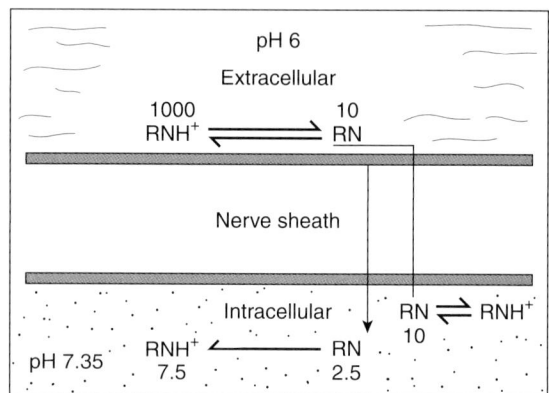

Figure 23-4 Dissociation of a local anesthetic at decreased tissue pH. (From Malamed SF: *Handbook of local anesthesia*, ed 4, St. Louis, 1997, Mosby.)

LOCAL ANESTHESIA

For the patient who is not in respiratory distress, local anesthesia can be used to achieve adequate pain control so that incision and drainage are possible. This technique takes advantage of the conscious patient's naturally protective airway reflexes. Most clinicians agree that adequate local anesthesia is difficult when acute inflammation or infection is present.

Biological Basis for Failure of Local Anesthesia   Local anesthetics are weak acids that in their un-ionized form (the base, or RN) are able to diffuse rapidly through cell membranes and other tissue barriers to reach nerve tissue. However, the ionized form, the cation or RNH^+, is the active form of the molecule. When a local anesthetic is injected into human tissue, it exists in an equilibrium between two states, a nonionized free base for diffusion and an ionized cation for clinical effect. This equilibrium is governed by the dissociation constant (pKa) of the anesthetic and the pH of the surrounding tissues (Figure 23-3). The chemical equation for this equilibrium reaction is:

$$RNH^+ \leftrightarrow RN + H^+$$

An infected area is likely to have a lower pH than normal tissues because of the products of inflammation (e.g., pus has a pH of 5 to 6). Therefore infected tissues have an excess of the hydrogen ion, H^+, that drives the equilibrium reaction toward the left, resulting in a greater proportion of the local anesthetic molecule in the cationic form (RNH^+) than in the RN form. The clinical effect of this shift in equilibrium is that the local anesthetic is less able to diffuse through infected tissues than through normal tissues, resulting in delayed onset and decreased intensity of local anesthesia (Figure 23-4). However, this process does not explain why a nerve block proximal to the site of infection may be unsuccessful.

Another possible mechanism for the failure to establish adequate regional anesthesia in the presence of infection has been proposed.[90] In a histochemical study of nerve tissues at sites proximal to the area of infection, degenerative inflammatory changes were found in nerve structures and their protein constituents. Brown[24] reported diminished local anesthetic effect at neutral pH using nerve preparations that had been exposed to inflammatory cells for 18 hours or longer. This finding suggests that inflammatory changes may travel along the nerves innervating a site of infection and support the use of nerve block techniques rather than infiltration for infected sites. The work of Kimberly and Byers[69] and others[110] clearly indicates that morphological changes occur in inflamed nerves, including axonal sprouting, that may explain the hyperalgesia in infected sites.

Local Anesthesia in Infected Sites

Nerve Block Techniques   The nerve block technique for establishment of local anesthesia of infected areas has several advantages over infiltration. First, it avoids passing a needle directly into an infected region. Nerve blocks avoid problems associated with the decreased pH of infected tissues, prevent contamination of the local anesthetic needle, and minimize trauma to the inflamed friable infected tissues. Second, a regional nerve block provides more profound anesthesia over a broader area for a greater duration. During an incision and drainage procedure, the surgeon frequently must explore an entire fascial space for loculations of pus. Successful local anesthesia for these spaces depends on a greater depth and distribution of anesthesia than infiltration alone typically provides.

Accessory Innervation   The oral cavity is one of the most highly innervated areas of the body. At several sites in the oral cavity, accessory innervation can interfere with successful local anesthesia for surgical procedures, even in uninfected cases. Mandibular molars often receive additional sensory nerve supply from the mylohyoid and lingual nerves.[31] Infiltration of the soft tissues just medial to the retromolar pad and posterior to the last molar can block the accessory mylohyoid and lingual innervation of the mandibular molars. The mild discomfort associated with the injection soon is followed by profound anesthesia of the mandibular molar teeth as a result of blocking accessory nerve fibers in this region. Similar techniques can be used for the mandibular anterior region, where crossover innervation from the other side can be problematic, and for maxillary teeth, where maxillary anterior teeth can receive nerve fibers from the middle superior alveolar nerve through the superior dental plexus (Bochdalek's plexus). Similarly, overlapping innervation can occur in the palate between the nasopalatine and greater palatine nerves.

Anesthetic Volume By increasing the total amount of local anesthetic in proximity to the nerve tissues, the local anesthetic dissociation equation is driven to the right. Therefore the amount of the nonionized base form (RN) of the local anesthetic would be increased, which is critical to diffusion of the anesthetic molecule through tissues toward the nerve structures. Once the local anesthetic molecule has diffused through the nerve membrane into the nerve cell, the equilibrium reaction is reestablished at the intracellular pH, which should be much closer to normal (see Figure 23-4).

Techniques for increasing the volume of local anesthetic in the infected site include (1) reinjection at the site of nerve block, (2) periodontal ligament injection, (3) intraseptal injection, (4) intrapulpal injection, and (5) local infiltration.[99,116] Two precautions must be observed if local anesthesia is used. First, the toxic dose of the local anesthetic used must not be exceeded. Because infected areas are hyperemic, local anesthetics injected into them are likely to reach the systemic circulation more rapidly than in uninfected tissues. Second, a contaminated needle and syringe must not be reused later in an uninfected site because it can spread the infection into a deeper fascial space.

Supplemental Intraoral and Extraoral Nerve Blocks Successful use of local anesthesia in infected cases depends primarily on the accurate deposition of local anesthetic in close proximity to the nerve to be anesthetized. Precisely placed nerve blocks can overcome the obstacles to successful local anesthesia imposed by the acidic pH of infected tissues and the possible inflammatory nerve degeneration progressing proximal to the infected site. The most common intraoral nerve block techniques are described in textbooks of dental local anesthesia.[13,64,81]

In addition, several other special intraoral nerve block techniques that are advantageous in odontogenic infections are the intraoral second division nerve block through the palatine approach and the anterior extraoral approach to maxillary nerve block.[84,97] Other intraoral and extraoral techniques for maxillary and mandibular nerve blocks also have been described.[13,113]

Sanders[101] described modifications of the inferior alveolar nerve block technique in children. An alternative open-mouth technique for inferior alveolar nerve block, described originally by Gow-Gates,[51] has been popularized by Malamed.[80] Levy[76] reported superior local anesthesia for mandibular third molars using the Gow-Gates injection compared with conventional inferior alveolar nerve block, perhaps as a result of blocking accessory innervation. However, the Gow-Gates technique may not be effective in infected sites. The closed-mouth mandibular block technique, first described by Vazirani,[115] was popularized by Akinosi[3] and is well illustrated by Gustainis and Peterson.[55] The closed-mouth technique is useful in patients with trismus; however, the clinician must be careful not to pass the local anesthetic needle through an infected site into an uninfected one such as the pterygomandibular space. Correct technique is important because a misdirected needle may pass into the infratemporal or lateral pharyngeal space.

PATIENT COMMUNICATION

Several options exist if satisfactory anesthesia has not been achieved despite use of the aforementioned techniques. These include proceeding with the surgery without use of additional drugs, using sedation and analgesia, or using general anesthesia. Partial local anesthesia may be achieved, or the patient may react to the mechanical stimuli of surgical manipulation and not to truly painful stimuli. A good rapport is established with the patient by this time, and after discussion of the options, the surgeon may be able to proceed as rapidly as possible. This approach often is effective with an extraction because the pain rapidly ceases once the dental nerve has been severed. In turn, the surgeon should promise to stop the procedure instantly on the patient's request and allow either a rest period or use of another form of pain control.

This technique requires that the patient never be overstressed. Sedation and analgesia techniques establish a quiet, relaxed state, often accompanied by analgesia, especially when a narcotic is used. If local anesthesia has been unsuccessful, sedation and analgesia also may not provide adequate pain relief.

General anesthesia is the final option in the management of failed local anesthesia. As with any outpatient general anesthesia the usual precautions and contraindications are important in the case of inadequate local anesthesia. Fasting and no liquid intake must be strictly observed, especially because gastric emptying time is delayed and gastric pH reduced by pain and anxiety. Several additional contraindications to ambulatory general anesthesia may occur in the presence of maxillofacial infections. They are trismus, swelling encroaching on the airway, and the possibility of discharge of infected material into the airway. Other techniques, whether conscious or unconscious, should be considered if these contraindications are present.

SEDATION AND ANALGESIA TECHNIQUES

Parenteral conscious sedation provides analgesia, anxiolysis, and sedation. Although conscious sedation can be done safely, overly deep sedation may cause airway obstruction, depress the hypoxic or hypercapnic respiratory drive, and obtund the protective airway reflexes. Airway swelling as a result of infection may increase the susceptibility to airway obstruction. Obtunded airway reflexes may increase the susceptibility to pulmonary aspiration of purulent discharge from an abscess. The surgeon must be aware that airway reflexes may be obtunded at the same time that a nominally conscious state has been maintained.[72]

Strict attention to patient preparation and case selection is essential. Impingement of the infected fascial space on the airway, the ability of the patient to open the mouth, and the location of the incision for surgical drainage are important factors. Infection of the buccal space infection, space of the body of the mandible, or submasseteric space does not impinge directly on the airway and the placement of the incision is such that an adequate pharyngeal curtain can be placed to protect against pulmonary aspiration. Alternatively, an infection involving the lateral pharyngeal space or lingual soft tissues compromises the airway. Administration of sedative and analgesic medications may jeopardize the integrity of the airway.

Infections affecting the muscles of mastication cause trismus. One benefit of a combined sedative-analgesic technique is that increased mouth opening may occur with the relief of pain. However, the patient who is debilitated may be extremely sensitive to the respiratory depressant effects of the anesthetic medication; thus extra caution is necessary.

The surgeon or anesthesiologist must proceed slowly and with extreme diligence in considering administration of sedative and analgesic medications. An appropriate fasting period before the procedure is essential. For a scheduled anesthetic an appropriate period of no oral intake requires at least an 8-hour fast of solid food (6 hours is the suggested guidelines in some countries) and at least a 2-hour abstinence from clear liquids. For a patient who has been in distress for the past several hours this period may be inadequate. However, these guidelines are satisfactory for patients with mild infection when an office or emergency department incision and drainage is feasible. Sometimes a patient has not fasted according to the above guidelines. Administration of opioids to increase the pain threshold may allow the necessary surgical intervention. This technique can be considered comparable with postoperative analgesia. Generally less medication would be administered than used for a sedative and analgesic technique. However, monitoring must be consistent with anesthesia guidelines.

Before administering sedative and analgesic medications, the surgeon must be able to control the airway. If trismus is present, insertion of a ratchet-type (molt) mouth prop between the upper and lower canines and premolars is prudent. The stability of these teeth should be checked to ensure that force applied to them will facilitate mouth opening and not compromise their integrity. The mouth prop is opened until slight pressure against the teeth makes the mouth prop stay in place. As the sedative and analgesic medications are titrated, the ratchet-type mouth prop gradually is opened by one-tooth increments on the ratchet until adequate access is achieved. The patient should be instructed before the procedure that a brief period of pain might ensue with each increment of opening the mouth prop. If the surgeon is unable to overcome the trismus, administration of sedative and analgesic medications should be discontinued.

Benzodiazepines and opioids are an appropriate combination for sedation and analgesia. Benzodiazepines provide anxiolysis, sedation, and amnesia. Opioids provide analgesia. They are beneficial especially when optimal local anesthesia cannot be achieved. Alternatively, opioids have a proportionately greater degree of respiratory depressant effects compared with benzodiazepines. Despite the respiratory depressant effects of opioids and benzodiazepines, both drugs have specific antagonists.[22,53,54,93] Appropriate anesthetic management should avoid the need for reversal agents. Sedation and analgesia should be titrated slowly; maximal anesthetic effect may require several minutes. If the surgeon intends to titrate the medication to achieve partial ptosis of the upper eyelids (Verrill's sign), the patient may become too deeply sedated.

Failure to achieve complete local anesthesia is not uncommon in the management of orofacial infections. Therefore the patient experiences some degree of discomfort unless a greater anesthetic depth is achieved. In select situations when the infection does not impinge directly on the airway, the surgeon has complete control of the airway, and the patient has fasted appropriately, the surgeon may consider administration of methohexital or propofol to increase anesthetic depth. Propofol may be a more appropriate choice because of its analgesic properties compared with methohexital's hyperalgesic effects. Subhypnotic doses (not deep sedation or general anesthetic doses) of methohexital also may be considered. Its analgesic and anxiolytic effects are of shorter duration compared with benzodiazepines or opioids. Regardless of the agent, increased airway compromise is a risk and neither agent can be recommended as a first choice for sedation and analgesia in patients with oromaxillofacial infections.

The respiratory depressant effects of the anesthetic medication persist into the recovery period. Generally supplemental oxygen should be administered into the postoperative period. Despite the administration of supplemental oxygen the patient still may experience periods of oxygen desaturation. This desaturation alerts the individual monitoring the patient to intervene. Intervention may entail simple stimulation of the patient. A greater concern should be the lack of recognizing an impending respiratory problem because the patient has satisfactory oxygen saturation. This situation is less likely if the patient is not receiving supplemental oxygen. Therefore respiratory rate and depth and oxygen saturation should be monitored during the postoperative period.

INTUBATION TECHNIQUES

Nasotracheal Versus Orotracheal Intubation Except when awake intubation is indicated, nasoendotracheal intubation should not be used to establish emergency control of the airway in patients with maxillofacial infection. Oral endotracheal intubation is quicker and has a greater success rate than endotracheal intubation. The less experienced anesthetist may require multiple attempts at nasotracheal intubation requiring additional minutes. In the obtunded or paralyzed patient (and even in the awake patient), multiple attempts increase the risk of complications including iatrogenic perforation of an abscess and tracheal soilage.

However, nasotracheal intubation may be beneficial for patients in whom prolonged intubation is anticipated. Patients generally can tolerate a nasal tube more easily and thus require less sedative medication. In addition, the tube can be secured more safely with less chance of accidental extubation. When nasoendotracheal intubation ultimately is preferred, a later conversion to nasal intubation can be established after the airway is protected emergently with an oral endotracheal tube. Chronic sinusitis is a disadvantage of prolonged nasal endotracheal intubation.[77] The primary contraindication to a nasotracheal intubation is a lateral pharyngeal or retropharyngeal space infection. However, in many situations, when the infection is not bilateral, nasotracheal intubation may be considered through the naris on the uninfected side provided care is taken to manually guide the tip of the tube past the area of infection.

Nasotracheal Intubation Stoelting[108] described nasotracheal intubation without laryngoscopy in the awake or sedated patient. It may be the safest technique when initial evaluation of the patient suggests that ventilation or intubation will be difficult or impossible once anesthesia is induced. One advantage is protection of the airway and minimized risk of pulmonary aspiration from purulent discharge or gastric regurgitation.[37] The alternative to awake nasotracheal intubation may be establishment of a surgical airway with or without sedation.

Success of awake intubation depends on patient comfort and cooperation, which includes careful explanation of the procedure to the patient. Sedation also minimizes potentially detrimental hemodynamic fluctuations.

Sedation that is too deep may compromise the integrity of the patient's airway, which may cause airway obstruction, oxygen desaturation, or increased risk of pulmonary aspiration. If the patient becomes agitated or combative during airway manipulation, the clinician must determine whether these are manifestations of hypoxia. Monitoring of oxygen saturation is mandatory. Supplemental oxygen administered during awake intubation also minimizes hypoxemia. Ventilatory monitoring with capnography can be accomplished similarly. A nasopharyngeal airway attached to an endotracheal tube adaptor can be connected to the anesthetic circuit allowing oxygenation and capnographic monitoring[98] (Figure 23-5).

Intubation in the awake individual can be a stimulating process. In the patient with underlying cardiovascular disease, stimulation may have significant detrimental effects. Anesthetizing the upper airway can improve patient com-

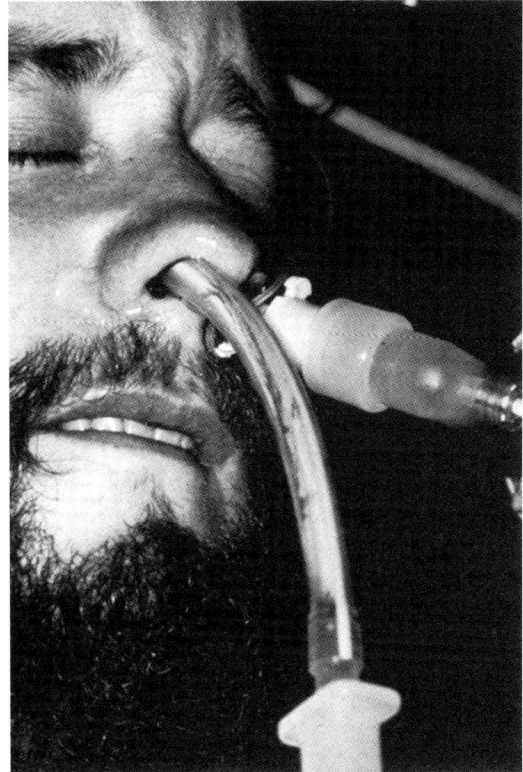

Figure 23-5 Fiberoptic intubation in a patient with a pterygomandibular space abscess. A nasopharyngeal airway in the left naris is attached to the anesthetic circuit. This allows the administration of supplemental oxygen in addition to ventilatory monitoring using capnography. The patient is intubated simultaneously with a fiberoptic laryngoscope through the other nostril. (From Flynn TR: Odontogenic infections, *Oral Maxillofac Clin North Am* 3:311, 1991.)

fort and lessen the stimulation associated with the procedure. The gag reflex can be controlled effectively with a nerve block of the lingual branch of the glossopharyngeal nerve, the superior laryngeal nerve, or both nerves. Both nerve blocks are relatively straightforward techniques. The glossopharyngeal nerve block requires bilateral deposition of 1 to 2 mL of local anesthetic agent into the inferior aspect of the anterior tonsillar pillar. The superior laryngeal nerve block is accomplished by the bilateral percutaneous deposition of 1 to 2 mL of local anesthetic agent into the thyrohyoid membrane along the inferior lateral margin of the hyoid bone. A needle should not be inserted through an infected site. Therefore the location of the infection may preclude the administration of these nerve blocks. Local anesthetic agents also can be topically administered orally (as swish, spray, or atomizer) or transtracheally. Transtracheal administration is achieved by inserting a needle into the trachea through the cricothyroid membrane. Approximately 4 mL of lidocaine 4% is injected into the trachea after a positive aspiration of air confirming appropriate needle placement. The patient generally coughs and the lidocaine is dispersed anesthetizing the mucosa of the trachea and upper airway. Topical application of lidocaine is as effective as nerve blocks in blunting the response to an awake intubation.[104] Although these techniques are relatively safe, the local anesthetic may blunt the protective reflexes against pulmonary aspiration. For nasal intubation, additional preparation includes topical application of a local anesthetic and a vasoconstrictor to the nasal mucosa.[37,72]

Nasoendotracheal intubation may be accomplished blindly or with the aid of a fiberoptic stylet or fiberoptic laryngoscope. Difficulty with the technique results when the posterior nasopharynx does not align directly with the glottic opening. Inflation of the cuff of the endotracheal tube has been reported as a technique to align the tip of the endotracheal tube with the glottic opening. After the tip of the tube is advanced past the epiglottis, the cuff is deflated and the tube is advanced between the vocal cords and into the trachea.[1,50] Rotation and flexion of the head and neck also can facilitate intubation. Persistent attempts at nasoendotracheal intubation without laryngoscopy and direct visualization of the glottis can result in nasal bleeding, mucosal lacerations, abscess rupture, and false passage of the endotracheal tube, with or without stimulation of the gag reflex. Therefore blind awake intubation should be used cautiously when the possibility of discharge of infected material into the airway exists, such as an infection medial to the mandible.

Lighted Stylet Tracheal Intubation   The American Society of Anesthesiologists recognizes lighted stylet tracheal intubation in its guidelines for management of the difficult airway.[7,34] The lighted stylet provides a fiberoptic light source at the tip of the endotracheal tube. When the device is inserted, the transillumination of the external neck indicates the position of the tip of the endotracheal tube. The device may be used to facilitate blind nasoendotracheal and oroendotracheal intubation. In a study comparing lighted stylet tracheal intubation with blind nasal intubation, the lighted stylet technique was favored because it required fewer attempts and less time.[44] For an anticipated difficult intubation the device also may optimize the laryngoscopic view when used in conjunction with direct laryngoscopy.[20]

Fiberoptic Intubation   Fiberoptic endoscopic nasal intubation is the technique of choice for the awake patient. An excellent review of this technique has been published recently.[46] The advantage of this technique is that the fiberoptic laryngoscope can be directed at its tip, under vision through the fiberoptic cable, and navigate the distorted anatomy of the edematous infected airway. The success of the technique depends on the skill and experience of the anesthesiologist. To improve the conditions for a successful intubation, the intensity of the room lights should be decreased, allowing the intubating team to determine the position of the endoscope as the fiberoptic light is transilluminated through the anterior neck. This technique may be difficult in the patient with an oromaxillofacial infection that distorts normal anatomical structure.[107] If the trachea is deviated to one side, the nostril on the side toward which the deviation has occurred may be used (Figure 23-6).

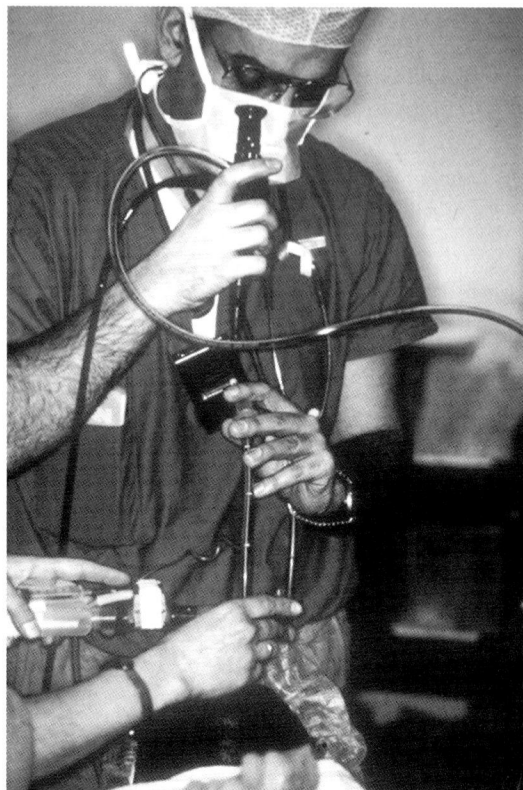

Figure 23-6 Fiberoptic intubation technique.

GENERAL ANESTHESIA

Preoxygenation   In preparation for intubation the patient should be preoxygenated to minimize the potential for hypoxemia. Preoxygenation is accomplished by administration of 100% oxygen for 3 minutes or 4 "vital capacity" breaths with 100% oxygen.[19]

Trismus   Limitation of the interincisal opening to 30 mm or less likely will cause difficulty with direct laryngoscopy for intubation. When a physical effect such as muscle spasm or the actual mass effect of the infection causes the mechanical obstruction of the oral opening, it may persist despite the induction of general anesthesia. When the trismus is caused by pain or mild inflammation, it may disappear or at least partially resolve after the administration of anesthetic medication.[23,78] An indication that of the potential for resolution of the trismus may be the degree of resistance encountered when attempting to open the patient's mouth during the initial examination. If a "spongy soft" stop is detected, the ability to substantially increase the mouth opening may be possible after achieving an appropriate anesthetic depth. In such situations, if no other factors compromise the integrity of the airway, the clinician may plan to sedate the patient as discussed in the sedation and analgesia section. As the patient becomes more sedate an attempt is made to further open the mouth. When adequate opening occurs, general anesthesia may be induced and intubation may be performed. If adequate mouth opening does not occur after the administration of sedative and analgesic medications, the patient should still be conscious with a patent airway and alternative plans may be pursued.

Sellick Maneuver The Sellick maneuver (cricoid pressure) consists of downward pressure on the cricoid cartilage causing temporary esophageal occlusion between the cricoid cartilage and the cervical vertebrae. The Sellick maneuver prevents gastric regurgitation and insufflation during anesthetic induction and positive-pressure ventilation. Its efficacy depends on application of adequate pressure to the cricoid cartilage. The technique is considered the gold standard for prevention of aspiration of gastric contents in obtunded and anesthetized patients. The Sellick maneuver does not prevent aspiration of purulent discharge from a head and neck infection.

Mask Induction of General Anesthesia Although artificially securing the airway before induction of general anesthetic may be preferred in patients with potentially compromised airways, extenuating circumstances may preclude the doctor's ability to intubate or achieve a surgical airway until the patient is asleep. Inhalation induction with a potent volatile agent is a recognized technique. A primary advantage of an inhalation induction compared with an intravenous induction is the ability to maintain spontaneous ventilations as anesthetic depth is increased. The spontaneous ventilation of the patient maintains airway patency and is the means by which the anesthetic depth may be reversed, ensuring a degree of safety. Alternatively the respiratory-depressant effects of intravenous drugs may compromise airway patency and are not as readily reversed. In a patient who is debilitated, even a low dose of an induction agent may have a profound respiratory-depressant effect potentially increasing the risk of such an occurrence.

The technique of inhalational induction depends on the selection of a volatile agent that does not irritate the airway. Historically, halothane has been the preferred agent. However, sevoflurane has since supplanted halothane. Both agents have fewer respiratory-depressant effects and less airway irritability compared with isoflurane (Forane) and desflurane. Sevoflurane is less irritating with less coughing and breath holding than halothane. Compared with halothane, sevoflurane has a significantly lower blood-gas partition coefficient, which is clinically manifested as a more rapid ability to change anesthetic depth.[21,36,102,121]

Brown and Sataloff[23] described an inhalation induction technique using halothane followed by endotracheal intubation. Patients are preoxygenated followed by induction of anesthesia with a combination of nitrous oxide and incremental increases of halothane. Nitrous oxide is used to take advantage of the second-gas effect and increase the rapidity of induction. Mostafa and Atherton[89] discussed the use of sevoflurane for difficult tracheal intubation. Although sevoflurane provided a smooth and rapid induction, in one case maintenance of a clear airway was diffi-

cult. Respiratory difficulty during an inhalational induction may result from airway irritability (e.g., breath holding, laryngospasm) unrelated to infection or airway distortion and edema directly associated with the infection. Advantages of sevoflurane are the decreased incidence of airway irritability with decreased respiratory distress and its low blood-gas partition coefficient, which allows rapid reversal and lightening of anesthetic depth. Induction with sevoflurane can be achieved satisfactorily without nitrous oxide. The ability to use 100% oxygen provides a safety margin. If obstruction occurs, oxygen desaturation is delayed. Although induction of general anesthesia with halothane can be accomplished similarly without nitrous oxide, the second-gas effect of nitrous oxide is of greater importance to facilitate a smooth, rapid induction because of the lower blood solubility of halothane.[91]

Preservation of spontaneous ventilations is not always possible. As the patient becomes anesthetized, the possibility of airway obstruction exists. Regardless of the cause, progression from a patent to an obstructed airway may be sudden. If the anesthesiologist cannot correct the airway obstruction, the exhalation of the anesthetic gases cannot reverse the anesthetic depth. The anesthesiologist should identify the most likely cause of the obstruction. If it is upper airway obstruction, the first step should be to carefully establish an oral airway to prevent iatrogenic disruption of the mucosa resulting in purulent drainage into the airway. If the patency of the airway is reestablished, the decision can be made to alter the anesthetic depth and at the appropriate time proceed with intubation. If the oral airway is not effective, alternative airway devices to facilitate ventilation may be considered depending on the location of the infection. If the airway remains obstructed, laryngoscopy and intubation may be attempted. However, if the airway cannot be immediately secured by intubation and the patient's lungs cannot be ventilated, a surgical airway is required. If the cause of the obstruction is believed to be laryngospasm, administration of succinylcholine may be considered. Succinylcholine should be administered only if the anesthesiologist believes that the administration of a neuromuscular blocking agent will result in relaxation and a high likelihood that the airway can be intubated, and airway patency will be reestablished and the patient's lungs can be ventilated if intubation fails. If any concerns exist, succinylcholine should not be administered; the anesthesiologist may make one attempt at laryngoscopy and intubation. However, if the airway cannot be secured immediately by intubation and the patient's lungs cannot be ventilated, a surgical airway is required.

Mask induction with an inhalational agent generally is not the first choice of the anesthesiologist. It may be selected when the patient is uncooperative or other techniques cannot be used. This technique was successful in 9 of 10 patients with Ludwig's angina.[5] Most anesthesiologists would prefer the patient to be in the supine or semi-supine position. However, the patient may not tolerate these positions because of an adverse effect of positioning on respirations or on the patient's cognitive abilities. Induction may be achieved with the patient sitting or in the lateral decubitus position on the operating table. As the anesthetic depth is increased, the patient may be repositioned into the supine or semisupine position. The airway may be more patent with the patient in the lateral decubitus position.

When discharge of pus into the airway is a possibility, the patient is placed in the lateral decubitus position or midway between the lateral and prone positions with no pillow or support under the head to facilitate gravity drainage of secretions or pus from the oral cavity. Adjusting the operating table to a few degrees of the Trendelenburg position may prevent passage of any pus down the trachea. When an adequate depth of anesthesia has been achieved, laryngoscopy may be performed with the patient in full lateral (right or left, according to the anesthesiologist's preference) position with no support under the head. Some anesthesiologists prefer the patient to be supine on the operating table in a slight Trendelenburg position. High-volume suction must be available with a Yankauer suction tip to evacuate any pus or secretions.

Laryngeal Mask Airway   The laryngeal mask airway (LMA) is designed to form an airtight seal in the hypopharynx. It establishes a direct connection with the patient's airway providing a possible route of ventilation in rare situations when ventilation is not possible with a face mask or tracheal intubation. The LMA can be inserted blindly with the head and neck in any position. Its disadvantage over the endotracheal tube is that it provides a direct conduit between the esophagus and the trachea. Therefore it does not protect against pulmonary aspiration. Increased pulmonary resistance tends to cause gastric insufflation, which is associated with an increased risk of pulmonary aspiration.[17]

Once the LMA is inserted and satisfactory ventilation is achieved, a more definitive airway should be secured. The LMA is designed to enhance intubation. The 30-degree angle at the junction of the mask and tube of the LMA is designed to facilitate visualization of the glottis when a fiberoptic endoscope is inserted through the LMA. With direct fiberoptic intubation a No. 6.0 or No. 6.5 endotracheal tube can be passed through a No. 3 or No. 4 LMA, respectively.

Use of the LMA may not be possible in a patient with an oromaxillofacial infection. Because the LMA sits within the hypopharynx, it cannot be used if the patient has a pathological condition impinging on the pharyngeal space. It also is placed orally and thus cannot be used if significant trismus is present.

SURGICAL AIRWAY: CRICOTHYROTOMY VERSUS TRACHEOTOMY

Unlike elective oral intubations in uncomplicated cases, failure to achieve oral intubation in a patient with an oromaxillofacial infection may require the establishment of an emergency surgical airway. The advantage of a surgical airway accomplished under local anesthesia (with or without sedation and analgesia) is that control of the airway can be established in the cooperative patient by sealing off the lower airway from the upper airway by a cuffed endotracheal or tracheotomy tube. Some consider this approach the gold standard for severe airway infections such as Ludwig's angina.[35,106] The patient remains conscious until the airway is secured; therefore the protective reflexes are maintained throughout the procedure. Traumatic rupture of an abscess with discharge of infected material into the airway is less likely. However, a surgical airway is not risk-free. Incision into an infected area may result in contamination of the lower airways and spread of infection into the mediastinum.[5]

When the airway must be secured surgically, cricothyrotomy or tracheotomy can be effective.[43,105] Table 23-1 summarizes the advantages and disadvantages of each technique. Cricothyrotomy provides the fastest airway access but is not satisfactory for long-term airway management. Tracheotomy technically is more complex and requires more time but can be left in position for an extended period.

Complications of Cricothyrotomy and Tracheotomy

If the infection extends to the cervicofacial region, the risk of aspiration of purulent material is increased. The higher location of entry into the airway associated with a cricothyrotomy may be a disadvantage, although this potential is probably more theoretical than clinically significant. Despite the risk of airway contamination an alternative to a surgical airway may not exist in certain situations.

Because of the anatomical location of a cricothyrotomy, short-term complications are unlikely unless the surgical

---

TABLE 23-1

Tracheotomy versus Cricothyrotomy: Advantages and Disadvantages

Procedure	Advantages	Disadvantages
Tracheotomy	Long-term airway access Prevention of damage to larynx	More time needed to perform procedure Neck extension required, with potential of worsening airway obstruction Potential bleeding from thyroid isthmus or nearby vessels
Cricothyrotomy	Rapid airway access Less likelihood of bleeding Neck extension not required	Short-term airway access Potential damage to subglottic larynx Possible impingement on infection because of higher location in neck

Modified from Bennett J, Spiro J: Anesthetic considerations in the acutely injured patient, *Oral Maxillofac Surg Clin North Am* 11:185; 1990.

landmarks are confused or the procedure is performed significantly off the midline. If the endotracheal tube or tracheotomy tube remains in a cricothyrotomy site for an extended period, significant damage to the subglottic region of the larynx may occur, but this complication can be avoided easily by conversion to a standard tracheotomy if the need for more extended airway access is anticipated.

Short-term complications of standard tracheotomy are bleeding, displacement of the tracheotomy tube, or creation of a "false passage" anterior or lateral to the trachea in the process of inserting the tracheotomy tube. Pneumothorax or pneumomediastinum may occur from positive-pressure ventilation through a false passage or direct injury to the apex of the pleura. Long-term complications of tracheotomy include formation of a tracheocutaneous fistula after decannulation or tracheal stenosis at the site of the tracheotomy. If cartilage is removed from the anterior tracheal wall during the tracheotomy, the likelihood of a symptomatic long-term stenosis at the level of the tracheotomy is increased. Symptomatic tracheal stenosis does not occur in adult patients until a significant proportion of the trachea is obstructed. Milder stenosis probably occurs after many tracheotomies but remains undetected because no serious problems ensue.

Jet Ventilation   An alternative technique to open tracheotomy or cricothyrotomy is the use of transtracheal ventilation or jet ventilation. A preformed or large-gauge intravenous catheter attached to a syringe is used to enter the trachea. Aspiration of air from the trachea confirms placement of the needle tip. The catheter is advanced and the needle withdrawn from the airway. Plastic tubing with a Luer adaptor is used to connect the ventilation apparatus to the hub of the catheter. Manual ventilation with this technique can provide adequate oxygenation on a temporary basis but carbon dioxide is not eliminated efficiently.[6,66,86] Alternatively, jet ventilation provides adequate gaseous exchange.[18] Jet ventilation also can protect against pulmonary aspiration.[6,59,65,71] Any type of jet ventilation entails risk and must be performed with caution to avoid pneumothorax or pneumomediastinum.[10] Most hospital operating rooms are equipped for jet ventilation when a difficult airway is anticipated. The technique is a rapid and safe method of providing ventilation in a patient with a difficult airway.

Needle aspiration before airway management is achieved is an important adjunct when an abscess threatens to rupture or drain into the airway. An 18-gauge needle can be inserted into a fluctuant abscess cavity to aspirate as much pus as possible into the syringe. This technique decompresses the abscess before induction of anesthesia and manipulation of the airway and drains the abscess into the oral cavity or onto the skin rather than into the oropharynx or hypopharynx. A further advantage of this technique is that a good culture specimen can be obtained, allowing the institution of antibiotic therapy immediately thereafter.

The surgeon must stand by the patient at all times during airway management procedures if infection threatens the airway. All tracheotomy instruments should be readily available. If the anesthesiologist encounters difficulty in maintaining the airway, an immediate emergency tracheotomy or cricothyroidotomy should be considered.

CRITERIA FOR EXTUBATION

The advantage of intubation in the patient with a compromised airway is assurance of airway patency. However, intubation has complications, including obstruction, collapse, displacement or kinking of the tube, dehydration of respiratory mucosa by dry gases, hemorrhage, necrosis, scarring or granuloma formation in the upper airway and trachea, and sinusitis from prolonged intubation.[45,77,114] Therefore extubation of patients recovering from an infection as soon as safely possible is important. Serious adverse events resulting from airway extubation have been documented in the literature; these accounted for 7% of the respiratory complaints reported in the American Society of Anesthesiologists Closed Claims Study.[27] The potential for such problems would be anticipated to be greater in the compromised airway such as in patients with oromaxillofacial infections. The determination of when to perform extubation may be as challenging as the decision as to when and how to perform intubation.

For this discussion, satisfaction of the essential requirements for extubation, such as adequate negative inspiratory pressure is assumed. The patency of the patient's airway is unique to this situation. Patients frequently receive maintenance anesthetic medications for comfort and tolerance of the endotracheal tube, and these sedative medications decrease the electromyographic activity of the strap muscles.[38] Decreased electromyographic activity of the strap muscles leads to clinical obstruction of the airway. Therefore residual sedation in the patient with a narrowed airway may cause unfavorable consequences.

The surgical team must understand airway evaluation. The most important aspect is clinical inspection of the airway. An intraoral and extraoral examination should be performed to evaluate edema, erythema, trismus, and lingual mobility and displacement. The pharynx should be inspected. In selected situations, administration of a bolus of a short-acting anesthetic (e.g., propofol) may facilitate adequate assessment of the pharynx. Alternatively, a fiberoptic examination may be beneficial in providing a good view of the airway to the level of the glottis. Postoperative CT scans sometimes are obtained to assess the adequacy of surgical intervention. If available, these radiographs should be assessed. The CT scan may demonstrate the need for further surgical drainage; if so, extubation would be delayed. The scan may indicate significant airway edema to suggest a delay in extubation. However, the supine positioning of the patient and the relaxation of the soft tissue around the endotracheal tube may show an airway that appears more compromised than actual (Figure 23-7). Finally, the surgeon may consider deflation of the cuff of the endotracheal tube and assessment if the patient can breathe around the tube (Figure

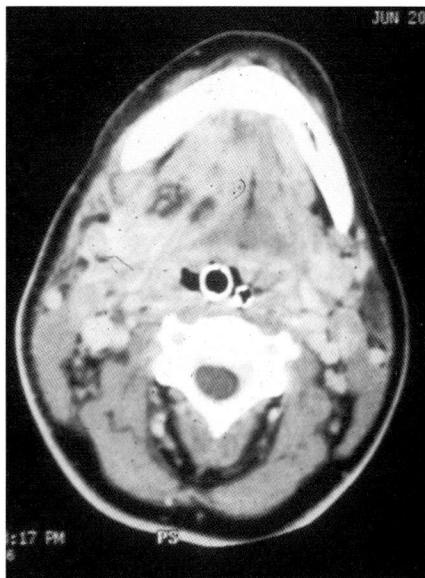

Figure 23-7 This CT scan shows a patient with an incision and drainage performed approximately 48 hours before reimaging. The scan demonstrate soft tissue encroachment on the endotracheal tube. The CT findings influenced the decision to maintain intubation. The patient removed the tube herself approximately 4 hours later and reintubation was not required.

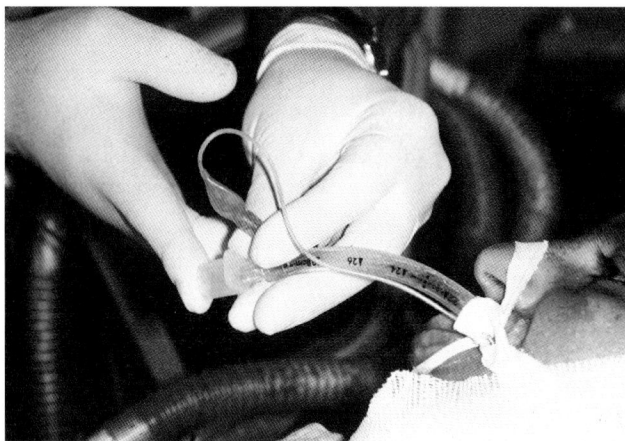

Figure 23-9 An endotracheal tube with a tube changer passed through it demonstrating the length and diameter of the tube changer relative to the endotracheal tube.

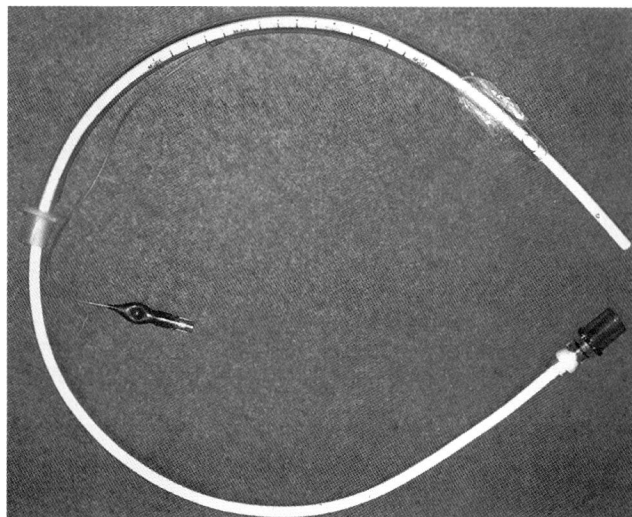

Figure 23-8 Occlusion of the endotracheal tube to determine whether the patient can breathe around the tube before extubation.

markings that identify the depth of insertion. The device must be stabilized while the endotracheal tube is being removed. At first the endotracheal tube may be withdrawn to the level of the pharynx. However, once initial airway patency is ensured, the endotracheal tube can be removed fully. If reintubation is necessary and the endotracheal tube has been removed completely, intubation should be accomplished with a new endotracheal tube. The tube changer then can be left in place for several hours. In some instances the device has been left in place for up to 72 hours. Generally the guide is removed within 1 hour of extubation.[85] The tube changer is not risk-free. If the airway is compromised, the tube changer may act as a conduit for the passage of purulent material. The tube changer is not always successful. Therefore the surgeon should not consider extubation until he or she is confident that the patient can maintain the airway.

The surgeon may consider using a fiberoptic laryngoscope as a tube changer. This practice requires another individual to hold the fiberoptic laryngoscope in place. In addition, the size of the internal lumen is significantly less than the lumen within the tube changer, which limits the ability to use jet ventilation if necessary. Alternatively, when the bronchoscope is inserted parallel to the tube changer (either through the opposing naris or orally), it may provide a visual aid in passing an endotracheal tube over the tube changer when the endotracheal tube does not pass easily into the trachea.[87]

EFFECT OF ANESTHETICS ON THE IMMUNE SYSTEM

No single anesthetic agent or technique is associated with depression of the immune system.[39] Associated hypoxia, uremia, and metabolic and respiratory acidosis all increase the severity of infection. When associated with anesthesia,

23-8). The practitioner must use all available information establish the plan of action.

The American Society of Anesthesiologists Task Force on Management of the Difficult Airway provided recommendations for extubation strategy.[26] These guidelines suggest the use of a device that can serve as a guide to facilitate reintubation. The endotracheal tube changer (guide) should be semirigid with a hollow core that will allow jet ventilation. The rigidity is required so that the guide maintains its form throughout the period of intubation (Figure 23-9). Several endotracheal tube changers are available.[15,32] The device should be inserted below the level of the tip of the endotracheal tube just above the carina. Commercial devices have these conditions may modify the clinical course of an infection. Despite the results of some animal studies that imply that anesthesia can decrease the survival rate in experimental infections, studies of human postoperative infections provide little information on the role of anesthetic factors in the development of these infections. Therefore few conclusions can be drawn about whether individual anesthetic agents affect perioperative infection.[28]

PULMONARY ASPIRATION OF INFECTED MATERIAL

The true incidence of aspiration of infected material from deep space odontogenic infections is unknown. Hought et al.[62] reported airway obstruction and pulmonary arrest but not aspiration pneumonia as a cause of death. Toews and de la Rocha[112] reported two cases of retropharyngeal abscess with mediastinal involvement. One of these patients aspirated pus from the ruptured abscess but survived. Toews and de la Rocha also reviewed 16 cases of oropharyngeal infection with endothoracic spread. Ten patients had odontogenic infection; three of these patients died. Of the seven patients with reported aspiration pneumonia, only one died. The true mortality rate of aspiration of pus from odontogenic infections probably is underreported.

The aspiration of large amounts of pus undoubtedly carries a grave prognosis. LeFrock et al.[74] reported a 70% mortality rate as a result of massive aspiration of any sort, and studies of aspiration pneumonia in general report a mortality rate of 35% to 80%.[48]

The oral flora is the common thread in most cases of aspiration pneumonia.[103] Gorbach and Bartlett[49] found that *Fusobacterium nucleatum, Bacteroides melaninogenicus, Bacteroides oralis, Peptostreptococcus, Peptococcus,* and *Veillonella,* all of which are components of the flora of maxillofacial infections, were the most common anaerobic isolates from the lungs in aspiration pneumonia.[12,49,79]

The prevention and treatment of aspiration in general have been reviewed.[63,70] The role of steroids in the treatment of aspiration remains unsupported[25,74]; therefore their use is not recommended.

Clindamycin is the empirical antibiotic of choice in nonallergic patients. Specific antibiotic therapy should be directed to the organisms isolated from the odontogenic abscess that has ruptured into the airway. However, because aspiration-induced pneumonia or lung abscess can be protracted, periodic reculturing of the infected lung should be performed to detect changes in the bacterial flora of the pulmonary infection. The most reliable technique for culture of pulmonary infections is transtracheal aspiration.[103]

REFERENCES

1. Ackerman WE, Phero JC: An aid to nasotracheal intubation, *Oral Maxillofac Surg* 47:1341, 1989.
2. Aiello G, Metcalf I: Anaesthetic implications of temporomandibular joint disease, *Can J Anaesth* 39:610, 1992.
3. Akinosi JO: A new approach to the mandibular nerve block, *Br J Oral Surg* 15:83, 1977.
4. Alexander RE, Throndson RR: A review of perioperative corticosteroid use in dentoalveolar surgery, *Oral Surg* 90:406, 2000.
5. Allen D, Loughnan TE, Ord RD: A reevaluation of the role of tracheostomy in Ludwig's angina, *J Oral Maxillofac Surg* 43:436, 1985.
6. American Heart Association: *Textbook of advanced cardiac life support,* Dallas, 1987, American Heart Association.
7. The American Society of Anesthesiologists Task Force on Management of the Difficult Airway: Practice guidelines for management of the difficult airway, *Anesthesiology* 78:597, 1993.
8. Anene O, Meert KL, Uy H, et al: Dexamethasone for the prevention of postextubation airway obstruction: a prospective, randomized, double-blind, placebo-controlled trial, *Crit Care Med* 24:1666, 1996.
9. Arne J, Desoins P, Fusciardi J, et al: Preoperative assessment for difficult intubation in general and ENT surgery: predictive value of a clinical multivariate risk index, *Br J Anaesth* 80:140, 1998.
10. Attia RR, Battit GE, Murphy JD: Transtracheal ventilation, *JAMA* 234:1152, 1975.
11. Barret A: Dexamethasone as an adjunct in oropharyngeal obstruction in a patient with leukemia, *Oral Surg Oral Med Oral Pathol* 70:741, 1990.
12. Bartlett JG, O'Keefe P: The bacteriology of perimandibular space infections, *J Oral Surg* 37:407, 1979.
13. Bennett CR: Monheim's local anesthesia and pain control in dental practice, ed 7, St Louis, 1984, Mosby.
14. Bennett J, Spiro J: Anesthetic considerations in the acutely injured patient, *Oral Maxillofac Surg Clin North Am* 11:185, 1999.
15. Benumof JL: Management of the difficult airway, *Anesthesiology* 75:1087, 1991.
16. Benumof JL: Difficult laryngoscopy: obtaining the best view, *Can J Anaesth* 41:361, 1994 (editorial).
17. Benumof JL: Laryngeal mask airway and the ASA difficult airway algorithm, *Anesthesiology* 84:686, 1996.
18. Benumof JL, Scheller MS: The importance of transtracheal jet ventilation in the management of the difficult airway, *Anesthesiology* 71:769, 1989.
19. Berthoud M, Read DH, Norman J: Preoxygenation—how long? *Anesthesia* 38:96, 1983.
20. Biehl JW, Bourke DL: Use of a lighted stylet to aid direct laryngoscopy, *Anesthesiology* 86:1012, 1997 (letter).
21. Black A, Sury MRJ, Hemington L, et al: A comparison of the induction characteristics of sevoflurane and halothane in children, *Anaesthesia* 51:539, 1996.
22. Blouin RT, Conard PF, Perreault S, et al: The effect of flumazenil on midazolam-induced depression of the ventilatory response to hypoxia during isohypercarbia, *Anesthesiology* 78:635, 1993.
23. Brown AC, Sataloff RT: Special anesthetic techniques in head and neck surgery, *Otolaryngol Clin North Am* 14:587, 1981.
24. Brown RD: The failure of local anesthesia in acute inflammation: some recent concepts, *Br Dent J* 151:47, 1981.
25. Bynum LJ, Pierce AK: Pulmonary aspiration of gastric contents, *Am Rev Respir Dis* 114:1129, 1976.
26. Caplan RA, Benumof JL, Berry FA, et al: Practice guidelines for management of the difficult airway: a report by the American Society of Anesthesiologists Task Force on management of the difficult airway, *Anesthesiology* 78:597, 1993.

27. Caplan RA, Posner KL, Ward RJ, et al: Adverse respiratory events in anesthesia: a closed claims analysis, *Anesthesiology* 72:828, 1990.

28. Cascorbi HF: Effect of anesthetics on the immune system, *Int Anesthesiol Clin* 19:69, 1981.

29. Cesar L, Gonzalez C, Calia FM: Bacteriologic flora of aspiration-induced pulmonary infections, *Arch Intern Med* 135:711, 1975.

30. Chou H-C, Wu T-L: Mandibulohyoid distance in difficult intubation, *Br J Anaesth* 71:335, 1991.

31. Coleman RD, Smith RA: The anatomy of mandibular anesthesia: review and analysis, *Oral Surg* 54:148, 1982.

32. Cooper RM: The use of an endotracheal ventilation catheter in the management of difficult extubations, *Can J Anaesth* 43:90, 1996.

33. Coyle PK: Glucocorticoids in central nervous system bacterial infection, *Arch Neurol* 56:796, 1999.

34. Davis L, Cook-Sather SD, Schreiner MS: Lighted stylet tracheal intubation: a review, *Anesth Analg* 90:745, 2000.

35. Demas PN, Sotereanos GC: The use of tracheotomy in oral and maxillofacial surgery, *J Oral Maxillofac Surg* 46:483, 1988.

36. D'Hollander AA, Monteny E, Dewachter B, et al: Intubation under typical supraglottic analgesia in unpremedicated and non-fasting patients: amnesic effects of subhypnotic doses of diazepam and Innovar, *Can Anesth Soc J* 21:467, 1974.

37. Doi M, Ikeda K: Airway irritation produced by volatile anaesthetics during brief inhalation: comparison of halothane, enflurane, isoflurane, and sevoflurane, *Can J Anaesth* 40:122, 1993.

38. Drummond GB: Influence of thiopentone on upper airway muscles, *Br J Anaesth* 63:12, 1989.

39. Duncan PG, Cullen BF: Anesthesia and immunology, *Anesthesiology* 45:522, 1976.

40. Eden AN, Kaufman A, Yu R: Corticosteroids and croup: controlled double-blind study, *JAMA* 200:133, 1967.

41. Eisenberg MS, Bergner L, Hallstrom A: Cardiac resuscitation in the community: importance of rapid provision and implications for program planning, *JAMA* 241:1905, 1979.

42. El-Ganzouri AR, McCarthy RJ, Tuman KJ, et al: Preoperative airway assessment: predictive value of a multivariate risk index, *Anesth Analg* 82:1197, 1996.

43. Feinberg SE, Peterson LJ: Use of cricothyroidostomy in oral and maxillofacial surgery, *J Oral Maxillofac Surg* 45:873, 1987.

44. Fox DJ, Castro T, Rastrelli AJ: Comparison of intubation techniques in the awake patient: the Flexi-lum surgical light (light wand) versus blind nasal approach, *Anesthesiology* 66:69, 1987.

45. Frerk CM: Predicting difficult intubation, *Anaesthesia* 46:1005, 1991.

46. Fulling PD, Roberts JT: Fiberoptic intubation, *Int Anesth Clin* 38:190, 2000.

47. Gersema L, Baker K: Use of corticosteroids in oral surgery, *J Oral Maxillofac Surg* 50:270, 1992.

48. Goldman E, McDonald JS, Peterson SS, et al: Transtracheal ventilation with oscillatory pressure for complete upper airway obstruction, *J Trauma* 28:611, 1988.

49. Gorbach SL, Bartlett JG: Anaerobic infections (second of three parts), *N Engl J Med* 290:1237, 1974.

50. Gorback MS: Inflation of the endotracheal tube cuff as an aid to blind nasal endotracheal intubation, *Anesth Analg* 66:916, 1987 (letter).

51. Gow-Gates GAE: Mandibular conduction anesthesia: a new technique using extraoral landmarks, *Oral Surg* 36:321, 1973.

52. Grodinsky M: Ludwig's angina: an anatomical and clinical study with review of the literature, *Surgery* 5:678, 1939.

53. Gross JB, Blouin RT, Zandsberg S, et al: Effect of flumazenil on ventilatory drive during sedation with midazolam and alfentanil, *Anesthesiology* 85:713, 1996.

54. Gross JB, Weller RS, Conard P: Flumazenil antagonism of midazolam-induced ventilatory depression, *Anesthesiology* 75:179, 1991.

55. Gustainis JF, Peterson LJ: An alternative method of mandibular nerve block, *J Am Dent Assoc* 103:33, 1981.

56. Hawkins DB, Crockett DM, Shum TK: Corticosteroids in airway management, *Otolaryngol Head Neck Surg* 91:593, 1983.

57. Haynes RC: Adrenocorticotrophic hormones: adrenocortical steroids and their synthetic analogs: inhibitors of the synthesis and actions of adrenocortical hormones. In Gilman AG, Rall TW, Nies AS, et al, editors: *Pharmacological basis of therapeutics,* ed 8, Elmsford, NY, 1990, Pergamon Press.

58. Hebert PC, Ducic Y, Boisvert D, et al: Adult epiglottitis in a Canadian setting, *Laryngoscope* 108:64, 1998.

59. Hess D, Keeports R, Didyoung R, et al: Use of high-frequency jet ventilation to prevent aspiration in a patient with an uncuffed tracheostomy tube, *Crit Care Med* 112:918, 1984.

60. Ho LI, Harn HJ, Lien TC, et al: Postextubation laryngeal edema in adults: risk factor evaluation and prevention by hydrocortisone, *Intensive Care Med* 22:933, 1996.

61. Hollinshead WH: Anatomy for surgeons, vol I, *Head and neck,* ed 2, New York, 1968, Harper & Row.

62. Hought RT, Fitzgerald BE, Latta JE, et al: Ludwig's angina: report of two cases and review of the literature from 1945 to January 1979, *J Oral Surg* 38:849, 1980.

63. Hupp JR, Peterson LJ: Aspiration pneumonitis: etiology, therapy, and prevention, *J Oral Surg* 39:430, 1981.

64. Jastak JT, Yagiela JA, Donaldson D: *Local anesthesia of the oral cavity,* ed 1, Philadelphia, 1995, WB Saunders.

65. Jawan B, Cheung HK, Chong ZK, et al: Aspiration and transtracheal jet ventilation with different pressures and depths of chest compression, *Crit Care Med* 27:142, 1999.

66. Jorden RC: Percutaneous transtracheal ventilation, *Emerg Med Clin North Am* 6:745, 1988.

67. Kairys SW, Olmstead EM, O'Connor GT: Steroid treatment or laryngotracheitis: a meta-analysis of the evidence from randomized trials, *Pediatrics* 83:683, 1989.

68. Karkouti K, Keith-Rose D, Wigglesworth D, et al: Predicting difficult intubation: a multivariate analysis, *Can J Anaesth* 47:730, 2000.

69. Kimberly CL, Byers MR: Inflammation of rat molar pulp and periodontium causes increased calcitonin gene-related peptide and axonal sprouting, *Anat Rec* 222:289, 1988.

70. Kinni ME, Stout MM: Aspiration pneumonitis: predisposing conditions and prevention, *J Oral Maxillofac Surg* 44:378, 1986.

71. Klain M, Keszler H, Stool S: Transtracheal high frequency jet ventilation prevents aspiration, *Crit Care Med* 11:170, 1983.

72. Kopriva CJ, Eltringham RJ, Siebert PE: A comparison of intravenous Innovar and topical spray on the laryngeal closure reflex, *Anesthesiology* 40:596, 1974.

73. Kuusela A-L, Vesikari T: A randomized double-blind, placebo-controlled trial of dexamethasone and racemic epinephrine in the treatment of croup, *Acta Pediatr Scand* 77:99, 1988.

74. LeFrock JL, Clark TS, Davies B, et al: Aspiration pneumonia: a ten-year review, *Am Surg* 45:305, 1979.

75. Leipzig B, Oski FA, Cummings CW, et al: A prospective randomized study to determine the efficacy of steroids in treatment of croup, *J Pediatr* 94:194, 1979.

76. Levy TP: An assessment of the Gow-Gates mandibular block for third molar surgery, *J Am Dent Assoc* 103:37, 1981.

77. Linden BE, Aguilar EA, Allen SJ: Sinusitis in the nasotracheally intubated patient, *Arch Otolaryngol Head Neck Surg* 114:860, 1988.

78. Loughnan TE, Allen DE: Ludwig's angina: the anaesthetic management of nine cases, *Anaesthesia* 40:295, 1985.

79. Macdonald JB, Socransky SS, Gibbons RJ: Aspects of the pathogenesis of mixed anaerobic infections of the mucous membranes, *J Dent Res* 42:529, 1963.

80. Malamed SF: The Gow-Gates mandibular block: evaluation after 4,275 cases, *Oral Surg* 51:463, 1981.

81. Malamed SF: *Handbook of local anesthesia,* ed 4, St Louis, 1997, Mosby.

82. Mallampati SR, Gatt SP, Gugino LD, et al: A clinical sign to predict difficult tracheal intubation: a prospective study, *Can Anaesth Soc J* 32:429, 1985.

83. McIntyre JWR: The difficult tracheal intubation, *Can J Anaesth* 34:204, 1987.

84. Mercuri LG: Intraoral second division nerve block, *Oral Surg* 47:109, 1979.

85. Miller J, Lovino W, Fine J, et al: High-frequency jet ventilation in oral and maxillofacial surgery, *J Oral Maxillofac Surg* 40:790, 1982.

86. Miller KA, Harkin CP, Bailey PL: Postoperative tracheal extubation, *Anesth Analg* 80:149, 1995.

87. Montgomery MT, Hogg JP, Roberts DL, et al: The use of glucocorticosteroids to lessen the inflammatory sequelae following third molar surgery, *J Oral Maxillofac Surg* 48:179, 1990.

88. Moreland LW, Corey J, McKenzie R: Ludwig's angina: report of a case and review of the literature, *Arch Intern Med* 148:461, 1988.

89. Mostafa SM, Atherton AMJ: Sevoflurane for difficult tracheal intubation, *Br J Anaesth* 79:393, 1997.

90. Najjar TA: Why can't you achieve adequate regional anesthesia in the presence of infection? *Oral Surg* 44:7, 1977.

91. Neff SPW, Merry AF, Anderson, B: Airway management in Ludwig's angina, *Anaesth Intensive Care* 27:659, 1999.

92. Oates JDL, MacLeod AD, Oates PD, et al: Comparisons of two methods for predicting difficult intubation, *Br J Anaesth* 66:305, 1991.

93. Ochs MW, Tucker MR, Owsley TG, et al: The effectiveness of flumazenil in reversing the sedation and amnesia produced by intravenous midazolam, *J Oral Maxillofac Surg* 48:240, 1990.

94. Ovassapian A: Fiberoptic airway endoscopy in anesthesia and critical care, New York, 1990, Raven Press.

95. Ovassapian A: The difficult airway. In Ovassapian A, editor: *Fiberoptic endoscopy and the difficult airway,* Philadelphia, 1996, Lippincott-Raven.

96. Ovassapian A: Management of the difficult airway. In Ovassapian A, editor: *Fiberoptic endoscopy and the difficult airway,* ed 2, Philadelphia, 1996, Lippincott-Raven.

97. Poore TE, Carney FMT: Maxillary nerve block: a useful technique, *J Oral Surg* 31:749, 1973.

98. Roelofse JA, Joubert JJ DeV, Payne KA: The Luomanen oral airway and endotracheal tube holder as an aid to pediatric fiberoptic endoscopy, *J Oral Maxillofac Surg* 48:533, 1990.

99. Saadoun AP, Malamed S: Intraseptal anesthesia in periodontal surgery, *J Am Dent Assoc* 111:249, 1985.

100. Samsoon GLT, Young JRB: Difficult tracheal intubation: a retrospective study, *Anaesthesia* 42:487, 1987.

101. Sanders B: *Pediatric oral and maxillofacial surgery,* St Louis, 1979, Mosby.

102. Sarner JB, Leveine M, Davis PJ, et al: Clinical characteristics of sevoflurane in children: a comparison with halothane, *Anesthesiology* 82:38, 1995.

103. Schreiner A: Anaerobic pulmonary infections, *Scand J Infect Dis* 19:77, 1979.

104. Sitzman BT, Rich GF, Rockwell JJ, et al: Local anesthetic administration for awake direct laryngoscopy, *Anesthesiology* 86:34, 1997.

105. Sparks CJ: Ludwig's angina causing respiratory arrest in the Solomon Islands, *Anaesth Intensive Care* 21:460, 1993.

106. Spitalnic SJ, Sucov A: Ludwig's angina: a case report and review, *J Emerg Med* 13:499, 1995.

107. Stella JP, Kageler W, Epker BN: Fiberoptic endotracheal intubation in oral and maxillofacial surgery, *J Oral Maxillofac Surg* 44:923, 1986.

108. Stoelting RK: Endotracheal intubation. In Miller RD, editor: *Anesthesia,* New York, 1981, Churchill Livingstone.

109. Super DM, Cartelli NA, Brooks LJ, et al: A prospective randomized double-blind study to evaluate the effect of dexamethasone in acute laryngotracheitis, *J Pediatr* 115:323, 1989.

110. Taylor PE, Byers MR: An immunocytochemical study of the morphological reaction of nerves containing calcitonin gene-related peptide to microabscess formation and healing in rat molars, *Arch Oral Biol* 35:629, 1990.

111. Tellez DW, Galvis AG, Storgion SA, et al: Dexamethasone in the prevention of postextubation stridor in children, *J Pediatr* 118:289, 1991.

112. Toews A, de la Rocha AG: Oropharyngeal sepsis with endothoracic spread, *Can J Surg* 23:265, 1980.

113. Topazian RG, Simon GT: Extra-oral mandibular and maxillary nerve block techniques, *Oral Surg* 15:206, 1962.

114. Uram J, Hauser MS: Deep neck and mediastinal necrotizing infection secondary to a traumatic intubation: report of a case, *J Oral Maxillofac Surg* 46:788, 1988.

115. Vazirani SJ: Closed mouth mandibular block, *Dent Digest* 66:10, 1960.

116. Walton RE, Torabine M: Managing local anesthesia problems in the endodontic patient, *J Am Dent Assoc* 123:97, 1992.

117. Wheeler M: Management strategies for the difficult pediatric airway, *Anesth Clin North Am* 16:743, 1998.

118. Williams AC: Ludwig's angina, *Surg Gynecol Obstet* 70:140, 1940.

119. Wilson ME, John R: Problems with the Mallampati sign, *Anaesthesia* 45:486, 1990.

120. Wilson ME, Spiegelhalter D, Roberson JA, et al: Predicting difficult intubation, *Br J Anaesth* 61:211, 1988.

121. Yurino M, Kimura H: Vital capacity rapid inhalation induction technique: comparison of sevoflurane and halothane, *Can J Anaesth* 40:440, 1993.

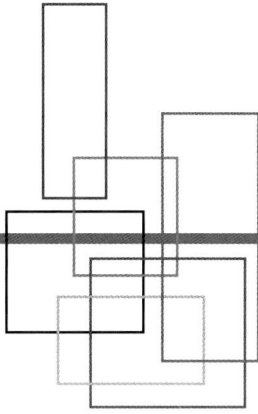

Immunocompromised Host and Infection

Samuel J. McKenna

The interaction between the human host and pathogenic microorganisms defines the manifestations of infection. The outcome of this interaction may be clinical resolution, some form of chronic infection, or rarely, in the oral and maxillofacial region, death. Characteristics of the invading pathogen and the host determine the outcome of infection. This chapter discusses the importance of host factors in modulating the course of infection. The immunocompromised host has one or more defects in natural defense functions that predispose to infection, and virtually any organism may become invasive if host defenses are severely impaired.[93] This chapter reviews clinically relevant host defense defects that may affect the prevention and management of infection in the maxillofacial region.

HOST RESPONSE TO INFECTION

The first line of defense to an invading microorganism is the mechanical barrier afforded by skin and mucosa. Surface products such as sebaceous gland secretions and lysozymes and lactoperoxidase in mucus, saliva, and tears enhance the function of these barriers. IgA provides a more specific surface defense. When surface barriers are breached, the next defense to microbial invasion is characterized by the activation of complement and recruitment of phagocytic cells (neutrophilic granulocytes, eosinophilic granulocytes, and mononuclear phagocytes) and augmented through macrophage release of cytokines. The presence of opsonizing antibodies from previous challenge by the microorganism enhances complement and phagocyte activation.

More specific defense against invading microorganisms is provided by humoral and cellular immune activity (see Chapter 1). In cellular immunity a microbial antigen presented to T lymphocytes by monocytes leads to clonal proliferation of T lymphocytes. The subset of T lymphocytes that interact with antigens is referred to as *helper* or *inducer lymphocytes* (CD4 lymphocytes). Therefore T lymphocytes are important in conferring immunological memory to the host. Other populations of T lymphocytes can lyse infected host cells and regulate (often suppress) the immune system (CD8 lymphocytes).

The humoral immune system comprises immunoglobulins, elaborated by B-lymphocytes, and complement. Antibodies bind with high specificity to microbial antigens to which the host has previously mounted an immune response. Activated B lymphocytes also serve a memory function by providing an accelerated response to repeat challenge by the pathogen. Chapter 1 includes a more thorough discussion of normal defense functions.

PRIMARY IMMUNODEFICIENCY STATES

Defects in host defense mechanisms may occur at any level of the host-pathogen interaction. Immune system deficiencies may be primary (congenital) or acquired. More than 70 primary immunodeficiency syndromes have been described. The prevalence of primary immunodeficiency cases of clinical importance is 1 in 10,000 population.[79] Rarely encountered primary immunodeficiency may affect any component of the inflammatory or immune system. Approximately half of these deficiencies involve B-lymphocyte function, one third T-lymphocyte disorders, and the balance are neutrophil and complement abnormalities. Primary antibody immunodeficiency may affect all or selected immunoglobulins. Deficiency of IgG is associated with recurrent respiratory and sinus infections by encapsulated bacteria.[104] Primary cellular immune deficiencies may include defective response to antigenic stimulation or T-lymphocyte proliferation, with or without cytokine production. Chronic mucocutaneous *Candida* spp. infection has been associated with primary cellular immune defects.[16] Individuals with combined primary immunodeficiency disorders have important defects in both humoral and cellular immune defense. Examples of combined deficiencies include severe combined immunodeficiency, Wiskott-Aldrich syndrome, ataxia-telangiectasia, and Job syndrome. Primary complement deficiency states also occur and are associated with increased risk of infection by encapsulated bacteria. Primary phagocyte disorders such as congenital neutropenia, Chédiak-Higashi syndrome, leukocyte actin deficiency, lazy leukocyte syndrome, and chronic granulomatous disease predispose to infection with pyogenic bacteria and fungi. The role for prophylactic antimicrobials with elective oral or facial surgery in primary immunodeficiency is not defined. However, the theoretical benefit of minimizing the bacterial challenge may outweigh the risk of an untoward drug reaction or development of microbial resistance. Treatment of established infection in these individuals should include the application of sound surgical principles in consultation with an infectious disease consultant.

ACQUIRED IMMUNODEFICIENCY STATES

Of greater clinical importance in facial surgery is acquired immunodeficiency, which may result from the natural expression of underlying disease, as a consequence of therapy for malignancy, or deliberate immunosuppressive therapy. Acquired immune system defects may impair host defenses at any point in the immune system, and the features of the defect determine the clinical manifestations of the immunodeficiency state (Box 24-1).

GRANULOCYTE DISORDERS

An increasing number of acquired conditions are associated with qualitative granulocyte defects such as hematological

disorders (e.g., acute and chronic leukemia, myelodysplasia, paroxysmal nocturnal hemoglobinuria, sickle cell disease), diabetes mellitus, uremia, cirrhosis, burns, certain infections, and drugs. Granulocyte dysfunction may be demonstrated at the level of adherence, chemotaxis/locomotion, phagocytosis, and microbicidal activity.

Granulocytopenia, defined as an absolute neutrophil count less than 1000 cells/mL, is an important risk factor for infection.[9] Granulocytopenia may be a result of the natural expression of a disease (e.g., marrow involvement by hematological malignancy or solid tumor, myelofibrosis, Felty's syndrome), pharmacological marrow suppression, or radiation therapy. In contrast to qualitative granulocyte disorders the risk of infection with granulocytopenia is quantifiable by absolute neutrophil count. When the absolute neutrophil count drops below 500 cells/mm^3, the risk of life-threatening infection increases substantially.[9] Neutrophil counts less than 100 cells/mm^3 are associated with bacteremia-seeded sepsis from colonizing flora, especially from the gastrointestinal tract.[24] Causes of infection in the setting of granulocytopenia or granulocyte dysfunction include the pyogenic bacteria and fungi (Box 24-2).

BOX **24-1**

Acquired Immunodeficiency States

General
Phagocyte
Humoral
Cellular

Specific, Nonneoplastic
Diabetes mellitus
Chronic renal failure
Alcoholism/chronic liver disease/cirrhosis
Splenectomy
Protein-calorie malnutrition
Aging
Organ transplantation
Collagen vascular disease
Corticosteroids
HIV/AIDS

Specific, Neoplastic
Acute lymphocytic leukemia
Lymphoma
Multiple myeloma
Antineoplastic chemotherapy/radiation therapy

BOX **24-2**

Distribution of Pathogens by Host Defect

Phagocytic Defects
Bacteria
Gram-negative bacilli
  Escherichia coli
  Pseudomonas aeruginosa
  Klebsiella pneumoniae
Gram-positive cocci
  Staphylococcus epidermidis
  Staphylococcus aureus
  α-*Streptococcus* spp.
Fungi—*Candida* spp.

Cellular Defects
Bacteria
  Listeria monocytogenes
  Salmonella spp.
  Mycobacterium spp.
  Nocardia
Fungi
  Candida spp.
  Aspergillus spp.
  Cryptococcus neoformans,
    Coccidioides immitis,
    Histoplasma capsulatum
Viruses
  Herpes simplex/varicella-zoster
  Epstein-Barr
  Cytomegalovirus
Parasites
  Pneumocystis carinii
  Toxoplasma gondii
  Strongyloides stercoralis

Humoral Defects
Bacteria
  Streptococcus pneumoniae
  Haemophilus influenzae
  Neisseria meningitidis
  Enterobacteriaceae
  Pseudomonas aeruginosa

HUMORAL IMMUNODEFICIENCY

Immunoglobulins and complement are important components in the defense against circulating encapsulated bacteria and viruses (see Box 24-2). Defects in the humoral immune system predispose patients to respiratory and gastrointestinal infections. Hypogammaglobulinemia may occur in the setting of chronic lymphocytic leukemia, multiple myeloma, lymphoma, allogeneic bone marrow transplantation, chronic graft-versus-host disease (GVHD), and burns.[4] Patients with chronic lymphocytic leukemia or multiple myeloma may produce an abnormal monoclonal protein that is defective in opsonization of encapsulated bacteria.[3] Hypocomplementemia occurs in a number of acquired immunodeficiency states.

CELLULAR IMMUNODEFICIENCY

Acquired defects in cellular immunity impair a host's ability to eliminate intracellular pathogens including bacteria, fungi, viruses, and parasites (see Box 24-2). Acquired cellular immune system defects may result from lymphoproliferative malignancies, especially Hodgkin's disease. Administration of therapeutic immunosuppressive drugs (e.g., corticosteroids, cyclophosphamide, azathioprine, cyclosporine, tacrolimus) also impairs T-lymphocyte function. Viral infection with the immunomodulating viruses, cytomegalovirus (CMV), Epstein-Barr virus (EBV), hepatitis B and C, and most notably human immunodeficiency virus (HIV) also may induce cellular immunodeficiency.[121]

NONNEOPLASTIC CONDITIONS ASSOCIATED WITH ACQUIRED IMMUNODEFICIENCY

From the standpoint of recognizing patients who may be immunodeficient, a classification based on underlying cause, as opposed to underlying defect, is most applicable to clinical practice. A diverse group of acquired defects result from nonneoplastic conditions (see Box 24-1).

SPLENECTOMY

Splenectomy may be the result of trauma or a variety of hematological disorders including staging for lymphoma. Many underlying conditions have been associated with diminished splenic function, including sickle cell disease, rheumatoid arthritis (RA), systemic lupus erythematosus (SLE), ulcerative colitis, and GVHD.[18] Functions of the spleen include IgM synthesis and intrasplenic mononuclear phagocytic activity. T-cell and granulocyte function depend on an intact spleen. Decreased or absent splenic function leads to deficiency of tuftsin, a phagocyte-stimulating peptide,[77] and properdin, important in opsonization.[12] Antibody response to new antigens also is compromised.[26] Common pathogens in splenic dysfunction include, but are not limited to, the encapsulated bacteria (e.g., *Streptococcus pneumoniae, Haemophilus influenzae,* and *Neisseria meningitidis*).[18] The risk of infection is greatest

during the first 6 months after splenectomy, especially from a malignant process.[40]

Of interest in the setting of maxillofacial trauma management is the potential for infection after an animal bite in patients who have undergone splenectomy. *Capnocytophaga canimorsus,* carried in the mouths of dogs and some cats, may cause sepsis in the setting of splenectomy.[54] These patients should receive 3 to 5 days of penicillin therapy after minor bites, and amoxicillin-clavulanate for deep wounds. In general, prophylactic antibiotics should be administered before elective oral and facial surgical procedures in the first 6 months after splenectomy. The role for prophylactic antibiotics after this point or in hyposplenic states has not been defined. In general, when a large bacterial inoculum is anticipated from manipulation of oral structures, prophylactic antibiotics should be considered.

DIABETES MELLITUS

Individuals with diabetes mellitus are subject to the same infections as those without diabetes and more characteristic infections such as rhinocerebral mucormycosis. Furthermore, infections in patients with diabetes may be more severe and recalcitrant.[19] Immunoglobulin response appears to be normal, although impaired activation of complement may impair opsonization.[44] In the setting of poor glycemic control, granulocyte adherence, chemotaxis, phagocytosis, and bactericidal activity are impaired. The magnitude of hyperglycemia required for impairment in phagocytic function is in the range of 11 to 15 mmol/L (198 to 270 mg/dL).[67] Insulin administration reverses granulocyte dysfunction.[48] T-lymphocyte dysfunction also occurs in patients with poorly controlled diabetes,[30] possibly accounting for infection by intracellular pathogens. Cellular immune function also is restored with insulin administration.[65]

The practical implications of diabetic-associated immunodeficiency is that serum glucose control is important in the management of established infection and the prevention of infection in the surgical patient. Patients with serum glucose levels in excess of 12.2 mmol/L (220 mg/dL) on the first postoperative day have a 2.7 times greater risk of infection than those with serum glucose levels less than 12.2 mmol/L.[6] Therefore optimization of glucose homeostasis in the early postoperative period should substantially reduce the risk of infectious complications and facilitate control of established infection. Prophylactic antibiotics generally are not required in patients with diabetes. However, when surgery is necessary in patients with poor glycemic control, prophylactic antibiotics should be provided.

Diabetic patients are at risk for more severe forms of head and neck infection, such as Ludwig's angina, orbital cellulitis, and chronic sinusitis.[116] They also are predisposed to rhinocerebral mucormycosis (RCM) and malignant external otitis (MOE). RCM is a life-threatening fungal infection of the Morales order (e.g., *Rhizopus, Absidia, Mucor*). Between 40% and 50% of patients with mucormycosis have diabetes, many with ketoacidosis.[85] Vasculopathy and poor glycemic control predispose the diabetic patient to infection by inhaled spores. Infection begins intranasally, spreading to the paranasal sinuses with possible extension into the orbit, central nervous system (CNS), or both. RCM manifests with facial or ocular pain. Necrotic lesions in the nose or on the palate are pathognemonic.[116] Orbital involvement manifests with pain, proptosis, and ophthalmoplegia. Evaluation should include CT with or without MR imaging of the paranasal sinuses, orbits, and brain. Diagnosis is based on the demonstration of branching hyphae in a soft tissue biopsy. Treatment consists of surgical debridement of infected, necrotic tissue and parenteral antifungal agents such as amphotericin.

MOE (also known as invasive external otitis) is an infection of the ear canal, adjacent soft tissues and, when fully expressed, involves the skull base. Between 90% and 100% of patients with MOE have diabetes and usually are elderly.[27] Unlike RCM, ketoacidosis is not a common presentation. Vasculopathy is believed to be a more important factor than glycemic control.[101] MOE almost always is caused by *Pseudomonas aeruginosa,* presenting with otalgia, otorrhea, hearing loss, occasional temporomandibular joint pain, and limited oral opening. Physical findings include ear canal swelling, erythema, and extensive granulation tissue formation. Symptoms of more extensive disease include cranial nerve VII neuropathy, CNS infection, or both. Suspected bony involvement should be evaluated with CT, MR, or possibly bone scan imaging. Treatment consists of surgical debridement and antipseudomonal antimicrobials. Even with treatment, MOE has a 10% to 20% mortality rate.[101]

ALCOHOL ABUSE AND LIVER DISEASE

Many facets of the immune system may be compromised by alcohol consumption. Acute intoxication with serum alcohol greater than 100 mg/dL inhibits granulocyte margination and adherence and thus delivery to the site of infection.[62] Humoral and cellular immunity are unaffected by acute ethanol exposure.[63]

Patients with alcoholism overlap among the toxic effects of alcohol consumption, malnutrition, and chronic liver disease. Chronic excessive ethanol exposure is associated with increased colonization of the upper respiratory tract and oral cavity by gram-negative bacilli[64] and malnutrition. Chronic ethanol use also has toxic bone marrow effects with maturation arrest of granulocyte precursors causing a delayed or even neutropenic response to infection.[62] Antibody response to new antigens is also defective.[35] Impaired cellular immunity is characterized by fewer T lymphocytes and decreased mitogenic response.[62]

Because of chronic liver disease, patients with alcoholism are at additional risk of infection. With the development of cirrhosis and portal hypertension, blood is shunted away from the liver, which allows pathogens to bypass liver-fixed macrophages. This process may explain the increased incidence of spontaneous pneumococcal and enteric bacteremia in chronic liver disease.[63] Although leukocyte functions are normal in the setting of cirrhosis, in vitro leukocyte chemotaxis and locomotor function are impaired because of the presence of chemotactic and cell-directed inhibitors.[94] Cellular immunity also is defective in alcoholic cirrhosis.[79] No consistent defect exists in humoral immunity in the nondrinking alcoholic patient with chronic liver disease.[62] The risk of infection from maxillofacial surgery procedures in chronic liver disease is unknown. However, because of the risk of spontaneous peritonitis, prophylactic antibiotics should be considered in the individual with end-stage liver disease.

RENAL DISEASE

Local defense may be impaired by skin and cutaneous sensory changes in the patient with chronic renal failure. Impaired cellular immunity is marked by lymphopenia and defective delayed-type-hypersensitivity that does not improve with hemodialysis.[120] Humoral immunity is largely unaffected, although antibody response may be reduced.[79] Neutrophil accumulation and chemotaxis are compromised and may improve with peritoneal dialysis.[36] Hemodialysis causes neutrophil sequestration and transient neutropenia from complement activation.[120] Although prophylactic antibiotic use is guided primarily by the need to protect vascular access for hemodialysis,[59] consultation with a nephrologist provides insight into the overall risk assessment, indications, and administration of prophylactic antibiotics.

INTRAVENOUS DRUG ABUSE

Infection is the most common cause of death in the setting of intravenous drug abuse (IVDA).[51] Immunological defects probably play a minor role compared with repeated injection of nonsterile substances.[25] Abnormal skin colonization by *S. aureus* is common,[8] possibly from repeated skin puncture or from self-administration of β-lactam antibiotics.[81] Skin and soft tissue infections represent a common reason for hospital admission in IVDA.[82]

No evidence exists of depressed humoral immunity in IVDA. In fact, immunoglobulin levels may be elevated.[11] On the other hand, cellular immunity is impaired with decreased lymphocyte proliferation.[52] However, in the absence of acquired immunodeficiency syndrome (AIDS), opportunistic infections characteristic of T-lymphocyte dysfunction are rare.[57] Although of uncertain clinical significance, in vitro phagocytic function may be impaired with chronic opioid exposure.[117]

Bacterial and fungal bone and joint infections, usually from hematogenous spread, are common in IVDA.[15] The axial skeleton is the favored site for bone infection. Polymicrobial infective endocarditis often from group A, B, or G streptococci is the most common cause of bacteremia in IVDA.[108] The extent of the involvement of the oral and maxillofacial region in any of the aforementioned infection patterns is unknown. However, knowledge of the impact of IVDA on immune function, microbiological patterns of infections, and the practice of self-administration of antibiotics affect the approach to the management of established infection and prevention of infection.

MALNUTRITION

Many infections are influenced by nutritional status.[13] Protein-calorie deficiency has several adverse effects on immune function. For example, barrier integrity may be compromised by mucosal thinning and decrease lysozyme and IgA production. Other defects include decreased cytokine production, lymphoid tissue atrophy, and lymphopenia, specifically with a smaller proportion of CD4 lymphocytes. T-lymphocyte response to antigen challenge also is decreased. Humoral immunity is impaired with decreased production of IgA, impaired complement activity, and decreased response to new antigens.[56,79] Granulocyte migration, phagocytosis, and microbicidal activity also are impaired.[105] Deficiencies of micronutrients such as vitamin A,[123] zinc,[114] and iron[14] further impair immune function.

In developed countries a number of chronic diseases are associated with protein-calorie malnutrition (e.g., diabetes mellitus, chronic renal failure, depression, alcoholism, gastrointestinal conditions). Cancer chemotherapy is associated with malnutrition as a result of nausea, diarrhea, and oral mucositis. Management of oral or maxillofacial infections is compromised further by the adverse effect of oral infection on enteral nutrition (e.g., oral swelling, pain, trismus).

AGING

A decline in the quality of skin and mucous membrane barriers, impaired circulation, and compromised wound healing contribute to increased susceptibility to infection in the elderly.[7] Further, decreased humoral[97] and cellular[106] immune function has been described. The higher incidence of herpes zoster in elderly individuals is an example of the deleterious effect of aging on cell-mediated immunity. Evidence exists also of decreased neutrophil function with aging.[124] Other factors that likely contribute to increased susceptibility to infection in the elderly include malnutrition, chronic illness, and communal living.

The microbiology of infection in the elderly may differ from that of the younger individual. For example, in either community- or hospital-acquired pneumonia, gram-negative and staphylococcal infection is more common than in younger individuals.[17] Frequent use of antimicrobial drugs almost certainly influences the identity of a pathogen and antimicrobial susceptibility in the institutionalized elderly individual.

Inflammatory and febrile response to pathogens may be attenuated in the elderly. Clinical infection may therefore manifest with blunted clinical features.[80] Thus mental status changes may be a better indicator of significant infection than more frequently applied markers such as fever. Although largely unstudied, advanced age alone probably is not an indication for prophylactic antibiotic use before

oral surgical procedures. Rather, the decision to use prophylactic antibiotics should include a global assessment of the elderly patient's status, the anticipated microbial exposure from surgery, and the potential effect of infection on other coexisting compromising condition, should infectious complication occur.

ORGAN TRANSPLANT RECIPIENT

Because of advances in the management of allograft rejection, long-term survival after organ transplantation has increased over the past 20 years.[119] Increasing numbers of individuals are living with functioning grafts, but with the trade-off of increased host susceptibility to infection. The risk of infection is determined by the magnitude of immunosuppression and exposure to potential pathogens. Therefore infection, not rejection, is the leading cause of death at all times after transplantation. Two thirds of transplant recipients have at least one significant infection.[103] Notwithstanding the risk of infection from therapeutic immunosuppression, the rejection response, associated with increased cytokine production, contributes to compromised host resistance.[72] Posttransplant infection with immunomodulatory viruses (cytomegalovirus, EBV, hepatitis B and C, and HIV) magnifies the risk of host infection with opportunistic pathogens such as *Pneumocystis, Listeria,* and fungi and alter histocompatibility antigen expression and therefore allograft rejection.[53]

A variety of immunosuppressive agents may be used to control graft rejection. Corticosteroids, especially in supraphysiological doses, affect all aspects of the immune system.[42,109] Cytotoxic immunosuppressant agents (e.g., methotrexate, cyclophosphamide, azathioprine, and actinomycin-D) cause bone marrow depression, leukopenia, and increase the risk of posttransplant infection.[3] Use of cyclosporine, introduced in 1980, and more recently potent agents such as tacrolimus, have facilitated lower corticosteroid and cytotoxic agent doses in antirejection protocols. Lower rates of infection have been described in kidney and heart transplant recipients managed with cyclosporine compared with cytotoxic agents.[29] Antilymphocyte serums and antithymocyte globulins are immunosuppressive adjuncts for the prevention and treatment of rejection. However, their use is associated with increased activation of latent viral infection.[43]

Transplant recipients are at greatest risk of infection during periods of aggressive immunosuppressive therapy. Although with greater consequences, infection during the first month after transplantation is comparable to postoperative infection in the immunocompetent patient undergoing surgery of similar magnitude.[102] Despite aggressive immunosuppressive therapy at this time, opportunistic infection is not common. Apparently prolonged immunosuppressive therapy, rather than short-term, high-dose administration determines the risk of infection.[103] Infection by an immunomodulating virus (CMV, EBV, hepatitis B and C, and HIV) coupled with ongoing immunosuppressive therapy increases the risk of opportunistic infection during the 1- and 6-month period after organ transplantation.[102] After 6 months, graft recipients receiving maintenance immunosuppression, with good organ function, and free of chronic viral infection are subject to the same infections as the general public and rarely suffer opportunistic infection.[103]

Although the true incidence of oral or maxillofacial infection in the setting of immunosuppressive therapy is unknown, control, if not elimination, of sources of oral infection before planned immunosuppression is important. Oral and facial surgeons may be called on to evaluate the immunosuppressed patient with fever of unknown origin. Fever is a sensitive indicator of underlying infection in the immunosuppressed patient.[89] However, fever also may be a manifestation of graft rejection. Physical and radiographic findings of periodontal or odontogenic infection should be treated aggressively to eliminate the source of infection.

Elective maxillofacial surgery in the organ transplant recipient should be deferred until maintenance immunosuppression and satisfactory graft function are achieved. Further, elective surgery in the individual with chronic viral infection and marginal or poor graft function should be critically evaluated in view of the increased risk of infection. In the latter scenario, prophylactic antibiotics should be administered before facial and oral surgical procedures.

COLLAGEN VASCULAR DISEASE

Immune function may be impaired in individuals with collagen vascular disease (CVD) such as RA and SLE from both the underlying disease and treatments. For example, hypocomplementemia has been noted in both RA and SLE,[74] increasing the risk of infection with encapsulated organisms. Dysfunctional immunoglobulins, including antileukocyte antibodies in SLE, predispose patients to infection.[88] Splenic dysfunction also occurs in some patients with SLE.[92] Granulocytopenia, impaired in vitro chemotaxis, opsonization, phagocytosis, and microbicidal activity are characteristic of SLE.[88] In Felty's syndrome (RA with neutropenia and splenomegaly), infection from neutropenia, neutrophil dysfunction, and hypocomplementemia is the most common cause of death.[74] In SLE and to a lesser extent in RA, numerous abnormalities in cellular immunity have been described in addition to the effects of immunosuppressive therapy.[99]

Measures to treat CVD further compromise host defenses. For example, corticosteroids have numerous effects on host defense mechanisms. Cytotoxic agents such as cyclophosphamide impair B-lymphocyte function and immunoglobulin production[112] and cause bone marrow suppression and neutropenia.[23] Gold compounds suppress immune function through inactivation of complement and lysosomal enzymes, altered phagocytic activity, and suppression of lymphocytic proliferation.[88]

The occurrence of cardiac valvular abnormalities and the risk of infective endocarditis in SLE is important in the setting of elective maxillofacial surgery.[98] Some believe that the risk of infective endocarditis in this setting is similar to that associated with a prosthetic valve and recommend prophylactic antibiotics for dental treatments in patients with SLE.[60,127] A more selective approach to prophylactic antibiotic administration, consistent with American Heart Association guidelines,[20] is to reserve prophylactic antibiotics to those patients with SLE who have an abnormal echocardiogram.[74,100]

Although controversial, in 1997 an advisory statement adopted by the American Academy of Orthopaedic Surgeons and the American Dental Association concluded that prophylactic antibiotics were not required routinely for dental treatment in patients with prosthetic joint replacement.[2] However, patients with a history of SLE or RA (or other source of immune compromise) are considered at increased risk of hematogenous prosthetic joint infection with dental treatments and should receive prophylactic antibiotics.[2]

CORTICOSTEROID USE

Corticosteroids are administered for many inflammatory and immunological conditions. Their effectiveness is paralleled by the theoretical risk of infectious complications. The most important mechanism by which corticosteroids suppress inflammation and increase susceptibility to infection is through impaired recruitment of leukocytes and monocyte-macrophages to sites of inflammation.[69,86] Corticosteroids also decrease levels of several cytokines essential to the production and function of T lymphocytes,[10] which increases the risk of infection to intracellular pathogens. The risk of clinically important immunosuppression and infection is related to the dose, frequency, and duration of corticosteroid administration. Clinically important impairment in cellular immune function is most likely to occur with chronic (less than 2 weeks' duration) use of daily supraphysiological doses (e.g., 40 to 60 mg prednisone or equivalent).[19] Alternate-day therapy has been associated with fewer infectious complications and preservation of delayed-type hypersensitivity.[21] Chronic high-dose corticosteroid use is associated with a more difficult clinical course, which requires longer courses of treatment for established infection and disseminated viral and fungal infection.[19] Corticosteroid administration for up to 2 weeks has little effect on delayed hypersensitivity, and daily doses equivalent to 20-mg prednisone are unlikely to cause significant immunosuppression.[74] However, the antiinflammatory effects of even low-dose corticosteroids may mask the clinical signs of infection, and clinical evaluation may be further confused by neutrophilic leukocytosis induced by corticosteroid administration. Prophylactic antibiotics are not necessary in the usual patient receiving chronic low-dose corticosteroids. In contrast, prophylactic antibiotics should be considered in the setting of chronic, supraphysiological corticosteroid doses, especially when a large microbial inoculum is anticipated.

HIV AND AIDS

In 2000, estimates totaled nearly 900,000 people living with HIV/AIDS in North America.[118] Morbidity and mortality from AIDS has decreased because of aggressive antiretroviral therapy and decreased AIDS opportunistic infections and other AIDS-related complications.[84] Transmission of HIV-1 to CD4 lymphocytes leads to cell death and a decreased CD4 lymphocyte count.[49] Individuals with CD4 counts greater than 500/mm³ generally have no symptoms, whereas CD4 counts of 50 to 200/mm³ reflect advanced immunodeficiency. Viral load, measured by plasma HIV-1 ribonucleic acid (RNA), is the single most useful predictor of the risk of disease progression to AIDS and death from AIDS.[122] For example, only 1.7% of patients with CD4 cell counts greater than 750/mm³ and HIV RNA less than 500 copies/mL develop AIDS within 6 years.[68]

AIDS is associated with several immunological defects. In addition to T-lymphocyte deficiency, B-lymphocyte, macrophage, and neutrophil dysfunction occur.[122] Individuals with AIDS may have decreased salivary lactoferrin and IgA production, which may account for the high incidence of oral infection.[75] With the decline in immune function, individuals with AIDS are subject to recurrent, life-threatening opportunistic infection. When the CD4 cell count decreases below 200/mm³, the risk of opportunistic infection increases dramatically.[111] Conversely, with CD4 cell counts greater than 200/mm³, *Pneumocystis carinii* pneumonia is unlikely.[90] The role of antibiotic administration before surgical procedures has not been established. However, extrapolating from established practice for the prevention of opportunistic infection such as *P. carinii* pneumonia, consideration of prophylactic antibiotics is reasonable when the CD4 cell count is less than 200/mm³. Prophylactic antibiotics are also a consideration in the patient with rising RNA titers and falling CD4 cell counts in the 200/mm³ to 400/mm³ range.

Depending on the magnitude of immune compromise, oral and maxillofacial manifestations of AIDS are common.[73] Bacillary angiomatosis (BA) appears as 2- to 3-mm red vascular cutaneous papules and nodules that can occur anywhere, usually sparing the oral mucosa. Two gram-negative rods, *Bartonella henselae* and *Bartonella quintana*, may be identified by Warthin-Starry silver staining technique and polymerase chain reaction methods in BA lesions. Treatment is with macrolide antibiotics[41] or doxycycline.[28] BA can mimic Kaposi's sarcoma. Although this infection is usually limited to the skin, osseous, visceral, or central nervous system involvement may occur.[76] Kaposi's sarcoma is associated with infection with human herpesvirus-8.[107]

Reactivation of herpes simplex and varicella-zoster infection is closely coupled to CD4 cell count. CMV infection is associated with CD4 cell counts less than 50/mm³.[76] CMV may manifest with large oral mucosal ulcerations but, more importantly, also may involve the retina or be disseminated with CNS involvement.

Oral hairy leukoplakia (OHL) occurs in 25% of individuals with HIV infection; it resembles candidiasis that does not rub off, most often affects the lateral tongue, is believed to be associated with EBV infection,[38] is associated with CD4 cell counts 300/mm³ or less,[34] and is therefore an early sign of HIV infection. OHL regresses in response to acyclovir,[37] gangciclovir,[78] and foscarnat[1] and with an

tiretroviral therapy,[50] although treatment usually is not necessary.

Human papilloma virus (HPV) infection also may involve the oral mucosa with multiple squamous papillomas on any mucosal surface, especially the lips, tongue, and gingiva. Treatment usually is not necessary unless function, aesthetics, or both are impaired by multiple or large lesions. Treatment, when indicated, consists of surgical excision with cauterization of the lesion base. Unfortunately, recurrence is common.

Oral candidiasis, an early manifestation of HIV/AIDS, occurs in up to 30% of HIV-positive individuals and 90% of adults with AIDS and CD4 cell counts below 400/mm³.[66] Although at least four different types of oral candidiasis are recognized, the most common, and probably the precursor of the hyperplastic form, is erythematous (atrophic) candidiasis.[96] Erythematous candidiasis is characterized by red, atrophic areas on the palate, buccal mucosa, and tongue. Hyperplastic candidiasis produces white lesions that cannot be rubbed off, may be mistaken for hairy leukoplakia, and is associated with long-standing AIDS and severe immune system deterioration.[34] Treatment consists of topical or systemic antifungal agents. Recurrence is common, and fluconazole-resistant and dose-dependent strains may develop after prolonged drug exposure in those with severe immunosuppression.[45] Candidiasis usually manifests as mucosal ulceration; infection with *Histoplasma capsulatum, Coccidioides immitis,* and *Aspergillus* spp. also has been described and represents disseminated fungal infection. Diagnosis requires tissue biopsy and special staining for fungal elements. Treatment is with systemic antifungal agents.[91] (See Chapter 11 for treatment considerations in fungal infections.)

Necrotizing ulcerative periodontitis, analogous to acute necrotizing ulcerative gingivitis in the non-AIDS population, is marked by rapid destruction of periodontal structures. It is associated with CD4 cell counts less than 100/mm³.[34] Treatment consists of systemic antimicrobial drugs and topical cleansing with 0.12% chlorhexidine. Necrotizing ulcerative gingivitis is an analogous process with sparing of the deeper periodontal structures.[87] A possible precursor of necrotizing ulcerative gingivitis may be linear gingival erythema, characterized by erythema of the incisor region marginal gingival. Treatment of this condition is also aggressive oral hygiene and 0.12% chlorhexidine application.

NEOPLASTIC CONDITIONS ASSOCIATED WITH ACQUIRED IMMUNODEFICIENCY

Immune system dysfunction in patients with cancer may be a consequence of intrinsic immune deficits associated with the malignancy, disruption of physical barriers, such as oral mucosa, and intensive antineoplastic therapy regimens.

Neutropenia is an important host defect in acute leukemia, bone marrow invasion by solid tumor, and myelosuppressive chemotherapy and radiation therapy. The incidence of infection increases linearly as the neu trophil count decreases below 1000/mm³.⁹ Most severe infections and nearly all bacteremias occur when the granulocyte count is below 100/mm³.²⁴ Both the rapidity of onset and the duration of neutropenia influence the risk of infection. For example, a precipitous decrease in neutrophil count for more than 10 days portends a high risk for infectious complications.⁵⁵ The duration of neutropenia varies with the chemotherapeutic regimen. At one extreme, bone marrow transplant recipients are at high risk for infection and generally require 3 weeks of intensive support for few or no circulating granulocytes.

Defects in surface barriers such as oral mucosa and other aerodigestive tract sites are important predisposing factors for infection in the neutropenic patient.¹¹⁰ Apart from the effects of cancer therapy, gingivostomatitis and oral and oropharyngeal mucosal infection are common in the setting of leukemia⁸³ and neutropenia.³¹ Barrier defects coupled with local colonization by pathogens and granulocytopenia predispose patients to septicemia and life-threatening infection. Oral herpes simplex infection is common in patients with neutropenia as a result of reactivation of latent infection,⁹⁵ also predisposing to bacterial and fungal colonization and invasion. Important oropharyngeal pathogens are listed in Box 24-3.⁷⁰ An increased contribution of gram-negative, aerobic bacteria to the normal oropharyngeal flora is expected in association with severe or chronic illness such as cancer.⁴⁷ However, through the liberal use of prophylactic and empirical antimicrobials directed toward gram-negative organisms, indwelling intravenous catheters, mucositis, a shift in infection pattern from gram-negative bacilli to gram-positive pathogens, especially coagulase-negative staphylococci, has been noted.¹²⁶

Qualitative granulocyte defects also may result from certain cancer chemotherapeutic agents such as daunorubicin, methotrexate, and vincristine, corticosteroids, and radiation therapy. Recombinant hematopoietic growth factors, granulocyte colony-stimulating factor (G-CSF) and granu-

locyte-macrophage colony-stimulating factor (GM-CSF) stimulate myeloid progenitors and have been used clinically in bone marrow transplantation to shorten the duration of neutropenia.²²,¹²⁵

Bone marrow transplantation is followed by approximately 1 month of profound bone marrow dysfunction and pancytopenia. During this period mucosal breakdown from pretransplant chemoradiotherapy and reactivation of herpes simplex exposes the recipient to oral pathogens. With successful engraftment granulocyte populations are replenished. However, during the second and third month after transplantation the greatest risk to infection is dysfunctional cellular and humoral immunity from acute GVHD.⁶¹ Defective cellular immunity is marked by decreased T-helper lymphocytes, increased T-suppressor lymphocytes, and impaired T-lymphocyte cytotoxicity. Humoral immune deficiency is marked by impaired antibody response to antigen challenge and decreased numbers of B lymphocytes. Immunosuppressive therapy for GVHD further subjects the bone marrow transplant patient to infection. With successful management of acute GVHD, gradual immune function recovery begins in the third month after transplantation and is complete by 1 to 2 years.⁶¹ Chronic GVHD may produce persistent immune compromise and ongoing risk of late infection.⁵

Cellular immune dysfunction may be innate to a malignancy (e.g., Hodgkin's disease, chronic lymphocytic leukemia, hairy-cell leukemia)¹²¹ or a consequence of immunosuppressive therapy (e.g., corticosteroids, cytotoxic agents) and radiation therapy. These individuals are at increased risk of opportunistic infections from a variety of intracellular pathogens that rarely cause life-threatening infection in the immunocompetent individual.

Humoral immune deficiency also may be innate to a neoplasm. For example, in multiple myeloma, immunoglobulin deficiency increases the risk of infection from encapsulated bacteria.⁴⁶ Immunoglobulin deficiency also may occur in chronic lymphocytic leukemia and some lymphomas. Staging splenectomy, when necessary, also contributes to the humeral defect.

Measures to optimize oral hygiene before and during antineoplastic therapy are important.³⁹ Prophylactic removal of third molars before the initiation of cancer chemotherapy may decrease infectious complications resulting from preservation of these teeth.¹¹⁵ In patients with neutropenia, fever is often the principal indicator of infection as the usual signs of infection are muted.³³ The accumulation of purulent exudate may be absent, making localization of an infectious process in the head and neck region more uncertain. Even in the absence of a collection of purulent fluid, surgical drainage of the suspected cellulitic process may hasten resolution of infectious process by altering favorably the oxidation-reduction potential of the local environment. Procurement of infected specimens for culture and sensitivity may provide useful information for modifying antimicrobial therapy in the immunocompromised cancer patient. The basic surgical principle of removal of the source of the infection is particularly important in the neutropenic patient. Notwithstanding the

---

BOX 24-3

Oral Sources of Pathogenic Organisms in the Immunocompromised Host

Bacteria
Streptococcus spp.
Capnocytophaga spp.
Eikenella corodens
Stomatococcus mucilaginosus
Rothia dentocariosus
Bacteroides spp.
Pseudomonas aeruginosa

Fungi
Candida spp.
Aspergillus spp.
Histoplasma capsulatum

Viruses
Herpes simplex
Cytomegalovirus

problem of immunosuppression, thrombocytopenia may complicate surgical management of the infected cancer patient. Close communication between the surgeon and oncologist is crucial to the successful management of the infected cancer patient.

PREVENTION AND MANAGEMENT OF INFECTION IN THE IMMUNOCOMPROMISED HOST

Few published recommendations exist for prevention of maxillofacial infections in the immunocompromised patient.[58,59,71,113,115] Prevention of infection depends partly on the nature of the immune system defect. The nature and severity of the host defense defects determine the type and risk of infection, respectively. Although gathering data to estimate the risk of systemic infection from an oral source in most immunocompromised states is not feasible, obvious sources of oral infection, especially odontogenic or periodontal, should be eliminated or controlled in the individual with existing or planned impaired immune system dysfunction. For example, immunosuppression resulting from therapeutic interventions to treat an underlying disease or prevent organ rejection can be anticipated and measures taken to optimize oral health before the nadir of immune function. Mucositis associated with malignancy and aggressive cancer chemotherapy is an important defect in natural host defenses, and measures to maintain optimal oral hygiene during periods of neutropenia are important. Optimizing oral health is particularly important in bone marrow transplantation and the associated profound and protracted neutropenia. Apart from eliminating potential sources of oral infection, measures to improve immune function may be beneficial. These may be as fundamental as meticulous perioperative glycemic control in the diabetic surgical patient to the administration of growth factors such as GM-CSF or G-CSF in the setting of profound neutropenia.

Violation of natural host barriers should be minimized in the individual whose immune system is compromised. Oral surgical procedures, for example, should be undertaken principally to prevent or treat active infection. However, when oral barriers must be surgically breached in the immunocompromised patient, the indications for prophylactic antibiotic administration remain unanswered in most clinical scenarios. Although the magnitude of most host defense defects is not readily quantifiable, the absolute neutrophil count in the neutropenic patient and the CD4+ count in the patient with AIDS may be of practical value in the determination of the magnitude of immunosuppression and the role for prophylactic antibiotics in oral and maxillofacial surgery. Determination of serum glucose and glycosylated hemoglobin levels quantifies poorly controlled diabetes, and these patients may benefit from administration of prophylactic antibiotics before surgery. Clinical judgment in these and other immune deficiencies that are not readily quantified (e.g., alcoholism, chronic liver disease, uremia, therapeutic immunosuppression), must guide the prudent use of prophylactic antibiotics before surgery. When surgery is necessary, sound surgical principles, including control of wound contamination, careful handling of soft and hard tissues, debridement of nonviable tissues, and prevention of seroma and hematoma formation, should be observed.

In established oral or facial infection in the immunocompromised host, treatment should be directed toward minimization of the magnitude and duration of pathogen exposure. Therefore treatment directed at removal of the source of infection and nonviable tissue is imperative. Especially in patients with neutropenia, local signs of inflammation and infection may be muted, increasing the difficulty of localization of the source. Because of the greater likelihood of resistant organisms or atypical infection, procurement of infected fluid, tissue, or both specimens for culture and sensitivity evaluation should be attempted. The response to therapy should be monitored carefully and treatments modified accordingly (Box 24-4).

BOX 24-4

Recommendations for Management of the Immunocompromised Host

Prevention of Infection
- Meticulous oral hygiene
  - Eliminate source(s) of oral infection before planned immunosuppression
- Candidiasis, herpes simplex, cytomegalovirus chemoprophylaxis
- Avoid mucosal barrier violation
- Consider prophylactic antibiotic administration before anticipated bacteremia from oral procedure
  - Neutropenia: neutrophil count <1000/mm^3
  - AIDS: CD4 <200/mm^3
    CD4 200-400/mm^3 *plus* decreasing CD4, rising HIV-1 RNA
  - Organ transplant
    - Acute rejection
    - Poorly functioning transplanted organ
    - Chronic viral infection
  - Diabetes mellitus: persistent serum glucose >200 mg/dL
  - Chronic supraphysiological corticosteroid use
  - Splenectomy (especially first 6 months after removal and malignant disease)
  - Combined host defects
- Careful surgical technique
  - Wound decontamination
  - Gentle tissue manipulation
  - Debridement of nonviable tissue
  - Avoidance of seroma/hematoma formation

Treatment of Established Infection
- Establish surgical drainage
- Remove source and nonviable tissue
- Local specimen(s) collection for microbiological, histological evaluation
- Antibiotics
- Monitor response—modify treatment accordingly

REFERENCES

1. Albrecht H, Stellbrink HJ, Brewster D, et al: Resolution of oral hairy leukoplakia during treatment with foscarnet, *AIDS* 8:1014, 1994.
2. American Dental Association; American Academy of Orthopaedic Surgeons: Antibiotic prophylaxis for dental patients with total joint replacements, *J Am Dent Assoc* 128:1004, 1997.
3. Anderson RJ, Schafer LA, Olin DB, et al: Infection risk factors in the immunosuppressed host, *Am J Med* 54:453, 1973.
4. Aoun M, Klaterasky J: Infection in the immunodeficient patient. In Root RK, Waldvogel F, Corey L, et al, editors: *Clinical infectious diseases: a practical approach,* New York, 1996, Oxford University Press.
5. Atkinson K, Farewell V, Storb R, et al: Analysis of late infections after human bone marrow transplantation: role of genotype nonidentity between marrow donor and recipient and of nonspecific suppression cells in patients with chronic graft-versus-host disease, *Blood* 60:714, 1982.
6. Baxter JK, Babineau TJ, Apovian CM, et al: Perioperative glucose control predicts increased nosocomial infection in diabetics, *Crit Care Med* 18:5707, 1980.
7. Ben-Yehuda A, Weksler ME: Host resistance and the immune system, *Clin Geriatr Med* 8:701, 1992.
8. Berman DS, Schaefler J, Simbenkoff M, et al: *Staphylococcus aureus* colonization in intravenous drug abusers, dialysis patients and diabetics, *J Infect Dis* 155:829, 1987.
9. Bodey GP, Buckley M, Sathe YS, et al: Quantitative relationship between circulating leukocytes and infection in patients with acute leukemia, *Ann Intern Med* 64:328, 1966.
10. Boumpas DT, Paliogianni F, Anastassiou ED, et al: Glucocorticoid action on the immune system: molecular and cellular aspects, *Clin Exp Rheumatol* 92:223, 1993.
11. Brown SM, Stimmel B, Taub RN, et al: Immunologic dysfunction in heroin addicts, *Arch Intern Med* 134:1001, 1974.
12. Carlisle HN, Saslaw S: Properdin levels in splenectomized persons, *Proc Soc Exp Biol Med* 102:150, 1959.
13. Chandra RK: Nutrition, immunity and infection: present knowledge and future directions, *Lancet* 1:688, 1983.
14. Chandra RK, Au B, Woodford G, et al: Iron status, immunocompromise and susceptibility to infection. In *Iron metabolism.* Amsterdam, Ciba Foundation Symp, No 51, 1977, Elsevier.
15. Chandrasekar PH, Narula AP: Bone and joint infections in intravenous drug abusers, *Rev Infect Dis* 8:904, 1986.
16. Christenson JC, Hill HR: Infections complicating congenital immunodeficiency syndromes. In Rubin RH, Young LS, editors: *Clinical approach to infection in the compromised host,* ed 3, New York, 1994, Plenum.
17. Crossley KB, Thurn JR: Nursing home acquired pneumonia, *Semin Respir Infect* 4:64, 1989.
18. Cunha BA: Infections and asplenia, *Infect Dis Pract* 21:48, 1997.
19. Cunha BA: Infection in non-leukopenic compromised hosts (diabetes mellitus, SLE, steroids and asplenia) in critical care, *Crit Care Med* 14:263, 1998.
20. Dajani AS, Bisno AL, Chung KJ, et al: Prevention of bacterial endocarditis: recommendations of the American Heart Association, *JAMA* 264:2919, 1990.
21. Dale DC, Fauci AS, Wolff SM: Alternate-day prednisone: leukocyte kinetics susceptibility to infection, *N Engl J Med* 291:1154, 1974.
22. Dale DC: Potential role of colony stimulating factors in the prevention and treatment of infectious disease, *Clin Infect Dis* 18(suppl):180, 1994.
23. Decker JL: Toxicity of immunosuppressive drugs in man, *Arthritis Rheum* 16:89, 1973.
24. De Jongh CA, Joshi JH, Newman KA, et al: Antibiotic synergism and response in gram-negative bacteremia in granulocytopenic cancer patients, *Am J Med* 80:96, 1986.
25. Des Jarlais FC, Friedman SR, Stoneburner RL: HIV infection and intravenous drug use: critical issues in transmission dynamics, infection outcome and prevention, *Rev Infect Dis* 10:151, 1988.
26. Di Padova F, Durig M, Harden F, et al: Impaired antipneumococcal antibody production in patients without spleens, *Br Med J* 290:14, 1985.
27. Doroghazi RM, Nadol JB, Hyslop NE, et al: Invasive external otitis: report of 21 cases and review of the literature, *Am J Med* 71:603, 1981.
28. Dover JS, Johnson RA: Cutaneous manifestations of HIV infection. Part II, *Arch Dermatol* 27:1549, 1992.
29. Dummer JS, Herdy A, Ho M, et al: Early infections in kidney, heart and liver transplant recipients on cyclosporine, *Transplantation* 36:259, 1983.
30. Eliashiv A, Olumida F, Norton L, et al: Depression of cell mediated immunity in diabetics, *Arch Surg* 113:1180, 1978.
31. Epstein JB, Chow AW: Oral complications associated with immunosuppression and cancer therapies, *Infect Dis Clin North Am* 13:901, 1999.
32. Fahey JL, Scroggins R, Utz JP, et al: Infection, antibody response and gammaglobulin components in multiple myeloma and macroglobulinemia, *Am J Med* 35:698, 1963.
33. Giamarello H: Empiric therapy for infections in the febrile, neutropenic, compromised host, *Med Clin North Am* 79:559, 1995.
34. Glick M, editor: *Clinician's guide to treatment of HIV-infected patients,* ed 2, Baltimore, Md, 1996, American Academy of Oral Medicine.
35. Gluckman SJ, Dvorak VC, MacGregor RR: Host defenses during prolonged alcohol consumption in a controlled environment, *Arch Intern Med* 137:1539, 1977.
36. Goldblum SE, Reed WP: Host defenses and immunologic alteration associated with chronic hemodialysis, *Ann Intern Med* 93:597, 1980.
37. Greenspan JS, Greenspan D: Oral hairy leukoplakia: diagnosis and management, *Oral Surg Oral Med Oral Pathol* 67:396, 1989.
38. Greenspan JS, Greenspan D, Lannette ET, et al: Replication of Epstein-Barr virus within epithelial cells of oral "hairy" leukoplakia, an AIDS-associated lesion, *N Engl J Med* 313:1564, 1985.
39. Greenberg MA, Cohen SG, McKitrick JC, et al: The oral flora as a source of septicemia in patients with acute leukemia, *Oral Surg Oral Med Oral Pathol* 53:32, 1982.
40. Grieco MH: Approach to the immunocompromised patient. In Gorbach SL, Bartlett JG, Blacklow NR, editors: *Infectious diseases,* Philadelphia, 1988, WB Saunders.
41. Guerra LG, Neira CJ, Boman D, et al: Rapid response of AIDS-related bacillary angiomatosis to azithromycin, *Clin Infect Dis* 17:264, 1993.
42. Haynes BF, Fauci AS: The differential effect of in vivo hydrocortisone on the kinetics of subpopulations of human peripheral blood-derived lymphocytes, *Blood* 46:235, 1975.

43. Hibberd P, Tolkoff-Rubin N, Conti D, et al: Preemptive ganciclovir therapy to prevent cytomegalovirus disease in cytomegalovirus antibody-positive renal transplant recipients, *Ann Intern Med* 18:123, 1995.

44. Hosteller MK: Effects of hyperglycemia on C3 and *Candida albicans, Diabetes* 39:211, 1990.

45. Hunter KD, Gibson J, Lockhart PB, et al: Fluconazole-resistant *Candida* species in the oral flora of fluconazole-exposed HIV positive patients, *Oral Surg Oral Med Oral Pathol* 85:558, 1998.

46. Jacobson DR, Zolla-Prazner S: Immunosuppression and infection in multiple myeloma, *Semin Oncol* 13:282, 1986.

47. Johanson WG, Pierce AK, Stanford JP: Changing oropharyngeal bacterial flora of hospitalized patients, emergence of gram-negative bacilli, *N Engl J Med* 281:1137, 1969.

48. Joshi NJ, Gregory MC, Weitkamp MR, et al: Infections in patients with diabetes mellitus, *N Engl J Med* 341:1906, 1999.

49. Kahn JO, Walker BD: Acute immunodeficiency virus type 1 infection, *N Engl J Med* 339:33, 1998.

50. Kessler HA, Benson CH, Urbanski P: Regression of oral hairy leukoplakia during zidovudine therapy, *Arch Intern Med* 148:2496, 1988.

51. Klatt EC, Mills NZ, Noguchi TT: Cause of death in hospitalized intravenous drug abusers, *J Forensic Sci* 35:1143, 1990.

52. Klimas NG, Blauey NT, Morgan RO, et al: Immune function and anti-HTLV I/II status in anti-HIV negative intravenous drug abusers receiving methadone, *Am J Med* 90:163, 1991.

53. Kontoyiannis DP, Rubin RH: Infection in the organ transplant recipient: an overview, *Infect Dis Clin North Am* 9:811, 1995.

54. Kullberg BJ, Westerndorp RG, van't Wout JW, et al: Purpura fulminans and symmetrical peripheral gangrene caused by *Capnocytophaga canimorsus* (formerly DF-2) septicemia: a complication of dog bite, *Medicine (Baltimore)* 70:287, 1991.

55. Lee JW, Pizzo PA: Management of the cancer patient with fever and prolonged neutropenia, *Hematol Oncol Clin North Am* 7:937, 1993.

56. Lepage P, Schwenk A, DeMol P, et al: Infection in the malnourished patient. In Root RK, Waldvogel F, Corey L, et al, editors: *Clinical infectious diseases: a practical approach,* New York, 1996, Oxford University Press.

57. Levine DP, Sobel JD: Infection in intravenous drug abusers. In Mandell GL, Bennett JE, Dolin R, editors: *Principles and practice of infectious diseases,* ed 4, New York, 1995, Churchill Livingstone.

58. Lockhart PB, Schmidtke MA: Antibiotic considerations in medically compromised patients, *Dent Clin North Am* 38:381, 1994.

59. Longmen LP, Martin MV: A practical guide to antibiotic prophylaxis in restorative dentistry, *Dent Update* 26:7, 1999.

60. Luce EB, Montgomery MT, Redding SW: The prevalence of cardiac valvular pathosis in patients with systemic lupus erythematosus, *Oral Surg Oral Med Oral Pathol* 70:590, 1990.

61. Lum LG: Immune recovery after bone marrow transplantation, *Hematol Oncol Clin North Am* 4:659, 1990.

62. Macgregor RR: Alcohol and immune defense, *JAMA* 256:1474, 1986.

63. Macgregor RR: Alcohol abuse, host defenses, and infection. In Root RK, Waldvogel F, Corey L, et al, editors: *Clinical infectious diseases: a practical approach,* New York, 1996, Oxford University Press.

64. Mackowaik PA, Jones SR, Martin RM, et al: Oropharyngeal colonization of chronic alcoholics by gram negative bacilli and other potential pathogens (abstract), *Clin Res* 24:349A, 1976.

65. Mahmoud AAF, Waren KS, Rodman HM, et al: Effects of diabetes mellitus on cellular immunity, *Surg Forum* 26:548, 1975.

66. McCarthy GM, Mackie ID, Koval J, et al: Factors associated with increased frequency of HIV-related oral candidiasis, *J Oral Pathol Med* 20:332, 1991.

67. McMahon MM, Bistrain BR: Host defenses and susceptibility to infection in patients with diabetes mellitus, *Infect Dis Clin North Am* 9:1, 1995.

68. Mellors JW, Munoz A, Giorgi JV, et al: Plasma viral load and CD4-4+ T-lymphocytes as a prognostic marker in HIV-1 infection, *Ann Intern Med* 126:946, 1997.

69. Meuleman J, Ketz P: The immunologic effects, kinetics, and used of glucocorticoids, *Med Clin North Am* 69:805, 1985.

70. Meunier F: Infections in patients with acute leukemia and lymphoma. In Mandell GL, Bennett JE, Dolin R, editors: *Principles and practice of infectious diseases,* ed 4, New York, 1995, Churchill Livingstone.

71. Meurman JH: Dental infection and general health, *Quintessence Int* 28:807, 1997.

72. Meyers JD, Spencer HC, Watts JC, et al: Cytomegalovirus pneumonia after human marrow transplantation, *Ann Intern Med* 82:181, 1975.

73. Monaici D, Greco D, Flecchia G, et al: Epidemiology, clinical features and prognostic value of HIV-1 related oral lesions, *J Oral Pathol Med* 19:477, 1990.

74. Mounzer KC, DiNubile MJ: Prophylactic use of antibiotics and vaccines in patients with rheumatologic disorders, *Rheum Clin North Am* 23:259, 1997.

75. Muller F, Holberg-Petersen M, Rolleg H: Non-specific oral immunity in individuals with HIV infection, *J Acquir Immune Defic Syndr* 5:46, 1992.

76. Myskowski PL, Ahkami R: Dermatologic complications of HIV infection, *Med Clin North Am* 80:1414, 1996.

77. Najjar VA, Fridkin M: Antineoplastic, immunogenic, and other effects of the tetrapeptide tuftsin: a natural macrophage activator, *Ann NY Acad Sci* 419:1, 1983.

78. Newman C, Polk F: Resolution of oral hairy leukoplakia during therapy with 9-(1,3-dihydroxy-2-propoxymethyl) guanine (DHPG), *Ann Intern Med* 107:348, 1987.

79. Nohr C: Non-AIDS immunosuppression. In Wilmore DW, Cheung LY, Harken AH, et al, editors: *Scientific American surgery,* section VII, subsection 3, New York, 1995, WebMD.

80. Norman DC, Toledo SD: Infections in elderly persons, *Clin Geriatr Med* 8:713, 1992.

81. Novik DM, Ness GL: Abuse of antibiotics by abusers of heroin or cocaine, *South Med J* 77:302, 1984.

82. Orangio GR, Pitlick SD, Della Latta P, et al: Soft tissue infection in parenteral drug abusers, *Am Surg* 199:97, 1984.

83. Overholser CD, Peterson DE, William LT, et al: Periodontal infections in patients with acute nonlymphocytic leukemia: prevalence of acute exacerbations, *Arch Intern Med* 142:551, 1982.

84. Palella FJ, Delaney KM, Moorman AC, et al: Declining morbidity and mortality among patients with advanced human immunodeficiency virus infection. HIV Outpatient Study Investigators, *N Engl J Med* 338:853, 1998.

85. Parfrey NA: Improved diagnosis and prognosis of mucormycosis: a clinico-pathologic study of 35 cases, *Medicine* 65:113, 1986.

86. Parillo JE, Fauci AS: Mechanisms of glucocorticoid action on immune processes, *Ann Rev Pharmacol Toxicol* 19:179, 1979.

87. Patton LL, Van der Horst C: Oral infection and other manifestations of HIV disease, *Infect Dis Clin North Am* 13:879, 1999.

88. Payan DG: Evaluation and management of patients with collagen vascular disease. In Rubin RH, Young LS, editors: *Clinical approach to infections in the compromised host,* New York, 1994, Plenum.

89. Peterson PK, Anderson RC: Infection in renal transplant recipients: current approaches to diagnosis, therapy and prevention, *Am J Med* 81(suppl 1A):2, 1986.

90. Phair J, Munoz A, Detels R, et al: The risk of *Pneumocystis carinii* pneumonia among men infected with human immunodeficiency virus type 1, *N Engl J Med* 322:161, 1990.

91. Phelan JA: Oral manifestations of HIV infection, *Med Clin North Am* 81:511, 1997.

92. Piliero P, Furie R: Functional asplenia in systemic lupus erythematosus, *Semin Arthritis Rheum* 20:185, 1990.

93. Pizzo PA: Current concepts: Fever in the immunocompromised patient, *N Engl Med* 341:893, 1999.

94. Quintilaini R, Maderazo EG: Infections in the compromised host. In Topazian RG, Goldberg MH, editors: *Oral and maxillofacial infections,* ed 3, Philadelphia, 1994, WB Saunders.

95. Rand KH, Kramer B, Johnson AC: Cancer chemotherapy associated symptomatic stomatitis: role of herpes simplex virus, *Cancer* 50:1262, 1982.

96. Reisacher WR, Finn DG, Stern J, et al: Manifestations of AIDS in the head and neck, *South Med J* 92:684, 1999.

97. Roberts-Thomson IC, Wittingham S, Youngchaiyud U, et al: Aging, immune response and mortality, *Lancet* 2:363, 1974.

98. Roldan AC, Shivley KB, Crawford HM: Echocardiographic study of valvular heart disease associated with SLE, *N Engl J Med* 335:1424, 1996.

99. Rosenthal CJ, Franklin DC: Depression of cellular mediated immunity in systemic lupus erythematosus, *Arthritis Rheum* 18:208, 1975.

100. Rossi SS, Glick M: Lupus erythematosus: considerations for dentistry, *J Am Dent Assoc* 129:330, 1998.

101. Rubin J, Yu VL: Malignant external otitis: insights into pathogenesis, clinical manifestations, diagnosis, and therapy, *Am J Med* 85:391, 1988.

102. Rubin RH: Infectious disease complications of renal transplantation, *Kidney Int* 44:221, 1993.

103. Rubin RH: Infection in organ transplant recipients. In Rubin RH, Young LS, editors: *Clinical approach to infection in the compromised host,* ed 3, New York, 1994, Plenum.

104. Rubin RH: Infection in the immunosuppressed host. In Dale CD, Federman DD, editors: *Scientific American Medicine,* section 7, subsection X, New York, 1998, WebMD.

105. Salimonu LS, Ojo-Amaize E, Wiliams AIO, et al: Depressed natural killer cell activity in children with protein-calorie malnutrition, *Clin Immunol Immunopathol* 24:1, 1982.

106. Saltzman RL, Peterson PK: Immunodeficiency in the elderly, *Rev Infect Dis* 9:1127, 1987.

107. Samouis G, Mautadakis E, Marakis S: Orofacial infection in the immunocompromised host, *Oncol Rep* 7:1389, 2000.

108. Saravolatz LD, Burch KH, Quinn EL, et al: Polymicrobial infective endocarditis: an increasing clinical entity, *Am Heart J* 95:163, 1978.

109. Saxon A, Stevens RH, Ramer SJ, et al: Glucocorticoids administered in vivo inhibit human suppressor T-lymphocyte function and diminished B-lymphocyte responsiveness in in vivo immunoglobulin synthesis, *J Clin Invest* 61:922, 1973.

110. Schimpff SC: Infections in the cancer patient: diagnosis, prevention, and treatment. In Mandell GL, Bennett JE, Dolin R, editors: *Principles and practice of infectious diseases,* ed 4, New York, 1995, Churchill Livingstone.

111. Schooley RT: Acquired immunodeficiency syndrome. In Dale CD, Federman DD, editors: *Scientific American Medicine,* section 7, subsection XI, New York, 2000, WebMD.

112. Shand FL: The immunopharmacology of cyclophosphamide, *Int J Pharmacol* 1:165, 1979.

113. Shuman SK, McCusker ML, Owen MK: Enhancing infection control for elderly and medically compromised patients, *J Am Dent Assoc* 124:76, 1993.

114. Sugarman B: Zinc and infection, *Rev Infect Dis* 5:137, 1983.

115. Tai C-C E, Precious DS, Wood RE: Prophylactic extraction of third molars in cancer patients, *Oral Surg Oral Med Oral Pathol* 78:151, 1994.

116. Tierney MR, Baker AS: Infection of head and neck in diabetes mellitus, *Infect Dis Clin North Am* 9:195, 1995.

117. Tubara E, Borelli G, Croce C, et al: Effect of morphine resistance to infection, *J Infect Dis* 148:656, 1983.

118. UNAIDS: Report on the global HIV/AIDS epidemic: June 2000, Geneva, 2000, World Health Organization.

119. United Network for Organ Sharing (UNOS): UNOS Critical Data: Milestones, 2001. Available from: http://www.unos.org

120. Van Der Meer JWN: Defects in host defense mechanisms. In Rubin RH, Young LS, editors: *Clinical approach to infection in the compromised host,* ed 3, New York, 1994, Plenum.

121. Vartivarian S, Bodey G: Infection associated with malignancy. In Gorbach SL, Bartlett JG, Blacklow NR, editors: *Infectious diseases,* ed 2, Philadelphia, 1998, WB Saunders.

122. Vergis EN, Mellors JW: Natural history of HIV-1 infection, *Infect Dis Clin North Am* 14:809, 2000.

123. West CE, Rombout JHW, Van Der Zijp AJ, et al: Vitamin A and immune function, *Proc Nutr Soc* 50:251, 1991.

124. Wiederman CJ, Niedermuhlbichler M, Beimpold H, et al: In vitro activation of neutrophils of the aged by recombinant growth hormone, *J Infect Dis* 164:1017, 1991.

125. Wingard JR, Elfenbein GJ: Host immunologic augmentation for the control of infection, *Infect Dis Clin North Am* 10:345, 1996.

126. Winston DJ: Prophylaxis and treatment of infection in the bone marrow transplant recipient, *Curr Clin Top Infect Dis* 13:293, 1993.

127. Zysset MK, Montgomery MT, Redding SW, et al: SLE: a consideration for antimicrobial prophylaxis, *Oral Surg Oral Med Oral Pathol* 64:30, 1987.

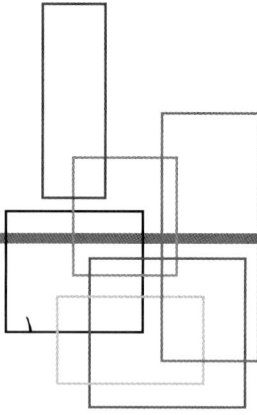

Control and Prevention of Infection in the Surgical Patient

Morton H. Goldberg

NOSOCOMIAL INFECTIONS IN THE INTENSIVE CARE UNIT

Nosocomial infections, those acquired in the hospital, have become a modern plague, often defeating the best efforts of surgeons and physicians to use contemporary technology and pharmacology to save lives and preserve the quality of life of their patients. The intensive care unit (ICU), where the most seriously ill, infirm, and injured patients who have undergone major surgery are clustered, is also the home of some of the most virulent, antibiotic-resistant pathogenic microorganisms.

In 1988 the Centers for Disease Control and Prevention reported that ICU patients accounted for 5% to 10% of all hospital patients but represented 20% of nosocomial infections, at a cost of $1 billion annually for therapy and for prolongation of hospital stay. One in five ICU patients had an acquired infection.

By 1991, although the incidence of ICU infections remained stable, the cost had increased to $7 billion annually. The risk of death doubles for an ICU patient who acquires a nosocomial infection, and the annual deaths from ICU infections have risen to 80,000, more than are killed on U.S. highways annually, and more than were killed in either the Vietnam or the Korean conflicts.

These risks are related to age, preexisting illness, extensive surgery, and invasive techniques such as central lines, endotracheal tubes, and urinary catheters. Furthermore, selective evolutionary pressures compound the problem by eliciting genetic survival mechanisms for many bacterial species, especially those that are frequently exposed to multiple broad-spectrum antibiotics. These organisms, the sites most commonly infected, and risk factors are summarized in Table 25-1.

The problem of ICU nosocomial infections is compounded by the transfer of microorganisms from patient to patient, and from the ICU to other areas of hospitals by hospital staff and inanimate objects. The transfer of infectious disease by the hands of medical personnel has been recognized for 150 years.

Maimonides (circa 1135-1204) was the first physician to recommend hand washing between patients. A documented historical perspective of this problem extends from the early nineteenth century, when Ignaz Philipp Semmelweis, the "Magnificent Magyar," first noticed that infections were transmitted within hospitals (Figure 25-l). While on staff of the Allgemeine Krankenhaus in Vienna in 1846, Semmelweis observed the epidemics of puerperal (childbed) fever among thousands of young healthy women after childbirth at the institution. Now known to be streptococcal and staphylococcal septicemia originating in the postpartum uterus, the disease was a mystery in that era; only the horrendous number of deaths was obvious. Having observed that the problem was far greater in the hospital than after home deliveries, Semmelweis reasoned that the disease was caused by the hospital and possibly by the physicians, who often rushed directly from autopsies to the delivery room. He further reasoned that infectious materials could be carried from the dead to the living and from the diseased or purulent processes of infected patients to otherwise healthy ones.

Without benefit of the knowledge of microorganisms as a cause of disease, Semmelweis postulated that washing of the hands by physicians between examinations and between visits to the autopsy room and the delivery room could prevent the spread of disease. Despite an immediate reduction of the mortality rate on his ward from 17% to 1% by washing hands in chlorinated water, Semmelweis was ridiculed by those who firmly believed that infection was caused by atmospheric, cosmic, and telluric influences; even the great Virchow condemned him. Semmelweis paid a heavy price for having discovered the cause and cure for iatrogenic nosocomial infection that was the scourge of his era: dismissal from the hospital and incarceration in a mental institution. Released years later after the independent

National Nosocomial Infection Surveillance System ICU (1986-1995)

Infection	Risk Factors	Common Organisms	Rate (%)
Pneumonia	Old age	*Staphylococcus aureus*	18.1
	Chronic lung disease	*Pseudomonas aeruginosa*	17.9
	Endotracheal intubation	*Klebsiella pneumoniae*	6.9
	Abdominal thoracic surgery	*Acinetobacter* spp.	5.1
	Nasogastric tube	*Enterobacter* spp.	4.6
	Immunosuppression	*Haemophilus influenzae*	4.6
	Prior antibiotic use	*Escherichia coli*	4.1
	Aspiration	*Serratia* spp.	3.9
Urinary tract infection	Female	*E. coli*	18.2
	Old age	*Enterococci*	14.0
	Diabetes mellitus	*Pseudomonas aeruginosa*	10.9
	Renal failure	*Klebsiella pneumoniae*	6.2
	Indwelling bladder catheter	*Enterobacter* spp.	5.3
		S. aureus	1.6
		Candida albicans	1.5
Bloodstream sepsis	Old age	Coagulase-negative *Staphylococcus*	35.5*
	Vascular catheterization	*Enterococci*	12.7†
	Parenteral nutrition	*S. aureus*	12.6‡
	Frequent dressing change	*Enterobacter* spp.	5.1
	Changes a catheter site	*P. aeruginosa*	3.9
		Candida spp.	5.9
		Bacteroides spp.	0.7
Surgical site infection	Old age		
	Obesity		
	Diabetes		
	Cancer	Coagulase-negative *Staphylococcus*	13§, 9‖
	Poor nutritional status	*S. aureus*	56§, 55‖
	Duration of surgery	Methicillin-resistant *Staphylococcus*	13§
	Prolonged preoperative hospitalization	*P. aeruginosa*	—
	Infection at another site	*E. coli*	—

*Mortality rate 21%.
†Mortality rate 32%.
‡Mortality rate 25%.
§Orthopedic site; Hartford Hospital, 1999.
‖Neurosurgery site.

corroboration of his hypothesis by Oliver Wendell Holmes in Boston, he died at age 46, ironically, of general suppuration secondary to a small finger cut sustained during a dissection.

Following the principles of Semmelweis and the later germ theory of infection, physicians of the late nineteenth century could control the spread of hospital gangrene, erysipelas, and other hospital contagions. Strict aseptic techniques, isolation of patients, and personal hygiene among surgical and nursing personnel controlled the threat of hospital-transmitted infections. The work of Lister and other early surgeons of the modem era led to hospital and operating room behavior that was highly intricate, compulsive, and stylistic, but uniquely successful (Figure 25-2).

By 1890 Koch had demonstrated that bacteria entering a wound could cause infection. Later, events at Johns Hopkins Medical School demonstrated that the use of

gloves created a valuable safety barrier for both the patient and the surgeon. One of the Hopkins "Big Four" (Osler, Halsted, Kelly, Welch), pathologist William Welch began to wear gloves while performing autopsies so as not to meet the same unfortunate demise as Semmelweis. Halsted provided rubber (latex) gloves for his surgical nurse, who was suffering from contact dermatitis of her hands from exposure to intraoperative antiseptics (carbolic acid and mercury). Finally, in one of the few controlled studies of the efficacy of surgical gloves, the herniorrhaphy infection rate at Johns Hopkins was reduced from 90% to 2% when the hands of the entire surgical team were sheathed in latex.

During 1990, two oral and maxillofacial surgery patients in the Hartford Hospital Surgical ICU almost simultaneously developed postoperative wound infections. One developed sepsis at his tracheostomy site, the other in the incision overlying a bone graft. Cultures from both wound

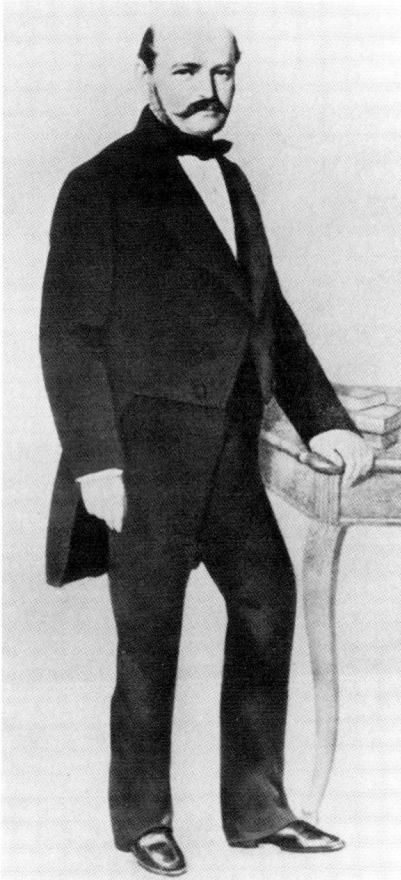

Figure 25-1 Ignaz Philipp Semmelweis (1818-1865). In 1847 Semmelweis discovered the role of surgeon's unclean hands in spreading obstetrical and surgical infections. (From Steingrueben Archives, Stuttgart.)

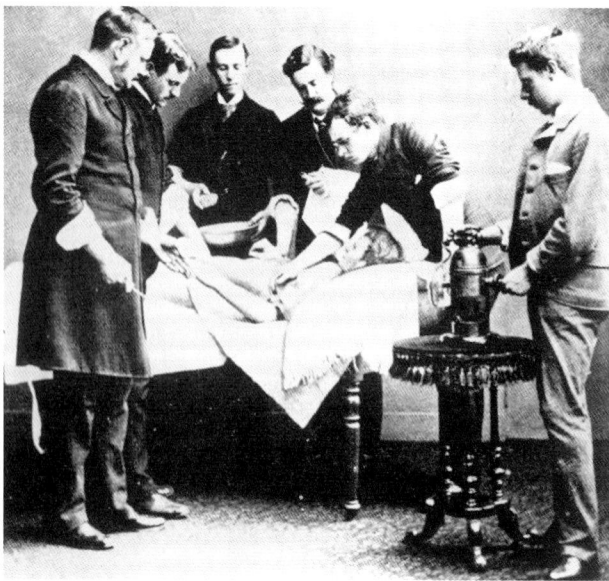

Figure 25-2 Lister's carbolic-acid spray machine during surgery, about 1870. Gloves, gowns, caps and masks were not yet in use. (From Bettman Archive, New York.)

infections revealed the gram-negative pathogen *Serratia,* an organism not commonly found in infection of the face, mouth, or neck. Because of the unusual and seemingly co-incidental nature of the infections, an infectious disease-epidemiology consultation was requested and resulted in the following elementary observations and conclusion:

1. Of the 20 patients in that intensive care unit (ICU) during the period of the *Serratia* spp. mini-epidemic, only two were on the oral and maxillofacial surgery service.
2. These two patients were the only ICU patients with *Serratia* spp. infections.
3. The two oral and maxillofacial surgery patients never came in contact with each other.
4. The two attending oral and maxillofacial surgeons were never in contact with each other's patients.
5. The ICU surgeons, residents, nurses, respiratory therapists, and phlebotomists had been in contact with all 20 patients.
6. Only the oral and maxillofacial surgery residents were in contact with both patients, but none of the other 18 patients in the ICU.

Therefore the single common denominator (and transmitter) in the *Serratia* spp. outbreak had to be the oral and maxillofacial residents, who on careful questioning admitted to "occasionally" changing dressings and examining incisions without benefit of hand washing or wearing sterile gloves. These residents were advised that reports of any subsequent *Serratia* spp. infections would result in hand culturing and disciplinary action against the identified offenders. The "epidemic" ended. Apparently, 150-year-old lessons must be relearned in each new generation.

Only recently has the role of the patient's environment been recognized also as a major factor in the chain of ICU sepsis. *Pseudomonas* spp., notoriously resistant to antibiotics, can survive and multiply on plastic intravenous catheters, in bedside carafes, air conditioning vents, and antiseptic solutions, and within the nasopharynges of ICU personnel. Vancomycin-resistant enterococci (VRE), easily spread from the colon and anus to the skin and bed of an ICU patient, then can be transferred by ICU personnel to objects within the ICU, including telephones, intravenous poles, light switches, doorknobs, computer keyboards, bed rails, bed pans, and even the walls and floors. These inanimate intermediate vectors thus are implicated in the transfer of VRE to other patients, hospital workers, and other areas of the hospital. The density of VRE in the stool of colonized hospitalized patients increases dramatically when antianaerobic antibiotics (clindamycin, metronidazole, amoxicillin-clavulanate, Cefotan, vancomycin) are administered. Limiting the use of these agents may decrease the spread of VRE. The National Nosocomial Infection Surveillance System has reported that the incidence of VRE nosocomial infections increased from 0.4% in 1989, to 13.6% in 1993, and the problem continues to escalate. With 30 million admissions to American hospitals annually, a large percentage of the population has been exposed to VRE; the outcome remains unknown and uncertain (Box 25-1).

Although statistics vary among hospitals and from study to study, apparently the predominant organisms responsible for severe nosocomial infections in North American hospitals are *Staphylococcus aureus, Pseudomonas* spp., and enterococci, all of which have proved remarkably capable of developing resistance to antibiotics.

Alexander Fleming's original serendipitous discovery of penicillin's antibacterial properties occurred during laboratory research on staphylococci in 1928. First used clinically during the early years of World War II, penicillin was effective against staphylococci, but by 1948 Fleming and others had observed that a remarkable resistance to penicillin had developed. This resistance in *S. aureus* by the production of β-lactamase quickly decreased the usefulness of the "wonder drug," especially among hospitalized patients.

The "staph epidemic" of the late 1950s and early 1960s, which included serious wound infections, fatal pneumonia, and generalized sepsis in otherwise healthy patients prompted the chemical modification of penicillin and aminoglycosides.

However, many bacterial species overcome antibiotics by a variety of biological pathways. Genetic mutation is an ancient and ongoing constant in evolution. A contemporary example is the development of *Staphylococcus* and *Pseudomonas* spp. resistance to fluoroquinolones by alteration in their deoxyribonucleic acid (DNA) topoisomerase.

BOX 25-1

Centers for Disease Control and Prevention Recommendations

> **Standard precautions:** recommended for all patients
> *Wash hands* between patients and after removing gloves.
> *Wear gloves* when direct contact with blood, bodily fluids, or secretions is anticipated.
> *Wear a gown* when clothing is likely to be soiled by a body fluid.
> *Wear a mask and goggles/glasses* when splashes of a body fluid are anticipated (e.g., during most invasive procedures).
> **Contact precautions:** used in addition to standard precautions for patients infected or colonized with epidemiologically significant organisms transmitted by direct contact (e.g., multidrug-resistant organisms [e.g., VRE], viral hemorrhagic fevers, scabies).
> *Place patient in private room* or cohort patients with identical infections.
> *Wear gown and gloves to enter room.*
> *Use dedicated stethoscope and thermometer* and other patient care equipment when possible.
> *Remove gown and gloves before leaving room.*
> *Wash hands with antimicrobial soap before leaving room.*

From Recommendations for preventing the spread of vancomycin resistance. Recommendations of the Hospital Infection Control Practices Advisory Committee (HICPAC), *MMWR Morb Mortal Wkly Rep* 44(RR-12):1, 1995.

Other bacteria (e.g., *Pneumococcus* spp.) also may acquire multidrug resistance from other species as they incorporate foreign DNA (transferable plasmids or transposons) by means of conjugation. Some plasmids or transposons have genetic substances, integrons, that absorb exogenous genes, which result in resistance to multiple antimicrobial agents. This transference of genetic material may be responsible for the emergence of vancomycin resistance in enterococci.

One of the most serious contemporary threats to health worldwide is the phenomenon of clinical infection caused by bacteria resistant to multiple antibiotics and the rapid spread of this resistance. Certainly the overuse, misuse, and abuse of antibiotics in medicine, veterinary medicine, and agriculture-husbandry has created the genetically selective pressure that has produced this problem.

STAPHYLOCOCCUS RESISTANCE

S. aureus, an aerobic gram-positive coccus that produces golden-pigmented colonies in the laboratory and characteristic clumping of cocci on Gram stain, produces coagulase, which is both a species marker and an indication of virulence. Coagulase-negative staphylococci, including *Staphylococcus epidermidis,* usually are nonpathogenic commensals except when associated with a foreign body or blood stream infection. Numerous extracellular toxins may be produced by staphylococci, including hemolysins, and have been associated with toxic shock, even of odontogenic origin. Epidermal necrolysis is induced also by staphylococcal toxins.

Although staphylococci inhabit the oral cavity in relatively small numbers, they have been reported in studies of the microbiology of oral infections to be as high as 10% of polymicrobial isolates in deep space infection of odontogenic origin. Significant oral staphylococci infections have been observed in a series of pediatric oral infections. Typically, *S. aureus* infections are localized, with abscess formation containing purulent exudate and necrotic tissue, as in traumatic skin and postoperative wound infections of the face and other areas. These usually require surgical drainage and appropriate antibiotic therapy.

Seeding of staphylococci to distant sites is a well-recognized phenomenon, including cardiac valves, prosthetic valves, and metal joint prostheses. The ability to adhere to foreign materials (trophism) is characteristic of staphylococci.

Methicillin, oxacillin, dicloxacillin, β-lactamase–stable penicillins, cephalothin, and cefazolin became available in the 1960s and controlled the "staph epidemic." Nonetheless, more than 15% of contemporary nosocomial infections are *S. aureus* in origin. However, by 1968 American hospitals were observing the appearance of methicillin-resistant staphylococci, a problem described even earlier in Europe. By the late 1970s many hospital (nosocomial) outbreaks of methicillin-resistant *S. aureus* (MRSA) had been reported, as had the development of resistance to cephalosporins and aminoglycosides, in MRSA. Nasal carriage as a source of *S. aureus* (including MRSA) bacteremia in the 1990s was an increasing and unsolved problem. Up to 40% of people tested as outpatients or on hospital admission have been colonized by *S. aureus*.

Even newer drugs, the quinolones, once encouragingly successful against MRSA, now have been observed to be increasingly ineffective. Since the emergence of MRSA, vancomycin has been the only reliable therapy for serious MRSA infections.

However, one case of reduced vancomycin effectiveness against MRSA was reported from Japan in 1997 and by 1999 two additional cases had been reported from Michigan and New Jersey, the latter two confirmed by the National Center for Infection Diseases. These strains of MRSA are classified as having intermediate resistance to vancomycin, with MICs between 4 μg/mL (susceptible) and 32 μg/mL (resistant). Intermediate resistance to vancomycin develops incrementally when MRSA are exposed to vancomycin, as in long-term therapy for renal infections, sepsis, or heart surgery. Urinary catheters and Gore-tex arteriovenous grafts also have been implicated as selective environmental factors, which contributed to the development of vancomycin-resistant MRSA. In animal models, vancomycin resistance decreases when the foreign material is removed.

The appearance of vancomycin-resistant MRSA in 1999 was not surprising. It had been predicted because *S. aureus* has been in close proximity to vancomycin-resistant enterococci in ICUs and because enterococcal vancomycin-resistant genetic material had been experimentally transferred to *S. aureus* in vitro.

The seriousness of the health menace of vancomycin-resistant MRSA cannot be overemphasized and the outlook has been described as "rather grim" and as "a chronicle of death foretold." A few new and investigational antimicrobial drugs, such as oxazolidinone quinolones (Linezolid) and quinapristin-dalfopristin (Synercid) may hold promise for efficacy against VRS. Toxicity and drug-drug interactions are being investigated. A 1999 investigation suggests that in vitro combination of vancomycin and commonly available β-lactams (oxacillin) may have an effective synergism against VRSA.

Guidelines for isolation and control of vancomycin-resistant staphylococci (VRSA) are similar to those used when MRSA first appeared and include barrier precautions and periodic surveillance cultures of at-risk patients and selected (ICU) hospital staff. Serious nosocomial staphylococcal infections account for almost 25% of the total length of all hospital in-patient stays, resulting in high rates of morbidity and mortality, and millions of dollars of added costs. The appearance of orofacial vancomycin-resistant staphylococci in facial trauma, postoperative wounds, or odontogenic infections appears inevitable.

ENTEROCOCCAL RESISTANCE

Enterococci are the second most common organism causing nosocomial and hospital-acquired wound infections and urinary tract infections in the United States and the third most common cause of nosocomial bacteremia in the late 1990s. These microorganisms are facultatively anaerobic gram-positive cocci, which until 1937 were classified as streptococci. They produce surface adhesives that facilitate adherence to cells of the urinary tract and endocardium. Enterococci exhibit both intrinsic and extrinsic antibiotic resistance; the former is demonstrated in enterococci isolated from aboriginal groups never exposed to antibiotics. The latter has been demonstrated often as enterococci have acquired resistance to a wide range of antibiotics, including macrolides, tetracyclines, quinolones, and even glycopeptides and chloramphenicol. Resistance has occurred by mutation or by transfer of DNA through plasmids and transposons. Until recently vancomycin has been used to treat infection caused by multidrug-resistant enterococci.

Because of the widespread use of vancomycin against MRSA and as therapy for *Clostridium difficile* colitis, DNA transference and selective genetic pressure have resulted in the appearance of vancomycin-resistant enterococci (VREF). Enterococcal bloodstream sepsis has a morality rate of 32%, and vancomycin-resistant enterococcal bacteremia has a mortality rate of 50%, a serious threat especially to hospitalized, compromised, and postoperative patients. The time and origin of vancomycin-resistant enterococci is unknown, but these glycopeptide-resistant organisms have been recovered from animals treated with vancomycin and from sewage.

Therapy of glycopeptide-resistant enterococci remains difficult, but the enforcement of infection control protocols is essential, especially the education or reeducation of each new hospital rotation of residents, surgeons, and students. Drug therapy includes ampicillin plus aminoglycoside or chloramphenicol, which have limited value because of resistance or a fluoroquinolone that may be equally ineffective and is not bactericidal.

In September 1999 the Food and Drug Administration granted accelerated approval to the experimental drug Synercid for the treatment of VREF when no alternative treatment is available. The use of Synercid resulted in negative blood culture results in 90% of patients with VREF bacteremia.

PSEUDOMONAS AERUGINOSA AND *PSEUDOMONAS CEPACIA* RESISTANCE

Pseudomonas, the only bacterial species known to produce a blue pigment, pyocyanin, has long been problematic for compromised hosts and ICU patients. It has numerous genetic virulence and survival factors that enable it to resist antibiotics. *Pseudomonas* can survive many commonly used antiseptics and can grow and multiply on and in plastic catheters, air conditioning units, bedside carafes, flower vases, and the nasopharynges of ICU personnel.

Although *Pseudomonas* usually exists as an opportunistic nosocomial pathogen in patients with indwelling catheters, organ transplants, intravascular monitoring devices, and neutropenia, it also causes malignant otitis externa in elderly patients with insulin-dependent diabetes. Recently *Pseudomonas* spp. have been recognized as a cause of acute sinusitis in ICU patients with endotracheal tubes or nasogastric tubes. It is the third most common pathogen in surgical site infections (10.9%), including tracheotomy sites. Odontogenic infections, although uncommon, have been reported.

Antibiotic therapy is difficult and has a high failure rate because of the propensity of *Pseudomonas* spp. to rapidly develop resistance. Monotherapy therefore rarely is used. Combination therapy, including a β-lactam (piperacillin or ticarcillin) and an aminoglycoside (gentamicin, tobramycin) is used frequently, as is the addition of rifampin. Sensitivity studies and susceptibility data of individual hospital isolates of *Pseudomonas* are important in the appropriate selection of therapy. Ciprofloxin and other quinolones, which initially were useful against *Pseudomonas* spp., have become increasingly impotent, perhaps because of widespread general use of these drugs, which should have been reserved for serious or life-threatening infections.

Nosocomial *Pseudomonas* spp. sinusitis was described first in 1982 and usually is associated with ICU patients who are nasally intubated and receiving ventilatory mechanical assistance or with the prolonged use of nasogastric tubes. An increased incidence of *Pseudomonas* spp. sinusitis also has been observed in patients with acquired immunodeficiency syndrome (AIDS), and *Pseudomonas* spp. have been implicated in sinusitis in patients with cystic fibrosis, at a rate of up to 38%. Corticosteroids may be a predisposing factor, especially in neurosurgical patients. Unexplained fever, nasal discharge, and a high index of suspicion, in addition to sinus imaging should be useful in diagnosis. Although most patients respond well to removal of the endotracheal or nasogastric tube, antibiotic therapy based on sensitivity testing may be necessary, although ironically the use of broad-spectrum antibiotics may have been the initial source of the problem. Topical antibiotic therapy for recalcitrant *Pseudomonas* spp. sinusitis has been described. The worst scenario, usually in compromised hosts, is the development of orbitocerebral complications, mimicking mucormycosis, an example of the aggressive potential of *Pseudomonas* spp. infections in the ICU.

SURGICAL INFECTION CONTROL

Modern concern with control and prevention of surgical infection stems from the great advances in surgical technique of the last 50 years. This contemporary resurgence of interest is derived from the increase in types and numbers of surgical infections, which has paralleled the expansion of surgical science and, paradoxically, the availability of antimicrobial agents. This interest has encouraged the contributions of epidemiologists, bacteriologists, immunologists, surgeons, engineers, and hospital administrators to focus clinical and laboratory research on postoperative infections. The Centers for Disease Control and Prevention (CDC), in a 10-year survey, Project SENIC (Study for the Efficacy of Nosocomial Infection Control), reported that up to 25% of all nosocomial infections develop from surgical wounds.

Surgical infection may be defined as any infection that occurs in a patient who has undergone a surgical procedure. Specifically, wound sepsis may occur as a result of surgery or trauma. The following criteria are necessary for wound infection: a bacterial inoculum of sufficient quantity and virulence, the availability of nutrients for bacterial growth, and a host who is compromised locally or systemically. Other important factors relating to wound sepsis include the surgeon, the assistant, the nursing and technical personnel, the type and length of the surgical procedure, invasive technology and the implantation of foreign (xenogenic) devices, equipment, and even the air circulating through the operating room.

The attitudes and self-discipline of surgeons always have been and remain the key to surgical infection control. The compulsive self-discipline of the surgeons of the early modern surgical era controlled surgical infection adequately to permit great surgical advances, even before the luxury of antibiotics.

Laufman has stated this truism quite succinctly: "The success of the elegant and lofty work of surgery depends on disciplined performance of the menial labors and the regimented drudgery of aseptic techniques." Since the decline in the death rate on Semmelweis' ward, no technique, apparatus, antiseptic, antibiotic, conference, or committee meeting has accomplished as much control of surgical infection as the simple ritual of washing hands.

The ready availability and efficacy of antibiotics have tempted a generation of surgeons to disregard the petty details of aseptic surgical behavior. Regarding surgical asepsis as an unnecessary ritual, young surgical residents or attending surgeons are overheard to state, "A 2-minute scrub is adequate; this is an intraoral approach," or "Don't worry about that old ritual; this patient was given prophylactic antibiotics." Forgetting the experience of Semmelweis, some may be fulfilling the prophecy of Thomas Henry Huxley: "It is the customary fate of new truths to begin as heresies and to end as superstitions."

A study comparing hand washing by personnel in ICUs of university and community hospitals revealed considerable disregard or ignorance of the principle of hand hygiene by physicians. Physicians washed their hands only 42% of the time between patient contacts in the university hospital and less in the community hospital. The morbidity, mortality, and medicolegal implications represent a staggering condemnation of the health professions.

Surgeons easily disregard the fact that they represent a source of exogenous bacterial contamination for the patient, even for such a microbial-laden environment as the oral cavity. This potential contamination is intensified by the presence of antibiotic-resistant bacteria that have colonized the surgeon's hospital-acclimated body.

Surgical aseptic discipline starts with surgical education. The surgical trainee must be taught to accept certain simplistic ritualistic maneuvers, learned and relearned by many generations of surgeons, designed to prevent contamination of surgical patients and their wounds. The proven wisdom of hand washing must be stressed constantly, and teaching surgical scrubbing techniques (all surfaces for 5 minutes with detergent antiseptic solution) should not be delegated to junior residents. No precaution is overly intellectual, arcane, or unique in the maintenance of surgical asepsis. Rather, it is simple, lucid, and repetitive. Self-discipline, taught by example and rigidly enforced if necessary, is the key to asepsis.

Most endemic infections are transmitted by the hands of health care workers. Pathogenic gram-negative bacilli can survive on the hands for more than 2 hours. The hands of health care workers can be reservoirs for *Pseudomonas* growth and have been responsible for colonizing patients in neonatal ICUs, where onychomycosis and otitis externa have been traced to the original source in the workers.

Chlorhexidine is superior to alcohol-soap combinations in decreasing microbial flora on the hands, especially staphylococci, and appears to have greater residual activity. A dose-response effect has been demonstrated, indicating that the volume of antiseptic agent used by the surgeon may be a determining factor in reducing the number of microorganisms on the hands. Yet another paradox has been identified recently. Bacteria can become resistant to antiseptics and antibiotics. The use of commercial liquid hand soaps in offices and homes may be creating resistance when used routinely for hand washing or dishwashing. Advertising has led to the widespread use of "disinfectant" soaps by creating a false market for their need.

However, over time chlorhexidine has been shown to be less effective against *Serratia* and *Pseudomonas* spp. than previously. Povidone-iodine (10%) solution currently is the safest and most efficacious skin preparation for the maxillofacial patient, and povidone-iodine surgical scrub (7.5%) is widely used as a presurgical hand scrub by surgeons. However, both preparations can be contaminated with *P. cepacia*.

The efficacy of preoperative antiseptic, decontamination of the oral cavity remains uncertain, but evidence exists that the normal quantity of potentially pathogenic microorganisms in salivary flora (ranging from 10^7/mL to 10^8/mL, and higher in florid periodontal disease) may be reduced substantially by preoperative oral rinses (povidone-iodine) or chlorhexidine (Peridex) to a level of 10^4/mL. Some studies have demonstrated that this technique correlates with a decreased incidence of postoperative wound complication particularly in oncological surgery. Its usefulness in trauma surgery and craniofacial surgery remains uncertain; in procedures in which the infection rate is small (e.g., orthognathic surgery), more study is needed to determine when the usual prophylactic parenteral bolus of antibiotic could be withheld if oral decontamination had been performed.

As Laufman notes, discipline in surgical attire is as important as clean hands. Lapses in aseptic technique in the area of gloves, gowns, head coverings, and surgical masks can lead to septic misfortune, because microorganisms easily are harbored by or shed from hair, contaminated gowns, or shoes. Hair is grossly contaminated; one large outbreak of staphylococcal wound infections was traced to the sideburns of a single surgical resident. All head and beard hair should be covered.

The use of gloves during surgery and during postoperative wound care is as important as hand washing and is essential for the protection of the surgeons, who may have small abrasions or cuts on their hands. However, the medical literature on glove reliability reveals that pinholes exist in 2% to 9% of unused latex gloves, and almost 19,000 bacteria can pass through a single pinhole in 20 minutes. Obviously blood also can pass through pinholes, a major consideration in preventing the spread of human immunodeficiency virus (HIV) infection. Therefore gloves should be changed when perforations are observed, after prolonged use (2 hours) and during procedures likely to cause perforations (intermaxillary wire fixation). Wearing double layers of gloves when handling infected tissue or treating patients with known HIV or hepatitis is a prudent preventive measure.

The nasopharynges of most hospital habitues have been colonized by hospital bacteria. Misuse of the face mask, which acts as a bacterial filter, especially lowering and raising it between cases rather than disposing of it, disseminates organisms in the operating room. The surgeon must insist on face mask discipline—full coverage of mouth and nose—among all operating room personnel, including the anesthesiologist.

Unfortunately, the ability of commercially available surgical masks to filter bacterial emissions from the nose and mouth varies greatly. Some investigators have suggested that the surgical infection rate remains unchanged regardless of whether masks are worn. However, *S. aureus* (including MRSA) organisms inhabit the nasopharynges of hospital personnel (and many patients, especially those admitted from extended-care facilities); thus sneezing or coughing into an open wound without a mask seems unwise medically and medicolegally. As procedures become longer and more invasive, exposing wide areas of tissue to potential contamination, complacency in traditional barrier techniques is inappropriate. Masks and protective eye shields are defenses against blood splashes, which occur most frequently when power-driven saws and drills are used.

The number of bacteria released into the operating room environment has been demonstrated to be directly proportional to the amount of talking during the procedure. Unnecessary chatter should be minimized, although occasional amenities and anecdotes are permissible.

Operating room attire and drapes should be kept dry, if possible. When moistened by blood or irrigation fluids, cloth permits the ingress and migration of bacteria into the sterile area, a phenomenon known as strike-through. Wearing scrub suits outside the operating room and into heavily contaminated areas such as ICUs should be forbidden. Discipline in surgical attire must be maintained.

Personnel traffic through the operating suite must be

reduced to the essential minimum. Airborne bacterial concentrations are related directly to the number and activity of people in the operating room. All unnecessary traffic into and out of an operating room while the wound is open must be prevented. During a demonstration of a craniofacial procedure at a large metropolitan hospital, 21 surgeons, residents, nurses, anesthesiologists, and other surgical guests were in the room; the operating room door was opened more than 100 times for personnel traffic during the operation. The infection rate for this series of cases was 18%, including wound sepsis, osteomyelitis, meningitis, and brain abscess, despite the use of antibiotic prophylaxis. Although many factors may have been involved in the high infection rate, the overcrowding and lack of traffic control were obvious abuses of the surgical environment. These factors may substantiate the sage observation that "the chances for success of a surgical procedure are inversely related to the number of people watching."

Scheduling of cases also requires self-discipline. The temptation to yield to personal convenience and squeeze short, dirty cases into a busy schedule of clean ones should be resisted. Contaminated cases should be isolated in special operating rooms, or surgery on such cases should be performed at the end of the surgical schedule. Maxillofacial surgeons should refuse to perform open procedures in rooms that are used routinely for bowel surgery or other "dirty" procedures.

Air contamination in the operating room is a potential source of wound infection. The technical specifications for reducing the bioparticulate content of operating room air, as in laminar airflow systems or other high-efficiency particulate air-filtered systems (HEPAs), are beyond the scope of this chapter. However, surgeons should be aware of the availability of such technology if its use becomes necessary. Total hip replacement surgery has used these techniques for some time with the expectation that exogenous bacterial contamination would be decreased, and results have been encouraging. Expenditures for installation of such preventative measures usually lie outside the control of any individual surgeon, and a convincing case usually must be made for their need. At Hartford Hospital, a spate of knee infections with *S. epidermidis* after arthroscopy was traced to an air vent in an operating room. The sterile arthroscope routinely had been left uncovered for a few minutes before its insertion. An exhaust vent near the personnel in the room caused a flow of contaminated air past the instrument. The problem was solved by moving the table and keeping the arthroscope covered.

HOST FACTORS

Various host factors contributing to surgical infection have been discussed in detail elsewhere. Corticosteroid therapy, the effects of cytotoxic and immunosuppressive drugs, diabetes, hypoproteinemia, malnutrition, malignancies, myeloma and abnormal neutrophil or lymphocyte function (HIV) are considered causes of diminished host resistance.

The search for these deficiencies in host defenses is the responsibility of the surgeon. Surgical judgment, especially in the realm of elective surgery, weighs heavily on the surgeon when dealing with the potential for infection in such high-risk patients. The prudent surgeon routinely seeks the advice, and occasionally the consent, of knowledgeable medical consultants in such cases.

LOCAL FACTORS

Local wound factors are as important as general host factors and are amenable to control by the surgeon. The surgeon has direct influence over the temporary breach of host defense known as the wound in such matters as preparation of the surgical site, local contamination, duration of surgery, hemostasis, elimination of dead space, vascular supply and tissue necrosis, use of drains, use of antibiotics, and postoperative wound care.

Classically the operative site has been prepared by shaving the skin and then coating it with a solution of iodophor or chlorhexidine. This attempt to rid the skin surface of bacteria has been criticized because of the fear of increasing the risk of infection by injuring the upper layer of dermis during shaving. Nevertheless, most experienced surgeons fear bacteria found in human hair and prefer gentle shaving of the operative site. Modern surgical prep antiseptic solutions are superior to Lister's carbolic phenol aerosol, but the principle remains valid.

These principles of surgical site preparation should be applied somewhat equivocally to oral and maxillofacial surgery, however. Although the ritual of preparation of the skin of the face and neck should follow these well-established concepts, their application is less meaningful in the domain of intraoral surgery. The use of antiseptic solutions in the mouth generally is frivolous, but an exception is a dilute oral rinse of povidone-iodine (Betadine or chlorhexidine), which significantly lowers the bacterial colony count of the gingival sulcus.

Because of the great potential for deep infection after intraoral orthognathic or reconstructive procedures that involve exposure of large areas of muscle, bone, and fascial spaces, the surgeon should perform oral hygiene and deep gingival scaling, in addition to elimination of pockets and pericoronal flaps, before surgery. A noncompromising philosophy toward the preoperative elimination of all oral sepsis (existing and potential) in these cases is an exemplary demonstration of surgical discipline.

Local contamination of the wound is an obvious consideration in the problem of wound sepsis. The species and the numbers of contaminating bacteria may be important factors in the predictability of wound infection. The work of Krizek and Robson and others in obtaining biopsies and performing quantitative swab cultures of surgical and traumatic wounds has revealed that the number of bacteria required to produce an invasive tissue infection is 10^5 per gram of tissue or per milliliter of body fluid. This number remains a constant, although many variables may be present in the wound. The marked contrast between the common presence of bacteria in a wound and the relatively uncommon occurrence of gross infection suggest that successful establishment of sepsis depends on basic host factors that permit a critical number of bacteria to persist or multiply.

The presence of devitalized tissue within a surgical or traumatic wound is a factor that clearly predisposes a patient to infection. Dead or dying tissue obviously does not possess the resistance to infection as does healthy tissue and may represent nutrient culture media for bacterial growth within a wound. In a traumatic wound, meticulous mechanical and hydrodebridement are more important than the use of antibiotics for prevention of infection. However, the fibrin layer on any fresh wound surface prevents irrigation debridement from being totally effective.

In an otherwise clean surgical wound, the surgeon must prevent tissue damage from impaired vascular flow (either arterial or venous), intolerable pressure from retractors, or unnecessary damage from clamps, ligatures, or cautery. The student surgeon should be reminded to "Treat the tissue gently, and it will reward you by healing quickly."

If contamination of a traumatic or surgical wound is obvious, or even suspected, several actions may be required, including short-term use of drains placed through separate stab wounds, antibiotic therapy, and leaving the skin or mucosa open for delayed healing or closure. The success of delayed primary wound closure may be the result of the prolonged exposure of anaerobes to atmospheric oxygen. Prolonged use of drains or open wet dressings, however, extends the period of wound exposure to exogenous bacterial invasion. Even dry dressings may become contaminated; fungal growth in heavyweight stretch (Elastoplast) bandages has been reported.

The location and duration of wounds also influence the rate of infection. In general, lacerations of the face and mouth are prone to heal with low rates of infection because of their excellent vascular supply. If wounds of the face communicate with the mouth or oropharynx, however, infection is much more likely. Blunt trauma to the lips, causing the skin, muscle, and mucosa to be lacerated or crushed by the incisor teeth, represents such a common situation. Involving the flora of the skin and the oral cavity, these lip wounds become readily infected if poorly debrided or left untreated for more than 6 hours.

The duration of surgery as a factor in wound sepsis has been well studied (Table 25-2). Tissue drying, tissue trauma, and external contamination increase with the length of the surgical procedure. In clean, elective surgery, the infection rate increases from 5.9% in procedures lasting less than 1 hour to 9% at 3 hours and 15% at 5 to 6 hours. Many maxillofacial, orthognathic, and reconstructive procedures now require considerable operating time, exposing tissue for durations compatible with high infection rates. That such high rates have not been observed is a reflection of the inherent resistance of oral tissue and the profuse vascularity of the face. The common use of antibiotic prophylaxis for major intraoral surgery, rational flap design, and the prevention of tissue desiccation by con-

TABLE 25-2

Incidence of Infection Related to Duration of Operation (General Surgery)

Duration of Surgery (min)	Infection Rate (%)
0-29	3.5
30-59	5.9
60-119	6.4
120-179	9.0
180-239	10.0
240-299	10.9
300-359	15.4

stant intraoperative irrigation are other factors contributing to the low infection rate. A study of 140 intraoral orthognathic cases by Gallagher and Epker revealed an infection rate of only 2.8% after intraoral cleansing and penicillin prophylaxis. Three of the four infections were caused by gram-negative bacilli, including *Klebsiella* and *Enterobacter* spp.

The presence of foreign bodies in a wound enhances bacterial growth. Meticulous debridement is the key to preventing infection in traumatic wounds, in addition to the therapeutic (not prophylactic) use of antibiotics and drains in grossly contaminated wounds, such as those caused by gunshots. Once a wound has become infected, sutures, wire ligatures, metal mesh, and other implants may act as infected foreign bodies and often must be removed. Large metallic or alloplastic foreign bodies implanted into the bone or soft tissue of the face and temporomandibular joints may become an added burden on the host's defense mechanisms. The term *xenogenic infection* describes infection related to implanted foreign bodies, inasmuch as the implant tilts the delicate balance between host defense and bacterial virulence. Rejection of the infected foreign implant is the body's natural response, and most require removal. Antibiotic therapy alone rarely suffices to salvage a contaminated implant. The prolonged use of an antibiotic or polyantibiotic therapy to attempt to salvage an infected dental implant may carry more risk than benefit.

Other local factors influencing wound sepsis that are controllable by the surgeon are the presence of large blood clots and surgical dead space. Clotted blood or seromas accumulating within the wound enhance bacterial growth and are impenetrable by antibiotics. Deep fascial spaces opened by trauma or during surgical dissection also can acquire a considerable volume of fluid or blood. Therefore meticulous hemostasis, fastidious wound closure, and judicious use of drains rank equally in importance with debridement in prevention of wound infection (Box 25-2).

SUMMARY

Many factors influence the control of infection in the surgical or trauma patient. The incidence of surgical infection

BOX 25-2

Factors in Wound Infection

Local Factors
Number of bacteria
Virulence of bacteria
Devitalized tissue
Decreased blood supply
Foreign bodies (traumatic or implants)

Systemic Factors
Generalized sepsis
Decreased host defenses
    Diabetes
    Malnutrition
    Cytotoxic-immunosuppressive drugs
    Malignancies
Extremes of age

Environmental Factors
Operating room traffic
Defective air system
Inadequate sterilization techniques
The surgeon as a source of infection

Endogenous Factors
Patient's skin and hair
Presence of infected tissue at time of surgery (cellulitis, abscess, fistula)
Presence of resistant or opportunistic organisms in the patient's oral cavity, nasopharynx, or on skin

Surgical Factors
Insufficient hemostasis
Presence of dead space
Insufficient debridement
Tissue necrosis from sutures, retractors, or dressings
Inappropriate or long-term use of drains
Excessive operating time
Primary closure of infected wounds

TABLE 25-3

Nosocomial Fungal Infection

Disease or Condition	Most Common Fungi
Acute leukemia	*Candida, Aspergillus* spp. *Phycomycetes (Mucor)* spp.
Lymphoma	*Cryptococcus, Nocardia* spp.
Kidney transplant	*Candida, Aspergillus, Nocardia, Cryptococcus* spp.
Diabetes	*Phycomycetes (Mucor), Candida, Cryptococcus* spp.
Intensive antibiotic therapy	*Candida, Aspergillus* spp.
Steroid therapy	*Candida, Aspergillus, Nocardia* spp.
Fungal subacute Bacterial endocarditis during intravenous therapy	*Candida, Rhodotorula, Aspergillus* spp.
Drug addiction	*Candida* spp.
Major surgery	*Candida* spp.
Burns	*Phycomycetes (Mucor)* spp.
Tape (Elastoplast) or wet dressing	*Candida, Phycomycetes* spp.
Hyperalimentation	*Candida* spp.
AIDS/HIV	All of the above

has waxed and waned during the past 150 years as surgeons have discovered, neglected, and then relearned the fundamental concepts of asepsis and aseptic technique. Modern technology has provided an armamentarium ranging from antibiotics to laminar airflow, but these drugs and devices have only augmented the daily repetitive performance of the aseptic technique of surgery. Constant vigilance and personal discipline are the keystones of infection control in surgery.

NOSOCOMIAL FUNGAL INFECTION

Mycotic superinfection, especially fungal septicemia, has become a serious nosocomial problem during the past 40 years. Hospitals with the greatest incidence of fungemia have been those with large population of patients with neoplastic disease, particularly hematological malignancies. The use of steroids, antibiotics, and chemotherapeutic agents has contributed to the problem, as has the use of indwelling catheters and parenteral hyperalimentation. The rapid spread of HIV in the last decade has led to greater numbers of nosocomial fungal infections. Oropharyngeal-esophageal fungal infection is one of the stigmata of AIDS and a sequela and prognostic marker of the disease. The use of multiple antibiotics to control overwhelming bacterial infections in severely immunocompromised hosts further suppresses their normal flora, thus creating an ideal environment for the mycotic infections so frequently seen in hospitalized patients who are HIV positive. Penicillin, cephalosporins, and aminoglycosides are the antibiotics most commonly implicated in secondary fungal infections.

Disseminated candidiasis, aspergillosis, and *Nocardia* spp. infections are those most frequently encountered in severe nosocomial fungal infections, but many other organisms have been described as secondary invaders of the hospitalized immune-depleted host. Wound infections and mucocutaneous fungal growth also may occur, and the mortality rate may reach almost 30% as a result of fungemia. Table 25-3 lists the underlying disease or condition most frequently associated with specific fungi. Both *Candida* spp. prosthetic valve endocarditis and *Aspergillus* spp. (fungus ball) endocarditis have been reported.

The first indication of potential disseminated fungal infection, especially candidiasis, may be the clinical appearance of oral thrush. The high incidence of oral candidiasis associated with steroid therapy has been recognized for many years. Oropharyngeal candidiasis occurs in 50% of patients with asthma treated with steroid aerosol.

Frequent oral examination therefore is necessary in a patient with asthma or leukemia or who is undergoing chemotherapy, including removal of dentures and fungal cultures of the mouth. The initial appearance of oral candidiasis may be that of patchy or diffuse mucosal erythema rather than the classic white lesions.

In approximately half the cases of systemic candidemia the organism gains access to the blood through the gastrointestinal tract, but equally often it enters through intravenous or bladder catheters. Thus if oral or esophageal candidiasis develops in the compromised host, caution is needed to prevent contamination of intravenous sites and catheters.

Other early clinical signs of fungemia include a change in fever pattern, lethargy, and hypotension, signs indistinguishable from those of bacteremia. Erythematous macronodular skin lesions may result from fungemia, and inflammation with a cheesy exudate may be observed at infected intravenous sites. A white, raised, retinal exudate known as fungal endophthalmitis is pathognomonic of fungemia, but unfortunately, funduscopic examination usually is not performed until well after the onset of the disseminated fungal infection. The diagnosis of fungemia can be made with certainty only by blood culture. At least one bottle in each set of blood cultures should be vented to facilitate laboratory growth of yeast from the blood.

Unfortunately, the mechanisms of fungal superinfection are not fully understood. *Candida albicans* is phagocytosed readily by white blood cells in vitro, but only one third of the ingested fungi are killed by leukocytes from patients with lymphomas, suggesting that susceptibility to *Candida* spp. infection is related directly to the poor killing ability of polymorphonuclear leukocytes in some compromised host states. Defects in the delayed immune system are believed to result in mucocutaneous candidiasis related to qualitative or quantitative defects in circulatory or secretory IgA. The main target organ in systemic candidiasis is the kidney, because the yeast-phase *Candida* spp. can move from interstitial areas to the renal tubular lumen, where they grow unhindered by host cellular defense mechanisms.

Conservative treatment of nosocomial fungal infections may be indicated if the patient's clinical condition remains satisfactory. Thus discontinuation of antibiotics, steroids, and hyperalimentation and replacement of all intravenous catheters and indwelling bladder catheters is indicated early in the course of the disease. However, clinical studies indicate that early, aggressive use of amphotericin B, fluconazole, or flucytosine results in a higher survival rate than does withholding the drug until the fungemia has reached an overwhelming state.

Daily or weekly antifungal prophylaxis with fluconazole, itraconazole, or nystatin reduces the incidence of oropharyngeal candidiasis in patients with HIV. Most benefit occurs in patients with AIDS who have a low CD4 count (<200 mm^3) and a history of recurrent oropharyngeal candidiasis. Apparently no significant difference exists between continuous and intermittent antifungal prophylaxis and just intermittent antifungal therapy in terms of emergence of antifungal resistance.

INFECTION CONTROL IN OUTPATIENT OROMAXILLOFACIAL SURGERY FACILITIES

The discipline of infection control extends to the office and outpatient clinics. The rate of exposure to hepatitis among oral-facial surgical personnel is so high that it threatens healthy patients who may be exposed to infection from carriers or other infected patients, especially if aseptic precautions are not taken to control the spread of the virus. Inadequate sterilization of surgical and anesthetic instruments contributes to this problem.

Sterilization is the complete destruction or removal of all forms of microbial life. In the modern operatory the use of disposable equipment and supplies has drastically reduced the potential for cross-contamination between patients or between surgical personnel and patients. Maximum use of commercially sterilized disposable supplies decreases the incidence of bacterial and viral infection; the use of nondisposable needles and scalpel blades is no longer an acceptable practice. For example, disposable local anesthetic cartridges are now standard, but they must be placed in a sterilized, dry container and withdrawn only with sterile forceps. The common habit of entering the container with fingers or blood-stained gloves represents gross cross-contamination.

In the past an overdependence existed on so-called cold-sterilization disinfectant solutions in dental offices. The use of these solutions often bred a false sense of security because cold sterilization does not kill all forms of life, such as viruses. Additional problems with cold-sterilization solutions include their inactivation by soaps and oils, and the disconcerting fact that some sterilization solutions support the growth of certain bacterial species (e.g., *Pseudomonas* spp.).

Excellent viricidal disinfectants are available and used routinely for countertops and other potential fomites. The disinfectants, which contain akyldimethyl benzyl ammonium chloride or variations as their active ingredients, kill bacteria and viruses but may require up to 10 minutes on a surface, an important fact for personnel responsible for cleaning operating rooms and countertops (office or hospital) between patients. Tables 25-4 and 25-5 list the killing activity of commonly used solutions. Although inadequate for sterilization of surgical instruments, many of these disinfectants may control the spread of viral and bacterial infection in the operating room or office by their application to countertops, dental chairs, surgical light handles, and even floors and walls. For example, the hepatitis B virus (HBV) can survive on inanimate objects for prolonged periods, and the estimated 0.5 to 1 million infection carriers of HBV in the United States represent a serious potential threat to practicing dentists and, through cross-contamination, to other patients in outpatient dental facilities. Inani-

TABLE 25-4

Activity of Some Common Disinfectants

Disinfectant	Vegetative Bacteria	Spores	Fungi	Viruses
Alcohol (ethyl), 70%-90%	Good	None	Fair	Fair
Alcohol (isopropyl), 70%-90%	Very good	None	Good	Fair
Alcohol (isopropyl), 70% + iodine 0.5%-2%	Very good	Fair	Good	Good
Benzalkonium Cl (Zephiran), 1:750-1:1000	Very good	None	Good	None
Chlorine (hypochlorites) 1%-5%	Very good	Fair	Fair	Good
Cresols, 1%-5%	Good	Poor	Good	Poor
Ethylene oxide gas mixture	Very good	Good	Good	Good
Formaldehyde solution, USP 37%	Good	Good	Good	Good
Formaldehyde, 20% + alcohol, 50% (Bard-Parker solution)	Very good	Very good	Good	Good
Glutaraldehyde, 2% (Cidex)	Very good	Very good	Good	Good
Hexachlorophene, 3%-4%	Fair	None	Good	Not known
Iodine (aqueous), 2%-5%	Very good	Poor	Good	Good
Iodophors, 1%	Good	Poor	Poor	Good
Quaternary ammonium	Good	Good	Good	Good
chlorides (fifth-generation)	Good	Good	Good	Good
Phenols, 1%-3%	Good	Poor	Good	Fair

TABLE 25-5

Office Sterilization of Countertops and Light Handles

Organism	Cidal Contact Time
Staphylococcus aureus	10 minutes
Hepatitis B virus	10 minutes
HIV 1	30 seconds
Herpes-virus types 1 and 2	30 seconds
Pseudomonas aeruginosa	10 minutes

mate vectors (fomites) have been implicated in the spread of both viral and bacterial (staphylococcal) infection. Disinfectants include hypochlorite (bleach), sodium dichloroisocyanurate dihydrate, iodophores, glutaraldehydes, phenols, and quaternary ammonium chlorides (quats). Combining new, fifth-generation quats with alcohol results in lower required contact-kill time for microbes on office surfaces.

Reliable, time-tested methods of instrument sterilization that are viricidal and bactericidal should be used in outpatient office facilities, as they are in the hospital operating room. The standard technique remains the steam autoclave, either at 121° C (250° F) for 15 minutes, or the "flash" technique at 131° C (270° F) for 3 minutes. All surgical instruments must be adequately scrubbed clean of dried blood and tissue debris before autoclaving. Dry-heat ovens require 160° to 175° C (320° to 347° F) for 1 to 1.5 hours for sterilization. Inexpensive ethylene oxide sterilizers are available for office use, but most require overnight exposure of instruments.

BARRIER TECHNIQUES

The efficacy of hand washing in the prevention of bacterial infection has been discussed previously, but the effectiveness of washing for removal of viruses is not known. Gross blood contamination can be removed by adequate mechanical scrubbing and cleaning under the fingernails. The use of disposable surgical gloves in dental offices should be universal, now 20 years into the AIDS pandemic. The refusal to wear gloves and other forms of noncompliance still exist and are exposed whenever the Occupational Safety and Health Administration (OSHA) imposes an impressive monetary fine on a practitioner, which is then duly reported by the communication media.

Needle safety remains an ongoing and serious problem for both health workers and patients because of the potential for transmission of both viral and bacterial infection. "Safe needles" or "engineered sharps protection" has become an issue for OSHA and some state legislatures (California, New Jersey, Tennessee, Texas, West Virginia, Minnesota) in an attempt to prevent needle stick disease transmission, although percutaneous injury rates appear to be declining. Dental anesthetic needles have smaller bores than those used for other medical purposes and therefore seldom carry a significant inoculum of blood, but with HIV and hepatitis B and C, the term "significant" is difficult to define. Resheathing devices are available for dental and intravenous needles and should be considered part of universal precautions.

Other barrier techniques, such as protective face masks and glasses, should be used to prevent mucosal and conjunctival exposure during oral surgery procedures with high-speed instruments that may cause aerosol droplet contamination. Herpetic whitlow, a painful, chronic infection of the fingers that occurs most frequently in medical personnel, is caused by herpes simplex virus type 1, spread by direct contact, and preventable by the routine use of gloves, as is the spread of varicella-zoster virus from its rash and vesicles. The medical history is undependable in detecting the presence of hepatitis, herpes, or AIDS, and all patients should be approached with a high index of suspicion and with the best defense—gloves.

The increased use of disposable surgical supplies has created the problem of disposal of these materials. Careless disposal of sharp instruments such as needles and blades creates an occupational hazard for trash handlers and environmental problems. Spread of hepatitis B from the operating room or office to the community by careless disposal can be controlled with the use of closed containers and commercial incineration.

The problem of disease and death from HIV is discussed in Chapter 24. In the office-outpatient facility and in the hospital, the problems for the surgeon include the subtle, frightening, and costly issues of identification of high-risk patients, application of universal barrier techniques, sterilization, disposal of medical-surgical waste, employee education, record keeping, behavior modification, ethics, legal concerns, and somewhat rigid and uncompromising OSHA regulations. Adherence to these regulations is essential for the safety of the public and medical personnel and creation of confidence in the face of the fear of communicable diseases engendered by the AIDS epidemic. The OSHA handbook of regulations or a hospital infection control manual provides a level of compliance that, as much as possible, protects the office team from the patients and the patients from medical personnel (hepatitis and HIV may be transmitted in either direction). Although transmission of HIV to patients during office procedures has been limited to a few unfortunate, fatal, and well-publicized cases, numerous outbreaks of hepatitis B (including lethal hepatitis) have occurred. Common denominators in these cases were surgeons who were asymptomatic and unaware of their status as carriers and who did not wear gloves.

The OSHA core regulations include the following:

1. Patients with HIV cannot be refused necessary health care treatment.
2. Universal barrier techniques are mandatory, including gloves, mask, and protective eye wear.
3. Instruments must be cleaned mechanically and heat sterilized between patients.
4. Environmental disinfection (countertops, lights, and so on) must be performed between patients.
5. Physicians must offer hepatitis B vaccine to employees.
6. Training records in infection control must be kept for each employee.
7. Medical records of employees (including needle sticks) must be kept.
8. Infectious waste disposal (including disposable sharps) must follow specific OSHA guidelines.

All OSHA regulations are subject to change. They may seem overwhelming, impractical, and costly, but each has its own rationale and merit. For example, universal precautions are important because not all patients with hepatitis or HIV are readily or voluntarily identifiable. The stress and risk to health care workers and patients could be ameliorated, however, if known patients with HIV could be clearly identified on hospital charts, as are those with other communicable diseases such as hepatitis, syphilis, and tuberculosis, none of which have created the social or legislative reactions seen with AIDS. With time, reason and education may prevail over emotion, media hype, and fear. In the interim, common sense and the application of universal precautions are the best and only defenses.

Dental office waterline safety is currently an issue where dental hand pieces use municipal water for irrigation. The American Dental Association has established goals for the improvement of the microbiological quality of water used in therapy in dental offices. Irrigation tubes have been identified as sources of a biofilm in their lumens, which consists of colonies of microorganisms that adhere to the tube lining. Although not considered a threat to the general population, biofilm may represent a threat to immunocompromised patients. Two immunocompromised patients in the United Kingdom developed localized infections with *P. aeruginosa* in oral treatment sites. The strain of *Pseudomonas* spp. in these infections was identical in both patients and to that isolated from the waterlines. Prevention of waterline contamination includes the use of an independent water source. Chemical treatment of office water used in therapy includes sodium hypochlorite, hydrogen peroxide compounds, and povidone-iodine, all of which can be used in accordance with manufacturers' protocols.

SUGGESTED READINGS

1. Abubaker AO: Discussion: antibiotic prophylaxis in orthognathic surgery: a one-day versus a five-day regimen, *J Oral Maxillofac Surg* 57:230, 1999.
2. Adair FW, Geftic SG, Gelzer I: Resistance of *Pseudomonas* to quaternary ammonium compounds: growth in benzalkonium chloride solution, *Appl Microbiol* 18:225, 1969.
3. Aebert H, Hünefeld G, Regal G: Paranasal sinusitis and sepsis in ICU patients with nasotracheal intubation, *Intens Care Med* 15:27, 1988.
4. Allen AL, Organ RJ: Occult blood accumulation under the fingernails: a mechanism for the spread of blood-borne infection, *J Am Dent Assoc* 105:455, 1982.
5. Anneroth G, Anneroth, I, Lynch D: Acquired immune deficiency syndrome (AIDS) in the United States in 1986: etiology, epidemiology, clinical manifestations, and dental implications, *J Maxillofac Surg* 44:956, 1986.
6. Archer GL, Climo MW: *Staphylococcus aureus* bacteremia—consider the source, *N Engl J Med* 344:55, 2001.
7. Autio KL, Rosen R, Reynolds NI, et al: Studies of cross-contamination in the dental clinic, *J Am Dent Assoc* 100:358, 1980.

8. Avery CMF, Johnson DA: Surgical glove perforation and maxillofacial trauma: to plate or wire? *Br J Oral Maxillofac Surg* 30:31, 1992.

9. Balfom HH: Varicella zoster virus infections, *Barrier* 2:1, 1988.

10. Bauer TM, Ofner E, Just HM, et al: An epidemiological study assessing the relative importance of airborne and direct contact transmission of microorganisms in a medical intensive care unit, *J Hosp Infect* 15:301, 1990.

11. Beck WC: Xenogenic infection, *Guthrie Bull* 45:79, 1975.

12. Beck WC: Handwashing, Semmelweis, and chlorine, *Infect Control Hosp Epidemiol* 9:366, 1988.

13. Beck WC: Two-way asepsis, *Complications Surg* 10:4, 1991.

14. Beck WC, Frank F: The open door in the operating room, *Am J Surg* 125:592, 1973.

15. Bodey GP, Luma M: Skin lesions associated with disseminated candidiasis, *JAMA* 229:1466, 1974.

16. Broderick A, Mori M, Nettleman MD, et al: Nosocomial infections: validation of surveillance and computer modeling to identify patients at risk, *Am J Epidemiol* 131:734, 1990.

17. Budtz-Jurgensen E: Clinical aspects of candidiasis infection in denture wearers, *J Am Dent Assoc* 96:474, 1978.

18. Burke FJT, Bagget FJ, Lomax AM: Assessment of the risk of glove puncture during oral surgery procedures, *Oral Surg Oral Med Oral Pathol* 82:18, 1996.

19. Centers for Disease Control, US DREW: Surveillance Survey, National Nosocomial Infection Study, US, 1975-1976, *MMWR Morb Mortal Wkly Rep* 26(46):377, 1977.

20. Centers for Disease Control, US DREW: Recommended infection control practices for dentistry, *MMWR Morb Mortal Wkly Rep* 35:237, 1986.

21. Centers for Disease Control, US DREW: Guidelines for prevention of transmission of HIV and HBV for health care and public safety workers, *MMWR Morb Mortal Wkly Rep* 38(Suppl 6), 1989.

22. Crawford JJ: New light on the transmissibility of viral hepatitis in dental practice and its control, *J Am Dent Assoc* 91:829, 1975.

23. Cruse DI, Foord R: A five year prospective study of 23,649 surgical wounds, *Arch Surg* 107:206, 1973.

24. Dineen P, Drusin L: Epidemics of postoperative wound infections associated with hair carriers, *Lancet* 2:1157, 1973.

25. Doebbling BN, Stanley GL, Sheetz CT, et al: Comparative efficacy of alternative handwashing agents in reducing nosocomial infections in intensive care units, *N Engl J Med* 327:88, 1992.

26. Donskey CJ, Chowdhry TK, Hecker MT, et al: Effect of antibiotic therapy on the density of vancomycin resistant Enterococci in the stool of colonized patients, *N Engl J Med* 348:1925, 2001.

27. Edlich RF, Smith QT, Edgerton MT: Resistance of the surgical wound to antimicrobial prophylaxis and its mechanisms of development, *Am J Surg* 126:583, 1973.

28. Farr BM: Hospital wards spreading vancomycin-resistant enterococci to intensive care units: returning coals to Newcastle, *Crit Care Med* 26:1942, 1998.

29. Fishman LS, Griffin IR, Sapico FL, et al: Hematogenous *Candida* endophthalmitis—a complication of candidemia, *N Engl J Med* 286:675, 1972.

30. Fridkin SK, Welbel SF, Weinstein RA: Magnitude and prevention of nosocomial infections in the intensive care unit, *Infect Dis Clin North Am* 11:479, 1997.

31. Friedman RB: Protecting the surgeon against infection, *Oral Maxillofac Clin North Am* 3:445, 1991.

32. Gallagher DM, Epker BM: Infection following intra-oral surgical correction of dentofacial deformities, *J Oral Surg* 38:117, 1980.

33. Games ID, Remington IS: Disseminated candidiasis in the surgical patient, *Surgery* 72:730, 1972.

34. Gartenberg G, Bottone EI, Keusch GT, et al: Hospital-acquired *mucormycosis (Rhizopus rhizopodiformis)* of the skin and subcutaneous tissue, *N Engl J Med* 299:1115, 1979.

35. Goldberg MH: Antibiotics and oral-cutaneous lacerations, *J Oral Surg* 23:117, 1965.

36. Goldberg MH: Postoperative oral infection with *Pseudomonas aeruginosa*, *J Oral Surg* 24:334, 1966.

37. Goldberg MH: Gram-negative bacteremia following exodontias, *J Oral Surg* 26:180, 1968.

38. Goldberg MH: Antibiotics—old friends and new acquaintances. A clinician's view, *Oral Maxillofac Surg Clin North Am* 13:15, 2001.

39. Goldman DA, Weinstein RA, Wenzel RD, et al: Strategies to prevent and control the emergence and spread of antimicrobial-resistant microorganisms in hospitals: a challenge to hospital leadership, *JAMA* 275:234, 1996.

40. Gori F, Nesi G, Pedemonte E: *Aspergillus* fungus balls on the mitral valve, *N Engl J Med* 344:310, 2001.

41. Hart PD, Russell E, Jr, Remington JS: The compromised host and infection. I. Deep fungal infection, *J Infect Dis* 120:169, 1969.

42. Hogan B, Samaranayake LP: The surgical mask unmarked: a review, *Oral Surg* 70:34, 1990.

43. Holbrook WP, Rodgers GD: Candidal infections: experience in a British dental hospital, *Oral Surg* 49:122, 1980.

44. Holmes OW: On the contagiousness of puerperal fever, *N Engl Quart J Med Surg* 1843.

45. Horan T, Culver D, Jarvis W: Pathogens causing nosocomial infections: preliminary data from the Nosocomial Infections Surveillance System, *Antimicrob Newsl* 5:65, 1988.

46. Hospital Infection Control Practice Advisory Committee (HICPAC): Recommendations for preventing the spread of vancomycin resistance, *MMWR Morb Mortal Wkly Rep* 44:1(RR-12), 1995.

47. Howe CW: Experimental studies on determinants of wound infection, *Surgery* 60:72, 1966.

48. Hurst V: Reducing the risk of transmitting viral hepatitis via dental instruments, *J Dent Res* 51(special issue):150, 1972 (abstract no. 408).

49. Infection control in the dental office: a realistic approach, *J Am Dent Assoc* 122:459, 1986.

50. Klein II, Watanakunakorn C: Hospital-acquired fungemia: its natural course and clinical significance, *Am J Med* 67:51, 1979.

51. Klein RS, Harris CA, Small CB, et al: Oral candidiasis in high risk patients as the initial manifestations of the acquired immunodeficiency syndrome, *N Engl J Med* 311:354, 1984.

52. Klimek J, Marsik F, Bartlett RC, et al: Clinical, epidemiologic and bacteriologic observations of an outbreak of methicillin-resistant *Staphylococcus aureus* at a large community hospital, *Am J Med* 61:340, 1976.

53. Klimek J, Quintiliani R: Resistant staphylococci in hospitals, *Lancet* 2:255, 1977.

54. Knight L, Fletcher J: Growth of *Candida albicans* in saliva: stimulation by glucose associated with antibiotics, corticosteroids, and diabetes mellitus, *J Infect Dis* 123:371, 1971.

55. Koch R: 19th Century discoverers and discoveries. In Wagenstein OW, Wagenstein SD, editors: *The rise of surgery*, Minneapolis, 1978, University of Minnesota Press, 1978.

56. Krizek TI, Robson MC: Evolution of quantitative bacteriology in wound management, *Am J Surg* 130:579, 1971.

57. Larson E: A causal link between handwashing and risk of infection? Examination of the evidence, *Infect Control* 9:28, 1988.

58. Laufman H: Surgical personnel and operating room efficiency, *Resid Staff Phys* 19:1S, 1973.

59. Laufman H: Infection hazard of intensive care, *Surg Gynecol Obstet* 139:413, 1974 (editorial).

60. Laufman H: The control of operating room infection: discipline, defense mechanisms, drugs, design and devices, *Bull NY Acad Med* 54:465, 1978.

61. Laufman H: Operating room air, *J Surg Pract* 8:12, 1979.

62. Leonard DW, Bolger WE: Topical antibiotic therapy for recalcitrant sinusitis, *Laryngoscope* 109:668, 1999.

63. Levine NS, Lindberg RB, Mason AD, et al: The quantitative swab culture and smear: a quick, simple method for determining the number of viable aerobic bacteria on open wounds, *J Trauma* 16:89, 1976.

64. Levitz RE, Ehren Krantz NJ: Herpetic whitlow: a misunderstood syndrome, *Infect Surg* 3:832, 1984.

65. Levy SB: Antibiotic resistance: an ecological imbalance. In Chadwick DJ, editor: *Antibiotic resistance: origins, evolution, selection and spread,* Ciba Foundation Symposium 207, Chichester, England, John Wiley & Sons, 1997.

66. MacLean LD, Meakins IL: A physiological basis for development of opportunistic infections, *Ann Surg* 176:273, 1972.

67. Mills SE: The dental unit waterline controversy, *J Am Dent Assoc* 131:1427, 2000.

68. Morgan JP, Hang RH, Kosman JW: Antimicrobial skin preparations for the maxillofacial region, *J Oral Maxillofac Surg* 54:89, 1996.

69. Moskow BS, Crikelair GF, Wheaton EA: Severe oral infection associated with prolonged steroid therapy, *Oral Surg* 34:590, 1972.

70. Nake DG, Goldman DA, Rhane FS: Infection control in intravenous therapy, *Ann Intern Med* 79:867, 1973.

71. OSAP: Update on Needle-Safety Legislation. Practice Management Notes, *Am Assoc Oral Maxillofacial Surg* May-June: 11, 2001.

72. OSHA Instruction CPD2-2.44B: Enforcement for occupational exposure to hepatitis B virus (HBV) and human immunodeficiency virus (HIV), Washington, DC, Feb 27, 1990, Occupational Safety and Health Administration.

73. Otis LL, Cottone IA: Prevalence of perforations in disposable latex gloves, *J Am Dent Assoc* 118:321, 1989.

74. Paries SE, Gamelle RL, Mead PB: The epidemiologic features of nosocomial-infections in patients with trauma, *Arch Surg* 126:97, 1991.

75. Parkhurst C: Oropharyngeal candidiasis. In *Clinical Evidence* No. 4 BMJ Pub, London, 762, Dec, 2000.

76. Pigadas N, Avery CME: Precautions against cross-infection during operations for maxillofacial trauma, *Br J Oral Maxillofac Surg* 38:110, 2000.

77. Polk HC: Operating room-based iatrogenic infections—types, sources and treatment. Presented at the Third Symposium on Control of Surgical Infections. American College of Surgeons, Washington, DC, January 10, 1972.

78. Proceedings, National Conference on Infection Control in Dentistry, US Department of Health and Human Services, Centers for Disease Control, Atlanta, October, 1986.

79. Quintilliani R: Combination therapy in post-traumatic infections, *Bull N Y Acad Med* 55:257, 1979.

80. Samaranayake LP, Scully C: Oral candidosis in HIV infection, *Lancet* 2:1491, 1989.

81. Sanders CV Jr, Luby JP, Johanson WG Jr, et al: *Serratia marcescens* infections from inhalation therapy medications: nosocomial outbreak, *Ann Intern Med* 73:15, 1970.

82. Scully C, Laskaris G, Pindborg J, et al: Oral manifestations of HIV infection and their management. I. More common lesions, *Oral Surg* 71:158, 1991.

83. Semmelweis IP: The etiology, the concept, and the prophylaxis of childbed fever, *Pest* 1861. Translated by Frank P. Murphy in *Medicine Classics* 5:350, 1941.

84. Shaw FE, Barrett CL, Hamm R, et al: Lethal outbreak of hepatitis B in dental practice, *JAMA* 255:3260, 1986.

85. Sholes DM, Gerding DN, John JF Jr, et al: Society for Healthcare Epidemiology of America and Infectious Diseases, Society of America Joint Committee on the Prevention of Antimicrobial Resistance: guidelines for the prevention of antimicrobial resistance in hospitals, *Infect Control Hosp Epidemiol* 18:275, 1997.

86. Slaughter FG: *Immortal Magyar: Semmelweis, conqueror of childhood fever*, New York, Schuman, 1950.

87. Smith FT: The germ fix, *Dent Economics* Nov:11, 1999.

88. Solomkin JS: Therapy of *Candida* infections in surgical patients, *J Surg Pract* 8:18, 1979.

89. Sproat LI, Inglis TI: A multi-center survey of hand hygiene practice in intensive care units, *J Hosp Infect* 26:137, 1994.

90. Stamm WE: Guidelines for prevention of catheter-associated urinary tract infections, *Ann Intern Med* 83:386, 1975.

91. Steere AC, Mallison GF: Handwashing practices for the prevention of nosocomial infections, *Ann Intern Med* 83:683, 1975.

92. Summers AN, Larson DL, Edmiston CE, et al: Efficacy of preoperative decontamination of the oral cavity, *J Plast Reconst Surg* 106:895, 2000.

93. Thomas LE III, Sydiskis RJ, DeVore DT, et al: Survival of herpes simplex virus and other selected microorganisms on patients' charts: potential source of infections, *J Am Dent Assoc* 111:461, 1985.

94. Thorwald J: *The century of the surgeon*, New York, 1957, Pantheon Books.

95. Tuna IC, Harrison MR: Fungal prosthetic valve endocarditis, *N Engl J Med* 344:275, 2001.

96. Von Eiff C, Becker K, Machka K, et al: Nasal carriage as a source of *Staphylococcus* bacteremia, *N Engl J Med* 344:11, 2001

97. Wangensteen OH, Wangensteen SD, Klinger CF: Some pre-Listerian and post-Listerian antiseptic wound practices and emergence of asepsis, *Surg Gynecol Obstet* 137:677, 1973.

98. Ward R, Borchert P, Wright A, et al: Hepatitis B antigen in saliva and mouth washings, *Lancet* 2:726, 1972.

99. Webb BC, Thomas CT, Wilcox MD, et al: Candida-associated denture stomatitis. Aetiology and management: a review. Part 3 Treatment of oral candidosis, *Aust Dent J* 43:244, 1988.

100. Weiss SH, Saxinger WC, Rechtman D, et al: HTLV-III infection among health care workers: association with needlestick injuries, *JAMA* 254:2089, 1985.

101. Wenzel RP: The economics of nosocomial infection, *J Hosp Infect* 31:79, 1995.

102. Wenzel RP, Edmond MB: Managing antibiotic resistance, *N Engl J Med* 343:1961, 2000.

103. White E, Mosley JW, Edwards VM, et al: Type B hepatitis: the occupational risk for dentists, *J Dent Res* 54(special issue):178, 1975 (abstract No. 531).

104. Whitney CG, Farley MM, Hadler J, et al: Increasing prevalence of multi drug resistant *Streptococcus pneumoniae* in the United States, *N Engl J Med* 343:1917, 2000.

105. Woeltje KF, Fraser V: Preventing nosocomial infections in the intensive care unit: lessons learned from outcomes research, *New Horizons* 6:84, 1998.

106. Yu VL, Goetz A, Wagener M, et al: Staphylococcus aureus nasal carriage and infection in patients on hemodialysis: efficacy of antibiotic prophylaxis, *N Engl J Med* 315:91, 1986.

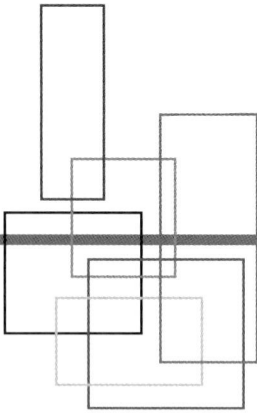

Medicolegal Aspects of Infection

James R. Hupp
Morton H. Goldberg

Patients with infections in or related to the oral and maxillofacial regions rarely bring legal actions against care providers. However, when legal problems occur, certain circumstances are common. These include endocarditis after dental care resulting from organisms found in the oropharyngeal region, alleged failure to diagnose an infection in a timely manner, alleged failure to adequately treat an infection, and postoperative infection resulting from alleged inappropriate care. This chapter reviews the essential elements of medical malpractice laws, with subsequent discussion regarding methods to avoid satisfying those tort elements. A brief presentation of the informed consent process, particularly as it applies to infection, is included. Finally, a review of some of the situations that may lead to legal problems when an infection occurs is provided.

TORT LAW

Liability (or tort) law represents a theory of legal thought that attempts to compensate an injured party for the non-criminal wrongdoing of another. The legal system is designed to identify potential wrongdoers and then determine whether the wrong they did caused the injured party's damages. In other words, the legal system represents a formal method to prove someone civilly liable for another person's injury. If liability is determined, the liable party is required to pay damages to the injured party.

The search for the identity of a potentially liable person involves determining the persons, institution, or both that owed an injured party a duty to provide care falling within the standards of acceptable medical care. In the case of medical malpractice the parties that owe a duty typically include the patient's treating physician and any corporation in which they delivered care. Identifying the individual, corporation, or other parties that owed the patient a duty is typically clear, although a few cases can hinge on this element.

Once the identity of the doctor owing the patient a duty is established, the injured party must show, by a preponderance (more than 50%) of the evidence that the duty was breached. Namely, that the doctor, institution, or both parties provided care (or lack of care) beneath the standards of acceptable medical/dental practice. This is usually accomplished during the discovery process, in which the attorneys and their experts subpoena medical records for review. Discovery also includes depositions in which the attorneys question the parties and various fact and expert witnesses. Most cases rely on the willingness of a doctor serving as an expert witness to conclude that the plaintiff's injuries were caused by treatment falling beneath the standard of care.

The tort law requirement that any breach of duty be shown to have caused the patient's injury is usually not at issue. However, in some cases in which a patient is seen by a series of providers, it can be a useful defense.

If a party's liability for causing an injury is determined to be present, damages are assessed in proportion to the degree of liability in cases with multiple defendants, and/or patients must bear part of the responsibility for damages if they are shown to be in part responsible for their injury.

Rare cases are heard by only a judge; most cases are decided by a jury. The majority of jury members are lay people with little, if any, advanced medical knowledge. The critical importance of recognizing the composition of most juries is discussed during the presentation of information about the informed consent process, patient instructions and compliance, and record keeping.

DOCTOR-PATIENT INTERACTIONS

In general, patients are poorly compliant with medications and other aspects of their own care. Use of antibiotics is in particular one of the worst areas for patient compliance. Poor compliance includes failure to fill a prescription, missing doses during the period of administration, or premature discontinuation of the antibiotic.

Patient instructions given verbally and in writing should emphasize the critical importance of following the doctor's recommendations, including antibiotic usage. A realistic description of the consequences of failure to follow the prescription's exact language is useful. In addition, patients can be reminded that if for some reason they cannot tolerate a particular drug, they should alert their health care provider so that an alternative medication may be substituted.

Rarely are patients who are facing a medical procedure ever as informed as their care provider about the available options and the attendant risks. In many counties and cultures, this imbalance of knowledge is accepted and patients are expected to simply trust that the doctor will make all decisions in the patient's best interest. However, in "Western" cultures, particularly in the United States, the legal system and much of society is no longer willing to completely accept the imbalance of knowledge. Instead, care providers planning procedures known to carry significant risks are expected to provide patients or their guardians enough information to make patients capable of reaching "informed" decisions about their care. This desire by patients to participate in making decisions affecting their physical and mental well-being reflects a now long-standing trend of patients' personal responsibility for their own futures. This trend is unlikely to reverse itself.

Thus surgeons in particular, but all health care providers in general, are expected to provide patients information and obtain their consent before proceeding with care. The practice of giving patients information before gaining their permission to receive care is called the "informed consent process." Informed consent does not rest exclusively on the often legalistic document that patients are expected to sign before certain procedures. Informed consent instead should consist of a series of interactions. These interactions are intended to give patients sufficient information about their condition, possible treatment options, and the risks and benefits of those options to allow patients to decide how to proceed.

The informed consent process has four key characteristics. It provides information (1) about the treatment options and risks, (2) given in adequate detail, (3) using a means and style of communication likely to be effective, (4) with a reasonable opportunity for the decision-maker to ask for any needed clarification. Included in a well-designed informed consent process is information about the reasonably predictable outcome should no procedure be done.

Not all conceivable options need to be presented. In many cases this more likely will confuse a patient rather than assist in reaching an informed decision. Only options reasonably likely to be successful and options reasonably likely that most patients would wish to know before making a decision should be included in the informed consent process. The amount of detail needed during the informed consent process varies directly proportionally to the severity and likelihood of occurrence of problems because of a certain treatment option. Typically the more complex the planned procedure, the more time is needed to present the information. Similarly, the more complex or risky the procedure will be, the greater time needed for the patient to consider the information provided in the informed consent process.

Almost all surgical procedures carry the risk of infection; therefore patients should be advised of this possibility. In addition, any attempt to cure an infection carries the risk that the infection may not be cured or can worsen despite proper care. This information is important to relay to patients.

The means of communication may vary. Because some people are more visually oriented, brochures, videos, and written forms are more effective. Others who gain information more effectively through listening benefit from conversations with the doctor and staff. Nonetheless, although videos, brochures, and verbal communications are useful means of communication, the written consent form document listing the planned procedure, provider or providers giving the care, risks of the procedure, and options to the procedure remains the most effective legal means of showing consent was received after information was provided.

The style of communication also is important and pertains to issues such as the amount of time available to patients to digest the information provided and the ease provided for them to seek any needed clarifications. Thus the process should not be rushed, particularly for complex cases. The doctor must take time to explain the information and then listen and answer any questions presented by the patient.

Most patients lack the educational background or experience to fully understand the various clinical options provided by a doctor during the informed consent process. Therefore the health professional bears a responsibility to provide guidance when helping a patient decide among viable treatment options or whether to undergo a procedure at all. For example, a patient with a chronically infected tooth and associated osteomyelitis may be given an option of a limited resection of bone or more aggressive approach in which a large portion of infected mandible is removed. Without some guidance, a patient may opt for the more limited procedure with the mistaken impression that the surgeon can always go back and remove more bone later. However, the surgeon may realize that a less invasive approach is unlikely to be successful and that a second surgical attempt to attempt to cure the infection will be much more difficult for the patient than performing the more definitive resection initially. Such cases are instances when doctors should adopt the philosophy of treating all patients as if they were members of their immediate family, rather than acting like salespersons, and treating clinical options as variations of styles or colors. Ultimately, doctors who adopt the philosophy that they are uncomfortable and unwilling to provide care to patients who are poorly informed or who do not truly understand what they are signing when given a consent form are unlikely to be sued successfully for failure to obtain their informed permission.

RECORDS AND COMMUNICATION

The American legal system involves many proceedings that regularly delay the speedy resolution of disputes. In addition, because patients have 2 or sometimes more years to lodge a complaint, many years may elapse before the legal discovery process is under way. During this delay, memories of details erode, particularly for the busy practitioner who often treats hundreds of patients each month.

The legal system and juries recognize that memories fade and therefore tend to disbelieve the ability of anyone to remember small details of events years or even months later. Thus if several years after an event a doctor claims to remember telling a patient about a particular risk or something specific during a certain patient encounter, the doctor's statement is unlikely to be accepted as true. Good record keeping therefore becomes legally, rather than just clinically, important. Judges, lawyers, and juries are much more likely to believe a recollection corroborated by a written notation than only a mental memory.

This raises the issue of how many details are necessary in documentation. For procedures done in hospital operating suites, the dictated operative notes typically are detailed and become important documents when surgical techniques are questioned. However, rarely do office procedures receive the same attention when written records are made. Ideally, each procedure or patient encounter, including telephone consultations, should prompt a reasonably detailed notation. However, when something unusual is done during a procedure or encounter, or when an unexpected outcome occurs, detailed record keeping becomes even more critical. Legally defensible health care benefits by keeping contemporaneous records of all events that transpire, including, when appropriate, a description in the records of why certain decisions were made, consultations obtained, and documentation of continued efforts to mitigate any patient problems.

The need to maintain close communication with patients until resolution of the health problem for which they sought care is obvious. However, this concept often is forgotten. Patients with health concerns are already in a vulnerable position and usually rely on their care provider for emotional support. When an unwanted outcome occurs, the patient's emotional support needs increase, requiring even more doctor empathy and clinical assistance than usual. When patients believe are they not receiving the appropriate attention of their care provider, they commonly feel betrayed, concluding that the confidence they put in another's hands to affect their body was poorly placed. At this point, many patients seek a legal remedy. Conversely, when a health professional sincerely works hard to help patients overcome any difficulties after a procedure, lawsuits are rare.

Several chapters in this book discuss means for effectively limiting the chance of infection, expeditiously recognizing infection, and properly managing infections. These are useful guidelines to clinical care, although they do not necessarily establish the standard of care for legal disputes. Legal problems occur in patients with infections in three alleged situations: failure to prevent infection, failure to properly diagnose an infection, or failure to appropriately manage an infection.

Failure to prevent an infection when preventative measures might have been helpful can occur in several circumstances. Surgery in the facial region almost always requires disruption of skin or mucosa, interrupting this primary barrier to microbes. In many situations, prophylactic antibiotics lower the incidence of postoperative infection, especially when the appropriate agent is given in adequate amounts in proper proximity to the contamination. However, some widely used protocols for purported prevention of infections are not well supported by scientific evidence, such as antibiotics before dental surgery to prevent infective endocarditis or antibiotics before removal of impacted teeth. Therefore simple failure to give antibiotics before surgery is not automatically a negligent act even if an infection eventually occurs. Other means of preventing infections include the use of aseptic techniques, removal of loose implants, and changing vascular access sites on a regular basis.

Failure to diagnose an infection can become a legal issue if the delay in reaching the proper diagnosis is believed to have prolonged the patient's illness or led to more serious problems than would have otherwise occurred. Deep abscesses, rapidly progressing infections, and smoldering osteomyelitis can be difficult situations to recognize. A heightened index of suspicion is usually the best defense when signs point to these circumstances.

Lawsuits charging a failure to properly manage an infection often include an alleged failure to recognize the presence or severity of an infectious process. Following guidelines in various chapters of this book helps limit this possibility. Philosophies such as "never let the sun set on pus" and recognition of the rapidity with which the oropharyngeal airway can be compromised by a regional infection are important for all clinicians. Another important factor in the minimization of problems managing infections is the value of consultation with other health professionals. Infectious disease specialists commonly have the latest information on antibiotic spectrums and the means to detect the extent of an infection. Practitioners who are uncomfortable managing infections beyond their area of anatomical expertise often benefit from consulting with or transferring patients to surgeons specializing in care for other areas of the head, neck, or thorax.

ANTIBIOTICS

The miracle of antibiotics is a double-edged sword wielded by both the surgeon and the plaintiff's attorney. The principles of antibiotic therapy, if followed, should prevent most harmful sequelae of facial infections if coupled with timely and appropriate surgery (incision and drainage, sequestrectomy, and so on) (see Chapter 5). Failure to use antibiotics or poor selection of an antibiotic is a common basis for lawsuits against surgeons.

As noted in other chapters, culture and sensitivity studies are not necessary for ordinary odontogenic infections in the otherwise healthy host. Empirical knowledge of the most frequent flora and their probable antibiotic susceptibility suffice scientifically, ethically, and legally in 80% to 90% of cases. Recalcitrant, recurrent infections and those in compromised hosts should be cultured, both to select an appropriate drug and to deflect later allegations of mismanagement. Defensive medical practice is a well-recognized strategy in this litigious society, but antibiotics should never be prescribed or administered solely for that purpose.

Noncompliance is a major factor in nonresponse to antibiotics. The patient must be questioned carefully about the frequency, timing, and duration of dosing, or indeed if the prescription was filled. Careful recording of patient noncompliance is an excellent example of practicing defensively.

THE COMPROMISED HOST

Poorly controlled diabetes frequently is associated with infection, including acute and chronic periodontitis and pericoronitis. Although antibiotics may not be necessary in mild to moderate infections in an otherwise healthy patient, failure to prescribe antibiotics in the treatment of infection in a patient with diabetes (be it a gangrenous foot or an infected tooth) may lead to rapid and diffuse spread of sepsis.

Even in a patient with well-controlled diabetes, infection should be treated aggressively, inasmuch as infection can alter the patient's metabolic state and insulin requirements, leading to a vicious downhill cycle of infection: infection—acidosis—worsening infection—hospitalization—continued deterioration of the patient's condition as a result of the worsening infection and diabetic state—litigation. Recalcitrant infections should alert the practitioner to the possibility of host compromise, justifying a medical diagnostic evaluation. Any compromised host may harbor uncommon or arcane microorganisms, especially if the patient has been hospitalized recently (see Chapter 24).

DEEP SPACE INFECTIONS

The spread of odontogenic infection into deep fascial spaces frequently leads to hospitalization, anesthesia, surgery, visible scarring, and loss of time from gainful employment. Failure to diagnose infection, including use of contemporary imaging, or failure to treat surgically in a timely manner may initiate litigation. Certainly in third molar surgery, the risk of infection should be included in the preoperative consent process.

Litigation in instances of Ludwig's angina is a special situation. Because of the decline of this disease in the era of antibiotics and improved dental care, its rapid course may catch the inexperienced surgeon unaware. Early consultation with an anesthesiologist is essential, and either fiberoptic intubation or tracheotomy may be necessary. The surgeon should obtain the assistance of another surgeon if he or she is not confident with this procedure. Timidity or delay may lead to airway obstruction and "evidence of poor clinical judgment" when presented to a jury.

OSTEOMYELITIS

Osteomyelitis is a common precipitating infection in malpractice litigation in surgery. Chronic pain, hospitalization, expensive and inconvenient therapies (intravenous antibiotics and hyperbaric oxygen), and reconstructive surgery are sequelae of infection that may lead the patient to consult an attorney. The best defense (and treatment) remains an early and high index of suspicion. Osteomyelitis is often insidious and easily masked by concomitant infection of overlying soft tissue or deep fascial spaces. Contemporary imaging and nuclear scanning are as well known to attorneys and their expert witnesses as they are to surgeons. Culturing is important, and lack of obtaining a culture presents a challenge during courtroom examination or cross-examination.

Treatment of osteomyelitis should be early and aggressive. Infectious disease consultation may be useful. However, experience suggests that internists' concepts of osteomyelitis often are based on osteomyelitis of long bones, vertebra, skull, and the pelvis, in which the clinical course and flora are only marginally similar to those of the mandible. The testimony of such experts for the plaintiff can be devastating to the defense yet impressive to the jury; however, on cross-examination, most admit to only minimal experience with osteomyelitis of the jaw.

The diagnosis of osteomyelitis must be conclusive. In one case, a 0.2-mm × 0.3-mm fragment of bone from an extraction site sent to a pathologist with a preliminary diagnosis of "rule out osteomyelitis" was returned with a diagnosis of "compatible with osteomyelitis." An unfortunate series of events then ensued with hospitalization, months of intravenous antibiotic therapy, and multiple surgeries terminating in a hemimaxillectomy. The defendant's oral and maxillofacial expert contended that true osteomyelitis had never existed, despite positive bone scan results (even dentoalveolar and periodontal infection will "light up" a scan). A determined plaintiff's attorney, a disfigured patient, and an insurance carrier fearful of a multimillion-dollar jury award resulted in a substantial pretrial settlement.

SUMMARY

Infection-related problems are not a common source of litigation. Following the guidelines for prevention and management of infections presented in this text should help minimize legal liability problems. In addition, communication and a close working relationship with patients who have infections, good record keeping, and treatment of all patients with respect and empathy lessen the chances of lawsuits or their possibility of success.

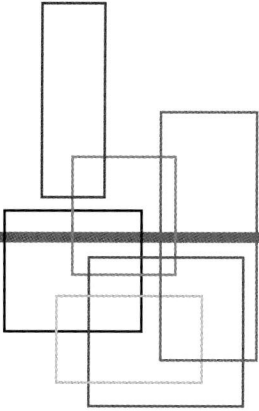

INDEX

A

Abducens nerve in cavernous sinus thrombosis, 212
Abelcet. *See* Amphotericin B
Abiotrophia, Gram stain identification of, 49b
Abrasions
  antibiotic therapy for, 367t
  maxillofacial, 371
Abscess
  brain. *See* Brain abscess
  of buccal root, 167f
  of buccal space, as complication of Crohn's disease,
      170-171
  versus cellulitis, 162
  cellulitis and, 100
  characteristics of, 297
  combination therapy for, 107
  as complication of orbital cellulitis, 336
  of deep temporal space, 203f
  dentoalveolar, 193, 196f
  epidural, management of, 357
  intracranial, pediatric, 413
  localization of, 166t
  of masticator space, 87, 87f
  of maxillary incisor, 167f
  in maxillofacial surgery, 110
  orbital, in ethmoid sinusitis, 315f
  palatal, 209f
  parapharyngeal, 88, 88f
  parotid, 285-286, 286f
  periapical, 85f
  periodontal. *See* Periodontal abscess
  periorbital, in sinusitis, 317
  peritonsillar, 324, 324f
  of pharyngeal space, 206f
  phoenix, 150
  of premolar root, 167f
  of pterygomandibular space, 203f, 205f
  retropharyngeal, 89, 89f
  septal, 313

Abscess—cont'd
  of submasseteric space, 202f
  subperiosteal, in orbital cellulitis, 335, 335f
Absidia
  in mucormycosis, 426
  in rhinoorbital-cerebral mucormycosis, 336
  sinusitis due to, 76
Accessory innervation, 444-445
Accutane. *See* Isotretinoin therapy
Acidaminococcus, Gram stain identification of, 49b
Acid-fast stains, 48-50
Acinetobacter
  Gram stain identification of, 49b
  life-threatening infection from, 159f
Acinetobacter baumanii, percent susceptibility of, 55t
Acne vulgaris, characteristics of, 301, 302f
Acquired immunodeficiency disorder. *See* AIDS
Actinobacillus
  Gram stain identification of, 49b
  infections due to, 35
Actinobacillus actinomycetemcomitans, 34t
  adherence by, 39
  attachment patterns of, 32
  in HACEK group, 47
  in HIV-associated periodontal disease, 145
  in pericoronitis, 143
  in periodontitis, 132, 133-134
Actinomadura, Gram stain identification of, 49b
Actinomyces
  in actinomycosis of salivary glands, 290
  characteristics and disorders associated with, 35
  disease due to, 35
  first-choice and alternative antibiotics for, 113t
  Gram stain identification of, 49b
  in immunocompromised host, 356
  in infants, 30
  in osteomyelitis, 216-217, 217
  in soft tissue infections, 188
  in tonsillitis, 323
Actinomyces baudetii in cervicofacial actinomycosis,
      232
Actinomyces bovis in cervicofacial actinomycosis,
      232

Page numbers followed by *f* indicate illustrations; *t* indicates
tables; *b* indicates boxes.

Actinomyces israelii
  in cervicofacial actinomycosis, 232, 305-306
  characteristics and disorders associated with, 35
  disease due to, 35
Actinomyces meyeri in cervicofacial actinomycosis, 36t, 232
Actinomyces naeslundii, 36t
  in cervicofacial actinomycosis, 232
  disease due to, 35
  in plaque, 132
Actinomyces odontolyticus, 36t
  in cervicofacial actinomycosis, 232
  disease due to, 35
Actinomyces viscosus, 36t
  disease due to, 35
  in plaque, 132
Actinomycosis
  cervicofacial, 231-234, 232f, 233f, 234f, 305-306
  cultures in, 103
  of pulpal tissue, 148
  of salivary glands, 290
Acute bacterial parotitis, 279, 283-287
  clinical signs of, 285-286, 285f
  diagnosis of, 285-286
  nosocomial *versus* community-acquired, 284-285
  predisposing factors in, 284-285
  treatment of, 286-287, 287f
Acute bacterial submandibular sialadenitis, 279, 287-289, 288f
Acute necrotizing ulcerative gingivitis, noma due to, 431
Acute necrotizing ulcerative gingivitis-periodontitis, 140-142
  clinical features and diagnosis of, 140-141
  etiology of, 141
  in HIV/AIDS patients, 144-145
  treatment of, 141-142
Acyclovir
  for herpes simplex infection, 123
  for HSV infections, 396
Adenitis, pediatric, 421t
Adenovirus
  immunofluorescent assay of, 50
  pediatric, 420
Adhesion molecules, inflammatory role of, 21
Adnexal structures, staphylococcal infections of, 298-302, 299f, 300f, 301f, 302f
Adult respiratory distress syndrome, sepsis and, 309-310
Advanced Trauma Life Support, 363
Adverse reactions, development of, 108-109
Aerobes, susceptibility testing of, 57-58, 57f, 58f
Aerococcus, Gram stain identification of, 49b
Aeromonas, Gram stain identification of, 49b
Afipia felis in cat-scratch disease, 290, 308, 432
Agglutination, latex, 50-51
Aggressin, 22
Aging, immune deficiency due to, 460
AIDS
  aspergillosis in, 251-253
  candidiasis in, 250
  cryptococcosis in, 256, 257
  fungal infections associated with, 477t
  immune deficiency due to, 461-462
  infection and, 356
  management of patients with, 357
  oral/maxillofacial manifestations of, 462

AIDS—cont'd
  pediatric, 420-421
  Pneumocystis carinii pneumonia in, 252
  Pneumocystis infection in, 255
  postoperative wound infections and, 401
Air, contamination of, 475
Air-fluid levels, Waters' view of, 71, 71f
Airway compromise
  assessing, 441-442
  in maxillofacial infections, 439-440, 439f
  treatment of, 440
Airway management, 442-451
  for children, 443
  with corticosteroids, 443
  with cricothyrotomy/tracheotomy, 450-451, 450t
  extubation in, 451-452, 452f
  general anesthesia in, 448-450
    with laryngeal mask airway, 450
    mask induction of, 449-450
    preoxygenation for, 448
    Sellick maneuver and, 449
    trismus and, 448-449
  intubation techniques in, 446-448
    fiberoptic, 448
    lighted stylet, 448, 448f
    nasotracheal, 447, 447f
      versus orotracheal, 446-447
  with jet ventilation, 451
  local anesthesia in, 444-445, 444f
  patient communication in, 445
  physical examination in, 440-441
  sedation and analgesia techniques in, 445-446
  surgical, 450-451, 450t
  of total/near-total obstruction, 442-443
  triage in, 442-443
Akyldimethyl benzyl ammonium chloride, antiseptic activity of, 478
Alcaligenes, Gram stain identification of, 49b
Alcaligenes xylosoxidans, percent susceptibility of, 55t
Alcohol, disinfectant activity of, 479t
Alcohol abuse
  immune deficiency due to, 459
  postoperative wound infections and, 401
Allergic fungal sinusitis, 341
Allergic reactions
  antibiotic selection and, 104
  versus immunity, 26
  to penicillin, 100-101
Allergic sialadenitis, acute, 290
Alloiococcus, Gram stain identification of, 49b
Alloplastic implants
  infections and, 397
  selection criteria for, 395
Alternaria in allergic fungal sinusitis, 341
Alternative pathway, initiation of, 8f, 9
AmBisome. *See* Amphotericin B
Amikacin
  microbes susceptible to, 56t
  pediatric dosages for, 415t
Aminoglycosides
  for maxillofacial infections, 121
  pediatric dosages for, 415t
Ammonium, quaternary, disinfectant activity of, 479t

Amoebic meningoencephalitis, pediatric, 421
Amoxicillin
    absorption of, 116
    antimicrobial spectrum of, 117t
    for implant surgery, 382b
    indications for, 113t
    microbial susceptibility to, 56t
    pediatric dosages for, 415t
    pharmacology of, 117t
Amoxicillin-clavulanate
    antimicrobial spectrum of, 117t
    blood-brain barrier and, 357
    pediatric dosages for, 415t
    pharmacology of, 117t
Amoxicillin-clavulanic acid
    antimicrobial spectrum of, 115b
    for odontogenic infections, 164
Amphotec. *See* Amphotericin B
Amphotericin B
    antimicrobial spectrum of, 121-122
    dosage of, 122
    nephrotoxicity of, 357
    side effects of, 122
Ampicillin
    absorption of, 116
    with amoxicillin, antimicrobial spectrum of, 115b
    antimicrobial spectrum of, 117t
    as first-choice antibiotic, 113t
    microbial susceptibility to, 55t, 56t
    pediatric dosages for, 415t
    pharmacology of, 114t, 117t
Ampicillin-amoxicillin, antibiotic-associated colitis due to, 109
Ampicillin-sulbactam
    antimicrobial spectrum of, 117t
    bacterial susceptibility to, 55t
    pediatric dosages for, 415t
    pharmacology of, 117t
Anachoresis, pulpal infection and, 147
Anaerobes, 36t
    Gram stains of, 48
    in odontogenic infections, 164
    in osteomyelitis, 216-217
    in pulpal tissue, 148
    susceptibility testing of, 58-59, 58f
Anaerobiospirillium, Gram stain identification of, 49b
Anaerohabdus, Gram stain identification of, 49b
Anaphylatoxin inactivator, conditions affecting, 11
Anaphylaxis, 26
Ancef. *See* Cefazolin
Ancobon. *See* Flucytosine
Anergy, defined, 15
Anesthesia, 439-455
    airway considerations in, 439-440, 439f
    airway exam preceding, 440-442
    airway management strategies and, 442-443
    communicating with patient about, 445
    for extubation, 451-452, 452f
    general, 445, 448-450
    immune system effects of, 452-453
    intubation techniques and, 446-448, 447f, 448f
    local, 439, 444-445, 444f
    and pulmonary aspiration of infected material, 453
    respiratory depressant effects of, 446

Anesthesia—cont'd
    surgical airway under, 450-451, 450t
    techniques for, 445-446
Angina, Ludwig's, 84, 177-181, 178f, 179f
    case reports of, 180
Anginosus aginosus, 34t
Anginosus constellatus, 34t
Anginosus cricetus, 34t
Anginosus intermedius, 34t
Anginosus mutans, 34t
Anginosus rattus, 34t
Anginosus sobrinus, 34t
Angle syndrome, neurological exam for, 348
Animal bites. *See also* Cat bites; Dog bites
    antibiotic therapy for, 366
    management of, 374, 374f
    maxillofacial infections from, 308
    pathogens in, 366
    splenic dysfunction and, 458
Ankylosis, TMJ, in infectious arthritis, 436-437, 436f
Anosmia, assessment for, 347
Anspor. *See* Cephradine
Anthrax, characteristics and treatment of, 305
Antibiotic therapy. *See also* specific agents
    for anaerobes, 103
    for animal bites, 366
    bactericidal, 103b
        versus bacteriostatic, 104-105
    bacteriostatic, 103b
    β-lactam. *See also* Carbapenems; Cephalosporins; Monobactams; Penicillin(s)
        viridans streptococci resistance and, 103
    blood levels of, 106
    choosing agents for, 101-106
        antibiotic history and, 105
        antibiotic sensitivity and, 103
        bacterial identification and, 101-103, 102t
        bactericidal *versus* bacteriostatic, 104-105
        cost and, 105
        patient compliance and, 105-106
        patient drug history and, 103
        spectrum and, 103
        toxicity and, 103
    combination, 107
    deciding to use, 100-101
    determining sensitivity to, 103
    in endodontics, 148
    enterococcal resistance to, 472
    fungal infections associated with, 477t
    immune suppression and, 38
    least toxic, 104
    for maxillofacial trauma, 366-368, 367t, 368t
    medicolegal aspects of, 486-487
    microbial resistance to, 471
    narrow-spectrum, 104
    for odontogenic infections, 163-165
    pediatric dosages for, 121b
    for periodontal disease, 136-137
    prophylactic. *See* Prophylactic antibiotics
    Pseudomonas resistance to, 472-473
    resistance to, 104
    risks of, 100-101
    with surgery, indications for, 165

Antibiotic-associated colitis, 109
Antibodies
    immunoglobulin functions as, 6-7
    monoclonal, immunologic function of, 10
Antifungal agents for maxillofacial infections, 121-123, 122t, 123tf
Antigen(s)
    binding of, 12-13
    leukocyte surface, 10
    lymphocyte response to, 13
Antigen testing, 15
Antimicrobial agents. *See also* Antibiotic therapy; specific agents
    microbial susceptibility to, 55t, 56t
    selective reporting of, 57
Antimicrobial peptides, characteristics and functions of, 3-4
Antimicrobial susceptibility testing, 54-59
    broth dilution, 57, 57f
    with disk diffusion procedure, 57, 58f
    empirical therapy and, 54
    with E-test method, 57-58, 58f
    methods for, 57-59
    rationale for, 54-57
Antiseptics, preoperative, 474
Antiviral agents for maxillofacial infections, 123-124
ANUGP. *See* Acute necrotizing ulcerative gingivitis-periodontitis
Aponeurosis of Zuckerkandl and Testut, 204
Appendix, immunoglobulin concentrations in, 5t
Arachidonic acid, metabolites of, inflammatory effects of, 19-20
Arcanobacterium, Gram stain identification of, 49b
Arcobacter, Gram stain identification of, 49b
Arestin for periodontal disease, 137
Arthritis, infectious, of TMJ, 436-437, 436f
Arthrobacter, Gram stain identification of, 49b
Aseptic technique, nosocomial infection and, 473-474
Aspergilloma, 252
Aspergillosis, 251-253
    allergic, 252
    invasive, 252-253, 423
    maxillofacial manifestations of, 423-426, 424f, 425f
    nasoorbital, 423
    nosocomial, 477-478
    paranasal, 424
    of sinuses, 316
    superficial, 252, 253f
Aspergillus, 38
    in allergic fungal sinusitis, 341
    azoles for treating, 122
    in immunocompromised host, 356
    sinusitis due to, 76
Aspergillus flavus in aspergillosis of sinuses, 316
Aspergillus fumigatus
    in aspergillosis, 251-253
    in aspergillosis of sinuses, 316
    in necrotizing external otitis, 318
Aspiration, pulmonary, of infected material, 453
Ataxia-telangiectasia, 457
Atherosclerosis
    P. gingivalis and, 40
    postoperative wound infections and, 401
Atridox for periodontal disease, 137
Attenuation, defined, 38
Auditory canal, external, infections of, 318-319
Augmentin for implant surgery, 382b

Aureobacterium, Gram stain identification of, 49b
Autoimmune disease of ear, 322
Avulsions
    antibiotic therapy for, 367t
    maxillofacial, 373, 373f
Azathioprine, immune suppression due to, 100
Azithromycin
    contraindications to, 222
    dosages for, 120t
    for maxillofacial infections, 120-121
    for odontogenic infections, 164
    pediatric dosages for, 415t
Azole antibiotics
    for maxillofacial infections, 122
    pharmacology of, 123t
Aztreonam
    indications for, 119
    microbes susceptible to, 56t
    pediatric dosages for, 415t

B

B lymphocytes
    differential characteristics of, 13, 13t
    functions of, 13, 456
    in HIV/AIDS, 462
    in Ig synthesis, 5
Bacampicillin
    antimicrobial spectrum of, 117t
    pharmacology of, 117t
Bacilli, gram-negative, infection occurrence of, 102b
Bacillus, Gram stain identification of, 49b
Bacillus anthrax, 305
Bacillus fusiformis in noma, 431
Bacitracin zinc for maxillofacial trauma patient, 367t
Bacteremia, diagnosis of, 46
Bacteria
    aerobic
        infections due to, 101-102
        susceptibility testing of, 57-58, 57f, 58f
    anaerobic, 36t, 110-111. *See also* Anaerobes
        in infants, 30
        infections found in, 102
        susceptibility testing of, 58, 58f
    antibiotic sensitivity of, 103
    attachment of, 39
    filamentous, 35
    gram-negative, penicillins for, 116
    gram-positive rod-shaped, 35
    identification of, 101-103, 102t
        with Gram stain, 49b
    mechanical removal of, 4
    normal
        in conjunctivae, 330
        in nasal cavities, 330, 349
        in oral cavity, 43, 283, 330, 349
    processing, isolation, and identification of, 51-52
    resistant, 101, 104
    susceptibility of, with common antibiotics, 55t
Bacterial infections, hydrostatic pressure in spread of, 188
Bacterial parotitis, chronic recurrent, 289
Bacterial toxins, 22-25
    endogenous pyrogens, 24-25
    endotoxin, 22-23
    fever due to, 24-25

Bacterial toxins—cont'd
    in pathogenicity, 39-40
    in sepsis and systemic inflammatory response syndrome, 23-24, 23b
    streptococcal/staphylococcal superantigens, 23
Bacteriocins, characteristics and functions of, 3-4
Bacterionema matruchotii, 34t
Bacteroides. See also Porphyromonas; Prevotella
    in animal bites, 110
    in cervicofacial actinomycosis, 232
    in children with primary dentition, 30
    enteric, 102
    Gram stain identification of, 49b
    infections due to, 35, 102
    life-threatening infection from, 159f
    in Ludwig's angina, 178
    in mediastinitis, 184
    oropharyngeal, 102
    penicillin resistance of, 164
    in plaque, 132
    in postoperative wounds, 400, 400t
    in pulpal tissue, 148
    in submental space infection, 176
    in tonsillitis, 323
Bacteroides distasonis, 36t
Bacteroides forsythus, 36t
    in periodontitis, 132
Bacteroides fragilis
    first-choice and alternative antibiotics for, 113t
    infection occurrence of, 102b
    in odontogenic infections, 164
    penicillin resistance of, 110, 116
    percent susceptibility of, 55t
    susceptibility testing of, 58
Bacteroides gingivalis in periodontal abscess, 139
Bacteroides melaninogenicus in aspiration pneumonia, 453
Bacteroides oralis in aspiration pneumonia, 453
Bacteroides ureolyticum, 36t
Balanitis, *Candida in,* 251
Barrier techniques, 479-480
Bartonella
    in cat-scratch disease, 432
    Gram stain identification of, 49b
Bartonella hensellae, PCR assays for, 51
Betadine. *See* Povidone-iodine
β-Lactam antibiotics. *See also* Carbapenems; Cephalosporins; Monobactams; Penicillin(s)
    for maxillofacial infections, 112-119
    viridans streptococci resistance and, 103
β-Lactamase inhibitors, blood-brain barrier and, 357
Bell's phenomenon, 343
Benzalkonium, disinfectant activity of, 479t
Benzathine penicillin G, pharmacology of, 117t
Benzodiazepines for sedation/alangesia, 446
Biaxin. *See* Clarithromycin
Bifidobacterium, Gram stain identification of, 49b
Bifidobacterium dentium, 36t
Bile, immunoglobulin concentrations in, 5t
Bilophila, Gram stain identification of, 49b
Biocef. *See* Cephalexin
Biopsy, fine-needle aspiration, *versus* surgical, 45
Bipolaris in allergic fungal sinusitis, 341

Bites. *See also* Cat bites; Dog bites; Human bites
    animal
        maxillofacial infections from, 308
        pathogens in, 366
    human
        antibiotic therapy for, 366
        maxillofacial infections from, 307
    wounds due to, 110
Bladder, neurogenic, urinary tract infections and, 4
Blastomyces, processing, isolation, and identification of, 53
Blastomyces dermatitidis
    in North American blastomycosis, 247
    processing, isolation, and identification of, 54
Blastomycosis
    North American, 247, 247b
    South American, 247-248, 248b
Blepharoplasty, infection after, 392-393, 393f
Blindness after blepharoplasty, 392-393
Blood, collecting specimens of, 46-47
Blood pressure, pediatric, 411t
Blood-brain barrier
    antimicrobials and, 356-357
    function of, 349
Bloodstream sepsis, nosocomial
    causative organisms in, 469t
    risk factors for, 469t
Bockhart's folliculitis, 299-300, 301f
Body fluids, IgG in, 7
Boils, characteristics of, 299
Bone
    infections of. *See* Osteomyelitis
    specimen collection from, 44-45, 45f
Bone grafts in infected fracture management, 377-378
Bone infections
    epidural abscess due to, 353
    intravenous drug use and, 459
Bone marrow transplantation, infection after, 463
Bone scans, radionuclide, 64-65, 64f
Bony orbit. *See also* Infraorbital space
    diagram of, 210f
Bordetella, Gram stain identification of, 49b
Bordetella pertussis
    immunofluorescent assay of, 50
    PCR assays for, 51
Borrelia burgdorferi
    in Lyme disease, 308-309, 355
    PCR assays for, 51
Borrelia vincentii in noma, 419, 431
Borreliosis, Lyme, 308-309
Bradykinin, formation and functions of, 17
Brain, pathogen habitat in, 348-349
Brain abscess, 350, 350f
    CT changes in, 351, 351t
    epidural, 354, 354f
    management of, 357
    MRI changes in, 351-352, 352f
    radionuclide imaging of, 352, 352f, 353f
    sinusitis associated with, 76
    ultrasonographic changes in, 351-352
Brain infection
    in AIDS patient, 357
    ascending midface infection and, 356, 356f
    factors protecting against, 348, 349

Brain infection—cont'd
    in immunocompromised hosts, 355-356
    immunological privilege and, 349, 357
    management of, 356-357
        in brain abscess, 357
        in cavernous sinus thrombosis, 357
        in epidural abscess, 357
        medical, 356-357
        in meningitis, 357
        in osteomyelitis, 357
        in subdural empyema, 357
        surgical, 357
    medical predisposition to, 354-355
    routes of, 349-350
        cranial nerves, 350
        hematogenous, 349
        meningitis, 350
        osteomyelitis, 350
        thrombophlebitis, 349
        ventricular seeding, 350
    vulnerability to, 348
Breast milk, immunoglobulin concentrations in, 5t
Brevibacterium, Gram stain identification of, 49b
Bronchial secretions, immunoglobulin concentrations in, 5t
Broth dilution testing, 57, 57f
Brown-Brenn Gram stain, 48
Brucella
    Gram stain identification of, 49b
    isolation of, 47
Buccal space
    borders of, 194t
    infection of, 170-171, 170f
        causes, contents, and neighboring spaces of, 195t
    in odontogenic infections, 195-197, 197f
Buccinator muscle, in spread of infection, 196
Buccopharyngeal fascia, 191
Buccopharyngeal gap, 82
    infection and, 198
Bullae, characteristics of, 296
Burkholderia, Gram stain identification of, 49b
Burkholderia cepacia, percent susceptibility of, 55t
Burkitt's lymphoma, pediatric, 420
Burns
    antibiotic therapy for, 367t
    fungal infections associated with, 477t
    infection risk after, 2
    maxillofacial, management of, 374-375, 374f

C

Calculus
    in periodontal disease, 132-133
    salivary, 281, 281f
Caldwell's view of paranasal sinuses, 69-70, 69f
Campylobacter, 34t
    in children with primary dentition, 30
    Gram stain identification of, 49b
    infections due to, 35
    in pulpal tissue, 148
Cancer
    immune dysfunction in, 462-464
    maxillofacial, radiation therapy for, 236-237
Cancer chemotherapy, granulocyte defects due to, 463
Cancrum oris. *See* Noma

Candida
    antibiotic therapy and, 4
    azole for treating, 122
    diagnosis of, 45
    overgrowth of, 109
        after tetracycline therapy, 38
Candida albicans
    adherence of, 39
    attachment patterns of, 32
    in candidiasis, 248-251
    characteristics and pathogenicity of, 37
    in HIV-associated periodontal disease, 145
    in neonates, 30
    processing, isolation, and identification of, 53
    in vaginitis, 250-251
Candida dubliniensis, characteristics and pathogenicity of, 37
Candida famata, characteristics and pathogenicity of, 37
Candida guillermondii, characteristics and pathogenicity of, 37
Candida krusei, characteristics and pathogenicity of, 37
Candida parapsilosis
    characteristics and pathogenicity of, 37
    in neonates, 30
Candida zeylanoides, characteristics and pathogenicity of, 37
Candidiasis, 109, 248-251
    in AIDS patients, 274
    angular cheilitis, 250, 250f
    atrophic, 250, 250f
    clinical characteristics of, 249-251, 250f
    cutaneous, 251
    deep organ, 251
    diagnosis and treatment of, 251
    hyperkeratotic, of tongue, 250, 250f
    leukoplakia, 250, 250f
    mucocutaneous, 251
    nosocomial, 477-478
    oral, 249-250, 249f, 462
    pathogenesis of, 249
    pediatric, 421
    primary cellular immune defects and, 456
    pseudomembranous, 249, 249f
    skin resurfacing and, 396
Capnocytophaga, 34t
    in children with primary dentition, 30
    Gram stain identification of, 49b
    in HIV-associated periodontal disease, 145
    in infants, 30
    infections due to, 35
    in pericoronitis, 143
    in periodontal abscess, 139
    in periodontitis, 132
    in plaque, 132
Capnocytophaga carnivorsus, animal bites and, 458
Carbapenems for maxillofacial infections, 119
Carbenicillin, microbial susceptibility to, 56t
Carbenicillin indanyl, pharmacology of, 117t
Carbohydrates, dietary, oral microbes and, 32
Carbol-fuchsin method, 48-49
Carbuncle, characteristics of, 299, 299f
Carbunculosis, nasal, 313
    of external ear, 317
Carcinoma, neck swelling due to, 310-311
Cardiobacterium, Gram stain identification of, 49b
Cardiobacterium hominis in HACEK group, 47

Caries, pulpal pain due to, 149
Carotid cavernous fistula *versus* orbital cellulitis, 334, 334f
Carotid occlusion as complication of orbital cellulitis, 336
Carotid sheath
    anatomy of, 190f, 191
    infections of, 207
Cat bites
    management of, 374
    splenic dysfunction and, 458
Catheters
    infections associated with, 38
    preventing contamination of, 368-369
Catonella, Gram stain identification of, 49b
Cat-scratch disease, 366
    head and neck infections from, 308
    maxillofacial manifestations of, 432-433, 433f, 434f
    salivary gland involvement in, 290
Cavernous sinus
    anatomy of, 211-212, 212f
    function of, 211
Cavernous sinus syndrome, neurological exam for, 348
Cavernous sinus thrombosis, 169-170, 211-213
    as complication of infraorbital space abscess, 209
    as complication of orbital cellulitis, 336, 338
    management of, 357
    mortality from, 354, 355f
    neurological impacts of, 356
    versus orbital cellulitis, 334
    pediatric, 413
    septic, 338-340, 339f
CD nomenclature, 10
CD4 T lymphocytes, 456
    in HIV/AIDS, 462
CD4+ T lymphocytes
    helper, 13
        differentiation of, 14
        immunologic role of, 14-15
CD8+ suppressor T lymphocytes, 13
Ceclor. *See* Cefaclor
Cefaclor
    antimicrobial spectrum of, 115b, 118t
    indications for, 113t
    pediatric dosages for, 415t
    pharmacology of, 114t, 119t
Cefadroxil
    antimicrobial spectrum of, 118t
    pediatric dosages for, 415t
    pharmacology of, 119t
Cefadyl. *See* Cephapirin
Cefalexin, pharmacology of, 114t
Cefamandole
    microbes susceptible to, 56t
    pharmacology of, 119t
Cefaroxime, indications for, 113t
Cefazolin
    antimicrobial spectrum of, 115b, 118t
    for maxillofacial trauma patient, 367t
    microbial susceptibility to, 55t, 56t
    pediatric dosages for, 415t
    pharmacology of, 114t, 119t
Cefdinir
    antimicrobial spectrum of, 118t
    pharmacology of, 119t

Cefditoren
    antimicrobial spectrum of, 118t
    pharmacology of, 119t
Cefepime
    antimicrobial spectrum of, 118t
    microbial susceptibility to, 55t, 56t
    pediatric dosages for, 415t
    pharmacology of, 119t
Cefixime
    antimicrobial spectrum of, 118t
    pharmacology of, 119t
Cefizox. *See* Ceftizoxime
Cefmetazole
    antimicrobial spectrum of, 118t
    microbial susceptibility to, 56t
    pharmacology of, 119t
Cefobid. *See* Cefoperazone
Cefonicid
    antimicrobial spectrum of, 118t
    microbial susceptibility to, 56t
    pharmacology of, 119t
Cefoperazone
    antimicrobial spectrum of, 118t
    microbial susceptibility to, 56t
    pharmacology of, 119t
Cefotan. *See* Cefotetan
Cefotaxime
    antimicrobial spectrum of, 118t
    as first-choice antibiotic, 113t
    microbial susceptibility to, 55t, 56t
    pediatric dosages for, 415t
    pharmacology of, 119t
Cefotetan
    antimicrobial spectrum of, 118t
    microbial susceptibility to, 56t
    pharmacology of, 119t
Cefoxitin
    antimicrobial spectrum of, 115b, 118t
    indications for, 113t
    microbial susceptibility to, 56t
    organisms effective against, 222
    pediatric dosages for, 415t
    for penicillin-allergic patients, 222
    pharmacology of, 114t, 119t
Cefpodoxime
    antimicrobial spectrum of, 118t
    pediatric dosages for, 415t
Cefpodoxime proxetil, pharmacology of, 119t
Cefprozil
    antimicrobial spectrum of, 118t
    pediatric dosages for, 415t
    pharmacology of, 119t
Ceftazidime
    antimicrobial spectrum of, 118t
    microbial susceptibility to, 55t, 56t
    pediatric dosages for, 415t
    pharmacology of, 119t
Ceftibuten
    antimicrobial spectrum of, 118t
    pediatric dosages for, 415t
Ceftin. *See* Cefuroxime axetil
Ceftizoxime
    antimicrobial spectrum of, 118t
    as first-choice antibiotic, 113t

Ceftizoxime—cont'd
    microbial susceptibility to, 56t
    pediatric dosages for, 415t
    pharmacology of, 119t
Ceftriaxone
    antimicrobial spectrum of, 118t
    as first-choice antibiotic, 113t
    pediatric dosages for, 415t
    pharmacology of, 119t
Cefuroxime
    antimicrobial spectrum of, 118t
    microbial susceptibility to, 56t
    pediatric dosages for, 415t
    pharmacology of, 119t
Cefuroxime axetil, pharmacology of, 119t
Cefzil. *See* Cefprozil
Cell surface receptors, 9-10
Cell-mediated immunity, 13
    mechanisms in, 14-15
    T cell roles in, 14
Cellular defense mechanisms, 9-15
    cell surface receptors, 9-10
    cellular myoskeleton, 10-11
    lymphocytes, 13-15, 13t
    phagocytes, 11-13
    signal transduction, 10
Cellular myoskeleton, immunologic function of, 10-11
Cellulitis
    versus abscess, 162
    abscess formation and, 100
    antibiotic therapy for, 103
    characteristics of, 297
    combination therapy for, 107
    H. influenzae
        in children, 417-418, 418f
        maxillofacial manifestations of, 435-436, 435f
    in infantile osteomyelitis of jaw, 228
    invasive fungal orbital, 336-338
    masticator space, MRI scan of, 64f
    of maxillofacial region, 302-303, 303f
    in odontogenic infection, 193, 193t
    orbital, 332-336, 332f
        after blepharoplasty, 392
        causes of, 332
        classification of, 330
        complications of, 336, 338
        differential diagnosis of, 333-334, 334f
        imaging of, 334-335, 335f
        in mucormycosis, 427f
        symptoms/signs of, 332-333, 333f
        treatment of, 335-336
    versus osteomyelitis, 65
    periorbital
        as complication of dacryocystitis, 340-341
        in sinusitis, 317
    preseptal, 330-332, 331f
Cellulomonas, Gram stain identification of, 49b
Centers for Disease Control and Prevention, prophylaxis recommendations of, 471
Centipeda, Gram stain identification of, 49b
Centipeda periodontii, 36t
Central nervous system, mucormycosis of, 254

Cephalexin
    antimicrobial spectrum of, 115b, 118t
    bacterial sensitivity to, 103
    for implant surgery, 382b
    for maxillofacial trauma patient, 367t
    for osteomyelitis of jaw, 222
    pediatric dosages for, 415t
    pharmacology of, 119t
Cephalosporins
    allergy to, 104
    antibiotic-associated colitis due to, 109
    generations of, 118t
    hypersensitivity reactions to, 108
    indications for, 113t, 222
    for maxillofacial infections, 118-119, 118f, 118t, 119t
    pediatric dosages for, 415t
    pharmacology of, 119t
    resistant microbes and, 4
    structure of, 118f
Cephalothin, microbes susceptible to, 56t
Cephapirin
    antimicrobial spectrum of, 118t
    pharmacology of, 119t
Cephradine
    antimicrobial spectrum of, 118t
    pharmacology of, 119t
Cerebritis, radionuclide imaging of, 352, 353f
Cerebrospinal fluid
    leakage of, 110
    protective function of, 349
Cerebrospinal fluid fistulas, 353
Cervical fascia, 189-192, 190f
Cervical nodes, cancer of, in children, 421t
Cervicofacial actinomycosis, 231-234, 232f, 233f, 234f
Chédiak-Higashi cells, 10
Chemokines, 21
Chemosis from septic cavernous sinus thrombosis, 338
Chemotactic factor inactivator, conditions affecting, 11
Chemotherapy
    cancer, granulocyte defects due to, 463
    for periodontal disease, 136-137
    superimposed infections and, 38
Chickenpox, 264-266, 420. *See also* Varicella-zoster virus
    ocular complications of, 342
    pathogenesis, clinical characteristics, diagnosis, treatment of, 259t
Children
    airway management in, 443
    maxillofacial infections in. *See* Pediatric maxillofacial infections
    vital signs/hematology values in, 411t
Chlamydia, processing, isolation, and identification of, 54
Chlamydia trachomatis
    immunofluorescent assay of, 50
    nucleic acid amplification strategies for, 51
    nucleic acid probe for detecting, 51
Chloramphenicol
    antimicrobial spectrum of, 115b
    for brain infections, 357
    indications for, 113t
    for maxillofacial infections, 120
    microbial susceptibility to, 56t
    pediatric dosages for, 415t

Chloramphenicol—cont'd
    pharmacology of, 114t
    toxicity of, 104
Chlorhexidene gluconate rinses after implant surgery, 382
Chlorhexidine
    hand washing with, 474
    for oral cavity decontamination, 403
    organisms resistant to, 474
Chlorhexidine oral rinse, antiplaque effects of, 136
Chlorine, disinfectant activity of, 479t
Cholesteatoma, 321, 321f
Chondritis of external ear, 317-318
Chromobacterium, Gram stain identification of, 49b
Chryseobacterium, Gram stain identification of, 49b
Chryseomonas, Gram stain identification of, 49b
Cicatricial ectropion, 344, 344f
Ciprofloxacin
    dosage of, with normal/impaired renal function, 122t
    indications, absorption, and side effects of, 121
    microbial susceptibility to, 55t, 56t
    pediatric dosages for, 415t
    pharmacology of, 114t
Citrobacter freundii, percent susceptibility of, 55t
Citrobacter koseri
    meningitis due to, 51
    percent susceptibility of, 55t
Claforan. *See* Cefotaxime
Clarithromycin
    contraindications to, 222
    dosages for, 120t
    for maxillofacial infections, 121
    pediatric dosages for, 415t
Classic pathway, initiation of, 8-9, 8f
Clindamycin
    antibiotic-associated colitis due to, 109
    antimicrobial spectrum of, 115b
    for chronic suppurative osteomyelitis, 223
    indications for, 113t, 222
    for maxillofacial infections, 120
    microbial susceptibility to, 55t, 103
    for odontogenic infections, 164
    for oral cavity decontamination, 403
    for osteomyelitis of jaw, 222
    pediatric dosages for, 415t
    pharmacology of, 114t
Clivus, transoral approaches to, 354
Closed wound irrigation-suction for osteomyelitis of jaw, 223-224, 223f
Clostridium
    first-choice and alternative antibiotics for, 113t
    Gram stain identification of, 49b
    in infants, 30
Clostridium difficile
    colitis due to, 109, 472
    immunoassay of, 51
Clostridium tetani
    immunization against, 368
    in tetanus, 306-307
Clotrimazole for maxillofacial infections, 122, 123
Clotting. *See* Coagulation system
Cloxacillin
    pediatric dosages for, 415t
    pharmacology of, 117t

Coagulation factors. *See* Factors; specific factors
Coagulation mediators, inflammatory role of, 21-22
Coagulation system, 17
    inflammation and fibrinolysis links with, 17-18
    interrelationships of, 15, 16f
    in severe infection, 24
Cocci
    Gram stain of, 49b
    gram-negative, 35, 36t
        staining of, 48
    gram-positive, 34-35, 36t
        infection occurrence of, 102b
Coccidioides, processing, isolation, and identification of, 53
Coccidioides immitis
    azole for treating, 122
    in coccidioidomycosis, 245-246
    processing, isolation, and identification of, 54
Coccidioidomycosis, 245-247, 246b
Cold sterilization, 478
Colitis
    antibiotic-associated, 109
    Clostridium difficile, 472
Collagen sialadenitis, 292
Collagen vascular disease, immune deficiency due to, 461
Colon, immunoglobulin concentrations in, 5t
Colony-stimulating factors, 3
Color vision, optic nerve damage and, 329
Colostrum, immunoglobulin concentrations in, 5t
Communication
    medicolegal issues in, 486
    methods of, 485
    patient, in airway management, 445
Complement receptors, 9-10
Complement system
    components and activation of, 8-9, 8f
    interrelationships of, 15, 16f
Compliance, patient, 105-106
Compromised host. *See* Immunocompromised host
Computed tomography
    diagnostic uses of, 62-63
    in osteomyelitis of jaw, 220
Condensing osteitis, 231, 231f
Condensing sclerosing osteitis, 150
Condylomata acuminata, 268
Congenital rubella syndrome of newborn, 273
Conjunctivae, normal flora of, 330
Conjunctivitis
    Parinaud's oculoglandular, 341-342
    with positive lymph node findings, 341
Consciousness, level of, assessment of, 347
Contusions
    antibiotic therapy for, 367t
    maxillofacial, 371-372
Cornea, infections of, 343-344
Corticosteroids
    in airway management, 443
    immune deficiency due to, 461
    for preventing graft rejection, 460
Corynebacterium
    Gram stain identification of, 49b
    isolation of, 47
    life-threatening infection from, 159f
    in maxillofacial/neck infections, 295

Corynebacterium—cont'd
  in odontogenic infections, 164
  in pulpal tissue, 148
Corynebacterium diphtheriae
  in laryngotracheal diphtheria, 326
  microbial interference with, 4
  pharyngitis due to, 45
Cosmetic plastic surgery. *See* Esthetic facial surgery
Cotrimoxazole, bacterial susceptibility to, 55t
Coxsackievirus infections
  mumps, 290
  pathogenesis, characteristics, diagnosis, treatment of, 269t
  pediatric, 420
Coxsackieviruses group a, 268-269
Cranial nerves
  brain infection and, 349
  in cavernous sinus thrombosis, 212, 212f
  dysfunction of, exam for, 347-348
  paralysis of, in mucormycosis, 428
Crepitus, characteristics of, 297
Cresols, disinfectant activity of, 479t
Cricoid pressure, intubation and, 449
Cricothyrotomy *versus* tracheotomy, 450-451, 450t
Crohn's disease, buccal space abscess as complication of, 170-171
Croup, 94, 95f, 325-326, 325f
Cryptococcosis, 255-257, 256b
  clinical characteristics of, 256
  cutaneous, 256
  diagnosis of, 256-257
  pathogenesis of, 255-256
  pulmonary, 256, 257
  treatment of, 257
Cryptococcus in immunocompromised host, 356
Cryptococcus neoformans
  in cryptococcosis, 255-257
  processing, isolation, and identification of, 53
Cryptosporidium parvum, immunofluorescent assay of, 50
Cultures
  blood, 46-47
  indications for, 103
Curvularia in allergic fungal sinusitis, 341
Cyclooxygenase pathway, 19
Cyclosporine, immune suppression due to, 100
Cysts
  mucous retention, 75, 75f
  neck swelling due to, 310
  periradicular, 150
  sebaceous, 301
  ultrasound in diagnosis of, 65-66, 65f
Cytokines, 18
  altered levels of, 39
  endotoxin and, 22
  inflammatory effects of, 20-21, 21
  production of, 14
  protective function of, 3
  in sepsis, 24
  in wound healing, 25-26, 26t
Cytomegalovirus, 266-267
  characteristics and pathogenicity of, 38
  nucleic acid amplification strategies for, 51
  pathogenesis, clinical characteristics, diagnosis, treatment of, 260t
  in salivary gland inclusion disease, 291

D

Dacryocystitis, 340-341, 340f
Danger space, 192
  infections of, 207
Dark-field microscopy, 50
Debridement
  in head and neck surgery, 404
  of necrotic tissue, 365
Decortication, mandibular, 225-226, 225f
Defense mechanisms. *See also* Immune response; Immune system
  cellular components of, 9-15, 12f, 13t
    cell surface receptors, 9-10
    cellular myoskeleton, 10-11
    lymphocytes, 13-15, 13t
    phagocytes, 11-13, 12f
    signal transduction, 10
  components of, 2-5, 2f
  determining status of, 99-100
  host, 1, 2f
    innate *versus* acquired, 40
  humoral, 6-9
    complement system in, 8-9, 8f
    immunoglobulins, 6-8, 6t, 7f
  local, 2-5, 2f
    antimicrobial peptides, 3-4
    epithelial lining, 2-3
    microbial interference, 4-5
    mucosal immune system, 5, 5t
    secretion and drainage system, 4
α-Defensins, production and characteristics of, 3
β-Defensins, production and characteristics of, 3
Delayed hypersensitivity reaction, cutaneous, 14
  anergy and, 15
Dental caries. *See* Caries
Dental implants. *See* Implants
Dental offices, waterline safety in, 480
Dental plaque in periodontal disease, 132
Dentoalveolar abscess, 193, 196f
Dermatobacter, Gram stain identification of, 49b
Dermatophilus, Gram stain identification of, 49b
Dermis, anatomy of, 294
Desulfomonas, Gram stain identification of, 49b
Desulfovibrio, Gram stain identification of, 49b
Diabetes mellitus
  as complication of mumps pancreatitis, 291
  fungal infections associated with, 477t
  immune deficiency due to, 458-459
  infection and, 356
  necrotizing external otitis and, 318
  postsurgical infection and, 396, 401
Diagnosis, medicolegal aspects of, 486
Diagnostic imaging, 62-98
  with computed tomography, 62-63
  of fascial spaces, 77-89
    anatomic considerations in, 77-78, 78f
    with CT, 79, 80f, 81
    in masticator space, 86-87, 86f, 87f
    with MRI, 81-82, 81f
    for osteomyelitis of jaw, 84-86, 85f, 86f
    in parapharyngeal and retropharyngeal spaces, 88-89, 88f, 89f
    in parotid space, 87-88
    with plain film, 78-79, 79f

Diagnostic imaging—cont'd
  of fascial spaces—cont'd
    in space of mandibular body, 84-86
    submandibular, 82, 83f-84f, 84
  in lymph node evaluation, 89-91, 90f
  with magnetic resonance imaging, 63, 64f
  maxillofacial/fascial space anatomic considerations in, 66, 66f, 67f, 68-69, 68f, 69f
  of midface/paranasal sinuses, 69-72
    with CT and MRI, 70-72, 71f, 72f, 73f
    for infectious sinusitis, 73-75
    with plain film studies, 69-70
    for sinusitis complications, 75-77, 75f
  with nuclear medicine, 63-65, 64f
  of orbital inflammatory processes, 91
  of orbital pseudotumors, 91-92
  of pediatric maxillofacial infections, 93-94
    croup, 94, 95f
    epiglottitis, 94, 94f
    periorbital/orbital, 93-94, 93f
    tonsillar/peritonsillar, 94, 94f
  with plain film examination, 62, 63f
  of salivary inflammatory disorders, 92-93, 92f
  with ultrasonography, 65-66, 65f
Diagnostic techniques, 43-61
  antimicrobial susceptibility testing, 54-59
    empirical therapy and, 54, 55t
    methods for, 57-59
    rationale for, 54-57
  direct methods of, 47-51
    for microbial antigens and nucleic acids, 50-51
    staining, 47-50
  for processing, isolation, identification, 51-54
    of bacteria, 51-52
    of mycobacteria, 52-54
    of viruses/*Chlamydia* spp., 54
  specimen collection for, 43-47
    from aspirate, 44, 44f
    from superficial sites, 45-46, 46f
    from tissue/bone, 44-45, 45f
Dialister, Gram stain identification of, 49b
Dichelobacter, Gram stain identification of, 49b
Dicloxacillin
  antimicrobial spectrum of, 115b
  pediatric dosages for, 415t
  pharmacology of, 114t, 117t
Diet, oral microbes and, 32
Diflucan. *See* Fluconazole
Diphtheria, laryngotracheal, 326
Diphtherial pharyngitis, 323
Diphtheroids, 34t. *See also Corynebacterium*
  disease due to, 35
  in maxillofacial/neck infections, 295
  in periodontal abscess, 139
Dirithromycin, dosages for, 120t
Disease
  host defenses and, 100
  systemic, oral infections and, 40
Disinfectants
  activity of, 479t
  viricidal, 478-479, 479t
Disseminated intravascular coagulation, mechanism of, 22
DNA, bacterial *versus* mammalian, 23

Dog bites. *See also* Animal bites
  management of, 374, 374f
  splenic dysfunction and, 458
Dose, proper, 106
Doxycycline
  pediatric dosages for, 416t
  for periodontal disease, 137
  pharmacology of, 114t
Drainage, guidelines for, 163
Drains, placement of, 365
Dressings, fungal infections associated with, 477t
Drug abuse
  fungal infections associated with, 477t
  intravenous
    immune deficiency due to, 459-460
    postoperative infection and, 377
Drug history, antibiotic selection and, 104
Drugs
  immunosuppressive, 100
  pediatric dosages for, 415t
  pharmacokinetics of, 106-107
  plasma half-life of, 106
Duodenum, immunoglobulin concentrations in, 5t
Dural sinus thrombosis, 354
Duricef. *See* Cefadroxil
Dysphagia, 440
  with odontogenic infection, 182
Dysplasia, florid osseous, 231, 231f
Dyspnea, 440

E

Ear infections, 317-322
  of external canal, 318-319
    acute otitis externa, 318, 318f
    bullous external otitis, 319
    chronic otitis externa, 318
    herpes simplex, 319
    herpes zoster, 319
    necrotizing external otitis, 318-319
  external noncanalicular
    furunculosis/carbunculosis, 317
    perichondritis/chondritis, 317-318
    relapsing polychondritis, 318
  of inner ear, 321-322
    autoimmune disease, 322
    labyrinthitis, 321-322
  of middle ear, 319-321
    otitis media, 320-321, 320f, 321f
  pediatric, 419
ECHO. *See* Enteric cytopathic human orphan virus
Ecthyma, characteristics of, 297-298
Ectropion, cicatricial, 344, 344f
Eggerthella lenta, 36t
Ehrlichia, PCR assays for, 51
Eicosanoids, 18
  inflammatory effects of, 19
Eikenella
  Gram stain identification of, 49b
  life-threatening infection from, 159f
  in odontogenic infections, 164
Eikenella corrodens, 34t
  in cervicofacial actinomycosis, 232
  first-choice and alternative antibiotics for, 113t
  in HACEK group, 47

Eikenella corrodens—cont'd
  in HIV-associated periodontal disease, 145
  in human bites, 110
  infection occurrence of, 102b
  in osteomyelitis, 217
  in periodontitis, 132
  in postoperative wounds, 400, 400t
Empedobacter, Gram stain identification of, 49b
Empyema
  epidural, sinusitis associated with, 76
  subdural, 350
    management of, 357
Endodontics, antibiotic therapy in, 148
Endophthalmitis, endogenous, 342-343, 343f
Endothelial cells, inflammatory role of, 21-22
Endotoxins
  in pathogenesis, 39-40
  in pulpal disease, 148
  structure and effects of, 22-23
Enophthalmos, 329
Enteric cytopathic human orphan virus in mumps, 290
Enterobacter in postoperative wounds, 400, 400t
Enterobacter aerogenes, percent susceptibility of, 55t
Enterobacter cloacae, percent susceptibility of, 55t
Enterococcus, 34t
  antibiotic resistance of, 472
  antimicrobials affecting, 56
  characteristics and disorders associated with, 34-35
  glycopeptide-resistant, 472
  Gram stain identification of, 49b
  methicillin-resistant, 158
  in nosocomial ICU infections, 471
  percent susceptibility of, 55t
  susceptibility testing of, 54
  vancomycin-resistant, 470-471
Enterococcus faecalis, 34t
Enterococcus faecium, 34t
Enterotoxin D, 40
Enteroviruses, 268-269
  nucleic acid amplification strategies for, 51
Enzyme-linked immunoassays, uses of, 51
Enzymes
  for Ig fragmentation, 6
  in pathogenesis, 40
Epidemic parotitis, 290-291
Epidermis, anatomy of, 294
Epidermodysplasia verruciformis, 268
Epididymoorchitis, mumps-related, 271
Epidural abscess, management of, 357
Epidural empyema, sinusitis associated with, 76
Epiglottitis, 94, 94f
  acute
    in adults, 325
    in children, 324-325, 325f
Epithelial hyperplasia, 268
Epithelial lining, protective function of, 2-3
Epithelialization in wound healing, 25-26
Epstein-Barr virus
  in mumps, 290
  in pediatric infections, 420
Erysipelas
  maxillofacial manifestations of, 434-435, 435f
  pediatric, 419

Erysipelas—cont'd
  signs of, 162
  streptococcal, of maxillofacial region, 298, 298f
Erysipeloid *versus* erysipelas, 298
Erysipelothrix, Gram stain identification of, 49b
Erysipelothrix rhusiopathiae, 298
Erythema migrans in Lyme disease, 308-309
Erythromycin
  bacterial sensitivity to, 103
  bacterial susceptibility to, 55t
  with clarithromycin, antimicrobial spectrum of, 115b
  contraindications to, 222
  dosages for, 120t
  as first-choice antibiotic, 113t
  indications for, 113t
  for maxillofacial infections, 120
  for odontogenic infections, 164
  pediatric dosages for, 415t
  pharmacology of, 114t
Escherichia coli
  first-choice and alternative antibiotics for, 113t
  infection occurrence of, 102b
  life-threatening infection from, 159f
  in Ludwig's angina, 178
  in osteomyelitis, 216-217
  in otoplasty-related infection, 397
  percent susceptibility of, 55t
  in periodontal abscess, 139
  in postoperative wounds, 400, 400t
Esophagitis, candidal, 250
Esthetic facial surgery, 392-398
  infections associated with
    after blepharoplasty, 392-393, 393f
    after facelift, 395-396
    after genioplasty, 397
    after otoplasty, 397
    after rhinoplasty, 393, 393f-394f, 395
    after skin resurfacing, 396-397
E-test method, 57-58, 58f
Ethmoid bone, anatomy of, 68, 69f
Ethmoid infundibulum, 69
Ethmoid sinus, 68
  infection of, 315, 315f
  mucoceles of, 75-76
Ethmoiditis, orbital complications of, 76
Ethmomaxillary plate, 69f, 70
Ethylene oxide gas mixture, disinfectant activity of, 479t
Eubacterium
  disease due to, 35
  Gram stain identification of, 49b
  in infants, 30
  in periodontitis, 132
Eubacterium brachy, disease due to, 35
Eubacterium combesii, 36t
  disease due to, 35
Eubacterium contortum, 36t
Eubacterium lentum, disease due to, 35
Eubacterium moniliforme, 36t
Eubacterium nitrogenes, locael of, 36t
Eubacterium nodatum, disease due to, 35
Eubacterium saburreum, 36t
  disease due to, 35
Eubacterium tenue, 36t
Eubacterium timidum, disease due to, 35

Eustachian tube, dysfunction of, in middle ear infections, 319-320
Ewing's tumor *versus* osteomyelitis of jaw, 218
Exophthalmos, 329, 329f
Exotoxins
    in pathogenicity, 40
    streptococcal/staphylococcal, 23
Exposure keratopathy, 343-344, 343f
Exserohilum in allergic fungal sinusitis, 341
Extraocular movements, assessment of, 329
Extubation, 451-452, 452f
Eye(s). *See also* Ophthalmic considerations
    anatomy of, 328-329
    examination of, 329-330
    infections of, with simulataneous head/neck infections, 341-342

F

Face. *See also* Midface
    infections of, 370
        posttraumatic, 370
    lower, pediatric infections of, 412t, 413-414, 413f, 414f
    skin, fascia, and muscles of, anatomy of, 294, 295f
    upper, pediatric infections of, 411-412, 412b, 412f, 412t
Facelift, infection after, 395-396
Facial muscles, 209f, 294
Facial nerve palsy, 343, 343f
Facial surgery
    esthetic. *See* Esthetic facial surgery
    and risk of infection, 353-354
Factor XII (Hageman factor)
    inflammation mediators and, 15
    in intrinsic coagulation cascade, 17
    mediator role of, 17
Factor XIIa
    action of, 17
    mediator role of, 17
Factors, macrophage-activating, 12
Famciclovir for HSV infections, 396
Fasciae
    buccopharyngeal, 191
    cervical, 189-192, 190f
    definition and function of, 188
    facial, anatomy of, 294
    head/neck
        anatomy of, 189-192, 190f, 191f
        infections in, 188-189
    parotideomasseteric, 189, 200, 204, 205f
    prevertebral, 191
    temporal, 189
Fascial spaces
    anatomy of, 77-78, 78f
    clinically significant, 168
    diagnostic imaging of, 77-89
        with CT, 79, 80f, 81
        in mandibular body space, 84-86, 85f
        in masticator space, 86-87, 86f, 87f
        with MRI, 81-82
        in parapharyngeal/retropharyngeal spaces, 88-89, 88f, 89f
        in parotid space, 87-88
        with plain film, 78-79, 79f
        in pretracheal space, 89
        submandibular, 82, 83, 83f-84f
    of head and neck, clinical anatomy of, 193, 195-197
    infections of, 168-169
        in canine space, 168-169, 169f

Fasciitis, necrotizing. *See* Necrotizing fasciitis
Fat pad, retroantral, 71, 71f
Fc receptors, 10
Fever
    mechanisms of, 24-25
    pharyngeal conjunctival, 341
    uveoparotid, 292
Fibrin, inflammatory effects of, 17-18
Fibrinogen, inflammatory effects of, 17-18
Fibrinolysis, coagulation and inflammation links with, 17-18
Fibrinolytic system, 17
    interrelationships of, 15, 16f
Fibrobacter, Gram stain identification of, 49b
Fibroblast growth factor, 3
Fibrous dysplasia *versus* osteomyelitis of jaw, 218
Filariasis, salivary gland infestation with, 291
Fistulas
    in canine space, 169, 169f
    cerebrospinal fluid, 353
Flagyl. *See* Metronidazole
Flap reconstruction in head and neck surgery, 399
Flavimonas, Gram stain identification of, 49b
Fleming, Alexander, 100, 471
Florid osseous dysplasia, 231, 231f
Fluconazole
    for maxillofacial infections, 122
    pharmacology of, 123t
Fluctuance, defined, 193
Flucytosine, administration and dosage of, 122
Fluorescent antibody stains, 50
Folliculitis
    Bockhart's, 299-300, 301f
    characteristics of, 299, 299f
Folliculitis cheloidalis, characteristics of, 300-301, 301f
Foreign bodies
    removal of, 364-365
    in wounds, 476
Formaldehyde, disinfectant activity of, 479t
Fortaz. *See* Ceftazidime
Fractures
    antibiotics in management of, 110
    craniofacial, 371
        antibiotic therapy for, 367t
        management of, 376, 376f
    facial, antibiotic use and, 366
    fixation/immobilization of, 365
    infected, 377-378
        management of, 371b
    mandibular, 370-371, 370f
        management of, 375, 375b, 376f
    mandibular/maxillary, antibiotic therapy for, 367t
    midface, 371
        management of, 375-376, 376f
    osteomyelitis associated with, 226-227, 227f, 228f
    preventing infection after, 375b
Francisella, Gram stain identification of, 49b
Frontal sinuses, infection of, 314-315, 315f
Fungal infections, 243-258
    in immunocompromised host, 356, 423
    maxillofacial manifestations of
        in aspergillosis, 423-426, 424f, 425f
        in noma, 430-432, 430f, 431f, 432f
        in rhinocerebral mucormycosis, 426-429, 426f, 427f, 428f, 429f

Fungal infections–cont'd
　nosocomial, 477-478, 477t
　opportunistic, 248-258
　　aspergillosis, 251-253, 252b, 253f
　　candidiasis, 248-251, 249b, 249f, 250f
　　cryptococcosis, 255-257, 256f
　　mucormycosis, 253-254, 254b, 254f
　　pneumocystosis, 254-255, 255b
　　sporotrichosis, 257-258, 257f, 258f
　pathogenic, 243-248
　　coccidioidomycosis, 245-247, 246b
　　histoplasmosis, 243-245
　　North American blastomycosis, 247, 247b
　　South American blastomycosis, 247-248, 248b
　pediatric, 421
　prophylaxis of, 478
Fungal orbital infections, 336-338
Fungal sinusitis, allergic, 341
Fungal stains, 48
Fungemia, nosocomial, 478
Fungi
　characteristics and pathogenicity of, 37-38
　immunofluorescent assay of, 50
　opportunistic, 243
　pathogenic, *versus* opportunistic, 243
　processing, isolation, and identification of, 53-54
　sinusitis due to, 76-77
　susceptibility testing of, 59
　virulent, 243
Furuncle, characteristics of, 299, 299f
Furunculosis
　of external ear, 317
　of nasal hair follicles, 313
Fusobacterium
　in animal bites, 110
　antibiotic sensitivity of, 103
　in ANUGP, 141
　in cervicofacial actinomycosis, 232
　in children with primary dentition, 30
　first-choice and alternative antibiotics for, 113t
　infections due to, 35, 102
　life-threatening infection from, 159f
　occurrence frequence of, in infections, 102b
　in odontogenic infections, 164
　in osteomyelitis, 217
　penicillin resistance of, 222
　percent susceptibility of, 55t
　in periodontal abscess, 139
　in plaque, 132
　in postoperative wounds, 400, 400t
　in pulpal tissue, 148
　in retropharyngeal space infection, 183
　with *Streptococcus milleri,* 102-103
　in submental space infection, 176
Fusobacterium nucleatum, 36t
　in aspiration pneumonia, 453
　in HIV-associated periodontal disease, 145
　in infants, 30
　noma due to, 419, 431
　in pericoronitis, 143
　in periodontitis, 132
Fusobacterium periodonticum, 36t

G

Gag reflex, controlling, 447
Gallbladder, immunoglobulin concentrations in, 5t
Gallium 67 citrate, diagnostic uses of, 65
Gangrene, characteristics of, 297
Gangrenous stomatitis, 418-419, 419f. *See also* Noma
Gardnerella, Gram stain identification of, 49b
Garfield, James, 283
Garré's sclerosing osteomyelitis, 229-230, 229f
　pediatric, 416, 417f
Gastric secretions, immunoglobulin concentrations in, 5t
Gastrointestinal mucormycosis, 254
Gastrointestinal tract, IgA synthesis in, 7
Gemella
　in children with primary dentition, 30
　Gram stain identification of, 49b
Gemella morbillorum, 34t
Genioplasty, infection after, 397
Genitourinary tract, IgA synthesis in, 7
Gentamicin
　bacterial susceptibility to, 55t
　microbes susceptible to, 56t
　pediatric dosages for, 415t
　with ticarcillin, as first-choice antibiotic, 113t
Geoptrichum, 38
German measles, 272-273
　pathogenesis, characteristics, diagnosis, treatment of, 269t
Giardia lamblia, immunofluorescent assay of, 50
Gilchrist's disease, 247, 247b
Gingivae, immunoglobulin concentrations in, 5
Gingival disease, classification of, 127b
Gingival pockets, 129, 129f
Gingivectomy, 135
Gingivitis, 128-137
　acute necrotizing ulcerative. *See* Acute necrotizing ulcerative
　　　gingivitis-periodontitis
　clinical features of, 128-130, 129f, 130f
　epidemiology of, 131-132
　HIV-associated, 144-145
　hormonal influences on, 130
　simple, 130
　treatment of, 134-137
Globicatella, Gram stain identification of, 49b
Gloves
　disposable, 479-480
　effectiveness of, 474
　in preventing nosocomial infection, 469
Glucocorticoids, immune suppression due to, 100
Glutaraldehyde, disinfectant activity of, 479t
Gonococcal pharyngitis, 323
Gordona
　acid fastness in, 50
　Gram stain identification of, 49b
Gradenigo's syndrome, neurological exam for, 348
Graft rejection, preventing, 460
Gram stain
　bacterial identification with, 49b
　Brown-Brenn, 48
　methods for, 47-48, 49t
Granulocyte disorders
　in cancer patient, 463
　immune deficiency due to, 457
Granulocyte-macrophage CSF, 3

Granulocytopenia, definition and causes of, 457, 457b
Granulomatous disease of nose and paranasal sinuses, 77
Grodinsky, numbered spaces of, 191-192
Growth factors, 3
  inflammatory role of, 21

H

HAART. *See* Highly active antiretroviral treatment
HACEK group, identification of, 47
Haemophilus
  Gram stain identification of, 49b
  processing, isolation, and identification of, 52
Haemophilus aprophilus in HACEK group, 47
Haemophilus influenzae
  ampicillin-resistant, 120
  buccal cellulitis due to, 170, 170f
  cellulitis due to, in children, 417-418, 418f
  first-choice and alternative antibiotics for, 113t
  infection occurrence of, 102b
  in labyrinthitis, 322
  in maxillary sinusitis, 314
  in maxillofacial cellulitis, 302-303, 303f
  in otitis media, 320
  in pediatric upper face infections, 412
  penicillin resistance of, 116
  in preseptal cellulitis, 330-332, 331f
  susceptibility testing of, 55
  in tonsillitis, 323
  type b
    in epiglottitis, 324-325
    meningitis due to, 50
Haemophilus influenzae cellulitis, maxillofacial manifestations of, 435-436, 435f
Haemophilus parainfluenzae in postoperative wounds, 400, 400t
Hageman factor (Factor XII). *See* Factor XII (Hageman factor)
Hair follicles
  anatomy of, 294-295
  furunculosis of, 313
  infections of, 299
Hairy leukoplakia in HIV/AIDS, 462
Half-life, plasma, 106
Halitosis in ANUGP, 140
Hand washing
  neglect of, 473
  in preventing nosocomial infection, 468
  as protection against viruses, 479
Hand-foot-mouth disease, 268-269
  pediatric, 420
Head
  deep spaces of, 189b
    borders of, 194t
  fasciae of, anatomy of, 189-192, 190f
  fascial infections in, 188-189
  infections of, with simultaneous eye/neck infections, 341-342
  skin of, 295-296
  venous drainage of, 212f
Head and neck cancer, postoperative infections and, 406
Head and neck infections
  in diabetic patients, 458-459
  pediatric, 412b
Head and neck surgery. *See also* Surgical wounds, head and neck
  infections after, 399-409
    antibiotic selection for, 403
    oral cavity decontamination and, 402-403

Head and neck surgery—cont'd
  infections after—cont'd
    patient factors in, 401
    prophylaxis of, 402
    reoperation and, 405-406
    treatment factors in, 402
    tumor factors in, 401-402
Headache, neurological exam for, 347
Health care workers, HIV infection risk of, 480
Hearing loss
  infection-induced, 347
  sensorineural, 322
Heart, septal defect of, and predisposition to infection, 354
Heart rate, pediatric, 411t
Heavy chains, immunoglobulin, 6
Heck's disease, 268
Heerfordt's syndrome, 292
Helcococcus, Gram stain identification of, 49b
Helicobacter, Gram stain identification of, 49b
Helicobacter pylori, 34t
  plaque and, 31
Helper lymphocytes, 456
Hematocrit, pediatric values for, 411t
Hematology, pediatric, 411t
Hematomas
  antibiotic therapy for, 367t
  maxillofacial, 371-372
  in neck dissection, 404f
  septal, 313
Hemispora, 38
Hemoglobin, pediatric values for, 411t
Hemorrhagic bullous otitis externa, 319
Hemostasis
  components of, 18
  in wound management, 364
Hepatitis B virus
  nucleic acid amplification strategies for, 51
  spread of, 478-479
Hepatitis C virus, nucleic acid amplification strategies for, 51
Herald bleeds, 207
Herpangina, 268-269
  pediatric, 420
Herpes laryngitis, 326
Herpes simplex infections
  antibiotics for, 123-124
  of brain, 350
  CD4 count in, 462
  characteristics and pathogenicity of, 38
  diagnosis of, 45
  of external ear canal, 319
  in herpetic whitlow, 479-480
  immunofluorescent assay of, 50
  oral, in neutropenic patient, 463
  PCR assays for, 51
  pediatric, 419-420
  skin resurfacing and, 396-397
Herpes zoster ophthalmicus, 342-343, 342f, 343f
Herpes zoster oticus, 319
Herpes zoster virus, 265-266
  pathogenesis, clinical characteristics, diagnosis, treatment of, 259t
Herpesvirus infections, 258, 259t-260t, 261-268
  cytomegalovirus, 260t, 266-267
  Epstein-Barr virus, 259t, 263-264

Herpesvirus infections—cont'd
    herpes simplex, 259t, 261-263, 261f, 262f
    papillomavirus, 260t, 267-268
    pediatric, 419-420
    varicella-zoster virus, 259t, 264-266
Herpetic whitlow, 479-480
Hexachlorophene, disinfectant activity of, 479t
Hiatus semilunaris, 69
High-efficiency particulate air-filtered systems, 475
Highly active antiretroviral treatment for AIDS, 255, 274-275
Histamine, inflammatory effects of, 18-19
Histatins, characteristics and functions of, 3
Histoplasma, processing, isolation, and identification of, 53
Histoplasma capsulatum
    in histoplasmosis, 245
    processing, isolation, and identification of, 54
Histoplasmosis, 243-245, 244b
    pediatric, 421
HIV. *See* Human immunodeficiency virus
HIV-associated gingivitis, 144-145
HIV-associated periodontitis, 144-145
H₂O₂, bactericidal effect of, 4
Hollinshead, nomenclature of, 189
Holmes, Oliver Wendell, 469
Holyoke, numbered spaces of, 191-192, 191f
Hormodendrum, 38
Hormones
    gingivitis and, 130
    in periodontal disease, 133
Horner's syndrome, 207
Host. *See also* Patient
    defense mechanisms of. *See* Defense mechanisms
    immunocompromised. *See* Immunocompromised host
    microbial interactions with, 1-2, 1f, 38-39
    resistance of, 40
    role of, in surgical infection, 475
Human bites
    antibiotic therapy for, 366
    maxillofacial infections from, 307
Human immunodeficiency virus, 273-275
Human immunodeficiency virus infection
    fungal infections associated with, 477t
    gingivitis associated with, 144-145
    health worker protection against, 480
    immune deficiency due to, 461-462
    mumps and, 290
    nucleic acid amplification strategies for, 51
    opportunistic infections and, 39, 144
    pathogenesis, characteristics, diagnosis, treatment of, 269t
    periodontal disease and, 144-145
    pneumocytosis in, 255
    postoperative, 376
    salivary gland infection and, 291
Human papillomavirus, 267-268
    nucleic acid probe for detecting, 51
    oral manifestations of, 462
    pathogenesis, clinical characteristics, diagnosis, treatment of, 260t
Human T-cell lymphotrophic virus, nucleic acid amplification strategies for, 51
Humoral defenses, 6-9
    complement system in, 8-9, 8f
    immunoglobulins in, 6-8, 7f

Humoral immune system, 456
Huxley, Thomas Henry, 473
Hydroxyapatite implants, bacteria retention by, 387
Hyperalimentation, fungal infections associated with, 477t
Hyperbaric oxygen for osteomyelitis of jaw, 224, 238-239, 238f
Hyperglycemia, postoperative wound infections and, 401
Hypersensitivity reaction, delayed cutaneous, 14
    anergy and, 15
Hypersensitivity reactions, 108
    delayed, 108-109
Hypersensitivity *versus* immunity, 26
Hypoglobus, 329

I

IFN-γ. *See* γ-Interferon
Ileum, immunoglobulin concentrations in, 5t
Imaging techniques. *See* Diagnostic imaging
Imipenem
    with aminoglycoside, indications for, 113t
    indications for, 119
    microbes susceptible to, 56t
    pediatric dosages for, 415t
Immediators, function of, 15
Immotile-cilia syndrome, immune system impacts of, 4
Immune complex injury, 27
Immune response
    antibiotic-induced suppression of, 38
    compromised, 100. *See also* Immunocompromised host; Immunodeficiency states
        conditions causing, 355
        odontogenic infection and, 165
    to organ transplants, 460-461
    status of, periodontal disease and, 144
Immune system
    anesthesia effects on, 452-453
    humoral, 456
    mucosal, 5, 5t
Immunity
    cell-mediated, 13
    versus hypersensitivity, 26
    transfer of, 14
Immunizations
    for *C. tetani,* 368
    rabies, 308
    tetanus, 307, 307t
Immunocompromised host, 456-457, 456-467
    causes of deficiency in, 456-457
        acquired, 457-458, 457b
        neoplastic, 462-464
        nonneoplastic, 458-462
            aging, 460
            alcoholism/liver disease, 459
            collagen vascular disease, 461
            corticosteroids, 461
            diabetes, 458-459
            HIV/AIDS, 461-462
            IV drug use, 459-460
            malnutrition, 460
            organ transplant, 460-461
            renal disease, 459
            splenectomy, 458
    infection in, 355-356
    infection prevention/management in, 464, 464b

Immunocompromised host—cont'd
    medicolegal issues with, 487
    nomalike lesions in, 432
    oral pathogens in, 463b
    Pseudomonas infections in, 472-473
    response to infection of, 456
Immunodeficiency states
    acquired, 457-464, 457b
        aging-related, 460
        from alcohol abuse/liver disease, 459
        from collagen vascular disease, 461
        corticosteroid-related, 461
        from diabetes mellitus, 458-459
        granulocyte disorders, 457, 457b
        from HIV/AIDS, 461-462
        from IV drug use, 459-460
        from malnutrition, 460
        in organ transplant recipient, 460-461
        from renal disease, 459
        from splenectomy, 458
    cellular, 457b, 458
    humoral, 457b, 458
    primary, 456-457
Immunoglobulin(s)
    classes of, 6, 6t
    concentrations of, in secretory organs, 5t
    in humoral defense, 6-8, 7f
    properties of, 6t
    protective mechanism of, 5
    receptors for, 10
    secretory, microbial interference by, 5
    synthesis of, 6
Immunoglobulin A
    properties of, 6t
    in secretions, 5
    structure of, 7
    subclasses of, 7
    synthesis of, 5
Immunoglobulin D
    immunological activity of, 8
    properties of, 6t
    structure of, 6-7
Immunoglobulin E
    immunological activity of, 8
    properties of, 6t
    structure of, 6-7
    synthesis of, 5
Immunoglobulin G
    classic pathway activation by, 8
    immunological activity of, 8
    properties of, 6t
    structure of, 6-7
    subclasses of, 7
    synthesis of, 5
Immunoglobulin M
    classic pathway activation by, 8
    immunological activity of, 8
    properties of, 6t
    structure of, 7
Immunological injury, mechanisms of, 26-27
    in type I reaction, 26
    in type II reaction, 26
    in type III reaction, 26-27
Immunological privilege, 340, 349

Immunosuppression
    candidiasis and, 248-249
    cytomegalovirus infection and, 266-267
    P. carinii pneumonia and, 255
Immunosuppressive drugs, 100
Impaction, tooth removal for, in compromised hosts, 165-166
Impetigo
    bullous, 302
    staphylococcal, 302, 418
    streptococcal, 418
        of maxillofacial region, 297-298, 298f
Implantitis, apical, 384-386, 385b, 385f, 386f
Implants, 381-391
    adjacent endodontic lesions and, 382
    alloplastic
        infections and, 397
        selection criteria for, 395
    classification of, 382
    craniofacial, 387, 388f, 389
    endosseous, 381
        in craniofacial reconstruction, 387, 388f, 389
        versus transosseous, 382
    failures of, 383-384
    immediate placement of, 382-383
    infections associated with, 383
        apical implantitis, 384-386, 385f
        early, 383-384, 384f
        iatrogenic, 384, 385f
        miscellaneous, 389, 389f
        periimplantitis, 386-387, 388f, 389
        sequestrum/involucrum formation and, 389, 389f
    periodontal disease and, 383
    polytetrafluoroethylene, 395
    preparation for, prophylaxis in, 381-383
Incisions
    guidelines for, 163
    surgical, infection management and, 100
Indium 111, white blood cells tagged with, 65
Infants
    microbes found in, 30
    osteomyelitis of jaw in, 227-228, 228f
Infection(s), 1-29
    bacterial
        hydrostatic pressure in spread of, 188
    deep space, medicolegal issues with, 487
    diagnosis of, 99
    effects of
        from bacterial toxins, 22-25
        nonspecific, 15-21
        vascular, 21-22
    factors involved in, 1
    identifying causative organism in, 101-103, 102t
    in immunocompromised host, 26-27, 456-467. *See also*
        Immunocompromised host
    microbe attachment in, 39
    nosocomial. *See* Nosocomial infections
    odontogenic. *See* Odontogenic infections
    ophthalmic considerations in. *See* Ophthalmic
        considerations
    opportunistic, 39. *See also* Immunocompromised host
        HIV and, 144
    pathogenicity of, 39
    postoperative, management of host factors in, 376-378, 377b,
        377f

Infection(s)—cont'd
  recurrent, 109
  response to
    arachidonic acid metabolites and, 19-20
    cell-derived mediators of inflammation and, 18-19
    coagulation system and, 17-18
    cytokines in, 20-21
    fibrinolytic system and, 17-18
    kinin system and, 15, 16f, 17
    lysosomal granule contents in, 20
    plasma-derived mediators in, 15
  secondary, 109
  superimposed, 38
  virulence of, 39
  wounds and, 25-26, 26t
Infection control
  barrier techniques in, 479-480
  medicolegal aspects of, 486
  OSHA guidelines for, 480-481
Infection management, 99-111
  antibiotic administration in, 106-107
    combination, 107
    determining dose for, 106
    route for, 107
    time interval for, 106-107
  antibiotic cost and, 105
  antibiotic history and, 105
  antibiotic therapy in, 100-111
    choosing agent for, 101-106
  assessment in, 99
  bactericidal *versus* bacteriostatic drugs in, 104-105
  causes of failure of, 108b
  determining antibiotic sensitivity in, 103
  host defenses and, 99-100
  least toxic antibiotic for, 104
  in outpatient facilities, 478-479, 479t
  patient compliance in, 105-106
  patient drug history and, 104
  patient monitoring in, 107-111
    for adverse reactions, 108-109
    in maxillofacial surgery, 109-111
    for response to treatment, 107-108
    for superinfection/recurrent infection, 109
  specific, narrow-spectrum agents in, 104
  surgical drainage and incision in, 100
Infectious mononucleosis, 266
Inflammation
  cell-derived mediators of, 18-19
  coagulation and fibrinolysis links with, 17-18
  mechanisms of, 16f
  plasma-derived mediators of, 15
Inflammatory conditions, 73-77
  cat-scratch disease, 432-433, 433f-434f
  erysipelas, 434-435, 435f
  fungal, 423-429
    aspergillosis, 423-426, 424f, 425f
    noma, 430-432, 430f, 431f, 432f
    rhinocerebral mucormycosis, 426-429, 426f, 427f, 428f, 429f
  Haemophilus influenzae cellulitis, 435-436, 435f
  infectious arthritis of TMJ, 436-437, 436f
  infectious sinusitis, 73-74, 73f
    complications of, 75-77
  orbital, 91-92
  uncommon, 423-438

Inflammatory system in severe infection, 24
Influenza virus
  immunoassay of, 51
  immunofluorescent assay of, 50
  in mumps, 290
Informed consent, process for, 485
Infraorbital space
  borders of, 194t
  infection of, causes, contents, and neighboring spaces of, 195t
Infratemporal space, infection of, causes, contents, and neighboring spaces of, 195t
Instruments, sterilization of, 479
Intensive care unit, nosocomial infections in, 468-471, 469t
γ-Interferon, immunologic functions of, 10
Interleukin(s)
  immunologic functions of, 14
  in sepsis, 24
Interleukin-1
  endotoxin and, 22
  in fever, 24-25
  inflammatory effects of, 21
Interleukin-3, 3
Interleukin-8, antimicrobial peptide interaction with, 3
Intermediate Restorative Material procedure, 151
Intermediators, function of, 15
Intraorbital space, infections of, 209, 209f, 210f
Intrinsic coagulation cascade, 17
Intubation, difficulties with, 442
Iodine, disinfectant activity of, 479t
Iodophors, disinfectant activity of, 479t
Irrigation, wound, 364-365
Irrigation-suction, closed wound, for osteomyelitis of jaw, 223-224, 223f
Ishihara color test, 329
Isotretinoin therapy, 302
Itraconazole
  for maxillofacial infections, 122
  pharmacology of, 123t
  side effects of, 123

J

J protein, 7
Jaws, osteomyelitis of, 214-242. *See also* Osteomyelitis
JC polyoma virus
  in immunocompromised host, 356
  PCR assays for, 51
Jejunum, immunoglobulin concentrations in, 5t
Jet ventilation, 451
Job syndrome, 457
Johnsonella, Gram stain identification of, 49b
Joint infections, intravenous drug use and, 459

K

Kaposi's sarcoma in AIDS patients, 274
Keflex. *See* Cephalexin
Keftab. *See* Cephalexin
Kefurox. *See* Cefuroxime
Kefzol. *See* Cefazolin
Keratin, protective function of, 2
Keratinocytes, regulatory proteins of, 3
Keratopathy
  exposure, 343-344, 343f
  neurotrophic, 344, 344f

Ketaconazole
    for maxillofacial infections, 122
    pharmacology of, 123t
Kidney transplant, fungal infections associated with, 477t
Kingella, Gram stain identification of, 49b
Kingella kingae in HACEK group, 47
Kinin system, 15, 17
    interrelationships of, 15, 16f
Kinyoun carbol-fuschin method, 48-49
Klebsiella
    infection occurrence of, 102b
    life-threatening infection from, 159f
    in necrotizing external otitis, 318
    in osteomyelitis, 217
Klebsiella oxytoca, percent susceptibility of, 55t
Klebsiella pneumoniae
    first-choice and alternative antibiotics for, 113t
    percent susceptibility of, 55t
    in postoperative wounds, 400, 400t
Kurthia, Gram stain identification of, 49b

L

Laboratory. *See also* Diagnostic techniques
    role of, 43
Labyrinthitis, 321-322
    labyrinthine fistula, 322
    luetic, 322
    serous, 321
    suppurative, 321-322
    toxic, 322
    varicella-zoster, 322
Lacerations
    antibiotic therapy for, 367t
    maxillofacial, 372-373
    traumatic, maxillofacial infections of, 306
Lacrimal sac, infection of, 340-341, 340f
Lacrimal secretions, immunoglobulin concentrations in, 5t
Lactam antibiotics. *See* β-Lactam antibiotics
Lactobacilli in pulpal tissue, 148
Lactobacillus, 34t
    caries due to, 35
    Gram stain identification of, 49b
Lactococcus, Gram stain identification of, 49b
Lactoferrin, function of, 3
Lagophthalmos, 343, 343f
Langerhans cells, regulatory proteins of, 3
Lanthionine, 4
Lantibiotics, characteristics of, 4
Laryngeal carcinoma, neck swelling due to, 310
Laryngeal mask airway in airway management, 450
Laryngitis
    acute, 324
    herpes, 326
Laryngoscopy, contraindications to, 443
Laryngotracheal diphtheria, 326
Laryngotracheitis, acute, 325-326, 325f
Larynx, anatomy of, 324
Latex agglutination, 50-51
Laufman, H., 473, 474
Lectin, mannose-binding, 9
Legionella
    Gram stain identification of, 49b
    susceptibility testing of, 54
Legionella pneumophila, immunofluorescent assay of, 50

Leishmaniasis, 275-276
    diffuse cutaneous, 275, 276f
    localized cutaneous, 275
    mucocutaneous, 275-276
    visceral, 276
Leptotricha buccalis, 36t
Leptotrichia
    Gram stain identification of, 49b
    in infants, 30
Leukemia, fungal infections associated with, 477t
Leukocidin, 22
Leukocyte surface antigens, 10
Leukocytes
    mobilization of, 11
    myoskeleton of, 10
Leukocytosis, diagnostic significance of, 46
Leukoplakia, 250, 250f
    in AIDS patients, 274
Leukotrienes, inflammatory effects of, 20
Level of consciousness, assessment of, 347
Levofloxacin, microbes susceptible to, 56t
Liability, physician, 484
Lid retraction, 344, 344f
Ligase chain reaction, diagnostic uses of, 51
Light chains, immunoglobulin, 6
Linezolid. *See* Oxazolidinone
Lipopolysaccharide-binding protein, 22
Lipopolysaccharides in pulpal disease, 148
Lipoteichoic acid, microbial interference by, 4
Lipoxins, inflammatory effects of, 20
Lipoxygenase pathway, 19
Lister, Joseph, 469, 470f
Listeria
    bacteriocin activity against, 4
    Gram stain identification of, 49b
Listeria monocytogenes, meningitis due to, 50-51
Liver disease, immune deficiency due to, 459
Lomefloxacin
    dosage of, with normal/impaired renal function, 122t
    microbes susceptible to, 56t
Lorabid. *See* Loracarbef
Loracarbef
    microbes susceptible to, 56t
    pediatric dosages for, 415t
    pharmacology of, 119t
Ludwig's angina, 84, 177-181, 178f, 179f, 188
    case reports of, 180
    in pediatric maxillofacial infections, 414, 414f
    submandibular/sublingual spaces and, 198-199
Luetic labyrinthitis, 322
Lumbar puncture, meningitis diagnosis with, 352-353
Lyme disease
    head and neck infections from, 308-309
    and predisposition to infection, 355
Lyme meningitis, 353
    MRI changes in, 351, 351f
Lymph nodes
    cervical, 89
    diagnostic imaging of, 89-91, 90f
    jugulodigastric, 90
    juguloomohyoid, 90
    parotid, 89
    positive findings in, with conjunctivitis, 341

Lymph nodes—cont'd
    retropharyngeal, 90
    spinal accessory, 90
    submandibular, 89, 90f
    submental, 89-90
Lymphadenitis
    defined, 297
    neck swelling due to, 311
    pediatric, 421t
Lymphangioma *versus* orbital cellulitis, 334, 334f
Lymphocytes
    B. *See* B lymphocytes
    cytokines of, 20-21
    defensive role of, 9-10
    differential characteristics of, 13t
    in Ig synthesis, 5
    immunologic function of, 13-15
    T. *See* T lymphocytes
Lymphocytic choriomeningitis virus, in mumps, 290
Lymphokines, 21
    activities of, 13-14
    nonimmunoglobulin, 13
Lymphoma
    Burkitt's, in children, 420
    fungal infections associated with, 477t
    versus orbital cellulitis, 334, 334f
Lymphosarcoma *versus* osteomyelitis of jaw, 218
Lysosomal granules, inflammatory effects of, 20
Lysosome, components of, 18

M

M protein, bacterial adherence and, 39
Macrolides
    contraindications to, 222
    dosages for, 120t
    for maxillofacial infections, 120-121, 120t
    for odontogenic infections, 164
    pediatric dosages for, 415t
Macrophage CSF, 3
Macrophage-activating factors, 12
Macrophages, immunologic function of, 12-13
Macule, characteristics of, 296
Magnetic resonance imaging
    diagnostic uses of, 63
    in osteomyelitis of jaw, 220
Maimonides, 468
Major histocompatibility complex, 13
Malignant external otitis in diabetic patient, 458-459
Mallampati distance test, 442
Malnutrition
    immune deficiency due to, 460
    noma associated with, 430
    in periodontal disease, 133
    postoperative infections and, 401
Mandible
    ascending ramus of, 205f
    fracture of, infection after, 370-371, 370f
    lingual surface of, 166f
    osteomyelitis of, 84-86, 85f, 215
        imaging of, 218-219, 218f, 219f
    space of body of, infections of, 197, 198f
Mandibular body space, diagnostic imaging of, 84-86, 85f

Mandibular odontogenic infections, deep spaces associated
        with, 197-208
    carotid sheath, 207
    danger, 207
    lateral pharyngeal, 204-205, 205f
    in mandibular body, 197, 198f
    masticator, 200-204, 201f, 202f, 203f
    mediastinum, 207-208, 208f
    parotid, 204, 204f
    pretracheal, 207
    retropharyngeal, 205-206
    sublingual, 197-198, 198f, 199f
    submandibular, 198-200, 199f
    submental, 200, 200f
    visceral, 207, 207f
Mandol. *See* Cefamandole
Mannose receptors, 9, 13
Mannose-binding lectin pathway, initiation of, 8f, 9
Mask ventilation, difficulties with, 442
Masks, surgical, 474
Mastication, muscles of, infections affecting, 446
Mastication sensitivity
    with pulpal necrosis, 147
    treatment of, 151
Masticator space
    cellulitis of, MRI scan of, 64f
    diagnostic imaging of, 86-87, 86f, 87f
    infections of, 171-173, 171f, 172f, 173f, 200-204
        deep temporal, 203-204, 203f
        pterygomandibular, 201-202, 202f, 203f
        submasseteric, 200-201, 201f, 202f
        superficial temporal, 202-203
Maxillae
    anatomy of, 66
    osteomyelitis of, 215
Maxillary odontogenic infections, 209-213
    in cavernous sinus thrombosis, 211-213, 212f, 213f
    of infraorbital space, 209, 209f, 210f
    of orbital space, 210-211, 210f, 211f
    of palatal space, 209
    of periorbital space, 210
Maxillary sinuses, 66, 66f, 67f, 68, 68f
    infection of, 314, 314f
        neurological aspects of, 356
Maxillofacial infections, 112-125. *See also* Maxillofacial
        trauma
    airways in, 439-440, 439f
    antifungal agents for, 121-123, 123t
    antiviral agents for, 123-124
    β-lactams for, 112
    cabapenems for, 119
    cephalosporins for, 118-119, 118t, 119t
    chloramphenicol for, 120
    contiguous spread of, 330
    macrolides for, 120-121, 120t
    monobactams for, 119
    nitroimidazoles for, 121
    pediatric. *See* Pediatric maxillofacial infections
    penicillins for, 112, 116, 116f, 117t, 118
    quinolones for, 121, 122t
    tetracyclines for, 119-120
    vancomycin for, 120

Maxillofacial soft tissue infections
  after trauma, 369-370
    facial, 370
    periauricular, 370
    perinasal, 369-370
    perioral, 369
    periorbital, 370
    of scalp, 370
  manifestations of, 296-297, 296b
  neck swelling in, 310-311
  nontraumatic, 305-306
    anthrax, 305
    cervicofacial actinomycosis, 305-306
  pathogenesis of, 296, 296b
  postoperative, 378
  pyogenic bacterial, 297-305
    staphylococcal
      of adnexal structures, 298-302, 299f, 300f, 301f
      cellulitis, 302-303, 303f
      impetigo, 302, 303f
      necrotizing fasciitis, 303-305, 304f
    streptococcal, 297-298
      erysipelas, 298, 298f
      impetigo, 297-298, 298f
      scarlet fever, 297
  from sepsis, 309-310
  traumatic, 306-309
    from animal bites, 308
    from cat-scratch disease, 308
    from human bites, 307
    from Lyme disease, 308-309
    from rabies, 308
    from tetanus, 306-307, 307t
Maxillofacial soft tissues, trauma to, 369-370
  infection prevention after, 372b
  management of, 372b
Maxillofacial surgery, antibiotic therapy in, 109-111
  for abscess, 110
  with fractures, 110
  for osteomyelitis, 110
  for pericoronitis, 110
  for soft tissue wounds, 110
Maxillofacial trauma, infection after, 359-380
  antibiotic therapy in, 366-368, 367t, 368t, 369t
  cardiovascular response to, 359
  debridement of necrotic tissue in, 365
  drain placement in, 365
  endocrine/metabolic response to, 360
  focused wound exam in, 364
  fracture fixation/immobilization in, 365
  hemostasis in, 364
  imaging evaluation in, 364
  irrigation/foreign body removal in, 364-365
  pathophysiology of, 359-363
  preventing secondary contamination in, 368-369
  pulmonary response to, 359-360
  soft tissue repair in, 365-366
  systemic history in, 363-364
  wound culture in, 364
  wound response and, 360-363, 360f, 362f
Maxipime. *See* Cefepime
Measles, 420
  German, 272-273
    pathogenesis, characteristics, diagnosis, treatment of, 269t

Measles virus, 272
  pathogenesis, characteristics, diagnosis, treatment of, 269t
Mediastinitis, 184-185, 184f
Mediastinum, infections of, 207-208, 208f
Medications. *See* Antibiotic therapy; Drugs; specific agents
Medicolegal issues, 484-487
  antibiotic-related, 486-487
  with compromised host, 487
  with deep space infections, 487
  with osteomyelitis, 487
  in physician-patient interactions, 484-485
  in records and communication, 486
  tort law, 484
Mefoxin. *See* Cefoxitin
Megamonas, Gram stain identification of, 49b
Megasphaera, Gram stain identification of, 49b
Melanocytes, regulatory proteins of, 3
Meningeal irritation, neurological exam for, 347
Meningitis
  bacterial, diagnosis of, 50
  as complication of orbital cellulitis, 336
  in cryptococcosis, 256
  lumbar puncture in diagnosis of, 352-353
  Lyme, 353
    MRI changes in, 351, 351f
  management of, 357
  mumps-related, 271
  pediatric, 413
  sinusitis associated with, 76
Meningoencephalitis
  amoebic, pediatric, 421, 421t
  as complication of viral mumps, 291
Menstruation, pH changes during, 4
Meomycin sulfate for maxillofacial trauma patient, 367t
Meropenem
  indications for, 119
  microbes susceptible to, 56t
  pediatric dosages for, 415t
Methanol, specimen fixation with, 47
Methicillin
  antimicrobial spectrum of, 117t
  indications for, 105
  staphylococcal resistance to, 471-472
Methylobacterium, Gram stain identification of, 49b
Metronidazole
  for anaerobic bacterial infections, 111
  antimicrobial spectrum of, 115b
  bacterial sensitivity to, 103
  bacterial susceptibility to, 55t
  blood brain barrier and, 357
  as first-choice antibiotic, 113t
  indications for, 113t
  for maxillofacial infections, 121
  for osteomyelitis of jaw, 222
  pediatric dosages for, 415t
  pharmacology of, 114t
Mezlin. *See* Mezlocillin
Mezlocillin
  antimicrobial spectrum of, 117t
  limitations of, 116, 118
  microbial susceptibility to, 56t
  pediatric dosages for, 415t
  pharmacology of, 117t
Microbacterium, Gram stain identification of, 49b

Microbes. *See also* specific classes; specific microbes
    attachment of, 39
    commensal, 53
    pathogenic potential of, 1
    quantity of, 1
    relationships with host, 1-2, 1f
    virulence of, 1
Microbial interference, 4-5
Microbiological diagnostic techniques. *See* Diagnostic techniques
Micrococcus, Gram stain identification of, 49b
Microfilaments, immunologic function of, 10-11
Microscopy, dark-field, 50
Microstatin. *See* Nystatin
Microtubules, immunologic function of, 10-11
Midface
    ascending infection of, 356, 356f
    fractures of, infection after, 371
Mikulicz's disease, 93
Miller, W. D., 132
Minimum inhibitory concentration, 106
Minocycline
    indications for, 113t
    for periodontal disease, 137
Mitsuokella, Gram stain identification of, 49b
Molars
    extraction of, chronic sinusitis and, 316
    impacted, infections of, 176-177, 176f, 177f
    maxillary, sinus infections and, 68
Molecular testing, 59
Monobactams for maxillofacial infections, 119
Monocid. *See* Cefonicid
Monoclonal antibodies, immunologic function of, 10
Monocytes
    complement receptors on, 9-10
    Fc receptors in, 10
    immunologic function of, 12-13
Monokines, 21
Mononuclear phagocytes, 12-13
Mononucleosis, infectious, 266
Moraxella
    in animal bite infections, 308
    Gram stain identification of, 49b
Moraxella catarrhalis, 34t
    in maxillary sinusitis, 314
Morganella morganii, percent susceptibility of, 55t
Motor paresis, neurological assessment of, 348
Mouth. *See also* Oral cavity
    normal flora of, 330
Moxifloxacin
    administration of, 121
    dosage of, with normal/impaired renal function, 122t
    indications for, 121
99mTc phosphate. *See* Technetium 99m phosphate
Mucocele, 75-76
    as complication of sinusitis, 316-317, 317f
    sinus, 71, 71f
Mucopyocele, 317
Mucor
    azoles for treating, 122
    in immunocompromised host, 356
    in mucormycosis, 426
    in rhinoorbital-cerebral mucormycosis, 336
    sinusitis due to, 76-77

Mucoralis in mucormycosis, 253-254
Mucormycosis, 76-77, 253-254, 254b, 254f
    case report of, 428-429
    CNS, 254
    cutaneous, 254, 254f
    in diabetic patient, 458-459
    gastrointestinal, 254
    paralysis due to, 347
    pediatric, 421
    pulmonary, 254
    rhinocerebral, 253-254, 254f, 426-429, 426f, 427f, 428f, 429f
    rhinoorbital-cerebral, 336-338
    of sinuses, 316
Mucosal immune system, 5, 5t
Mucous membrane, immune functions of, 5, 5t
Mucous retention cysts, 75, 75f
Mumps, 420
    causes and complications of, 290-291
    diagnostic imaging of, 92
    pathogenesis, characteristics, diagnosis, treatment of, 269t
Mumps virus, 271-272
Muscles, facial, anatomy of, 209f, 294
Mycelex. *See* Clotrimazole
Mycobacterium
    infections due to, atypical, 291
    processing, isolation, and identification of, 52-53
    in salivary gland infections, 291
    susceptibility testing of, 59
Mycobacterium avium-intracellulare in salivary gland infection, 291
Mycobacterium catarrhalis in tonsillitis, 323
Mycobacterium genavense, PCR assays for, 51
Mycobacterium tuberculosis
    nucleic acid amplification strategies for, 51
    in osteomyelitis, 217
    salivary gland infection with, 291
Mycoplasma bucalle, 37t
Mycoplasma catarrhalis, in otitis media, 320
Mycoplasma hominis, 37t
Mycoplasma in bullous external otitis, 319
Mycoplasma orale, 37t
Mycoplasma penetrans, 37t
    characteristics and pathogenicity of, 37
Mycoplasma pneumoniae
    characteristics and pathogenicity of, 37
    first-choice and alternative antibiotics for, 113t
Mycoplasma salivarium, 37t
    characteristics and pathogenicity of, 37
Mycotic infections. *See* Fungal infections
Myroides, Gram stain identification of, 49b

N

Nafcil. *See* Nafcillin
Nafcillin
    antimicrobial spectrum of, 117t
    limitations of, 116, 118
    for maxillofacial trauma patient, 367t
    pediatric dosages for, 416t
    pharmacology of, 117t
Nasal cavities, bacteria colonizing, 349
Nasal infections, 313-317. *See also* Sinus infections
    furunculosis/carbunculosis, 313
    pediatric, 419
    septal abscess, 313

Nasal secretions, immunoglobulin concentrations in, 5t
Nasolacrimal duct, obstruction of, 340-341
Nasopharynx
    anatomy of, 322
    bacterial colonization of, 474
    commensal organisms of, 53
    normal flora of, 330
Nasoseptal surgery, infection after, 393, 393f-394f, 395
Nasotracheal intubation, 447
    fiberoptic, 448, 448f
    with lighted stylet guidance, 448
    versus orotracheal, 446-447
National Nosocomial Infection Surveillance System, 400, 401,
        469t, 470-471
National Research Council, wound classification of, 400
Natural killer cells, 13
Neck
    deep fascial spaces of, 189b
    deep spaces of, borders of, 194t
    fasciae of, anatomy of, 189-192, 190f, 191f
    fascial infections in, 188-189
    infections of, with simultaneous eye/head infections,
        341-342
    skin of, 295-296
    swelling of, differential diagnosis of, 310-311
Necrotic tissue, debridement of
    conservative, 365
    in head and neck surgery, 404
Necrotizing fasciitis, 195, 196f
    after dacryocystorhinostomy surgery, 331, 331f
    after implant surgery, 389
    maxillofacial, 303-305, 304f
    pediatric, 419
Necrotizing ulcerative periodontitis in HIV/AIDS, 462
Needles, disease transmission by, 479
Neisseria
    in animal bite infections, 308
    Gram stain identification of, 49b
    in periodontal abscess, 139
    processing, isolation, and identification of, 52
Neisseria gonorrhoeae
    first-choice and alternative antibiotics for, 113t
    nucleic acid amplification strategies for, 51
    nucleic acid probe for detecting, 51
    in pharyngitis, 323
    pharyngitis due to, 45
    susceptibility testing of, 54, 55
Neisseria meningitidis
    in labyrinthitis, 322
    meningitis due to, 50
    susceptibility testing of, 54
Neisseria sicca, 34t
    disease due to, 35
Neisseriasubflava, 34t
Neomycin sulfate for maxillofacial trauma patient, 367t
Neonates
    acute bacterial parotitis in, 283-284
    congenital rubella syndrome of, 273
    microbes found in, 30
Neoplasms, neck swelling due to, 310-311
Nerve blocks, 444-445
    for controlling gag reflex, 447
Nervous system, pathways to, 349-350
Neuralgia, postherpetic, 265

Neurogenic bladder, urinary tract infections and, 4
Neurological considerations, 347-358. *See also* Nervous system
    and facial soft tissue, bone, sinus infections, 354, 354f
    physical exam for, 347-349. *See also* Neurological examination
Neurological examination
    for cranial nerve dysfunction, 347-348
    for headache, 347
    for level of consciousness, 347
    for meningeal irritation, 347
    for motor paresis, 348
Neurological infection
    diagnosis of, 350-353
        tools for, 350-353, 351f, 352f, 353f
    oral/facial surgery and, 353-354
    trauma-related, 353
Neurotrophic keratopathy, 344, 344f
Neutropenia, 462-463
Nisin, 4
Nitrofurantoin, microbes susceptible to, 56t
Nitroimidazoles for maxillofacial infections, 121
Nizoral. *See* Ketaconazole
Nocardia
    acid fastness in, 49
    Gram stain identification of, 49b
    in immunocompromised host, 356
    in maxillofacial soft tissue infections, 306
    in nosocomial infections, 477
Nocardia asteroides in osteomyelitis of jaw, 235
Nocardia brasiliensis in osteomyelitis of jaw, 235
Nocardia farcinica in osteomyelitis of jaw, 235
Nocardia nova in osteomyelitis of jaw, 235
Nocardia otitidiscaviarum in osteomyelitis of jaw, 235
Nocardia transvalensis in osteomyelitis of jaw, 235
Nocardiopsis, Gram stain identification of, 49b
Nocardium in osteomyelitis of jaw, 234-235, 235f
Nodules, characteristics of, 297
Noma, 418-419, 419f
    maxillofacial manifestations of, 430-432, 430f, 431f, 432f
Nomenclature, Hollinshead's, 189
Noncompliance, patient, 487
Norfloxacin, microbes susceptible to, 56t
North American blastomycosis, 247, 247b
Nose. *See also* Nasal cavities
    commensal organisms of, 53
    infections of. *See* Nasal infections
    normal flora of, 330
Nosocomial infections
    deaths caused by, 468
    fungal, 477-478, 477t
    in ICU, 468-471, 469t
    NNIS program for, 400-401, 401t
    preventing, 368-369
    from surgical wounds, 473
Nuclear medicine, diagnostic uses of, 63-65, 64f
Nucleic acid probes, 51
Nutritional deficiencies. *See* Malnutrition
Nystatin for maxillofacial infections, 123

O

Occlusal loading in periodontal disease, 133
Occupational Safety and Health Administration, infection
        control guidelines of, 480-481
Oculoglandular conjunctivitis, Parinaud's, 341-342

Odontogenic infections, 158-168, 192-213
    of buccal space, 170-171, 170f
    of canine space, 168-169, 169f
    cavernous sinus thrombosis, 169-170
    deep spaces associated with, 193, 194t, 195-197, 195t,
            196f, 197f
        buccal, 195-197, 197f
        subcutaneous, 195, 196f
        vestibular, 193, 195, 196f
    examination for, 159
    historical perspective on, 158
    of impacted third molar teeth, 176-177, 176f, 177f
    life-threatening, 158-159
    Ludwig's angina, 177-181, 178f, 179f
    mandibular, 197-208. *See also* Mandibular odontogenic
            infections
    of masticator spaces, 171-173, 171f, 172f, 173f
    maxillary, 209-213. *See also* Maxillary odontogenic infections
    mediastinitis, 184-185, 184f
    pathophysiology of, 159, 192, 192f
    pathways of, 161-162, 161f
    patient history and system review in, 160
    pediatric, 413, 414, 416-417
    of pharyngeal space, 181-182, 181f, 182f
    physical examination in, 161
    of retropharyngeal space, 182-183, 182f
    signs of, 159-160
    spread of, medicolegal aspects of, 487
    stages of, 192-193, 193t
    of submandibular/sublingual spaces, 173-175, 173f,
            174f, 175f
    of submental space, 175-176, 176f
    treatment of, 162-166
        anatomical considerations in, 166-168
        antibiotic therapy in, 162-164
        case reports of, 164-166
        incision and drainage in, 162
Odontoid, transoral approaches to, 354
Oerskovia, Gram stain identification of, 49b
Ofloxacin
    dosage of, with normal/impaired renal function, 122t
    microbes susceptible to, 56t
Omnicef. *See* Cefdinir
Oophoritis, mumps-related, 271
Operating room
    bioparticulate content of, 475
    decontamination of, 474-475
Ophthalmic considerations. *See also* Orbit, infections of
    in complications of maxillofacial infections, 343-345
    in orbital infections, 330-341
    in simultaneous infections of eye, head, neck, 341-343
Ophthalmicus, herpes zoster, 342-343, 342f, 343f
Ophthalmological examination, 161
Ophthalmoscopy, 330
Opioids for sedation/alangesia, 446
Opsonin
    deficiencies of, 11
    in phagocytosis, 11
Optic nerve
    assessment of, 329, 330
    in orbital cellulitis, 336
Oral cavity
    bacteria colonizing, 349
    decontamination of, in head and neck surgery, 402-403

Oral cavity—cont'd
    impaired drainage in, 4
    infections of, systemic disease and, 40
    of neonates/infants, 30
    normal flora of, 43
        changes in, 283
Oral hairy leukoplakia in HIV/AIDS, 462
Oral hygiene in immunocompromised host, 463, 464
Oral surgery and risk of infection, 353-354
Orbit. *See also* Eye(s); Ophthalmic considerations
    abnormalities of, 71-72, 72f
    anatomy of, 328-329
    cellulitis of, 76, 332-336, 332f
        causes of, 332
        complications of, 336, 338
        differential diagnosis of, 333-334, 334f
        imaging of, 334-335, 335f
        symptoms/signs of, 332-333, 333f
        treatment of, 335-336
    examination of, 329-330
    infections of
        allergic fungal sinusitis, 341
        cellulitis/abscess, 332-336, 332f, 333f, 334f, 335f
        classification of, 330
        dacryocystitis, 340-341, 340f
        fungal, 336-338
        posttraumatic, 370
        preseptal cellulitis, 330-332, 331f
        septic cavernous sinus thrombosis, 338-340, 339f
    inflammatory disorders of, 91-92
    pseudotumors of, 91-92
    in sinusitis, 317
    in spread of sinus infection, 328-329
Orbital apex syndrome, 338-339, 339f
Orbital space, infections of, 210-211, 210f, 211f
Orchitis as complication of mumps parotitis, 291
Organ transplants
    fungal infections associated with, 477t
    immune deficiency and, 460-461
Orofacial microbes. *See also* Bacteria; specific microbes
    acquisition and variation of, 30-31
    aerobic, 33t-34t
    anaerobic, 36t
    classification of, 33, 33t-34t
    in edentulous individuals, 30-31
    enterococci, 34, 34t
    factors regulating, 31-32, 31t
        dietary, 31t, 32
        saliva, 31-32, 31t
    fungi/yeasts, 37-38
    gram-negative cocci, 34t, 35
    gram-positive cocci, 34-35, 34t
    gram-positive rods and filaments, 35, 36t
    host interactions with, 38-40
        in parasitism, 38-39
        pathogenicity/virulence of, 39
        toxins and virulence factors in, 39-40
    host resistance to, 40
    mycoplasma, 37, 37t
    normal, 43, 283, 330, 349
    retention of, 32
    spirochetes, 37, 37t
    staphylococci, 33t, 34
    streptococci, 33-34

Orofacial microbes—cont'd
  taxa of, 30
  viruses, 38
Orofacial region, microbiology of, 30-42
Oropharynx
  anatomy of, 322
  commensal organisms of, 53
  normal flora of, 330
Osseointegration, 381
Osseous dysplasia, florid, 231, 231f
Osteitis
  condensing, 231, 231f
  condensing sclerosing, 150
Osteoid osteoma *versus* osteomyelitis of jaw, 218
Osteomyelitis
  brain infections due to, 349, 354
  versus cellulitis, 65
  chronic, 86, 86f
  conditions associated with, 215
  cultures in, 103
  development of, 162
  implant site susceptibility to, 389
  internal fixation hardware and, 378, 378f
  of jaw, 84-86, 85f, 214-242
    actinomycotic, 231-234, 232f, 233f, 234f
    acute suppurative, 217-218
    causative organisms in, 214
    chronic sclerosing, 230-231, 230f, 231f
    classification of, 214-215
    clinical findings in, 217-218
    condensing osteitis, 231
    defined, 214
    differential diagnosis of, 218-219
    etiology and pathogenesis of, 215-216
    with fractures, 226-227, 227f
    imaging techniques in, 218-220, 218f, 219f, 220f
    infantile, 227-228, 228f
    versus malignancy, 235
    microbiology of, 216-217
    nocardial, 234-235, 235f
    versus osteoradionecrosis, 236-237, 236f, 237f
    pathogenesis of, 216f
    pediatric, chronic, recurrent, multifocal, 228-229
    predisposing factors in, 215
    proliferative periostitis, 229-230, 229f
    treatment of, 221-226, 221b
      acute suppurative, 221
      with antibiotic-impregnated beads, 224, 224f
      antibiotics in, 221-224, 222b, 223f, 224f
      chronic suppurative, 222-223
      with closed wound irrigation-suction, 223-224, 223f
      decortication in, 225-226, 225f
      with hyperbaric oxygen, 238-239, 239f
      resection/reconstruction in, 226, 226f
      saucerization in, 225, 225f
      sequestrectomy in, 224-225
      surgery in, 224
  management of, 357
  in maxillofacial surgery, 110
  medicolegal issues with, 487
  pediatric, 416-417, 417f
  sinusitis associated with, 76
  specimen collection in, 46
Osteoradionecrosis of mandible, treatment protocol for, 239f

Osteoradionecrosis, 236-237, 236f, 237f
  prevention of, 239-240
Osteosarcoma *versus* osteomyelitis of jaw, 218
Ostiomeatal complex
  anatomy of, 69
  evaluation of, 72
Otitis externa
  acute, 318
  chronic, 318, 318f
  malignant, in diabetic patient, 458-459
  necrotizing, 318-319
Otitis media, 320-321
  acute, 320, 320f
  chronic
    complications of, 321, 321f
    with perforation, 320-321, 320f
    without perforation, 321
  serous, 320
Otoplasty, infection after, 397
Outpatient facilities, infection control in, 478-479, 479t
Oxacillin
  antimicrobial spectrum of, 115b, 117t
  microbial susceptibility to, 55t, 56t
  pediatric dosages for, 416t
  pharmacology of, 114t, 117t
Oxazolidinone quinolones for vancomycin-resistance staphylococci, 472
Oxygen, hyperbaric. *See* Hyperbaric oxygen
Oxygenation, assessing, 440

P

Paget's disease *versus* osteomyelitis of jaw, 218
Pain
  in pericoronitis, 142
  from periodontal abscess, 137-138
  pulpal, 149
Palatal space, infections of, 209
Palatectomy in mucormycosis, 429, 429f
Pancreatitis, mumps, 290-291
Papain for Ig fragmentation, 6
Papillomavirus, human. *See* Human papillomavirus
Papules, characteristics of, 296
Paracoccidioides, processing, isolation, and identification of, 53
Paracoccidioides brasiliensis in South American blastomycosis, 247-248
Paracoccidioidomycosis, 247-248, 248b
Parainfluenza virus
  immunofluorescent assay of, 50
  in mumps, 290
Paramyxovirus infection
  pathogenesis, characteristics, diagnosis, treatment of, 269t
  pediatric, 420
Paramyxoviruses, 271-272
  in mumps, 290
Paranasal sinuses, 66, 66f, 67f, 68-69, 68f, 69f
  acute noninfectious sinusitis of, 74-75
  CT and MRI of, 70-72, 71f, 72f
  granulomatous disease of, 77
  infectious sinusitis of, 73-74, 73f
  pathology of, 73-77
  sinusitis complications in, 75-77, 75f
    fungal, 76-77
    mucocele, 75-76

Paranasal sinuses—cont'd
  sinusitis complications in—cont'd
    mucous retention cysts, 75, 75f
    orbital/extrasinus, 76
Parapharyngeal space, diagnostic imaging of, 88-89, 88f, 89f
Parasites, attenuation of, 38
Parasitism, 38-39
  aberrant, 38
  attenuated, 38
Paresis, motor, neurological assessment of, 348
Parinaud's oculoglandular conjunctivitis, 341-342
Parinaud's oculoglandular syndrome, 433, 434f
Parotid gland
  benign hypertrophy of, 93
  immunoglobulin concentrations in, 5t
  infections of, 279
Parotid space
  diagnostic imaging of, 87-88
  infections of, 204, 204f
Parotideomasseteric fascia, 189, 200, 204, 205f
Parotitis, 420
  bacterial, impaired oral drainage and, 4
  chronic recurrent bacterial, 289
  epidemic, 290-291
  radiological, 290
  viral, 92
Pasteurella, Gram stain identification of, 49b
Pasteurella multocida in animal bite infections, 110, 308, 366
Pathogen, defined, 39
Pathogenesis, endotoxins in, 39-40
Pathogenicity
  defined, 39
  exotoxins in, 40
Patient. *See also* Host
  communication with, in airway management, 445
  compliance of, 105-106, 376-377
  drug history of, 104
  immunocompromised. *See* Immunocompromised host
  informed consent by, 485
  instructions for, medicolegal aspects of, 485
  medical history of, 354-355
  monitoring of, 107-108
  noncompliance by, 487
  role of, in surgical infection, 475
  surgical. *See* Surgical patient
Pattern recognition receptors, 9
Pectobacterium, Gram stain identification of, 49b
Pediatric maxillofacial infections, 93-94, 410-422
  croup, 94, 95f
  diagnostic issues in, 410
  of ear, nose, and throat, 419
  epiglottitis, 94, 94f
  erysipelas/necrotizing fasciitis, 419
  Haemophilus influenzae, 417-418, 418f
  impetigo, 418
  laboratory testing in, 410
  of lower face, 411-413, 412b, 412t, 413-414, 413f, 414f
  mycotic/protozoal, 421
  noma, 418-419, 419f
  odontogenic/bacterial, 414, 416-417, 417f
  patient history in, 410
  periorbital/orbital, 93-94, 93f
  physical exam in, 411, 411t
  scalded skin syndrome, 418, 418f

Pediatric maxillofacial infections—cont'd
  tonsillar/peritonsillar, 94, 94f
  of upper face, 411-413, 412b, 412f, 412t, 413f
  viral, 419-421
    DNA, 419-420
    RNA, 420-421
Pediococcus, Gram stain identification of, 49b
Penicillin(s)
  allergy to, 100-101, 104, 222
  antimicrobial spectrum of, 117t
  contraindications to, 112
  destruction of, by penicillinase and amidase, 116f
  extended-spectrum, 116, 118
    antimicrobial spectrum of, 117t
  as first-choice antibiotic, 113t
  hypersensitivity reactions to, 108
  for maxillofacial infections, 112, 114t, 115b, 116, 116f, 117t, 118
  microbial susceptibility to, 55t, 56t, 110, 217
  for odontogenic infections, 164
  pediatric dosages for, 415t
  penicillinase-resistant, as first-choice antibiotic, 113t
  prophylactic, for third molar surgery, 177
  resistance to, 116, 164, 471
    in osteomyelitis, 222
    staphylococcal, 158, 298-299
  structure of, 116f
Penicillin G
  antimicrobial spectrum of, 117t
  bacterial sensitivity to, 103
  blood-brain barrier and, 357
  as first-choice antibiotic, 113t
  for maxillofacial trauma patient, 367t
  pediatric dosages for, 416t
  pharmacology of, 114t, 117t
  pharmacology/pharmacokinetics of, 116
Penicillin V
  antimicrobial spectrum of, 117t
  for implant surgery, 382b
  pharmacology of, 114t, 117t
  pharmacology/pharmacokinetics of, 116
Penicillium, 38
Pepsin for Ig fragmentation, 6
Peptides, antimicrobial, characteristics and functions of, 3-4
Peptidoglycan, 23
Peptococcus. See also Peptostreptococcus
  in aspiration pneumonia, 453
  in pulpal tissue, 148
  in tonsillitis, 323
Peptococcus niger, 36t
Peptostreptococcus. See also Peptococcus
  antibiotic sensitivity of, 103
  in aspiration pneumonia, 453
  characteristics and disorders associated with, 34
  in children with primary dentition, 30
  first-choice and alternative antibiotics for, 113t
  Gram stain identification of, 49b
  in Ludwig's angina, 178
  in odontogenic infections, 164
  in osteomyelitis, 217
  pericoronitis due to, 110
Peptostreptococcus anaerobius, 36t
Peptostreptococcus asaccharolyticus, 36t
Peptostreptococcus magnus, 36t

Peptostreptococcus micros, 36t
in HIV-associated periodontal disease, 145
in pericoronitis, 143
Periauricular infections, 370
Perichondritis of external ear, 317-318
Pericoronitis, 142-144
clinical features and diagnosis of, 142-143
etiology of, 143
in maxillofacial surgery, 110
treatment of, 143-144
Peridex. *See* Chlorhexidine
Periimplantitis, 386-389, 388f
bacterial causes of, 387, 387b
Perinasal infections, 369-370
Periodontal abscess, 137-140
chronic, 137
clinical features and diagnosis of, 137-138, 138f
etiology of, 138-139
treatment of, 137-140
Periodontal disease
implant survival and, 383
necrotizing, classification of, 127b-128b
opportunistic infections and, 39
Periodontal infections, 126-145. *See also* Periradicular disease;
Pulpal infections
acute, 137-145. *See also* Abscess(es); Acute necrotizing ulcerative gingivitis-periodontitis; Pericoronitis
HIV and, 144-145
bacteria associated with, 133, 133b
chronic inflammatory, 128-137, 130f. *See also* Gingivitis;
Periodontitis
epidemiology of, 131-132
treatment of, 134-137
classification of, 126, 127b-128b
Periodontitis
aggressive, 128, 130
chronic, 130
classification of, 127b
clinical features of, 128-130, 129f, 130f
epidemiology of, 131-132
HIV-associated, 144-145, 274
juvenile, 131
necrotizing ulcerative, in HIV/AIDS, 462
nonplaque factors in, 132-133
periradicular
acute, 149
asymptomatic chronic, 149-150
chronic suppurative, 150
symptomatic chronic, 150
plaque factors in, 132
prepubertal, 130
rapidly progressive, 131
systemic-disease-associated, classification of, 127b
treatment of, 134-137
Periodontium
functional aspects of, 126, 128, 129f
in health, gingivitis, and periodontitis, 129f
Periodontosis, 131
Perioral infections, 369
Periorbital infections, 210, 370
Periostitis, proliferative, 229-230, 229f
Periradicular disease
acute periodontitis, 149
asymptomatic periodontitis, 149-150

Periradicular disease—cont'd
chronic suppurative periodontitis, 150
chronic symptomatic periodontitis, 150
classification of, 149-150
condensing sclerosing osteitis, 150
phoenix abscess, 150
treatment of, 151-152
Peritonsillar space, infections of, 207, 207f
pH, bacterial control and, 4
Phagocytes
cytokines of, 20-21
defensive role of, 9-10
immunologic function of, 11-13, 12f
mononuclear, 12-13
Phagocytosis, initiation of, 11-12
Pharmacokinetics, 106-107
Pharyngeal conjunctival fever, 341
Pharyngeal space
infections of, 181-182, 181f, 182f
lateral
borders of, 194t
infection of, causes, contents, and neighboring spaces of,
195t
infections of, 204-205, 205f
Pharyngitis, 322-323
diagnosis of, 45
diphtherial, 323
gonococcal, 323
staphylococcal, 323
streptococcal, 323
uveitis after, 345
Phlebitis
brain infection due to, 354
midface infection and, 356
Phoenix abscess, 150
Phycomycosis
pediatric, 421
rhinocerebral, 426-429, 426f, 427f, 428f, 429f
Physical examination, ophthalmological, 161
Physician, liability of, 484. *See also* Medicolegal issues
Physician-patient interactions, medicolegal aspects of, 484-485
Picornavirus infections, 268-269, 420-421
Piperacillin
antimicrobial spectrum of, 117t
limitations of, 116, 118
microbial susceptibility to, 55t, 56t
pediatric dosages for, 416t
pharmacology of, 117t
Piperacillin-tazobactam
antimicrobial spectrum of, 117t
bacterial susceptibility to, 55t
Pipracil. *See* Piperacillin
Plague, 366
Plaque
dental, in periodontal disease, 132
Helicobacter pylori associated with, 31
mechanical removal of, 135
Plasma half-life, 106
Platelet-activating factor in wound healing, 26t
Platelet-derived growth factor in wound healing, 26t
Platelet-derived growth factors, 3
Platelets, activation of, 25
Plesiomonas, Gram stain identification of, 49b
PMNs. *See* Polymorphonuclear neutrophils

Pneumocystis carinii
immunofluorescent assay of, 50
in pneumocystosis, 254-255
Pneumocystis carinii pneumonia in HIV/AIDS, 462
Pneumocystosis, 254-255, 255b
Pneumonia
aspiration, 453
impaired oral drainage and, 4
nosocomial
causative organisms in, 469t
risk factors for, 469t
pneumocystis carinii, in HIV/AIDS, 462
Pockets, gingival, 129, 129f
Polychondritis, relapsing, of ear, 318
Polymerase chain reaction, diagnostic uses of, 51
Polymorphonuclear neutrophils, complement receptors on, 9-10
Polymyxin B for maxillofacial trauma patient, 367t
Polytetrafluoroethylene implants, 395
Porphyromonas
in children with primary dentition, 30
Gram stain identification of, 49b
infection occurrence of, 102b
infections due to, 35
in odontogenic infections, 164
penicillin resistance of, 217, 222
Porphyromonas asaccharolyticus, 36t
Porphyromonas asacchrolyticus, 102
Porphyromonas catoniae in infants, 30
Porphyromonas endodontalis, 36t, 102
Porphyromonas gingivalis, 36t, 102
adherence of, 39
attachment patterns of, 32
in HIV-associated periodontal disease, 145
in periodontitis, 132
in systemic disease, 40
Porphyromonas intermedia in HIV-associated periodontal disease, 145
Postherpetic neuralgia, 265
Pott's puffy tumor, 76, 315, 315f
Povidone-iodine
as oral rinse, 475
as surgical scrub, 474
Pregnancy
gingivitis during, 130
pH changes in, 4
Pretracheal space
borders of, 194t
diagnostic imaging of, 89
infections of, 207
Prevotella
antibiotic sensitivity of, 103
attachment of, 39
in children with primary dentition, 30
first-choice and alternative antibiotics for, 113t
Gram stain identification of, 49b
infection occurrence of, 102b
infections due to, 35
metalloproteinases of, 40
in odontogenic infections, 164
in osteomyelitis, 217
penicillin resistance of, 110, 217, 222
percent susceptibility of, 55t
pericoronitis due to, 110

Prevotella buccae, 102
Prevotella buccalis, 36t
Prevotella corrodens in Ludwig's angina, 178
Prevotella dentalis, 36t
Prevotella denticola, 36t, 102
Prevotella heparinolytica, 36t
Prevotella intermedia, 36t, 102
in ANUGP, 141
in infants, 30
in pericoronitis, 143
in periodontitis, 132
Prevotella loescheii, 36t, 102
attachment patterns of, 32
Prevotella melaninogenica, 36t, 102
in infants, 30
in Ludwig's angina, 178
noma due to, 419
in periodontal abscess, 139
Prevotella nigrescens, 36t
Prevotella oralis, 36t, 102
in Ludwig's angina, 178
Prevotella oris, 36t
Prevotella ruminicola, 102
Prevotella tannerae, 36t
Priapism as complication of mumps orchitis, 291
Procaine penicillin G, pharmacology of, 117t
Proliferative periostitis, 229-230, 229f
Prophylactic antibiotics
after soft tissue trauma, 372b
with esthetic facial surgery, 392
hand washing as adjunct to, 473
for head and neck surgery, 402
in implant surgery, 381-383
with implants, 381-382, 382b
with maxillofacial trauma, 366-368
for postoperative wounds, 401, 401t
for rabies, 368, 369t
with skin resurfacing, 396
for tetanus, 368, 368t
in third molar surgery, 177
Prophylactic antifungal therapy, 478
Propionibacterium
Gram stain identification of, 49b
isolation of, 47
in odontogenic infections, 164
Propionibacterium acnes, shunt colonization with, 350
Propionibacterium propionicum in cervicofacial actinomycosis, 232
Proptosis, 329
aspergillos-related, 424, 424f, 425f, 426
from septic cavernous sinus thrombosis, 338
Prostaglandins, inflammatory effects of, 19-20
Protein(s)
alternative pathway activation by, 9
dietary, oral microbes and, 32
lipopolysaccharide-binding, 22
mannose-binding lectin pathway activation by, 9
membrane, in complement activation, 9
regulatory, 3
Protein C, 17
Protein J, 7
Protein M, bacterial adherence and, 39
Proteus
aztreonam for, 119
first-choice and alternative antibiotics for, 113t

Proteus—cont'd
    life-threatening infection from, 159f
    in necrotizing external otitis, 318
    in osteomyelitis, 217
Proteus mirabilis
    in otitis externa, 318
    percent susceptibility of, 55t
Proteus vulgaris, percent susceptibility of, 55t
Protozoal infections, 275-276
    leishmaniasis, 275-276
    pediatric, 421, 421t
Pseudofolliculitis barbae, differential diagnosis of, 299, 300f
Pseudo-Ludwig's angina, 178
Pseudomonas
    aztreonam for, 119
    in bullous external otitis, 319
    chlorhexidine resistance of, 474
    Gram stain identification of, 49b
    health workers as carriers of, 474
    life-threatening infection from, 159f
    in Ludwig's angina, 178
    in nosocomial ICU infections, 470-471
    in osteomyelitis, 217
    in otitis media, 321
    susceptibility testing of, 54, 55
Pseudomonas aeruginosa
    after otoplasty, 397
    antibiotic resistance of, 472-473
    antimicrobials affecting, 56
    carbapenems for, 119
    first-choice and alternative antibiotics for, 113t
    in MOE, 459
    in noma, 419, 431
    in otitis externa, 318
    percent susceptibility of, 55t
    in perichondritis/chondritis of ear, 317-318
    skin resurfacing and, 396
Pseudomonas cepacia, antibiotic resistance of, 472-473
Pseudopockets, 129, 129f
Pseudosialectasis, 93
Pseudotumors, orbital, 91-92
Pterygomandibular space
    borders of, 194t
    infection of, causes, contents, and neighboring spaces of, 195t
Pulmonary mucormycosis, 254
Pulp
    microorganisms found in, 148-149
    necrotic, 146-147
        treatment of, 152
    normal, 146
    portals of entry to, 147
Pulpal infections, 145-149. *See also* Periodontal infections; Periradicular disease
    antibiotic therapy for, 148
    classification of, 145-146
    irreversible pulpitis, 146
    microbial virulence factors in, 147-148
    necrotic pulp, 146-147
    pain in, 149
    portals of entry for, 147
    reversible pulpitis, 146
Pulpectomy, indications for, 151

Pulpitis
    irreversible, 146
        treatment of, 150-151
    reversible, 146
        treatment of, 150
Puncture wounds
    antibiotic therapy for, 367t
    maxillofacial, 306, 374, 374f
Pupillary reaction, assessment of, 33
Pustules, characteristics of, 296
Pyoceles, 75
Pyrogens
    endogenous, 19
    mechanisms of, 24-25

Q

Q beta replicase system, diagnostic uses of, 51
Quaternary ammonium, disinfectant activity of, 479t
Quinapristin-dalfopristin for vancomycin-resistance staphylococci, 472
Quinolones
    adverse effects of, 165
    dosage of, with normal/impaired renal function, 122t
    for maxillofacial infections, 121
    oxazolidinone, for vancomycin-resistance staphylococci, 472
    staphylococcal resistance to, 472

R

Rabies
    characteristics, management, prevention of, 308
    prophylaxis algorithm for, 309f
    prophylaxis of, 368, 369t
Rabies virus, immunofluorescent assay of, 50
Radiation
    dental care after, 240
    for osteomyelitis of jaw, osteoradionecrosis due to, 236-237, 236f, 237f
Radiation therapy, postoperative infections and, 402
Radiographs, diagnostic uses of, 62
Radiological parotitis, 290
Radionuclide imaging
    diagnostic uses of, 64-65, 64f
    in osteomyelitis of jaw, 219-220, 219f
Radiopharmaceuticals for bone scans, 64
Ramsay Hunt syndrome, 319
Rashes, 108
    in scarlet fever, 323
Rat-bite fever, 366
Receptors
    cell surface, 9-10
    complement, 9-10
    Fc, 10
    histamine, 18
    for immunoglobulins, 10
    mannose, 9, 13
    pattern recognition, 9
Records, medicolegal issues in, 486
Rectum, immunoglobulin concentrations in, 5t
Red saturation test, 329
Renal disease, immune deficiency due to, 459
Respiration rate, pediatric, 411t
Respiratory syncytial virus
    immunoassay of, 51
    immunofluorescent assay of, 50

Respiratory tract, IgA synthesis in, 7
Retina, septic emboli to, 330
Retin-A. *See* Tretinoin therapy
Retropharyngeal space
    borders of, 194t
    diagnostic imaging of, 88-89, 88f, 89f
    infections of, 204, 205-206
Retropharyngeal space infection, 182-183, 182f
Retroviruses, 273-275
    pathogenesis, characteristics, diagnosis, treatment of, 269t
Rhinitis, viral, acute sinusitis and, 314
Rhinocerebral mucormycosis, 253-254, 254f
    in diabetic patient, 458-459
Rhinoorbital-cerebral mucormycosis, 336-338
Rhinoplasty, infection after, 393, 393f-394f, 395
Rhizopus
    azoles for treating, 122
    in mucormycosis, 253-254, 426
    in rhinoorbital-cerebral mucormycosis, 336
    sinusitis due to, 76
Rhodamine-auramine stain, 49
Rhodococcus
    acid fastness in, 50
    Gram stain identification of, 49b
Rhytidectomy, skin-flap, infection after, 396
Ribonucleic acid viruses, 268, 269t, 270-275
    coxsackieviruses group A, 268, 269t, 270
    HIV, 269t, 273-275
    measles virus, 269t, 272
    mumps virus, 269t, 271-272
    paramyxoviruses, 269t, 271
    retroviruses, 269t, 273-275
    rubella virus, 269t, 272-273
Rickettsia, immunofluorescent assay of, 50
Rickettsia rickettsii, vascular invasion by, 22
Rifampin
    microbes susceptible to, 56t
    pediatric dosages for, 416t
Rikenella, Gram stain identification of, 49b
Ritter's disease, 302, 303f
RNA retroviruses, pathogenesis, characteristics, diagnosis, treatment of, 269t, 273-275
Rocephin. *See* Ceftriaxone
Rocky Mountain spotted fever, 22
ROCM. *See* Rhinoorbital-cerebral mucormycosis
Rods
    Gram stain of, 49b
    gram-negative, 36t
        antimicrobials affecting, 56
        in immunocompromised host, 355-356
        infections due to, 35, 37
        in pulpal tissue, 148
        staining of, 48
    gram-positive, 35, 36t
Roseomonas, Gram stain identification of, 49b
Rothia, Gram stain identification of, 49b
Rothia dentocariosa, 34t
    disease due to, 35
    in plaque, 132
Roth's spots, 342
Rubella, 272-273
    pathogenesis, characteristics, diagnosis, treatment of, 269t
    pediatric, 420

Rubeola, 272
    pathogenesis, characteristics, diagnosis, treatment of, 269t
Ruminobacter, Gram stain identification of, 49b

S
Saliva
    antimicrobial system in, 4
    histatin production in, 3
    HIV disease transmission by, 291
    immunoglobulin concentrations in, 5t
    in regulation of oral microbiota, 31-32, 31t
Salivarius salivarius, 33t
Salivarius vestibularis, 33t
Salivary gland infections, 279-293
    bacterial, 283-290
        actinomycosis, 290
        acute allergic sialadenitis/radiological parotitis, 290
        acute parotitis, 283-287, 285f, 286f, 287f
        acute submandibular sialadenitis, 287-289, 288f
        cat-scratch disease, 290
        chronic recurrent parotitis, 289, 289f
        chronic recurrent submandibular sialadenitis, 289-290
    classification of, 279b
    diagnosis of, 280-282, 281f, 282f
    differential diagnosis of, 279, 282, 283b
    general considerations in, 279-282
    immunological
        collagen sialadenitis, 292
        sarcoidosis, 292
    medications associated with, 280b
    mycobacterial
        atypical, 291
        tuberculosis, 291
    parasitic (filariasis), 291
    patient history in, 279-280
    risk factors for, 280b
    viral, 290-291
        cytomegalovirus, 291
        epidemic parotitis, 290-291
        HIV-associated, 291
        mumps, 290-291
        sialadenitis, 290-291
Salivary glands
    enlargement of, assessment algorithm for, 284f
    inflammatory disorders of, 92-93, 92f
Salmonella, first-choice and alternative antibiotics for, 113t
Sarcoidosis, salivary gland involvement in, 292
Sarcoma, Kaposi's, in AIDS patients, 274
Saucerization for osteomyelitis of jaw, 225, 225f
Scalded skin syndrome, staphylococcal, 302, 418, 418f
Scales, characteristics of, 297
Scalp, infections of, 370
    posttraumatic, 370
Scarlatiniform staphylococcal scalded skin syndrome, 302
Scarlet fever
    maxillofacial manifestations of, 297
    with pharyngitis, 323
Scintigraphy, salivary, 282
Sclerosing osteomyelitis
    chronic diffuse, 230-231, 230f
    focal, 231, 231f
    Garré's, 229-230, 229f
Scopulariopsis, 38
Sebaceous cysts, 301

Sebaldella, Gram stain identification of, 49b
Secretion and drainage system, protective functions of, 4
Secretions
  IgA in, 7
  immunoglobulins in, 5, 5t
Selenomonas
  in children with primary dentition, 30
  Gram stain identification of, 49b
  in infants, 30
  infections due to, 35
Selenomonas noxia, 36t
Selenomonas sputigena, 36t
Sellick maneuver, intubation and, 449
Semmelweis, Ignaz Philipp, 468-469, 470f, 473
Sepsis
  blood, nosocomial, 469t
  duration of surgery and, 476, 476t
  in head and neck infections, 309-310
  mortality from, 24
  systemic inflammatory response syndrome and, 23-24
  types of, 23, 23b
  of wound, 475-476
Septal abscess, 313
Septal defect of heart and predisposition to infection, 354
Septic cavernous sinus thrombosis, 338-340, 339f
Septic shock, 23, 23b
Septorhinoplasty, infection after, 395
Sequestrectomy
  for chronic suppurative osteomyelitis, 222-223
  for osteomyelitis of jaw, 224-225
Serotonin, inflammatory effects of, 19
Serratia
  chlorhexidine resistance of, 474
  first-choice and alternative antibiotics for, 113t
  life-threatening infection from, 159f
  in nosocomial ICU infections, 470
Serratia marcescens, percent susceptibility of, 55t
Serum
  IgM in, 8
  immunoglobulin concentrations in, 5t
Severe combined immunodeficiency, 457
Shaving
  contraindications to, 372
  controversy over, 475
Shewanella, Gram stain identification of, 49b
Shigella, first-choice and alternative antibiotics for, 113t
Shingles, 265-266, 420. *See also* Varicella-zoster virus
  pathogenesis, clinical characteristics, diagnosis, treatment of, 259t
Shock, septic, 23, 23b
Sialadenitis
  acute allergic, 290
  acute bacterial submandibular, 279, 287-289, 288f
  acute nonobstructive, 92
  autoimmune, 93
  causes of, 279, 280
  chronic, 93
  chronic recurrent submandibular, 289-290, 289f
  collagen, 292
  submandibular, 85f
  viral, 290-291
Sialoceles, formation of, 280
Sialochemistry, 282
Sialoendoscopy, 281

Sialography, 281-282, 282f
Sialosis, 93
Signal transduction, immunologic function of, 10
Silent sinus syndrome, 345
Sinus
  cavernous. *See* Cavernous sinus
  intercavernous, 213
Sinus infections
  acute sinusitis, complications of, 316-317
  brain infection due to, 354
  chronic sinusitis, complications of, 316-317
  fungal
    aspergillosis, 316
    mucormycosis, 316
  orbital involvement in, 328-329
  paranasal, 313-317
    acute sinusitis, 313-315, 314f
    chronic sinusitis, 315-316
  from septic thrombosis, 356
  silent sinus syndrome, 345
Sinuses
  commensal organisms of, 53
  ethmoid, 68
  fractures of, infection after, 371
  maxillary, 66, 66f, 67f, 68, 68f
  midface/paranasal, anatomy of, 66, 66f, 67f, 68-69, 68f, 69f
  paranasal. *See* Paranasal sinuses
  sphenoid, 69, 69f
Sinusitis
  acute, 71, 71f
    management of, 369
  allergic fungal, 341
  chronic, 73f
  complications of, 75-77
    mucocele, 75-76
    mucous retention cysts, 75, 75f
    orbital and extrasinus, 76
  fungal, 76-77
  granulomatous, 77
  infectious, 73-74
  noninfectious, 74-75
  nosocomial *Pseudomonas,* 473
  odontogenic, 316
Sjögren's syndrome, 93
  versus collagen sialadenitis, 292
Skin
  appendages of, 294-295
  commensal organisms of, 53
  facial, anatomy of, 294, 295f
  lipids of, bacterial growth and, 4
  microbiology of, 295-296
  physiology of, 294-295
Skin resurfacing, infection after, 396-397
Skin-flap rhytidectomy, infection after, 396
Smears
  acid-fast, 48
  Gram-stained direct, 47b
Smoking
  postoperative wound infections and, 401
Smoking, periodontal disease and, 133
Soft tissues
  actinomyces infections of, 188
  maxillofacial. *See* Maxillofacial soft tissues
  necrotic, conservative debridement of, 365

South American blastomycosis, 247-248, 248b
Specimen collection
    from aspirates, 44, 44f
    of blood, 46-47
    guidelines for, 43-44, 44b
    with swabs, 45-46, 46f
    from tissue/bone, 44-45, 45f
Specimens
    dark-field microscopy of, 50
    examination of, 47-51
        direct methods of, 47-51
        staining methods for, 47-50
    staining of, 47-50
        with acid-fast stains, 48-50
        with Brown-Brenn Gram stain, 48
        fluorescent antibody, 50
        with fungal stains, 48
        with Gram stain, 47-48, 49t
    transport of, 43-44
    wet preparations of, 50
Spectinomycin, indications for, 113t
Spectracef. *See* Cefditoren
Sphenoid sinuses, 69, 69f
    infection of, 315
    mucoceles of, 76
Sphingobacterium, Gram stain identification of, 49b
Sphingomonas, Gram stain identification of, 49b
Spinal fluid, serological tests of, 353
Spirochetes, 37t
    infections due to, 37
Splenectomy, immune deficiency due to, 458
Sporanox. *See* Itraconazole
Sporothrix, processing, isolation, and identification of, 53
Sporothrix schenckii in sporotrichosis, 257-258
Sporotrichosis, 257-258, 257b
    cutaneous, 257-258
    disseminated, 258, 258f
    extracutaneous, 258
    mucosal, 258
Squamous cell carcinoma, intraosseous, *versus* osteomyelitis of
        jaw, 218
Stains, fluorescent antibody, 50
Staph epidemic, 471
Staphylococcal impetigo, 302, 418, 418f
Staphylococcal scalded skin syndrome, 302
Staphylococcal superantigens, 23
Staphylococcus
    in animal bites, 110
    antibiotic resistance of, 471-472
    antimicrobials affecting, 56
    in cervicofacial actinomycosis, 232
    Gram stain identification of, 49b
    infection occurrence of, 102b
    in Ludwig's angina, 178
    methicillin-resistant, 120
    microbial interference by, 4
    in otitis media, 320
    penicillin-resistant, 158, 298-299, 471
    percent susceptibility of, 55t
    in postoperative wounds, 400, 400t
    skin resurfacing and, 396
    susceptibility testing of, 54
Staphylococcus albus in periodontal abscess, 139
Staphylococcus asaccharolyticus, 33t

Staphylococcus aureus, 33t, 35
    in animal bite infections, 308
    antibiotic sensitivity of, 103
    in dacryocystitis, 340
    in epiglottitis, 325
    in facial infections, 298-299
    first-choice and alternative antibiotics for, 113t
    in furunculosis/carbunculosis, 313
    in head/neck infections, 295-296
    nasal carriers of, 395
    in nosocomial ICU infections, 471
    in odontogenic infections, 164
    in osteomyelitis, 216-217
    in otoplasty-related infections, 397
    pathogenicity of, 40
    in pediatric upper face infections, 412
    penicillin resistance of, 116
    penicillinase-producing, prophylaxis against, 366
    percent susceptibility of, 55t
    in pharyngitis, 323
    in septal abscess, 313
    in tonsillitis, 323
Staphylococcus epidermidis, 33t
    antibiotic sensitivity of, 103
    in dacryocystitis, 340
    first-choice and alternative antibiotics for, 113t
    in head/neck infections, 295
    in odontogenic infections, 164
    in osteomyelitis, 216-217
    shunt colonization with, 350
Staphylococcus pneumoniae in labyrinthitis, 322
Staphylococcus salivarius in pharyngitis, 323
Stenotrophomonas, Gram stain identification of, 49b
Stenotrophomonas maltophilia, percent susceptibility of, 55t
Stensen's duct
    in acute bacterial parotitis, 285, 285f
    calculi in, 281
    in chronic recurrent bacterial parotitis, 289
Sterilization
    cold, 478
    of countertops/handles, 479t
    defined, 478
    of instruments, 479
Steroid therapy
    fungal infections associated with, 477t
    immune suppression due to, 100
Stomach, candidiasis of, 250
Stomatitis, gangrenous, 418-419, 419f. *See also* Noma
Stomatococcus, Gram stain identification of, 49b
Stomatococcus mucilaginosus, 33t
Stratum corneum, 294
Streptococcal superantigens, 23
Streptococcus
    α, first-choice and alternative antibiotics for, 113t
    α-hemolytic, in osteomyelitis, 217
    β-hemolytic, 33t
        infection occurrence of, 102b
    in animal bites, 110
    antibiotic sensitivity of, 103
    attachment of, 39
    in cervicofacial actinomycosis, 232
    characteristics and disorders associated with, 33-34
    in children with primary dentition, 30
    first-choice and alternative antibiotics for, 113t

Streptococcus—cont'd
  Gram stain identification of, 49b
  group A
    immunoassay of, 51
    susceptibility testing of, 54
  group A β-hemolytic
    in erysipelas, 435
    in pharyngitis, 323
  group B, in neonates, 30
  group D, infection occurrence of, 102b
  in impetigo, 418
  in maxillofacial/neck infections, 297-298
    erysipelas, 298, 298f
    impetigo, 297-298, 298f
    scarlet fever, 297
  in neonates, 30
  in odontogenic infections, 164
  in otitis media, 320
  in plaque, 132
  in postoperative wounds, 400, 400t
  skin resurfacing and, 396
  Veillonella interaction with, 32
  viridans
    antibiotic sensitivity of, 103
    infection occurrence of, 102b
    opportunistic infections due to, 39
Streptococcus crista, 33t
Streptococcus gordonii, 33t
Streptococcus intermedius in periodontal abscess, 139
Streptococcus milleri
  with *Fusobacterium,* 102-103
  infections due to, 102
Streptococcus mitis, 33t
  in neonates, 30
Streptococcus mutans
  attachment patterns of, 32
  infections found in, 102
Streptococcus oralis, 33t
  in neonates, 30
Streptococcus parasanguis, 33t
Streptococcus pneumoniae, 33t
  antibiotic treatment of, 121
  first-choice and alternative antibiotics for, 113t
  in maxillary sinusitis, 314
  meningitis due to, 50
  in pharyngitis, 323
  susceptibility testing of, 54
  susceptibility to, 55t
  in tonsillitis, 323
Streptococcus pyogenes, 34t
  in epiglottitis, 325
  first-choice and alternative antibiotics for, 113t
  infections found in, 102
  pharyngitis due to, 45
Streptococcus salivarius
  infections found in, 102
  in neonates, 30
Streptococcus sanguis, 33t
  attachment patterns of, 32
  in infants, 30
  infections found in, 102
Streptococcus viridans in periodontal abscess, 139
Streptomyces, Gram stain identification of, 49b
Stye, characteristics of, 300

Subcutaneous space in odontogenic infections, 195, 196f
Subdural empyema, 350
  management of, 357
Sublingual space
  borders of, 194t
  infections of, 173-175, 174f, 197-198, 198f, 199f
    causes, contents, and neighboring spaces of, 195t
Submandibular fascial space, diagnostic imaging of, 82, 83, 83f-84f
Submandibular gland, infections of, 279
Submandibular sialadenitis
  acute bacterial, 287-289, 288f
  chronic recurrent, 289-290, 289f
Submandibular space
  borders of, 194t
  infections of, 173-175, 174f, 175f, 198-200, 198f, 199f, 200f
    causes, contents, and neighboring spaces of, 195t
Submasseteric space
  borders of, 194t
  infections of, causes, contents, and neighboring spaces of, 195t
Submaxillary space, 198
Submental space
  borders of, 194t
  infections of, 175-176, 176f, 200
Sugar, refined, oral microbes and, 32
Sulfisoxazole, pediatric dosages for, 416t
Superantigens, streptococcal/staphylococcal, 23
Superficial musculoaponeurotic system elevation procedure, 396
Superinfections
  causes of, 38-39, 109
  fungal, 478
  minimizing risk of, 104
Superior ophthalmic vein thrombosis, 338, 339f
Superior orbital fissure syndrome, 338-339
Suprax. *See* Cefixime
Surface antigens, leukocyte, 10
Surgery
  antibiotic prophylaxis in, 100
  aseptic technique and, 473-474
  duration of, wound sepsis and, 476, 476t
  fungal infections associated with, 477t
  of head and neck. *See* Head and neck surgery
  maxillofacial. *See* Maxillofacial surgery
  and risk of infection, 353-354
Surgical drainage, infection management and, 100
Surgical masks, 474
Surgical patient, control and prevention of infection in, 468-483. *See also* Nosocomial infections
  enterococcal resistance and, 472
  host factors in, 475
  in ICU, 468-471, 469t
  local factors in, 475-476
  Pseudomonas resistance and, 472-473
  Staphylococcus resistance and, 471-472
  surgical practices and, 473-475
Surgical scrubs, agents for, 474
Surgical supplies, disposable, 480
Surgical wounds
  categories of, 399-400
  clean, 399
  with exposed hardware, 405

Surgical wounds—cont'd
head and neck. *See also* Head and neck surgery
cost of, 406
grading scale for, 403-404, 403t
infection management for, 404-405
isolates found in, 400, 400t
microbes in, 400, 400t
nosocomial infections of, 473
risk prediction for, 400-401
Susceptibility testing, antimicrobial. *See* Antimicrobial susceptibility testing
Swabs, specimen collection with, 45-46, 46f
Swelling
facial, 161
of neck, differential diagnosis of, 310-311
from necrotic pulp, 152
Swimmer's ear, 318, 318f
Sycosis vulgaris, 299, 300f
Synercid. *See* Quinapristin-dalfopristin
Syphilis, luetic labyrinthitis in, 322
Systemic inflammatory response syndrome, sepsis and, 23-24
Systemic lupus erythematosus, salivary gland involvement in,
292

T

T lymphocytes
CD4, 13-15, 456, 462
in cell-mediated immunity, 14
cytotoxic, 13
differential characteristics of, 13, 13t
functions of, 13, 456
in HIV/AIDS, 462
in Ig synthesis, 5
Tazicef. *See* Ceftazidime
Tazidime. *See* Ceftazidime
Tears, immunoglobulin concentrations in, 5t
Technetium 99m phosphate for bone scans, 64-65
Teeth
impacted, in compromised hosts, 165-166
spread of infection from. *See* Odontogenic infections
Temporal fascia, 189
Temporal space
deep infection of, 195t
superficial infection of, 195t
Temporomandibular joint, infectious arthritis of, 436-437, 436f
Testut, aponeurosis of, 204
Tetanus
characteristics, treatment, and prevention of, 306-307, 307t
prophylaxis of, 368, 368t
Tetracycline
antimicrobial spectrum of, 115b
Candida overgrowth and, 38
contraindications to, 164
indications for, 113t
for maxillofacial infections, 119-120
microbial susceptibility to, 56t
pediatric dosages for, 416t
pharmacology of, 114t
side effects of, 119-120
Third molar, impacted, infections of, 176-177, 176f, 177f
Throat infections, 322-326
laryngeal, 324-326
acute epiglottitis in adults, 325
acute epiglottitis in children, 324-325, 325f

Throat infections—cont'd
laryngeal—cont'd
acute laryngitis, 324
acute laryngotracheitis, 325-326, 325f
herpes laryngitis, 326
laryngotracheal diphtheria, 326
oropharyngeal/nasopharyngeal, 322-324
pharyngitis, 322-323
tonsillitis, 323-324, 324f
pediatric, 419
Thrombin, formation of, 17
Thrombophlebitis
brain infections and, 349, 354
and spread to cavernous sinus, 203
Thrombosis
cavernous sinus. *See* Cavernous sinus thrombosis
dural sinus, 354
superior ophthalmic vein, 338, 339f
Thrush, 109, 249-250, 249f
Th1/Th2 cells, immunologic roles of, 14
Thumb sign, 325, 325f
Thymocytes, differentiation of, 14
Thyroid cartilage, deviation of, 441
Thyroid disease, neck swelling due to, 310
Thyromental distance test, 442
Ticarcillin
antimicrobial spectrum of, 117t
limitations of, 116, 118
microbes susceptible to, 56t
pediatric dosages for, 416t
pharmacology of, 117t
Ticarcillin-clavulanate, antimicrobial spectrum of, 117t
Timentin. *See* Ticarcillin
Tinea barbae, differential diagnosis of, 299
Tissierella, Gram stain identification of, 49b
Tissue, specimen collection from, 44-45, 45f
Titanium, bone attachment to, 381
TMX/SMX. *See* Trimethoprim/sulfamethoxazole
TNF receptor-associated periodic syndrome, 10
Tobacco use
periodontal disease and, 133
postoperative wound infections and, 401
Tobramycin
microbial susceptibility to, 55t, 56t
pediatric dosages for, 415t
Togaviruses, 272
pathogenesis, characteristics, diagnosis, treatment of, 269t
Tolosa-Hunt syndrome, neurological exam for, 347-348
Tongue, cleavage planes in, 439, 439f
Tonsillar infections, 94, 94f
Tonsillitis
acute, 323
chronic, 324
Tonsilloliths, 324
Tort law, 484
Toxic shock syndrome I, 40
Toxins, bacterial. *See* Bacterial toxins
Toxoplasma in immunocompromised host, 356
Toxoplasmosis in AIDS patients, 357
Trachea, deviation of, 441
Tracheobronchitis, *Aspergillus,* 253
Tracheotomy *versus* cricothyrotomy, 450-451, 450t
Transforming growth factor-α, 3

Transforming growth factor-β, 3
in wound healing, 25, 26t
Trauma
brain abscess due to, 353
maxillofacial. *See* Maxillofacial trauma
Treponema amylovorum, 37t
characteristics and pathogenicity of, 37
Treponema denticola, 37t
characteristics and pathogenicity of, 37
Treponema in periodontitis, 132
Treponema maltophilum, 37t
characteristics and pathogenicity of, 37
Treponema medium, 37t
attachment patterns of, 32
characteristics and pathogenicity of, 37
Treponema pallidum
dark-field microscopy of, 50
immunofluorescent assay of, 50
in labyrinthitis, 322
in osteomyelitis, 217
Treponema pectinovorum, characteristics and pathogenicity of, 37
Treponema socranskii, 37t
characteristics and pathogenicity of, 37
Treponema vincentii
in ANUGP, 141
characteristics and pathogenicity of, 37
Tretinoin therapy, 302
Trichomonas, metronidazole for, 111
Trimethoprim/sulfamethoxazole
as first-choice antibiotic, 113t
indications for, 113t
microbial susceptibility to, 56t
pediatric dosages for, 416t
pharmacology of, 114t
Trismus
assessment for, 161, 441
intubation and, 448-449
in masticator space infection, 171, 171f
in pediatric lower face infections, 413-414, 413f
in pharyngeal space infection, 181-182
sedative/analgesic technique and, 446
in submasseteric space abscess, 202f
in tetanus, 307
Tropheryma whippelii, PCR assays for, 51
Trovafloxacin
bacterial susceptibility to, 55t
dosage of, with normal/impaired renal function, 122t
Trumpet blower's syndrome, 280
Tsukamurella
acid fastness in, 50
Gram stain identification of, 49b
Tuberculosis, salivary gland involvement in, 291
Tuftsin
disorders associated with, 12
in phagocytosis, 11-12
Tumor necrosis factor-α, 3
Tumor staging
postoperative wounds infections and, 401-402
wound infections and, 401
Tumor-necrosis factor
endotoxin and, 22
in fever, 24-25
in sepsis, 24

Tumor-necrosis factor-α, inflammatory effects of, 21
Tumor-necrosis factor-β, inflammatory effects of, 21
Tumors
head and neck, surgery on. *See* Head and neck surgery
Pott's puffy, 76
Turicella, Gram stain identification of, 49b
Tympanic membrane, perforation of, 320-321, 320f

U

Ulcers
in AIDS patients, 274
characteristics of, 296-297
Ultracef. *See* Cefadroxil
Uncinate process, 69
Ureters, dyskinesia of, 4
Urinary bladder, neurogenic, urinary tract infections and, 4
Urinary tract infections
nosocomial
causative organisms in, 469t
risk factors for, 469t
ureteral dyskinesia in, 4
Urticaria, 108
Uterine fluid, antimicrobial system in, 4
Uveitis, poststreptococcal, 345
Uveoparotid fever, 292

V

Vaginitis, *Candida,* 250-251
Valacyclovir
for herpes simplex infection, 123
for HSV infections, 396
Valtrex. *See* Valacyclovir
Vancomycin
administration and side effects of, 120
antimicrobial spectrum of, 115b
bacterial susceptibility to, 55t
enterococcal resistance to, 472
indications for, 113t
for maxillofacial infections, 120
pharmacology of, 114t
staphylococcal resistance to, 472
Vancomycin-resistant enterococci, 470-471
Vantin. *See* Cefpodoxime proxetil
Varicella-zoster infections
CD4 count, 462
of external ear canal, 319
pathogenesis, clinical characteristics, diagnosis, treatment of, 259t
PCR assays for, 51
pediatric, 420
Varicella-zoster labyrinthitis, 322
Varicella-zoster virus, immunofluorescent assay of, 50
Vascular system, inflammatory role of, 21-22
Vasculitis, mechanism of, 22
Vasoactive amines, 18
Vasoactive mediators, inflammatory role of, 21
Veillonella
in aspiration pneumonia, 453
Gram stain identification of, 49b
in infants, 30
in pericoronitis, 143
in pulpal tissue, 148
streptococcal interaction with, 32

Veillonella atypica, 36t
  disease due to, 35
Veillonella dispar, 36t
  disease due to, 35
Veillonella parvula, 36t
  disease due to, 35
Velosef. *See* Cephradine
Ventilation, jet, 451
Ventricular seeding, brain infection and, 349
Ventricular shunt, infection predisposition and, 354-355
Ventriculitis, trauma-induced, 353
Vesicles, characteristics of, 296
Vestibular space in odontogenic infections, 193, 195, 196f
Vibrio, Gram stain identification of, 49b
Viral infections, 258-275. *See also* specific viruses
  herpesvirus, 258, 259t-260t, 261-268
    cytomegalovirus, 266-267
    Epstein-Barr virus, 263-264
    herpes simplex virus, 261-263, 261f, 262f
    papillomaviruses, 267-268
    pathogenesis, characteristics, diagnosis, treatment of, 259t-260t
    varicella-zoster virus, 264-266
  pediatric, 419-421
    DNA, 419-420
    RNA, 420-421
  RNA, 268, 269t, 270-275
    coxsackieviruses group A, 268, 269t, 270
    HIV, 273-275
    measles, 272
    mumps, 271-272
    paramyxoviruses, 271
    retroviruses, 273
    rubella, 272-273
    togaviruses, 272
Viral sialadenitis, 290-291
Viricidal disinfectants, 478-479, 479t
Virulence, defined, 1
Virulence factors
  defined, 39
  in pathogenicity, 39-40
  in pulpal disease, 147-148
Viruses
  characteristics and pathogenicity of, 38
  immunofluorescent assay of, 50
  processing, isolation, and identification of, 54
  susceptibility testing of, 59
  in tonsillitis, 323
Visceral space, infections of, 207, 207f
Vision, assessment of, 329
Visual fields, assessment of, 329
Visual loss from septic cavernous sinus thrombosis, 338
Visual pathways, examination of, 329-330
Vital signs, pediatric, 411t

W

Waldeyer's ring, infection and, 206
Warts
  anogenital, 268
  cutaneous, 267-268

Waterlines, contamination of, 480
Waters' view of paranasal sinuses, 68f, 69-70
Weeksella, Gram stain identification of, 49b
Wegener's granulomatosis *versus* orbital cellulitis, 334, 334f
Welch, William, 469
Wet preparations, 50
Wharton's duct
  obstruction of, acute bacterial submandibular sialadenitis and, 287-288
  salivary calculus in, 281, 281f
Wheal, characteristics of, 297
White blood cell count, pediatric values for, 411t
White blood cells, tagging, 65
Williams, Ashbel, 188, 199
Wiskott-Aldrich syndrome, 457
Wolinella recta
  in HIV-associated periodontal disease, 145
  in periodontitis, 132
Wound healing, 25-26, 26t
Wounds. *See also* Maxillofacial trauma; Trauma
  antibiotics in management of, 110
  devitalized tissue in, 476
  focused exam of, 364
  foreign bodies in, 476
  Gram stain culture of, 364
  hemostasis and, 364
  infections of
    criteria for, 473
    factors in, 477b
  irrigation of, 364-365
  placing drains in, 365
  preventing secondary contamination of, 368-369
  puncture, maxillofacial, 374, 374f
  removing foreign bodies from, 364-365
  repair of, 365-366
  sepsis of, 475-476
  surgical. *See* Surgical wounds
  traumatic, maxillofacial infections of, 306

X

Xerostomia
  in acute bacterial parotitis, 283
  microbe effects of, 31

Y

Yeast infection, implant-associated, 389
Yeasts
  characteristics and pathogenicity of, 37-38
  in infants, 30

Z

Zefazone. *See* Cefmetazole
Zenacef. *See* Cefuroxime
Ziehl-Neelsen method, 48-49
Zithromax. *See* Azithromycin
Zoster sine herpete, 265
Zovirax. *See* Acyclovir
Zuckerkandl, aponeurosis of, 204
Zygomycosis, rhinocerebral, 426-429, 426f, 427f, 428f, 429f

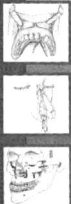

Here's a sample of the coverage you can expect!

Oral and Maxillofacial Surgery Clinics

February	Emerging Biomaterials
May	Surgical Endodontics
August	Obstructive Sleep Apnea
November	Secondary Cleft Palate

Atlas of Oral and Maxillofacial Clinics

March	Craniofacial Surgery
September	An Atlas of Head and Neck Images

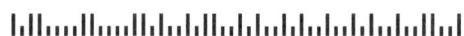